Emergency Treatment

**Comprehensive Evaluation & Treatment:** Provides a step-wise approach to the evaluation and treatment of coma, seizures, shock, and other common complications of poisoning and to the proper use of gastric decontamination and dialysis procedures.

Common Poisons & Drugs

**Specific Poisons & Drugs: Diagnosis & Treatment:** Alphabetical listing of specific drugs and poisons, including the pathophysiology, toxic dose and level, clinical presentation, diagnosis, and specific treatment associated with each substance.

Antidotes & Drug Therapy

**Therapeutic Drugs & Antidotes:** Descriptions of therapeutic drugs and antidotes discussed in the two preceding sections, including their pharmacology, indications, adverse effects, drug interactions, recommended dosage, and formulations.

Industrial Chemicals

**Environmental & Occupational Toxicology:** Approach to hazardous materials incidents; evaluation of occupational exposures; and the toxic effects, physical properties, and workplace exposure limits for over 500 common industrial chemicals.

Index

**Index:** Includes generic drug and chemical names and numerous brand name drugs and commercial products.

fifth edition

# POISONING & DRUG OVERDOSE

by the faculty, staff and associates of
the California Poison Control System


Edited by
**Kent R. Olson, MD, FACEP, FACMT, FAACT**
Clinical Professor of Medicine, Pediatrics, and Pharmacy,
University of California, San Francisco;
Medical Director, California Poison Control System,
San Francisco Division

**Associate Editors**

**Ilene B. Anderson, PharmD**
Clinical Professor of Pharmacy, University of California, San Francisco;
Senior Toxicology Management Specialist,
California Poison Control System,
San Francisco Division

**Neal L. Benowitz, MD**
Professor of Medicine
and Chief, Division of Clinical Pharmacology and Toxicology,
University of California, San Francisco;
Associate Medical Director,
California Poison Control System,
San Francisco Division

**Paul D. Blanc, MD, MSPH**
Professor of Medicine and Chief, Division of Occupational and Environmental Medicine,
University of California, San Francisco

**Richard F. Clark, MD, FACEP**
Professor of Medicine,
University of California, San Diego;
Director, Division of Medical Toxicology
and Medical Director,
California Poison Control System,
San Diego Division

**Thomas E. Kearney, PharmD, ABAT**
Professor of Clinical Pharmacy,
University of California, San Francisco;
Managing Director,
California Poison Control System,
San Francisco Division

**John D. Osterloh, MD, MS**
Chief Medical Officer,
Division of Laboratory Sciences
National Center for Environmental Health,
Centers for Disease Control and Prevention,
Atlanta, Georgia



**Lange Medical Books/McGraw-Hill**
Medical Publishing Division
New York Chicago San Francisco Lisbon London Madrid Mexico
New Delhi San Juan Seoul Singapore Sydney Toronto

The McGraw·Hill Companies

**Poisoning & Drug Overdose, Fifth Edition**



1 2 3 4 5 6 7 8 9 0 DOC/DOC 0 9 8 7 6

ISBN-13: 978-0-07-144333-3
ISBN: 0-07-144333-9
ISSN: 1048-8847



The book was set by Silverchair Science + Communications, Inc.
The editors were Martin Wonsiewicz, Karen Edmonson, and Barbara Holton.
The production supervisor was Phil Galea.
The index was prepared by Kathy Pitcoff.
Cover design by Mary McKeon
Photo credit: Leonard Lessin / Photo Researchers, Inc.
Cover: *Cocaine preparation. Anhydrous ammonia crystallization. The illegal drug cocaine is derived from the leaves of the Coca plant that have peen pulverized into a paste. Anhydrous ammonia is added to remove alkaloids from the paste. The crystallized cocaine is then dried under heating lamps or in microwave ovens to produce Cocaine hydrochloride, cocaine in its powdered form.*
RR Donnelly was printer and binder.

This book is printed on acid-free paper.

INTERNATIONAL EDITION ISBN-13: 978-0-07-110469-2; ISBN-10: 0-07-110469-0

# Contents

**Authors** .......... **vi**
**Preface** .......... **xv**
**Section I. Comprehensive Evaluation & Treatment** .......... **1**
This section provides a step-wise approach to the evaluation and treatment of coma, seizures, shock, and other common complications of poisoning and to the proper use of gastric decontamination and dialysis procedures.

**Section II. Specific Poisons & Drugs: Diagnosis & Treatment** .......... **68**
Organized alphabetically, this section lists specific drugs and poisons, as well as the pathophysiology, toxic dose and level, clinical presentation, diagnosis, and specific treatment associated each substance.

**Section III. Therapeutic Drugs & Antidotes** .......... **406**
This section provides descriptions of therapeutic drugs and antidotes discussed in Sections I and II, including their pharmacology, indications, adverse effects, drug interactions, recommended dosage, and formulations.

**Section IV. Environmental & Occupational Toxicology** .......... **520**
This section describes the approach to hazardous materials incidents; the evaluation of occupational exposures; and the toxic effects, physical properties, and workplace exposure limits for over 500 common industrial chemicals.

**Index** .......... **641**
The index includes generic drug and chemical names and numerous brand name drugs and commercial products.

# Authors

**Timothy E. Albertson, MD, PhD**
Professor of Medicine, Medical Pharmacology and Toxicology, University of California Medical Center, Davis; Medical Director, California Poison Control System, Sacramento Division
tealbertson@ucdavis.edu
*Section II: Amphetamines; Barbiturates; Dextromethorphan; Opiates and Opioids*

**Judith A. Alsop, PharmD, DABAT**
Associate Clinical Professor, School of Pharmacy, University of California, San Francisco; Clinical Professor of Medicine, School of Medicine, University of California, Davis
jalsop@calpoison.org
*Section II: Plants; Section III: Metoclopramide; Ondansetron; Potassium*

**Ilene B. Anderson, PharmD**
Clinical Professor, School of Pharmacy, University of California, San Francisco; Senior Toxicology Management Specialist, California Poison Control System, San Francisco Division
iba@calpoison.org
*Section II: Botulism; Camphor and Other Essential Oils; Ethylene Glycol and Other Glycols; Lomotil and Other Antidiarrheals; Methanol; Warfarin and Related Rodenticides*

**John Balmes, MD**
Professor, Department of Medicine, University of California, San Francisco; Chief, Division of Occupational and Environmental Medicine, San Francisco General Hospital
jbalmes@medsfgh.ucsf.edu
*Section II: Asbestos; Formaldehyde; Gases, Irritant; Molds; Phosgene; Sulfur Dioxide*

**Neal L. Benowitz, MD**
Professor of Medicine and Chief, Division of Clinical Pharmacology and Toxicology, University of California, San Francisco; Associate Medical Director, California Poison Control System, San Francisco Division
nbenowitz@medsfgh.ucsf.edu
*Section II: Anesthetics, Local; Antiarrhythmic Drugs; Antidepressants, General (Noncyclic); Antidepressants, Tricyclic; Beta-Adrenergic Blockers; Calcium Antagonists; Cardiac Glycosides; Chloroquine and Other Aminoquinolines; Cocaine; Ergot Derivatives; Lithium; Marijuana; Monoamine Oxidase Inhibitors; Nicotine; Nitrates and Nitrites; Nitroprusside; Phencyclidine (PCP) and Ketamine; Pseudoephedrine, Phenylephrine and Other Decongestants; Quinidine and Other Type IA Antiarrhythmic Drugs; Quinine; Vacor (PNU); Section III: Dopamine; Epinephrine; Norepinephrine*

**David P. Betten**
Assistant Clinical Professor, Department of Emergency Medicine, College of Human Medicine, Michigan State University, East Lansing
davebetten@yahoo.com
*Section II: Colchicine*

**Kathleen Birnbaum, PharmD**
Toxicology Management Specialist, Department of Clinical Pharmacy, University of California, San Francisco
kbirnbaum@calpoison.org
*Section III: Insulin; Leucovorin Calcium*

**Paul D. Blanc, MD, MSPH**
Professor of Medicine, and Chief, Division of Occupational and Environmental Medicine, University of California, San Francisco
Paul.blanc@ucsf.edu
*Section II: Carbon Disulfide; Cyanide; Isocyanates; Manganese; Metal Fume Fever; Methemoglobinemia; Nitrogen Oxides; Section IV: Evaluation of the Patient with Occupational Chemical Exposure; The Toxic Hazards of Industrial and Occupational Chemicals*

**Stephen C. Born, MD, MPH**
Associate Clinical Professor, Division of Occupational and Environmental Medicine, University of California, San Francisco
sborn@sfghoem.ucsf.edu
*Section II: Dioxins, Ethylene Oxide*

**Alan Buchwald, MD**
Consultant in Medical Toxicology and Medical Director, Occupational Health Center, Dominican Santa Cruz Hospital, Santa Cruz, California
albuchwald955@pol.net
*Section II: Copper*

**Cindy Burkardt**
Toxicology Management Specialist, California Poison Control System, San Francisco Division
cburkhardt@calpoison.org
*Section III: DTPA; Thiosulfate, Sodium*

**Chris Camilleri, DO**
Attending Physician, University of California Davis Medical Center, Sacramento.
*Section II: Benzene*

**F. Lee Cantrell, PharmD**
Assistant Clinical Professor, School of Pharmacy, University of California, San Diego and San Francisco; Interim Director, California Poison Control System, San Diego Division
fcantrel@ucsd.edu
*Section II: Thyroid Hormone; Section III: Cyproheptadine; Folic Acid; Inamrinone (formerly Amrinone)*

**Terry Carlson, PharmD**
Toxicology Management Specialist, California Poison Control System, Fresno/Madera Division
tcarlson@calpoison.org
*Section III: Naloxone and Nalmefene*

**Richard F. Clark, MD**
Professor of Medicine, University of California, San Diego; Director, Division of Medical Toxicology, University of California Medical Center, San Diego; Medical Director, California Poison Control System, San Diego Division
rfclark@ucsd.edu
*Section II: Hymenoptera; Lionfish and Other Scorpaenoidea; Scorpions; Snakebite; Section III: Antivenom, Crotalinae (Rattlesnake); Antivenom, Latrodectus Mactans (Black Widow Spider); Antivenom, Micrurus Fulvius (Coral Snake), and Exotic Antivenoms*

**Matthew D. Cook**
Assistant Clinical Professor, Medical Toxicology Fellow, and Attending Physician, Department of Emergency Medicine, University of California Medical Center, San Diego
mattkook@yahoo.com
*Section II: Phosphorus*

**Delia A. Dempsey, MD, MS**
Assistant Adjunct Professor of Pediatrics, Medicine, and Clinical Pharmacy, University of California, San Francisco; Assistant Medical Director, California Poison Control System, San Francisco Division
ddempsey@medsfgh.ucsf.edu
*Section I: Special Considerations in Pediatric Patients; Section II: Bromides; Methyl Bromide; Pentachlorophenol and Dinitrophenol*

**Jo Ellen Dyer, PharmD**
Clinical Professor, Department of Pharmacy, University of California, San Francisco; Senior Toxicology Management Specialist, California Poison Control System, San Francisco Division
jdyer@calpoison.org
*Section I: Special Considerations in the Evaluation of Drug-Facilitated Assault; Section II: Azide, Sodium; Gamma-Hydroxybutyrate (GHB)*

**Andrew Erdman, MD**
Clinical Pharmacology Fellow, University of California, San Francisco
andrewerdman@sbcglobal.net
*Section II: Isoniazid (INH)*

**Gary W. Everson, PharmD**
Toxicology Management Specialist, California Poison Control System, Fresno/Madera Division
geverson@calpoison.org
*Section II: Phenol and Related Compounds; Section III: Mannitol*

**Jeffrey Fay, PharmD**
Assistant Clinical Professor, Department of Pharmacy, University of California, San Francisco; Toxicology Management Specialist, California Poison Control System, Fresno/Madera Division
jfay@calpoison.org
*Section II: Vasodilators*

**Thomas J. Ferguson, MD, PhD**
Associate Clinical Professor of Internal Medicine, University of California, Davis; Medical Director, Cowell Student Health Center, University of California, Davis
tjferguson@ucdavis.edu
*Section II: Chromium; Thallium*

**Frederick Fung, MD, MS**
Clinical Professor of Occupational Medicine, University of California, Irvine; Medical Director, Occupational Medicine Department and Toxicology Services, Sharp Rees-Stealy Medical Group, San Diego, California
fred.fung@sharp.com
*Section II: Carbon Tetrachloride and Chloroform*

**Mark J. Galbo, MS**
Environmental Toxicologist, School of Pharmacy, University of California, San Francisco; Poison Information Specialist, California Poison Control System, San Francisco Division
mjgalbo@calpoison.org
*Section II: Naphthalene and Paradichlorobenzene; Warfare Agents—Chemical*

**Fabian Garza, PharmD**
School of Pharmacy, University of California, San Francisco; Toxicology Management Specialist, California Poison Control System, Fresno/Madera Division
fgarza@calpoison.org
*Section III: Methylene Blue*

**Richard J. Geller, MD, MPH**
Associate Clinical Professor of Emergency Medicine, University of California, San Francisco; Medical Director, California Poison Control System, Fresno/Madera Division
*Section II: Disulfiram; Paraquat and Diquat; Selenium; Section III: Atropine and Glycopyrrolate; Pralidoxime (2-PAM) & Other Oximes*

**Robert L. Goldberg, MD, FACOEM**
Director, Occupational and Environmental Medicine Residency Program; Health Sciences Associate Clinical Professor of Medicine, Department of Medicine, University of California, San Francisco
robert.goldberg@ucsf.edu
*Section II: Polychlorinated Biphenyls (PCBs)*

**Colin S. Goto, MD**
Assistant Clinical Professor of Pediatrics, University of California, San Diego; Attending Physician, Division of Emergency Medicine, Children's Hospital and Health Center, San Diego, California
cgoto@chsd.org
*Section II: Hydrocarbons*

**Christine A. Haller, MD**
Assistant Professor of Medicine and Laboratory Medicine, University of California, San Francisco; California Poison Control System, San Francisco Division; San Francisco General Hospital
dchaller@worldnet.att.net
*Section II: Caffeine; Herbal and Alternative Products; Section III: L-Carnitine (Levocarnitine); Silymarin or Milk Thistle (Silybum Marianum)*

**Jennifer Hannum, MD**
Medical Toxicology Fellow, Department of Emergency Medicine, University of California Medical Center, San Diego
jhannum@ucsd.edu
*Section II: Hydrogen Fluoride and Hydrofluoric Acid; Methylene Chloride; Section III: Calcium*

**Sandra Hayashi, PharmD**
Assistant Clinical Professor, School of Pharmacy, University of California, San Francisco; Toxicology Management Specialist, California Poison Control System, San Francisco Division
shayashi@calpoison.org
*Section II: Angiotensin Blockers and ACE Inhibitors; Section III: Prussian Blue*

**Patricia Hess Hiatt, BS**
Administrative Operations Manager, California Poison Control System, San Francisco Division
phiatt@calpoison.org
*Section IV: The Toxic Hazards of Industrial and Occupational Chemicals*

**Raymond Ho, PharmD**
Toxicology Management Specialist, California Poison Control System, San Francisco Division
rho@calpoison.org
*Section III: Botulinum Antitoxin*

**David L. Irons, PharmD**
Toxicology Management Specialist, Department of Clinical Pharmacy, University of California, San Francisco
dirons@calpoison.org
*Section II: Vitamins; Section III: Deferoxamine*

**Leslie M. Israel, DO, MPH**
Associate Clinical Professor of Occupational Medicine, University of California, Irvine
lisrael@uci.edu
*Section II: Cadmium*

**Thomas E. Kearney, PharmD, DABAT**
Professor of Clinical Pharmacy, University of California, San Francisco; Managing Director, California Poison Control System, San Francisco Division
pcctk@calpoison.org
*Section II: Carbamazepine and Oxcarbazepine; Valproic Acid; Section III: Introduction; Acetylcysteine (N-Acetylcysteine [NAC]); Apomorphine; Benzodiazepines (Diazepam, Lorazepam, and Midazolam); Benztropine; Bicarbonate, Sodium; Botulinum Antitoxin; Bretylium; Bromocriptine; Charcoal, Activated; Cimetidine and Other H2 Blockers; Dantrolene; Diazoxide; Digoxin-Specific Antibodies; Diphenhydramine; Esmolol; Ethanol; Fomepizole (4-Methylpyrazole, 4-MP); Glucagon; Glucose; Haloperidol and Droperidol; Isoproterenol; Labetalol; Lidocaine; Methocarbamol; Morphine; Neuromuscular Blockers; Nicotinamide (Niacinamide); Nitroprusside; Octreotide; Penicillamine; Pentobarbital; Phenobarbital; Phentolamine; Physostigmine and Neostigmine; Propranolol; Protamine; Pyridoxine (Vitamin B6); Thiamine (Vitamin B1); Vitamin K1 (Phytonadione)*

**Susan Kim, PharmD**
Professor of Clinical Pharmacy, University of California, San Francisco; Senior Toxicology Management Specialist, California Poison Control System, San Francisco Division
susank@calpoison.org
*Section II: Antidiabetic Agents; Antineoplastic Agents; Beta-2 Adrenergic Stimulants; Food Poisoning: Bacterial; Food Poisoning: Fish and Shellfish; Jellyfish and Other Cnidaria; Salicylates; Skeletal Muscle Relaxants*

**Lada Kokan, MD**
Attending Physician, Emergency Department, Kaiser Permanente, San Francisco, California
lada.kokan@telus.net
*Section II: Monoamine Oxidase Inhibitors*

**Michael J. Kosnett, MD, MPH**
Associate Clinical Professor of Medicine, Department of Clinical Pharmacology and Toxicology, University of Colorado Health Sciences Center, Denver
michael.kosnett@uchsc.edu
*Section II: Arsenic; Arsine; Lead; Mercury; Section III: BAL (Dimercaprol); EDTA, Calcium (Calcium Disodium EDTA, Calcium Disodium Edetate, Calcium Disodium Versenate); Succimer (DMSA); Unithiol (DMPS)*

**Grant D. Lackey, PharmD, PhD, CSPI, FASCP**
Assistant Clinical Professor of Medicine, University of California, Davis; Assistant Clinical Professor of Medicine, University of California, San Francisco; Toxicology Management Specialist, California Poison Control System, Sacramento Division
glackey@calpoison.org
*Section II: Antipsychotic Drugs, Including Phenothiazines; Section III: Phenytoin and Fosphenytoin*

**Chi-Leung Lai, PharmD**
Assistant Clinical Professor of Pharmacy, University of California, San Francisco; Assistant Clinical Professor of Medicine, University of California Medical Center, Davis; Toxicology Management Specialist, California Poison Control System, Sacramento Division
clai@calpoison.org
*Section II: Boric Acid, Borates, and Boron*

**John P. Lamb, PharmD**
Clinical Professor of Medicine, University of California, Davis; Assistant Clinical Professor of Pharmacy, University of California, San Francisco; Toxicology Management Specialist, California Poison Control System, Sacramento Division
jlamb@calpoison.org
*Section II: Pyrethrins and Pyrethroids*

**Darren H. Lew, PharmD**
Toxicology Management Specialist, California Poison Control System, Fresno/Madera Division
dlew@calpoison.org
*Section II: Chlorinated Hydrocarbon Pesticides*

**Jon Lorett, PharmD**
Toxicology Management Specialist, Department of Clinical Pharmacy, University of California, San Francisco
jlorett@calpoison.org
*Section II: Ipecac Syrup; Section III: Ipecac Syrup*

**Binh T. Ly, MD**
Associate Clinical Professor of Medicine; Associate Director, Emergency Medicine Residency Program; Associate Director, Medical Toxicology Fellowship Program, Division of Medical Toxicology, Department of Emergency Medicine, University of California, San Diego
bly@ucsd.edu
*Section II: Hydrogen Fluoride and Hydrofluoric Acid; Methylene Chloride; Section III: Calcium*

**Richard Lynton, MD**
Staff Physician, VA Medical Center, Sacramento; Assistant Clinical Professor, University of California, Davis School of Medicine
richard.lynton@med.va.gov
*Section III: Propofol*

**Beth H. Manning, PharmD**
Assistant Clinical Professor, School of Pharmacy, University of California, San Francisco; Toxicology Management Specialist, California Poison Control System, San Francisco Division
bmanning@calpoison.org
*Section II: Anticholinergics; Antihistamines*

**Anthony S. Manoguerra, PharmD**
Professor of Clinical Pharmacy and Associate Dean, University of California, San Diego
amanoguerra@ucsd.edu
*Section II: Iron*

**Kathy Marquardt, PharmD, DABAT**
Associate Clinical Professor, School of Pharmacy, University of California, San Francisco; Associate Clinical Professor, School of Medicine, University of California, Davis; Senior Toxicology Management Specialist, California Poison Control System, Sacramento Division
kmarquardt@calpoison.org
*Section II: Mushrooms; Mushrooms, Amatoxin-Type*

**Michael J. Matteucci, MD**
Assistant Clinical Professor and Medical Toxicology Fellow, Department of Medicine, University of California, San Diego; Attending Physician, University of California Medical Center, San Diego; Attending Physician, Naval Medical Center, San Diego
mmatteucchi@ucsd.edu
*Section II: Isopropyl Alcohol*

**Kathryn H. Meier, PharmD**
Assistant Clinical Professor, School of Pharmacy, University of California, San Francisco; Toxicology Management Specialist, California Poison Control System, San Francisco Division
kmeier@calpoison.org
*Section II: Dapsone; Fluoride; Magnesium; Section III: Hydroxocobalamin*

**Eileen Morentz**
Poison Information Provider, California Poison Control System, San Francisco Division
morentz@calpoison.org
*Section II: Nontoxic or Minimally Toxic Household Products*

**Walter H. Mullen, PharmD**
Assistant Clinical Professor of Pharmacy, University of California, San Francisco; Toxicology Management Specialist, California Poison Control System, San Francisco Division
wmullen@calpoison.org
*Section II: Caustic and Corrosive Agents; Iodine; Section III: Flumazenil; Nitrite, Sodium and Amyl*

**Stephen W. Munday, MD, MPH, MS**
Assistant Clinical Professor, Department of Family and Preventative Medicine, University of California, San Diego; Assistant Director of Outpatient Medicine, Medical Toxicologist, Sharp Rees-Stealy Medical Group, San Diego, California
stephen.munday@sharp.com
*Section II: Hydrogen Sulfide*

**Nancy G. Murphy, MD**
Medical Toxicology Fellow, Department of Clinical Pharmacology and Experimental Therapeutics, University of California, San Francisco
nancy.murphy@iwk.nshealth.ca
*Section II: Anesthetics, Local; Calcium Antagonists; Cocaine*

**Steve Offerman, MD**
Assistant Professor, Department of Emergency Medicine, University of California, Davis
steve.offerman@gmail.com
*Section II: Fluoroacetate*

**Kent R. Olson, MD, FACEP, FACMT, FAACT**
Clinical Professor of Medicine, Pediatrics, and Pharmacy, University of California, San Francisco; Medical Director, California Poison Control System, San Francisco Division
olson@calpoison.org
*Section I: Emergency Evaluation and Treatment; Section II: Acetaminophen; Carbon Monoxide; Oxalic Acid; Phosphine and Phosphides; Smoke Inhalation; Theophylline; Section III: Oxygen & Hyperbaric Oxygen; Section IV: Emergency Medical Response to Hazardous Materials Incidents; The Toxic Hazards of Industrial and Occupational Chemicals*

**Michael A. O'Malley, MD, MPH**
Associate Clinical Professor, School of Medicine, University of California, Davis
maomalley@ucdavis.edu
*Section II: Chlorophenoxy Herbicides*

**Cyrus Rangan, MD**
Assistant Medical Director, California Poison Control System, San Francisco Division; Director, Toxics Epidemiology Program, Los Angeles County Department of Health Services; Attending Staff, Children's Hospital, Los Angeles
crangan@calpoison.org
*Section II: Clonidine and Related Drugs*

**Freda M. Rowley, PharmD**
Assistant Clinical Professor of Pharmacy, University of California, San Francisco; Toxicology Management Specialist, California Poison Control System, San Francisco Division
frowley@calpoison.org
*Section II: Anticonvulsants, Newer; Section III: Iodide (Potassium Iodide, KI)*

**Thomas R. Sands, PharmD**
Assistant Clinical Professor, School of Pharmacy, University of California, San Francisco; Associate Clinical Professor, School of Medicine, University of California, Davis; Toxicology Management Specialist, California Poison Control System, Sacramento Division
tsands@calpoison.org
*Section II: Bromates; Chlorates*

**Aaron Schneir, MD**
Assistant Professor, Division of Medical Toxicology, Department of Emergency Medicine, University of California Medical Center, San Diego
aschneir@ucsd.edu
*Section II: Nitrous Oxide*

**Jay Schrader, CPhT**
Poison Information Provider, California Poison Control System, San Francisco Division
jschrader@calpoison.org
*Section II: Nontoxic or Minimally Toxic Household Products*

**Kerry Schwarz, PharmD**
Toxicology Management Specialist, California Poison Control System, San Diego Division
kschwarz@calpoison.org
*Section II: Antiseptics and Disinfectants*

**Craig Smollin, MD**
Medical Toxicology Fellow, California Poison Control System, San Francisco Division
*Section II: Glysophate; Phenytoin*

**Karl A. Sporer, MD**
Associate Clinical Professor, University of California, San Francisco; Attending Physician, San Francisco General Hospital
ksporer@sfghed.ucsf.edu
*Section II: Tetanus*

**Jeffrey R. Suchard, MD, FACEP**
Assistant Clinical Professor, Director of Medical Toxicology, Department of Emergency Medicine, University of California Medical Center, Irvine
jsuchard@uci.edu
*Section II: Spiders*

**Winnie W. Tai, PharmD**
Assistant Clinical Professor of Pharmacy, University of California, San Francisco; Toxicology Management Specialist, California Poison Control System, San Francisco Division
tai@calpoison.org
*Section II: Metaldehyde; Nonsteroidal Anti-Inflammatory Drugs*

**David A. Tanen, MD**
Assistant Program Director and Research Director, Emergency Medicine Department, Naval Medical Center, San Diego, California
dtanen@yahoo.com
*Section II: Organophosphorus and Carbamate Insecticides; Warfare Agents–Biological; Warfare Agents–Chemical*

**John H. Tegzes, VMD**
Associate Professor, College of Veterinary Medicine, Western University of Health Sciences, Pomona, California
jtegzes@westernu.edu
*Section III: Tetanus Toxoid and Immune Globulin*

**R. Steven Tharratt, MD, MPVM**
Professor of Medicine and Anesthesiology, University of California, Davis; Associate Medical Director, California Poison Control System, Sacramento Division
rstharratt@ucdavis.edu
*Section II: Ammonia; Chlorine; Section IV: Emergency Medical Response to Hazardous Materials Incidents*

**Josef G. Thundiyil, MD, MPH**
Medical Toxicology Fellow, California Poison Control System, San Francisco Division
*Section II: Freons and Halons; Trichloroethane, Trichloroethylene, and Tetrachloroethylene*

**Ben T. Tsutaoka, PharmD**
Assistant Clinical Professor, School of Pharmacy, University of California, San Francisco; Toxicology Management Specialist, California Poison Control System, San Francisco Division
btsutaoka@calpoison.org
*Section II: Benzodiazepines; Sedative-Hypnotic Agents; Section III: Vasopressin*

**Rais Vohra, MD**
Toxicology Fellow, Department of Emergency Medicine, University of California Medical Center, San Diego; California Poison Control System, San Diego Division
raisvohra@hotmail.com
*Section II: Antimony and Stibine*

**Michael J. Walsh, PharmD**
Assistant Clinical Professor, School of Pharmacy, University of California, San Francisco; Toxicology Management Specialist, California Poison Control System, Sacramento Division
mwalsh@calpoison.org
*Section II: Detergents*

**Janet Weiss, MD**
Director of Toxicology, TheToxDoc, Berkeley, California
toxdoc@yahoo.com
*Section II: Ethylene Dibromide; Toluene and Xylene*

**R. David West, PharmD**
Toxicology Management Specialist, California Poison Control System, Fresno/Madera Division
dwest@calpoison.org
*Section III: Magnesium*

**Timothy J. Wiegand, MD**
Medical Toxicology Fellow, California Poison Control System, San Francisco Division
*Section II: Diuretics; Lithium; Phencyclidine (PCP) and Ketamine*

**Saralyn R. Williams, MD**
Associate Clinical Professor of Medicine, Division of Medical Toxicology, University of California, San Diego; Assistant Medical Director, California Poison Control System, San Diego Division
srwilliams@ucsd.edu
*Section II: Ethanol; Strychnine*

**Olga F. Woo, PharmD**
Associate Clinical Professor of Pharmacy, University of California, San Francisco
2tao.olga@gmail.com
*Section II: Antibacterial Agents; Antiviral and Antiretroviral Agents; Barium*

**Lisa Wu, MD**
Medical Toxicology Fellow, Department of Clinical Pharmacology, University of California, San Francisco
lisawu5@hotmail.com
*Section II: Amantadine; Lysergic Acid Diethylamide (LSD) and Other Hallucinogens*

**Evan T. Wythe, MD**
Associate Director, Eden Emergency Medical Group, Castro Valley, California
wythe@sbcglobal.net
*Section II: Radiation (Ionizing)*

# Preface

*Poisoning & Drug Overdose* provides practical advice for the diagnosis and management of poisoning and drug overdose and concise information about common industrial chemicals.

The manual is divided into four sections and an index, each identified by a black tab in the right margin. **Section I** leads the reader through initial emergency management, including treatment of coma, hypotension, and other common complications; physical and laboratory diagnosis; and methods of decontamination and enhanced elimination of poisons. **Section II** provides detailed information for approximately 150 common drugs and poisons. **Section III** describes the use and side effects of approximately 60 antidotes and therapeutic drugs. **Section IV** describes the medical management of chemical spills and occupational chemical exposures and includes a table of over 500 chemicals. The **Index** is comprehensive and extensively cross-referenced.

The manual is designed to allow the reader to move quickly from section to section, obtaining the needed information from each. For example, in managing a patient with isoniazid intoxication, the reader will find specific information about isoniazid toxicity in **Section II,** practical advice for gut decontamination and management of complications such as seizures in **Section I,** and detailed information about dosing and side effects for the antidote pyridoxine in **Section III.**


## ACKNOWLEDGMENTS

The success of the first and second editions of this manual would not have been possible without the combined efforts of the staff, faculty, and fellows of the San Francisco Bay Area Regional Poison Control Center, to whom I am deeply indebted. From its inception, this book has been a project by and for our poison center; as a result, all royalties from its sale have gone to our center's operating fund and not to any individual editor or author.

In January 1997, four independent poison control centers joined their talents to become the California Poison Control System, administered by the University of California, San Francisco. With the third and fourth editions, the manual became a project of our statewide system, bringing in new authors and editors.

On behalf of the authors and editors of the fifth edition, my sincere thanks go to all those who contributed to the first four editions:

Timothy E. Albertson, MD, PhD (3rd and 4th ed.)
Judith A. Alsop, PharmD (3rd and 4th ed.)
Ilene Brewer Anderson, PharmD (1st, 2nd, 3rd and 4th ed.)
Margaret Atterbury, MD (1st ed.)
Georgeanne M. Backman (1st ed.)
John Balmes, MD (2nd, 3rd and 4th ed.)
Shireen Banerji, PharmD (4th ed.)
James David Barry, MD (4th ed.)
Charles E. Becker, MD (1st and 2nd ed.)
Neal L. Benowitz, MD (1st, 2nd, 3rd and 4th ed.)
Bruce Bernard, MD (1st ed.)
Kathleen Birnbaum, PharmD (4th ed.)
Paul D. Blanc, MD, MSPH (1st, 2nd, 3rd and 4th ed.)
Stephen Born, MD (4th ed.)
Christopher R. Brown, MD (3rd ed.)
Randall G. Browning, MD, MPH (3rd ed.)
James F. Buchanan, PharmD (1st ed.)
Alan Buchwald, MD (3rd and 4th ed.)
F. Lee Cantrell, PharmD (4th ed.)
Terry Carlson, PharmD (4th ed.)
Gregory Cham, MD (4th ed.)
Chulathida Chomchai, MD (4th ed.)
Summon Chomchai, MD (4th ed.)
Richard F. Clark, MD (3rd and 4th ed.)
Delia Dempsey, MD (2nd, 3rd and 4th ed.)
Chris Dutra, MD (1st ed.)
Jo Ellen Dyer, PharmD (2nd, 3rd and 4th ed.)
Brent R. Ekins, PharmD (3rd ed.)
Andrew Erdman, MD (4th ed.)
Gary Everson, PharmD (4th ed.)
Thomas J. Ferguson, MD, PhD (3rd and 4th ed.)

Donna E. Foliart, MD, MPH (1st ed.)
Frederick Fung, MD (4th ed.)
Mark J. Galbo, MS (2nd, 3rd and 4th ed.)
Fabian Garza, PharmD (4th ed.)
Rick Geller, MD (3rd and 4th ed.)
Colin Goto, MD (4th ed.)
Gail M. Gullickson, MD (1st ed.)
Christine A. Haller, MD (3rd and 4th ed.)
Patricia H. Hiatt, BS
(1st, 2nd, 3rd and 4th ed.)
B. Zane Horowitz, MD (3rd ed.)
Yao-min Hung, MD (4th ed.)
Leslie Isreal, DO, MPH (4th ed.)
Gerald Joe, PharmD (2nd and 3rd ed.)
Jeffrey R. Jones, MPH, CIH (1st ed.)
Thomas E. Kearney, PharmD
(2nd and 3rd ed.)
Kathryn H. Keller, PharmD
(1st, 2nd, 3rd and 4th ed.)
Michael T. Kelley, MD (1st ed.)
Susan Y. Kim, PharmD
(1st, 2nd, 3rd and 4th ed.)
Michael Kosnett, MD
(2nd, 3rd and 4th ed.)
Amy Kunihiro, MD (4th ed.)
Grant D. Lackey, PharmD (4th ed.)
Chi-Leung Lai, PharmD (4th ed.)
Rita Lam, PharmD (4th ed.)
Shelly Lam, PharmD (4th ed.)
John P. Lamb, PharmD (4th ed.)
Belle L. Lee, PharmD (1st ed.)
Darrem Lew, PharmD (4th ed.)
Diane Liu, MD, MPH (2nd and 3rd ed.)
Binh T. Ly, MD (4th ed.)
Richard Lynton, MD (4th ed.)
Beth Manning, PharmD (4th ed.)
Anthony S. Manoguerra, PharmD (3rd ed.)
Kathy Marquardt, PharmD (4th ed.)
Timothy D. McCarthy, PharmD
(1st, 2nd and 3rd ed.)
Howard E. McKinney, PharmD (1st ed.)
Kathryn H. Meier, PharmD
(2nd, 3rd and 4th ed.)
Michael A. Miller, MD (4th ed.)
Eileen Morentz (4th ed.)
Walter Mullen, PharmD (3rd and 4th ed.)
Stephen W. Munday, MD, MPH, MS
(4th ed.)
Frank J. Mycroft, PhD, MPH
(1st, 2nd and 3rd ed.)
Steve Offerman, MD (4th ed.)
Kent R. Olson, MD
(1st, 2nd, 3rd and 4th ed.)
Michael O'Malley, MD, MPH
(3rd and 4th ed.)
Gary Joseph Ordog, MD (3rd ed.)
John D. Osterloh, MD
(1st, 2nd and 3rd ed.)
Gary Pasternak, MD (1st ed.)
Manish Patel, MD (4th ed.)
Paul D. Pearigen, MD (3rd ed.)
Cyrus Rangan, MD (4th ed.)
Brett A. Roth, MD (3rd ed.)
Freda M. Rowley, PharmD (4th ed.)
Thomas R. Sands, PharmD (4th ed.)
Aaron Schnier, MD (4th ed.)
Jay Schrader (4th ed.)
Kerry Schwarz, PharmD (4th ed.)
Dennis J. Shusterman, MD, MPH
(3rd and 4th ed.)
Karl A. Sporer, MD (2nd, 3rd and 4th ed.)
Jeffrey R. Suchard, MD (4th ed.)
Winnie W. Tai, PharmD (4th ed.)
David A. Tanen, MD (4th ed.)
S. Alan Tani, PharmD (2nd and 3rd ed.)
John H. Tegzes, VMD (4th ed.)
R. Steven Tharratt, MD (4th ed.)
Ben Tsutaoka, PharmD (4th ed.)
Mary Tweig, MD (1st ed.)
Peter H. Wald, MD, MPH
(1st, 3rd and 4th ed.)
Michael J. Walsh, PharmD (4th ed.)
Jonathan Wasserberger, MD (3rd ed.)
Janet S. Weiss, MD (3rd and 4th ed.)
R. David West, PharmD (4th ed.)
Saralyn R. Williams, MD (3rd and 4th ed.)
Olga F. Woo, PharmD
(1st, 2nd, 3rd and 4th ed.)
Evan T. Wythe, MD
(1st, 2nd, 3rd and 4th ed.)
Peter Yip, MD (1st ed.)
Shoshana Zevin, MD (3rd ed.)

We are also grateful for the numerous comments and suggestions received from colleagues, students, and the editorial staff at McGraw-Hill, which helped us to improve the manual with each edition.

**Kent R. Olson, MD, FACEP, FACMT, FAACT**

San Francisco, California
July 2006

# SECTION I. **Comprehensive Evaluation and Treatment**

## ▶ EMERGENCY EVALUATION AND TREATMENT

*Kent R. Olson, MD*

Even though they may not appear to be acutely ill, all poisoned patients should be treated as if they have a potentially life-threatening intoxication. Figure I–1 provides a checklist of emergency evaluation and treatment procedures. More detailed information on diagnosis and treatment for each emergency step is referenced by page and presented immediately after the checklist.

When treating suspected poisoning cases, **quickly review the checklist** to determine the scope of appropriate interventions and **begin needed life-saving treatment.** If further information is required for any step, turn to the cited pages for a detailed discussion of each topic. Although the checklist is presented in a **sequential format,** many steps may be performed **simultaneously** (eg, airway management, naloxone and dextrose administration, and gastric lavage).

### AIRWAY

**I. Assessment.** The most common factor contributing to death from drug overdose or poisoning is loss of airway-protective reflexes with subsequent airway obstruction caused by the flaccid tongue, pulmonary aspiration of gastric contents, or respiratory arrest. All poisoning patients should be suspected of having a potentially compromised airway.

- **A. Patients who are awake** and talking are likely to have intact airway reflexes but should be monitored closely because worsening intoxication can result in rapid loss of airway control.
- **B. In lethargic or obtunded patients,** the gag or cough reflex may be an indirect indication of the patient's ability to protect the airway. If there is any doubt, it is best to perform endotracheal intubation (see below).

**II. Treatment.** Optimize the airway position and perform endotracheal intubation if necessary. Early use of naloxone (see p 477) or flumazenil (see p 452) may awaken a patient intoxicated with opioids or benzodiazepines, respectively, and obviate the need for endotracheal intubation. (***Note:*** Flumazenil is ***not*** recommended except in very select circumstances, as its use may precipitate seizures.)

- **A. Position the patient and clear the airway**
  - **1. Optimize the airway position** to force the flaccid tongue forward and maximize the airway opening. The following techniques are useful. ***Caution:*** Do ***not*** perform neck manipulation if you suspect a neck injury.
    - **a.** Place the neck and head in the **"sniffing" position,** with the neck flexed forward and the head extended
    - **b.** Apply the **"jaw thrust"** maneuver to create forward movement of the tongue without flexing or extending the neck. Pull the jaw forward by placing the fingers of each hand on the angle of the mandible just below the ears. (This motion also provides a painful stimulus to the angle of the jaw, the response to which indicates the patient's depth of coma.)
    - **c.** Place the patient in a **head-down, left-sided position** that allows the tongue to fall forward and secretions or vomitus to drain out of the mouth.
  - **2.** If the airway is still not patent, examine the oropharynx and **remove any obstruction or secretions** by suction, by a sweep with the finger, or with Magill forceps.

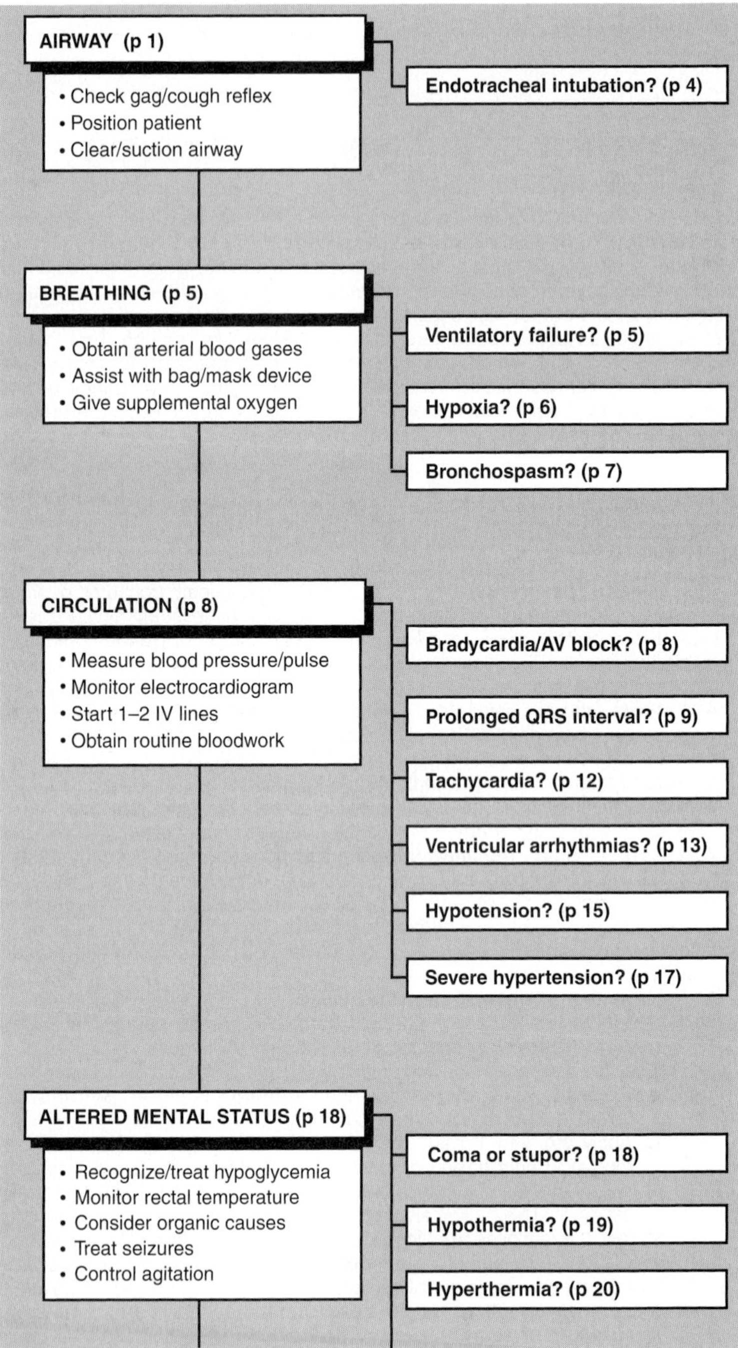
AIRWAY (p 1)
• Check gag/cough reflex
• Position patient
• Clear/suction airway
Endotracheal intubation? (p 4)
BREATHING (p 5)
• Obtain arterial blood gases
• Assist with bag/mask device
• Give supplemental oxygen
Ventilatory failure? (p 5)
Hypoxia? (p 6)
Bronchospasm? (p 7)
CIRCULATION (p 8)
• Measure blood pressure/pulse
• Monitor electrocardiogram
• Start 1–2 IV lines
• Obtain routine bloodwork
Bradycardia/AV block? (p 8)
Prolonged QRS interval? (p 9)
Tachycardia? (p 12)
Ventricular arrhythmias? (p 13)
Hypotension? (p 15)
Severe hypertension? (p 17)
ALTERED MENTAL STATUS (p 18)
• Recognize/treat hypoglycemia
• Monitor rectal temperature
• Consider organic causes
• Treat seizures
• Control agitation
Coma or stupor? (p 18)
Hypothermia? (p 19)
Hyperthermia? (p 20)

**FIGURE I–1.** Checklist of emergency evaluation and treatment procedures.

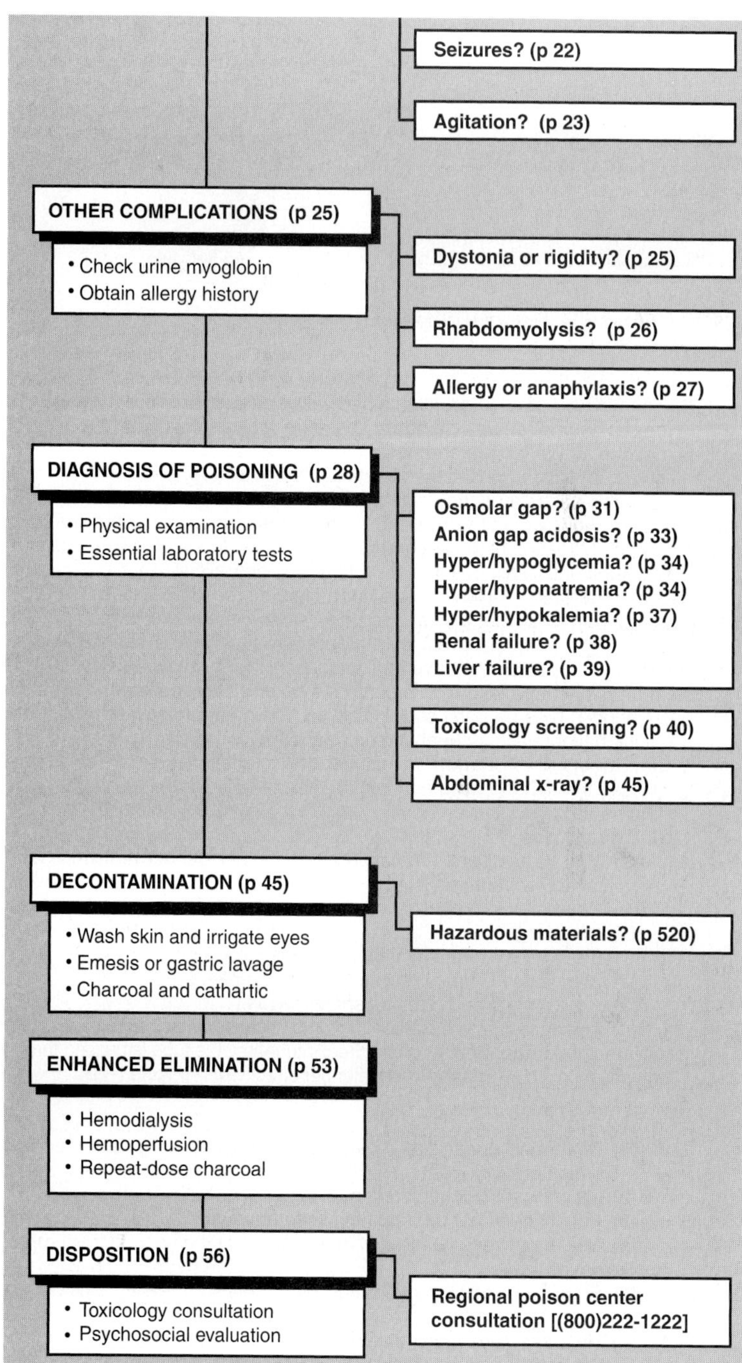
Seizures? (p 22)
Agitation? (p 23)
OTHER COMPLICATIONS (p 25)
• Check urine myoglobin
• Obtain allergy history
Dystonia or rigidity? (p 25)
Rhabdomyolysis? (p 26)
Allergy or anaphylaxis? (p 27)
DIAGNOSIS OF POISONING (p 28)
• Physical examination
• Essential laboratory tests
Osmolar gap? (p 31)
Anion gap acidosis? (p 33)
Hyper/hypoglycemia? (p 34)
Hyper/hyponatremia? (p 34)
Hyper/hypokalemia? (p 37)
Renal failure? (p 38)
Liver failure? (p 39)
Toxicology screening? (p 40)
Abdominal x-ray? (p 45)
DECONTAMINATION (p 45)
• Wash skin and irrigate eyes
• Emesis or gastric lavage
• Charcoal and cathartic
Hazardous materials? (p 520)
ENHANCED ELIMINATION (p 53)
• Hemodialysis
• Hemoperfusion
• Repeat-dose charcoal
DISPOSITION (p 56)
• Toxicology consultation
• Psychosocial evaluation
Regional poison center
consultation [(800)222-1222]

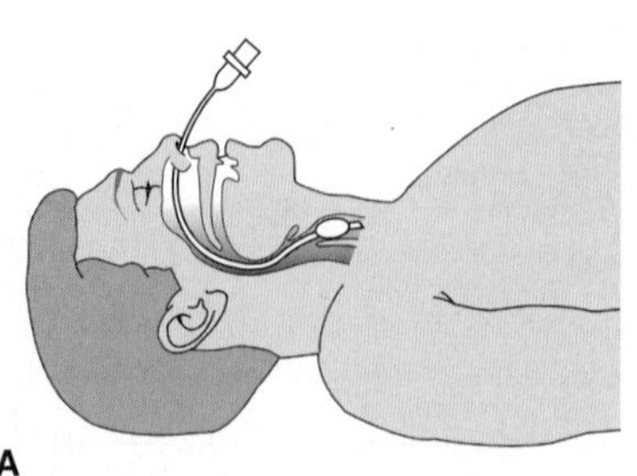


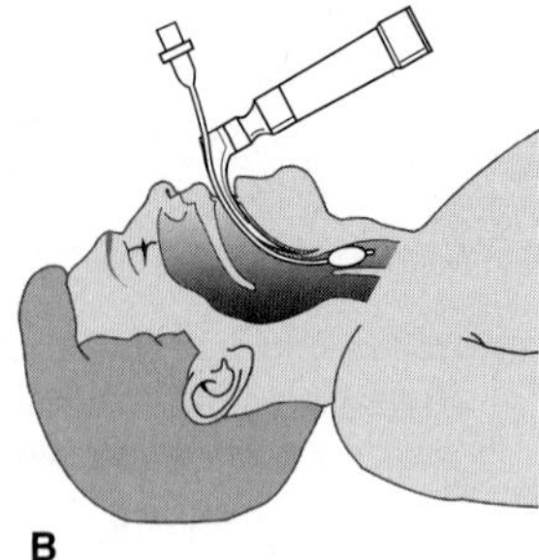


**FIGURE I–2.** Two routes for endotracheal intubation. A: Nasotracheal intubation. B: Orotracheal intubation.

3. The airway can also be maintained with **artificial oropharyngeal or nasopharyngeal airway devices.** These devices are placed in the mouth or nose to lift the tongue and push it forward. They are only temporary measures. A patient who can tolerate an artificial airway without complaint probably needs an endotracheal tube.

**B.** **Perform endotracheal intubation** if personnel trained in the procedure are available. Intubation of the trachea provides the most reliable protection of the airway, preventing aspiration and obstruction and allowing for mechanically assisted ventilation. However, it is not a simple procedure and *should be attempted only by those with training and experience.* Complications include vomiting with pulmonary aspiration; local trauma to the oropharynx, nasopharynx, and larynx; inadvertent intubation of the esophagus or a mainstem bronchus; and failure to intubate the patient after respiratory arrest has been induced by a neuromuscular blocker. There are two routes for endotracheal intubation: nasotracheal and orotracheal.

1. **Nasotracheal intubation.** In nasotracheal intubation, a soft flexible tube is passed through the nose and into the trachea by using a "blind" technique (Figure I–2A).
   a. **Advantages**
      **(1)** May be performed in a conscious patient without requiring neuromuscular paralysis.
      **(2)** Once placed, it is usually better tolerated than an orotracheal tube.
   b. **Disadvantages**
      **(1)** Perforation of the nasal mucosa with epistaxis.
      **(2)** Stimulation of vomiting in an obtunded patient.
      **(3)** Patient must be breathing spontaneously.
      **(4)** Anatomically more difficult in infants because of their anterior epiglottis.
2. **Orotracheal intubation.** In orotracheal intubation, the tube is passed through the patient's mouth into the trachea under direct vision (Figure I–2B).
   a. **Technique**
   b. **Advantages**
      **(1)** Performed under direct vision, making accidental esophageal intubation unlikely.
      **(2)** Insignificant risk of bleeding.
      **(3)** Patient need not be breathing spontaneously.
      **(4)** Higher success rate than that achieved via the nasotracheal route.
   c. **Disadvantages**
      **(1)** Frequently requires neuromuscular paralysis, creating a risk of fatal respiratory arrest if intubation is unsuccessful.
      **(2)** Requires neck manipulation, which may cause spinal cord injury if the patient has also had neck trauma.

## BREATHING

Along with airway problems, breathing difficulties are the major cause of morbidity and death in patients with poisoning or drug overdose. Patients may have one or more of the following complications: ventilatory failure, hypoxia, or bronchospasm.

**I. Ventilatory failure.**

**A. Assessment.** Ventilatory failure has multiple causes, including failure of the ventilatory muscles, central depression of respiratory drive, and severe pneumonia or pulmonary edema. Examples of drugs and toxins that cause ventilatory failure and the causative mechanisms are listed in Table I–1.

**B. Complications.** Ventilatory failure is the most common cause of death in poisoned patients.

1. Hypoxia may result in brain damage, cardiac arrhythmias, and cardiac arrest.
2. Hypercarbia results in acidosis, which may contribute to arrhythmias, especially in patients with salicylate or tricyclic antidepressant overdoses.

**C. Differential diagnosis.** Rule out the following:

1. Bacterial or viral pneumonia.
2. Viral encephalitis or myelitis (eg, polio).
3. Traumatic or ischemic spinal cord or central nervous system (CNS) injury.
4. Tetanus, causing rigidity of chest wall muscles.
5. Pneumothorax.

**D. Treatment.** Obtain measurements of arterial blood gases. Quickly estimate the adequacy of ventilation from the $pCO_2$ level; obtundation with an elevated or rising $pCO_2$ (eg, > 60 mm Hg) indicates a need for assisted ventilation. Do ***not*** wait until the patient is apneic or until the $pCO_2$ is above 60 mm to begin assisted ventilation.

1. Assist breathing manually with a bag-valve-mask device or bag-valve-endotracheal tube device until the mechanical ventilator is ready for use.
2. If not already accomplished, **perform endotracheal intubation.**
3. **Program the ventilator** for tidal volume (usually 15 mL/kg), rate (usually 12–15 breaths/min), and oxygen concentration (usually 30–35% to start). Monitor the patient's response to ventilator settings frequently by obtaining arterial blood gas values.
   a. If the patient has some spontaneous ventilation, the machine can be set to allow the patient to breathe spontaneously with only intermittent mandatory ventilation (usually 10–12 breaths/min).
   b. If the endotracheal tube has been placed only for airway protection, the patient can be left to breathe entirely spontaneously with blow-by oxygen mist (T-piece).

**TABLE I–1. SELECTED DRUGS AND TOXINS CAUSING VENTILATORY FAILURE[a]**

| Paralysis of ventilatory muscles | Depression of central respiratory drive |
|---|---|
| Botulinum toxin (botulism) | Antihistamines |
| Neuromuscular blockers | Barbiturates |
| Nicotine | Clonidine and other sympatholytic agents |
| Organophosphates and carbamates | Ethanol and alcohols |
| Saxitoxin ("red tide") | Gamma hydroxybutyrate (GHB) |
| Snakebite | Opioids |
| Strychnine and tetanus (muscle rigidity) | Phenothiazines and antipsychotic drugs |
| Tetrodotoxin | Sedative-hypnotics |
| Warfare nerve gases | Tricyclic antidepressants |

[a]Adapted in part, with permission, from Olson KR, Pentel PR, Kelly MT: Physical assessment and differential diagnosis of the poisoned patient. *Med Toxicol* 1987;2:52.

**II. Hypoxia.**

**A. Assessment.** Examples of drugs or toxins causing hypoxia are listed in Table I–2. Hypoxia can be caused by the following conditions:

1. **Insufficient oxygen** in ambient air (eg, displacement of oxygen by inert gases).
2. **Disruption of oxygen absorption** by the lung (eg, resulting from pneumonia or pulmonary edema).
   - a. **Pneumonia.** The most common cause of pneumonia in overdosed patients is pulmonary aspiration of gastric contents. Pneumonia may also be caused by intravenous injection of foreign material or bacteria, aspiration of petroleum distillates, or inhalation of irritant gases.
   - b. **Pulmonary edema.** All agents that can cause chemical pneumonia (eg, irritant gases and hydrocarbons) can also cause pulmonary edema. This usually involves an alteration of permeability in pulmonary capillaries, resulting in **noncardiogenic** pulmonary edema (adult respiratory distress syndrome [ARDS]). In noncardiogenic pulmonary edema, the pulmonary capillary wedge pressure (reflecting filling pressure in the left ventricle) is usually normal or low. In contrast, **cardiogenic** pulmonary edema caused by cardiac-depressant drugs is characterized by low cardiac output with elevated pulmonary wedge pressure.
3. **Cellular hypoxia**, which may be present despite a normal arterial blood gas value.
   - a. **Carbon monoxide** poisoning (see p 151) and **methemoglobinemia** (p 262) may severely limit oxygen binding to hemoglobin (and, therefore, the oxygen-carrying capacity of blood) without altering the $pO_2$, because routine blood gas determination measures dissolved oxygen in the plasma but does not measure actual oxygen content. In such cases, only the direct measurement of oxygen saturation using a co-oximeter (not its calculation from the $pO_2$) will reveal decreased oxyhemoglobin saturation. ***Note:*** Pulse oximetry gives falsely normal or nearly normal results and is not reliable.
   - b. **Cyanide** (p 176) and **hydrogen sulfide** poisoning (p 224) interfere with cellular oxygen utilization, resulting in decreased oxygen uptake by the tissues, and may cause abnormally high venous oxygen saturation.

**TABLE I–2. SELECTED CAUSES OF HYPOXIA[a]**

| | |
|---|---|
| **Inert gases** | **Pneumonia or noncardiogenic pulmonary edema** |
| Carbon dioxide | Aspiration of gastric contents |
| Methane and propane | Aspiration of hydrocarbons |
| Nitrogen | Chlorine and other irritant gases |
| **Cardiogenic pulmonary edema** | Cocaine |
| Beta receptor antagonists | Ethchlorvynol (IV and oral) |
| Quinidine, procainamide, and disopyramide | Ethylene glycol |
| | Mercury vapor |
| Tricyclic antidepressants | Metal fumes ("metal fumes fever") |
| Verapamil | Nitrogen dioxide |
| **Cellular hypoxia** | Opioids |
| Carbon monoxide | Paraquat |
| Cyanide | Phosgene |
| Hydrogen sulfide | Salicylates |
| Methemoglobinemia | Sedative-hypnotic drugs |
| Sulfhemoglobinemia | Smoke inhalation |

[a]See also Table I–1.

**B. Complications.** Significant or sustained hypoxia may result in brain damage and cardiac arrhythmias.

**C. Differential diagnosis.** Rule out the following:

1. Erroneous sampling (eg, inadvertently measuring venous blood gases rather than arterial blood gases).
2. Bacterial or viral pneumonia.
3. Pulmonary contusion caused by trauma.
4. Acute myocardial infarction with pump failure.

**D. Treatment**

1. **Correct hypoxia**. Administer supplemental oxygen as indicated, based on arterial $pO_2$. Intubation and assisted ventilation may be required.
   - a. If carbon monoxide poisoning is suspected, give 100% oxygen and consider hyperbaric oxygen (see p 490).
   - b. See also treatment guides for cyanide (p 176), hydrogen sulfide (p 224), and methemoglobinemia (p 262).
2. **Treat pneumonia.** Obtain frequent sputum samples and initiate appropriate antibiotic therapy when there is evidence of infection.
   - a. There is no basis for prophylactic antibiotic treatment of aspiration- or chemical-induced pneumonia.
   - b. Although some physicians recommend corticosteroids for chemical-induced pneumonia, there is little evidence of their benefit.
3. **Treat pulmonary edema.**
   - a. Avoid excessive fluid administration. Pulmonary artery cannulation and wedge pressure measurements may be necessary to guide fluid therapy.
   - b. Administer supplemental oxygen to maintain a $pO_2$ of at least 60–70 mm Hg. Endotracheal intubation and use of positive end-expiratory pressure (PEEP) ventilation may be necessary to maintain adequate oxygenation.

**III. Bronchospasm**

**A. Assessment.** Examples of drugs and toxins that cause bronchospasm are listed in Table I–3. Bronchospasm may result from the following:

1. **Direct irritant injury** from inhaled gases or pulmonary aspiration of petroleum distillates or stomach contents.
2. **Pharmacologic effects** of toxins, eg, organophosphate or carbamate insecticides or beta-adrenergic antagonists.
3. **Hypersensitivity** or allergic reactions.

**B. Complications.** Severe bronchospasm may result in hypoxia and ventilatory failure. Exposure to high concentrations of irritant gases can lead to asthma ("reactive airway dysfunction syndrome" [RADS]).

**C. Differential diagnosis.** Rule out the following:

1. Asthma or other preexisting bronchospastic disorders.
2. Stridor caused by upper-airway injury and edema (progressive airway edema may result in acute airway obstruction).
3. Airway obstruction by a foreign body.

**D. Treatment**

1. Administer supplemental oxygen. Assist ventilation and perform endotracheal intubation if needed.

**TABLE I–3. SELECTED DRUGS AND TOXINS CAUSING BRONCHOSPASM**

| | |
|---|---|
| Beta receptor antagonists | Isocyanates |
| Brevetoxin | Organophosphates and other anticholinesterases |
| Chlorine and other irritant gases | Particulate dusts |
| Drugs causing allergic reactions | Smoke inhalation |
| Hydrocarbon aspiration | Sulfites (eg, in foods) |

2. Remove the patient from the source of exposure to any irritant gas or other offending agent.
3. Immediately discontinue any beta-adrenergic antagonist treatment.
4. Administer bronchodilators:
   a. Aerosolized beta-2 receptor stimulant (eg, albuterol [2.5–5 mg] in nebulizer). Repeat as needed or give 5–15 mg as a continuous nebulizer treatment over 1 hour (children: 0.3–0.5 mg/kg/h).
   b. Aerosolized ipratropium bromide, 0.5 mg every 4–6 hours, especially if excessive cholinergic stimulation is suspected.
   c. For reactive airways, consider inhaled or oral steroids.
5. For patients with bronchospasm and bronchorrhea caused by organophosphorus or other cholinesterase inhibitor poisoning, give atropine (see p 415) intravenously. Ipratropium bromide (see 4.b above) may also be helpful.

## CIRCULATION

I. **General assessment and initial treatment**
   A. **Check blood pressure and pulse rate and rhythm.** Perform cardiopulmonary resuscitation (CPR) if there is no pulse and perform advanced cardiac life support (ACLS) for arrhythmias and shock. Note that some ACLS drugs may be ineffective or dangerous in patients with drug- or poison-induced cardiac disorders. For example, procainamide is contraindicated in patients with tricyclic antidepressant overdose, and atropine and isoproterenol are ineffective in patients with beta receptor antagonist poisoning.
   B. **Begin continuous electrocardiographic (ECG) monitoring.** Arrhythmias may complicate a variety of drug overdoses, and all patients with potentially cardiotoxic drug poisoning should be monitored in the emergency department or an intensive care unit for at least 6 hours after the ingestion.
   C. **Secure venous access.** Antecubital or forearm veins are usually easy to cannulate. Alternative sites include femoral, subclavian, internal jugular, and other central veins. Access to central veins is technically more difficult but allows measurement of central venous pressure and placement of a pacemaker or pulmonary artery lines.
   D. **Draw blood** for routine studies (see p 31).
   E. **Begin intravenous infusion** of normal saline (NS), 5% dextrose in NS (D5-NS), 5% dextrose in half NS ($D_5W$ 0.45% sodium chloride), or 5% dextrose in water ($D_5W$) at a keep-open rate; for children, use 5% dextrose in quarter NS ($D_5W$ 0.25% sodium chloride). If the patient is hypotensive (see p 15), NS or another isotonic crystalloid solution is preferred.
   F. In seriously ill patients (eg, those who are hypotensive, obtunded, convulsing, or comatose), **place a Foley catheter** in the bladder, obtain urine for routine and toxicologic testing, and measure hourly urine output.

II. **Bradycardia and atrioventricular (AV) block**
   A. **Assessment.** Examples of drugs and toxins causing bradycardia or AV block and their mechanisms are listed in Table I–4.
      1. Bradycardia and AV block are common features of intoxication with calcium antagonists (see p 143) and drugs that depress sympathetic tone or increase parasympathetic tone. These conditions may also result from severe intoxication with membrane-depressant drugs (eg, tricyclic antidepressants, quinidine, and other type Ia and Ic antiarrhythmic agents).
      2. Bradycardia or AV block may also be a reflex response (baroreceptor reflex) to hypertension induced by alpha-adrenergic agents such as phenylpropanolamine and phenylephrine.
      3. In children, bradycardia is commonly caused by respiratory compromise and usually responds to ventilation and oxygenation.

**TABLE I–4. SELECTED DRUGS AND TOXINS CAUSING BRADYCARDIA OR ATRIOVENTRICULAR BLOCK[a]**

| | |
|---|---|
| **Cholinergic or vagotonic agents** | **Sympatholytic agents** |
| Digitalis glycosides | Beta receptor antagonists |
| Organophosphates and carbamates | Clonidine |
| Physostigmine, neostigmine | Opioids |
| | **Other** |
| **Membrane-depressant drugs** | Calcium antagonists |
| Propranolol | Carbamazepine |
| Encainide and flecainide | Lithium |
| Quinidine, procainamide, and disopyramide | Phenylpropanolamine and other alpha-adrenergic agonists |
| Tricyclic antidepressants | |
| | Propoxyphene |

[a]Adapted in part, with permission, from Olson KR et al. *Med Toxicol* 1987;2:71.

**B. Complications.** Bradycardia and AV block frequently cause hypotension, which may progress to asystolic cardiac arrest.

**C. Differential diagnosis.** Rule out the following:

1. Hypothermia.
2. Myocardial ischemia or infarction.
3. Electrolyte abnormality (eg, hyperkalemia).
4. Metabolic disturbance (eg, hypothyroidism).
5. Physiologic origin, owing to an intrinsically slow pulse rate (common in athletes) or an acute vaso-vagal reaction.
6. Cushing reflex (caused by severe intracranial hypertension).

**D. Treatment.** Do ***not*** treat bradycardia or AV block unless the patient is symptomatic (eg, exhibits signs of syncope or hypotension). ***Note:*** Bradycardia or even AV block may be a protective reflex to lower the blood pressure in a patient with life-threatening hypertension (see item VII below).

1. Maintain an open airway and assist ventilation (see pp 1–4) if necessary. Administer supplemental oxygen.
2. Rewarm hypothermic patients. A sinus bradycardia of 40–50/min is normal when the body temperature is 32–35°C (90–95°F).
3. Administer atropine, 0.01–0.03 mg/kg IV (see p 415). If this is not successful, use isoproterenol 1–10 mcg/min IV (see p 465), titrated to the desired rate, or use an emergency transcutaneous or transvenous pacemaker.
4. Use the following specific antidotes if appropriate:
   - **a.** For beta receptor antagonist overdose, give glucagon (see p 456).
   - **b.** For digitalis intoxication, use Fab antibody fragments (see p 440).
   - **c.** For tricyclic antidepressant or membrane-depressant drug overdose, administer sodium bicarbonate (see p 423).
   - **d.** For calcium antagonist overdose, give calcium (see p 428).

**III. QRS interval prolongation**

**A. Assessment.** Examples of drugs and toxins causing QRS interval prolongation are listed in Table I–5.

1. QRS interval prolongation of greater than 0.12 second in the limb leads (Figure I–3) strongly indicates serious poisoning by tricyclic antidepressants (see p 91) or other membrane-depressant drugs (eg, quinidine [p 326], flecainide [p 79], chloroquine [p 165], and propranolol [p 131]). Rightward axis deviation of the terminal 40 msec of the ECG, which is easily recognized as a late R wave in the aVR lead, may precede QRS widening in patients with tricyclic antidepressant intoxication. (See Figure I–4.)
2. QRS interval prolongation may also result from a ventricular escape rhythm in a patient with complete heart block (eg, from digitalis, calcium antagonist poisoning, or intrinsic cardiac disease).

**TABLE I–5. SELECTED DRUGS AND TOXINS CAUSING QRS INTERVAL PROLONGATION[a]**

| | |
|---|---|
| Chloroquine and related agents | Lamotrigine |
| Cocaine (high-dose) | Phenothiazines (thioridazine) |
| Digitalis glycosides (complete heart block) | Propoxyphene |
| Diphenhydramine (high-dose) | Propranolol |
| Encainide and flecainide | Quinidine, procainamide, and disopyramide |
| Hyperkalemia | Tricyclic antidepressants |

[a]Adapted, in part, with permission, from Olson KR et al. *Med Toxicol* 1987;2:71.

**B. Complications.** QRS interval prolongation in patients with tricyclic antidepressant or similar drug poisonings is often accompanied by hypotension, AV block, and seizures.

**C. Differential diagnosis.** Rule out the following:

1. Intrinsic conduction system disease (bundle branch block or complete heart block) caused by coronary artery disease. Check an old ECG if available.
2. Hyperkalemia with critical cardiac toxicity may appear as a "sine wave" pattern with markedly wide QRS complexes. These are usually preceded by peaked T waves (Figure I–5).
3. Hypothermia with a core temperature of less than 32°C (90°F) often causes an extraterminal QRS deflection (J wave or Osborne wave), resulting in a widened QRS appearance (Figure I–6).

**D. Treatment**

1. Maintain the airway and assist ventilation if necessary (see pp 1–4). Administer supplemental oxygen.

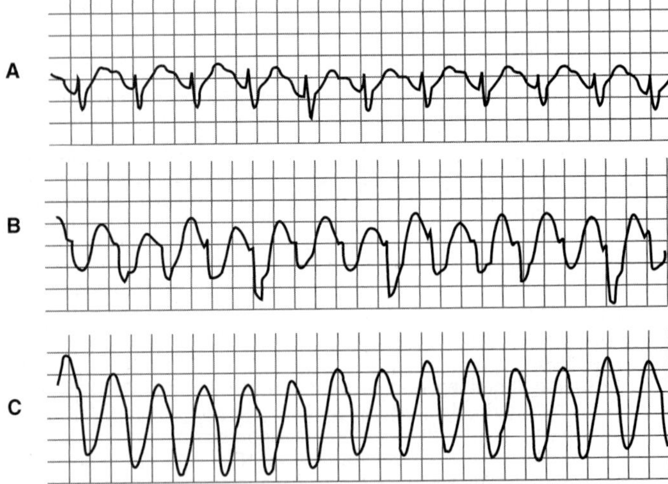


**FIGURE I–3.** Widened QRS interval caused by tricyclic antidepressant overdose. A: Delayed intraventricular conduction results in prolonged QRS interval (0.18 s). B and C: Supraventricular tachycardia with progressive widening of QRS complexes mimics ventricular tachycardia. (Modified and reproduced, with permission, from Benowitz NL, Goldschlager N. Cardiac disturbances in the toxicologic patient. Page 71 in Clinical Management of Poisoning and Drug Overdose. Haddad LM, Winchester JF [editors]. Saunders, 1983.)

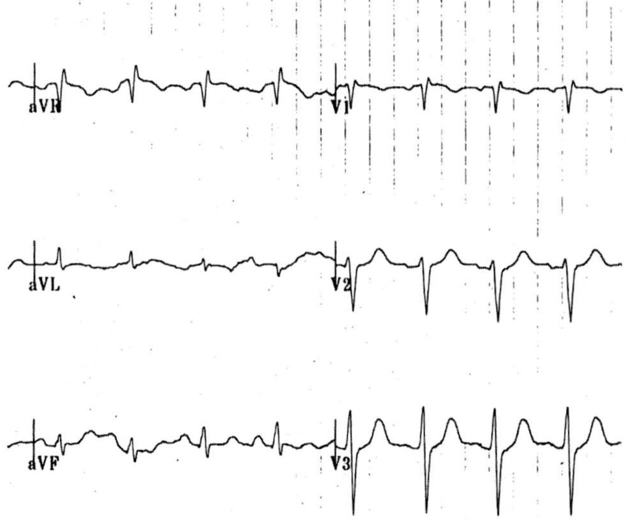


**FIGURE I–4.** Right axis deviation of the terminal 40 msec, easily recognized as a late R wave in aVR.

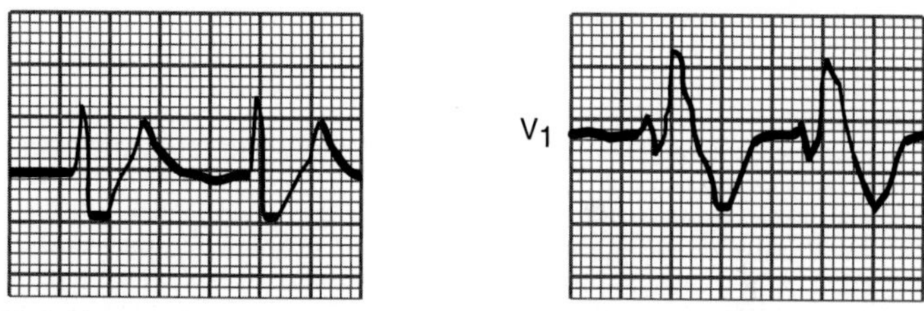


**FIGURE I–5.** Electrocardiogram of patient with hyperkalemia. (Modified and reproduced, with permission, from Goldschlager N, Goldman MJ: Effect of drugs and electrolytes on the electrocardiogram, p 199. In: Electrocardiography: Essentials of Interpretation. Goldschlager N, Goldman MJ [editors]. Lange, 1984.)

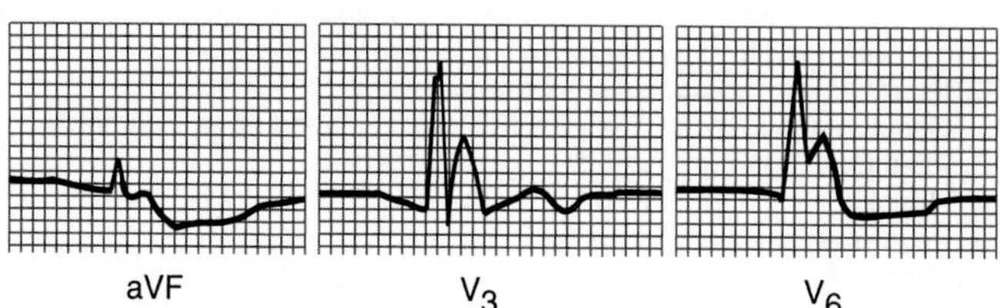


**FIGURE I–6.** Electrocardiogram of patient with hypothermia, showing prominent J waves. (Modified and reproduced, with permission, from Goldschlager N, Goldman MJ: Miscellaneous abnormal electrocardiogram patterns, p 227. In: Electrocardiography: Essentials of Interpretation. Goldschlager N, Goldman MJ [editors]. Lange, 1984.)

**TABLE I–6. SELECTED DRUGS AND TOXINS CAUSING TACHYCARDIA**[a]

| | |
|---|---|
| **Sympathomimetic agents** | **Anticholinergic agents** |
| Amphetamines and derivatives | *Amanita muscaria* mushrooms |
| Caffeine | Antihistamines |
| Cocaine | Atropine and other anticholinergics |
| Ephedrine and pseudoephedrine | Phenothiazines |
| Phencyclidine (PCP) | Plants (many: see p 390) |
| Theophylline | Tricyclic antidepressants |
| **Agents causing cellular hypoxia** | **Other** |
| Carbon monoxide | Ethanol or sedative-hypnotic drug withdrawal |
| Cyanide | |
| Hydrogen sulfide | Vasodilators (reflex tachycardia) |
| Oxidizing agents (methemoglobinemia) | Thyroid hormone |

[a]Adapted, with permission, from Olson KR et al. *Med Toxicol* 1987;2:71.

2. Treat hyperkalemia (see p 37) and hypothermia (p 19) if they occur.
3. Treat AV block with atropine (see p 415), isoproterenol (p 465), and a pacemaker if necessary.
4. For tricyclic antidepressant or other sodium channel–blocking drug overdose, give sodium bicarbonate, 1–2 mEq/kg IV bolus (see p 423); repeat as needed.
5. Give other antidotes if appropriate:
   a. Digoxin-specific Fab antibodies for complete heart block induced by digitalis (see p 440).
   b. Glucagon for beta receptor antagonist intoxication (see p 456).
   c. Calcium for calcium antagonist poisoning (see p 428).

**IV. Tachycardia**

**A. Assessment.** Examples of drugs and toxins causing tachycardia and their mechanisms are listed in Table I–6.

1. Sinus tachycardia and supraventricular tachycardia are often caused by excessive sympathetic stimulation or inhibition of parasympathetic tone. Sinus tachycardia may also be a reflex response to hypotension or hypoxia.
2. Sinus tachycardia and supraventricular tachycardia accompanied by QRS interval prolongation (eg, with tricyclic antidepressant poisoning) may have the appearance of ventricular tachycardia (see Figure I–3).

**B. Complications.** Simple sinus tachycardia (heart rate < 140/min) is rarely of hemodynamic consequence; children and healthy adults easily tolerate rates up to 160–180/min. However, sustained rapid rates may result in hypotension, chest pain, myocardial ischemia, or syncope.

**C. Differential diagnosis.** Rule out the following:

1. Occult blood loss (eg, from gastrointestinal bleeding or trauma).
2. Fluid loss (eg, from gastritis or gastroenteritis).
3. Hypoxia.
4. Fever and infection.
5. Myocardial infarction.
6. Anxiety.
7. Intrinsic conduction system disease (eg, Wolff-Parkinson-White syndrome).

**D. Treatment.** If tachycardia is not associated with hypotension or chest pain, observation and sedation (especially for stimulant intoxication) are usually adequate.

1. For sympathomimetic-induced tachycardia, give esmolol, 0.025–0.1 mg/kg/min IV (p 449).

2. For anticholinergic-induced tachycardia, give physostigmine, 0.01–0.03 mg/kg IV (see p 497), or neostigmine, 0.01–0.03 mg/kg IV. ***Caution:*** Do not use these drugs in patients with tricyclic antidepressant overdose, because additive depression of conduction may result in asystole.

## V. Ventricular arrhythmias

**A. Assessment.** Examples of drugs and toxins causing ventricular arrhythmias are listed in Table I–7.

**TABLE I–7. SELECTED DRUGS AND TOXINS CAUSING VENTRICULAR ARRHYTHMIAS[a]**

| | |
|---|---|
| **Ventricular tachycardia or fibrillation** | |
| Amphetamines and other sympathomimetic agents | Digitalis glycosides |
| Aromatic hydrocarbon solvents | Fluoride |
| Caffeine | Phenothiazines |
| Chloral hydrate | Theophylline |
| Chlorinated or fluorinated hydrocarbon solvents | Tricyclic antidepressants |
| Cocaine | |
| **QT prolongation or torsade de pointes[b]** | |
| Alfuzosin | Methadone |
| Amiodarone | Moexipril |
| Arsenic | Moxifloxacin |
| Astemizole and terfenadine | Nicardipine |
| Azithromycin | Octreotide |
| Bepridil | Ofloxacin |
| Chloral hydrate | Ondansetron |
| Chloroquine, quinine, and related agents | Paroxetine |
| Cisapride | Pentamidine |
| Citrate | Pimozide |
| Clarithromycin | Procainamide |
| Clozapine | Organophosphate insecticides |
| Disopyramide | Quetiapine |
| Dofetilide | Quinidine |
| Dolasetron | Risperidone |
| Domperidone | Roxithromycin |
| Droperidol | Salmeterol |
| Erythromycin | Sertraline |
| Felbamate | Sotalol |
| Flecainide | Sparfloxacin |
| Fluoride | Tacrolimus |
| Fluoxetine | Tamoxifen |
| Foscarnet | Telithromycin |
| Fosphenytoin | Thallium |
| Gatifloxacin | Thioridazine |
| Gemifloxacin | Tizanidine |
| Granisetron | Tricyclic antidepressants |
| Halofantrine | Vardenafil |
| Haloperidol | Venlafaxine |
| Ibutilide | Voriconazole |
| Indapamide | Ziprasidone |
| Isradipine | |
| Levofloxacin | |
| Levomethadyl | |
| Lithium | |
| Mesoridazine | |

[a]References: Olson KR et al. *Med Toxicol* 1987;2:71; and Woolsey RL: Drugs that prolong the QT interval and/or induce torsade de pointes. Internet: http://www.torsades.org.

[b]Torsade de pointes can deteriorate into ventricular fibrillation and cardiac arrest.

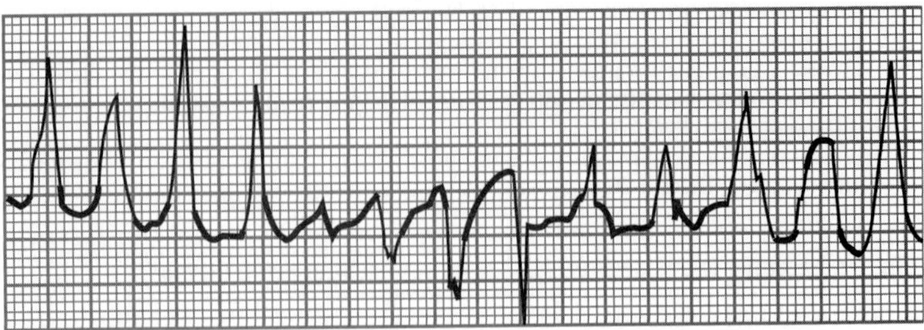

**FIGURE I–7.** Polymorphic ventricular tachycardia (Torsade de pointes). (Modified and reproduced, with permission, from Goldschlager N, Goldman MJ: Effect of drugs and electrolytes on the electrocardiogram, p 197. In: Electrocardiography: Essentials of Interpretation. Goldschlager N, Goldman MJ [editors]). Lange, 1984.)

1. Ventricular irritability is commonly associated with excessive sympathetic stimulation (eg, from cocaine or amphetamines). Patients intoxicated by chlorinated, fluorinated, or aromatic hydrocarbons may have heightened myocardial sensitivity to the arrhythmogenic effects of catecholamines.
2. Ventricular tachycardia may also be a manifestation of intoxication by a tricyclic antidepressant or another sodium channel–blocking drug, although with these drugs true ventricular tachycardia may be difficult to distinguish from sinus or supraventricular tachycardia accompanied by QRS interval prolongation (see Figure I-3).
3. Agents that cause **QT interval prolongation** (QTc > 0.42 second) may produce "atypical" ventricular tachycardia (torsade de pointes). **Torsade de pointes** is characterized by polymorphous ventricular tachycardia that appears to rotate its axis continuously (Figure I–7). Torsade de pointes may also be caused by hypokalemia, hypocalcemia, or hypomagnesemia.

B. **Complications.** Ventricular tachycardia in patients with a pulse may be associated with hypotension or may deteriorate into pulseless ventricular tachycardia or ventricular fibrillation.

C. **Differential diagnosis.** Rule out the following possible causes of ventricular premature beats, ventricular tachycardia, or ventricular fibrillation:
1. Hypoxemia.
2. Hypokalemia.
3. Metabolic acidosis.
4. Myocardial ischemia or infarction.
5. Electrolyte disturbances (eg, hypocalcemia or hypomagnesemia) or congenital disorders that may cause QT prolongation and torsade de pointes.

D. **Treatment.** Perform CPR if necessary and follow standard guidelines for management of arrhythmias, with the exception that procainamide and bretylium should ***not*** be used, especially if tricyclic antidepressant or sodium channel–blocking drug overdose is suspected.
1. Maintain an open airway and assist ventilation if necessary (see pp 1–4). Administer supplemental oxygen.
2. Correct acid-base and electrolyte disturbances.
3. **For ventricular fibrillation**, immediately apply direct-current countershock at 3–5 J/kg. Repeat twice if no response. Continue CPR if the patient is still without a pulse and administer epinephrine, repeated countershocks, amiodarone, and/or lidocaine as recommended in advanced cardiac life support (ACLS) guidelines.
4. **For ventricular tachycardia in patients without a pulse**, immediately give a precordial thump or apply synchronized direct-current countershock at 1–3 J/kg. If this is not successful, begin CPR and apply countershock at

3–5 J/kg; administer amiodarone and/or lidocaine and repeated countershocks as recommended in ACLS guidelines.

5. **For ventricular tachycardia in patients with a pulse**, use lidocaine, 1–3 mg/kg IV (see p 469), or amiodarone, 300 mg IV or 5 mg/kg in children. Do ***not*** use procainamide or other type Ia antiarrhythmic agents. For suspected myocardial sensitivity caused by chloral hydrate or halogenated or aromatic hydrocarbons, use esmolol, 0.025–0.100 mg/kg/min IV (see p 449), or propranolol, 0.5–3 mg IV (p 504).
6. **For tricyclic antidepressant or other sodium channel–blocking drug overdose,** administer sodium bicarbonate, 1–2 mEq/kg IV (see p 423), in repeated boluses until the QRS interval narrows or the serum pH exceeds 7.7.
7. **For "atypical" or polymorphic ventricular tachycardia (torsade de pointes),** do the following:
   - **a.** Use overdrive pacing or isoproterenol, 1–10 mcg/min IV (see p 465), to increase the heart rate (this makes repolarization more homogeneous and abolishes the arrhythmia).
   - **b.** Alternatively, administer intravenous magnesium sulfate, 1–2 g in adults, over 20–30 minutes (see p 470).

## VI. Hypotension

**A. Assessment.** Examples of drugs and toxins causing hypotension and their mechanisms are listed in Table I–8.

1. Physiologic derangements resulting in hypotension include volume loss because of vomiting, diarrhea, or bleeding; apparent volume depletion caused by venodilation; arteriolar dilation; depression of cardiac contractility; arrhythmias that interfere with cardiac output; and hypothermia.

**TABLE I–8. SELECTED DRUGS AND TOXINS CAUSING HYPOTENSION[a]**

| HYPOTENSION WITH RELATIVE BRADYCARDIA | HYPOTENSION WITH TACHYCARDIA |
|---|---|
| **Sympatholytic agents** | **Fluid loss or third spacing** |
| Beta receptor antagonists | Amatoxin-containing mushrooms |
| Bretylium | Arsenic |
| Clonidine and methyldopa | Colchicine |
| Hypothermia | Copper sulfate |
| Opioids | Hyperthermia |
| Reserpine | Iron |
| Tetrahydrozoline and oxymetazoline | Rattlesnake envenomation |
| **Membrane-depressant drugs** | Sedative-hypnotic agents |
| Encainide and flecainide | **Peripheral venous or arteriolar dilation** |
| Quinidine, procainamide, and disopyramide | Alpha antagonists (doxazosin, prazosin, terazosin) |
| Propoxyphene | Beta-2 receptor agonists (eg, albuterol) |
| Propranolol | Caffeine |
| Tricyclic antidepressants | Calcium antagonists (nifedipine, amlodipine, nicardipine) |
| **Others** | Hydralazine |
| Barbiturates | Hyperthermia |
| Calcium antagonists (verapamil, diltiazem) | Minoxidil |
| Fluoride | Nitrites |
| Organophosphates and carbamates | Sodium nitroprusside |
| Sedative-hypnotic agents | Phenothiazines |
| Tilmicosin | Theophylline |
| | Tricyclic antidepressants |

[a]Adapted, in part, with permission, from Olson KR et al. *Med Toxicol* 1987;2:57.

2. Volume loss, venodilation, and arteriolar dilation are likely to result in hypotension with reflex tachycardia. In contrast, hypotension accompanied by bradycardia should suggest intoxication by sympatholytic agents, membrane-depressant drugs, calcium antagonists, or cardiac glycosides or the presence of hypothermia.

**B. Complications.** Severe or prolonged hypotension can cause acute renal tubular necrosis, brain damage, and cardiac ischemia. Metabolic acidosis is a common finding.

**C. Differential diagnosis.** Rule out the following:

1. Hypothermia, which results in a decreased metabolic rate and lowered blood pressure demands.
2. Hyperthermia, which causes arteriolar dilation and venodilation and direct myocardial depression.
3. Fluid loss caused by gastroenteritis.
4. Blood loss (eg, from trauma or gastrointestinal bleeding).
5. Myocardial infarction.
6. Sepsis.
7. Spinal cord injury.

**D. Treatment.** Fortunately, hypotension usually responds readily to empiric therapy with intravenous fluids and low doses of vasopressor drugs (eg, dopamine). When hypotension does not resolve after simple measures, a systematic approach should be followed to determine the cause of hypotension and select the appropriate treatment.

1. Maintain an open airway and assist ventilation if necessary (see pp 1–4). Administer supplemental oxygen.
2. Treat cardiac arrhythmias that may contribute to hypotension (heart rate < 40–50/min or > 180–200/min [see pp 10–13, 15]).
3. Hypotension associated with hypothermia often will not improve with routine fluid therapy but will normalize rapidly upon rewarming of the patient. A systolic blood pressure of 80–90 mm Hg is expected when the body temperature is 32°C (90°F).
4. Give a fluid challenge using NS, 10–20 mL/kg, or another crystalloid solution.
5. Administer dopamine, 5–15 mcg/kg/min (see p 443). Note that dopamine may be ineffective in some patients with depleted neuronal stores of catecholamines (eg, from disulfiram [p 184], reserpine, or tricyclic antidepressant [p 91] overdose) or in cases where alpha-adrenergic receptors may be blocked (tricyclic antidepressants, phenothiazines). In such cases norepinephrine, 0.1 mcg/kg/min IV (p 448), or phenylephrine may be more effective.
6. Consider specific antidotes:
   a. Sodium bicarbonate (see p 423) for tricyclic antidepressant or other sodium channel–blocking drug overdose.
   b. Glucagon (see p 458) for beta receptor antagonist overdose.
   c. Calcium (see p 428) for calcium antagonist overdose.
   d. Propranolol (see p 504) or esmolol (p 449) for theophylline, caffeine, or metaproterenol or other beta-agonist overdose.
7. If the above measures are unsuccessful, insert a central venous pressure (CVP) monitor or pulmonary artery catheter to determine whether further intravenous fluids are needed and to measure the cardiac output (CO) and calculate the systemic vascular resistance (SVR) as follows:

$$SVR = \frac{80(MAP - CVP)}{CO}$$

   where MAP is the mean arterial pressure and normal SVR = 770–1500. Select further therapy on the basis of the following:
   a. If the central venous pressure or pulmonary artery wedge pressure remains low, give more intravenous fluids.

b. If the cardiac output is low, give more dopamine or dobutamine.
c. If the systemic vascular resistance is low, administer norepinephrine, 4–8 mcg/min (see p 487), or phenylephrine.
d. If adrenal insufficiency is suspected, administer corticosteroids (eg, hydrocortisone, 100 mg IV every 8 hours).

## VII. Hypertension

A. **Assessment.** Hypertension is frequently overlooked in drug-intoxicated patients and often goes untreated. Many young persons have normal blood pressures in the range of 90/60 mm Hg to 100/70 mm Hg; in such a person an abrupt elevation to 170/100 mm Hg is much more significant (and potentially catastrophic) than the same blood pressure elevation in an older person with chronic hypertension. Examples of drugs and toxins causing hypertension are listed in Table I–9. Hypertension may be caused by a variety of mechanisms:

1. Amphetamines and other related drugs cause hypertension and tachycardia through generalized sympathetic stimulation.
2. Selective alpha-adrenergic agents cause hypertension with reflex (baroreceptor-mediated) bradycardia or even AV block.
3. Anticholinergic agents cause mild hypertension with tachycardia.
4. Substances that stimulate nicotinic cholinergic receptors (eg, organophosphates) may initially cause tachycardia and hypertension, followed later by bradycardia and hypotension.
5. Withdrawal from sedative-hypnotic drugs, ethanol, opioids, or clonidine can cause hypertension and tachycardia.

B. **Complications.** Severe hypertension can result in intracranial hemorrhage, aortic dissection, myocardial infarction, and congestive heart failure.

C. **Differential diagnosis.** Rule out the following:

1. Idiopathic hypertension (which is common in the general population). However, without a prior history of hypertension, it should not be initially assumed to be the cause of the elevated blood pressure.
2. Increased intracranial pressure caused by spontaneous hemorrhage, trauma, or other causes. This may result in hypertension with reflex bradycardia (Cushing reflex).

D. **Treatment.** Rapid lowering of the blood pressure is desirable as long as it does not result in hypotension, which can potentially cause an ischemic cere-

**TABLE I–9. SELECTED DRUGS AND TOXINS CAUSING HYPERTENSION**[a]

| | |
|---|---|
| **HYPERTENSION WITH TACHYCARDIA** | |
| **Generalized sympathomimetic agents** | **Anticholinergic agents**[b] |
| Amphetamines and derivatives | Antihistamines |
| Cocaine | Atropine and other anticholinergics |
| Ephedrine and pseudoephedrine | Tricyclic antidepressants |
| Epinephrine | **Other** |
| Levodopa | Ethanol and sedative-hypnotic drug withdrawal |
| LSD (lysergic acid diethylamide) | Nicotine (early stage) |
| Marijuana | Organophosphates (early stage) |
| Monoamine oxidase inhibitors | |
| **HYPERTENSION WITH BRADYCARDIA OR ATRIOVENTRICULAR BLOCK** | |
| Clonidine, tetrahydrozoline, and oxymetazoline[c] | Norepinephrine |
| Ergot derivatives | Phenylephrine |
| Methoxamine | Phenylpropanolamine |

[a]Adapted, in part, with permission, from Olson KR et al. *Med Toxicol* 1987;2:56.
[b]Hypertension usually mild and associated with therapeutic or slightly supratherapeutic levels. Overdose may cause hypotension, especially with tricyclics.
[c]Hypertension often transient and followed by hypotension.

bral infarction in older patients with cerebrovascular disease. For a patient with chronic hypertension, lowering the diastolic pressure to 100 mm Hg is acceptable. However, for a young person whose normal diastolic blood pressure is 60 mm Hg, the diastolic pressure should be lowered to 80 mm Hg.

1. **For hypertension with little or no tachycardia**, use phentolamine, 0.02–0.1 mg/kg IV (see p 495), or nitroprusside, 2–10 mcg/kg/min IV (p 485).
2. **For hypertension with tachycardia**, add to the treatment in item 1 above propranolol, 0.02–0.1 mg/kg IV (p 504), or esmolol, 0.025–0.1 mg/kg/min IV (p 449), or labetalol, 0.2–0.3 mg/kg IV (p 459). ***Caution:*** Do not use propranolol or esmolol without a vasodilator to treat hypertensive crisis; beta receptor antagonists may paradoxically worsen hypertension, because any alpha-mediated vasoconstriction is unopposed when beta-2-mediated vasodilation is blocked.
3. **If hypertension is accompanied by a focally abnormal neurologic examination** (eg, hemiparesis), perform a computed tomography (CT) scan as quickly as possible. In a patient with a cerebrovascular accident, hypertension should generally not be treated unless specific complications of the elevated pressure (eg, heart failure or cardiac ischemia) are present. Consult a neurologist.

## ALTERED MENTAL STATUS

**I. Coma and stupor**

**A. Assessment.** A decreased level of consciousness is the most common serious complication of drug overdose or poisoning. Examples of drugs and toxins that cause coma are listed in Table I–10.

1. Coma is most often a result of global depression of the brain's reticular activating system, caused by anticholinergic agents, sympatholytic drugs, generalized CNS depressants, or toxins that result in cellular hypoxia.
2. Coma sometimes represents a postictal phenomenon after a drug- or toxin-induced seizure.
3. Coma may also be caused by brain injury associated with infarction or intracranial bleeding. Brain injury is suggested by the presence of focal neurologic deficits and is confirmed by a CT scan.

**TABLE I–10. SELECTED DRUGS AND TOXINS CAUSING COMA OR STUPOR[a]**

| | |
|---|---|
| **General CNS depressants** | **Cellular hypoxia** |
| Anticholinergics | Carbon monoxide |
| Antihistamines | Cyanide |
| Barbiturates | Hydrogen sulfide |
| Benzodiazepines | Methemoglobinemia |
| Carbamazepine | Sodium azide |
| Ethanol and other alcohols | **Other or unknown mechanisms** |
| GHB (gamma hydroxybutyrate) | Bromide |
| Phenothiazines | Diquat |
| Sedative-hypnotic agents | Disulfiram |
| Tricyclic antidepressants | Hypoglycemic agents |
| Valproic acid | Lithium |
| **Sympatholytic agents** | Nonsteroidal anti-inflammatory drugs (NSAIDs) |
| Clonidine, tetrahydrozoline, and oxymetazoline | Phencyclidine |
| Methyldopa | Salicylates |
| Opioids | |

[a]Adapted, in part, with permission, from Olson KR et al. *Med Toxicol* 1987;2:61.

B. **Complications.** Coma frequently is accompanied by respiratory depression, which is a major cause of death. Other conditions that may accompany or complicate coma include hypotension (see p 15), hypothermia (p 19), hyperthermia (p 20), and rhabdomyolysis (p 26).

C. **Differential diagnosis.** Rule out the following:
1. Head trauma or other causes of intracranial bleeding.
2. Abnormal levels of blood glucose, sodium, or other electrolytes.
3. Hypoxia.
4. Hypothyroidism.
5. Liver or renal failure.
6. Environmental hyperthermia or hypothermia.
7. Serious infections such as encephalitis and meningitis.

D. **Treatment**
1. Maintain the airway and assist ventilation if necessary (see pp 1–4). Administer supplemental oxygen.
2. Give dextrose, thiamine, and naloxone.
   a. **Dextrose.** All patients with depressed consciousness should receive concentrated dextrose unless hypoglycemia is ruled out with an immediate bedside glucose determination. Use a secure vein and avoid extravasation; concentrated dextrose is highly irritating to tissues. Initial doses include the following:
      (1) Adults: 50% dextrose, 50 mL (25 g) IV.
      (2) Children: 25% dextrose, 2 mL/kg IV.
   b. **Thiamine.** Thiamine is given to prevent or treat Wernicke's syndrome resulting from thiamine deficiency in alcoholic patients and others with suspected vitamin deficiencies. It is not given routinely to children. Give thiamine, 100 mg, in the IV bottle or intramuscularly (see p 513).
   c. **Naloxone.** All patients with respiratory depression should receive naloxone (see p 477); if a patient is already intubated and is being artificially ventilated, naloxone is not immediately necessary and can be considered a diagnostic rather than therapeutic drug. ***Caution:*** Although naloxone has no CNS depressant activity of its own and normally can be given safely in large doses, it may precipitate abrupt opioid withdrawal. If an amphetamine or cocaine has been injected along with heroin, reversal of the opioid-induced sedation may unmask stimulant-mediated hypertension, tachycardia, or psychosis. In addition, acute pulmonary edema is sometimes temporally associated with abrupt naloxone reversal of opioid intoxication.
      (1) Give naloxone, 0.4 mg IV (may also be given intramuscularly [IM]).
      (2) If there is no response within 1–2 minutes, give naloxone, 2 mg IV.
      (3) If there is still no response and opioid overdose is highly suspected by history or clinical presentation (pinpoint pupils, apnea, or hypotension), give naloxone, 10–20 mg IV.
   d. Consider **flumazenil** if benzodiazepines are the only suspected cause of coma and there are no contraindications (see p 452). ***Caution:*** Use of flumazenil can precipitate seizures in patients who are addicted to benzodiazepines or who have co-ingested a convulsant drug or poison.
3. Normalize the body temperature (see hypothermia, p 19, and hyperthermia, p 20).
4. If there is any possibility of CNS trauma or cerebrovascular accident, perform a CT scan.
5. If meningitis or encephalitis is suspected, perform a lumbar puncture and treat with appropriate antibiotics.

II. **Hypothermia**

A. **Assessment.** Hypothermia may mimic or complicate drug overdose and should be suspected in every comatose patient. Examples of drugs and toxins that cause hypothermia are listed in Table I–11.

**TABLE I–11. SELECTED DRUGS AND TOXINS ASSOCIATED WITH HYPOTHERMIA**[a]

| | |
|---|---|
| Barbiturates | Phenothiazines |
| Ethanol and other alcohols | Sedative-hypnotic agents |
| Hypoglycemic agents | Tricyclic antidepressants |
| Opioids | Vasodilators |

[a]Adapted, in part, with permission, from Olson KR et al. *Med Toxicol* 1987;2:60.

1. Hypothermia is usually caused by exposure to low ambient temperatures in a patient with blunted thermoregulatory response mechanisms. Drugs and toxins may induce hypothermia by causing vasodilation, inhibiting the shivering response, decreasing metabolic activity, or causing loss of consciousness in a cold environment.
2. A patient whose temperature is lower than 32°C (90°F) may appear to be dead, with a barely detectable pulse or blood pressure and without reflexes. The ECG may reveal an abnormal terminal deflection (J wave or Osborne wave; see Figure I–6).

**B. Complications.** Because there is a generalized reduction of metabolic activity and less demand for blood flow, hypothermia is commonly accompanied by hypotension and bradycardia.

1. Mild hypotension (systolic blood pressure of 70–90 mm Hg) in a patient with hypothermia should not be treated aggressively; excessive intravenous fluids may cause fluid overload and further lowering of the temperature.
2. Severe hypothermia (temperature < 28–30°C) may cause intractable ventricular fibrillation and cardiac arrest. This may occur abruptly, such as when the patient is moved or rewarmed too quickly or when CPR is performed.

**C. Differential diagnosis.** Rule out the following:

1. Sepsis.
2. Hypoglycemia.
3. Hypothyroidism.
4. Environmental hypothermia caused by exposure to a cold environment.

**D. Treatment**

1. Maintain the airway and assist ventilation if necessary (see pp 1–4). Administer supplemental oxygen.
2. Because the pulse rate may be profoundly slow (10/min) and weak, perform careful cardiac evaluation before assuming that the patient is in cardiac arrest. Do ***not*** treat bradycardia; it will resolve with rewarming.
3. Unless the patient is in cardiac arrest (asystole or ventricular fibrillation), rewarm slowly (using blankets, warm intravenous fluids, and warmed-mist inhalation) to prevent rewarming arrhythmias.
4. For patients in cardiac arrest, usual antiarrhythmic agents and direct-current countershock are frequently ineffective until the core temperature is above 32–35°C (90–95°F). Provide gastric or peritoneal lavage with warmed fluids and perform CPR. For ventricular fibrillation, bretylium, 5–10 mg/kg IV (see p 426), may be effective.
5. Open cardiac massage, with direct warm irrigation of the ventricle, or a partial cardiopulmonary bypass may be necessary in hypothermic patients in cardiac arrest who are unresponsive to the above treatment.

**III. Hyperthermia**

**A. Assessment.** Hyperthermia (temperature > 40°C or 104°F) may be a catastrophic complication of intoxication by a variety of drugs and toxins (Table I–12). It may be caused by excessive heat generation because of sustained seizures, rigidity, or other muscular hyperactivity; an increased metabolic rate; impaired dissipation of heat secondary to impaired sweating (eg, anticholinergic agents); or hypothalamic disorders.

TABLE I–12. SELECTED DRUGS AND TOXINS ASSOCIATED WITH HYPERTHERMIA[a]

| Excessive muscular hyperactivity, rigidity, or seizures | Impaired heat dissipation or disrupted thermoregulation |
|---|---|
| Amoxapine | Amoxapine |
| Amphetamines and derivatives (including MDMA) | Anticholinergic agents |
| Cocaine | Antihistamines |
| Lithium | Phenothiazines and other antipsychotic agents |
| LSD (lysergic acid diethylamide) | Tricyclic antidepressants |
| Maprotiline | **Other** |
| Monoamine oxidase inhibitors | Exertional heatstroke |
| Phencyclidine | Malignant hyperthermia |
| Tricyclic antidepressants | Metal fume fever |
| **Increased metabolic rate** | Neuroleptic malignant syndrome (NMS) |
| Dinitrophenol and pentachlorophenol | Serotonin syndrome |
| Salicylates | Withdrawal from ethanol or sedative-hypnotic drugs |
| Thyroid hormone | |

[a]Adapted, with permission, from Olson KR et al. *Med Toxicol* 1987;2:59.

1. **Neuroleptic malignant syndrome (NMS)** is a hyperthermic disorder seen in some patients who use antipsychotic agents and is characterized by hyperthermia, muscle rigidity (often so severe as to be called "lead-pipe" rigidity), metabolic acidosis, and confusion.
2. **Malignant hyperthermia** is an inherited disorder that causes severe hyperthermia, metabolic acidosis, and rigidity after certain anesthetic agents (most commonly halothane and succinylcholine) are used.
3. **Serotonin syndrome** occurs primarily in patients taking monoamine oxidase (MAO) inhibitors (see p 269) who also take serotonin-enhancing drugs such as meperidine (Demerol™), fluoxetine (Prozac™), or other serotonin reuptake inhibitors (SSRIs; see Antidepressants, p 89) and is characterized by irritability, muscle rigidity and myoclonus (especially of the lower extremities), diaphoresis, autonomic instability, and hyperthermia. It may also occur in people taking an overdose of or combinations of SSRIs even without concurrent use of MAO inhibitors.

**B. Complications.** Untreated, severe hyperthermia is likely to result in hypotension, rhabdomyolysis, coagulopathy, cardiac and renal failure, brain injury, and death. Survivors often have permanent neurologic sequelae.

**C. Differential diagnosis.** Rule out the following:

1. Sedative-hypnotic drug or ethanol withdrawal (delirium tremens).
2. Exertional or environmental heat stroke.
3. Thyrotoxicosis.
4. Meningitis or encephalitis.
5. Other serious infections.

**D. Treatment. Immediate rapid cooling** is essential to prevent death or serious brain damage.

1. Maintain the airway and assist ventilation if necessary (see pp 1–4). Administer supplemental oxygen.
2. Administer glucose-containing intravenous fluids and give concentrated glucose bolus (p 457) if the patient is hypoglycemic.
3. Rapidly gain control of seizures (see below), agitation (p 22), or muscular rigidity (p 25).
4. Begin external cooling with tepid (lukewarm) sponging and fanning. This evaporative method is the most efficient method of cooling.
5. Shivering often occurs with rapid external cooling, and it may generate even more heat. Some physicians recommend chlorpromazine to abolish shivering, but this agent can lower the seizure threshold, inhibit sweating,

and cause hypotension. It is preferable to use a benzodiazepine such as diazepam, 0.1–0.2 mg/kg IV; lorazepam, 0.05–0.1 mg/kg IV; or midazolam, 0.05–0.1 mg/kg IV or IM (see p 419) or use neuromuscular paralysis (see below).

6. The most rapidly effective and reliable means of lowering the temperature is neuromuscular paralysis. Administer a nondepolarizing agent (see p 480) such as pancuronium, 0.1 mg/kg IV, or vecuronium, 0.1 mg/kg IV. ***Caution:*** The patient will stop breathing; be prepared to ventilate and intubate endotracheally.
7. **Malignant hyperthermia.** If muscle rigidity persists despite administration of neuromuscular blockers, a defect at the muscle cell level (ie, malignant hyperthermia) should be suspected. Give dantrolene, 1–10 mg/kg IV (see p 436).
8. **Neuroleptic malignant syndrome.** Consider bromocriptine (see p 427).
9. **Serotonin syndrome.** Anecdotal case reports suggest benefit with cyproheptadine (Periactin™), 4 mg orally (PO) every hour for 3–4 doses (see p 435).

## IV. Seizures

**A. Assessment.** Seizures are a major cause of morbidity and mortality from drug overdose or poisoning. Seizures may be single and brief or multiple and sustained and may result from a variety of mechanisms (Table I–13).

**TABLE I–13. SELECTED DRUGS AND TOXINS CAUSING SEIZURES[a]**

| **Adrenergic-sympathomimetic agents** | **Antidepressants and antipsychotics** |
|---|---|
| Amphetamines and derivatives (including MDMA) | Amoxapine |
| Caffeine | Bupropion |
| Cocaine | Haloperidol and butyrophenones |
| Ephedrine | Loxapine, clozapine, and olanzapine |
| Phencyclidine | Phenothiazines |
| Phenylpropanolamine | Tricyclic antidepressants |
| Theophylline | Venlafaxine other serotonin reuptake inhibitors (SSRIs) |
| **Others** | |
| Antihistamines (diphenhydramine, hydroxyzine) | GHB (gamma hydroxybutyrate) |
| Beta receptor antagonists (primarily propranolol; not reported for atenolol, metoprolol, pindolol, or practolol) | Isoniazid (INH) |
| | Lamotrigine |
| | Lead and other heavy metals |
| Boric acid | Lidocaine and other local anesthetics |
| Camphor | Lithium |
| Carbamazepine | Mefenamic acid |
| Cellular hypoxia (eg, carbon monoxide, cyanide, hydrogen sulfide) | Meperidine (normeperidine metabolite) |
| | Metaldehyde |
| Chlorinated hydrocarbons | Methanol |
| Cholinergic agents (carbamates, nicotine, organophosphates) | Methyl bromide |
| | Phenols |
| Cicutoxin (water hemlock) and other plant toxins | Phenylbutazone |
| Citrate | Piroxicam |
| DEET (diethyltoluamide) (rare) | Salicylates |
| Ethylene glycol | Strychnine (opisthotonus and rigidity) |
| Fipronil | Tiagabine |
| Fluoride | Withdrawal from ethanol or sedative-hypnotic drugs |
| Foscarnet | |

[a]Adapted, in part, with permission, from Olson KR et al. *Med Toxicol* 1987;2:63.

1. Generalized seizures usually result in loss of consciousness, often accompanied by tongue biting and fecal and urinary incontinence.
2. Other causes of muscular hyperactivity or rigidity (see p 25) may be mistaken for seizures, especially if the patient is also unconscious.

**B. Complications**

1. Any seizure can cause airway compromise, resulting in apnea or pulmonary aspiration.
2. Multiple or prolonged seizures may cause severe metabolic acidosis, hyperthermia, rhabdomyolysis, and brain damage.

**C. Differential diagnosis.** Rule out the following:

1. Any serious metabolic disturbance (eg, hypoglycemia, hyponatremia, hypocalcemia, or hypoxia).
2. Head trauma with intracranial injury.
3. Idiopathic epilepsy.
4. Withdrawal from alcohol or a sedative-hypnotic drug.
5. Exertional or environmental hyperthermia.
6. CNS infection such as meningitis or encephalitis.
7. Febrile seizures in children.

**D. Treatment**

1. Maintain an open airway and assist ventilation if necessary (see pp 1–4). Administer supplemental oxygen.
2. Administer naloxone (see pp 22 and 447) if seizures are thought to be caused by hypoxia resulting from opioid-associated respiratory depression.
3. Check for hypoglycemia and administer dextrose and thiamine as for coma (see p 18).
4. Use one or more of the following anticonvulsants. ***Caution:*** Anticonvulsants can cause hypotension, cardiac arrest, or respiratory arrest if administered too rapidly.
   a. Diazepam, 0.1–0.2 mg/kg IV (see p 419).
   b. Lorazepam, 0.05–0.1 mg/kg IV (see p 419).
   c. Midazolam, 0.1–0.2 mg/kg IM (useful when intravenous access is difficult) or 0.05–0.1 mg/kg IV (see p 419).
   d. Phenobarbital, 10–15 mg/kg IV; slow infusion over 15–20 minutes (see p 494).
   e. Pentobarbital, 5–6 mg/kg IV; slow infusion over 8–10 minutes, then continuous infusion at 0.5–3 mg/kg/h titrated to effect (p 493).
   f. Propofol, 2–2.5 mg/kg IV (children: 2.5–3.5 mg/kg); infused in increments (40 mg at a time in adults) IV every 10–20 seconds until desired effect (see p 502).
   g. Phenytoin, 15–20 mg/kg IV; slow infusion over 25–30 minutes (see p 496). ***Note:*** Phenytoin is ineffective for convulsions caused by theophylline and is considered the anticonvulsant of *last* choice for most drug-induced seizures.
5. Immediately check the rectal or tympanic **temperature** and cool the patient rapidly (see p 20) if the temperature is above 40°C (104°F). The most rapid and reliably effective method of temperature control is neuromuscular paralysis with pancuronium, 0.1 mg/kg IV (p 480) or another nondepolarizing neuromuscular blocker. ***Caution:*** If paralysis is used, the patient must be intubated and ventilated; in addition, monitor the electroencephalogram (EEG) for continued brain seizure activity because peripheral muscular hyperactivity is no longer visible.
6. Use the following specific antidotes if available:
   a. Pyridoxine (see p 508) for isoniazid (INH; p 233).
   b. Pralidoxime (2-PAM; see p 500) or atropine (p 415) or both for organophosphate or carbamate insecticides (p 292).

**V. Agitation, delirium, or psychosis**

**A. Assessment.** Agitation, delirium, or psychosis may be caused by a variety of drugs and toxins (Table I–14). In addition, such symptoms may result from a

**TABLE I–14. SELECTED DRUGS AND TOXINS CAUSING AGITATION, DELIRIUM, OR CONFUSION[a]**

| Predominant confusion or delirium | Predominant agitation or psychosis |
|---|---|
| Amantadine | Amphetamines and derivatives |
| Anticholinergic agents | Caffeine |
| Antihistamines | Cocaine |
| Bromide | Cycloserine |
| Carbon monoxide | Dextromethorphan |
| Cimetidine | LSD (lysergic acid diethylamide) |
| Disulfiram | Marijuana |
| Lead and other heavy metals | Mercury |
| Levodopa | Phencyclidine (PCP) |
| Lidocaine and other local anesthetics | Procaine |
| Lithium | Serotonin reuptake inhibitors (SSRIs) |
| Salicylates | Steroids (eg, prednisone) |
| Withdrawal from ethanol or sedative-hypnotic drugs | Theophylline |

[a]Adapted, in part, with permission, from Olson KR et al. *Med Toxicol* 1987;2:62.

functional thought disorder or metabolic encephalopathy caused by medical illness.

1. Functional psychosis or stimulant-induced agitation and psychosis are usually associated with an intact sensorium, and hallucinations are predominantly auditory.
2. With metabolic encephalopathy or drug-induced delirium, there is usually alteration of the sensorium (manifested by confusion or disorientation). Hallucinations, when they occur, are predominantly visual.

**B. Complications.** Agitation, especially if accompanied by hyperkinetic behavior and struggling, may result in hyperthermia (see p 20) and rhabdomyolysis (p 26).

**C. Differential diagnosis.** Rule out the following:

1. Serious metabolic disturbance (hypoxia, hypoglycemia, or hyponatremia).
2. Alcohol or sedative-hypnotic drug withdrawal.
3. Thyrotoxicosis.
4. CNS infection such as meningitis or encephalitis.
5. Exertion-induced or environmental hyperthermia.

**D. Treatment.** Sometimes the patient can be calmed with reassuring words and reduction of noise, light, and physical stimulation. If this is not quickly effective, rapidly gain control of the patient to determine the rectal or tympanic temperature and begin rapid cooling and other treatment if needed.

1. Maintain an open airway and assist ventilation if necessary (see pp 1–4). Administer supplemental oxygen.
2. Treat hypoglycemia (see p 35), hypoxia (p 6), or other metabolic disturbances.
3. Administer one of the following sedatives:
   - **a.** Midazolam, 0.05–0.1 mg/kg IV over 1 minute, or 0.1–0.2 mg/kg IM (see p 419).
   - **b.** Lorazepam, 0.05–0.1 mg/kg IV over 1 minute (see p 419).
   - **c.** Diazepam, 0.1–0.2 mg/kg IV over 1 minute (see p 419).
   - **d.** Droperidol, 2.5–5 mg IV, or haloperidol, 0.1–0.2 mg/kg IM or IV over 1 minute (see p 458). ***Note:*** Do not give haloperidol *decanoate* salt intravenously. ***Caution:*** Both droperidol and haloperidol have caused prolongation of the QT interval and polymorphic ventricular tachycardia (torsade de pointes) and should be avoided or used with great caution in patients with preexisting QT prolongation or with toxicity from agents known to prolong the QT.

4. If hyperthermia occurs as a result of excessive muscular hyperactivity, skeletal-muscle paralysis is indicated. Use pancuronium, 0.1 mg/kg IV (see p 480), or another nondepolarizing neuromuscular blocker. ***Caution:*** Be prepared to ventilate and endotracheally intubate the patient after muscle paralysis.

## OTHER COMPLICATIONS

**I. Dystonia, dyskinesia, and rigidity**

**A. Assessment.** Examples of drugs and toxins causing abnormal movements or rigidity are listed in Table I–15.

1. **Dystonic reactions** are common with therapeutic or toxic doses of many antipsychotic agents and with some antiemetics. The mechanism triggering these reactions is thought to be related to central dopamine blockade. Dystonias usually consist of forced, involuntary, and often painful neck rotation (torticollis), tongue protrusion, jaw extension, or trismus. Other extrapyramidal or parkinsonian movement disorders (eg, pill rolling, bradykinesia, and masked facies) may also be seen with these agents.
2. In contrast, **dyskinesias** are usually rapid, repetitive body movements that may involve small localized muscle groups (eg, tongue darting, focal myoclonus) or may consist of generalized hyperkinetic activity. The cause is not dopamine blockade but, more commonly, increased dopamine effects or blockade of central cholinergic effects.
3. **Rigidity** may also be seen with a number of toxins and may be caused by CNS effects or spinal cord stimulation. Neuroleptic malignant syndrome and serotonin syndrome (see p 21) are characterized by rigidity, hyperthermia, metabolic acidosis, and an altered mental status. Rigidity seen with malignant hyperthermia (see p 20) is caused by a defect at the muscle cell level and may not reverse with neuromuscular blockade.

**B. Complications.** Sustained muscular rigidity or hyperactivity may result in rhabdomyolysis (see p 26), hyperthermia (p 20), ventilatory failure (p 5), or metabolic acidosis (p 33).

**C. Differential diagnosis.** Rule out the following:

1. Catatonic rigidity caused by functional thought disorder.

**TABLE I–15. SELECTED DRUGS AND TOXINS CAUSING DYSTONIAS, DYSKINESIAS, AND RIGIDITY[a]**

| | |
|---|---|
| **Dystonia** | **Dyskinesias** |
| Haloperidol and butyrophenones | Amphetamines |
| Metoclopramide | Anticholinergic agents |
| Phenothiazines (prochlorperazine) | Antihistamines |
| Ziprasidone and other atypical antipsychotic agents | Caffeine |
| | Carbamazepine |
| **Rigidity** | Carisoprodol |
| Black widow spider bite | Cocaine |
| Lithium | GHB (gamma hydroxybutyrate) |
| Malignant hyperthermia | Ketamine |
| Methaqualone | Levodopa |
| Monoamine oxidase inhibitors | Lithium |
| Neuroleptic malignant syndrome | Phencyclidine (PCP) |
| Phencyclidine (PCP) | Serotonin reuptake inhibitors (SSRIs) |
| Strychnine | Tricyclic antidepressants |
| Tetanus | |

[a]Adapted, in part, with permission, from Olson KR et al. *Med Toxicol* 1987;2:64.

2. Tetanus.
3. Cerebrovascular accident.
4. Postanoxic encephalopathy.
5. Idiopathic parkinsonism.

**D. Treatment**

1. Maintain the airway and assist ventilation if necessary (see pp 1–4). Administer supplemental oxygen.
2. Check the rectal or tympanic temperature and treat hyperthermia (see p 20) rapidly if the temperature is above 40°C (102.2°F).
3. **Dystonia.** Administer an anticholinergic agent such as diphenhydramine (Benadryl™; see p 442), 0.5–1 mg/kg IM or IV, or benztropine (Cogentin™; p 422), 1–4 mg IM in adults. Follow this treatment with oral therapy for 2–3 days.
4. **Dyskinesia.** Do not treat with anticholinergic agents. Instead, administer a sedative such as diazepam, 0.1–0.2 mg/kg IV (see p 419); lorazepam, 0.05–0.1 mg IV or IM; or midazolam, 0.05–0.1 mg/kg IV or 0.1–0.2 mg/kg IM (p 419).
5. **Rigidity.** Do not treat with anticholinergic agents. Instead, administer a sedative (see item 4, directly above) or provide specific pharmacologic therapy as follows:
   a. Intravenous calcium (see p 428) or *Latrodectus* antivenom for a black widow spider bite (p 346).
   b. Dantrolene (see p 436) for malignant hyperthermia (p 21).
   c. Bromocriptine (see p 427) for neuroleptic malignant syndrome (p 21).

**II. Rhabdomyolysis**

**A. Assessment.** Muscle cell necrosis is a common complication of poisoning. Examples of drugs and toxins that cause rhabdomyolysis are listed in Table I–16.

1. Causes of rhabdomyolysis include prolonged immobilization on a hard surface, excessive seizures or muscular hyperactivity, hyperthermia, and direct cytotoxic effects of the drug or toxin (eg, carbon monoxide, colchicine, *Amanita phalloides* mushrooms, and some snake venoms).
2. The diagnosis is made by finding Hematest-positive urine with few or no intact red blood cells or an elevated serum creatine phosphokinase (CPK) level.

**B. Complications.** Myoglobin released by damaged muscle cells may precipitate in the kidneys, causing acute tubular necrosis and renal failure. This is more likely when the serum CPK level exceeds several thousand IU/L and if

**TABLE I–16. SELECTED DRUGS AND TOXINS ASSOCIATED WITH RHABDOMYOLYSIS**

| Excessive muscular hyperactivity, rigidity, or seizures | Direct cellular toxicity |
|---|---|
| Amphetamines and derivatives | Amatoxin-containing mushrooms |
| Clozapine and olanzapine | Carbon monoxide |
| Cocaine | Colchicine |
| Lithium | Ethylene glycol |
| Monoamine oxidase inhibitors | **Other or unknown mechanisms** |
| Phencyclidine (PCP) | Chlorophenoxy herbicides |
| Seizures caused by a variety of agents | Ethanol |
| Strychnine | Gemfibrozil |
| Tetanus | Hemlock |
| Tricyclic antidepressants | Hyperthermia caused by a variety of agents |
| | Hypokalemia |
| | Sedative-hypnotic agents (prolonged immobility) |
| | "Statin" cholesterol drugs (eg, cerivastatin) |
| | Trauma |

the patient is dehydrated. With severe rhabdomyolysis, hyperkalemia, hyperphosphatemia, hyperuricemia, and hypocalcemia may also occur.

**C. Differential diagnosis.** Hemolysis with hemoglobinuria may also produce Hematest-positive urine.

**D. Treatment**

1. Aggressively restore volume in dehydrated patients. Then establish a steady urine flow rate (3–5 mL/kg/h) with intravenous fluids. For massive rhabdomyolysis accompanied by oliguria, also consider a bolus of mannitol, 0.5 g/kg IV (see p 471).
2. Alkalinize the urine by adding 100 mEq of sodium bicarbonate to each liter of 5% dextrose. (Acidic urine promotes deposition of myoglobin in the tubules.)
3. Provide intensive supportive care, including hemodialysis if needed, for acute renal failure. Kidney function is usually regained in 2–3 weeks.

**III. Anaphylactic and anaphylactoid reactions**

**A. Assessment.** Examples of drugs and toxins that cause anaphylactic or anaphylactoid reactions are listed in Table I–17. These reactions are characterized by bronchospasm and increased vascular permeability that may lead to laryngeal edema, skin rash, and hypotension.

1. **Anaphylaxis** occurs when a patient with antigen-specific immunoglobulin E (IgE) bound to the surface of mast cells and basophils is exposed to the antigen, triggering the release of histamine and various other vasoactive compounds.
2. **Anaphylactoid reactions** are also caused by release of active compounds from mast cells but do not involve prior sensitization or mediation through IgE.

**B. Complications.** Severe anaphylactic or anaphylactoid reactions can result in laryngeal obstruction, respiratory arrest, hypotension, and death.

**C. Differential diagnosis.** Rule out the following:

1. Anxiety with vasodepressor syncope or hyperventilation.
2. Pharmacologic effects of the drug or toxin (eg, procaine reaction with procaine penicillin).
3. Bronchospasm or laryngeal edema from irritant gas exposure.

**D. Treatment**

1. Maintain the airway and assist ventilation if necessary (see pp 1–4). Endotracheal intubation may be needed if laryngeal swelling is severe. Administer supplemental oxygen.
2. Treat hypotension with intravenous crystalloid fluids (eg, normal saline) and place the patient in a supine position.
3. Administer epinephrine (see p 448) as follows:
   a. For mild to moderate reactions, administer 0.3–0.5 mg subcutaneously (SC) (children: 0.01 mg/kg, maximum 0.5 mg).

**TABLE I–17. EXAMPLES OF DRUGS AND TOXINS CAUSING ANAPHYLACTIC OR ANAPHYLACTOID REACTIONS**

| Anaphylactic reactions (IgE-mediated) | Anaphylactoid reactions (not IgE-mediated) |
|---|---|
| Antisera (antivenins) | Acetylcysteine (when given intravenously) |
| Foods (nuts, fish, shellfish) | Blood products |
| Hymenoptera and other insect stings | Iodinated contrast media |
| Immunotherapy allergen extracts | Opioids (eg, morphine) |
| Penicillins and other antibiotics | Scombroid |
| Vaccines | Tubocurarine |
| **Other or unclassified** | |
| Exercise | |
| Sulfites | |
| Tartrazine dye | |

b. For severe reactions, administer 0.05–0.1 mg IV bolus every 5 minutes or give an infusion starting at a rate of 1–4 mcg/min and titrating upward as needed.

4. Administer diphenhydramine (Benadryl™; see p 442), 0.5–1 mg/kg IV over 1 minute. Follow with oral therapy for 2–3 days. An $H_2$ blocker such as cimetidine (Tagamet™; p 433), 300 mg IV every 8 hours, is also helpful.
5. Administer a corticosteroid such as hydrocortisone, 200–300 mg IV, or methylprednisolone, 40–80 mg IV.

## DIAGNOSIS OF POISONING

Diagnosis and treatment of poisoning often must proceed rapidly without the results of extensive toxicologic screening. Fortunately, in most cases the correct diagnosis can be made by using carefully collected data from the history, a directed physical examination, and commonly available laboratory tests.

I. **History.** Although frequently unreliable or incomplete, the history of ingestion may be very useful if carefully obtained.
   A. Ask the patient about all drugs taken, including nonprescription drugs, herbal medicines, and vitamins.
   B. Ask family members, friends, and paramedical personnel about any prescriptions or over-the-counter medications known to be used by the patient or others in the house.
   C. Obtain any available drugs or drug paraphernalia for later testing, but handle them very carefully to avoid poisoning by skin contact or an inadvertent needle stick with potential for hepatitis B or human immunodeficiency virus (HIV) transmission.
   D. Check with the pharmacy on the label of any medications found with the patient to determine whether other prescription drugs have been obtained there.

II. **Physical examination**
   A. **General findings.** Perform a carefully directed examination emphasizing key physical findings that may uncover one of the common "autonomic syndromes." Important variables in the autonomic physical examination include blood pressure, pulse rate, pupil size, sweating, and peristaltic activity. The autonomic syndromes are summarized in Table I–18.
      1. **Alpha-adrenergic syndrome.** Hypertension with reflex bradycardia is characteristic of alpha-adrenergic syndrome. The pupils are usually dilated. (Examples: phenylpropanolamine and phenylephrine.)
      2. **Beta-adrenergic syndrome.** Beta-2–mediated vasodilation may cause hypotension. Tachycardia is common. (Examples: albuterol, metaproterenol, theophylline, and caffeine.)
      3. **Mixed alpha- and beta-adrenergic syndrome.** Hypertension is accompanied by tachycardia. The pupils are dilated. The skin is sweaty, although mucous membranes are dry. (Examples: cocaine and amphetamines.)
      4. **Sympatholytic syndrome.** Blood pressure and pulse rate are both decreased (peripheral alpha receptor antagonists may cause hypotension with reflex tachycardia). The pupils are small, often of pinpoint size. Peristalsis is often decreased. (Examples: centrally acting alpha-2 agonists [clonidine and methyldopa], opioids, and phenothiazines.)
      5. **Nicotinic cholinergic syndrome.** Stimulation of nicotinic receptors at autonomic ganglia activates both parasympathetic and sympathetic systems, with unpredictable results. Excessive stimulation frequently causes depolarization blockage. Thus, initial tachycardia may be followed by bradycardia, and muscle fasciculations may be followed by paralysis. (Examples: nicotine; in addition, the depolarizing neuromuscular blocker succinylcholine, which acts on nicotinic receptors in skeletal muscle.)
      6. **Muscarinic cholinergic syndrome.** Muscarinic receptors are located at effector organs of the parasympathetic system. Stimulation causes brady-

**TABLE I–18. AUTONOMIC SYNDROMES[a,b]**

| | Blood Pressure | Pulse Rate | Pupil Size | Sweating | Peristalsis |
|---|---|---|---|---|---|
| Alpha-adrenergic | + | – | + | + | – |
| Beta-adrenergic | ± | + | ± | ± | ± |
| Mixed adrenergic | + | + | + | + | – |
| Sympatholytic | – | – | - - | – | – |
| Nicotinic | + | + | ± | + | + |
| Muscarinic | – | - - | - - | + | + |
| Mixed cholinergic | ± | ± | - - | + | + |
| Anticholinergic (antimuscarinic) | ± | + | + | - - | - - |

[a]Key to symbols: + = increased; ++ = markedly increased; – = decreased; - - = markedly decreased; ± = mixed effect, no effect, or unpredictable.
[b]Adapted, with permission, from Olson KR et al. *Med Toxicol* 1987;2:54.

cardia, miosis, sweating, hyperperistalsis, bronchorrhea, wheezing, excessive salivation, and urinary incontinence. (Example: bethanechol.)

7. **Mixed cholinergic syndrome.** Because both nicotinic and muscarinic receptors are stimulated, mixed effects may be seen. The pupils are usually miotic (of pinpoint size). The skin is sweaty, and peristaltic activity is increased. Fasciculations are a manifestation of nicotinic stimulation and may progress to muscle weakness or paralysis. (Examples: organophosphate and carbamate insecticides and physostigmine.)
8. **Anticholinergic (antimuscarinic) syndrome.** Tachycardia with mild hypertension is common. The pupils are widely dilated. The skin is flushed, hot, and dry. Peristalsis is decreased, and urinary retention is common. Patients may have myoclonic jerking or choreoathetoid movements. Agitated delirium is common, and hyperthermia may occur. (Examples: atropine, scopolamine, benztropine, antihistamines, and antidepressants; all of these drugs are primarily antimuscarinic.)

**B. Eye findings**

1. **Pupil size** is affected by a number of drugs that act on the autonomic nervous system. Table I–19 lists common causes of miosis and mydriasis.
2. Horizontal-gaze **nystagmus** is common with a variety of drugs and toxins, including barbiturates, ethanol, carbamazepine, phenytoin, and scorpion envenomation. Phencyclidine (PCP) may cause horizontal, vertical, and even rotatory nystagmus.

**C. Neuropathy.** A variety of drugs and poisons can cause sensory or motor neuropathy, usually after chronic repeated exposure (Table I–20). Some agents (eg, arsenic and thallium) can cause neuropathy after a single large exposure.

**D. Abdominal findings.** Peristaltic activity is commonly affected by drugs and toxins (see Table I–18 on autonomic syndromes).

1. Ileus may also be caused by **mechanical factors** such as injury to the gastrointestinal tract with perforation and peritonitis or mechanical obstruction by a swallowed foreign body.
2. Abdominal distension and ileus may also be a manifestation of acute **bowel infarction,** a rare but catastrophic complication that results from prolonged hypotension or mesenteric artery vasospasm (caused, for example, by ergot or amphetamines). Radiographs or CT scans may reveal air in the intestinal wall, biliary tree, or hepatic vein. The serum phosphorus and alkaline phosphatase levels are often elevated.

**TABLE I–19. SELECTED CAUSES OF PUPIL SIZE CHANGES[a]**

| CONSTRICTED PUPILS (MIOSIS) | DILATED PUPILS (MYDRIASIS) |
|---|---|
| **Sympatholytic agents** | **Sympathomimetic agents** |
| Clonidine | Amphetamines and derivatives |
| Opioids | Cocaine |
| Phenothiazines | Dopamine |
| Tetrahydrozoline and oxymetazoline | LSD (lysergic acid diethylamide) |
| Valproic acid | Monoamine oxidase inhibitors |
| **Cholinergic agents** | Nicotine[b] |
| Carbamate insecticides | **Anticholinergic agents** |
| Nicotine[b] | Antihistamines |
| Organophosphates | Atropine and other anticholinergics |
| Physostigmine | Carbamazepine |
| Pilocarpine | Glutethimide |
| **Others** | Tricyclic antidepressants |
| Heatstroke | |
| Pontine infarct | |
| Subarachnoid hemorrhage | |

[a]Adapted, in part, with permission, from Olson KR et al. *Med Toxicol* 1987;2:66.
[b]Nicotine can cause pupils to be dilated (rare) or constricted (common).

3. Vomiting, especially with hematemesis, may indicate the ingestion of a corrosive substance.

E. **Skin findings**

1. **Sweating** or absence of sweating may provide a clue to one of the autonomic syndromes (see Table I–18).

**TABLE I–20. SELECTED CAUSES OF NEUROPATHY**

| Cause | Comments |
|---|---|
| Acrylamide | Sensory and motor distal axonal neuropathy |
| Antineoplastic agents | Vincristine most strongly associated (see p 100) |
| Antiretroviral agents | Nucleoside reverse transcriptase inhibitors |
| Arsenic | Sensory predominant mixed axonal neuropathy (see p 115) |
| Buckthorn (*K humboldtiana*) | Livestock and human demyelinating neuropathy |
| Carbon disulfide | Sensory and motor distal axonal neuropathy |
| Dimethylaminopropionitrile | Urogenital and distal sensory neuropathy |
| Disulfiram | Sensory and motor distal axonal neuropathy |
| Ethanol | Sensory and motor distal axonal neuropathy (see p 189) |
| *n*-Hexane | Sensory and motor distal axonal neuropathy |
| Isoniazid (INH) | Preventable with co-administration of pyridoxine (see p 233) |
| Lead | Motor predominant mixed axonal neuropathy (see p 237) |
| Mercury | Organic mercury compounds (see p 253) |
| Methyl *n*-butyl ketone | Acts like *n*-hexane via 2,5-hexanedione metabolite |
| Nitrofurantoin | Sensory and motor distal axonal neuropathy |
| Nitrous oxide | Sensory axonal neuropathy with loss of proprioception (see p 283) |
| Organophosphate insecticides | Specific agents only (eg, triorthocresyl phosphate) |
| Pyridoxine (Vitamin $B_6$) | Sensory neuropathy with chronic excessive dosing |
| Selenium | Polyneuritis |
| Thallium | Sensory and motor distal axonal neuropathy (see p 354) |
| Tick paralysis | Ascending flaccid paralysis after bites by several tick species |

**TABLE I–21. SOME COMMON ODORS CAUSED BY TOXINS AND DRUGS[a]**

| Odor | Drug or Toxin |
|---|---|
| Acetone | Acetone, isopropyl alcohol |
| Acrid or pearlike | Chloral hydrate, paraldehyde |
| Bitter almonds | Cyanide |
| Carrots | Cicutoxin (water hemlock) |
| Garlic | Arsenic (arsine), organophosphates, selenium, thallium |
| Mothballs | Naphthalene, paradichlorobenzene |
| Pungent aromatic | Ethchlorvynol |
| Rotten eggs | Hydrogen sulfide, stibine, mercaptans, old sulfa drugs |
| Wintergreen | Methyl salicylate |

[a]Adapted, in part, with permission, from Olson KR et al. *Med Toxicol* 1987;2:67.

2. **Flushed red skin** may be caused by carbon monoxide poisoning, boric acid toxicity, chemical burns from corrosives or hydrocarbons, or anticholinergic agents. It may also result from vasodilation (eg, phenothiazines or disulfiram-ethanol interaction).
3. **Pale coloration** with diaphoresis is frequently caused by sympathomimetic agents. Severe localized pallor should suggest possible arterial vasospasm, such as that caused by ergot (see p 187) or some amphetamines (p 73).
4. **Cyanosis** may indicate hypoxia, sulfhemoglobinemia, or methemoglobinemia (see p 262).

**F. Odors.** A number of toxins may have characteristic odors (Table I–21). However, the odor may be subtle and may be obscured by the smell of emesis or by other ambient odors. In addition, the ability to smell an odor may vary; for example, only about 50% of the general population can smell the "bitter almond" odor of cyanide. Thus, the absence of an odor does not guarantee the absence of the toxin.

**III. Essential clinical laboratory tests.** Simple, readily available clinical laboratory tests may provide important clues to the diagnosis of poisoning and may guide the investigation toward specific toxicology testing.

**A. Routine tests.** The following tests are recommended for routine screening of the overdose patient:

1. Serum osmolality and calculation of the osmolar gap.
2. Electrolytes for determination of sodium, potassium, and anion gap.
3. Serum glucose.
4. Blood urea nitrogen (BUN) and creatinine for evaluation of renal function.
5. Hepatic transaminases and hepatic function tests.
6. Complete blood count or hemogram.
7. Urinalysis to check for crystalluria, hemoglobinuria, or myoglobinuria.
8. Electrocardiogram.
9. Stat serum acetaminophen level and serum ethanol level.
10. Pregnancy test (females of childbearing age).

**B. Serum osmolality and osmolar gap.** Serum osmolality may be measured in the laboratory with the freezing-point-depression osmometer or the heat-of-vaporization osmometer. Under normal circumstances the measured serum osmolality is approximately 290 mOsm/L and can be calculated from the results of the sodium, glucose, and BUN tests. The difference between the calculated osmolality and the osmolality measured in the laboratory is the osmolal gap, more commonly referred to as the osmolar gap (Table I–22). ***Note:*** Clinical studies suggest that the normal osmolar gap may vary from –14 to +10 mOsm/L. Thus, small osmolar gaps may be difficult to interpret.

**TABLE I–22. CAUSES OF ELEVATED OSMOLAR GAP[a]**

| | |
|---|---|
| Acetone | Mannitol |
| Dimethyl sulfoxide (DMSO) | Metaldehyde |
| Ethanol | Methanol |
| Ethyl ether | Osmotic contrast dyes |
| Ethylene glycol and other low-molecular-weight glycols | Propylene glycol |
| Isopropyl alcohol | Renal failure without dialysis |
| Magnesium | Severe alcoholic ketoacidosis, diabetic ketoacidosis, or lactic acidosis |

[a]Osmolar gap = measured - calculated osmolality. Normal = 0 ± 5-10 (see text).
Calculated osmolality = 2[Na] + [glucose]/18 + [BUN]/2.8 = 290 mOsm/L. Na (serum sodium) in mEq/L; glucose and BUN (urea nitrogen) in mg/dL.
***Note:*** The osmolality may be measured as falsely normal if a vaporization point osmometer is used instead of the freezing point device, because volatile alcohols will be boiled off.

1. **Causes of an elevated osmolar gap** (Table I–22)
   - **a.** The osmolar gap may be increased in the presence of low-molecular-weight substances such as ethanol, other alcohols, and glycols, any of which can contribute to the measured but not the calculated osmolality. Table I–23 describes how to estimate alcohol and glycol levels by using the osmolar gap.
   - **b.** An osmolar gap accompanied by anion gap acidosis should immediately suggest poisoning by methanol or ethylene glycol. ***Note:*** A falsely normal osmolar gap despite the presence of alcohols may result from using a heat-of-vaporization method to measure osmolality, because the alcohols will boil off before the serum boiling point is reached.
2. **Differential diagnosis**
   - **a.** Combined osmolar and anion gap elevation may also be seen with severe alcoholic ketoacidosis or diabetic ketoacidosis, owing to accumulation of unmeasured anions (beta-hydroxybutyrate) and osmotically active substances (acetone, glycerol, and amino acids).
   - **b.** Patients with chronic renal failure who are not undergoing hemodialysis may have an elevated osmolar gap owing to accumulation of low-molecular-weight solutes.
   - **c.** False elevation of the osmolar gap may be caused by the use of an inappropriate sample tube (lavender top, ethylenediaminetetraacetic acid [EDTA]; gray top, fluoride-oxalate; blue top, citrate; see Table I–33, p 44).
   - **d.** A falsely elevated gap may occur in patients with severe hyperlipidemia.

**TABLE I–23. ESTIMATION OF ALCOHOL AND GLYCOL LEVELS FROM THE OSMOLAR GAP[a]**

| Alcohol or Glycol | Molecular Weight (mg/mmol) | Conversion Factor[b] |
|---|---|---|
| Acetone | 58 | 5.8 |
| Ethanol | 46 | 4.6 |
| Ethylene glycol | 62 | 6.2 |
| Isopropyl alcohol | 60 | 6 |
| Methanol | 32 | 3.2 |
| Propylene glycol | 76 | 7.6 |

[a]Adapted, with permission, from *Current Emergency Diagnosis & Treatment*, 3rd ed. Ho MT, Saunders CE (editors). New York: Appleton & Lange, 1990.
[b]To obtain estimated serum level (in mg/dL), multiply osmolar gap by conversion factor.

**TABLE I–24. SELECTED DRUGS AND TOXINS CAUSING ELEVATED ANION GAP ACIDOSIS[a,b]**

| Lactic acidosis | Other than lactic acidosis |
|---|---|
| Acetaminophen (levels >600 mg/L) | Alcoholic ketoacidosis (beta hydroxybutyrate) |
| Antiretroviral drugs | Benzyl alcohol |
| Beta-adrenergic receptor agonists | Diabetic ketoacidosis |
| Caffeine | Ethylene glycol (glycolic and other acids) |
| Carbon monoxide | Exogenous organic and mineral acids |
| Cyanide | Formaldehyde (formic acid) |
| Hydrogen sulfide | Ibuprofen (propionic acid) |
| Iron | Metaldehyde |
| Isoniazid (INH) | Methanol (formic acid) |
| Metformin and phenformin | Salicylates (salicylic acid) |
| Salicylates | Valproic acid |
| Seizures, shock, or hypoxia | |
| Sodium azide | |
| Theophylline | |

[a]Anion gap = [Na] - [Cl] - $[HCO_3]$ = 8 -12 mEq/L.
[b]Adapted, in part, with permission, from Olson KR et al. *Med Toxicol* 1987;2:73.

3. **Treatment** depends on the cause. If ethylene glycol (see p 193) or methanol (p 260) poisoning is suspected, based on an elevated osmolar gap not accounted for by ethanol or other alcohols and on the presence of metabolic acidosis, antidotal therapy (eg, fomepizole [see p 454] or ethanol [see p 450]) and hemodialysis may be indicated.

C. **Anion gap metabolic acidosis.** The normal anion gap of 8–12 mEq/L accounts for unmeasured anions (eg, phosphate, sulfate, and anionic proteins) in the plasma. Metabolic acidosis is usually associated with an elevated anion gap.

1. **Causes of elevated anion gap** (Table I–24)
   a. An elevated anion gap acidosis is usually caused by an accumulation of lactic acid but may also be caused by other unmeasured acid anions such as formate (eg, methanol poisoning), glycolate or oxalate (eg, ethylene glycol poisoning), and beta-hydroxybutyrate (in patients with ketoacidosis).
   b. In any patient with an elevated anion gap, also check the osmolar gap; a combination of elevated anion and osmolar gaps suggests poisoning by methanol or ethylene glycol. ***Note:*** Combined osmolar and anion gap elevation may also be seen with severe alcoholic ketoacidosis and even diabetic ketoacidosis.
   c. A narrow anion gap may occur with an overdose by bromide or nitrate, both of which can increase the serum chloride level measured by some laboratory instruments. Also, high concentrations of lithium, calcium, and magnesium will narrow the anion gap due to lowering of the serum sodium concentration.
2. **Differential diagnosis.** Rule out the following:
   a. Common causes of lactic acidosis such as hypoxia and ischemia.
   b. False depression of the serum bicarbonate and $pCO_2$ measurements, which can occur from incomplete filling of the red-topped Vacutainer™ blood collection tube.
   c. False depression of the $pCO_2$ and calculated bicarbonate measurements, which can result from excess heparin when obtaining arterial blood gases (0.25 mL heparin in 2 mL blood falsely lowers $pCO_2$ by about 8 mm and bicarbonate by about 5 mEq/L).
3. **Treatment**
   a. Treat the underlying cause of the acidosis.
      (1) Treat seizures (see p 22) with anticonvulsants or neuromuscular paralysis.

(2) Treat hypoxia (see p 6) and hypotension (p 15) if they occur.

(3) Treat methanol (see p 260) or ethylene glycol (p 193) poisoning with fomepizole or ethanol and hemodialysis.

(4) Treat salicylate intoxication (see p 333) with alkaline diuresis and hemodialysis.

**b.** Treatment of the acidemia itself is not generally necessary unless the pH is less than 7–7.1. In fact, mild acidosis may be beneficial by promoting oxygen release to tissues. However, acidemia may be harmful in poisoning by salicylates or tricyclic antidepressants.

(1) In salicylate intoxication (see p 333), acidemia enhances salicylate entry into the brain and must be prevented. Alkalinization of the urine promotes salicylate elimination.

(2) In a tricyclic antidepressant overdose (see p 91), acidemia enhances cardiotoxicity. Maintain the serum pH at 7.45–7.5 with boluses of sodium bicarbonate.

**D. Hyperglycemia and hypoglycemia.** A variety of drugs and disease states can cause alterations in the serum glucose level (Table I–25). A patient's blood glucose level can be altered by nutritional state, endogenous insulin levels, and endocrine and liver functions and by the presence of various drugs or toxins.

**1. Hyperglycemia,** especially if severe (>500 mg/dL) or sustained, may result in dehydration and electrolyte imbalance caused by the osmotic effect of excess glucose in the urine; in addition, the shifting of water from the brain into plasma may result in hyperosmolar coma. More commonly, hyperglycemia in poisoning or drug overdose cases is mild and transient. Significant or sustained hyperglycemia should be treated if it is not resolving spontaneously or if the patient is symptomatic.

**a.** If the patient has altered mental status, maintain an open airway, assist ventilation if necessary, and administer supplemental oxygen (see pp 1–4).

**b.** Replace fluid deficits with intravenous normal saline (NS) or another isotonic crystalloid solution. Monitor serum potassium levels, which may fall sharply as blood glucose is corrected, and give supplemental potassium as needed.

**c.** Correct acid-base and electrolyte disturbances.

**d.** Administer regular insulin, 5–10 U IV initially, followed by infusion of 5–10 U/h, while monitoring the effects on serum glucose level (children: administer 0.1 U/kg initially and 0.1 U/kg/h). (See p 461.)

**TABLE I–25. SELECTED CAUSES OF ALTERATIONS IN SERUM GLUCOSE**

| Hyperglycemia | Hypoglycemia |
|---|---|
| Beta-2 adrenergic receptor agonists | Akee fruit |
| Caffeine intoxication | Endocrine disorders (hypopituitarism, Addison's disease, myxedema) |
| Corticosteroids | Ethanol intoxication (especially pediatric) |
| Dextrose administration | Fasting |
| Diabetes mellitus | Hepatic failure |
| Diazoxide | Insulin |
| Excessive circulating epinephrine | Oral sulfonylurea hypoglycemic agents |
| Glucagon | Pentamidine |
| Iron poisoning | Propranolol intoxication |
| Theophylline intoxication | Renal failure |
| Thiazide diuretics | Salicylate intoxication |
| Vacor | Streptozocin |
| | Valproic acid intoxication |

2. **Hypoglycemia,** if severe (serum glucose < 40 mg/dL) and sustained, can rapidly cause permanent brain injury. For this reason, whenever hypoglycemia is suspected as a cause of seizures, coma, or altered mental status, immediate empiric treatment with dextrose is indicated.
   a. If the patient has altered mental status, maintain an open airway, assist ventilation if necessary, and administer supplemental oxygen (see pp 1–4).
   b. If available, perform rapid bedside blood glucose testing (now possible in most emergency departments).
   c. If the blood glucose is low (<70 mg/dL) or if bedside testing is not available, administer concentrated 50% dextrose, 50 mL IV (25 g). In children, give 25% dextrose, 2 mL/kg (see p 457).
   d. In malnourished or alcoholic patients, also give thiamine, 100 mg IM or IV, to treat or prevent acute Wernicke's syndrome.
   e. For hypoglycemia caused by oral sulfonylurea drug overdose (see p 93), consider antidotal therapy with octreotide (p 488) or, if octreotide is not available, diazoxide (p 438).

E. **Hypernatremia and hyponatremia.** Sodium disorders occur infrequently in poisoned patients (see Table I–26). More commonly they are associated with underlying disease states. Antidiuretic hormone (ADH) is responsible for concentrating the urine and preventing excess water loss.
1. **Hypernatremia** (serum sodium > 145 mEq/L) may be caused by excessive sodium intake, excessive free water loss, or impaired renal concentrating ability.
   a. **Dehydration with normal kidney function.** Excessive sweating, hyperventilation, diarrhea, or osmotic diuresis (eg, hyperglycemia or mannitol administration) may cause disproportional water loss. The urine osmolality is usually greater than 400 mOsm/kg, and the ADH function is normal.
   b. **Impaired renal concentrating ability.** Excess free water is lost in the urine, and urine osmolality is usually less than 250 mOsm/L. This may be caused by hypothalamic dysfunction with reduced ADH production (diabetes insipidus [DI]) or impaired kidney response to ADH (nephrogenic DI). Nephrogenic DI has been associated with chronic lithium therapy.
2. **Treatment of hypernatremia.** Treatment depends on the cause, but in most cases, the patient is hypovolemic and needs fluids. ***Caution:*** Do ***not*** reduce the serum sodium level too quickly, because osmotic imbalance may cause excessive fluid shift into brain cells, resulting in cerebral edema. The correction should take place over 24–36 hours; the serum sodium should be lowered about 1 mEq/L/h.

**TABLE I–26. SELECTED DRUGS AND TOXINS ASSOCIATED WITH ALTERED SERUM SODIUM**

| Hypernatremia | Hyponatremia |
|---|---|
| Cathartic abuse | Beer potomania |
| Lactulose therapy | Cerebral salt wasting syndrome (eg, after trauma) |
| Lithium therapy (nephrogenic diabetes insipidus) | Diuretics |
| Mannitol | Iatrogenic (IV fluid therapy) |
| Severe gastroenteritis (many poisons) | Syndrome of inappropriate ADH (SIADH): |
| Sodium or salt overdose | Amitriptyline |
| Valproic acid (divalproex sodium) | Chlorpropamide |
| | Clofibrate |
| | MDMA (ecstasy) |
| | Oxytocin |
| | Phenothiazines |

a. **Hypovolemia.** Administer normal saline (0.9% sodium chloride, NS) to restore fluid balance, then half NS in dextrose ($D_5$W-0.45% sodium chloride).

b. **Volume overload.** Treat with a combination of sodium-free or low-sodium fluid (eg, 5% dextrose or $D_5$W-0.25% sodium chloride) and a loop diuretic such as furosemide (Lasix™), 0.5–1 mg/kg.

c. **Lithium-induced nephrogenic DI.** Administer fluids (see 2.a, above). Discontinue lithium therapy. Partial improvement may be seen with oral administration of indomethacin, 50 mg 3 times a day, and hydrochlorothiazide, 50–100 mg/d. (Note, however, that indomethacin may also impair renal lithium clearance.)

3. **Hyponatremia** (serum sodium < 130 mEq/L) is a common electrolyte abnormality and may result from a variety of mechanisms. Severe hyponatremia (serum sodium < 110–120 mEq/L) can result in seizures and altered mental status.

a. **Pseudohyponatremia** may result from a shift of water from the extracellular space (eg, hyperglycemia). Plasma sodium falls by about 1.6 mEq/L for each 100-mg/dL rise in glucose. Reduced relative blood water volume (eg, hyperlipidemia or hyperproteinemia) may produce pseudohyponatremia if older (flame emission) devices are used, but this is unlikely with current direct-measurement electrodes.

b. **Hyponatremia with hypovolemia** may be caused by excessive volume loss (sodium and water) that is partially replaced by free water. To maintain intravascular volume, the body secretes ADH, which causes water retention. A urine sodium level less than 10 mEq/L suggests that the kidney is appropriately attempting to compensate for volume losses. An elevated urine sodium level (>20 mEq/L) implies renal salt wasting, which can be caused by diuretics, adrenal insufficiency, or nephropathy. A syndrome of salt wasting has been reported in some patients with head trauma ("cerebral salt wasting syndrome").

c. **Hyponatremia with volume overload** occurs in conditions such as congestive heart failure and cirrhosis. Although the total body sodium is increased, baroreceptors sense an inadequate circulating volume and stimulate release of ADH. The urine sodium level is normally less than 10 mEq/L, unless the patient has been on diuretics.

d. **Hyponatremia with normal volume** occurs in a variety of situations. Measurement of serum and urine osmolalities may help determine the diagnosis.

(1) **Syndrome of inappropriate ADH secretion (SIADH).** In patients with SIADH, ADH is secreted independently of volume or osmolality. Causes include malignancies, pulmonary disease, severe head injury, and some drugs (see Table I–26). The serum osmolality is low, but the urine osmolality is inappropriately increased (>300 mOsm/L). The serum blood urea nitrogen (BUN) is usually low (<10 mg/dL).

(2) **Psychogenic polydipsia,** or compulsive water drinking (generally > 10 L/d), causes reduced serum sodium because of the excessive free water intake and because the kidney excretes sodium to maintain euvolemia. The urine sodium level may be elevated, but urine osmolality is appropriately low because the kidney is attempting to excrete the excess water and ADH secretion is suppressed.

(3) **Beer potomania** may result from chronic daily excessive beer drinking (>4 L/d). It usually occurs in patients with cirrhosis who already have elevated ADH levels.

(4) Other causes of euvolemic hyponatremia include hypothyroidism, postoperative state, and idiosyncratic reactions to diuretics (generally thiazides).

4. **Treatment of hyponatremia.** Treatment depends on the cause, the patient's volume status, and, most important, the patient's clinical condition. ***Caution:*** Avoid overly rapid correction of the sodium, because brain damage (central pontine myelinolysis) may occur if the sodium is increased by more than 25 mEq/L in the first 24 hours. Obtain frequent measurements of serum and urine sodium levels and adjust the rate of infusion as needed to increase the serum sodium by no more than 1–1.5 mEq/h. Arrange consultation with a nephrologist as soon as possible. **For patients with profound hyponatremia** (serum sodium < 110 mEq/L) accompanied by coma or seizures, administer hypertonic (3% sodium chloride) saline, 100–200 mL.
   a. **Hyponatremia with hypovolemia.** Replace lost volume with normal saline (0.9% sodium chloride, NS). If adrenal insufficiency is suspected, give hydrocortisone, 100 mg every 6–8 hours. Hypertonic saline (3% sodium chloride) is rarely indicated.
   b. **Hyponatremia with volume overload.** Restrict water (0.5–1 L/d) and treat the underlying condition (eg, congestive heart failure). If diuretics are given, do ***not*** allow excessive free water intake. Hypertonic saline is dangerous in these patients; if it is used, also administer furosemide, 0.5–1 mg/kg. Consider hemodialysis to reduce volume and restore the sodium level.
   c. **Hyponatremia with normal volume.** Asymptomatic patients may be treated conservatively with water restriction (0.5–1 L/d). Psychogenic compulsive water drinkers may have to be restrained or separated from all sources of water, including washbasins and toilets. Demeclocycline (a tetracycline antibiotic that can produce nephrogenic DI), 300–600 mg twice a day, can be used to treat mild chronic SIADH. (The onset of action may require a week.) For patients with coma or seizures, give hypertonic (3%) saline, 100–200 mL, along with furosemide, 0.5–1 mg/kg.

F. **Hyperkalemia and hypokalemia.** A variety of drugs and toxins can cause serious alterations in the serum potassium level (Table I–27). Potassium levels are dependent on potassium intake and release (eg, from muscles), diuretic use, proper functioning of the ATPase pump, serum pH, and beta-adrenergic activity. Changes in serum potassium levels do not always reflect overall body gain or loss but may be caused by intracellular shifts (eg, acidosis drives potassium out of cells, but beta-adrenergic stimulation drives it into cells).

1. **Hyperkalemia** (serum potassium > 5 mEq/L) produces muscle weakness and interferes with normal cardiac conduction. Peaked T waves and prolonged PR intervals are the earliest signs of cardiotoxicity. Critical hyper-

**TABLE I–27. SELECTED DRUGS AND TOXINS AND OTHER CAUSES OF ALTERED SERUM POTASSIUM**[a]

| Hyperkalemia | Hypokalemia |
|---|---|
| Acidosis | Alkalosis |
| Angiotensin-converting enzyme (ACE) inhibitors | Barium |
| Beta receptor antagonists | Beta-adrenergic drugs |
| Digitalis glycosides | Caffeine |
| Fluoride | Cesium |
| Lithium | Diuretics (chronic) |
| Potassium | Epinephrine |
| Renal failure | Theophylline |
| Rhabdomyolysis | Toluene (chronic) |

[a]Adapted in part, with permission, from Olson KR et al. *Med Toxicol* 1987;2:73.

kalemia produces widened QRS intervals, AV block, ventricular fibrillation, and cardiac arrest (see Figure I–5).

a. Hyperkalemia caused by **fluoride intoxication** (see p 199) is usually accompanied by hypocalcemia.

b. **Digitalis intoxication** associated with hyperkalemia is an indication for administration of digoxin-specific Fab antibodies (see p 440).

2. **Treatment of hyperkalemia.** A potassium level higher than 6 mEq/L is a medical emergency; a level higher than 7 mEq/L is critical.

a. Monitor the ECG. QRS prolongation indicates critical cardiac poisoning.

b. Administer calcium chloride, 10–20 mg/kg IV (see p 428), if there are signs of critical cardiac toxicity. ***Note:*** Use calcium with caution in patients with digitalis glycoside poisoning; intractable ventricular fibrillation may result.

c. Sodium bicarbonate, 1–2 mEq/kg IV (see p 423), rapidly drives potassium into cells and lowers the serum level.

d. Glucose plus insulin also promotes intracellular movement of potassium. Give 50% dextrose, 50 mL (25% dextrose, 2 mL/kg in children), plus regular insulin, 0.1 U/kg IV.

e. Inhaled beta-2 adrenergic agonists such as albuterol also enhance potassium entry into cells and can provide a rapid supplemental method of lowering serum potassium levels.

f. Kayexalate (sodium polystyrene sulfonate), 0.3–0.6 g/kg PO in 2 mL/kg 70% sorbitol, is effective but takes several hours.

g. Hemodialysis rapidly lowers serum potassium levels.

3. **Hypokalemia** (serum potassium < 3.5 mEq/L) may cause muscle weakness, hyporeflexia, and ileus. Rhabdomyolysis may occur. The ECG shows flattened T waves and prominent U waves. In severe hypokalemia, AV block, ventricular arrhythmias, and cardiac arrest may occur.

a. With **theophylline, caffeine, or beta-2 agonist** intoxication, an intracellular shift of potassium may produce a very low serum potassium level with normal total body stores. Patients usually do not have serious symptoms or ECG signs of hypokalemia, and aggressive potassium therapy is not required.

b. With **barium** poisoning (see p 126), profound hypokalemia may lead to respiratory muscle weakness and cardiac and respiratory arrest; therefore, intensive potassium therapy is necessary. Up to 420 mEq has been given in 24 hours.

c. Hypokalemia resulting from **diuretic therapy** may contribute to ventricular arrhythmias, especially those associated with chronic digitalis glycoside poisoning.

4. **Treatment of hypokalemia.** Mild hypokalemia (potassium 3–3.5 mEq/L) is usually not associated with serious symptoms.

a. Administer potassium chloride orally or intravenously. See p 499 for recommended doses and infusion rates.

b. Monitor serum potassium and the ECG for signs of hyperkalemia from excessive potassium therapy.

c. If hypokalemia is caused by diuretic therapy or gastrointestinal fluid losses, measure and replace other ions such as magnesium, sodium, and chloride.

G. **Renal failure.** Examples of drugs and toxins that cause renal failure are listed in Table I–28. Renal failure may be caused by a direct nephrotoxic action of the poison or acute massive tubular precipitation of myoglobin (rhabdomyolysis), hemoglobin (hemolysis), or calcium oxalate crystals (ethylene glycol), or it may be secondary to shock caused by blood or fluid loss or cardiovascular collapse.

1. **Assessment.** Renal failure is characterized by a progressive rise in the serum creatinine and blood urea nitrogen (BUN) levels, usually accompanied by oliguria or anuria.

**TABLE I–28. EXAMPLES OF DRUGS AND TOXINS AND OTHER CAUSES OF ACUTE RENAL FAILURE**

| | |
|---|---|
| **Direct nephrotoxic effect** | Foscarnet |
| Acetaminophen | Heavy metals (eg, mercury) salts |
| Acyclovir (chronic, high-dose treatment) | Indinavir |
| *Amanita phalloides* mushrooms | **Hemolysis** |
| *Amanita smithiana* mushrooms | Arsine |
| Analgesics (eg, ibuprofen, phenacetin) | Naphthalene |
| Antibiotics (eg, aminoglycosides) | Oxidizing agents (esp. with G6PD deficiency) |
| Bromates | **Rhabdomyolysis (see also Table I–16)** |
| Chlorates | Amphetamines and cocaine |
| Chlorinated hydrocarbons | Coma with prolonged immobility |
| *Cortinarius* sp. mushrooms | Hyperthermia |
| Cyclosporin | Phencyclidine (PCP) |
| EDTA | Status epilepticus |
| Ethylene glycol (glycolate, oxalate) | Strychnine |

   a. The serum creatinine level usually rises about 1–1.5 mg/dL/day after total anuric renal failure.
   b. A more abrupt rise should suggest rapid muscle breakdown (rhabdomyolysis), which increases the creatine load and also results in elevated creatine phosphokinase (CPK) levels that may interfere with determination of the serum creatinine level.
   c. Oliguria may be seen before renal failure occurs, especially with hypovolemia, hypotension, or heart failure. In this case, the BUN level is usually elevated out of proportion to the serum creatinine level.
2. **Complications.** The earliest complication of acute renal failure is hyperkalemia (see p 37); this may be more pronounced if the cause of the renal failure is rhabdomyolysis or hemolysis, both of which release large amounts of intracellular potassium into the circulation. Later complications include metabolic acidosis, delirium, and coma.
3. **Treatment**
   a. Prevent renal failure, if possible, by administering specific treatment (eg, acetylcysteine for acetaminophen overdose, British anti-Lewisite [BAL; dimercaprol] chelation for mercury poisoning, and intravenous fluids for rhabdomyolysis or shock).
   b. Monitor the serum potassium level frequently and treat hyperkalemia (see p 37) if it occurs.
   c. Do ***not*** give supplemental potassium, and avoid cathartics or other medications containing magnesium, phosphate, or sodium.
   d. Perform hemodialysis as needed.

H. **Hepatic failure.** A variety of drugs and toxins may cause hepatic injury (Table I–29). Mechanisms of toxicity include direct hepatocellular damage (eg, *Amanita phalloides* mushrooms [see p 272]), metabolic creation of a hepatotoxic intermediate (eg, acetaminophen [p 68] or carbon tetrachloride [p 153]), and hepatic vein thrombosis (eg, pyrrolizidine alkaloids; see Plants, p 309).
1. **Assessment.** Laboratory and clinical evidence of hepatitis usually does not become apparent until at least 24–36 hours after exposure to the poison. Then transaminase levels rise sharply and may fall to normal over the next 3–5 days. If hepatic damage is severe, measurements of hepatic function (eg, bilirubin and prothrombin time) will continue to worsen after 2–3 days, even as transaminase levels are returning to normal. Metabolic acidosis and hypoglycemia usually indicate a poor prognosis.

**TABLE I–29. EXAMPLES OF DRUGS AND TOXINS CAUSING HEPATIC DAMAGE**

| | |
|---|---|
| Acetaminophen | 2-Nitropropane |
| *Amanita phalloides* and similar mushrooms | Pennyroyal oil |
| Arsenic | Phenol |
| Carbon tetrachloride and other chlorinated hydrocarbons | Phosphorus |
| Copper | Polychlorinated biphenyls (PCBs) |
| Dimethylformamide | Pyrrolizidine alkaloids (see Plants, p 390) |
| Ethanol | Thallium |
| *Gyrometra* mushrooms | Troglitazone |
| Halothane | Valproic acid |
| Iron | |

2. **Complications**
   a. Abnormal hepatic function may result in excessive bleeding owing to insufficient production of vitamin K–dependent coagulation factors.
   b. Hepatic encephalopathy may lead to coma and death, usually within 5–7 days, from massive hepatic failure.
3. **Treatment**
   a. Prevent hepatic injury if possible by administering specific treatment (eg, acetylcysteine for acetaminophen overdose).
   b. Obtain baseline and daily transaminase, bilirubin, and glucose levels and prothrombin time.
   c. Provide intensive supportive care for hepatic failure and encephalopathy (eg, glucose for hypoglycemia, fresh frozen plasma for coagulopathy, or lactulose for encephalopathy).
   d. Liver transplantation may be the only effective treatment once massive hepatic necrosis has resulted in severe encephalopathy.

**IV. Toxicology screening.*** To maximize the utility of the toxicology laboratory, it is necessary to understand what the laboratory can and cannot do and how knowledge of the results will affect the patient. Comprehensive blood and urine screening is of little practical value in the initial care of the poisoned patient. However, specific toxicologic analyses and quantitative levels of certain drugs may be extremely helpful. Before ordering any tests, always ask these two questions: (i) How will the result of the test alter the approach to treatment? and (ii) Can the result of the test be returned in time to affect therapy positively?

A. **Limitations of toxicology screens.** Owing to long turnaround time, lack of availability, reliability factors, and the low risk of serious morbidity with supportive clinical management, toxicology screening is estimated to affect management in less than 15% of all cases of poisoning or drug overdose.
   1. Comprehensive toxicology screens or panels may look specifically for only 40–100 drugs out of more than 10,000 possible drugs or toxins (or 6 million chemicals). However, these 40–50 drugs (Tables I–30 and I–31) account for more than 80% of overdoses.
   2. To detect many different drugs, comprehensive screens usually include multiple methods with broad specificity, and sensitivity may be poor for some drugs (resulting in analytic false-negative results). However, some drugs present in therapeutic amounts may be detected on the screen even though they are causing no clinical symptoms (clinical false positives).
   3. Because many agents are neither sought nor detected during a toxicology screening (Table I–32), a negative result does not always rule out poisoning; the negative predictive value of the screen is only about 70%. In contrast, a positive result has a predictive value of about 90%.

*By John Osterloh, MD and Christine A. Haller, MS, MD

**TABLE I–30. DRUGS COMMONLY INCLUDED IN A COMPREHENSIVE URINE SCREEN[a]**

**Alcohols**
- Acetone
- Ethanol
- Isopropyl alcohol
- Methanol

**Analgesics**
- Acetaminophen
- Salicylates

**Anticonvulsants**
- Carbamazepine
- Phenobarbital
- Phenytoin
- Primidone

**Antihistamines**
- Benztropine
- Chlorpheniramine
- Diphenhydramine
- Pyrilamine
- Trihexyphenidyl

**Opioids**
- Codeine
- Dextromethorphan
- Hydrocodone
- Meperidine
- Methadone
- Morphine
- Oxycodone[b]
- Pentazocine
- Propoxyphene

**Phenothiazines**
- Chlorpromazine
- Prochlorperazine
- Promethazine
- Thioridazine
- Trifluoperazine

**Sedative-hypnotic drugs**
- Barbiturates[c]
- Benzodiazepines[c]
- Carisoprodol
- Chloral hydrate
- Ethchlorvynol
- Glutethimide
- Meprobamate
- Methaqualone

**Stimulants**
- Amphetamines[c]
- Caffeine
- Cocaine and benzoylecgonine
- Phencyclidine (PCP)
- Strychnine

**Tricyclic antidepressants**
- Amitriptyline
- Desipramine
- Doxepin
- Imipramine
- Nortriptyline
- Protriptyline

**Cardiac drugs**
- Diltiazem
- Lidocaine
- Procainamide
- Propranolol
- Quinidine and quinine
- Verapamil

[a]Newer drugs in any category may not be included in screening.
[b]Depends on the order of testing.
[c]Not all drugs in this class are detected.

4. The specificity of toxicologic tests is dependent on the method and the laboratory. The presence of other drugs, drug metabolites, disease states, or incorrect sampling may cause erroneous results (Table I–33).
5. **Adulteration** of urine may be attempted by persons undergoing enforced drug testing to evade drug detection. Methods used include dilution (ingested or added water) and addition of acids, baking soda, bleach, metal salts, nitrite salts, glutaraldehyde, or pyridinium chlorochromate. The intent is to inactivate, either chemically or biologically, the initial screening immunoassay to produce a negative test. Adulteration is variably successful depending on the agent used and the type of immunoassay. Laboratories that routinely perform urine testing for drug surveillance programs often have methods to test for some of the adulterants as well assay indicators that suggest possible adulterations.

**B. Uses for toxicology screens**

1. **Comprehensive screening** of urine and blood should be carried out whenever the diagnosis of brain death is being considered to rule out the presence of common depressant drugs that might result in temporary loss of brain activity and mimic brain death. Toxicology screens may be used to confirm clinical impressions during hospitalization and can be inserted in

**TABLE I–31. DRUGS COMMONLY INCLUDED IN A HOSPITAL "DRUGS OF ABUSE" PANEL[a]**

| Drug | Detection Time Window for Recreational Doses | Comments |
|---|---|---|
| Amphetamines | 2 days | Often misses MDA or MDMA. Many false positives (see Table I–33) |
| Barbiturates | Less than 2 days for most drugs, up to 1 week for phenobarbital | |
| Benzodiazepines | 2–7 days (varies with specific drug and duration of use) | May not detect triazolam, lorazepam, alprazolam |
| Cocaine | 2 days | Detects metabolite benzoylecgonine |
| Ethanol | Less than 1 day | |
| Marijuana (THC) | 2–5 days after single use (longer for chronic use) | |
| Opioids | 2–3 days | Synthetic opioids (meperidine, methadone, propoxyphene, oxycodone) are not detected. Separate testing for methadone is sometimes offered |
| Phencyclidine (PCP) | Up to 7 days | (see Table I–33) |

[a]Labs often perform only some of these tests, depending on what their emergency department requests and local patterns of drug use in the community. Also, positive results are usually not confirmed with a second, more specific test; thus, false positives may be reported.

the permanent medicolegal record. This may be important if homicide, assault, or child abuse is suspected.

2. **Selective screens** (eg, for "drugs of abuse") with rapid turnaround times are often used to confirm clinical impressions and may aid in disposition of the patient. Positive results should be subjected to confirmatory testing with a second method.

C. **Approach to toxicology testing**

1. Communicate clinical suspicions to the laboratory.

**TABLE I–32. DRUGS AND TOXINS NOT COMMONLY INCLUDED IN EMERGENCY TOXICOLOGIC SCREENING PANELS[a]**

| | |
|---|---|
| Anesthetic gases | Ethylene glycol |
| Antiarrhythmic agents | Fentanyl and other opiate derivatives |
| Antibiotics | Fluoride |
| Antidepressants (newer) | Formate (formic acid, from methanol poisoning) |
| Antihypertensives | Hypoglycemic agents |
| Antipsychotic agents (newer) | Isoniazid (INH) |
| Benzodiazepines (newer) | Lithium |
| Beta receptor antagonists other than propranolol | LSD (lysergic acid diethylamide) |
| Borate | MAO inhibitors |
| Bromide | Noxious gases |
| Calcium antagonists (newer) | Plant, fungal, and microbiologic toxins |
| Colchicine | Pressors (eg, dopamine) |
| Cyanide | Solvents and hydrocarbons |
| Digitalis glycosides | Theophylline |
| Diuretics | Valproic acid |
| Ergot alkaloids | Vasodilators |

[a]Many of these are available as separate specific tests.

**TABLE I–33. INTERFERENCES IN TOXICOLOGIC BLOOD OR URINE TESTS**

| Drug or Toxin | Method[a] | Causes of Falsely Increased Level |
|---|---|---|
| Acetaminophen | SC[b] | Salicylate, salicylamide, methyl salicylate (each will increase acetaminophen level by 10% of their level in mg/L); bilirubin; phenols; renal failure (each 1 mg/dL increase in creatinine can increase acetaminophen level by 30 mg/L). |
| | GC, IA | Phenacetin. |
| | HPLC[b] | Cephalosporins; sulfonamides. |
| Amitriptyline | HPLC, GC | Cyclobenzaprine. |
| Amphetamines (urine) | GC[c] | Other volatile stimulant amines (misidentified). GC mass spectrometry poorly distinguishes d-methamphetamine from l-methamphetamine (found in Vicks inhaler). |
| | IA[c], TLC[c] | Many false positives: cross-reacting stimulant drugs (ephedrine, fenfluramine, MDA, MDMA, phentermine, phenmetrazine, pseudoephedrine, and other amphetamine analogs); cross-reacting nonstimulant drugs (bupropion, chlorpromazine, labetalol, ranitidine, sertraline, trazodone, trimethobenzamide); drugs metabolized to amphetamines (benzphetamine, clobenzorex, famprofazone, fenproporex, selegiline). |
| Benzodiazepines | IA | Oxaprozin and many other NSAIDs may falsely lower the result. |
| Chloride | SC, EC | Bromide (variable interference) |
| Creatinine | SC[b] | Ketoacidosis (may increase Cr up to 2–3 mg/dL in non-rate methods); cephalosporins; creatine (eg, with rhabdomyolysis). |
| | EZ | Creatine, lidocaine metabolite, 5-fluorouracil, nitromethane "fuel" |
| Cyanide | SC | Thiosulfate |
| Digoxin | IA | Endogenous digoxinlike natriuretic substances in newborns and in patients with hypervolemic states (cirrhosis, heart failure, uremia, pregnancy) and renal failure (up to 0.5 ng/mL); plant or animal glycosides (bufotoxins; Chan Su; oleander); after digoxin antibody (Fab) administration (with tests that measure total serum digoxin); presence of heterophile or human antimouse antibodies (up to 45.6 ng/mL reported in one case). |
| | MEIA | **Falsely lowered** serum digoxin concentrations during therapy with spironolactone, canrenone. |
| Ethanol | SC[b] | Other alcohols, ketones (by oxidation methods). |
| | EZ | Isopropyl alcohol; patient with elevated lactate and LDH |
| Ethylene glycol | EZ | Other glycols; elevated triglycerides. |
| | GC | Propylene glycol (may also **decrease** the ethylene glycol level). |
| Glucose | EC, EZ | Acetaminophen (increases); ascorbate decreases urine glucose level (Medisense™ device). |
| | Any method | Glucose level may fall by up to 30 mg/dL/h when transport to lab is delayed. (Does not occur if specimen is collected in gray-top tube.) |
| Iron | SC | Deferoxamine causes 15% lowering of total iron-binding capacity (TIBC). Lavender-top Vacutainer tube contains EDTA, which lowers total iron. |

(*continued*)

**TABLE I–33. INTERFERENCES IN TOXICOLOGIC BLOOD OR URINE TESTS (CONTINUED)**

| Drug or Toxin | Method[a] | Causes of Falsely Increased Level |
|---|---|---|
| Isopropanol | GC | Skin disinfectant containing isopropyl alcohol used before venipuncture (highly variable, usually trivial, but up to 40 mg/dL). |
| Ketones | SC | Acetylcysteine; valproic acid; captopril; levodopa. |
| Lithium | FE, SC | Green-top Vacutainer specimen tube (may contain lithium heparin) can cause marked elevation (up to 6–8 mEq/L). |
| | SC | Procainamide, quinidine can produce 5–15% elevation. |
| Methadone (urine) | IA | Diphenhydramine, verapamil, disopyramide. |
| Methemoglobin | SC | Sulfhemoglobin (cross-positive ~10% by co-oximeter); methylene blue (2 mg/kg dose gives transient false-positive 15% methemoglobin level); hyperlipidemia (triglyceride level of 6000 mg/dL may give false methemoglobin of 28.6%). |
| | | **Falsely decreased level** with in vitro spontaneous reduction to hemoglobin in Vacutainer tube (~10%/h). Analyze within 1 hour. |
| Morphine/codeine (urine) | TLC[c] | Hydromorphone; hydrocodone; oxycodone (misidentification) |
| | IA[c] | Cross-reacting opioids: hydrocodone; hydromorphone; monoacetylmorphine; morphine from poppy seed ingestion. (Oxycodone usually not detected by IA except in overdose amounts.) Also rifampin and ofloxcin and other quinolones in different IAs. |
| Osmolality | Osm | Lavender-top (EDTA) Vacutainer specimen tube (15 mOsm/L); gray-top (fluoride-oxalate) tube (150 mOsm/L); blue-top (citrate) tube (10 mOsm/L); green-top (lithium heparin) tube (theoretically, up to 6–8 mOsm/L). |
| | | **Falsely normal** if vapor pressure method used (alcohols are volatilized). |
| Phencyclidine (urine) | IA[c] | Diphenhydramine; methadone; dextromethorphan; chlorpromazine. |
| Salicylate | SC | Phenothiazines (urine); diflunisal; ketosis[c]; salicylamide; accumulated salicylate metabolites in patients with renal failure (~10% increase). |
| | EZ | Acetaminophen (slight salicylate elevation). |
| | IA, SC | Diflunisal. |
| | SC | Decreased or altered salicylate level: bilirubin; phenylketones. |
| Theophylline | HPLC[b] | Acetazolamide; cephalosporins; endogenous xanthines and accumulated theophylline metabolites in renal failure (minor effect). |
| | IA | Caffeine overdose; accumulated theophylline metabolites in renal failure. |
| Tricyclic antidepressants | IA | Carbamazepine, quetiapine |

[a]GC = gas chromatography (interferences primarily with older methods); HPLC = high-pressure liquid chromatography; IA = immunoassay; SC = spectrochemical; TLC = thin-layer chromatography; EC = electrochemical; EZ = enzymatic; FE = flame emission; MEIA = microparticle enzymatic immunoassay.
[b]Uncommon methodology.
[c]More common with urine test. Confirmation by a second test is required. Note: urine testing is sometimes affected by intentional adulteration to avoid drug detection (see text).

**TABLE I–34. SPECIFIC QUANTITATIVE LEVELS AND POTENTIAL INTERVENTIONS[a]**

| Drug or Toxin | Potential Intervention |
|---|---|
| Acetaminophen | Acetylcysteine |
| Carbamazepine | Repeat-dose charcoal, hemoperfusion |
| Carboxyhemoglobin | 100% oxygen |
| Digoxin | Digoxin-specific antibodies |
| Ethanol | Low level indicates search for other toxins |
| Ethylene glycol | Ethanol or fomepizole therapy, hemodialysis |
| Iron | Deferoxamine chelation |
| Lithium | Hemodialysis |
| Methanol | Ethanol or fomepizole therapy, hemodialysis |
| Methemoglobin | Methylene blue |
| Salicylate | Alkalinization, hemodialysis |
| Theophylline | Repeat-dose charcoal, hemoperfusion |
| Valproic acid | Hemodialysis, repeat-dose charcoal |

[a]For specific guidance see individual chapters in Section II.

2. Obtain blood and urine specimens on admission in unusual cases and have the laboratory store them temporarily. If the patient recovers rapidly, they can be discarded.
3. Urine is usually the best sample for broad qualitative screening. Blood samples should be saved for possible quantitative testing, but blood is not a good specimen for screening for many common drugs, including psychotropic agents, opioids, and stimulants.
4. Decide if a specific quantitative blood level may assist in management decisions (eg, use of an antidote or dialysis; Table I–34). Quantitative levels are helpful only if there is a predictable correlation between the serum level and toxic effects.
5. A regional poison control center (1-800-222-1222) or toxicology consultant may provide assistance in considering certain drug etiologies and in selecting specific tests.

**V. Abdominal x-rays.** Abdominal x-rays may reveal radiopaque tablets, drug-filled condoms, or other toxic material.

**A.** The radiograph is useful only if positive; recent studies suggest that few types of tablets are predictably visible (Table I–35).

**B.** Do ***not*** attempt to determine the radiopacity of a tablet by placing it directly on the x-ray plate. This often produces a false-positive result because of an air contrast effect.

## DECONTAMINATION

### I. Surface decontamination

**A. Skin.** Corrosive agents rapidly injure the skin and must be removed immediately. In addition, many toxins are readily absorbed through the skin, and systemic absorption can be prevented only by rapid action. Table II–20 (p 158) lists several corrosive chemical agents that can have systemic toxicity, and many of them are readily absorbed through the skin.

1. Be careful not to expose yourself or other care providers to potentially contaminating substances. Wear protective gear (gloves, gown, and goggles) and wash exposed areas promptly. Contact a regional poison center for information about the hazards of the chemicals involved; in the majority of cases, health-care providers are not at significant personal risk for secondary contamination, and simple measures such as emer-

**TABLE I–35. RADIOPAQUE DRUGS AND POISONS[a]**

**Usually visible**
- Bismuth subsalicylate (Pepto-Bismol)
- Calcium carbonate (Tums)
- Iron tablets
- Lead and lead-containing paint
- Metallic foreign bodies
- Potassium tablets

**Sometimes/weakly visible**
- Acetazolamide
- Arsenic
- Brompheniramine and dexbrompheniramine
- Busulfan
- Chloral hydrate
- Enteric-coated or sustained-release preparations (highly variable)
- Meclizine
- Perphenazine with amitriptyline
- Phosphorus
- Prochlorperazine
- Sodium chloride
- Thiamine
- Tranylcypromine
- Trifluoperazine
- Trimeprazine
- Zinc sulfate

[a]Reference: Savitt DL, Hawkins HH, Roberts JR: The radiopacity of ingested medications. *Ann Emerg Med* 1987; 16:331.

gency department gowns and plain latex gloves provide sufficient protection. For radiation and other hazardous materials incidents, see also Section IV (p 520).

2. Remove contaminated clothing and flush exposed areas with copious quantities of tepid (lukewarm) water or saline. Wash carefully behind ears, under nails, and in skin folds. Use soap and shampoo for oily substances.
3. There is rarely a need for chemical neutralization of a substance spilled on the skin. In fact, the heat generated by chemical neutralization can potentially create worse injury. Some of the few exceptions to this rule are listed in Table I–36.

**B. Eyes.** The cornea is especially sensitive to corrosive agents and hydrocarbon solvents that may rapidly damage the corneal surface and lead to permanent scarring.

**TABLE I–36. SOME TOPICAL AGENTS FOR CHEMICAL EXPOSURES TO THE SKIN[a]**

| Chemical Corrosive Agent | Topical Treatment |
|---|---|
| Hydrofluoric acid | Calcium soaks |
| Oxalic acid | Calcium soaks |
| Phenol | Mineral oil or other oil; isopropyl alcohol |
| Phosphorus (white) | Copper sulfate 1% (colors embedded granules blue, facilitates removal) |

[a]Reference: Edelman PA; Chemical and electrical burns. In: *Management of the Burned Patient.* Achauer BM (editor). New York: Appleton & Lange, 1987, pp 183–202.

1. Act quickly to prevent serious damage. Flush exposed eyes with copious quantities of tepid tap water or saline. If available, instill local anesthetic drops in the eye first to facilitate irrigation. Remove the victim's contact lenses if they are being worn.
2. Place the victim in a supine position under a tap or use intravenous tubing to direct a stream of water across the nasal bridge into the medial aspect of the eye. Use at least 1 L to irrigate each eye.
3. If the offending substance is an acid or a base, check the pH of the victim's tears after irrigation and continue irrigation if the pH remains abnormal.
4. Do not instill any neutralizing solution; there is no evidence that such treatment works, and it may further damage the eye.
5. After irrigation is complete, check the conjunctival and corneal surfaces carefully for evidence of full-thickness injury. Perform a fluorescein examination of the eye by using fluorescein dye and a Wood's lamp to reveal corneal injury.
6. Patients with serious conjunctival or corneal injury should be referred to an ophthalmologist immediately.

**C. Inhalation.** Agents that injure the pulmonary system may be acutely irritating gases or fumes and may have good or poor warning properties (see p 212).

1. Be careful not to expose yourself or other care providers to toxic gases or fumes without adequate respiratory protection (see p 525).
2. Remove the victim from exposure and give supplemental humidified oxygen, if available. Assist ventilation if necessary (see pp 1–4).
3. Observe closely for evidence of upper respiratory tract edema, which is heralded by a hoarse voice and stridor and may progress rapidly to complete airway obstruction. Endotracheally intubate patients who show evidence of progressive airway compromise.
4. Also observe for late-onset noncardiogenic pulmonary edema resulting from slower-acting toxins, which may take several hours to appear. Early signs and symptoms include dyspnea, hypoxemia, and tachypnea (see p 212).

**II. Gastrointestinal decontamination.** There remains some controversy about the roles of emesis, gastric lavage, activated charcoal, and cathartics to decontaminate the gastrointestinal tract. There is little support in the medical literature for gut-emptying procedures, and studies have shown that after a delay of 60 minutes or more, very little of the ingested dose is removed by emesis or gastric lavage. Moreover, recent studies suggest that in the typical overdosed patient, simple oral administration of activated charcoal without prior gut emptying is probably just as effective as the traditional sequence of gut emptying followed by charcoal.

However, there are some circumstances where aggressive gut decontamination may potentially be life saving, even after more than 1–2 hours. Examples include ingestion of highly toxic drugs (eg, calcium antagonists, colchicine), ingestion of drugs not adsorbed to charcoal (eg, iron, lithium), ingestion of massive amounts of a drug (eg, 150–200 aspirin tablets), and ingestion of sustained-release or enteric-coated products.

**A. Emesis.** Syrup of ipecac–induced emesis is no longer the treatment of choice for any ingestions. It may be employed in rare situations when medical care is expected to be delayed more than 60 minutes *and if the ipecac can be given within a few minutes of the ingestion.* Ipecac is no longer used in emergency departments because of the ready availability of activated charcoal. After syrup of ipecac administration, vomiting usually occurs within 20–30 minutes. If the ingestion occurred more than 30–60 minutes before ipecac administration, emesis is not very effective. Moreover, persistent vomiting after ipecac use is likely to delay the administration of activated charcoal (see item C, below).

1. **Indications**
   a. Early prehospital management of selected (see Contraindications below) potentially serious oral poisonings, particularly in the home immediately after ingestion, when other measures (eg, activated charcoal) are not available and transport time to a medical facility may be prolonged (eg, more than 1 hour).
   b. Possibly useful to remove ingested agents not adsorbed by activated charcoal (eg, iron, lithium, potassium). However, most of these cases are preferably managed with whole-bowel irrigation (see below).
2. **Contraindications**
   a. Obtunded, comatose, or convulsing patient.
   b. Ingestion of a substance likely to cause onset of CNS depression or seizures within a short clinical time frame (eg, opioids, sedative-hypnotic agents, tricyclic antidepressants, camphor, cocaine, isoniazid, or strychnine).
   c. Ingestion of a corrosive agent (eg, acids, alkali, or strong oxidizing agents).
   d. Ingestion of a simple aliphatic hydrocarbon (see p 219). These hydrocarbons are likely to cause pneumonitis if aspirated but usually do not cause systemic poisoning once they enter the stomach. For hydrocarbons that do carry a potential for systemic toxicity, activated charcoal with or without gastric lavage is preferable.
3. **Adverse effects**
   a. Persistent vomiting may delay administration of activated charcoal or oral antidotes (eg, acetylcysteine).
   b. Protracted forceful vomiting may result in hemorrhagic gastritis or a Mallory-Weiss tear.
   c. Vomiting may promote passage of toxic material into the small intestine, enhancing absorption.
   d. Drowsiness occurs in about 20% and diarrhea in 25% of children.
   e. Repeated daily use (eg, by bulimic patients) may result in cardiac arrhythmias and cardiomyopathy owing to accumulation of cardiotoxic alkaloids.
4. **Technique.** Use only syrup of ipecac, not the fluid extract (which contains much higher concentrations of emetic and cardiotoxic alkaloids).
   a. Administer 30 mL of syrup of ipecac orally (15 mL for children under age 5 years, 10 mL for children under age 1 year; not recommended for children under age 6 months). After 10–15 minutes, give 2–3 glasses of water (there is no consensus on the quantity of water or the timing of administration).
   b. If emesis has not occurred after 20 minutes, a second dose of ipecac may be given. Repeat the fluid administration. Have the patient sit up or move around, because this sometimes stimulates vomiting.
   c. If the second dose of ipecac does not induce vomiting, use an alternative method of gut decontamination (eg, activated charcoal). It is not necessary to empty the stomach just to remove the ipecac.
   d. A soapy water solution may be used as an alternative emetic. Use only standard dishwashing liquid or lotion soap, two tablespoons in a glass of water. Do ***not*** use powdered laundry or dishwasher detergent or liquid dishwashing concentrate; these products are corrosive. There is no other acceptable alternative to syrup of ipecac. Manual digital stimulation, copper sulfate, salt water, mustard water, apomorphine, and other emetics are unsafe and should not be used.

B. **Gastric lavage.** Gastric lavage is only occasionally used in hospital emergency departments. Although there is little clinical evidence to support its use, gastric lavage is probably slightly more effective than ipecac, especially for recently ingested liquid substances. However, it does not reliably remove undissolved pills or pill fragments (especially sustained-release or enteric-coated products). In addition, the procedure may delay administration of activated charcoal and may hasten the movement of drugs and poisons into the small intestine, especially if the patient is supine or in the right decubitus position. Gastric lavage is not necessary for small to moderate ingestions of most substances if activated charcoal can be given promptly.

**1. Indications**

**a.** To remove ingested liquid and solid drugs and poisons when the patient has taken a massive overdose or a particularly toxic substance. Lavage is more likely to be effective if initiated within 30–60 minutes of the ingestion, although it may still be useful several hours after ingestion of agents that slow gastric emptying (eg, salicylates or anticholinergic drugs).

**b.** To administer activated charcoal and whole-bowel irrigation to patients unwilling or unable to swallow them.

**c.** To dilute and remove corrosive liquids from the stomach and to empty the stomach in preparation for endoscopy.

**2. Contraindications**

**a.** Obtunded, comatose, or convulsing patients. Because it may disturb the normal physiology of the esophagus and airway protective mechanisms, gastric lavage must be used with caution in obtunded patients whose airway reflexes are dulled. In such cases, endotracheal intubation with a cuffed endotracheal tube should be performed first to protect the airway.

**b.** Ingestion of sustained-release or enteric-coated tablets. (Owing to the size of most tablets, lavage is unlikely to return intact tablets, even through a 40F orogastric hose.) In such cases, whole-bowel irrigation (see below) is preferable.

**c.** Use of gastric lavage after ingestion of a corrosive substance is controversial; some gastroenterologists recommend that lavage be performed as soon as possible after liquid caustic ingestion to remove corrosive material from the stomach and to prepare for endoscopy.

**3. Adverse effects**

**a.** Perforation of the esophagus or stomach.

**b.** Nosebleed from nasal trauma during passage of the tube.

**c.** Inadvertent tracheal intubation.

**d.** Vomiting resulting in pulmonary aspiration of gastric contents in an obtunded patient without airway protection.

**4. Technique**

**a.** If the patient is deeply obtunded, protect the airway by intubating the trachea with a cuffed endotracheal tube.

**b.** Place the patient in the left lateral decubitus position. This helps prevent ingested material from being pushed into the duodenum during lavage.

**c.** Insert a large gastric tube through the mouth or nose and into the stomach (36–40F [catheter size] in adults; a smaller tube will suffice for liquid poisons or if simple administration of charcoal is all that is intended). Check tube position with air insufflation while listening with a stethoscope positioned on the patient's stomach.

**d.** Withdraw as much of the stomach contents as possible. If the ingested poison is a toxic chemical that may contaminate hospital personnel (cyanide, organophosphate insecticide, etc), take steps to isolate it immediately (eg, use a self-contained wall suction unit).

**e.** Administer activated charcoal, 60–100 g (1 g/kg; see item C, below), down the tube before starting lavage to begin adsorption of material that may enter the intestine during the lavage procedure.

**f.** Instill tepid (lukewarm) water or saline, 200- to 300-mL aliquots, and re-

**TABLE I–37. DRUGS AND TOXINS POORLY ADSORBED BY ACTIVATED CHARCOAL[a]**

| | |
|---|---|
| Alkali | Inorganic salts |
| Cyanide[b] | Iron |
| Ethanol and other alcohols | Lithium |
| Ethylene glycol | Mineral acids |
| Fluoride | Potassium |
| Heavy metals | |

[a]Few studies have been performed to determine in vivo adsorption of these and other toxins to activated charcoal. Adsorption may also depend on the specific type and concentration of charcoal.
[b]Charcoal should still be given because usual doses of charcoal (60–100 g) will adsorb usual lethal ingested doses of cyanide (200–300 mg).

move by gravity or active suction. Use repeated aliquots for a total of 2 L or until the return is free of pills or toxic material. ***Caution:*** Use of excessive volumes of lavage fluid or plain tap water can result in hypothermia or electrolyte imbalance in infants and small children.

**C. Activated charcoal** is a highly adsorbent powdered material made from a distillation of wood pulp. Owing to its very large surface area, it is highly effective in adsorbing most toxins when given in a ratio of approximately 10 to 1 (charcoal to toxin). Only a few toxins are poorly adsorbed to charcoal (Table I–37), and in some cases this requires a higher ratio (eg, for cyanide a ratio of about 100:1 is necessary). Studies in volunteers taking nontoxic doses suggest that activated charcoal given alone without prior gastric emptying is as effective as or even more effective than emesis and lavage procedures in reducing drug absorption. However, there are no well-designed clinical studies demonstrating its effectiveness in poisoned patients. As a result, some toxicologists advise against its routine use.

1. **Indications**
   - **a.** Used after ingestion to limit drug absorption from the gastrointestinal tract if it can be given safely and in a reasonable time period after the ingestion.
   - **b.** Charcoal is often given even if the offending substance may not be well adsorbed to charcoal in case other substances have been co-ingested.
   - **c.** Repeated oral doses of activated charcoal may enhance elimination of some drugs from the bloodstream (see p 50).
2. **Contraindications.** Ileus without distension is not a contraindication for a single dose of charcoal, but further doses should be withheld. Charcoal should not be given to a drowsy patient unless the airway is adequately protected.
3. **Adverse effects**
   - **a.** Constipation or intestinal impaction and bezoar are potential complications, especially if multiple doses of charcoal are given.
   - **b.** Distension of the stomach with a potential risk of pulmonary aspiration, especially in a drowsy patient.
   - **c.** Many commercially available charcoal products contain charcoal and the cathartic sorbitol in a premixed suspension. Even single doses of sorbitol often cause stomach cramps and vomiting, and repeated doses may cause serious fluid shifts to the intestine, diarrhea, dehydration, and hypernatremia, especially in young children and elderly persons.
   - **d.** May bind coadministered acetylcysteine (not clinically significant).
4. **Technique.** (See Table I-38 for guidelines on prehospital and hospital use.)
   - **a.** Give activated charcoal aqueous suspension (without sorbitol), 60–100 g (1 g/kg), orally or by gastric tube.
   - **b.** One or two additional doses of activated charcoal may be given at 1- or 2-hour intervals to ensure adequate gut decontamination, particularly

**TABLE I–38. GUIDELINES FOR ADMINISTRATION OF ACTIVATED CHARCOAL**

**General:**

The risk of the poisoning justifies the risk of charcoal administration

Activated charcoal can be administered within 60 minutes of the ingestion[a]

**Prehospital:**

The patient is alert and cooperative

Activated charcoal without sorbitol is readily available

Administration of charcoal will not delay transport to a health-care facility

**Hospital:**

The patient is alert and cooperative, or the activated charcoal will be given via gastric tube (assuming the airway is intact or protected)

[a]The time after ingestion during which charcoal remains an effective decontamination modality has not been established with certainty in clinical trials. For drugs with slow or erratic intestinal absorption, or those with anticholinergic or opioid effects or other pharmacological effects that may delay gastric emptying into the small intestine, or drugs in a modified-release formulation, or after massive ingestions that may produce a tablet mass or bezoar, it is appropriate to administer charcoal more than 60 minutes after ingestion, or even several hours after ingestion.

after large ingestions. In rare cases, as many as 8 or 10 repeated doses may be needed to achieve the desired 10:1 ratio of charcoal to poison (eg, after an ingestion of 200 aspirin tablets); in such circumstances, the doses should be given over a period of several hours.

**D. Cathartics.** Controversy remains over the use of cathartics to hasten elimination of toxins from the gastrointestinal tract. Some toxicologists still use cathartics routinely when giving activated charcoal even though few data exist to support their efficacy.

1. **Indications**
   a. To enhance gastrointestinal transit of the charcoal-toxin complex, decreasing the likelihood of desorption of toxin or development of a "charcoal bezoar."
   b. To hasten passage of iron tablets and other ingestions not adsorbed by charcoal.
2. **Contraindications**
   a. Ileus or intestinal obstruction.
   b. Sodium- and magnesium-containing cathartics should not be used in patients with fluid overload or renal insufficiency, respectively.
   c. There is no role for oil-based cathartics (previously recommended for hydrocarbon poisoning).
3. **Adverse effects**
   a. Severe fluid loss, hypernatremia, and hyperosmolarity may result from overuse or repeated doses of cathartics.
   b. Hypermagnesemia may occur in patients with renal insufficiency who are given magnesium-based cathartics.
   c. Abdominal cramping and vomiting may occur, especially with sorbitol.
4. **Technique**
   a. Administer the cathartic of choice (10% magnesium citrate, 3–4 mL/kg, or 70% sorbitol, 1 mL/kg) along with activated charcoal or mixed together as a slurry. Avoid using commercially available combination products containing charcoal plus sorbitol, as they have a larger than desirable amount of sorbitol (eg, 96 g sorbitol/50 g charcoal).
   b. Repeat with one-half the original dose if there is no charcoal stool after 6–8 hours.

**E. Whole-bowel irrigation.** Whole-bowel irrigation has become an accepted method for elimination of some drugs and poisons from the gut. The technique makes use of a surgical bowel-cleansing solution containing a nonabsorbable polyethylene glycol in a balanced electrolyte solution that is formulated to pass through the intestinal tract without being absorbed. This solution is given at high flow rates to force intestinal contents out by sheer volume.

1. **Indications**
   a. Large ingestions of iron, lithium, or other drugs poorly adsorbed to activated charcoal.
   b. Large ingestions of sustained-release or enteric-coated tablets containing valproic acid (eg, Depakote™), theophylline (eg, Theo-Dur™), aspirin (eg, Ecotrin™), verapamil (eg, Calan SR™), diltiazem (eg, Cardizem CD™), or other dangerous drugs.
   c. Ingestion of foreign bodies or drug-filled packets or condoms. Although controversy persists about the optimal gut decontamination for "body stuffers" (persons who hastily ingest drug-containing packets to hide incriminating evidence), prudent management involves several hours of whole-bowel irrigation accompanied by activated charcoal. Follow-up imaging studies may be indicated to search for retained packets if the amount of drug or its packaging is of concern.
2. **Contraindications**
   a. Ileus or intestinal obstruction.
   b. Obtunded, comatose, or convulsing patient unless the airway is protected.
3. **Adverse effects**
   a. Nausea and bloating.
   b. Regurgitation and pulmonary aspiration.
   c. Activated charcoal may not be as effective when given with whole-bowel irrigation.
4. **Technique**
   a. Administer bowel preparation solution (eg, CoLyte™ or GoLYTELY™), 2 L/h by gastric tube (children: 500 mL/h or 35 mL/kg/h), until rectal effluent is clear.
   b. Some toxicologists recommend administration of activated charcoal 25–50 g every 2–3 hours while whole-bowel irrigation is proceeding if the ingested drug is adsorbed by charcoal.
   c. Be prepared for large-volume stool within 1–2 hours. Pass a rectal tube or, preferably, have the patient sit on a commode.
   d. Stop administration after 8–10 L (children: 150–200 mL/kg) if no rectal effluent has appeared.

**F. Other oral binding agents.** Other binding agents may be given in certain circumstances to trap toxins in the gut, although activated charcoal is the most widely used effective adsorbent. Table I–39 lists some alternative binding

**TABLE I–39. SELECTED ORAL BINDING AGENTS**

| Drug or Toxin | Binding Agent(s) |
|---|---|
| Calcium | Cellulose sodium phosphate |
| Chlorinated hydrocarbons | Cholestyramine resin |
| Digitoxin[a] | Cholestyramine resin |
| Heavy metals (arsenic, mercury) | Demulcents (egg white, milk) |
| Iron | Sodium bicarbonate |
| Lithium | Sodium polystyrene sulfonate (Kayexalate) |
| Paraquat[a] | Fuller's earth, Bentonite |
| Potassium | Sodium polystyrene sulfonate (Kayexalate) |
| Thallium | Prussian blue |

[a]Activated charcoal is also very effective.

agents and the toxin(s) for which they may be useful.

**G. Surgical removal.** Occasionally, drug-filled packets or condoms, intact tablets, or tablet concretions persist despite aggressive gastric lavage or whole-gut lavage, and surgical removal may be necessary. Consult a regional poison control center or a medical toxicologist for advice.

## ENHANCED ELIMINATION

Measures to enhance elimination of drugs and toxins have been overemphasized in the past. Although a desirable goal, rapid elimination of most drugs and toxins is frequently not practical and may be unsafe. A logical understanding of pharmacokinetics as it applies to toxicology (toxicokinetics) is necessary for the appropriate use of enhanced removal procedures.

**I. Assessment.** Three critical questions must be answered:

**A. Does the patient need enhanced removal?** Ask the following questions: How is the patient doing? Will supportive care enable the patient to recover fully? Is there an antidote or another specific drug that might be used? Important indications for enhanced drug removal include the following:

1. Obviously severe or critical intoxication with a deteriorating condition despite maximal supportive care (eg, phenobarbital overdose with intractable hypotension).
2. The normal or usual route of elimination is impaired (eg, lithium overdose in a patient with renal failure).
3. The patient has ingested a known lethal dose or has a lethal blood level (eg, theophylline or methanol).
4. The patient has underlying medical problems that could increase the hazards of prolonged coma or other complications (eg, severe chronic obstructive pulmonary disease or congestive heart failure).

**B. Is the drug or toxin accessible to the removal procedure?** For a drug to be accessible to removal by extracorporeal procedures, it should be located primarily within the bloodstream or in the extracellular fluid. If it is extensively distributed to tissues, it is not likely to be easily removed.

1. **The volume of distribution (Vd)** is a numerical concept that provides an indication of the accessibility of the drug:

   Vd = apparent volume into which the drug is distributed
   = (amount of drug in the body)/(plasma concentration)
   = (mg/kg)/(mg/L) = L/kg

   A drug with a very large Vd has a very low plasma concentration. In contrast, a drug with a small Vd is potentially quite accessible by extracorporeal removal procedures. Table I–40 lists some common volumes of distribution.

2. **Protein binding** may affect accessibility; highly protein-bound drugs have low free drug concentrations and are difficult to remove by dialysis.

**TABLE I–40. VOLUME OF DISTRIBUTION OF SOME DRUGS AND POISONS**

| Large Vd (>5–10 L/kg) | Small Vd (<1 L/kg) |
|---|---|
| Antidepressants | Alcohols |
| Digoxin | Carbamazepine |
| Lindane | Lithium |
| Opioids | Phenobarbital |
| Phencyclidine (PCP) | Salicylate |
| Phenothiazines | Theophylline |

**C. Will the method work?** Does the removal procedure efficiently extract the toxin from the blood?

1. The **clearance (CL)** is the rate at which a given volume of fluid can be "cleared" of the substance.
   a. The CL may be calculated from the extraction ratio across the dialysis machine or hemoperfusion column, multiplied by the blood flow rate through the following system:

$$CL = \text{extraction ratio} \times \text{blood flow rate}$$

   b. A crude urinary CL measurement may be useful for estimating the effectiveness of fluid therapy for enhancing renal elimination of substances not secreted or absorbed by the renal tubule (eg, lithium):

$$\text{Renal CL} = \text{urine flow rate} \times \frac{\text{urine drug level}}{\text{serum drug level}}$$

   ***Note:*** The units of clearance are milliliters per minute. Clearance is not the same as elimination rate (milligrams per minute). If the blood concentration is small, the actual amount of drug removed is also small.

2. **Total clearance** is the sum of all sources of clearance (eg, renal excretion plus hepatic metabolism plus respiratory and skin excretion plus dialysis). If the contribution of dialysis is small compared with the total clearance rate, the procedure will contribute little to the overall elimination rate (Table I–41).
3. The **half-life** ($T_{1/2}$) depends on the volume of distribution and the clearance:

$$T_{1/2} = \frac{0.693 \times Vd}{CL}$$

   where the unit of measurement of Vd is liters (L) and that of CL is liters per hour (L/h).

**II. Methods available for enhanced elimination**

**A. Urinary manipulation.** These methods require that the renal route be a significant contributor to total clearance.

1. Forced diuresis may increase glomerular filtration rate, and ion trapping by urinary pH manipulation may enhance elimination of polar drugs.
2. Alkalinization is commonly used for salicylate overdose, but "forced" diuresis (producing urine volumes of up to 1 L/h) is generally not used because of the risk of fluid overload.

**B. Hemodialysis.** Blood is taken from a large vein (usually a femoral vein) with a double-lumen catheter and is pumped through the hemodialysis system. The patient must be anticoagulated to prevent clotting of blood in the dialyzer. Drugs and toxins flow passively across the semipermeable membrane down a concentration gradient into a dialysate (electrolyte and buffer) solution. Fluid and electrolyte abnormalities can be corrected concurrently.

1. Flow rates of up to 300–500 mL/min can be achieved, and clearance rates may reach 200–300 mL/min. Removal of drug is dependent on flow rate—insufficient flow (ie, due to clotting) will reduce clearance proportionately.
2. Characteristics of the drug or toxin that enhance its extractability include small size (molecular weight < 500 daltons), water solubility, and low protein binding.
3. ***Note:*** Smaller, portable dialysis units that utilize a resin column or filter to recycle a smaller volume of dialysate ("mini-dialysis") do not efficiently remove drugs or poisons and should not be used.

**C. Hemoperfusion.** Using equipment and vascular access similar to that for hemodialysis, the blood is pumped directly through a column containing an adsorbent material (either charcoal or Amberlite™ resin). Systemic anticoagulation is required, often in higher doses than for hemodialysis, and thrombocytopenia is

**TABLE I–41. ELIMINATION OF SELECTED DRUGS AND TOXINS[a]**

| Drug or Toxin | Volume of Distribution (L/kg) | Usual Body Clearance (mL/min) | Reported Clearance by: Dialysis (mL/min) | Reported Clearance by: Hemoperfusion[b] (mL/min) |
|---|---|---|---|---|
| Acetaminophen | 0.8–1 | 400 | 120–150 | 125–300 |
| Amitriptyline | 6–10 | 500–800 | NHD[c] | 240[d] |
| Bromide | 0.7 | 5 | 100 | NA[c] |
| Carbamazepine | 1.2 | 60–90 | 59–100[e] | 80–130 |
| Digitoxin | 0.6 | 4 | 10–26 | NA |
| Digoxin | 5–7 | 150–200 | NHD | 90–140 |
| Ethanol | 0.7 | 100–300 | 100–200 | NHP[c] |
| Ethchlorvynol | 2–4 | 120–140 | 20–80 | 150–300[d] |
| Ethylene glycol | 0.6–0.8 | 200 | 100–200 | NHP |
| Glutethimide | 2.7 | 200 | 70 | 300[d] |
| Isopropyl alcohol | 0.7 | 30 | 100–200 | NHP |
| Lithium | 0.6–1 | 25–30 | 50–150 | NHP |
| Meprobamate | 0.75 | 60 | 60 | 85–150 |
| Metformin | 26–1952 L[f] | 491–652[g] | 68–170 | |
| Methanol | 0.7 | 40–60 | 100–200 | NHP |
| Formic acid (methanol metabolite) | | | 198–248 | |
| Methaqualone | 5.8 | 130–175 | 23 | 150–270 |
| Methotrexate | 0.5–1 | 50–100 | NA | 54 |
| Nadolol | 2 | 135 | 46–102 | NA |
| Nortriptyline | 20–40 | 500–1000 | 24–34 | 216[d] |
| Paraquat | 2.8 | 30–200 | 10 | 50–155 |
| Pentobarbital | 0.8–1 | 27–36 | 23–55 | 200–300 |
| Phenobarbital | 0.8 | 2–15 | 144–188[h] | 100–300 |
| Phenytoin | 0.6 | 15–30 | NHD | 76–189 |
| Procainamide | 1.9 | 650 | 70 | 75 |
| *N*-acetylprocainamide (NAPA) | 1.4 | 220 | 48 | 75 |
| Salicylate | 0.15 | 30 | 35–80 | 57–116 |
| Theophylline | 0.3–0.6 | 80–120 | 30–50 | 60–225 |
| Thiocyanate (cyanide metabolite) | | | 83–102 | |
| Trichloroethanol (chloral hydrate) | 0.6–1.6 | 25 | 68–162 | 119–200 |
| Valproic acid | 0.15–0.4 | 10 | 23 | 55 |

[a]Adapted in part from Pond SM: Diuresis, dialysis, and hemoperfusion: Indications and benefits. *Emerg Med Clin North Am* 1984;2:29, and Cutler RE et al: Extracorporeal removal of drugs and poisons by hemodialysis and hemoperfusion. *Ann Rev Pharmacol Toxicol* 1987;27:169.
[b]Hemoperfusion data are mainly for charcoal hemoperfusion.
[c]Abbreviations: NHD = not hemodialyzable; NA = not available; NHP = not hemoperfusable.
[d]Data are for XAD-4 resin hemoperfusion.
[e]Lower clearance (14–59 mL/min) reported with older dialysis equipment; newer high-flux dialysis may produce clearances of 59 mL/min up to estimated 100 mL/min (based on case reports)
[f]Literature reports of metformin Vd vary widely
[g]Metformin clearance is markedly reduced in patients with renal insufficiency (108–130 mL/min)
[h]Lower clearance 60–75 mL/min reported with older dialysis equipment; newer high-flux dialysis may produce clearances of 144–188 mL/min (Palmer: *Am J Kid Dis* 2000;36:640).

**TABLE I–42. SOME DRUGS REMOVED BY REPEAT-DOSE ACTIVATED CHARCOAL[a]**

| | |
|---|---|
| Caffeine | Phenobarbital |
| Carbamazepine | Phenylbutazone |
| Chlordecone | Phenytoin |
| Dapsone | Salicylate |
| Digitoxin | Theophylline |
| Nadolol | |

[a]Note: based on volunteer studies. There are few data on clinical benefit in drug overdose.

a common complication. At the present time, few dialysis centers have the equipment for hemoperfusion and the procedure is rarely carried out.

1. Because the drug or toxin is in direct contact with the adsorbent material, drug size, water solubility, and protein binding are less important limiting factors.
2. For most drugs, hemoperfusion can achieve greater clearance rates than hemodialysis. For example, the hemodialysis clearance rate for phenobarbital is 60–80 mL/min, whereas the hemoperfusion clearance rate is 200–300 mL/min.

**D. Peritoneal dialysis.** Dialysate fluid is infused into the peritoneal cavity through a transcutaneous catheter and drained off, and the procedure is repeated with fresh dialysate. The gut wall and peritoneal lining serve as the semipermeable membrane.

1. Peritoneal dialysis is easier to perform than hemodialysis or hemoperfusion and does not require anticoagulation, but it is only about 10–15% as effective owing to poor extraction ratios and slower flow rates (clearance rates 10–15 mL/min).
2. However, peritoneal dialysis can be performed continuously, 24 hours a day; a 24-hour peritoneal dialysis with dialysate exchange every 1–2 hours is approximately equal to 4 hours of hemodialysis.

**E. Continuous renal replacement therapy.** Continuous arteriovenous or venovenous hemodiafiltration (CAVHD or CVVHD, respectively) has been suggested as an alternative to conventional hemodialysis when the need for rapid removal of the drug is less urgent. Like peritoneal dialysis, these procedures are associated with lower clearance rates but have the advantage of being minimally invasive, with no significant impact on hemodynamics, and can be carried out "continuously" for many hours. However, their role in management of acute poisoning remains uncertain.

**F. Repeat-dose activated charcoal.** Repeated doses of activated charcoal (20–30 g or 0.5–1 g/kg every 2–3 hours) are given orally or via gastric tube. The presence of a slurry of activated charcoal throughout several meters of the intestinal lumen reduces blood concentrations by interrupting enterohepatic or enteroenteric recirculation of the drug or toxin, a mode of action quite distinct from simple adsorption of ingested but unabsorbed tablets. This technique is easy and noninvasive and has been shown to shorten the half-life of phenobarbital, theophylline, and several other drugs (Table I–42). However, it has not been shown in clinical trials to alter patient outcome. ***Caution:*** Repeat-dose charcoal may cause serious fluid and electrolyte disturbance secondary to large-volume diarrhea, especially if premixed charcoal-sorbitol suspensions are used. Also, it should not be used in patients with ileus or obstruction.

## DISPOSITION OF THE PATIENT

**I. Emergency department discharge or intensive care unit admission?**

**A.** All patients with potentially serious overdose should be observed for at least 6–8 hours before discharge or transfer to a nonmedical (eg, psychiatric) facility. If signs or symptoms of intoxication develop during this time, admission for further observation and treatment is required. ***Caution:*** Beware of delayed complications from slow absorption of medications (eg, from a tablet concretion or bezoar or sustained-release or enteric-coated preparations). In these circumstances, a longer period of observation is warranted. If specific drug levels are determined, obtain repeated serum levels to be certain that they are decreasing as expected.

**B.** Most patients admitted for poisoning or drug overdose will need observation in an intensive care unit, although this depends on the potential for serious cardiorespiratory complications. Any patient with suicidal intent must be kept under close observation.

**II. Regional poison control center consultation: (800) 222-1222.** Consult with a regional poison control center to determine the need for further observation or admission, administration of antidotes or therapeutic drugs, selection of appropriate laboratory tests, or decisions about extracorporeal removal. An experienced clinical toxicologist is usually available for immediate consultation. A single toll-free number is now effective nationwide and will automatically connect the caller to the regional poison control center.

**III. Psychosocial evaluation**

**A. Psychiatric consultation for suicide risk.** All patients with intentional poisoning or drug overdose should have psychiatric evaluation for suicidal intent.

**1.** It is not appropriate to discharge a potentially suicidal patient from the emergency department without a careful psychiatric evaluation. Most states have provisions for the physician to place an emergency psychiatric hold, forcing involuntary patients to remain under psychiatric observation for up to 72 hours.

**2.** Patients calling from home after an intentional ingestion should always be referred to an emergency department for medical and psychiatric evaluation.

**B. Child abuse** (see also below) or **sexual abuse**

**1.** Children should be evaluated for the possibility that the ingestion was not accidental. Sometimes parents or other adults intentionally give children sedatives or tranquilizers to control their behavior.

**2.** Accidental poisonings may also warrant social services referral. Occasionally children get into stimulants or other abused drugs that are left around the home. Repeated ingestions suggest overly casual or negligent parental behavior.

**3.** Intentional overdose in a child or adolescent should raise the possibility of physical or sexual abuse. Teenage girls may have overdosed because of unwanted pregnancy.

**IV. Overdose in the pregnant patient**

**A.** In general, it is prudent to check for pregnancy in any young woman with drug overdose or poisoning. Unwanted pregnancy may be a cause for intentional overdose, or special concerns may be raised about treatment of the pregnant patient.

**B.** Inducing emesis with syrup of ipecac is probably safe in early pregnancy, but protracted vomiting is unwelcome, especially in the third trimester. Gastric lavage or oral activated charcoal is preferable in all trimesters.

**C.** Some toxins are known to be teratogenic or mutagenic (see below and Table I–45, p 62). However, adverse effects on the fetus are generally associated with chronic, repeated use as opposed to acute, single exposure.

## ► SPECIAL CONSIDERATIONS IN PEDIATRIC PATIENTS

*Delia A. Dempsey, MD, MS*

The majority of calls to poison control centers involve children under 5 years of age. Fortunately, children account for a minority of serious poisonings requiring emergency hospital treatment. Most common childhood ingestions involve nontoxic sub-

**TABLE I–43. EXAMPLES OF POTENT PEDIATRIC POISONS**

| Drug or Poison | Potentially Fatal Dose in a 10-kg Toddler | No. of Pediatric Deaths Reported to AAPCC 1983–1990 |
|---|---|---|
| Benzocaine | 2 mL of a 10% gel | |
| Camphor | 5 mL of 20% oil | |
| Chloroquine | One 500-mg tablet | 2 |
| Chlorpromazine | One or two 200-mg tablets | 1 |
| Codeine | Three 60-mg tablets | |
| Desipramine | Two 75-mg tablets | 4 |
| Diphenoxylate/atropine (Lomotil) | Five 2.5-mg tablets | 2 |
| Hydrocarbons (eg, kerosene) | One swallow (if aspirated) | 12 |
| Hypoglycemic sulfonylureas | Two 5-mg glyburide tablets | |
| Imipramine | One 150-mg tablet | 3 |
| Iron | Ten adult-strength tablets | 16 |
| Lindane | Two teaspoons (10 mL) | |
| Methyl salicylate | Less than 5 mL of oil of wintergreen | 4 |
| Quinidine | Two 300-mg tablets | 1 |
| Selenious acid (gun bluing) | One swallow | 4 |
| Theophylline | One 500-mg tablet | |
| Thioridazine | One 200-mg tablet | |
| Verapamil | One or two 240-mg tablets | 3 |

References: Koren G: Medications which can kill a toddler with one teaspoon or tablet. *Clin Toxicol* 1993;31(3):407; Osterhoudt K: Toxtalk 1997;8(7); Litovitz T, Manoguerra A: Comparison of pediatric poisoning hazards: An analysis of 3.8 million exposure incidents. *Pediatrics* 1992;89(6):999.

stances or nontoxic doses of potentially toxic drugs or products (see p 287). Important causes of serious or fatal childhood poisoning include iron supplements (p 230); tricyclic antidepressants (p 91); cardiovascular medications such as digitalis (p 155), beta receptor antagonists (p 131), or calcium antagonists (p 143); methylsalicylate (p 333); and hydrocarbons (p 219). See Table I–43.

**I. High-risk populations.** Two age groups are commonly involved in pediatric poisonings: children between 1 and 5 years old and adolescents.

**A. Ingestions in toddlers and young children** usually result from oral exploration. Unintentional ingestion in children under 6 months of age or between the ages of 5 and adolescence is rare. In young infants, consider the possibility of intentional administration by an older child or adult. In school-age children, suspect abuse or neglect as a reason for the ingestion, and in adolescents, suspect a suicide attempt.

**B. In adolescents and young adults**, overdoses are usually suicidal but may also result from drug abuse or experimentation. Common underlying reasons for adolescents' suicide attempts include pregnancy; sexual, physical, or mental abuse; school failure; conflict with peers; conflict with homosexual orientation; a sudden or severe loss; and alcoholism or illicit drug use. Any adolescent who makes a suicide attempt or gesture needs psychiatric evaluation and follow-up.

**II. Poisoning prevention.** Young children with an unintentional ingestion are at higher risk for a second ingestion than is the general pediatric population. After an incident, prevention strategies need to be reviewed. If the family does not understand the instructions or it is the second poisoning incident, consider a home evaluation for childproofing by a public health nurse or other health-care professional.

**A. Childproof** the home, day-care setting, and households the child commonly visits (eg, grandparents and other relatives). Store medicines, chemicals, and cleaning products out of the reach of children or in locked cabinets. Do not store chemicals in food containers, and do not store chemicals in the same cabinets as food. Common places children find medications include visitors' purses or backpacks and bedside tables.

**B. Use child-resistant containers** to store prescription and nonprescription medications. However, child-resistant containers are not childproof; they only lessen the time it takes a determined child to get into the container.

**III. Child abuse.** Consider the possibility that the child was intentionally given the drug or toxin. Most states require that all health-care professionals report suspected cases of child abuse or neglect, which means that this is not a discretionary decision but a ***legal obligation to report any suspicious incident.*** The parents or guardians should be informed in a straightforward, nonjudgmental manner that a report is being made under this legal obligation. In serious cases, the suspected abuse report should be made before the child is released, and the local child-protective services should decide whether it is safe to release the child to the parents or guardians. In unclear situations, the child can be admitted for "observation" to allow time for social services to make an expeditious evaluation. The following should alert medical personnel to the possibility of abuse or neglect:

**A.** The story does not make sense or does not ring true, or it changes over time, or different people give different stories.

**B.** The child is nonambulatory (eg, a child under 6 months of age). Carefully review how the child gained access to the drug or toxin.

**C.** The child is over 4–5 years old. Accidental ingestions are rare in older children, and ingestion may be a signal of abuse or neglect.

**D.** The drug ingested was a tranquilizer (eg, haloperidol or chlorpromazine), a drug of abuse (eg, cocaine or heroin), a sedative (eg, diazepam), or ethanol, or the parents are intoxicated.

**E.** There is a long interval between the time of ingestion and the time the child is taken for medical evaluation.

**F.** There are signs of physical or sexual abuse or neglect: multiple or unusual bruises; a broken bone or burns; a very dirty, unkempt child; or a child with a flat affect or indifferent or inappropriate behavior.

**G.** A history of repeated episodes of possible or documented poisonings or a history of prior abuse.

**H.** Munchausen syndrome by proxy: drugs or toxins are given to the child to simulate illness. Most perpetrators are mothers, often with a medical background. This is a rare diagnosis.

**IV. Clinical evaluation.** The physical and laboratory evaluation is essentially the same as for adults. However, normal vital signs vary with age (Table I–44).

**A. Heart rate.** Newborns may have normal heart rates as high as 190/min, and 2-year-olds up to 120/min. Abnormal tachycardia or bradycardia suggests the possibility of hypoxemia in addition to the numerous drugs and poisons that affect heart rate and rhythm (see Tables I–4 [p 9] through I–7 [p 13]).

**B. Blood pressure** is a very important vital sign in a poisoned child. The blood pressure cuff must be of the proper size; cuffs that are too small can falsely elevate the pressure. The blood pressures of infants are difficult to obtain by auscultation but are easily obtained by Doppler.

**1.** Many children normally have a lower blood pressure than adults. However, low blood pressure in the context of a poisoning should be regarded

**TABLE I–44. PEDIATRIC VITAL SIGNS**[a]

| Age | Respiratory Rate (/min) | Heart Rate (/min) | Blood Pressure (mm Hg) | | | |
|---|---|---|---|---|---|---|
| | | | Lower Limit | Average | Upper Limit | Severe |
| Newborn | 30–80 | 110–190 | 52/25 | 50–55[b] | 95/72 | 110/85 |
| 1 month | 30–50 | 100–170 | 64/30 | 85/50 | 105/68 | 120/85 |
| 6 months | 30–50 | 100–170 | 60/40 | 90/55 | 110/72 | 125/85 |
| 1 year | 20–40 | 100–160 | 66/40 | 90/55 | 110/72 | 125/88 |
| 2 years | 20–30 | 100–160 | 74/40 | 90/55 | 110/72 | 125/88 |
| 4 years | 20–25 | 80–130 | 79/45 | 95/55 | 112/75 | 128/88 |
| 8 years | 15–25 | 70–110 | 85/48 | 100/60 | 118/75 | 135/92 |
| 12 years | 15–20 | 60–100 | 95/50 | 108/65 | 125/84 | 142/95 |

[a]References: Dieckmann RA, Coulter K: Pediatric emergencies. Page 811 in *Current Emergency Diagnosis and Treatment,* 4th ed. Saunders CE, Ho MT (editors). Appleton & Lange, 1992; Gundy JH: The pediatric physical exam. Page 68 in: *Primary Pediatric Care.* Hoekelman RA et al (editors). Mosby, 1987; Hoffman JIE: Systemic arterial hypertension. Page 1438 in *Rudolph's Pediatrics.* 19th ed. Rudolph AM et al (editors). Appleton & Lange 1991; Liebman J, Freed MD: Cardiovascular system. Page 447 in: *Nelson's Essentials of Pediatrics.* Behrman RE, Kleigman R (editors). Saunders, 1990; Lum GM: Kidney and urinary tract. Page 624 in *Current Pediatric Diagnosis and Treatment,* 10th ed. Hathaway WE et al (editors). Appleton & Lange, 1991.
[b]Mean arterial pressure range on the first day of life.

as normal only if the child is alert, active, and appropriate and has normal peripheral perfusion.

2. Idiopathic or essential hypertension is rare in children. Elevated blood pressure should be assumed to indicate an acute condition, although the systolic blood pressure can be transiently elevated if the child is vigorously crying or screaming. Unless a child's baseline blood pressure is known, values at the upper limit of normal should be assumed to be "elevated." The decision to treat elevated blood pressure must be made on an individual basis, based on the clinical scenario and the toxin involved.

V. **Neonates** present specific problems, including unique pharmacokinetics and potentially severe withdrawal from prenatal drug exposure.

A. **Neonatal pharmacokinetics.** Newborns (birth to 1 month) and infants (1–12 months) are unique from a toxicologic and pharmacologic perspective. Drug absorption, distribution, and elimination are different from those of older children and adults. Incorrect dosing, transplacental passage proximate to the time of birth, breast-feeding, dermal absorption, and intentional poisoning are potential routes of toxic exposure. Of particular importance are enhanced skin absorption and reduced drug elimination, which may lead to toxicity after relatively mild exposure.

1. **Skin absorption.** Neonates have a very high ratio of surface area to body weight, which predisposes them to poisoning via percutaneous absorption (eg, hexachlorophene, boric acid, or alcohols).
2. **Elimination** of many drugs (eg, acetaminophen, many antibiotics, caffeine, lidocaine, morphine, phenytoin, and theophylline) is prolonged in neonates. For example, the half-life of caffeine is approximately 3 hours in adults but may be greater than 100 hours in newborns.

B. **Neonatal drug withdrawal** may occur in infants with chronic prenatal exposure to illicit or therapeutic drugs. The onset is usually within 72 hours of birth, but a postnatal onset as late as 14 days has been reported. Signs usually commence in the nursery, and infants are not discharged until clinically stable. However, with early discharge from nurseries becoming the norm, an infant in withdrawal may first present to an emergency department or acute care clinic. The presentation may be as mild as colic or as severe as withdrawal seizures or profound diarrhea.

1. **Opioids** (especially methadone and heroin) are the most common cause of serious neonatal drug withdrawal symptoms. Other drugs for which a withdrawal syndrome has been reported include phencyclidine (PCP), cocaine, amphetamines, tricyclic antidepressants, phenothiazines, benzodiazepines, barbiturates, ethanol, clonidine, diphenhydramine, lithium, meprobamate, and theophylline. A careful drug history from the mother should include illicit drugs, alcohol, and prescription and over-the-counter medications and whether she is breast-feeding.
2. **The manifestations of neonatal opioid withdrawal** include inability to sleep, irritability, tremulousness, inconsolability, high-pitched incessant cry, hypertonia, hyperreflexia, sneezing and yawning, lacrimation, disorganized suck, poor feeding, vomiting, diarrhea, tachypnea or respiratory distress, tachycardia, autonomic dysfunction, sweating, fevers, and seizures. Morbidity and mortality from untreated opioid withdrawal can be significant and commonly result from weight loss, metabolic acidosis, respiratory alkalosis, dehydration, electrolyte imbalance, and seizures. Withdrawal is a diagnosis of exclusion; immediately rule out sepsis, hypoglycemia, hypocalcemia, and hypoxia, and consider hyperbilirubinemia, hypomagnesemia, hyperthyroidism, and intracranial hemorrhage. Seizures do not usually occur as the only clinical manifestation of opioid withdrawal.
3. **Treatment of neonatal opioid withdrawal** is mainly supportive and includes swaddling, rocking, a quiet room, frequent small feedings with high-caloric formula, and intravenous fluids if necessary. A variety of drugs have been used, including morphine, paregoric, tincture of opium, diazepam, lorazepam, chlorpromazine, and phenobarbital. Numerous abstinence-scoring systems exist to evaluate opioid withdrawal objectively and treat it. The scoring and treatment of a neonate in withdrawal should be supervised by a neonatologist or a pediatrician experienced with neonatal withdrawal.

VI. **Pregnancy and drugs or chemicals.** Estimates of the percentage of congenital abnormalities and adverse pregnancy outcomes attributable to prescription medications, chemicals, hyperthermia, and ionizing radiation range from less than 1% to 5%, depending on the author.

A. The adverse effects of drugs and chemicals on pregnancy are dose- and time-dependent. Pregnancy termination should not be considered because of exposure to a contraindicated drug without careful consideration of the true risk. Even with exposure to well-documented teratogens, the majority of exposed fetuses are unaffected (eg, valproic acid).

B. The adverse effects of the drug or chemical on pregnancy or the fetus may include prevention of implantation (eg, nonsteroidal anti-inflammatory drugs [NSAIDs]), fetal death (eg, intra-amniotic methylene blue), malformations (eg, thalidomide), postnatal adverse physiologic effects (eg, oral hypoglycemics), and adverse outcomes apparent only years after birth (eg, diethylstilbestrol). Some drugs that have a very long half-life require cessation of exposure for months prior to conception (eg, ribavirin, retinoids).

C. For clinical assistance in determining the risk posed to a pregnancy by a specific exposure, contact **Motherisk** (*www.motherisk.org*, 416-813-6780). Motherisk is an evidence-based information and phone consultation service based in Toronto, Canada, devoted to the study of the safety or risk of drugs, chemicals, and disease during pregnancy and lactation.

D. Table I–45 lists drugs' and chemicals' **FDA Pregnancy Ratings** (see also Table III–1) Some drugs have more than one pregnancy category because the category changes with trimester or because different manufacturers/authorities are not in agreement. The best single source for data regarding the effect of drugs on pregnancy and lactation is *Drugs in Pregnancy and Lacta-*

**TABLE I–45. DRUGS AND CHEMICALS THAT POSE A RISK TO THE FETUS OR PREGNANCY**

| Drug Name | FDA[a] Category | Recommendation or Comments[b] |
|---|---|---|
| Amantadine | C | Contraindicated (first trimester) |
| Aminoglutethimide (anticonvulsant) | D | No data |
| Aminopterin | X | Contraindicated (any trimester) |
| Amiodarone | D | Risk (third trimester) |
| Amphetamine | C | Risk (third trimester) |
| Androgenic hormones | X | Contraindicated (any trimester) |
| Angiotensin-converting enzyme (ACE) inhibitors | C/D | Risk (second and third trimesters) |
| Angiotensin II receptor antagonists | C/D | Risk (second and third trimesters) |
| Antidepressants | C | Risk (third trimester) |
| Antineoplastic cytotoxic agents | C/D/X | Look up individual drugs. Only category X are given in table. Recommendations vary widely |
| Azathioprine | D | Risk (third trimester) |
| Barbiturates | C or D | Recommendation by drug varies from Probably Compatible to Risk (first and third trimesters) |
| Benzodiazepines | D/X | Recommendation varies by agent from Low Risk (animal data) to Contraindicated (any trimester). Look up individual agents |
| Benzphetamine | X | Contraindicated (any trimester) |
| Beta-adrenergic blockers | C/D | Risk (second and third trimesters) |
| Bexarotene | X | Contraindicated (any trimester) |
| Blue Cohosh (herb) | C | Risk (third trimester)—used to stimulate labor |
| Bromides, anticonvulsant | D | Risk (third trimester) |
| Carbamazepine | D | Compatible: benefits>>risks |
| Carbarsone, 29% arsenic | D | Contraindicated (any trimester) |
| Carbimazole | D | Risk (third trimester) (use propylthiouracil PTH) |
| Chenodiol | X | Contraindicated (any trimester) |
| Ciguatoxin | | Contraindicated (any trimester) |
| Clarithromycin | C | High risk (animal data) |
| Clomiphene (fertility agent) | X | Contraindicated (any trimester) |
| Clonazepam, anticonvulsant | D | Low risk (animal data) |
| Cocaine, systemic use | C/X | Contraindicated (any trimester) (topical use okay) |
| Colchicine | D | Risk (animal data) |
| Corticosteroids | C/D | Recommendation varies from compatible, to benefits>>risks, to risk in third trimester. Look up individual agents |
| Coumarin derivatives | D/X | Contraindicated (any trimester) |
| Diazoxide | C | Risk (third trimester) |
| Dihydroergotamine | X | Contraindicated (any trimester) |
| Diuretics | B-C/D | Compatible but do not use for gestational hypertension (Category D) |
| Ecstasy (MDMA) | C | Contraindicated (any trimester) |
| Edrophonium | C | Risk (third trimester) |
| Electricity | D | Risk (third trimester); still birth associated with relatively mild shocks |
| Epinephrine | C | Risk (third trimester) |
| Ergotamine | X | Contraindicated (any trimester) |
| Erythromycin (estolate salt) | | Hepatic toxicity in pregnant women. Other salts compatible. |
| Estrogenic hormones | X | Contraindicated (any trimester) |
| Ethanol | D/X | Contraindicated (any trimester) |
| Ethotoin | D | Compatible (benefits>>risks) |
| Fenfluramine | C | Contraindicated (any trimester) |

(*continued*)

**TABLE I–45. DRUGS AND CHEMICALS THAT POSE A RISK TO THE FETUS OR PREGNANCY (CONTINUED)**

| Drug Name | FDA[a] Category | Recommendation or Comments[b] |
|---|---|---|
| Fluconazole ≥ 400 mg/d | C | Risk (third trimester) |
| Flucytosine | C | Contraindicated (first trimester) |
| Fluorouracil | D/X | Contraindicated (first trimester) |
| Fluphenazine | C | Risk (third trimester) |
| HMG-CoA reductase inhibitors: all drugs in this class | X | Contraindicated (any trimester) |
| Iodide $^{125}$I and $^{131}$I (radiopharmaceuticals) | X | Contraindicated (any trimester)—ablates fetal thyroid |
| Iodine and iodide-containing compounds, including topicals, expectorants, and diagnostic agents | D/X | Varies from contraindicated (any trimester) to risk (second and third trimesters). Fetal and neonatal goiter and hypothyroidism |
| Kanamycin | D | Risk (third trimester) |
| Leflunomide | X | Contraindicated (any trimester) |
| Leuprolide | X | Contraindicated (any trimester) |
| Lithium | D | Risk (third trimester) |
| LSD (lysergic acid diethylamide) | C | Contraindicated (any trimester) |
| Marijuana | X | Contraindicated (any trimester) |
| Measles vaccine (live attenuated) | C | Contraindicated (any trimester)—avoid from 1–2 months before pregnancy until after delivery |
| Menadiol, Menadione, Vitamin K3 | C | Risk (third trimester) |
| Mephobarbital, anticonvulsant | D | Compatible: benefits>>risks |
| Meprobamate | D | Contraindicated (first trimester) |
| Metaraminol | C | Risk (second and third trimesters) |
| Methaqualone | D | No data |
| Methimazole | D | Risk (third trimester) (use propylthiouracil PTH) |
| Methotrexate | X | Contraindicated (any trimester) |
| Methylene blue, intra-amniotic | C/D | Contraindicated (second and third trimesters) |
| Methylergonovine maleate, ergot derivative | C | Contraindicated (any trimester) |
| Mifepristone, RU 486 | X | Contraindicated (any trimester) |
| Misoprostol (oral) | X | Contraindicated (any trimester) |
| Misoprostol: low dose for cervical ripening | X | Low risk (human data) |
| Mumps vaccine (live attenuated) | C | Contraindicated (any trimester) |
| Naloxone | B | Compatible |
| Narcotic agonist analgesics | B or C/D | Risk (third trimester): Category D—risk associated with prolonged use or high doses at term |
| Narcotic agonist-antagonist analgesics | B or C/D | Risk (third trimester) |
| Narcotic antagonists (except naloxone) | D | Risk (third trimester) or no data (use naloxone) |
| Nonsteroidal anti-inflammatory drugs (NSAIDs, COX-2 inhibitors, full-dose aspirin) | B-C/D | Risk (first and third trimesters) |
| Norepinephrine | D | Risk (third trimester) |
| Oral antidiabetic agents | C | Insulin is the preferred agent for management of diabetes during pregnancy. Oral antidiabetic agents cross placenta—risk of severe hypoglycemia in newborn |
| *p*-Aminosalicylic acid | C | Risk (third trimester) |
| Paramethadione | D | Contraindicated (first trimester) |
| Penicillamine | D | Risk (third trimester) |
| Phencyclidine | X | Contraindicated (any trimester) |
| Phensuximide | D | Risk (3rd trimester) |
| Phentermine | C | Contraindicated (any trimester) |
| Phenylephrine | C | Risk (third trimester) |
| Phenytoin | D | Compatible: benefits>>risks |

*(continued)*

**TABLE I–45. DRUGS AND CHEMICALS THAT POSE A RISK TO THE FETUS OR PREGNANCY (CONTINUED)**

| Drug Name | FDA[a] Category | Recommendation or Comments[b] |
|---|---|---|
| Plicamycin, mithramycin | X | Contraindicated (first trimester) |
| Podofilox, Podophyllum | C | Contraindicated (any trimester) |
| Primidone | D | Risk (third trimester) |
| Progestogenic hormones | D or X | Contraindicated (any trimester) |
| Quinine, antimalarial | D/X | Risk (third trimester) |
| Quinolone antibiotics | C | Arthropathy in immature animals |
| Retinoid agents | X | Contraindicated (any trimester) |
| Ribavirin, antiviral | X | Contraindicated (any trimester) |
| Rubella vaccine (live attenuated) | C/D | Contraindicated (any trimester)—avoid from 1–2 months before pregnancy until after delivery |
| Smallpox vaccine (live attenuated) | X | Epidemic: compatible (benefits>>risks); otherwise risk (third trimester) |
| Streptomycin | D | Risk (third trimester) |
| Sulfonamides | C/D | Risk (third trimester) |
| Tacrolimus | C | Risk (third trimester) |
| Tamoxifen | D | Contraindicated (any trimester) |
| Terpin hydrate | D | Contraindicated (any trimester) due to ethanol content |
| Tetracyclines, all | D | Contraindicated (second and third trimesters) |
| Thalidomide | X | Contraindicated (any trimester) |
| Tramadol | C | Risk (third trimester) |
| Tretinoin: topical doses | C | Low risk (human data) |
| Triamterene | C/D | Risk (any trimester)—weak folic acid antagonist, and Category D for gestational hypertension use |
| Trimethadione | D | Contraindicated (first trimester) |
| Trimethaphan | C | Contraindicated (any trimester) |
| Trimethoprim | C | Risk (third trimester) |
| Valproic acid | D | Risk (third trimester) |
| Varicella vaccine (live attenuated) | C | Contraindicated (any trimester)—avoid from 1–2 months before pregnancy until after delivery |
| Venezuelan equine encephalitis vaccine, VEE TC-84 (live attenuated) | X | Contraindicated (any trimester)—avoid from 1–2 months before pregnancy until after delivery |
| Vidarabine, antiviral | C | Teratogenic in animals |
| Vitamin A | A/X | Contraindicated (any trimester) in doses greater than FDA RDA |
| Vitamin D | A/D | Compatible except for doses greater than FDA RDA |
| Vitamin $K_3$, Menadiol, Menadione | C | Risk (third trimester) |
| Voriconazole | D | Teratogenic in animals |
| Warfarin | D/X | Contraindicated (any trimester) |
| Yellow fever vaccine (live attenuated) | D | Epidemic: compatible (Benefits>>Risks). Otherwise avoid from 1–2 months before pregnancy until after delivery |
| Zonisamide, anticonvulsant | C | Teratogenic in animals |

[a]**FDA Categories** (see also p 407): **A** = controlled study has shown no risk; **B** = no evidence of risk in humans; **C** = risk cannot be ruled out; **D** = positive evidence of risk; **X** = contraindicated in pregnancy.

[b]From *Drugs in Pregnancy and Lactation, 7th Edition, A Reference Guide to Fetal and Neonatal Risk* (Briggs GG, Freeman RK, Yaffe SJ). Lippincott, Philadelphia: Williams & Wilkins, 2005). All recommendations are based on human data. Animal data are cited only if human data are unavailable and animal data show serious toxicity in multiple species. Risk = Human data suggest risk; exposure during pregnancy should be avoided unless the benefits of the drug outweigh the risks. Contraindicated = Human exposure data indicate that the drug should not be used in pregnancy. Numbers in the parentheses indicate times during pregnancy when the drug is contraindicated or poses risk: All = any time during pregnancy.

*tion,* 7th Edition, *A Reference Guide to Fetal and Neonatal Risk* (Briggs GG, Freeman RK, Yaffe SJ. Lippincott, Williams & Wilkins. Philadelphia, 2005). The authors have assembled data for individual drugs into monographs. In addition to the FDA pregnancy categories, the authors make recommendations regarding use based on their review of the literature. Drugs that have a D or X category or have a "risk" or "contraindication" recommendation by Briggs et al, are included in Table I–45. Drugs that are labeled FDA category D or X may still be considered compatible with pregnancy if the benefits to the mother outweigh the risks to the fetus (maternal benefit >> fetal risk). Selected anticonvulsants fall into this category.

## ▶ SPECIAL CONSIDERATIONS IN THE EVALUATION OF DRUG-FACILITATED ASSAULT

*Jo Ellen Dyer, PharmD*

Since 1996, reports of drug-facilitated assault have been increasing. Drugs may be used to render the victim helpless or unconscious so that the assailant can commit a rape or robbery. The amnestic effects of many of the drugs used often leave little or no recollection of the events, making investigation and prosecution of the suspect more difficult.

I. **High-risk populations** include single women or men, traveling or new to an area, without companions. Drug administration may occur in a bar or club when the victim visits the restroom or accepts an opened bottle or drink. In one series of self-reported cases, half the victims reported meeting the assailant in a public place and over 70% of the victims knew the assailant (eg, a friend or colleague).

II. **Drugs utilized.** Contrary to the popular belief that specific "date rape drugs" are involved in these crimes, a variety of drugs with amnestic or CNS depressant effects can be used to facilitate assault, including benzodiazepines, other sedative-hypnotic drugs, skeletal muscle relaxants, anticholinergics, hallucinogens, and of course ethanol (Table I–46).
   - **A.** Note that many of these drugs are also commonly used to "get high" and might have been self-administered by the victim for this purpose.
   - **B.** Benzodiazepines are often selected for their anterograde amnestic effect, which is related to but distinct from sedation. The strength of amnestic effects can be predicted to increase with dose, rapidity of onset, lipophilic character, and slow redistribution from the CNS.

III. **Routes of surreptitious drug administration:**
   - **A.** Drink: tablet, ice, liquid in eyedropper.
   - **B.** Smoke: applied to a cigarette or joint.
   - **C.** Ingestion: brownie, gelatin, fruit.
   - **D.** Vaginal syringe: drug in contraceptive gel.
   - **E.** Represented as another drug.

IV. **Clinical evaluation.** If the victim presents early after the assault, he or she may still be under the influence of the drug and may appear inappropriately disinhibited or relaxed for the situation. Unfortunately, victims often present many hours, days, or even weeks after the assault, making collection of physical and biochemical evidence much more difficult. Determining the time course of drug effects with estimation of last memory and first recall may provide useful information to investigators.
   - **A. Use open-ended questions** to avoid suggesting symptoms to a victim who may be trying to fill in a lapse in memory.
   - **B.** Perform a thorough examination and maintain the legal chain of custody for any specimens obtained.

V. **Laboratory.** Timing of laboratory analysis may be crucial, as elimination rates of commonly used sedative and amnestic drugs vary and some may be extremely short. Immediate collection of toxicology specimens is important to avoid loss of

**TABLE I–46 EXAMPLES OF SUBSTANCES DETECTED IN URINE OF DRUG-FACILITATED ASSAULT VICTIMS**

| Drug | Usual Duration of Detection in Urine[a] |
|---|---|
| Amphetamines | 1–3 days |
| Barbiturates | 2–7 days |
| Benzodiazepines | 2–7 days |
| Benzoylecgonine | 1–2 days |
| Cannabinoids | 2–5 days (single use) |
| Carisoprodol | 1–2 days[b] |
| Chloral Hydrate | 1–2 days[b] |
| Clonidine | 1–2 days[b] |
| Cyclobenzaprine | 1–2 days[b] |
| Diphenhydramine | 1–2 days[b] |
| Ethanol | Less than 1 day |
| Gamma hydroxybutyrate (GHB) | Less than 1 day[b] |
| Ketamine | 1–2 days[b] |
| Meprobamate | 1–2 days[b] |
| Opioids | 2–3 days |
| Scopolamine | 1–2 days[b] |

[a]Estimate of the duration of detection, using methods more sensitive than typical drug screening. Actual detection will depend on individual metabolism, dose, and concentration in specimen. Also, assays vary in sensitivity and specificity depending on the laboratory, so it is important to consult with the lab for definitive information.
[b]Specific information not available; duration given is an estimate.

evidence. For a service that deals in assaults or sexual abuse, it is important to confer in advance with the laboratory so that it is clearly understood what type of testing will be performed; the laboratory can then develop a testing strategy (what tests to use, the sequence of tests and confirmations, and level of sensitivity and specificity). Such a service should ideally be part of law enforcement.

**A. Blood.** Collect a specimen as soon as possible and within 24 hours of the alleged assault. Have the specimen centrifuged and the plasma or serum frozen at –80°C for future analysis. Pharmacokinetic evaluation of multiple blood levels may allow estimations of time course, level of consciousness, and amount ingested.

**B. Urine.** Collect a specimen if it is within 72 hours of suspected ingestion and freeze for analysis. (***Note:*** Flunitrazepam [Rohypnol™] may be detected for up 96 hours.)

**C. Analysis.** (See Table I–46.) Hospital laboratories doing routine toxicology testing have different testing strategies and levels of detection and may not detect drugs used to facilitate sexual assault. Rapid toxicology screens (eg, "drugs of abuse" screens) *will not detect* all commonly available benzodiazepines or other CNS depressants (such as ketamine, gamma-hydroxybutyrate, and carisoprodol) that are popular drugs of abuse. It may be necessary to contract for special services through national reference laboratories, state laboratories, or a local medical examiner's office to identify less common drugs used for assault and to detect very low levels of drugs that remain in cases of late presentation.

**VI. Treatment** of the intoxication is based on the clinical effects of the drug(s) involved. Assessment and treatment of effects related to individual drugs is detailed in Section II of this book. In addition, victims often need psychological support and counseling and the involvement of law enforcement authorities. If the assault involves a minor, state law generally mandates reporting to child protective services and law enforcement officials.

## GENERAL TEXTBOOKS AND OTHER REFERENCES IN CLINICAL TOXICOLOGY

Dart RC et al (editors): *Medical Toxicology*, 3rd ed. Philadelphia: Lippincott Williams & Wilkins, 2004.

Ford M (editor): *Clinical Toxicology.* Philadelphia: WB Saunders, 2000.

Goldfrank LR et al (editors): *Goldfrank's Toxicologic Emergencies,* 8th ed. New York: McGraw-Hill, 2006.

Haddad LM, Winchester JF, Shannon M (editors): *Clinical Management of Poisoning and Drug Overdose,* 3rd ed. Philadelphia: WB Saunders, 1998.

Poisindex [computerized poison information system, available as CD-ROM or mainframe application, updated quarterly]. Micromedex [updated quarterly]. Medical Economics, Inc.

## SELECTED INTERNET SITES

American Academy of Clinical Toxicology: *http://www.clintox.org*
American Association of Poison Control Centers: *http://www.aapcc.org*
American College of Medical Toxicology: *http://www.acmt.net*
Agency for Toxic Substances & Disease Registry: *http://www.atsdr.cdc.gov/*
Animal Poison Control Center: *http://www.aspca.org*
Centers for Disease Control: *http://www.cdc.gov/*
Food and Drug Administration: *http://www.fda.gov/*
National Institute on Drug Abuse: *http://www.nida.nih.gov/*
National Pesticide Information Center: *http://www.npic.orst.edu/*
PubMed (Medline-made-easy): *http://www.ncbi.nlm.nih.gov/entrez*
QT Prolonging Drugs: *http://www.qtdrugs.org/*
Substance Abuse and Mental Health Services Administration: *http://workplace.samhsa.gov*
TOXNET Databases: *http://toxnet.nlm.nih.gov/index.html*

## SECTION II. **Specific Poisons and Drugs: Diagnosis and Treatment**

# ▶ ACETAMINOPHEN

*Kent R. Olson, MD*

Acetaminophen (Anacin-3, Liquiprin, Panadol, Paracetamol, Tempra, Tylenol, and many other brands) is a widely used drug found in many over-the-counter and prescription analgesics and cold remedies. When it is combined with another drug such as diphenhydramine, codeine, or propoxyphene, the more dramatic acute symptoms caused by the other drug may mask the mild and nonspecific symptoms of early acetaminophen toxicity, resulting in a missed diagnosis or delayed antidotal treatment. Common combination products containing acetaminophen include Darvocet, Excedrin ES, Lorcet, Norco, NyQuil, Percocet, Unisom Dual Relief Formula, Sominex 2, Tylenol with Codeine, Tylox, Vicks Formula 44-D, and Vicodin.

**I. Mechanism of toxicity**

- **A. Hepatic injury.** One of the products of normal metabolism of acetaminophen by cytochrome P-450 mixed-function oxidase enzymes is highly toxic; normally this reactive metabolite (NAPQI) is detoxified rapidly by glutathione in liver cells. However, in an overdose, production of NAPQI exceeds glutathione capacity and the metabolite reacts directly with hepatic macromolecules, causing liver injury.
- **B. Renal damage** may occur by the same mechanism, owing to renal P-450 metabolism.
- **C.** Overdose during **pregnancy** has been associated with fetal death and spontaneous abortion.
- **D. Pharmacokinetics.** Rapidly absorbed, with peak levels usually reached within 30–120 minutes (***Note:*** Absorption may be delayed after ingestion of sustained-release products or with co-ingestion of opioids or anticholinergics). Volume of distribution (Vd) = 0.8–1 L/kg. Elimination is mainly by liver conjugation (90%) to nontoxic glucuronides or sulfates; cytochrome P-450 mixed-function oxidase (CYP 2E1, 1A2) accounts for only about 3–8% but produces a toxic intermediate (see A, above). The elimination half-life is 1–3 hours after a therapeutic dose and may be greater than 12 hours after an overdose. (See also Table II–59, p 382.)

**II. Toxic dose**

- **A. Acute ingestion** of more than 200 mg/kg in children or 6–7 g in adults is potentially hepatotoxic.
  1. Children younger than 10–12 years of age appear to be less susceptible to hepatotoxicity because of the smaller contribution of cytochrome P-450 to acetaminophen metabolism.
  2. In contrast, the margin of safety is lower in patients with induced cytochrome P-450 microsomal enzymes, because more of the toxic metabolite may be produced. **High-risk patients** include alcoholics and patients taking inducers of CYP 2E1 such as isoniazid. Fasting and malnutrition also increase the risk of hepatotoxicity, presumably by lowering cellular glutathione stores.
- **B. Chronic toxicity** has been reported after daily consumption of supratherapeutic doses by alcoholic patients and persons taking isoniazid. Children have developed toxicity after receiving as little as 60–150 mg/kg/day for 2–8 days.

**III. Clinical presentation.** Clinical manifestations depend on the time after ingestion.

- **A. Early** after acute acetaminophen overdose, there are usually no symptoms other than anorexia, nausea, or vomiting. Rarely, a massive overdose may cause altered mental status and metabolic acidosis. Transient prolongation of the prothrombin time (PT/INR) in the absence of hepatitis has been noted in the first 24 hours; some, but not all, of these patients go on to develop liver injury.
- **B. After 24–48 hours,** when transaminase levels [aspartate aminotransferase (AST) and alanine aminotransferase (ALT)] begin to rise, hepatic necrosis becomes evident. If acute fulminant hepatic failure occurs, death may ensue. Encephalopathy,

metabolic acidosis, and a continuing rise in PT/INR indicate a poor prognosis. Acute renal failure occasionally occurs, with or without concomitant liver failure.

**IV. Diagnosis.** Prompt diagnosis is possible only if the ingestion is suspected and a serum acetaminophen level is obtained. However, patients may fail to provide the history of acetaminophen ingestion, because they are unable (eg, comatose from another ingestion), unwilling, or unaware of its importance. Therefore, many clinicians routinely order acetaminophen levels in all overdose patients regardless of the history of substances ingested.

**A. Specific levels**

1. After an acute overdose, obtain a 4-hour postingestion acetaminophen level and use the nomogram (Figure II–1) to predict the likelihood of toxicity. Do not attempt to interpret a level drawn before 4 hours unless it is "nondetectable." Obtain a second level at 8 hours if the 4-hour value is borderline or if delayed absorption is anticipated.
2. The nomogram should not be used to assess chronic or repeated ingestions.
3. Falsely elevated acetaminophen levels may occur in the presence of high levels of salicylate and other interferents by various methods (see Table I–33, p 43). This problem is rare with currently used analysis methods.

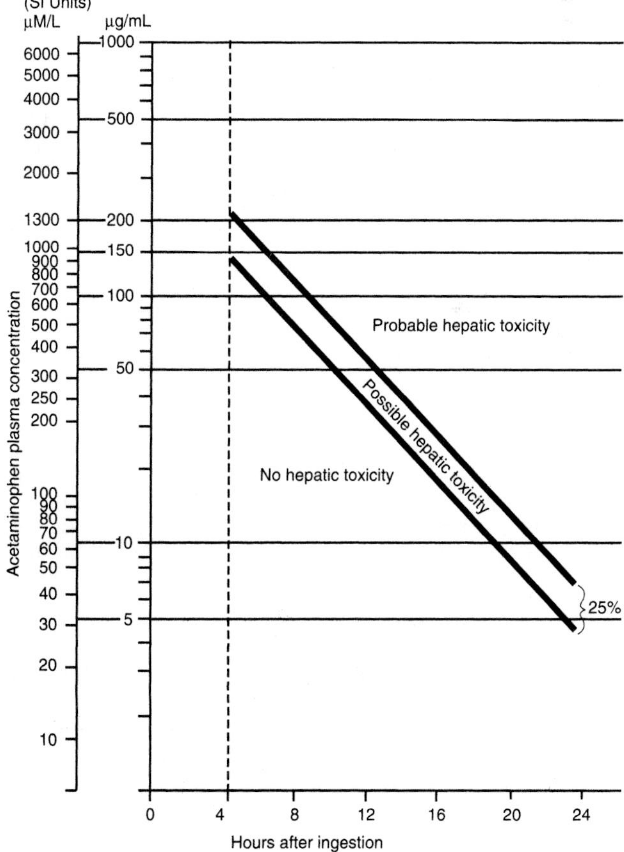


**FIGURE II–1.** Nomogram for prediction of acetaminophen hepatotoxicity after acute overdose. The upper line defines serum acetaminophen concentrations likely to be associated with hepatotoxicity; the lower line defines serum levels 25% below those expected to cause hepatotoxicity. (Courtesy of McNeil Consumer Products, Inc.)

B. **Other useful laboratory studies** include electrolytes, glucose, BUN, creatinine, liver transaminases, and PT/INR.

V. **Treatment**

A. **Emergency and supportive measures**

1. **Spontaneous vomiting** may delay the oral administration of antidote or charcoal (see below) and should be treated with metoclopramide (see p 475) or a 5-$HT_3$ receptor antagonist such as ondansetron (p 489).
2. Provide general supportive care for hepatic or renal failure if it occurs. Emergency **liver transplant** may be necessary for fulminant hepatic failure. Encephalopathy, metabolic acidosis, hypoglycemia, and progressive rise in the prothrombin time are indications of severe liver injury.

B. **Specific drugs and antidotes.** If the serum level falls above the upper ("probable toxicity") line on the nomogram or if stat serum levels are not immediately available, initiate antidotal therapy with ***N*-acetylcysteine** (NAC, p 407). The effectiveness of NAC depends on **early treatment,** before the metabolite accumulates; it is of maximal benefit if started within 8–10 hours and of diminishing value after 12–16 hours (however, treatment should not be withheld even if the delay is 24 hours or more). If vomiting interferes with or threatens to delay oral acetylcysteine administration, give the NAC intravenously.

1. If the serum level falls between the two nomogram lines, consider giving NAC if the patient is at increased risk for toxicity; eg, the patient is alcoholic, malnourished or fasting or is taking drugs that induce P-450 2E1 activity [(eg, isoniazid (INH)]; after multiple or subacute overdoses; or if the time of ingestion is uncertain or unreliable.
2. If the serum level falls below the lower nomogram line, treatment is not indicated unless the time of ingestion is uncertain or the patient is considered to be at particularly high risk.
3. ***Note:*** After ingestion of **extended-release** tablets (eg, Tylenol Arthritis Pain™), which are designed for prolonged absorption, there may be a delay before the peak acetaminophen level is reached. This can also occur after co-ingestion of drugs that delay gastric emptying, such as opioids and anticholinergics. In such circumstances, repeat the serum acetaminophen level at 8 hours and possibly 12 hours. In such cases, it may be prudent to initiate NAC therapy before 8 hours while waiting for subsequent levels.
4. **Duration of NAC treatment.** The conventional US protocol for treatment of acetaminophen poisoning calls for 17 doses of oral NAC given over approximately 72 hours. However, for decades successful protocols in Canada, the United Kingdom, and Europe have utilized intravenous NAC for only 20 hours. In uncomplicated cases, give NAC (orally or IV) for 20 hours and follow hepatic transaminase levels and the PT/INR until 36 hours have passed since the time of ingestion. If evidence of liver injury develops, NAC is continued until liver function tests are improving.
5. **Chronic** acetaminophen ingestions: Patients may give a history of several doses taken over 24 hours or more, in which case the nomogram cannot accurately estimate the risk of hepatotoxicity. In such cases, we advise NAC treatment if the amount ingested was more than 150–200 mg/kg or 6–7 g within a 24-hour period, if liver enzymes are elevated, or if the patient falls within a high-risk group (see above). Treatment may be stopped 24–36 hours after the last dose of acetaminophen if liver enzymes and PT/INR are normal.

C. **Decontamination** (see p 45). Administer activated charcoal orally if conditions are appropriate (see Table I–38, p 51). Gastric lavage is not necessary after small to moderate ingestions if activated charcoal can be given promptly.

1. Although activated charcoal adsorbs some of the orally administered antidote *N*-acetylcysteine, this effect is not considered clinically important.
2. Do not administer charcoal if more than 3–4 hours has passed since ingestion unless delayed absorption is suspected (eg, as with Tylenol Arthritis Pain™ or co-ingestants containing opioids or anticholinergic agents).

D. **Enhanced elimination.** Hemodialysis effectively removes acetaminophen from the blood but is not generally indicated because antidotal therapy is so effective. Dialysis should be considered for massive ingestions with very high levels (eg, >1000 mg/L) complicated by coma and/or hypotension.

## ► AMANTADINE

*Lisa Wu, MD*

Amantadine (Symmetrel) is an antiviral agent that is also effective in the treatment of Parkinson's disease and for prophylaxis against the parkinsonian side effects of neuroleptic agents. Recently, it has also been studied as a potential treatment for hepatitis C, Huntington's disease, brain injury or encephalopathy, and cocaine dependence. Although there is limited information about its effects in acute overdose, it has been associated with seizures, arrhythmias, and death. Withdrawal from amantadine has also been linked to neuroleptic malignant syndrome.

**I. Mechanism of toxicity**

**A.** Amantadine is thought to enhance the release of dopamine and prevent dopamine reuptake in the peripheral and central nervous systems. It also acts as a noncompetitive antagonist at the NMDA receptor. In addition, it has anticholinergic properties, especially in overdose.

**B. Pharmacokinetics.** Peak absorption = 1–4 hours; volume of distribution (Vd) = 4–8 L/kg. Eliminated renally with a half-life of 7–37 hours (see also Table II–59, p 382).

**II. Toxic dose.** The toxic dose has not been determined. Because the elimination of amantadine depends entirely on kidney function, elderly patients with renal insufficiency may develop intoxication with therapeutic doses.

**III. Clinical presentation**

**A. Amantadine intoxication** causes agitation, visual hallucinations, nightmares, disorientation, delirium, slurred speech, ataxia, myoclonus, tremor, and sometimes seizures. Anticholinergic manifestations include dry mouth, urinary retention, and mydriasis. Rarely, ventricular arrhythmias that include torsade de pointes (see p 13) and multifocal premature ventricular contractions may occur. Amantadine has also been reported to cause heart failure.

**B. Amantadine withdrawal,** either after standard therapeutic use or in the days after an acute overdose, may result in hyperthermia and rigidity (similar to neuroleptic malignant syndrome; see p 21).

**IV. Diagnosis** is based on a history of acute ingestion or is made by noting the abovementioned constellation of symptoms and signs in a patient taking amantadine.

**A. Specific levels** are not readily available. Serum levels above 1.5 mg/L have been associated with toxicity.

**B. Other useful laboratory studies** include electrolytes, BUN, creatinine, CPK, and ECG.

**V. Treatment**

**A. Emergency and supportive measures**

1. Maintain an open airway and assist ventilation if necessary (see p 1–4).
2. Treat coma (see p 18), seizures (p 22), arrhythmias (p 13), and hyperthermia (p 20) if they occur.
3. Monitor an asymptomatic patient for at least 8–12 hours after acute ingestion.

**B. Specific drugs and antidotes.** There is no known antidote. Although some of the manifestations of toxicity are caused by the anticholinergic effects of amantadine, physostigmine should not be used.

1. Treat **tachyarrhythmias** with beta blockers such as propranolol (see p 504) and esmolol (p 449).
2. **Hyperthermia** requires urgent cooling measures (see p 20) and may respond to specific pharmacologic therapy with dantrolene (p 436). When hyperthermia occurs in the setting of amantadine withdrawal, some have advocated using amantadine as therapy.

**C. Decontamination.** Administer activated charcoal orally if conditions are appropriate (see Table I–38, p 51). Gastric lavage is not necessary after small to moderate ingestions if activated charcoal can be given promptly.

D. **Enhanced elimination.** Amantadine is not effectively removed by dialysis, because the volume of distribution is very large (5 L/kg). The serum elimination half-life ranges from 12 hours to 34 days, depending on renal function. In a patient with no renal function, dialysis or hemoperfusion may be necessary.

# ▶ AMMONIA

*R. Steven Tharratt, MD, MPVM*

Ammonia is widely used as a refrigerant, a fertilizer, and a household and commercial cleaning agent. Anhydrous ammonia ($NH_3$) is a highly irritating gas that is very water-soluble. It is also a key ingredient in the illicit production of methamphetamine. Aqueous solutions of ammonia may be strongly alkaline, depending on the concentration. Solutions for household use are usually 5–10% ammonia, but commercial solutions may be 25–30% or more. The addition of ammonia to chlorine or hypochlorite solutions will produce chloramine gas, an irritant with properties similar to those of chlorine (see p 162).

I. **Mechanism of toxicity.** Ammonia gas is highly water-soluble and rapidly produces an alkaline corrosive effect on contact with moist tissues such as the eyes and the upper respiratory tract. Exposure to aqueous solutions causes corrosive alkaline injury to the eyes, skin, or gastrointestinal tract (see Caustic and Corrosive Agents, p 157).

II. **Toxic dose**

A. **Ammonia gas.** The odor of ammonia is detectable at 3–5 ppm, and persons without protective gear will experience respiratory irritation at 50 ppm and usually self-evacuate the area. Eye irritation is common at 100 ppm. The workplace recommended exposure limit (ACGIH TLV-TWA) for anhydrous ammonia gas is 25 ppm as an 8-hour time-weighted average and the OHSA Permissible Exposure Limit (as an 8-hour time-weighted average) is 50 ppm. The level considered immediately dangerous to life or health (IDLH) is 300 ppm. The Emergency Response Planning Guidelines (ERPG) suggest 25 ppm will cause no more than mild, transient health effects for exposures of up to 1 hour.

B. **Aqueous solutions.** Diluted aqueous solutions of ammonia (eg, < 5%) rarely cause serious burns but are moderately irritating. More concentrated industrial cleaners (eg, 25–30% ammonia) are much more likely to cause serious corrosive injury.

III. **Clinical presentation.** Clinical manifestations depend on physical state and route of exposure.

A. **Inhalation of ammonia gas.** Symptoms are rapid in onset owing to the high water solubility of ammonia and include immediate burning of the eyes, nose, and throat, accompanied by coughing. With serious exposure, upper-airway swelling may rapidly cause airway obstruction, preceded by croupy cough, hoarseness, and stridor. Bronchospasm with wheezing may occur. Massive inhalational exposure may cause noncardiogenic pulmonary edema.

B. **Ingestion of aqueous solutions.** Immediate burning in the mouth and throat is common. With more concentrated solutions, serious esophageal and gastric burns are possible, and victims may have dysphagia, drooling, and severe throat, chest, and abdominal pain. Hematemesis and perforation of the esophagus or stomach may occur. The absence of oral burns does not rule out significant esophageal or gastric injury.

C. **Skin or eye contact with gas or solution.** Serious alkaline corrosive burns may occur.

IV. **Diagnosis** is based on a history of exposure and description of the typical ammonia smell, accompanied by typical irritative or corrosive effects on the eyes, skin, and upper respiratory or gastrointestinal tract.

A. **Specific levels.** Blood ammonia levels may be elevated (normal 8–33 micromol/L) but are not predictive of toxicity.

B. **Other useful laboratory studies** may include electrolytes, arterial blood gases or pulse oximetry, and chest radiographs.

V. **Treatment**

A. **Emergency and supportive measures.** Treatment depends on the physical state of the ammonia and the route of exposure.

1. **Inhalation of ammonia gas**
   a. Observe carefully for signs of progressive upper-airway obstruction, and intubate early if necessary (see p 4).
   b. Administer humidified supplemental oxygen and bronchodilators for wheezing (see p 7). Treat noncardiogenic pulmonary edema (p 7) if it occurs.
   c. Asymptomatic or mildly symptomatic patients may be sent home after a brief (1- to 2-hour) observation.
2. **Ingestion of aqueous solution.** If a solution of 10% or greater has been ingested or if there are any symptoms of corrosive injury (dysphagia, drooling, or pain), perform flexible endoscopy to evaluate for serious esophageal or gastric injury. Obtain chest and abdominal radiographs to look for mediastinal or abdominal free air, which suggests esophageal or gastrointestinal perforation.
3. **Eye exposure.** After eye irrigation, perform fluorescein examination and refer the patient to an ophthalmologist if there is evidence of corneal injury.

B. **Specific drugs and antidotes.** There is no specific antidote for these or other common caustic burns. The use of corticosteroids in alkaline corrosive ingestions has been proved ineffective and may be harmful in patients with perforation or serious infection.

C. **Decontamination** (see p 45)

1. **Inhalation.** Remove immediately from exposure, and give supplemental oxygen if available.
2. **Ingestion.**
   a. Immediately give water by mouth to dilute the ammonia. Do ***not*** induce vomiting, as this may aggravate corrosive effects. Do ***not*** attempt to neutralize the ammonia (eg, with an acidic solution).
   b. Gastric lavage may be useful to remove liquid caustic in the stomach (in cases of deliberate ingestion of large quantities) and to prepare for endoscopy; use a small, flexible tube and pass it gently to avoid injury to damaged mucosa.
   c. Do ***not*** use activated charcoal; it does not adsorb ammonia, and it may obscure the endoscopist's view.
3. **Skin and eyes.** Remove contaminated clothing and wash exposed skin with water. Irrigate exposed eyes with copious amounts of tepid water or saline (see p 45).

D. **Enhanced elimination.** There is no role for dialysis or other enhanced elimination procedures.

## ► AMPHETAMINES

*Timothy E. Albertson, MD, PhD*

Dextroamphetamine (Dexedrine) and methylphenidate (Ritalin) are used for the treatment of narcolepsy and for attention-deficit disorders in children. Several amphetamine-related drugs (benzphetamine, diethylpropion, phendimetrazine, phenmetrazine, and phentermine) are marketed as prescription anorectic medications for use in weight reduction (Table II–1). Fenfluramine and dexfenfluramine were marketed as anorectic medications but were withdrawn from the market in 1997 because of concerns about cardiopulmonary toxicity with long-term use. Methamphetamine (crank, speed), 3,4-methylenedioxymethamphetamine (MDMA, ecstasy), paramethoxyamphetamine (PMA), and several other amphetamine derivatives (see Lysergic Acid Diethylamide [LSD] and Other Hallucinogens, p 247), as well as a number of prescription drugs, are used orally and intravenously as illicit stimulants and hallucinogens. "Ice" is a smokable form of methamphetamine. Phenylpropanolamine, ephedrine, and other over-the-counter decongestants are discussed on p 322.

TABLE II–1. AMPHETAMINE-LIKE PRESCRIPTION DRUGS[a] (SEE ALSO TABLE II–32, P 248)

| Drug | Clinical Indications | Typical Adult Dose (mg) | Half-Life (hrs)[b] |
|---|---|---|---|
| Benzphetamine | Anorectant | 25–50 | 6–12 |
| Dexfenfluramine (withdrawn from US market 1997) | Anorectant | 15 | 17–20 |
| Dextroamphetamine | Narcolepsy, hyperactivity (children) | 5–15 | 10–12 |
| Diethylpropion | Anorectant | 25, 75 (sustained-release) | 2.5–6 |
| Fenfluramine (withdrawn from US market 1997) | Anorectant | 20–40 | 10–30 |
| Mazindol | Anorectant | 1–2 | 10 |
| Methamphetamine | Narcolepsy, hyperactivity (children) | 5–15 | 4–5 |
| Methylphenidate | Hyperactivity (children) | 5–20 | 2–7 |
| Pemoline | Narcolepsy, hyperactivity (children) | 18.7–75 | 9–14 |
| Phendimetrazine | Anorectant | 35, 105 (sustained-release) | 5–12.5 |
| Phenmetrazine | Anorectant | 25,75 (sustained-release) | |
| Phentermine | Anorectant | 8, 30 (sustained-release) | 7–24 |

[a]See also Table II–32 (LSD and other hallucinogens).
[b]Half-life variable, dependent on urine pH.

**I. Mechanism of toxicity**

**A.** Amphetamine and related drugs activate the sympathetic nervous system via CNS stimulation, peripheral release of catecholamines, inhibition of neuronal reuptake of catecholamines, and inhibition of monoamine oxidase. Amphetamines, particularly MDMA, PMA, fenfluramine, and dexfenfluramine, also cause serotonin release and block neuronal serotonin uptake. The various drugs have different profiles of catecholamine and serotonin action, resulting in different levels of CNS and peripheral stimulation.

**B. Pharmacokinetics.** All these drugs are well absorbed orally and have large volumes of distribution (Vd = 3–33 L/kg, except pemoline, with Vd = 0.2–0.6 L/kg), and they are generally extensively metabolized by the liver. Excretion of most amphetamines is highly dependent on urine pH, with amphetamines being eliminated more rapidly in an acidic urine (see also Table II–59, p 382).

**II. Toxic dose.** These drugs generally have a low therapeutic index, with toxicity at levels only slightly above usual doses. However, a high degree of tolerance can develop after repeated use. Acute ingestion of more than 1 mg/kg of dextroamphetamine (or an equivalent dose of other drugs; see Table II–1) should be considered potentially life threatening.

**III. Clinical presentation**

**A. Acute CNS effects** of intoxication include euphoria, talkativeness, anxiety, restlessness, agitation, seizures, and coma. Intracranial hemorrhage may occur owing to hypertension or cerebral vasculitis.

**B. Acute peripheral manifestations** include sweating, tremor, muscle fasciculations and rigidity, tachycardia, hypertension, acute myocardial ischemia, and infarction (even with normal coronary arteries). Inadvertent intra-arterial injection may cause vasospasm resulting in gangrene; this has also occurred with oral use of DOB (2,5-dimethoxy-4-bromoamphetamine; see Lysergic Acid Diethylamide [LSD] and Other Hallucinogens, p 247).

C. **Death** may be caused by ventricular arrhythmia, status epilepticus, intracranial hemorrhage, or hyperthermia. **Hyperthermia** frequently results from seizures and muscular hyperactivity and may cause brain damage, rhabdomyolysis, and myoglobinuric renal failure (see p 20).

D. **Chronic effects** of amphetamine abuse include weight loss, cardiomyopathy, pulmonary hypertension, dental changes, stereotypic behavior (such as picking at the skin), paranoia, and paranoid psychosis. Psychiatric disturbances may persist for days or weeks. After cessation of habitual use, patients may suffer fatigue, hypersomnia, hyperphagia, and depression lasting several days.

E. Prolonged use (usually 3 months or longer) of fenfluramine or dexfenfluramine in combination with phentermine ("fen-phen") has been associated with an increased risk of pulmonary hypertension and fibrotic valvular heart disease (primarily aortic, mitral, and tricuspid regurgitation). The pathology of the valvular disease is identical to that seen with carcinoid syndrome.

F. Illicit manufacture of methamphetamine can expose the "chemist" and his or her family to various toxic chemicals, including corrosive agents, solvents, and heavy metals.

IV. **Diagnosis** is usually based on a history of amphetamine use and clinical features of sympathomimetic drug intoxication.

A. **Specific levels.** Amphetamines and many related drugs can be detected in urine and gastric samples, providing confirmation of exposure. However, quantitative serum levels do not correlate well with severity of clinical effects and are not generally available. Amphetamine derivatives and adrenergic amines may cross-react in immunoassays (see Table I–33, p 43), and distinguishing the specific drug requires confirmatory testing (eg, with thin-layer chromatography, gas chromatography, or mass spectrometry). Selegiline (a drug used in Parkinson's disease) is metabolized to *l*-amphetamine and *l*-methamphetamine, and Clobenzorex (an anorectic drug sold in Mexico) is metabolized to amphetamine; these drugs can produce a positive result on urine and blood tests for amphetamines. Amphetamine, methamphetamine, and MDMA can be screened for by using hair and liquid chromatography–mass spectrometry.

B. **Other useful laboratory studies** include electrolytes, glucose, BUN and creatinine, CPK, urinalysis, urine dipstick test for occult hemoglobin (positive in patients with rhabdomyolysis with myoglobinuria), ECG and ECG monitoring, and CT scan of the head (if hemorrhage is suspected). Echocardiogram and right heart catheterization may be useful for detecting valvular disease or pulmonary hypertension.

V. **Treatment**

A. **Emergency and supportive measures**

1. Maintain an open airway and assist ventilation if necessary (see p 1).
2. Treat agitation (see p 23), seizures (p 22), coma (p 18), and hyperthermia (p 20) if they occur. Benzodiazepines are usually satisfactory for treatment of agitation, although butyrophenones (eg, haloperidol, p 458) may also be used.
3. Continuously monitor the temperature, other vital signs, and the ECG for a minimum of 6 hours.

B. **Specific drugs and antidotes.** There is no specific antidote.

1. **Hypertension** (see p 17) is best treated with sedation and, if this is not effective, a parenteral vasodilator such as phentolamine (p 495) or nitroprusside (p 485).
2. Treat **tachyarrhythmias** (p 12) with propranolol (see p 504) or esmolol (p 449).
3. Treat **arterial vasospasm** as described for ergots (p 187).

C. **Decontamination**. Administer activated charcoal orally if conditions are appropriate (see Table I–38, p 51). Gastric lavage is not necessary after small to moderate ingestions if activated charcoal can be given promptly. Consider whole-bowel irrigation and repeated doses of charcoal after ingestion of drug-filled packets ("body stuffers").

D. **Enhanced elimination.** Dialysis and hemoperfusion are not effective. Repeat-dose charcoal has not been studied. Renal elimination of dextroamphetamine may be enhanced by acidification of the urine, but this is not recommended because of the risk of aggravating the nephrotoxicity of myoglobinuria.

## ► ANESTHETICS, LOCAL

*Nancy G. Murphy, MD, and Neal L. Benowitz, MD*

Local anesthetics are used widely to provide anesthesia via local subcutaneous injection; topical application to skin and mucous membranes; and epidural, spinal, and regional nerve blocks. In addition, lidocaine (see p 469) is used intravenously as an antiarrhythmic agent and cocaine (see p 170) is a popular drug of abuse. Commonly used agents are divided into two chemical groups: ester-linked and amide-linked (Table II–2).

**TABLE II–2. LOCAL ANESTHETICS**

| Anesthetic | Usual Half-Life | Maximum Adult Single Dose[a] (mg) |
|---|---|---|
| **Ester-linked** | | |
| Benzocaine[b] | | N/A |
| Benzonatate[c] | | 200 |
| Butacaine[b] | | N/A |
| Butamben[b] | | N/A |
| Chloroprocaine | 1.5–6 min | 800 |
| Cocaine[b] | 1–2.5 h | N/A |
| Hexylcaine[b] | | N/A |
| Procaine | 7–8 min | 600 |
| Proparacaine[b] | | N/A |
| Propoxycaine | | 75 |
| Tetracaine | 5–10 min | 15 |
| **Amide-linked** | | |
| Articaine | 1–2 h | 500 |
| Bupivacaine | 2–5 h | 400 |
| Dibucaine | | 10 |
| Etidocaine | 1.5 h | 400 |
| Levobupivacaine | 1-3 h | 300 |
| Lidocaine | 1.2 h | 300 |
| Lidocaine with epinephrine | 2 h | 500 |
| Mepivacaine | | 400 |
| Prilocaine | | 600 |
| Ropivacaine | | 225 |
| **Other** (neither ester- nor amide-linked) | | |
| Dyclonine[b] | | N/A |
| Pramoxine[b] | | N/A |

[a]Maximum single dose for subcutaneous infiltration. N/A: not applicable.
[b]Used only for topical anesthesia.
[c]Given orally as an antitussive.

Toxicity from local anesthetics (other than cocaine) is usually caused by therapeutic overdosage (ie, excessive doses for local nerve blocks), inadvertent acceleration of intravenous infusions (lidocaine), or accidental injection of products meant for dilution (eg, 20% lidocaine) instead of those formulated for direct administration (2% solution). Acute injection of lidocaine has also been used as a method of homicide.

**I. Mechanism of toxicity**

**A.** Local anesthetics bind to sodium channels in nerve fibers, blocking the sodium current responsible for nerve conduction and thereby increasing the threshold for conduction and reversibly slowing or blocking impulse generation. In therapeutic concentrations, this results in local anesthesia. In high concentrations, such actions may result in CNS and cardiovascular toxicity.

**B.** In addition, some local anesthetics (eg, benzocaine, prilocaine, lidocaine) have been reported to cause methemoglobinemia (see p 262).

**C. Pharmacokinetics.** With local subcutaneous injection, peak blood levels are reached in 10–60 minutes, depending on the vascularity of the tissue and whether a vasoconstrictor such as epinephrine has been added. **Ester-type** drugs are hydrolyzed rapidly by plasma cholinesterase and have short half-lives. **Amide-type** drugs are metabolized by the liver, have a longer duration of effect, and may accumulate after repeated doses in patients with hepatic insufficiency. For other kinetic values, see Table II–59, p 382.

**II. Toxic dose.** Systemic toxicity occurs when brain levels exceed a certain threshold. Toxic levels can be achieved with a single large subcutaneous injection, with rapid intravenous injection of a smaller dose, or by accumulation of drug with repeated doses. The recommended maximum single subcutaneous doses of the common agents are listed in Table II–2.

**III. Clinical presentation**

**A.** Toxicity owing to **local anesthetic effects** includes prolonged anesthesia and, rarely, permanent sensory or motor deficits. Spinal anesthesia may block nerves to the muscles of respiration, causing respiratory arrest, or may cause sympathetic blockade, resulting in hypotension.

**B.** Toxicity resulting from **systemic absorption** of local anesthetics affects primarily the CNS, with headache, confusion, perioral paresthesias, slurred speech, muscle twitching, convulsions, coma, and respiratory arrest. Cardiotoxic effects include sinus arrest, atrioventricular block, asystole, reentrant arrhythmias, ventricular tachycardia/fibrillation, and hypotension.

**C. Methemoglobinemia** (see also p 262) may occur after exposure to benzocaine, prilocaine, or lidocaine.

**D. Allergic reactions** (bronchospasm, hives, and shock) are uncommon and occur almost exclusively with ester-linked local anesthetics. Methylparaben, which is used as a preservative in some multidose vials, may be the cause of some reported hypersensitivity reactions.

**E.** Features of toxicity caused by **cocaine** are discussed on p 170.

**IV. Diagnosis** is based on a history of local anesthetic use and typical clinical features. Abrupt onset of confusion, slurred speech, or convulsions in a patient receiving lidocaine infusion for arrhythmias should suggest lidocaine toxicity.

**A. Specific levels.** Serum levels of some local anesthetics may confirm their role in producing suspected toxic effects, but these levels must be obtained promptly because they fall rapidly.

1. Serum concentrations of lidocaine greater than 6–10 mg/L are considered toxic.
2. Lidocaine is often detected in comprehensive urine toxicology screening as a result of use either as a local anesthetic (eg, for minor procedures in the emergency department) or as a cutting agent for drugs of abuse.

**B. Other useful laboratory studies** include electrolytes, glucose, BUN and creatinine, ECG monitoring, arterial blood gases or pulse oximetry, and methemoglobin level (benzocaine).

**V. Treatment**

**A. Emergency and supportive measures**

1. Maintain an open airway and assist ventilation if necessary (see pp 1–7).

2. Treat coma (see p 18), seizures (p 22), hypotension (p 15), arrhythmias (p 13), and anaphylaxis (p 27) if they occur. Extracorporeal circulatory assistance (eg, balloon pump or partial cardiopulmonary bypass) has been used for short-term support for patients with acute massive overdose with 20% lidocaine solution and inadvertent intravascular administration of bupivacaine.
3. Monitor vital signs and ECG for at least 6 hours.

**B. Specific drugs and antidotes.** There is no specific antidote.

**C. Decontamination**

1. **Parenteral exposure.** Decontamination is not feasible.
2. **Ingestion** (see p 47). Administer activated charcoal orally if conditions are appropriate (see Table I–38, p 51). Gastric lavage is not necessary after small to moderate ingestions if activated charcoal can be given promptly.

**D. Enhanced elimination.** Because lidocaine has a moderate volume of distribution, hemoperfusion is potentially beneficial, particularly after a massive overdose or when metabolic elimination is impaired because of circulatory collapse or severe liver disease.

## ▶ ANGIOTENSIN BLOCKERS AND ACE INHIBITORS

*Sandra Hayashi, PharmD*

The angiotensin-converting enzyme (ACE) inhibitors and angiotensin receptor (AR) blockers are widely used for the treatment of hypertension, heart failure, and patients who have had a myocardial infarction. Currently at least 10 ACE inhibitors and 7 AR blockers are marketed in the United States.

**I. Mechanism of toxicity**

**A.** ACE inhibitors reduce vasoconstriction and aldosterone activity by blocking the enzyme that converts angiotensin I to angiotensin II. Angiotensin receptor blockers directly inhibit the action of angiotensin II.

**B.** All the ACE inhibitors except captopril and lisinopril must be metabolized to their active moieties (eg, enalapril is converted to enalaprilat).

**C.** Angioedema and cough associated with ACE inhibitors are thought to be mediated by bradykinin, which normally is broken down by angiotensin-converting enzyme. However, it has also been reported with AR blockers, which do not alter bradykinin elimination.

**D. Pharmacokinetics.** (See also Table II–59.) The volume of distribution (Vd) of ACE inhibitors is fairly small (eg, 0.7 L/kg for captopril). The parent drugs are rapidly converted to their active metabolites, with half-lives of 0.75–1.5 hours. The active metabolites have elimination half-lives of 5.9–35 hours. The AR blockers have half-lives of 5–24 hours; losartan has an active metabolite.

**II. Toxic dose.** Only mild toxicity has resulted from most reported overdoses of up to 7.5 g of captopril, 440 mg of enalapril (serum level 2.8 mg/L at 15 hours), and 420 mg of lisinopril. A 75-year-old man was found dead after ingesting approximately 1125 mg of captopril, and he had a postmortem serum level of 60.4 mg/L. A 33-year-old survived a captopril level of 5.98 mg/L. A 45-year-old woman recovered without sequelae after intentional ingestion of 160 mg of candesartan cilexetil along with several other drugs.

**III. Clinical presentation**

**A. Hypotension,** usually responsive to fluid therapy, has been reported with acute overdose. Bradycardia may also occur.

**B. Hyperkalemia** has been reported with therapeutic use, especially in patients with renal insufficiency and those taking nonsteroidal anti-inflammatory drugs.

**C. Bradykinin-mediated effects** in patients taking therapeutic doses of ACE inhibitors include dry **cough** (generally mild but often persistent and annoying) and **acute angioedema,** usually involving the tongue, lips, and face, which may lead to life-threatening airway obstruction.

**IV. Diagnosis** is based on a history of exposure.

**A. Specific levels.** Blood levels are not readily available and do not correlate with clinical effects.

B. **Other useful laboratory studies** include electrolytes, glucose, BUN, and creatinine.

V. **Treatment**

A. **Emergency and supportive measures**

1. If hypotension occurs, treat it with supine positioning and intravenous fluids (see p 15). Vasopressors are rarely necessary.
2. Treat angioedema with usual measures (eg, diphenhydramine, corticosteroids) and discontinue the ACE inhibitor. Switching to an AR blocker may not be appropriate as angioedema has also been reported with these agents.
3. Treat hyperkalemia (see p 37) if it occurs.

B. **Specific drugs and antidotes.** No specific antidote is available.

C. **Decontamination** (see p 45). Administer activated charcoal orally if conditions are appropriate (see Table I–38, p 51). Gastric lavage is not necessary after small to moderate ingestions if activated charcoal can be given promptly.

D. **Enhanced elimination.** Hemodialysis may effectively remove these drugs but is not likely to be indicated clinically.

## ► ANTIARRHYTHMIC DRUGS

*Neal L. Benowitz, MD*

Because of their actions on the heart, antiarrhythmic drugs are extremely toxic, and overdoses are often life threatening. Several classes of antiarrhythmic drugs are discussed elsewhere in Section II: type Ia drugs (quinidine, disopyramide, and procainamide, p 326); type II drugs (beta blockers, p 131); type IV drugs (calcium antagonists, p 143); and the older type Ib drugs (lidocaine, p 79, and phenytoin, p 304). This section describes toxicity caused by type Ib (tocainide and mexiletine); type Ic (flecainide, encainide, propafenone, and moricizine) and type III (bretylium and amiodarone) antiarrhythmic drugs. Sotalol, which also has type III antiarrhythmic actions, is discussed in the section on beta-adrenergic blockers (see p 131).

I. **Mechanism of toxicity**

A. **Type I drugs** in general act by inhibiting the fast sodium channel responsible for initial cardiac cell depolarization and impulse conduction. Type Ia and type Ic drugs (which also block potassium channels) slow depolarization and conduction in normal cardiac tissue, and even at normal therapeutic doses the QT (types Ia and Ic) and QRS intervals (type Ic) are prolonged. Type Ib drugs slow depolarization primarily in ischemic tissue and have little effect on normal tissue or on the ECG. In overdose, all type I drugs have the potential to markedly depress myocardial automaticity, conduction, and contractility.

B. **Type II and type IV drugs** act by blocking beta-adrenergic receptors (type II) or calcium channels (type IV). Their actions are discussed elsewhere (type II, p 131; type IV, p 143).

C. **Type III drugs** act primarily by blocking potassium channels to prolong the duration of the action potential and the effective refractory period, resulting in QT interval prolongation at therapeutic doses.

1. Intravenous administration of **bretylium** initially causes release of catecholamines from nerve endings, followed by inhibition of catecholamine release.
2. **Amiodarone** is also a noncompetitive beta-adrenergic blocker and has calcium channel–blocking effects, which may explain its tendency to cause bradyarrhythmias. Amiodarone may also release iodine, and chronic use has resulted in altered thyroid function (both hyper- and hypothyroidism).

D. **Relevant pharmacokinetics.** All the drugs discussed in this section are widely distributed to body tissues. Most are extensively metabolized, but significant fractions of tocainide (40%), flecainide (30%), and bretylium (> 90%) are excreted unchanged by the kidneys. (See also Table II–59, p 382.)

II. **Toxic dose.** In general, these drugs have a narrow therapeutic index, and severe toxicity may occur slightly above or sometimes even within the therapeutic range, especially if combinations of antiarrhythmic drugs are taken together.

**TABLE II–3. ANTIARRHYTHMIC DRUGS**

| Class | Drug | Usual Half-life (hours) | Therapeutic Daily Dose (mg) | Therapeutic Serum Levels (mg/L) | Major Toxicity[a] |
|---|---|---|---|---|---|
| Ia | Quinidine and related (p 326) | | | | |
| Ib | Tocainide | 11–15 | 1200–2400 | 4–10 | S,B,H |
| | Mexiletine | 10–12 | 300–1200 | 0.8–2 | S,B,H |
| | Lidocaine (p 469) | | | | |
| | Phenytoin (p 304) | | | | |
| Ic | Flecainide | 14–15 | 200–600 | 0.2–1 | B,V,H |
| | Encainide[b, d] | 2–11 | 75–300 | [b] | S,B,V,H |
| | Propafenone[b] | 2–10[c] | 450–900 | 0.5–1 | S,B,V,H |
| | Moricizine | 1.5–3.5 | 600–900 | 0.02–0.18 | B,V,H |
| II | Beta blockers (p 131) | | | | |
| III | Amiodarone | 50 days | 200–600 | 1.0–2.5 | B,V,H |
| | Bretylium | 5–14 | 5–10 mg/kg (IV loading dose) | 1–3 | H |
| | Sotalol (p 131) | | | | |
| IV | Calcium antagonists (p 143) | | | | |

[a]Major toxicity: S = seizures H = hypotension
B = bradyarrhythmias V = ventricular arrhythmias
[b]Active metabolite may contribute to toxicity; level not established.
[c]Genetically slow metabolizers; may have half-lives of 10–32 hours. Also, metabolism is nonlinear, so half-lives may be longer in patients with overdose.
[d]Encainide no longer sold in the United States.

**A.** Ingestion of **twice the daily therapeutic dose** should be considered potentially life threatening (usual therapeutic doses are given in Table II–3).

**B.** An exception to this rule of thumb is amiodarone, which is distributed so extensively to tissues that even massive single overdoses produce little or no toxicity (toxicity usually occurs only after accumulation during chronic amiodarone dosing).

**III. Clinical presentation**

**A. Tocainide and mexiletine**

1. **Side effects** with therapeutic use may include dizziness, paresthesias, tremor, ataxia, and gastrointestinal disturbance.
2. **Overdose** may cause sedation, confusion, coma, seizures, respiratory arrest, and cardiac toxicity (sinus arrest, AV block, asystole, and hypotension). As with lidocaine, the QRS and QT intervals are usually normal, although they may be prolonged after massive overdose.

**B. Flecainide, encainide, propafenone, and moricizine**

1. **Side effects** with therapeutic use include dizziness, blurred vision, headache, and gastrointestinal upset. Ventricular arrhythmias (monomorphic or polymorphic ventricular tachycardia; see p 13) may occur at therapeutic levels, especially in persons receiving high doses and those with reduced ventricular function. Propafenone has been associated with cholestatic hepatitis.

2. **Overdose** causes hypotension, bradycardia, sinoatrial and AV nodal block, and asystole. The QRS and QT intervals are prolonged, and ventricular arrhythmias may occur.

C. **Bretylium**

1. The major toxic **side effect** of bretylium is hypotension caused by inhibition of catecholamine release. Orthostatic hypotension may persist for several hours.
2. After **rapid intravenous injection,** transient hypertension, nausea, and vomiting may occur.

D. **Amiodarone**

1. **Acute overdose** in a person not already on amiodarone is not expected to cause toxicity. Bradyarrhythmias have been observed during intravenous loading. Acute hepatitis has been associated with IV loading doses given over several days.
2. With **chronic use,** amiodarone may cause ventricular arrhythmias (monomorphic or polymorphic ventricular tachycardia; see p 12) or bradyarrhythmias (sinus arrest, AV block). Amiodarone may cause pneumonitis or pulmonary fibrosis, hepatitis, photosensitivity dermatitis, corneal deposits, hypothyroidism or hyperthyroidism, tremor, ataxia, and peripheral neuropathy.

IV. **Diagnosis** is usually based on a history of antiarrhythmic drug use and typical cardiac and electrocardiographic findings. Syncope in any patient taking these drugs should suggest possible drug-induced arrhythmia.

A. **Specific levels.** Serum levels are available for most type Ia and type Ib drugs (Table II–3); however, because toxicity is immediately life threatening, measurement of drug levels is used primarily for therapeutic drug monitoring or to confirm the diagnosis rather than to determine emergency treatment. The following antiarrhythmic drugs may be detected in *comprehensive* urine toxicology screening: diltiazem, lidocaine, metoprolol, phenytoin, propranolol, quinidine, and verapamil.

B. **Other useful laboratory studies** include electrolytes, glucose, BUN and creatinine, liver enzymes, thyroid panel (chronic amiodarone), and ECG and ECG monitoring.

V. **Treatment**

A. **Emergency and supportive measures**

1. Maintain an open airway and assist ventilation if necessary (see pp 1–7).
2. Treat coma (see p 18), seizures (p 22), hypotension (p 15), and arrhythmias (p 12) if they occur. ***Note:*** Type Ia antiarrhythmic agents should not be used to treat cardiotoxicity caused by type Ia, type Ic, or type III drugs.
3. Continuously monitor vital signs and ECG for a minimum of 6 hours after exposure, and admit the patient for 24 hours of intensive monitoring if there is evidence of toxicity.

B. **Specific drugs and antidotes.** In patients with intoxication by type Ia or type Ic drugs, QRS prolongation, bradyarrhythmias, and hypotension may respond to **sodium bicarbonate,** 1–2 mEq/kg IV (see p 423). The sodium bicarbonate reverses cardiac-depressant effects caused by inhibition of the fast sodium channel.

C. **Decontamination** (see p 47). Administer activated charcoal orally if conditions are appropriate (see Table I–38, p 51). Gastric lavage is not necessary after small to moderate ingestions if activated charcoal can be given promptly.

D. **Enhanced elimination.** Owing to extensive tissue binding with resulting large volumes of distribution, dialysis and hemoperfusion are not likely to be effective for most of these agents. Hemodialysis may be of benefit for tocainide or flecainide overdose in patients with renal failure, but prolonged and repeated dialysis would be necessary. No data are available on the effectiveness of repeat-dose charcoal.

# ▶ ANTIBACTERIAL AGENTS

*Olga F. Woo, PharmD*

The antibiotic class of drugs has proliferated immensely since the first clinical use of sulfonamide in 1936 and the mass production of penicillin in 1941. In general, harmful effects have resulted from allergic reactions or inadvertent intravenous overdose. Serious toxicity from a single acute ingestion is rare. Table II–4 lists common and newer antibacterial agents and their toxicities.

I. **Mechanism of toxicity.** The precise mechanisms underlying toxic effects vary with the agent and are not well understood. In some cases, toxicity is caused by an extension of pharmacologic effects, whereas in other cases allergic or idiosyncratic reactions are responsible. Also, be aware that some intravenous preparations may contain preservatives such as benzyl alcohol or large amounts of potassium or sodium. Finally, drug interactions may increase toxic effects by inhibiting metabolism of the antibiotic. Prolonged QT interval and torsade de pointes (atypical ventricular tachycardia) have emerged as serious effects of macrolides or quinolones when they are used alone or interact with other medications.

II. **Toxic dose.** The toxic dose is highly variable, depending on the agent. Life-threatening allergic reactions may occur after subtherapeutic doses in hypersensitive individuals.

III. **Clinical presentation.** After acute oral overdose, most agents cause only nausea, vomiting, and diarrhea. Specific features of toxicity are described in Table II–4.

IV. **Diagnosis** is usually based on the history of exposure.

   A. **Specific levels.** Serum levels for most commonly used antibiotics are usually available. These levels are particularly useful for predicting toxic effects of **aminoglycosides, chloramphenicol,** and **vancomycin.**

   B. **Other useful laboratory studies** include complete blood count (CBC), electrolytes, glucose, BUN and creatinine, liver function tests, urinalysis, ECG (QT interval), and methemoglobin level (for patients with dapsone overdose).

V. **Treatment**

   A. **Emergency and supportive measures**

      1. Maintain an open airway and assist ventilation if necessary (see pp 1–7).
      2. Treat coma (see p 18), seizures (p 22), hypotension (p 15), anaphylaxis (p 27), and hemolysis (see Rhabdomyolysis, p 26) if they occur.
      3. Replace fluid losses resulting from gastroenteritis with intravenous crystalloids.
      4. Maintain steady urine flow with fluids to alleviate crystalluria from overdoses of sulfonamides, ampicillin, and amoxicillin.

   B. **Specific drugs and antidotes**

      1. **Trimethoprim** poisoning: Administer **leucovorin** (folinic acid; see p 468). Folic acid is not effective.
      2. **Dapsone** overdose (see also p 178): Administer **methylene blue** (p 473) for symptomatic methemoglobinemia.
      3. Treat **isoniazid** (INH) overdose (see also p 233) with **pyridoxine** (p 508).

   C. **Decontamination** (see p 45). Administer activated charcoal orally if conditions are appropriate (see Table I–38, p 51). Gastric lavage is not necessary after small to moderate ingestions if activated charcoal can be given promptly.

   D. **Enhanced elimination.** Most antibiotics are excreted unchanged in the urine, so maintenance of adequate urine flow is important. The role of forced diuresis is unclear. Hemodialysis is not usually indicated, except perhaps in patients with renal dysfunction and a high level of a toxic agent.

      1. Charcoal hemoperfusion effectively removes **chloramphenicol** and is indicated after a severe overdose with a high serum level and metabolic acidosis.
      2. **Dapsone** undergoes enterohepatic recirculation and is eliminated more rapidly with repeat-dose activated charcoal (see p 50).

**TABLE II–4. ANTIBACTERIAL DRUGS**

| Drug | Half-Life[a] | Toxic Dose or Serum Level | Toxicity |
|---|---|---|---|
| Aminoglycosides | | | |
| Amikacin | 2–3 h | > 35 mg/L | Ototoxicity to vestibular and cochlear cells; nephrotoxicity causing proximal tubular damage and acute tubular necrosis; competitive neuromuscular blockade if given rapidly intravenously with other neuromuscular blocking drugs. Threshold for toxic effects varies with the drug and the dosage schedule. |
| Gentamicin | 2 h | > 12 mg/L | |
| Kanamycin | 2–3 h | > 30 mg/L | |
| Neomycin | | 0.5–1 g/d | |
| Streptomycin | 2.5 h | > 40–50 mg/L | |
| Tobramycin | 2–2.5 h | > 10 mg/L | |
| Bacitracin | | Unknown | Ototoxicity and nephrotoxicity. |
| Cephalosporins | | | |
| Cefazolin | 90–120 min | Unknown | Convulsions reported in patients with renal insufficiency; coagulopathy associated with cefazolin. |
| Cephalothin | | | |
| Cephaloridine | | 6 g/d | Proximal tubular necrosis. |
| Cefaclor | 0.6–0.9 h | | Neutropenia. |
| Cefoperazone | 102–156 min | 3–4 mg/L | One case of symptomatic hepatitis. All these antibiotics have the *N*-methyltetrazolethiol side chain, which may inhibit aldehyde dehydrogenase to cause a disulfiram-like interaction with ethanol (see p 189) and coagulopathy (inhibition of vitamin K production). |
| Cefamandole | 30–60 min | | |
| Cefotetan | 3–4.6 h | | |
| Moxalactam | 114–150 min | | |
| Cefmetazole | 72 min | | |
| Ceftriaxone | 4.3–4.6 h Extensive excretion in bile | Intravenous bolus over < 3–5 min | Pseudolithiasis ("gall-bladder sludge"). Should be administered IV over 30 min. |
| Chloramphenicol | 4 h | > 40 mg/L | Leukopenia, reticulocytopenia; circulatory collapse (gray baby syndrome). |
| Dapsone | 10–50 h | As little as 100 mg in an 18-month-old | Methemoglobinemia, sulfhemoglobinemia, hemolysis; metabolic acidosis; hallucinations, confusion; hepatitis (see p 178). |
| Daptomycin | 8–9 h | Chronic | A cyclic lipopeptide. Available only as an injection. May cause muscle pain, weakness, or asymptomatic elevation of the CPK level. |
| Ethambutol | | > 15 mg/kg/day | Optic neuritis, red/green color blindness, peripheral neuropathy. |
| Gramicidin | | Unknown | Hemolysis. |
| Isoniazid (INH) | 0.5–4 h | 1–2 g orally | Convulsions, metabolic acidosis (see p 33); hepatotoxicity and peripheral neuropathy with chronic use. |
| Lincomycin, clindamycin | 4.4–6.4 h<br>2.4–3 h | Unknown | Hypotension and cardiopulmonary arrest after rapid intravenous administration. |
| Linezolid | 4.5–5.5 h | Duration-related (more than 2 weeks) | Thrombocytopenia, anemia; peripheral neuropathy. Linezolid is an inhibitor of monoamine oxidase (see p 269). |

(*continued*)

**TABLE II–4. ANTIBACTERIAL DRUGS (CONTINUED)**

| Drug | Half-Life[a] | Toxic Dose or Serum Level | Toxicity |
|---|---|---|---|
| Macrolides | | | Can prolong the QT interval and lead to torsade de pointes (atypical ventricular tachycardia). |
| Azithromycin | 68 h | Chronic | Least likely of the macrolides to induce torsade in animal studies |
| Clarithromycin | 3–4 h | Chronic | |
| Erythromycin | 1.4 h | Unknown | Abdominal pain; idiosyncratic hepatotoxicity with estolate salt. Administration of more than 4 g/day may cause tinnitus, ototoxicity. |
| Metronidazole | 6–14 h | 5 g/d | Convulsions; at therapeutic doses may cause disulfiram-like interaction with ethanol (see p 189). |
| Nalidixic acid | 1.1–2.5 h | 50 mg/kg/d | Seizures, hallucinations, confusion; visual disturbances; metabolic acidosis; intracranial hypertension. |
| Nitrofurantoin | 20 min | Unknown | Hemolysis in G6PD-deficient patients. |
| Penicillins | | | |
| Penicillin | 30 min | 10 million units/d IV, or CSF > 5 mg/L | Seizures with single high dose or chronic excessive doses in patients with renal dysfunction. |
| Methicillin | 30 min | Unknown | Interstitial nephritis, leukopenia. |
| Nafcillin | 1.0 h | Unknown | Neutropenia. |
| Ampicillin, amoxicillin | 1.5 h<br>1.3 h | Unknown | Acute renal failure caused by crystal deposition. |
| Penicillins, anti-pseudomonal | | | |
| Carbenicillin | 1.0–1.5 | > 300 mg/kg/d or > 250 mg/L | Bleeding disorders due to impaired platelet function; hypokalemia. Risk of toxicity higher in patients with renal insufficiency. |
| Mezlocillin | 0.8–1.1 | > 300 mg/kg/d | |
| Piperacillin | 0.6–1.2 | > 300 mg/kg/d | |
| Ticarcillin | 1.0–1.2 | > 275 mg/kg/d | |
| Polymyxins | | | Nephrotoxicity and noncompetitive neuromuscular blockade. |
| Polymyxin B | 4.3–6 h | 30,000 units/kg/d | |
| Polymyxin E | | 250 mg IM in a 10-month-old | |
| Pyrazinamide | 9–10 h | 40–50 mg/kg/day for prolonged period | Hepatotoxicity, hyperuricemia. |
| Quinolones | | | May damage growing cartilage; hemolysis in patients with G6PD deficiency; exacerbation of myasthenia gravis; acute renal failure. Some agents can prolong the QT interval. |
| Ciprofloxacin | 4 h | | Crystalluria associated with doses above daily maximum and with alkaline urine. Inhibits cytochrome P450 1A2. |
| Gatifloxacin | 7–14 h | | Case report of induced cholestatic hepatitis. |
| Norfloxacin | 3–4 h | | Crystalluria associated with doses above daily maximum and with alkaline urine. |

(*continued*)

**TABLE II–4. ANTIBACTERIAL DRUGS (CONTINUED)**

| Drug | Half-Life[a] | Toxic Dose or Serum Level | Toxicity |
|---|---|---|---|
| Quinolones *(cont)* | | | |
| Sparfloxacin | 16–30 h | Chronic | Associated with prolonged QT and torsade de pointes. Photosensitivity (use at least SPF 15 in sun-exposed areas). |
| Trovafloxacin | 9.1–12.2 h | | Pancreatitis and acute hepatitis (deaths reported). Alatrofloxacin is the IV form of trovafloxacin. |
| Rifampin | 1.5–5 h | 100 mg/kg/d | Facial edema, pruritus; headache, vomiting, diarrhea; red urine and tears. Rifamycin class of antibiotics are inducers of hepatic cytochrome P-450, especially CYP3A. |
| Spectinomycin | 1.2–2.8 h | | Acute toxicity not reported. |
| Sulfonamides | | Unknown | Acute renal failure caused by crystal deposition. |
| Tetracyclines | 6–12 h | > 1g/d in infants | Benign intracranial hypertension. Degradation products (eg, expired prescription) are nephrotoxic, may cause Fanconi-like syndrome. Some products contain sulfites. May discolor/damage developing teeth. |
| | | > 4 g/d in pregnancy or > 15 mg/L | Acute fatty liver. |
| Demeclocycline | 10–17 h | Chronic | Nephrogenic diabetes insipidus. |
| Minocycline | 11–26 h | Chronic | Vestibular symptoms. |
| Tigecycline | 37–67 h | Chronic | A glycylcycline (analog of minocycline). May cause fetal harm. Available only as an IV injection. |
| Trimethoprim | 8–11 h | Unknown | Bone marrow depression; methemoglobinemia; hyperkalemia. |
| Vancomycin | 4–6 h | > 80 mg/L | Ototoxic and nephrotoxic. Hypertension, skin rash/flushing ("red-man syndrome") associated with rapid IV administration. |

[a]Normal renal function.

## ► ANTICHOLINERGICS

*Beth H. Manning, PharmD*

Anticholinergic intoxication can occur with a wide variety of prescription and over-the-counter medications and numerous plants and mushrooms. Common drugs that have anticholinergic activity include antihistamines (see p 97), antipsychotics (see p 107), antispasmodics, skeletal muscle relaxants (see p 341), and tricyclic antidepressants (see p 91). Common combination products containing anticholinergic drugs include Atrohist™, Donnagel™, Donnatal™, Hyland's Teething Tablets™, Lomotil™, Motofen™, Ru-Tuss™, Urised™, and Urispas™. Common anticholinergic medications are described in Table II–5. Plants and mushrooms containing anticholinergic alkaloids include jimsonweed (*Datura stramonium*), deadly nightshade (*Atropa belladonna*), and fly agaric (*Amanita muscaria*).

**TABLE II–5. ANTICHOLINERGIC DRUGS[a]**

| Tertiary Amines | Usual Adult Single Dose (mg) | Quaternary Amines | Usual Adult Single Dose (mg) |
|---|---|---|---|
| Atropine | 0.4–1 | Anisotropine | 50 |
| Benztropine | 1–6 | Clidinium | 2.5–5 |
| Biperiden | 2–5 | Glycopyrrolate | 1 |
| Darifenacin | 7.5–15 | Hexocyclium | 25 |
| Dicyclomine | 10–20 | Ipratropium bromide | N/A[b] |
| Flavoxate | 100–200 | Isopropamide | 5 |
| L-Hyoscyamine | 0.15–0.3 | Mepenzolate | 25 |
| Oxybutynin | 5 | Methantheline | 50–100 |
| Oxyphencyclimine | 10 | Methscopolamine | 2.5 |
| Procyclidine | 5 | Propantheline | 7.5–15 |
| Scopolamine | 0.4–1 | Tridihexethyl | 25–50 |
| Solifenacin succinate | 5–10 | Trospium chloride | 20 |
| Tolterodine | 2–4 | | |
| Trihexyphenidyl | 6–10 | | |

[a]These drugs act mainly at muscarinic cholinergic receptors, and sometimes are more correctly referred to as antimuscarinic drugs.
[b]Not used orally; available as metered-dose inhaler and 0.02% inhalation solution and 0.03% nasal spray.

**I. Mechanism of toxicity**

**A.** Anticholinergic agents competitively antagonize the effects of acetylcholine at peripheral muscarinic and central receptors. Exocrine glands, such as those responsible for sweating and salivation, and smooth muscle are mostly affected. The inhibition of muscarinic activity in the heart leads to a rapid heartbeat.

**B.** Tertiary amines such as atropine are well absorbed centrally, whereas quaternary amines such as glycopyrrolate have a less central effect.

**C. Pharmacokinetics.** Absorption may be delayed because of the pharmacologic effects of these drugs on gastrointestinal motility. The duration of toxic effects can be quite prolonged (eg, benztropine intoxication may persist for 2–3 days). (See also Table II–59, p 382.)

**II. Toxic dose.** The range of toxicity is highly variable and unpredictable. Fatal atropine poisoning has occurred after as little as 1–2 mg was instilled in the eye of a young child. Intramuscular injection of 32 mg of atropine was fatal in an adult. Doses up to 360 mg of trospium chloride produced increased heart rate and dry mouth but no other significant toxicity in healthy adults.

**III. Clinical presentation.** The anticholinergic syndrome is characterized by warm, dry, flushed skin; dry mouth; mydriasis; delirium; tachycardia; ileus; and urinary retention. Jerky myoclonic movements and choreoathetosis are common and may lead to rhabdomyolysis. Hyperthermia, coma, and respiratory arrest may occur. Seizures are rare with pure antimuscarinic agents, although they may result from other pharmacologic properties of the drug (eg, tricyclic antidepressants and antihistamines).

**IV. Diagnosis** is based on a history of exposure and the presence of typical features such as dilated pupils and flushed skin. A trial dose of physostigmine (see below) can be used to confirm the presence of anticholinergic toxicity; rapid reversal of signs and symptoms is consistent with the diagnosis.

A. **Specific levels.** Concentrations in body fluids are not generally available. Common over-the-counter (OTC) agents are usually detectable on comprehensive urine toxicology screening but are not found on hospital drugs of abuse panels.

B. **Other useful laboratory studies** include electrolytes, glucose, CPK, arterial blood gases or pulse oximetry, and ECG monitoring.

V. **Treatment**

A. **Emergency and supportive measures**

1. Maintain an open airway and assist ventilation if needed (see pp 1–7).
2. Treat hyperthermia (see p 20), coma (p 18), rhabdomyolysis (p 26), and seizures (p 22) if they occur.

B. **Specific drugs and antidotes**

1. A small dose of **physostigmine** (see p 497), 0.5–1 mg IV in an adult, can be given to patients with severe toxicity (eg, hyperthermia, severe delirium, or tachycardia). *Caution:* Physostigmine can cause AV block, asystole, and seizures, especially in patients with tricyclic antidepressant overdose.
2. **Neostigmine,** a peripherally acting cholinesterase inhibitor, may be useful in treating anticholinergic-induced ileus.

C. **Decontamination** (see p 45). Administer activated charcoal orally if conditions are appropriate (see Table I–38, p 51). Gastric lavage is not necessary after small to moderate ingestions if activated charcoal can be given promptly. Because of slowed gastrointestinal motility, gut decontamination procedures may be helpful even in late-presenting patients.

D. **Enhanced elimination.** Hemodialysis, hemoperfusion, peritoneal dialysis, and repeat-dose charcoal are not effective in removing anticholinergic agents.

## ▶ ANTICONVULSANTS, NEWER

*Freda M. Rowley, PharmD*

In the last decade a number of newer anticonvulsants have been introduced and are being used in a variety of treatment settings, including treatment of partial and generalized seizure disorders, chronic pain syndromes, bipolar disorders, and migraine prophylaxis. Characteristics of several of these drugs are listed in Table II–6.

I. **Mechanism of toxicity**

A. **Felbamate** has effects on sodium channels, enhances activity of the inhibitory neurotransmitter gamma-aminobutyric acid (GABA), and blocks *N*-methyl-D-aspartate (NMDA) receptors.

B. **Gabapentin** acts via unknown mechanisms. It has structural similarity to GABA but does not bind GABA receptors or alter normal levels of GABA in the brain.

C. **Lamotrigine** blocks voltage-sensitive sodium channels and inhibits the release of excitatory neurotransmitters.

D. **Levetiracetam** acts via unknown mechanisms. It is structurally a GABA derivative but does not appear to have activity at GABA receptors.

E. **Tiagabine** is thought to enhance GABA activity by binding to GABA recognition sites, and it blocks GABA reuptake at presynaptic neurons.

F. **Topiramate** acts via unknown mechanisms, possibly involving sodium channel blockade and potentiation of GABA effects.

G. **Vigabatrin** prevents inactivation of GABA by irreversible inhibition of GABA transaminase.

H. **Zonisamide** blocks sodium and calcium channels.

I. **Pharmacokinetics.** See Tables II–6 and II–59.

II. **Toxic dose.** There have been few reports of overdose. Toxic effects may be influenced by the presence of other medications with CNS activity.

III. **Clinical presentation.** Specific features of potential or reported toxicity of each agent are described in Table II–6.

**TABLE II–6. ANTICONVULSANT DRUGS (NEWER)**

| Drug | Usual Elimination Half-Life (hours) | Usual Daily Dose (mg/day) | Reported Potential Toxic Effects |
|---|---|---|---|
| Felbamate | 20–23 h | 1800–4800 mg | Mild CNS depression, nystagmus, ataxia; tachycardia; nausea and vomiting. Delayed (> 12 h) crystalluria, hematuria, renal dysfunction. Aplastic anemia, hepatic failure reported with therapeutic use (rare). |
| Gabapentin | 5–7 h | 900–3600 mg | Somnolence, dizziness, ataxia, mild tremor, slurred speech, diplopia; tachycardia, hypotension or hypertension; diarrhea. |
| Lamotrigine | 22–36 h | 200–500 mg | Lethargy, dizziness, ataxia, stupor, nystagmus, hypertonia, seizures; QRS prolongation; nausea and vomiting; hypokalemia; hypersensitivity: fever, rash (Stevens-Johnson syndrome), hepatitis, renal failure. |
| Levetiracetam | 6–8 h | 1000–3000 mg | Drowsiness. |
| Tiagabine | 7–9 h | 30–70 mg | Somnolence, confusion, agitation, dizziness, ataxia, weakness, tremor, clonus, seizures. |
| Topiramate | 21 h | 200–600 mg | Sedation, confusion, slurred speech, ataxia, tremor, anxiety, nervousness, seizures. |
| Vigabatrin | 4–8 h | 2000–4000 mg | Sedation, confusion, coma, agitation, delirium, psychotic disturbances (hallucinations, delusions, paranoia). |
| Zonisamide | 50–68 h | 100–400 mg | Somnolence, ataxia, agitation; bradycardia, hypotension; respiratory depression. |

**IV. Diagnosis** usually is based on the history of ingestion or is suspected in any patient on these medications who presents with altered mental status, ataxia, or seizures.

**A. Specific levels.** Serum levels are not routinely available and are not likely to be useful for emergency management.

**B. Other useful laboratory studies** include electrolytes, glucose, creatinine (gabapentin, topiramate), CBC (felbamate), liver transaminases, bilirubin (felbamate), and ECG monitoring (lamotrigine).

**V. Treatment**

**A. Emergency and supportive measures**

1. Maintain an open airway and assist ventilation if necessary (see pp 1–7). Administer supplemental oxygen.
2. Treat stupor and coma (see p 18) if they occur. Protect the patient from self-injury caused by ataxia.
3. Treat agitation and delirium (see p 23) if they occur.
4. Monitor asymptomatic patients for a minimum of 4–6 hours. Admit symptomatic patients for at least 24 hours after **lamotrigine, felbamate, topiramate,** or **zonisamide** ingestions.

**B. Specific drugs and antidotes.** There are no specific antidotes. Sodium bicarbonate (see p 423) has not been studied, but it has been recommended for lamotrigine-induced QRS interval prolongation.

**C. Decontamination (see p 45).** Administer activated charcoal orally if conditions are appropriate (see Table I–38, p 51). Gastric lavage is not necessary after small to moderate ingestions if activated charcoal can be given promptly.

**D. Enhanced elimination.** Hemodialysis is effective at removing **gabapentin** and **topiramate,** but clinical manifestations are usually responsive to supportive care, making enhanced removal procedures unnecessary.

# ▶ ANTIDEPRESSANTS, GENERAL (NONCYCLIC)

*Neal L. Benowitz, MD*

Many noncyclic antidepressants are now available, including trazodone (Desyrel™), fluoxetine (Prozac™), sertraline (Zoloft™), citalopram (Celexa™), escitalopram (Lexapro™), paroxetine (Paxil™), fluvoxamine (Luvox™), venlafaxine (Effexor™), and bupropion (Wellbutrin™). Bupropion is also marketed under the brand name Zyban™ for smoking cessation. Mirtazapine (Remeron™) is a tetracyclic antidepressant. Nefazodone (Serzone) was recently withdrawn from the U.S. market due to its risk of hepatotoxicity. In general, these drugs are much less toxic than the **tricyclic antidepressants** (see p 91) and the **monoamine oxidase (MAO) inhibitors** (p 269), although serious effects such as seizures and hypotension occasionally occur. Noncyclic and tricyclic antidepressants are described in Table II–7.

**I. Mechanism of toxicity**

**A.** Most agents cause CNS depression. Bupropion is a stimulant that can also cause seizures, presumably related to inhibition of reuptake of dopamine and norepinephrine.

**B.** Trazodone and mirtazapine produce peripheral alpha-adrenergic blockade, which can result in hypotension and priapism.

**C.** Serotonin uptake inhibitors (often called selective serotonin reuptake inhibitors or SSRIs) such as fluoxetine, citalopram, sertraline, paroxetine, fluvoxamine, venlafaxine, and trazodone may interact with each other or with chronic use of an MAO inhibitor (see p 269) to produce the **"serotonin syndrome"** (see below and p 21).

**D.** None of the drugs in this group has significant anticholinergic effects.

**E. Pharmacokinetics.** These drugs have large volumes of distribution (Vd = 12–88 L/kg, except trazodone [Vd = 1.3 L/kg]). Most are eliminated via hepatic metabolism (paroxetine is 65% renal). (See also Table II–59, p 382.)

**II. Toxic dose.** The noncyclic antidepressants generally have a wide therapeutic index, with doses in excess of 10 times the usual therapeutic dose tolerated without serious toxicity. Bupropion can cause seizures in some patients with moderate overdose or even in therapeutic doses.

**III. Clinical presentation**

**A. Central nervous system.** The usual presentation after overdose includes ataxia, sedation, and coma. Respiratory depression may occur, especially with co-ingestion of alcohol or other drugs. These agents, particularly bupropion, can cause restlessness, anxiety, and agitation. Tremor and seizures are common with bupropion but occur occasionally after overdose with SSRIs, particularly venlafaxine and citalopram.

**B. Cardiovascular** effects are usually not life-threatening, although trazodone can cause hypotension and orthostatic hypotension, bupropion can cause sinus tachycardia, and citalopram can cause sinus bradycardia with hypotension. Citalopram can also cause QT interval prolongation.

**C. Serotonin syndrome** (see p 21) is characterized by confusion, hypomania, restlessness, myoclonus, hyperreflexia, diaphoresis, shivering, tremor, incoordination, and hyperthermia. This reaction may be seen when a patient taking an MAO inhibitor (p 269) ingests a serotonin uptake blocker. Because of the long duration of effects of MAO inhibitors and most of the serotonin uptake blockers, this reaction can occur up to several days to weeks after either

**TABLE II–7. ANTIDEPRESSANTS**

| | Usual Adult Daily Dose (mg) | Neurotransmitter Effects[a] | Toxicity[b] |
|---|---|---|---|
| **Tricyclic antidepressants** | | | |
| Amitriptyline | 75–200 | NE, 5-HT | A, H, QRS, Sz |
| Amoxapine | 150–300 | NE, DA | A, H, Sz |
| Clomipramine | 100–250 | NE, 5-HT | A, H, QRS, Sz |
| Desipramine | 75–200 | NE | A, H, Sz |
| Doxepin | 75–300 | NE, 5-HT | A, H, QRS, Sz |
| Imipramine | 75–200 | NE, 5-HT | A, H, QRS, Sz |
| Maprotiline | 75–300 | NE | A, H, QRS, Sz |
| Nortriptyline | 75–150 | NE | A, H, QRS, Sz |
| Protriptyline | 20–40 | NE | A, H, QRS, Sz |
| Trimipramine | 75–200 | NE, 5-HT | A, H, QRS, Sz |
| **Newer, noncyclic drugs** | | | |
| Bupropion | 200–450 | DA, NE | Sz |
| Citalopram | 20–40 | 5-HT | Sz, SS |
| Fluoxetine | 20–80 | 5-HT | Sz, SS |
| Fluvoxamine | 50–300 | 5-HT | Sz, SS |
| Mirtazapine | 15–45 | Alpha-2 | |
| Nefazodone | 100–600 | 5-HT, alpha-2 | H |
| Paroxetine | 20–50 | 5-HT | Sz, SS |
| Sertraline | 50–200 | 5-HT | Sz, SS |
| Trazodone | 50–400 | 5-HT, alpha-2 | H, Sz, SS |
| Venlafaxine | 30–600 | 5-HT, NE | Sz, SS |
| **Monoamine oxidase inhibitors** | See p 269 | | |

[a]DA = dopamine reuptake inhibitor; NE = norepinephrine reuptake inhibitor; 5-HT = serotonin reuptake inhibitor; alpha-2 = central alpha-2-adrenergic receptor blocker.
[b]A = anticholinergic effects; H = hypotension; QRS = QRS prolongation; Sz = seizures. SS = serotonin syndrome.

treatment regimen has been discontinued. The syndrome has also been described in patients taking an overdose of a single SSRI or combinations of various SSRIs without concomitant MAO inhibitor use.

**IV. Diagnosis.** A noncyclic antidepressant overdose should be suspected in patients with a history of depression who develop lethargy, coma, or seizures. As these agents uncommonly affect cardiac conduction, QRS interval prolongation should suggest a tricyclic antidepressant overdose (see p 91).

**A. Specific levels.** Blood and urine assays are not routinely available and are not useful for emergency management. These drugs are unlikely to appear on a rapid "drugs of abuse" screen, and may or may not appear on comprehensive toxicology screening, depending on the laboratory.

**B. Other useful laboratory studies** include electrolytes, glucose, arterial blood gases or pulse oximetry, and ECG monitoring.

**V. Treatment**

**A. Emergency and supportive measures**

1. Maintain an open airway and assist ventilation if needed (see pp 1–7). Administer supplemental oxygen.
2. Treat coma (see p 18), hypotension (p 15), and seizures (p 22) if they occur.

**B. Specific drugs and antidotes.** For suspected serotonin syndrome, anecdotal reports claim benefit from cyproheptadine (Periactin), 4 mg orally every hour for 3 doses, or methysergide (Sansert), 2 mg orally every 6 hours for 3 doses, presumably because of the serotonin antagonist effects of these drugs.

**C. Decontamination** (see p 45). Administer activated charcoal orally, if conditions are appropriate (see Table I–38, p 51). Gastric lavage is not necessary after small to moderate ingestions if activated charcoal can be given promptly.

**D. Enhanced elimination.** Owing to extensive protein binding and large volumes of distribution, dialysis, hemoperfusion, peritoneal dialysis, and repeat-dose charcoal are not effective.

## ▶ ANTIDEPRESSANTS, TRICYCLIC

*Neal L. Benowitz, MD*

Tricyclic antidepressants are commonly taken in overdose by suicidal patients and represent a major cause of poisoning hospitalizations and deaths. Currently available tricyclic antidepressants are described in Table II–7. Amitriptyline also is marketed in combination with chlordiazepoxide (Limbitrol™) or perphenazine (Etrafon™ or Triavil™). **Cyclobenzaprine** (Flexeril™), a centrally acting muscle relaxant (see p 342), is structurally related to the tricyclic antidepressants but exhibits minimal cardiotoxic and variable CNS effects. **Newer, noncyclic antidepressants** are discussed on p 89. **Monoamine oxidase inhibitors** are discussed on p 269.

**I. Mechanism of toxicity.** Tricyclic antidepressant toxicity affects primarily the cardiovascular and central nervous systems.

**A. Cardiovascular effects.** Several mechanisms contribute to cardiovascular toxicity:

1. Anticholinergic effects and inhibition of neuronal reuptake of catecholamines result in tachycardia and mild hypertension.
2. Peripheral alpha-adrenergic blockade causes vasodilation and contributes to hypotension.
3. Membrane-depressant (quinidine-like) effects cause myocardial depression and cardiac conduction disturbances by inhibition of the fast sodium channel that initiates the cardiac cell action potential. Metabolic or respiratory acidosis may contribute to cardiotoxicity by further inhibiting the fast sodium channel.

**B. Central nervous system effects.** These effects result in part from anticholinergic toxicity (eg, sedation and coma), but seizures are probably a result of inhibition of reuptake of norepinephrine or serotonin in the brain or other central effects.

**C. Pharmacokinetics.** Anticholinergic effects of these drugs may retard gastric emptying, resulting in slow or erratic absorption. Most of these drugs are extensively bound to body tissues and plasma proteins, resulting in very large volumes of distribution and long elimination half-lives (Tables II–7 and II–59). Tricyclic antidepressants are metabolized primarily by the liver, with only a small fraction excreted unchanged in the urine. Active metabolites may contribute to toxicity; several drugs are metabolized to other well-known tricyclic antidepressants (eg, amitriptyline to nortriptyline, imipramine to desipramine).

**II. Toxic dose.** Most of the tricyclic antidepressants have a narrow therapeutic index so that doses of less than 10 times the therapeutic daily dose may produce severe intoxication. In general, ingestion of 10–20 mg/kg is potentially life threatening.

**III. Clinical presentation.** Tricyclic antidepressant poisoning may produce any of three major toxic syndromes: anticholinergic effects, cardiovascular effects, and seizures. Depending on the dose and the drug, patients may experience some or all of these toxic effects. Symptoms usually begin within 30–40 minutes of ingestion but may be delayed owing to slow and erratic gut absorption. Patients who are awake initially may abruptly lose consciousness or develop seizures without warning.

**A. Anticholinergic** effects include sedation, delirium, coma, dilated pupils, dry skin and mucous membranes, diminished sweating, tachycardia, diminished or absent bowel sounds, and urinary retention. Myoclonic or metonymic jerking is common with anticholinergic intoxication and may be mistaken for seizure activity.

**B. Cardiovascular** toxicity manifests as abnormal cardiac conduction, arrhythmias, and hypotension.

1. Typical electrocardiographic findings include sinus tachycardia with prolongation of the PR, QRS, and QT intervals. Various degrees of AV block may be seen. Prolongation of the QRS complex to 0.12 second or longer is a fairly reliable predictor of serious cardiovascular and neurologic toxicity (except in the case of moraine, which causes seizures and coma with no change in the QRS interval).
2. Sinus tachycardia accompanied by QRS interval prolongation may resemble ventricular tachycardia (see Figure I–4, p 11). True ventricular tachycardia and fibrillation may also occur. Atypical or polymorphous ventricular tachycardia (torsade de pointes; see Figure I–7, p 14) associated with QT interval prolongation may occur with therapeutic dosing but is actually uncommon in overdose. Development of bradyarrhythmias usually indicates a severely poisoned heart and carries a poor prognosis.
3. Hypotension caused by venodilation is common and usually mild. In severe cases, hypotension results from myocardial depression and may be refractory to treatment; some patients die with progressive intractable cardiogenic shock. Pulmonary edema is also common in severe poisonings.

**C. Seizures** are common with tricyclic antidepressant toxicity and may be recurrent or persistent. The muscular hyperactivity from seizures and myoclonic jerking, combined with diminished sweating, can lead to severe hyperthermia (see p 21), resulting in rhabdomyolysis, brain damage, multisystem failure, and death.

**D. Death** from tricyclic antidepressant overdose usually occurs within a few hours of admission and may result from ventricular fibrillation, intractable cardiogenic shock, or status epilepticus with hyperthermia. Sudden death several days after apparent recovery has been reported occasionally, but in all such cases there was evidence of continuing cardiac toxicity within 24 hours of death.

**IV. Diagnosis.** Tricyclic antidepressant poisoning should be suspected in any patient with lethargy, coma, or seizures accompanied by QRS interval prolongation. QRS interval prolongation greater than 0.12 second in the limb leads suggests severe poisoning. However, with amoxapine, seizures and coma may occur with no widening of the QRS interval.

**A. Specific levels**

1. Plasma levels of some of the tricyclic antidepressants can be measured by clinical laboratories. Therapeutic concentrations are usually less than 0.3 mg/L (300 ng/mL). Total concentrations of parent drug plus metabolite of 1 mg/L (1000 ng/mL) or greater usually are associated with serious poisoning. Generally, plasma levels are not used in emergency management because the QRS interval and clinical manifestations of overdose are reliable and more readily available indicators of toxicity.
2. Most tricyclics are detectable on comprehensive urine toxicology screening. Some rapid immunologic techniques are available and have sufficiently broad cross-reactivity to detect several tricyclics. However, use of these assays for rapid screening in the hospital laboratory is not recommended because they may miss some important drugs and give positive results for others that are present in therapeutic concentrations.

B. **Other useful laboratory studies** include electrolytes, glucose, BUN, creatinine, CPK, urinalysis for myoglobin, arterial blood gases or oximetry, 12-lead ECG and continuous ECG monitoring, and chest x-ray.

V. **Treatment**

A. **Emergency and supportive measures**

1. Maintain an open airway and assist ventilation if necessary (see pp 1–7). ***Caution:*** Respiratory arrest can occur abruptly and without warning.
2. Treat coma (see p 18), seizures (p 22), hyperthermia (p 20), hypotension (p 15), and arrhythmias (pp 13–15) if they occur. ***Note:*** Do **not** use procainamide or other type Ia or Ic antiarrhythmic agents for ventricular tachycardia, because these drugs may aggravate cardiotoxicity.
3. Consider cardiac pacing for bradyarrhythmias and high-degree AV block and overdrive pacing for torsade de pointes.
4. Mechanical support of the circulation (eg, cardiopulmonary bypass) may be useful (based on anecdotal reports) in stabilizing patients with refractory shock, allowing time for the body to eliminate some of the drug.
5. If seizures are not immediately controlled with usual anticonvulsants, paralyze the patient with a neuromuscular blocker such as pancuronium (see p 480) to prevent hyperthermia, which may induce further seizures, and lactic acidosis, which aggravates cardiotoxicity. ***Note:*** Paralysis abolishes the muscular manifestations of seizures but has no effect on brain seizure activity. After paralysis, ECG monitoring is necessary to determine the efficacy of anticonvulsant therapy.
6. Continuously monitor the temperature, other vital signs, and ECG in asymptomatic patients for a minimum of 6 hours, and admit patients to an intensive care setting for at least 24 hours if there are any signs of toxicity.

B. **Specific drugs and antidotes**

1. In patients with QRS interval prolongation or hypotension, administer **sodium bicarbonate** (see p 423), 1–2 mEq/kg IV, and repeat as needed to maintain arterial pH between 7.45 and 7.55. Sodium bicarbonate may reverse membrane-depressant effects by increasing extracellular sodium concentrations and by a direct effect of pH on the fast sodium channel.
2. Hyperventilation, by inducing a respiratory alkalosis (or reversing respiratory acidosis), may also be of benefit but works only transiently and may provoke seizures.
3. Although **physostigmine** was advocated in the past, it should ***not*** be administered routinely to patients with tricyclic antidepressant poisoning; it may aggravate conduction disturbances, causing asystole, further impair myocardial contractility, worsening hypotension, and contribute to seizures.

C. **Decontamination** (see p 45). Administer activated charcoal orally if conditions are appropriate (see Table I–38, p 51). Gastric lavage is not necessary after small to moderate ingestions if activated charcoal can be given promptly, but it should be considered for large ingestions (eg, >20–30 mg/kg).

D. **Enhanced elimination.** Owing to extensive tissue and protein binding with a resulting large volume of distribution, dialysis and hemoperfusion are not effective. Although repeat-dose charcoal has been reported to accelerate tricyclic antidepressant elimination, the data are not convincing.

## ► ANTIDIABETIC AGENTS

*Susan Kim, PharmD*

Agents used to lower blood glucose are divided into two main groups: oral drugs and insulin products. The oral agents include sulfonylureas, biguanides, glitazones, meglitinides, and alpha-glucosidase inhibitors, each with a different mechanism of action, potency, and duration of activity. All **insulin** products are given by the parenteral route, and all produce effects similar to those of endogenous insulin; they differ by antigenicity and by onset and duration of effect. Table II–8 lists the various available antidiabetic agents. Other drugs and poisons can also cause hypoglycemia (see Table I–25).

**I. Mechanism of toxicity**

**A. Oral agents**

1. **Sulfonylureas** lower blood glucose primarily by stimulating endogenous pancreatic insulin secretion and secondarily by enhancing peripheral insulin receptor sensitivity and reducing glycogenolysis.
2. **Meglitinides** also increase pancreatic insulin release and can cause hypoglycemia in overdose.
3. **Biguanides.** Metformin decreases hepatic glucose production and intestinal absorption of glucose while increasing peripheral glucose uptake and utilization. It does not stimulate insulin release and is not likely to produce acute hypoglycemia. Severe **lactic acidosis** is a rare but potentially fatal side effect of metformin (and its predecessor phenformin, no longer available in the United States). It occurs mainly in patients with renal insufficiency, alcoholism, and advanced age and has occurred after injection of iodinated contrast agents resulted in acute renal failure.
4. **Alpha-glucosidase inhibitors** delay the digestion of ingested carbohydrates, reducing postprandial blood glucose concentrations.
5. **Glitazones** decrease hepatic glucose output and improve target cell response to insulin. Hepatotoxicity has been reported with chronic therapy for all the drugs in this class and led to removal of troglitazone from the US market.
6. Although biguanides, alpha-glucosidase inhibitors, and glitazones are not likely to cause hypoglycemia after acute overdose, they may contribute to the hypoglycemic effects of sulfonylureas, meglitinides, or insulin.

**B. Insulin.** Blood glucose is lowered directly by the stimulation of cellular uptake and metabolism of glucose. Cellular glucose uptake is accompanied by an intracellular shift of potassium and magnesium. Insulin also promotes glycogen formation and lipogenesis.

**C. Pharmacokinetics** (see Tables II–8 and II–59)

**II. Toxic dose**

**A. Sulfonylureas.** Toxicity depends on the agent and the total amount ingested. Toxicity may also occur owing to drug interactions, resulting in impaired elimination of the oral agent.

1. **Ingestion of a single tablet** of chlorpropamide (250 mg), glipizide (5 mg), or glyburide (2.5 mg) each produced hypoglycemia in children 1–4 years old. Two 500-mg tablets of acetohexamide caused hypoglycemic coma in an adult. In a 79-year-old nondiabetic person, 5 mg of glyburide caused hypoglycemic coma.
2. **Interactions** with the following drugs may increase the risk of hypoglycemia: other hypoglycemics, sulfonamides, propranolol, salicylates, clofibrate, probenecid, pentamidine, valproic acid, dicumarol, cimetidine, MAO inhibitors, and alcohol. In addition, co-ingestion of alcohol may occasionally produce a disulfiram-like interaction (see p 184).
3. **Hepatic** or **renal insufficiency** may impair drug elimination and result in hypoglycemia.

**B. Repaglinide.** A 4-mg dose produced hypoglycemia in a nondiabetic 18-year-old patient.

**C. Metformin.** Lactic acidosis occurred 9 hours after ingestion of 25 g of metformin by an 83-year-old patient, and fatal lactic acidosis and cardiovascular collapse occurred 4 hours after ingestion of 35 g in a 33-year-old patient. Pediatric ingestions up to 1700 mg have been well tolerated.

**D. Insulin.** Severe hypoglycemic coma and permanent neurologic sequelae have occurred after injections of 800–3200 units of insulin. Orally administered insulin is not absorbed and is not toxic.

**TABLE II–8. ANTIDIABETIC DRUGS[a]**

| Agent | Onset (h) | Peak (h) | Duration[b] (h) |
|---|---|---|---|
| **Insulins** | | | |
| Regular insulin | 0.5–1 | 2–3 | 8–12 |
| Rapid insulin zinc (semilente) | 0.5 | 4–7 | 12–16 |
| Insulin lispro | 0.25 | 0.5–1.5 | 6–8 |
| Insulin aspart | 0.25 | 1–3 | 3–5 |
| Insulin glulisine | 0.3 | 0.6–1 | 5 |
| Isophane insulin (NPH) | 1–2 | 8–12 | 18–24 |
| Insulin zinc (lente) | 1–2 | 8–12 | 18–24 |
| Insulin glargine | 1.5 | Sustained effect | 22–24 |
| Extended zinc insulin (ultralente) | 4–8 | 16–18 | 36 |
| Protamine zinc insulin (PZI) | 4–8 | 14–20 | 36 |
| **Sulfonylureas** | | | |
| Acetohexamide | 2 | 4 | 12–24 |
| Chlorpropamide | 1 | 3–6 | 24–72[b] |
| Glimepiride | 2–3 | | 24 |
| Glipizide [extended-release form] | 0.5 [2–3] | 1–2 [6–12] | <24 [24] |
| Glyburide [micronized form] | 0.5 | 4 [2–3] | 24[b] |
| Tolazamide | 1 | 4–6 | 14–20 |
| Tolbutamide | 1 | 5–8 | 6–12 |
| **Meglitinides** | | | |
| Nateglinide | 0.25 | 1–2 | 1.5–3 |
| Repaglinide | 0.5 | 1–1.5 | 1–1.5 |
| **Biguanides** | | | |
| Metformin | | 2 | 2.5–6 |
| **Alpha glucosidase inhibitors** | | | |
| Acarbose | | N/A (less than 2% of an oral dose absorbed systemically) | |
| Miglitol | | 2–3 | 2 |
| **Glitazones (thiazolidinediones)** | | | |
| Pioglitazone | | 2–4 | 3–7 |
| Rosiglitazone | | 1–3.5 | 3–4 |

[a]See also Table II–55 (p 357).
[b]Duration of hypoglycemic effects after overdose may be much longer, especially with glyburide and chlorpropamide.

**III. Clinical presentation**

**A. Hypoglycemia** may be delayed in onset, depending on the agent used and the route of administration (ie, subcutaneous versus intravenous). Manifestations of hypoglycemia include agitation, confusion, coma, seizures, tachycardia, and diaphoresis. Serum potassium and magnesium levels may also be depressed. Note that in patients receiving beta-adrenergic blocking agents (see p 131), many of the manifestations of hypoglycemia (tachycardia, diaphoresis) may be blunted or absent.

**B. Lactic acidosis** from metformin or phenformin may begin with nonspecific symptoms such as malaise, vomiting, myalgias, and respiratory distress. The mortality rate for severe lactic acidosis is reportedly as high as 50%.

**IV. Diagnosis.** Overdose involving a sulfonylurea, meglitinide, or insulin should be suspected in any patient with hypoglycemia. Other causes of hypoglycemia that should be considered include alcohol ingestion (especially in children) and fulminant hepatic failure.

**A. Specific levels**

1. Serum concentrations of many agents can be determined in commercial toxicology laboratories but have little utility in acute clinical management.
2. Exogenously administered animal insulin can be distinguished from endogenous insulin (ie, in a patient with hypoglycemia caused by insulinoma) by determination of C peptide (present with endogenous insulin secretion).

**B. Other useful laboratory studies** include glucose, electrolytes, magnesium, and ethanol. If metformin or phenformin is suspected, obtain a venous blood lactate level (gray-top tube).

**V. Treatment.** Observe asymptomatic patients for at least 8 hours after ingestion.

**A. Emergency and supportive measures**

1. Maintain an open airway and assist ventilation if necessary (see pp 1–7).
2. Treat coma (see p 18) and seizures (p 22) if they occur.
3. Obtain fingerstick blood glucose levels every 1–2 hours until stabilized.

**B. Specific drugs and antidotes**

1. If the patient is hypoglycemic, administer concentrated **glucose** (see p 457). In adults, give 50% dextrose ($D_{50}W$), 1–2 mL/kg; in children, use 25% dextrose ($D_{25}W$), 2–4 mL/kg. Give repeated glucose boluses and administer 5–10% dextrose ($D_5$–$D_{10}$) as needed to maintain normal serum glucose concentrations (60–110 mg/dL).
2. For patients with a **sulfonylurea** or **meglitinide** overdose, consider intravenous **octreotide** (see p 488) or **diazoxide** (p 438) if 5% dextrose infusions do not maintain satisfactory glucose concentrations.
3. Maintaining serum glucose concentrations above 90–100 mg/dL for the first 12 hours of therapy or longer is often necessary to prevent recurrent hypoglycemia. However, once hypoglycemia resolves (usually 12–24 hours after the ingestion) and the patient no longer requires dextrose infusions, serum glucose concentrations should be allowed to normalize. Follow serum glucose levels closely for several hours after the last dose of dextrose.
4. Lactic acidosis caused by biguanides may be treated with judicious doses of sodium bicarbonate. Excessive bicarbonate administration may worsen intracellular acidosis.

**C. Decontamination** (see p 45)

1. **Oral agents.** Administer activated charcoal orally if conditions are appropriate (see Table I–38, p 51). Gastric lavage is not necessary after small to moderate ingestions if activated charcoal can be given promptly.
2. **Insulin.** Orally ingested insulin is not absorbed and produces no toxicity, so gut decontamination is not necessary.

**D. Enhanced elimination**

1. **Sulfonylureas.** Alkalinization of the urine (see p 54) increases the renal elimination of chlorpropamide. Forced diuresis and dialysis procedures are of no known value for other hypoglycemic agents. The high degree of protein binding of the sulfonylureas suggests that dialysis procedures would not generally be effective. However, charcoal hemoperfusion reduced the serum half-life of chlorpropamide in a patient with renal failure.
2. **Metformin** is removed by hemodialysis, which can also help correct severe lactic acidosis. Continuous venovenous hemodiafiltration has also been recommended.

# ▶ ANTIHISTAMINES

*Beth Manning, PharmD*

Antihistamines ($H_1$ receptor antagonists) are commonly found in over-the-counter and prescription medications used for motion sickness, control of allergy-related itching, and cough and cold palliation and as sleep aids (Table II–9). Acute intoxication with antihistamines results in symptoms very similar to those of anticholinergic poisoning. $H_2$ receptor blockers (cimetidine, ranitidine, and famotidine) inhibit gastric acid secretion but otherwise share no effects with $H_1$ agents, do not produce significant intoxication, and are not discussed here. Common combination products containing antihistamines include Actifed™, Allerest™, Contac™, Coricidin™, Dimetapp™, Dristan™, Drixoral™, Excedrin PM™, Nyquil™, Nytol™, Pamprin™, PediaCare™, Tavist™, Triaminic™, Triaminicol™, Unisom Dual Relief Formula™, and Vicks Pediatric Formula 44™.

**I. Mechanism of toxicity**

**A.** $H_1$ blocker antihistamines are structurally related to histamine and antagonize the effects of histamine on $H_1$ receptor sites. They have anticholinergic effects (except the "nonsedating" agents: cetirizine, desloratadine, fexofenadine, and loratadine). They may also stimulate or depress the CNS, and some agents (eg, diphenhydramine) have local anesthetic and membrane-depressant effects in large doses.

**B. Pharmacokinetics.** Drug absorption may be delayed because of the pharmacologic effects of these agents on the gastrointestinal tract. Volumes of distribution are generally large (3–20 L/kg). Elimination half-lives are highly variable, ranging from 1–4 hours for diphenhydramine to 7–24 hours for many of the others. (See also Table II–59, p 382.)

**II. Toxic dose.** The estimated fatal oral dose of diphenhydramine is 20–40 mg/kg. In general, toxicity occurs after ingestion of 3–5 times the usual daily dose. Children are more sensitive to the toxic effects of antihistamines than are adults. The nonsedating agents are associated with less toxicity. Up to 300 mg of loratadine is expected to cause only minor effects in pediatric patients.

**III. Clinical presentation**

**A.** An overdose results in many symptoms similar to anticholinergic poisoning: drowsiness, dilated pupils, flushed dry skin, fever, tachycardia, delirium, hallucinations, and myoclonic or choreoathetoid movements. Convulsions, rhabdomyolysis, and hyperthermia may occur with a serious overdose, and complications such as renal failure and pancreatitis have been reported.

**B. Massive diphenhydramine** overdoses have been reported to cause QRS widening and myocardial depression similar to tricyclic antidepressant overdoses (see p 91).

**C. QT interval prolongation** and torsade-type atypical ventricular tachycardia (see p 14) have been associated with elevated serum levels of **terfenadine** or **astemizole.** Both of these drugs have been removed from the US market.

**IV. Diagnosis** is generally based on the history of ingestion and can usually be readily confirmed by the presence of typical anticholinergic syndrome. Comprehensive urine toxicology screening will detect most common antihistamines.

**A. Specific levels** are not generally available or useful.

**B. Other useful laboratory studies** include electrolytes, glucose, CPK, arterial blood gases or pulse oximetry, and ECG monitoring (diphenhydramine, terfenadine, or astemizole).

**V. Treatment**

**A. Emergency and supportive measures**

1. Maintain an open airway and assist ventilation if necessary (see pp 1–7).
2. Treat coma (p 18), seizures (p 22), hyperthermia (p 20), and atypical ventricular tachycardia (p 15) if they occur.
3. Monitor the patient for at least 6–8 hours after ingestion.

**B. Specific drugs and antidotes.** There is no specific antidote for antihistamine overdose. As for anticholinergic poisoning (see p 85), **physostigmine** has

**TABLE II–9. ANTIHISTAMINES**

| Drug | Usual Duration of Action (hr) | Usual Single Adult Dose (mg) | Sedation |
|---|---|---|---|
| **Ethanolamines** | | | |
| Bromodiphenhydramine | 4–6 | 12.5–25 | +++ |
| Carbinoxamine | 3–4 | 4–8 | ++ |
| Clemastine | 10–12 | 0.67–2.68 | ++ |
| Dimenhydrinate | 4–6 | 50–100 | +++ |
| Diphenhydramine | 4–6 | 25–50 | +++ |
| Diphenylpyraline | 6–8 | 5 | ++ |
| Doxylamine | 4–6 | 25 | +++ |
| Phenyltoloxamine | 6–8 | 50 | +++ |
| **Ethylenediamines** | | | |
| Pyrilamine | 4–6 | 25–50 | ++ |
| Thenyldiamine | 8 | 10 | ++ |
| Tripelennamine | 4–6 | 25–50 | ++ |
| **Alkylamines** | | | |
| Acrivastine | 6–8 | 8 | + |
| Brompheniramine | 4–6 | 4–8 | + |
| Chlorpheniramine | 4–6 | 4–8 | + |
| Dexbrompheniramine | 6–8 | 2–4 | + |
| Dexchlorpheniramine | 6–8 | 2–4 | + |
| Dimethindene | 8 | 1–2 | + |
| Pheniramine | 8–12 | 25–50 | + |
| Pyrrobutamine | 8–12 | 15 | + |
| Triprolidine | 4–6 | 2.5 | + |
| **Piperazines** | | | |
| Buclizine | 8 | 50 | |
| Cetirizine | 24 | 5–10 | +/– |
| Cinnarizine | 8 | 15–30 | + |
| Cyclizine | 4–6 | 25–50 | + |
| Flunarizine | 24 | 5–10 | + |
| Hydroxyzine | 20–25 | 25–50 | +++ |
| Meclizine | 12–24 | 25–50 | + |
| **Phenothiazines** | | | |
| Methdilazine | 6–12 | 4–8 | +++ |
| Promethazine | 4–8 | 25–50 | +++ |
| Trimeprazine | 6 | 2.5 | +++ |
| **Others** | | | |
| Astemizole[a] | 30–60 days | 10 | +/– |
| Azatidine | 12 | 1–2 | ++ |
| Cyproheptadine | 8 | 2–4 | + |
| Desloratadine | 24 | 5 | +/– |
| Fexofenadine | 24 | 60 | +/– |
| Loratadine | >24 | 10 | +/– |
| Phenindamine | 4–6 | 25 | +/– |
| Terfenadine[a] | 12 | 60 | +/– |

[a]Withdrawn from the US market because of reports of prolonged QT syndrome and torsade-type atypical ventricular tachycardia.

been used for treatment of severe delirium or tachycardia. However, because antihistamine overdoses carry a greater risk for seizures, physostigmine is not recommended routinely. **Sodium bicarbonate** (see p 423), 1–2 mEq/kg IV, may be useful for myocardial depression and QRS interval prolongation after a massive diphenhydramine overdose.

**C. Decontamination** (see p 45). Administer activated charcoal orally if conditions are appropriate (see Table I–38, p 51). Gastric lavage is not necessary after small to moderate ingestions if activated charcoal can be given promptly. Because of slowed gastrointestinal motility, gut decontamination procedures may be helpful even in late-presenting patients.

**D. Enhanced elimination.** Hemodialysis, hemoperfusion, peritoneal dialysis, and repeat-dose activated charcoal are not effective in removing antihistamines.

## ► ANTIMONY AND STIBINE

*Rais Vohra, MD*

**Antimony** is widely used as a hardening agent in soft metal alloys and alloys of lead; for compounding rubber; as a major flame retardant component (5–20%) of plastics; and as a coloring agent in dyes, varnishes, paints, and glazes. Exposure to antimony dusts and fumes may also occur during mining and refining of ores and from the discharge of firearms. Organic antimony compounds are used as antiparasitic drugs. Foreign or folk remedies may contain antimony potassium tartrate ("tartar emetic") (1). **Stibine** (antimony hydride, $SbH_3$) is a colorless gas with the odor of rotten eggs that is produced as a by-product when antimony-containing ore or furnace slag is treated with acid.

**I. Mechanism of toxicity.** The mechanism of antimony and stibine toxicity is not known. Because these compounds are chemically related to arsenic and arsine, their modes of action may be similar.

**A. Antimony** compounds probably act by binding to sulfhydryl groups, enhancing oxidative stress, and inactivating key enzymes. Ingested antimonials are also corrosive to gastrointestinal mucosal membranes.

**B. Stibine,** like arsine, may cause hemolysis. It is also an irritant gas.

**II. Toxic dose**

**A.** The lethal oral dose of metallic **antimony** in rats is 100 mg/kg body weight; the trivalent and pentavalent oxides are less toxic, with $LD_{50}$ in rats ranging from 3200–4000 mg/kg body weight. The recommended workplace limit (ACGIH TLV-TWA) for antimony is 0.5 mg/$m^3$ as an 8-hour time-weighted average. The air level considered immediately dangerous to life or health (IDLH) is 50 mg/$m^3$.

**B.** The recommended workplace limit (ACGIH TLV-TWA) for **stibine** is 0.1 ppm as an 8-hour time-weighted average. The air level considered immediately dangerous to life or health (IDLH) is 5 ppm.

**III. Clinical presentation**

**A. Acute ingestion of antimony** causes nausea, vomiting, hemorrhagic gastritis, and diarrhea ("cholera stibie"). Hepatitis and renal insufficiency may occur. Death is rare if the patient survives the initial gastroenteritis. Cardiac dysrhythmias (including torsade), pancreatitis, and arthralgias have been associated with the use of the organic antimonial compounds for treatment of parasitic infections (e.g. leishmaniasis).

**B. Acute stibine inhalation** causes acute hemolysis, resulting in anemia, jaundice, hemoglobinuria, and renal failure.

**C. Chronic exposure to antimony dusts and fumes** in the workplace is the most common type of exposure and may result in headache, anorexia, pneumonitis, peptic ulcers, and dermatitis (antimony spots). Sudden death presumably resulting from a direct cardiotoxic effect has been reported in workers exposed to antimony trisulfide. Based on evidence of in vitro genotoxicity and limited rodent carcinogenicity testing, antimony trioxide is a suspected carcinogen (IARC 2B).

**IV. Diagnosis** is based on a history of exposure and typical clinical presentation.

**A. Specific levels.** Urine antimony levels are normally below 2 mcg/L. Serum and whole-blood levels are not reliable and are no longer used. Urine concentrations correlate poorly with workplace exposure, but exposure to air concentrations greater than the TLV-TWA will increase urinary levels. Urinary antimony is increased after firearm discharge exposure. There is no established toxic antimony level after stibine exposure.

**B. Other useful investigations** include CBC, plasma-free hemoglobin, serum lactate dehydrogenase (LDH), free haptoglobin, electrolytes, BUN, creatinine, urinalysis for free hemoglobin, liver transaminases, bilirubin, prothrombin time, and 12-lead ECG. Chest radiography is recommended for chronic respiratory exposures.

**V. Treatment**

**A. Emergency and supportive measures**

1. **Antimony.** Large-volume intravenous fluid resuscitation may be necessary for shock caused by gastroenteritis (see p 15). Electrolyte abnormalities should be corrected, and intensive supportive care may be necessary with multiple organ failure.
2. **Stibine.** Blood transfusion may be necessary after massive hemolysis. Treat hemoglobinuria with fluids and bicarbonate as for rhabdomyolysis (see p 26).

**B. Specific drugs and antidotes.** There is no specific antidote. BAL (dimercaprol), dimercaptosuccinic acid (DMSA), and dimercaptopropanesulfonic acid (DMPS) have been proposed as chelators for antimony, although data in human poisoning are conflicting. Chelation therapy is not expected to be effective for stibine.

**C. Decontamination** (see p 45)

1. **Inhalation.** Remove the patient from exposure, and give supplemental oxygen if available. Protect rescuers from exposure.
2. **Ingestion** of antimony salts. Activated charcoal is probably not effective in light of its poor adsorption of antimony. Gastric lavage may be helpful if performed soon after a large ingestion.

**D. Enhanced elimination.** Hemodialysis, hemoperfusion, and forced diuresis are ***not*** effective at removing antimony or stibine. Exchange transfusion may be effective in treating massive hemolysis caused by stibine.

## ▶ ANTINEOPLASTIC AGENTS

*Susan Kim, PharmD*

Because of the inherently cytotoxic nature of most chemotherapeutic antineoplastic agents, overdoses are likely to be extremely serious. These agents are classified into nine categories (Table II–10). Other than iatrogenic errors, relatively few acute overdoses have been reported for these agents. Radiologic agents are not included in this chapter, and arsenic is discussed on p 115.

**I. Mechanism of toxicity.** In general, toxic effects are extensions of the pharmacologic properties of these drugs.

**A. Alkylating agents.** These drugs attack nucleophilic sites on DNA, resulting in alkylation and cross-linking and thus inhibiting replication and transcription. Binding to RNA or protein moieties appears to contribute little to cytotoxic effects.

**B. Antibiotics.** These drugs intercalate within base pairs in DNA, inhibiting DNA-directed RNA synthesis. Another potential mechanism may be the generation of cytotoxic free radicals.

C. **Antimetabolites.** These agents interfere with DNA synthesis at various stages. For example, methotrexate binds reversibly to dihydrofolate reductase, preventing synthesis of purine and pyrimidine nucleotides.
D. **Hormones.** Steroid hormones regulate the synthesis of steroid-specific proteins. The exact mechanism of antineoplastic action is unknown.
E. **Mitotic inhibitors.** These agents act in various ways to inhibit orderly mitosis, thereby arresting cell division.
F. **Monoclonal antibodies** target antigens specific to or overexpressed in cancerous cells. The antibodies may be directly cytotoxic or may be used to deliver radionuclides or cytotoxins to the target cells.
G. **Platinum** containing complexes produce intra- and/or interstrand Pt-DNA cross-links.
H. **Topoisomerase inhibitors** inhibit topoisomerase I, an enzyme that relieves torsional strain during DNA replication. The cleavable complex normally formed between DNA and topoisomerase I is stabilized by these drugs, resulting in breaks in single-stranded DNA.
I. **Miscellaneous.** The cytotoxic actions of other antineoplastic drugs result from a variety of mechanisms, including blockade of protein synthesis and inhibition of hormone release.
J. **Pharmacokinetics.** Most oral antineoplastic agents are readily absorbed, with peak levels reached within 1–2 hours of ingestion. As a result of rapid intracellular incorporation and the delayed onset of toxicity, pharmacokinetic values are usually of little utility in managing acute overdose. (See also Table II–59.)

II. **Toxic dose.** Because of the highly toxic nature of these agents (except for hormones), exposure to even therapeutic amounts should be considered potentially serious.

III. **Clinical presentation.** The organ systems affected by the various agents are listed in Table II–10. The most common sites of toxicity are the hematopoietic and gastrointestinal systems.
A. **Leukopenia** is the most common manifestation of bone marrow depression. Thrombocytopenia and anemia may also occur. Death may result from overwhelming infections or hemorrhagic diathesis. With alkylating agents, the lowest blood counts occur 1–4 weeks after exposure, whereas with antibiotics, antimetabolites, and mitotic inhibitors, the lowest blood counts occur 1–2 weeks after exposure.
B. **Gastrointestinal** toxicity is also very common. Nausea, vomiting, and diarrhea often accompany therapeutic administration, and severe ulcerative gastroenteritis and extensive fluid loss may occur.
C. **Extravasation** of some antineoplastic drugs at the intravenous injection site may cause severe local injury, with skin necrosis and sloughing.

IV. **Diagnosis** is usually based on the history. Because some of the most serious toxic effects may be delayed until several days after exposure, early clinical symptoms and signs may not be dramatic.
A. **Specific levels.** Not generally available. For methotrexate, see Table II–10, p 103.
B. **Other useful laboratory studies** include CBC with differential, platelet count, electrolytes, glucose, BUN and creatinine, liver enzymes, and prothrombin time. ECG may be indicated for cardiotoxic agents, and pulmonary function tests are indicated for agents with known pulmonary toxicity.

V. **Treatment**
A. **Emergency and supportive measures**
1. Maintain an open airway and assist ventilation if necessary (see pp 1–7).
2. Treat coma (see p 18), seizures (p 22), hypotension (p 15), and arrhythmias (pp 10–15) if they occur.
3. Treat nausea and vomiting with metoclopramide (see p 475) and fluid loss caused by gastroenteritis with intravenous crystalloid fluids.

TABLE II–10. ANTINEOPLASTIC DRUGS

| Drug | Major Site(s) of Toxicity[a] | Comments |
|---|---|---|
| **Alkylating agents** | | |
| Altretamine | G+, N+, M+ | Reversible peripheral sensory neuropathy. |
| Busulfan | D+, En+, G+, M+, N+, P++ | Acute overdose of 2.4 g was fatal in a 10 yo, and 140 mg resulted in pancytopenia in a 4 yo. High doses cause coma, seizures. Hemodialysis may be effective. Pulmonary fibrosis, adrenal insufficiency with chronic use. |
| Carmustine (BCNU) | D+, Ex+, G+, H+, M+, P+ | Flushing, hypotension, and tachycardia with rapid IV injection. |
| Chlorambucil | D+, G+, H+, M+ N++ | Seizures, confusion, coma reported after overdose. Acute ODs of 1.5–6.8 mg/kg in children caused seizures up to 3–4 hours postingestion. Not dialyzable. |
| Cyclophosphamide | Al++, C+, D+, En+, G++, M++, R+ | Hemodialysis effective. Acetylcysteine and 2 mercaptoethanesulfonate have been used investigationally to reduce hemorrhagic cystitis. |
| Dacarbazine | Al+, An+, En+, G++, H+, M+, N+, Ex± | May produce flu-like syndrome. Photosensitivity reported. |
| Estramustine | En±, G±, H±, M± | Has weak estrogenic and alkylating activity. |
| Ifosfamide | M++, N+, Al++, G+, R++ | Hemorrhagic cystitis, somnolence, confusion, hallucinations, status epilepticus, coma seen during therapy. Combined hemodialysis and hemoperfusion reduced serum levels by 84%. Methylene blue may protect against and treat encephalopathy. |
| Lomustine (CCNU) | Al+, G+, H+, M+, P+ | Thrombocytopenia, leukopenia, liver and lymph node enlargement after overdose. 1400 mg taken over a week fatal in an adult. |
| Mechlorethamine | D+, G++, M++, N+, Ex+ | Lymphocytopenia may occur within 24 hours. Watch for hyperuricemia. |
| Melphalan | An+, G+, M+ | Hemodialysis may be effective although of questionable need (normal half-life only 90 minutes). |
| Thiotepa | An+, G++, M++ | Bone marrow suppression usually very severe. |
| Temozolomide | G+, M+, N+ | Relatively benign safety profile. |
| **Antibiotics** | | |
| Bleomycin | An++, D++, G+, P++ | Pulmonary fibrosis with chronic use. Febrile reaction in 20–25% of patients. |
| Dactinomycin | Al++, D+, G++, M++, Ex++ | A 10-fold overdose in a 1-year-old child resulted in pancytopenia, acute renal failure, choreoathetosis. Highly corrosive to soft tissue. |
| Daunorubicin | Al++, An+, C++, G++, M++, Ex++ | Congestive cardiomyopathy may occur after total cumulative dose > 600 $mg/m^2$. |

| | | |
|---|---|---|
| Doxorubicin | Al++, An+, C++, D+, Ex++, G++, M++, Ex++ | Cardiotoxicity and cardiomyopathy may occur after total cumulative dose > 550 mg/m$^2$. Arrhythmias after acute overdose. Hemoperfusion may be effective. Dexrazoxane is usually given for cardioprotection. |
| Epirubicin | C++, Ex++, G+, M++ | Death from multiorgan failure reported in a 63-year-old woman after a single 320 mg/m$^2$ dose. Risk of congestive heart failure increases steeply after cumulative dose of 900 mg/m$^2$. |
| Idarubicin | C++, G+, M++, Ex++ | Congestive heart failure, acute life-threatening arrhythmias may occur. |
| Mitomycin | Al+, D+, G++, H+, M+, P+, R+, Ex++ | Hemolytic uremic syndrome reported with therapeutic doses. |
| Mitoxantrone | An+, C+, G++, M++ | Four reported overdosed patients died from severe leukopenia and infection. Reversible cardiomyopathy in one overdose case. Hemoperfusion was ineffective. |
| **Antimetabolites** | | |
| Capecitabine | D+, G+, M+ | Prodrug, converted to 5-fluorouracil. |
| Cladribine | M++, N++, R++ | Irreversible paraparesis/quadriparesis seen in high doses. |
| Clofarabine | C+, D+, G++, H+, M++ | Systemic inflammatory response syndrome, capillary leak possible. |
| Cytarabine | An+, En+, G+, H+, M+, N++, P++ | "Cytarabine syndrome": fever myalgia, bone pain, rash, malaise. Fatal pulmonary edema seen during treatment. |
| Floxuridine | Al+, G++, M++ | |
| Fludarabine | G+, M++, N++, R+ | Blindness, coma, death at high doses. |
| 5-Fluorouracil | Al+, C+, D+, G++, M++, N+ | Acute cerebellar syndrome seen. Coronary vasospasm with angina may occur. |
| Gemcitabine | An+, D+, H+, M++, P++, R+ | Can cause bronchospasm, severe ARDS. |
| 6-Mercaptopurine | D+, G+, H++, M+ | Hemodialysis removes drug but of questionable need (half-life 20–60 minutes). A 22-month-old child who ingested 86 mg/kg had severe neutropenia. Nadir at 11 days. |
| Methotrexate | Al+, D+, G++, H+, M++, N+, P+,R+ | Peak serum level 1–2 hours after oral dose. Folinic acid (leucovorin; see p 468) is a specific antidote. Hemoperfusion questionably effective. Urinary alkalinization and repeat dose charcoal may be helpful. |
| Pemetrexed | An+, D+, G++, H+, M++, P+ | Folic acid antagonist. Leucovorin may be useful. Patients must take daily vitamin $B_{12}$, folic acid. |
| Pentostatin | D+, G+, M+, N++, R++, | Central nervous system depression, convulsions, coma seen at high doses. |
| Rasburicase | An++, G+, M+ | Hemolysis in G6PD-deficient pts. Methemoglobinemia reported. |
| 6-Thioguanine | G+, H+, M+, R+ | Hemodialysis probably ineffective owing to rapid intracellular incorporation. |

(*continued*)

TABLE II–10. ANTINEOPLASTIC DRUGS (CONTINUED)

| Drug | Major Site(s) of Toxicity[a] | Comments |
|---|---|---|
| **Hormones** | | |
| **Androgens** | | |
| Testolactone | En±, G± | Toxicity unlikely after single acute overdose. |
| **Antiandrogens** | | |
| Flutamide, bicalutamide, nilutamide | G+, H+, P+ (nilutamide) | Gynecomastia. Aniline metabolite of flutamide has caused methemoglobinemia (see p 262). Nilutamide 13 g ingestion resulted in no evidence of toxicity. |
| **Antiestrogens** | | |
| Tamoxifen, toremifene, fulvestrant | Al±, D±, En±, G± | Acute toxic effects unlikely. Tremors, hyperreflexia, unsteady gait, qt prolongation with high doses of tamoxifen. |
| **Progestins** | | |
| Medroxyprogesterone, megestrol | An±, En±, G± | Acute toxic effects unlikely. May induce porphyria in susceptible patients. |
| **Aromatase Inhibitors** | | |
| Anastrozole, exemestane, letrozole | G± | Acute toxic effects unlikely. |
| **Gonadotropin releasing hormone analogs** | | |
| Goserelin, histrelin, leuprolide, triptorelin | En+ | Acute toxic effects unlikely. Initial increase in luteinizing hormone, follicle-stimulating hormone. |
| **Mitotic inhibitors** | | |
| Docetaxel | An+, D+, G+, M++, N+ | Severe fluid retention in 6% of patients. |
| Etoposide | An+, G+, M++ | Myelosuppression major toxicity. Dystonic reaction reported. |
| Paclitaxel | Al++, An++, C+,G+, M++, N+ | Severe hypersensitivity reactions, including death, reported. Hypotension, bradycardia, ECG abnormalities, conduction abnormalities may occur. Fatal myocardial infarction 15 h into infusion reported. |

| | | |
|---|---|---|
| Teniposide | An+, G+, M++, Ex+ | One report of sudden death from hypotension, cardiac arrhythmias. Hypotension from rapid IV injection. |
| Vinblastine | G+, M++, N+, Ex++ | Myelosuppression, ileus, SIADH reported after overdose. Plasma exchange used after OD. Fatal if given intrathecally. |
| Vincristine sulfate | G+, M±, N++, Ex++ | Delayed (up to 9 days) seizures, delirium, coma reported after overdoses. Fatal if given intrathecally. Glutamic acid 500 mg TID orally may reduce the incidence of neurotoxicity. |
| Vinorelbine | G+, M++, N+, Ex++ | Severe granulocytopenia |
| **Monoclonal antibodies** | | |
| Alemtuzumab | An+, D+, G+, M++ | Can cause severe prolonged lymphopenia. Serious risk of fatal bacterial or opportunistic infections. |
| Bevacizumab | C+, G+, M+, N+, P+, R+ | Fatal GI perforation, wound dehiscence, hemorrhagic events including hemoptysis seen during therapy. |
| Cetuximab | An++, D++, G+, N+ | Potentially fatal infusion reaction in 3% of patients |
| Gemtuzumab ozogamicin | An+, H+, M++ | Associated with hepatic veno-occlusive disease. |
| Ibritumomab tiuxetan | An++, G+, M++, P+ | Given with radiolabeled drug. Severe, fatal infusion reactions reported. |
| Rituximab | An++, C+, D++, M+, P+, R++ | Severe, fatal hypersensitivity reaction possible. Tumor lysis syndrome has caused acute renal failure. Potentially fatal mucocutaneous reactions reported. |
| Tositumomab | An++, G+, M++ | Given with radiolabeled iodine-tositumomab complex. May cause hypothyroidism. |
| Trastuzumab | An++, C++, G+, P+ | Can precipitate congestive heart failure. Severe, fatal hypersensitivity and infusion reactions reported. |
| **Platinum complex** | | |
| Carboplatin | An+, G++, M++, R+ | Peripheral neuropathy in 4% of patients. Deaths from renal, hepatic failure, thrombocytopenia, thrombotic microangiopathic hemolytic anemia. |
| Cisplatin | An+, G++, M+, N+, P+, R++ | Ototoxic, nephrotoxic. A 750 mg acute overdose was fatal. Good hydration essential. Hemodialysis not effective. Fosfomycin, NAC, and sodium thiosulfate have been suggested for reducing cytotoxic effects. |
| Oxaliplatin | An+, Ex+, G+, M+, N++ | 74% experience neuropathy. OD of 500 mg resulted in fatality from respiratory failure, bradycardia. |
| **Topoisomerase inhibitors** | | |
| Irinotecan | G++, M+, P+ | Severe diarrhea. Cholinergic syndrome during infusion. |
| Topotecan | G+, M++, P+ | Severe thrombocytopenia, anemia common. Fourfold increase in clearance seen during hemodialysis. |
| **Miscellaneous** | | |
| Aldesleukin (Interleukin 2) | C++, G+, H+, M+, N+, P+, R+ | Commonly causes capillary leak syndrome resulting in severe hypotension. |

*(continued)*

TABLE I–10. ANTINEOPLASTIC DRUGS (CONTINUED)

| Drug | Major Site(s) of Toxicity[a] | Comments |
|---|---|---|
| Asparaginase | An++, En+, G+, H++, N++, R+ | Bleeding diathesis, hyperglycemia, pancreatitis. |
| Azacitidine | G+, H+, M+, R+ | |
| BCG (Intravesical) | G+ | Attenuated *Mycobacterium bovis*. Bladder irritation common. Risk of sepsis in immunocompromised patients. |
| Bexarotene | D+, G+, M+, N+ | Serious lipid and thyroid abnormalities, fatal pancreatitis during therapy. |
| Bortezomib | C+, G+, M+, N+ | Peripheral neuropathy, orthostatic hypotension reported. |
| Denileukin | An+, C+, D+, G+, N+ | Can cause vascular leak syndrome (hypoalbuminemia, edema, hypotension). |
| Erlotinib | D+, G+, H+, P++ | Fatal interstitial lung disease reported. |
| Gefitinib | D+, G+, H+, P++ | Interstitial lung disease reported in 1% of patients; fatal in 1/3 of cases. |
| Hydroxyurea | Al+, D+, G+,H,+ M++ | Leukopenia, anemia more common than thrombocytopenia. Peak serum level within 2 h of oral dose. |
| Imatinib | G+, H+, M+ | Fluid retention and edema, and muscle cramps. |
| Levamisole | G+, M+, N+ | May have nicotinic and muscarinic effects at cholinergic receptors. Gastroenteritis, dizziness, headache after 2.5 mg/kg dose reported. Fatality reported after ingestion of 15 mg/kg in a 3-year-old and 32 mg/kg in an adult. Disulfiram-like ethanol interaction may also occur. |
| Mitotane | Al+, D+, En++, G++, N++ | Adrenal suppression; glucocorticoid replacement essential during stress. |
| Pegaspargase | An++, G+, H+, N+ | Bleeding diathesis. |
| Porfimer | D+, G+ | Used in conjunction with phototherapy: risk of photosensitivity. |
| Procarbazine hydrochloride | An+, D+, En+, G++, M++, N++ | Monoamine oxidase inhibitor activity. Disulfiram-like ethanol interaction. Coma, seizures during therapy. |
| Streptozocin | En+, G+, H+, M+, R++ | Destroys pancreatic beta islet cells, may produce acute diabetes mellitus. Niacinamide (see p 483) may be effective in preventing islet cell destruction. Renal toxicity in two-thirds of patients. |
| Tretinoin | C+, D+, G+, M+, N+, P+ | Retinoic acid-APL syndrome seen in ~25% of patients with acute promyelocytic leukemia: fever, dyspnea, pulmonary infiltrates, and pleural or pericardial effusions. Fatal multiorgan thrombosis reported. |

[a]Al = alopecia; An = anaphylaxis, allergy or drug fever; C = cardiac; D = dermatologic; En = endocrine; Ex = extravasation risk; G = gastrointestinal; H = hepatic; M = myelosuppressive; N = neurologic; P = pulmonary; R = renal; + = mild to moderate severity; ++ = severe toxicity; ± = minimal.

4. **Bone marrow depression** should be treated with the assistance of an experienced hematologist or oncologist.
5. **Extravasation.** Immediately stop the infusion and withdraw as much fluid as possible by negative pressure on the syringe. Then give the following specific treatment:
   a. **Dactinomycin, daunorubicin, doxorubicin, idarubicin, and mitoxantrone.** Apply ice compresses to the extravasation site for 15 minutes 4 times daily for 3 days. For **mitomycin**, apply moderate heat. Topical application of dimethyl sulfoxide (DMSO) may be beneficial (commercially available 50% solution is less concentrated than those used in experimental studies but may be tried). There is no justification for injection of hydrocortisone or sodium bicarbonate.
   b. **Mechlorethamine** (and concentrated **dacarbazine** and **cisplatin**). Infiltrate the site of extravasation with 10 mL of sterile 2.5% sodium thiosulfate (dilute 1 mL of 25% thiosulfate with sterile water to a volume of 10 mL).
   c. **Etoposide, paclitaxel, vincristine,** or **vinblastine.** Place a heating pad over the area and apply heat intermittently for 24 hours; elevate the limb. Local injection of hyaluronidase (150–900 units) may be beneficial. Do not use ice packs.

B. **Specific drugs and antidotes.** Very few specific treatments or antidotes are available (Table II–10).

C. **Decontamination** (see p 45). Administer activated charcoal orally if conditions are appropriate (see Table I–38, p 51). Gastric lavage is not necessary after small to moderate ingestions if activated charcoal can be given promptly.

D. **Enhanced elimination.** Because of the rapid intracellular incorporation of most of these agents, dialysis and other extracorporeal removal procedures are generally not effective (see Table II–10 for exceptions).

## ► ANTIPSYCHOTIC DRUGS, INCLUDING PHENOTHIAZINES

*Grant D. Lackey, PharmD, PhD*

Phenothiazines, butyrophenones, and other related drugs are used widely to treat psychosis and agitated depression. In addition, some of these drugs (eg, prochlorperazine, promethazine, and droperidol) are used as antiemetic agents. Suicidal overdoses are common, but because of the high toxic-therapeutic ratio, acute overdose seldom results in death. A large number of newer agents that often are referred to as "atypical antipsychotics" have been developed. Atypical antipsychotics differ from other neuroleptics in their binding to dopamine receptors and their effects on dopamine mediated behaviors. Overdose experience with these agents is limited. Table II–11 describes available antipsychotic agents.

I. **Mechanism of toxicity.** A variety of pharmacologic effects are responsible for toxicity involving primarily the cardiovascular and central nervous systems.

A. **Cardiovascular.** Anticholinergic effects may produce tachycardia. Alpha-adrenergic blockade may cause hypotension, especially orthostatic hypotension. With very large overdoses of some agents, quinidinelike membrane-depressant effects on the heart may occur. Many of these agents can cause QT prolongation (see p 14).

B. **Central nervous system.** Centrally mediated sedation and anticholinergic effects contribute to CNS depression. Alpha-adrenergic blockade causes small pupils despite anticholinergic effects on other systems. Extrapyramidal dystonic reactions are relatively common with therapeutic doses and probably are caused by central dopamine receptor blockade. The seizure threshold

**TABLE II–11. ANTIPSYCHOTIC DRUGS**

| Drug | Type[a] | Usual Adult Daily Dose (mg) | Toxicity[b] |
|---|---|---|---|
| Aripiprazole | O | 10–30 | A, E, H, Q |
| Chlorpromazine | P | 200–2000 | A, E, H, Q |
| Chlorprothixene | T | 75–200 | E |
| Clozapine | D | 100–900 | A, H |
| Droperidol | B | 2–10 | E, Q |
| Ethopropazine | P | 50–400 | A, H |
| Fluphenazine | P | 2.5–20 | E, A |
| Haloperidol | B | 1–100 | E, Q |
| Loxapine | D | 60–100 | E |
| Mesoridazine | P | 150–400 | A, H, Q |
| Molindone | O | 50–225 | E |
| Olanzapine | D | 5–20 | A, E, H |
| Perphenazine | P | 10–30 | E |
| Pimozide | O | 2–10 | E, Q |
| Prochlorperazine[c] | P | 15–40 | E |
| Promethazine[c] | P | 25–200 | A, E |
| Quetiapine | D | 150–750 | A, E, H, Q |
| Risperidone | O | 4–16 | E, H, Q |
| Thioridazine | P | 150–300 | A, H, Q |
| Thiothixene | T | 5–60 | E |
| Trifluoperazine | P | 1–40 | E |
| Trimethobenzamide[c] | O | 600–1000 | A, E |
| Ziprasidone | O | 60–160 | A, E, H, Q |

[a]P = phenothiazine; T = thiothixine; B = butyrophenone; D = dibenzodiazepine; O = other.
[b]E = extrapyramidal reactions; A = anticholinergic effects; H = hypotension; Q = QT interval prolongation.
[c]Used primarily as an antiemetic.

may be lowered by unknown mechanisms. Temperature regulation is also disturbed, resulting in poikilothermia.

**C. Pharmacokinetics.** These drugs have large volumes of distribution (Vd = 10–30 L/kg), and most have long elimination half-lives (eg, chlorpromazine = 18–30 hours). Elimination is largely by hepatic metabolism. See Table II–55, p 357.

**II. Toxic dose.** Extrapyramidal reactions, anticholinergic side effects, and orthostatic hypotension are often seen with therapeutic doses. Tolerance to the sedating effects of the antipsychotics is well described, and patients on chronic therapy may tolerate much larger doses than other persons.

**A.** Typical daily doses are given in Table II–11.

**B.** The toxic dose after acute ingestion is highly variable. Serious CNS depression and hypotension may occur after ingestion of 200–1000 mg of chlorpromazine in children or 3–5 g in adults.

III. **Clinical presentation.** Major toxicity is manifested in the cardiovascular and central nervous systems. Also, anticholinergic intoxication (see p 85) may occur as a result of ingestion of benztropine (Cogentin) or other co-administered drugs.

A. **Mild intoxication** causes sedation, small pupils, and orthostatic hypotension. Anticholinergic manifestations include dry mouth, absence of sweating, tachycardia, and urinary retention. Paradoxically, clozapine causes hypersalivation through an unknown mechanism.

B. **Severe intoxication** may cause coma, seizures, and respiratory arrest. The ECG usually shows QT interval prolongation and occasionally QRS prolongation (particularly with thioridazine [Mellaril]). Hypothermia or hyperthermia may occur. Clozapine can cause a prolonged confusional state and rarely cardiac toxicity. Risperidone, aripiprazole, and quetiapine can cause QT interval prolongation, but delirium is less severe.

C. **Extrapyramidal** dystonic side effects of therapeutic doses include torticollis, jaw muscle spasm, oculogyric crisis, rigidity, bradykinesia, and pill-rolling tremor.

D. Patients on chronic antipsychotic medication may develop the **neuroleptic malignant syndrome** (see p 21), which is characterized by rigidity, hyperthermia, sweating, lactic acidosis, and rhabdomyolysis.

E. Clozapine use has been associated with agranulocytosis.

IV. **Diagnosis** is based on a history of ingestion and findings of sedation, small pupils, hypotension, and QT interval prolongation. Dystonias in children should always suggest the possibility of antipsychotic exposure, often as a result of intentional administration by parents. Phenothiazines are occasionally visible on plain abdominal x-rays (see Table I–35).

A. **Specific levels.** Quantitative blood levels are not routinely available and do not help in diagnosis or treatment. Qualitative screening may easily detect phenothiazines in urine or gastric juice, but butyrophenones such as haloperidol are usually not included in toxicologic screens (see Table I–30, p 40).

B. **Other useful laboratory studies** include electrolytes, glucose, BUN, creatinine, CPK, arterial blood gases or oximetry, abdominal x-ray (to look for radiopaque pills), and chest x-ray.

V. **Treatment.**

A. **Emergency and supportive measures**

1. Maintain an open airway and assist ventilation if necessary (see pp 1–7). Administer supplemental oxygen.
2. Treat coma (p 18), seizures (p 22), hypotension (p 15), and hyperthermia (p 20) if they occur.
3. Monitor vital signs and ECG for at least 6 hours and admit the patient for at least 24 hours if there are signs of significant intoxication. Children with antipsychotic intoxication should be evaluated for possible intentional abuse.

B. **Specific drugs and antidotes.** There is no specific antidote.

1. **Dystonic reactions.** Give diphenhydramine, 0.5–1 mg/kg IM or IV (see p 442), or benztropine (see p 422).
2. QRS interval prolongation. Treat quinidine-like cardiotoxic effects with bicarbonate, 1–2 mEq/kg IV (see p 423).
3. **Hypotension** from these dugs probably involves vasodilation caused by alpha-1 receptor blockade. Treat with IV fluids and, if needed, a vasoconstrictor such as norepinephrine or phenylephrine. Theoretically, drugs with beta-2 activity (eg, epinephrine, isoproterenol) may worsen hypotension.
4. **QT prolongation and torsade** may respond to magnesium infusion or overdrive pacing (see p 14).

C. **Decontamination** (see p 45). Administer activated charcoal orally if conditions are appropriate (see Table I–38, p 51). Gastric lavage is not necessary after small to moderate ingestions if activated charcoal can be given promptly.

D. **Enhanced elimination.** Owing to extensive tissue distribution, these drugs are not effectively removed by dialysis or hemoperfusion. Repeat-dose activated charcoal has not been evaluated.

# ▶ ANTISEPTICS AND DISINFECTANTS

*Kerry Schwarz, PharmD*

**Antiseptics** are applied to living tissue to kill or prevent the growth of microorganisms. **Disinfectants** are applied to inanimate objects to destroy pathogenic microorganisms. Despite their unproven worth, they are used widely in households, the food industry, and hospitals. This chapter describes toxicity caused by **chlorhexidine, glutaraldehyde, hexylresorcinol, hydrogen peroxide, ichthammol,** and **potassium permanganate.** These agents are often used as dilute solutions that usually cause little or no toxicity. Hexylresorcinol is commonly found in throat lozenges. Ichthammol is found in many topical salves. Descriptions of the toxicity of other antiseptics and disinfectants appear elsewhere in this book, including the following: hypochlorite (see p 162), iodine (p 227), isopropyl alcohol (p 234), mercurochrome (p 253), phenol (p 303), and pine oil (p 219).

**I. Mechanism of toxicity**

**A. Chlorhexidine** is commonly found in dental rinses, mouthwashes, skin cleansers, and a variety of cosmetics. Many preparations also contain isopropyl alcohol. Systemic absorption of chlorhexidine salts is minimal. Ingestion of products with a concentration less than 0.12% is not likely to cause more than minor irritation, but higher concentrations have caused corrosive injury.

**B. Glutaraldehyde** (pH 3–4) is used to disinfect medical equipment, as a tissue preservative, and topically as an antifungal and is found in some x-ray solutions. It is highly irritating to the skin and respiratory tract and has caused allergic contact dermatitis with repeated exposures.

**C. Hexylresorcinol** is related to phenol but is much less toxic, although alcohol-based solutions have vesicant properties.

**D. Hydrogen peroxide** is an oxidizing agent, but it is very unstable and readily breaks down to oxygen and water. Generation of oxygen gas in closed body cavities can potentially cause mechanical distension that results in gastric or intestinal perforation, as well as venous or arterial gas embolization. Hydrogen peroxide is found in many dental products, including mouth rinses and tooth whiteners, skin disinfectants, hair products, and earwax removers, and has many industrial uses. In veterinary medicine it is used to induce emesis.

**E. Ichthammol** (ichthyol, ammonium ichthosulfonate) contains about 10% sulfur in the form of organic sulfonates and is keratolytic to tissues.

**F. Potassium permanganate** is an oxidant, and the crystalline form and concentrated solutions are corrosive owing to the release of potassium hydroxide when potassium permanganate comes in contact with water.

**II. Toxic dose**

**A. Chlorhexidine** ingestions of less than 4% are expected to cause irritation, and ingestion of 150 mL of 20% solution caused esophageal damage and hepatic injury.

**B.** The lethal dose of **glutaraldehyde** is estimated to be from 50 mg/kg to 5 g/kg. Topical application of 10% solutions can cause dermatitis, and 2% solutions have caused ocular damage.

**C. Hexylresorcinol** is used in some antihelminthics, in doses of 400 mg (for children age 1–7 years) to 1 g (older children and adults). Most lozenges contain only about 2–4 mg.

**D. Hydrogen peroxide** for household use is available in 3–5% solutions and causes only mild throat and gastric irritation with ingestion of less than 1 oz. However, gas embolization has occurred with low concentrations used in surgical irrigations. Concentrations above 10% are found in some hair-bleaching solutions and are potentially corrosive. Most reported deaths have been associated with ingestion of undiluted 35% hydrogen peroxide, marketed as "hyperoxygen therapy" in health food stores or "food grade" in industry.

**E. Potassium permanganate** solutions of greater than 1:5000 strength may cause corrosive burns.

**III. Clinical presentation.** Most low-concentration antiseptic ingestions are benign, and mild irritation is self-limited. Spontaneous vomiting and diarrhea may occur, especially after a large-volume ingestion.

**A.** Exposure to **concentrated** antiseptic solutions may cause corrosive burns on the skin and mucous membranes, and oropharyngeal, esophageal, or gastric injury may occur. Glottic edema has been reported after ingestion of concentrated potassium permanganate.

**B.** Permanganate may also cause **methemoglobinemia** (see p 262).

**C. Hydrogen peroxide** ingestion may cause gastric distension and, rarely, perforation. Severe corrosive injury and **air emboli** have been reported with ingestion of the concentrated forms and may be caused by the entry of gas through damaged gastric mucosa or oxygen gas liberation within the venous or arterial circulation.

**IV. Diagnosis** is based on a history of exposure and the presence of mild gastrointestinal upset or frank corrosive injury. Solutions of potassium permanganate are dark purple, and skin and mucous membranes are often characteristically stained.

**A. Specific levels.** Drug levels in body fluids are not generally useful or available.

**B. Other useful laboratory studies** include electrolytes, glucose, methemoglobin level (for potassium permanganate exposure), and upright chest x-ray (for suspected gastric perforation).

**V. Treatment**

**A. Emergency and supportive measures**

1. In patients who have ingested concentrated solutions, monitor the airway for swelling and intubate if necessary.
2. Consult a gastroenterologist for possible endoscopy after ingestions of corrosive agents such as concentrated hydrogen peroxide and potassium permanganate. Most ingestions are benign, and mild irritation is self-limited.
3. Consider **hyperbaric oxygen** treatment for gas emboli associated with concentrated peroxide ingestion.

**B. Specific drugs and antidotes.** No specific antidotes are available for irritant or corrosive effects. If **methemoglobinemia** occurs, administer methylene blue (see p 473).

**C. Decontamination** (see p 45)

1. **Ingestion** of concentrated corrosive agents (see also p 157)
   - **a.** Dilute immediately with water or milk.
   - **b.** Do ***not*** induce vomiting because of the risk of corrosive injury. Perform gastric lavage cautiously.
   - **c.** Activated charcoal and cathartics are not effective.
2. **Eyes and skin.** Irrigate the eyes and skin with copious amounts of tepid water. Remove contaminated clothing.

**D. Enhanced elimination.** Enhanced elimination methods are neither necessary nor effective.

## ► ANTIVIRAL AND ANTIRETROVIRAL AGENTS

*Olga F. Woo, PharmD*

Human immunodeficiency virus (HIV) infection was first reported in 1981. The search for effective anti-HIV treatment began in 1987 with zidovudine (AZT) as a single-agent regimen. In 1994 the first protease inhibitor, saquinavir, was introduced. More agents and different classes of antiretroviral agents were developed later (Table II–12). Fusion inhibitors (a new class of agents) are usually reserved for treatment of advanced HIV infection; they interfere with HIV-1 entry into cells by inhibiting the fusion of viral and cellular membranes.

**TABLE II–12. ANTIVIRAL AND ANTIRETROVIRAL DRUGS**

| Drug | Half-Life | Toxic Dose or Serum Level | Toxicity |
|---|---|---|---|
| **Antiherpes drugs** | | | |
| Acyclovir | 2.5–3.3 h | Chronic | High-dose chronic therapy has caused crystalluria and renal failure, leukopenia. Coma, seizures, renal failure after large acute overdoses. Hallucinations and confusion after IV administration. |
| Cidofovir | | 16.3 and 17.4 mg/kg (case reports) | No renal dysfunction after treatment with probenecid and IV hydration. |
| Famciclovir | 2–2.3 h | — | Prodrug metabolized to active penciclovir. |
| Foscarnet | 3.3–4 h | 1.14–8 times recommended dose (average 4 times) | Seizures, renal impairment. One patient had seizures and died after receiving 12.5 g daily for 3 days. |
| Ganciclovir | 3.5 h (IV)<br>4.8 h (oral) | Adults: 5–7 g or 25 mg/kg IV | Neutropenia, thrombocytopenia, pancytopenia, increased serum creatinine; 9 mg/kg IV caused a seizure; 10 mg/kg IV daily caused hepatitis.<br>Children: 1 g instead of 31 mg in a 21-month-old had no toxic effect; an 18-month-old received 60 mg/kg IV, was treated with exchange transfusion, and had no effect; a 4-month-old received 500 mg, was treated with peritoneal dialysis and had no effect; 40 mg in a 2 kg infant caused hepatitis. |
| Penciclovir | | | Extensive intracellular metabolism. |
| Trifluridine | | 15–30 mg/kg IV | Reversible bone marrow toxicity reported after 3–5 courses of IV treatment. Systemic absorption is negligible after ophthalmic instillation. Ingestion of contents of one bottle (7.5 mL, 75 mg) unlikely to cause any adverse effects. |
| Valacyclovir | | | Prodrug promptly converted to acyclovir. |
| Vidarabine | Rapid deamination to ara-hypoxanthine metabolite, whose half-life is 2.4–3.3 h | Chronic 1–20 mg/kg/day IV for 10–15 days | Nausea, vomiting, diarrhea, dizziness, ataxia, tremor, confusion, hallucinations, psychosis; decreased Hct, Hgb, WBC, platelets; increased AST, ALT, LDH. Poorly absorbed orally; no toxicity expected if one tube (3.5 g, 105 mg) ingested. |
| **Nucleoside (or nucleotide) reverse transcriptase inhibitors (NRTI)** | | | Lactic acidosis, mitochondrial toxicity, hepatotoxicity. |
| Abacavir | 1.54 ± 0.63 h | Chronic | Diarrhea, nausea, vomiting; hypersensitivity (fatal reactions reported); perioral paresthesias. |
| Didanosine (ddI) | 1.5 ± 0.4 h | Chronic | Diarrhea, pancreatitis, peripheral neuropathy, salt overload with buffered product. |
| Emtricitabine (FTC) | 10 h | Chronic | Lactic acidosis and severe hepatomegaly with steatosis. |
| Lamivudine (3TC) | 5–7 h | Chronic | Headaches, nausea. |

| | | | |
|---|---|---|---|
| Stavudine (d4T) | 1.15 h IV<br>1.44 h PO | Chronic | Hepatic steatosis, lactic acidosis, peripheral neuropathy. |
| Tenofovir[a] | 17 h | Chronic | Diarrhea, flatulence, nausea, vomiting. |
| Zalcitabine (ddC) | 1–3 h | Chronic | Oral ulcers, peripheral neuropathy. |
| Zidovudine (AZT) | 0.5–1.5 h | Chronic | Anemia, fatigue, headaches, nausea, neutropenia, neuropathy, myopathy. |
| **Non-nucleoside reverse transcriptase inhibitors (NNRTI)** | | | Hepatotoxicity, rash. |
| Delavirdine | 5.8 h (range 2–11) | Chronic | Hepatotoxicity, rash. |
| Efavirenz | 40–76 h | Chronic | CNS effects: confusion, disengagement, dizziness, hallucinations, insomnia, somnolence, vivid dreams. |
| Nevirapine | 45 h single dose; 25–30 h multiple doses | Chronic | Hepatotoxicity, rash. |
| **Protease inhibitors (PI)** | | | Dyslipidemias, insulin resistance (diabetes mellitus), hepatotoxicity, lipodystrophy; osteoporosis. |
| Amprenavir | 7.1–10.6 h | Chronic | Diarrhea, nausea, perioral/oral paresthesias, rash. Liquid product contains propylene glycol. |
| Atazanavir | 6.5–7.9 h | Chronic | Commonly causes elevated bilirubin; concentration- and dose-dependent prolongation of PR interval. |
| Fosamprenavir | 7.7 h | Chronic | Contains a sulfonamide moiety. Skin rash commonly occurs: onset usually 11 days, duration of 13 days. One case of Stevens-Johnson syndrome. Spontaneous bleeding may occur in hemophiliacs. |
| Indinavir | 1.8 h | Chronic | Hyperbilirubinemia, kidney stones, nausea. |
| Lopinavir | 5–6 h | Chronic | Diarrhea, nausea, increased cholesterol and triglycerides, and GGT. Solution contains 42.4% alcohol. |
| Nelfinavir | 3–5 h | Chronic | Diarrhea, nausea, vomiting. |
| Ritonavir | 2–4 h | Chronic | Diarrhea, nausea, vomiting, significant drug interactions. |
| Saquinavir | ? | Chronic | Abdominal pain, diarrhea, nausea; fetal harm during first trimester of pregnancy. |
| Tipranavir | 5.5 h | Chronic | Increased risk for hepatotoxicity in patients with chronic hepatitis B or hepatitis C. |
| **Fusion inhibitors** | | | |
| Enfuvirtide | 3.8 ± 0.6 h | Chronic | Increased risk for a bacterial pneumonia to occur; infection at injection site (abscess, cellulitis). Does not inhibit CYP450 enzymes. |

[a]Tenofovir is a nucleotide reverse transcriptase inhibitor (NtRTI).

The use of combinations of antiviral drugs with different mechanisms of action in highly active antiretroviral therapy (HAART) regimens has dramatically improved survival in patients with HIV infection. Acute single ingestions are infrequent, and toxicity has been generally mild. Chronic toxicity, however, commonly occurs.

Antiviral/retroviral drugs that are metabolized mainly via the hepatic cytochrome P-450 isoenzyme system may be associated with clinically significant drug interactions involving other antiviral/retroviral, concomitant drugs, and complementary (dietary supplements-herbals) treatments (eg, St. John's Wort).

I. **Mechanism of toxicity.** The mechanism underlying toxic effects varies with the agent and is usually an extension of its pharmacologic effect.

   A. **Neurotoxicity** may be the result of inhibition of mitochondrial DNA polymerase and altered mitochondrial cell function.

   B. **Hepatic steatosis, severe lactic acidosis,** and **lipodystrophy** may be due to inhibition of DNA polymerase-gamma, which depletes mitochondrial DNA, causing mitochondrial dysfunction. Mitochondrial RNA formation may also be inhibited.

   C. Acyclovir crystal deposition in the tubular lumen leading to an obstructive nephropathy may cause **acute renal failure.** Indinavir is poorly water soluble and can precipitate in the kidney, causing kidney stones and interstitial nephritis.

   D. Other serious toxicities that develop after chronic use of many of these agents include bone marrow depression, diabetes mellitus, hepatotoxicity, lactic acidosis, lipodystrophy, lipoatrophy, pancreatitis, peripheral neuropathy, renal failure, and seizures.

II. **Toxic dose**

   A. **Acyclovir.** High-dose chronic therapy has caused crystalluria and renal failure. A patient who had an acute ingestion of 20 g recovered. A 1.5-day-old and a 2-year-old child recovered from accidental overdoses involving 100 mg/kg 3 times a day for 4 days and 800 mg intravenously, respectively.

   B. **Atazanavir**. Laboratory evidence of hyperbilirubinemia is common and is not dose-dependent. The abnormality is reversible when the drug is discontinued.

   C. **Cidofovir.** Two adults who received overdoses of 16.3 and 17.4 mg/kg, respectively, were treated with IV hydration and probenecid and had no toxic effects.

   D. **Efavirenz.** A 33-year-old female who ingested 54 g developed manic symptoms and recovered after 5 days

   E. **Enfuvirtide**. This drug is given by injection, and patients often develop local injection site reactions (eg, abscess, cellulitis, nodules, and cysts).

   F. **Fosamprenavir** is a water-soluble prodrug to amprenavir that commonly causes skin reactions. The drug contains a sulfonamide moiety, and caution should be exercised in patients with an allergy to sulfonamides. Life-threatening Stevens-Johnson syndrome has been reported to the manufacturer.

   G. **Foscarnet.** An adult receiving 12.5 g for 3 days developed seizures and died. Adults who received 1.14–8 times (average of 4 times) the recommended doses developed seizures and renal impairment.

   H. **Ganciclovir.** All toxic reports have been after intravenous administration. The doses producing toxic effects after high chronic or inadvertent acute IV overdose have been variable. No toxic effects were noted in two adults who were given 3.5 g and 11 mg/kg for 7 doses over 3 days, respectively. However, single doses of 25 mg/kg and 6 g, or daily doses of 8 mg/kg for 4 days or 3 g for 2 days, resulted in neutropenia, granulocytopenia, pancytopenia, and/or thrombocytopenia. An adult and a 2-kg infant developed hepatitis after 10 mg/kg and 40-mg doses, respectively. An adult developed seizures after a 9-mg/kg dose, and others have had increased serum creatinine levels after 5- to 7-g doses.

   I. **Indinavir.** Patients with acute and chronic overdoses, up to 23 times the recommended total daily dose of 2400 mg, resulting in interstitial nephritis, kidney stones, or acute renal dysfunction, have recovered after intravenous fluid therapy.

J. **Nevirapine.** An alleged 6-g ingestion in an adult was benign.

K. **Zidovudine.** Acute overdoses have been mild with ingestions of less than 25 g.

III. **Clinical presentation.** Gastrointestinal symptoms are common after therapeutic doses and are more remarkable after an acute overdose. Specific features of toxicity are described in Table II–12. **Lactic acidosis,** often severe and sometimes fatal, has been reported with antiretroviral drugs, particularly nucleoside reverse transcriptase inhibitors (NRTIs).

IV. **Diagnosis** is usually based on the history of exposure. Unexplained mental status changes, neurologic deficits, weight gain, and renal abnormalities occurred after erroneous administration of acyclovir, particularly in pediatric patients.

A. **Specific levels.** Serum levels are not commonly available for these agents and have not been particularly useful for predicting toxic effects.

B. **Other useful laboratory studies** include CBC, electrolytes, glucose, BUN, creatinine, liver function tests, and urinalysis. Lactic acid levels and arterial blood gases are recommended if lactic acidosis is suspected.

V. **Treatment**

A. **Emergency and supportive measures**

1. Maintain an open airway and assist ventilation if necessary.
2. Treat coma (see p 18), seizures (p 22), hypotension (p 15), and anaphylaxis (p 27) if they occur.
3. Replace fluid losses resulting from gastroenteritis with intravenous crystalloids.
4. Maintain steady urine flow with intravenous fluids to alleviate crystalluria and reverse renal dysfunction.
5. Treat lactic acidosis with judicious doses of sodium bicarbonate and by withdrawal of the offending drug.

B. **Specific drugs and antidotes.** There are no specific antidotes for these agents.

C. **Decontamination** (see p 45). Administer activated charcoal orally if conditions are appropriate (see Table I–38, p 51). Gastric lavage is not necessary after small to moderate ingestions if activated charcoal can be given promptly.

D. **Enhanced elimination.** The few reported overdoses with these agents have been benign or associated with mild toxicities. Hemodialysis may remove 60% of the total body burden of acyclovir and approximately 30% of emtricitabine over 3 hours. Enhanced elimination, however, has yet to be evaluated or employed after acute overdoses.

## ► ARSENIC

*Michael J. Kosnett, MD, MPH*

Arsenic compounds are found in a select group of industrial, commercial, and pharmaceutical products. Use of arsenic as a wood preservative in industrial applications (such as marine timbers and utility poles) accounts for two-thirds of domestic consumption, but former widespread use in new lumber sold for residential purposes (eg, decks, fencing, play structures) ended with a voluntary ban effective at the end of 2003. Arsenic-treated lumber used in residential structures and objects created prior to 2004 has not been officially recalled or removed. Arsenic-impregnated gels are used as ant baits, and a few organoarsenicals, such as methane arsonates and cacodylic acid, continue to be used as herbicides and defoliants. Phenylarsenic compounds are used as feed additives for poultry and swine, and intravenous arsenic trioxide, reintroduced to the US pharmacopoeia in 2000, is used as a drug for cancer chemotherapy. Inorganic arsenic is used in the production of nonferrous alloys, semiconductors, and certain types of glass. Inorganic arsenic is sometimes found in folk remedies and tonics, particularly from Asian sources. Artesian well water can be contaminated by inorganic arsenic from natural geologic deposits, and elevated levels of arsenic may be encountered in mine tailings and sediments and coal fly ash. Arsine, a hydride gas of arsenic, is discussed on p 119.

I. **Mechanism of toxicity.** Arsenic compounds may be organic or inorganic and may contain arsenic in either a pentavalent (arsenate) or a trivalent (arsenite) form. Once absorbed, arsenicals exert their toxic effects through multiple mechanisms, including inhibition of enzymatic reactions vital to cellular metabolism, induction of oxidative stress, and alteration in gene expression and cell signal transduction. Although arsenite and arsenate undergo in vivo biotransformation to less toxic pentavalent monomethyl and dimethyl forms, there is evidence that the process also forms more toxic trivalent methylated compounds.
   A. **Soluble arsenic compounds,** which are well absorbed after ingestion or inhalation, pose the greatest risk for acute human intoxication.
   B. **Inorganic arsenic dusts** (such as arsenic trioxide) may exert irritant effects on the skin and mucous membranes. Contact dermatitis has also been reported. Although the skin is a minor route of absorption for most arsenic compounds, systemic toxicity has resulted from industrial accidents involving percutaneous exposure to highly concentrated liquid formulations.
   C. The chemical warfare agent **lewisite** (dichloro [2-chlorovinyl] arsine) is a volatile vesicant liquid that causes immediate severe irritation and necrosis to the eyes, skin, and airways (see also p 373).
   D. Arsenate and arsenite are **known human carcinogens** by both ingestion and inhalation.

II. **Toxic dose.** The toxicity of arsenic compounds varies considerably with the valence state, chemical composition, and solubility. Humans are generally more sensitive than other animals to the acute and chronic effects of arsenicals.
   A. **Inorganic arsenic compounds.** In general, trivalent arsenic ($As^{3+}$) is 2–10 times more acutely toxic than pentavalent arsenic ($As^{5+}$). However, overexposure to either form produces a similar pattern of effects, requiring the same clinical approach and management.
      1. Acute ingestion of as little as 100–300 mg of a soluble trivalent arsenic compound (eg, sodium arsenite) could be fatal.
      2. The lowest observed acute effect level (LOAEL) for acute human toxicity is approximately 0.05 mg/kg, a dose associated with gastrointestinal distress in some individuals.
      3. Death attributable to malignant arrhythmias has been reported after days to weeks of cancer chemotherapy regimens in which 0.15 mg/kg/day of arsenic trioxide was administered intravenously.
      4. Repeated ingestion of approximately 0.04 mg/kg/day can result in gastrointestinal distress and hematologic effects after weeks to months and peripheral neuropathy after 6 months to several years. Lower chronic exposures, approximately 0.01 mg/kg/day, can result in characteristic skin changes (initially spotted pigmentation, followed within years by palmar-plantar hyperkeratosis) after intervals of 5–15 years.
      5. The US National Research Council (2001) estimated that chronic ingestion of drinking water containing arsenic at a concentration of 10 mcg/L could be associated with an excess lifetime cancer risk greater than 1 in 1000. The latency period for development of arsenic-induced cancer is probably a decade or longer.
   B. **Organic arsenic.** In general, pentavalent organoarsenic compounds are less toxic than either trivalent organoarsenic compounds or inorganic arsenic compounds. Marine organisms may contain large quantities of arsenobetaine, an organic trimethylated compound that is excreted unchanged in the urine and produces no known toxic effects. Arsenosugars (dimethylarsinoyl riboside de-

rivatives) are present in some marine and freshwater animals (eg, bivalve mollusks) and marine algae (eg, seaweeds often used in Asian foods).

**III. Clinical presentation**

**A. Acute exposure** most commonly occurs after accidental, suicidal, or deliberate poisoning by ingestion. A single, massive dose produces a constellation of multisystemic signs and symptoms that emerge over the course of hours to weeks.

1. **Gastrointestinal effects.** After a delay of minutes to hours, diffuse capillary damage results in hemorrhagic gastroenteritis. Nausea, vomiting, abdominal pain, and watery diarrhea are common. Although prominent gastrointestinal (GI) symptoms may subside within 24 to 48 hours, severe multisystemic effects may still ensue.
2. **Cardiovascular effects.** In severe cases, extensive tissue third spacing of fluids combined with fluid loss from gastroenteritis may lead to hypotension, tachycardia, shock, and death. Metabolic acidosis and rhabdomyolysis may be present. After a delay of 1–6 days, there may be a second phase of congestive cardiomyopathy, cardiogenic or noncardiogenic pulmonary edema, and isolated or recurrent cardiac arrhythmias. Prolongation of the QT interval may be associated with torsade de pointes ventricular arrhythmia.
3. **Neurologic effects.** Mental status may be normal, or there may be lethargy, agitation, or delirium. Delirium or obtundation may be delayed by 2–6 days. Generalized seizures may occur but are rare. Symmetric, sensorimotor axonal peripheral neuropathy may evolve 1–5 weeks after acute ingestion, beginning with painful distal dysesthesias, particularly in the feet. Ascending weakness and paralysis may ensue, leading in severe cases to quadriplegia and neuromuscular respiratory failure.
4. **Hematologic effects.** Pancytopenia, particularly leukopenia and anemia, characteristically develops within 1–2 weeks after acute ingestion. A relative eosinophilia may be present, and there may be basophilic stippling of red blood cells.
5. **Dermatologic effects.** Findings that occasionally appear after a delay of 1–6 weeks include desquamation (particularly involving palms and soles), a diffuse maculopapular rash, periorbital edema, and herpes zoster or herpes simplex. Transverse white striae in the nails (Aldrich-Mees lines) may become apparent months after an acute intoxication.

**B. Chronic intoxication** is also associated with multisystemic effects, which may include fatigue and malaise, gastroenteritis, leukopenia and anemia (occasionally megaloblastic), sensory predominant peripheral neuropathy, hepatic transaminase elevation, noncirrhotic portal hypertension, and peripheral vascular insufficiency. Skin disorders and cancer may occur (see below), and a growing body of epidemiologic evidence links chronic arsenic ingestion with an increased risk of hypertension, cardiovascular mortality, diabetes mellitus, and chronic nonmalignant respiratory disease.

1. **Skin lesions,** which emerge gradually over a period of 1–10 years, typically begin with a characteristic pattern of spotted ("raindrop") pigmentation on the torso and extremities, followed after several years by the development of hyperkeratotic changes on the palms and soles. Skin lesions may occur after lower doses than those causing neuropathy or anemia. Arsenic-related skin cancer, which includes squamous cell carcinoma, Bowen's disease, and basal cell carcinoma, is characteristically multicentric and occurs in non-sun-exposed areas.
2. **Cancer.** Chronic inhalation increases the risk of lung cancer. Chronic ingestion is an established cause of cancer of the lung, bladder, and skin.

**IV. Diagnosis** usually is based on a history of exposure combined with a typical pattern of multisystemic signs and symptoms. Suspect acute arsenic poisoning in a patient with abrupt onset of abdominal pain, nausea, vomiting, watery diarrhea, and hypotension, particularly when followed by an evolving pattern of delayed cardiac dysfunction, pancytopenia, and peripheral neuropathy. Metabolic acidosis and elevated CPK may occur early in the course of severe cases. Some arsenic compounds, particularly those of lower solubility, are radiopaque and may be visible on a plain abdominal x-ray.

A. **Specific levels.** In the first 2–3 days after acute symptomatic poisoning, total 24-hour urinary arsenic excretion is typically in excess of several thousand micrograms (spot urine greater than 1000 mcg/L) and, depending on the severity of poisoning, may not return to background levels (less than 50 mcg in a 24-hour specimen or less than 30 mcg/L in a spot urine) for several weeks. Spot urine analyses are usually sufficient for diagnostic purposes.
   1. **Ingestion of seafood,** which may contain very large amounts of nontoxic organoarsenicals such as arsenobetaine and arsenosugars, can "falsely" elevate measurements of *total* urinary arsenic for up to 3 days. Speciation of urinary arsenic by a laboratory capable of reporting the concentration of inorganic arsenic and its primary human metabolites, monomethylarsinic acid (MMA) and dimethylarsinic acid (DMA), may sometimes be helpful: Background urine concentration of the sum of urinary inorganic arsenic, MMA, and DMA is usually less than 20 mcg/L in the absence of recent seafood ingestion. It should be noted that although arsenobetaine is excreted unchanged in the urine, arsenosugars, which are abundant in bivalve mollusks and seaweed, are metabolized in part to DMA.
   2. **Blood levels** are highly variable and are rarely of value in the diagnosis or management in patients capable of producing urine. Although whole-blood arsenic, normally less than 5 mcg/L, may be elevated early in acute intoxication, it may decline rapidly to the normal range despite persistent elevated urinary arsenic excretion and continuing symptoms.
   3. **Elevated concentrations of arsenic in nails or hair** (normally less than 1 ppm) may be detectable in certain segmental samples for months after urine levels normalize but should be interpreted cautiously owing to the possibility of external contamination.

B. **Other useful laboratory studies** include CBC with differential and smear for basophilic stippling, electrolytes, glucose, BUN and creatinine, liver enzymes, CPK, urinalysis, ECG and ECG monitoring (with particular attention to the QT interval), and abdominal and chest x-rays.

V. **Treatment**

A. **Emergency and supportive measures**
   1. Maintain an open airway and assist ventilation if necessary (see pp 1–7)
   2. Treat coma (see p 18), shock (p 27), and arrhythmias (pp 10–15) if they occur. Because of the association of arsenic with prolonged QT intervals, avoid quinidine, procainamide, and other type Ia antiarrhythmic agents. Phenothiazines should not be given as antiemetics or antipsychotics because of their ability to prolong the QT interval and lower the seizure threshold.
   3. Treat hypotension and fluid loss with aggressive use of intravenous crystalloid solutions, along with vasopressor agents if needed, to support blood pressure and optimize urine output.
   4. Prolonged inpatient support and observation are indicated for patients with significant acute intoxication, because cardiopulmonary and neurologic complications may be delayed for several days. Continuous cardiac monitoring beyond 48 hours is warranted in patients with persistent symptoms or evidence of toxin-related cardiovascular disturbance, including electrocardiographic abnormalities, or any degree of congestive heart failure.

B. **Specific drugs and antidotes.** Treat seriously symptomatic patients with *chelating agents,* which have shown therapeutic benefit in animal models of acute arsenic intoxication when administered promptly (ie, minutes to hours) after exposure. Treatment should not be delayed during the several days often required to obtain specific laboratory confirmation.

1. **Unithiol** (2,3-dimercaptopropanesulfonic acid, DMPS, Dimaval; see p 515), a water-soluble analog of dimercaprol (BAL) that can be administered intravenously, has the most favorable pharmacologic profile for treatment of acute arsenic intoxication. Although published experience is sparse, 3–5 mg/kg every 4 hours by slow intravenous infusion over 20 minutes is a suggested starting dose. In the United States, the drug is available through compounding pharmacists.
2. **Dimercaprol** (BAL, British anti-Lewisite, 2-3 dimercaptopropanol; see p 417) is the chelating agent of second choice if unithiol is not immediately available. The starting dose is 3–5 mg/kg by deep intramuscular injection every 4–6 hours. Lewisite burns to the skin and eyes can be treated with topical inunctions of dimercaprol.
3. Once patients are hemodynamically stable and GI symptoms have subsided, parenteral chelation may be changed to oral chelation with either **oral unithiol,** or **oral succimer** (DMSA, 2-3 dimercaptosuccinic acid; see p 510). A suggested dose of unithiol is 4–8 mg/kg orally every 6 hours. Alternatively, give succimer, 7.5 mg/kg orally every 6 hours or 10 mg/kg orally every 8 hours.
4. The therapeutic endpoints of chelation are poorly defined. For chelation instituted to treat symptomatic acute intoxication, one empiric approach would be to continue treatment (initially parenterally, then orally) until total urinary arsenic levels are less than 500 mcg/24 hours (or spot urine < 300 mcg/L), levels below those associated with overt symptoms in acutely poisoned adults. Alternatively, oral chelation could be continued until total urinary arsenic levels reach background levels (< 50 mcg/24 hours or spot urine < 30 mcg/L). The value of chelation for treatment of an established neuropathy (or prevention of an incipient neuropathy) has not been proved.

C. **Decontamination** (see p 45). Administer activated charcoal orally if conditions are appropriate (see Table I–38, p 51). However, note that animal and in vitro studies suggest that activated charcoal has a relatively poor affinity for inorganic arsenic salts. Consider gastric lavage for large ingestions.

D. **Enhanced elimination.** Hemodialysis may be of possible benefit in patients with concomitant renal failure but otherwise contributes minimally to arsenic clearance. There is no known role for diuresis, hemoperfusion, or repeat-dose charcoal.

## ► ARSINE

*Michael Kosnett, MD, MPH*

Arsine is a colorless hydride gas ($AsH_3$) formed when arsenic comes in contact with hydrogen or with reducing agents in aqueous solution. Typically, exposure to arsine gas occurs in smelting operations or other industrial settings when arsenic-containing ores, alloys, or metallic objects come in contact with acidic (or occasionally alkaline) solutions and newly formed arsine is liberated. Arsine is also used as a dopant in the microelectronics industry.

I. **Mechanism of toxicity.** Arsine is a potent hemolytic agent. Recent investigations suggest that hemolysis occurs when arsine interacts with heme to form a reactive intermediate that alters transmembrane ion flux and greatly increases intracellular calcium. ***Note:*** Arsenite and other oxidized forms of arsenic do ***not*** cause hemolysis. Deposition of massive amounts of hemoglobin in the renal tubule can cause acute renal injury. Massive hemolysis also decreases systemic oxygen delivery and creates hypoxic stress, and arsine and/or its reaction products exert direct cytotoxic effects on multiple organs.

**II. Toxic dose.** Arsine is the most toxic form of arsenic. Acute exposure guideline levels (AEGL) recently developed by the US EPA and the National Research Council indicate that disabling effects (AEGL-2) may occur after 30 minutes of exposure to ≥ 0.21 ppm, 1 hour of exposure to ≥ 0.17 ppm, or 8 hours of exposure to ≥ 0.02 ppm. Lethal or life-threatening effects (AEGL-3) may occur from 30 minutes of exposure to ≥ 0.63 ppm, 4 hours of exposure to ≥ 0.13 ppm, or 8 hours of exposure to ≥ 0.06 ppm. The level considered by NIOSH (1994) as "immediately dangerous to life or health" (IDLH) is 3 ppm. The odor threshold of 0.5–1.0 ppm provides insufficient warning properties.

**III. Clinical presentation**

**A. Acute effects.** Because arsine gas is not acutely irritating, inhalation causes **no immediate symptoms.** Those exposed to high concentrations may sometimes detect a garlic-like odor, but more typically they are unaware of the presence of a significant exposure. In most industrial accidents involving arsine, the hazardous exposure occurred over the course of 30 minutes to a few hours.

**B.** After a **latent period of 2–24 hours** (depending on the intensity of exposure), massive hemolysis occurs, along with early symptoms that may include malaise, headache, fever or chills, and numbness or coldness in the extremities. There may be concomitant gastrointestinal complaints of nausea, vomiting, and crampy pain in the abdomen, flank, or low back. In severe exposures, abrupt cardiovascular collapse and death may occur within 1 or 2 hours.

**C. Hemoglobinuria** imparts a dark, reddish color to the urine, and the skin may develop a copper, bronze, or "jaundiced" discoloration that may be attributable to elevated plasma hemoglobin.

**D.** Oliguria and **acute renal failure** often occur 1–3 days after exposure and are a major aspect of arsine-related morbidity.

**E.** A minority of patients may develop agitation and delirium within 1–2 days of presentation.

**F. Chronic arsine poisoning,** a rarely reported condition, has been associated with headache, weakness, shortness of breath, nausea, vomiting, and anemia.

**IV. Diagnosis.** Arsine poisoning should be suspected in a patient who presents with the abrupt onset of hemolysis, hemoglobinuria, and progressive oliguria. A consistent work history or another likely source of exposure increases the index of suspicion but is not always apparent.

**A. Specific levels.** Urine and whole-blood arsenic levels may be elevated but are rarely available in time to assist with prompt diagnosis and management. Whole-blood arsenic concentrations in patients with severe arsine poisoning have ranged from several hundred to several thousand micrograms per liter.

**B. Other useful laboratory studies**

1. The complete blood count in the first few hours after acute exposure may be normal or reveal only moderate depression of the hematocrit or hemoglobin. However, within approximately 12–36 hours these values will decline progressively, with hemoglobin levels declining to 5–10 g/100 mL. The peripheral blood smear may reveal erythrocyte fragmentation and abnormal red blood cell forms, including characteristic "ghost cells" in which an enlarged membrane encloses a pale or vacant interior. Leukocytosis is common.
2. Initial urinalysis will typically be heme positive on dipstick, but with scant formed red blood cells on microscopic examination. Later, as oliguria progresses, an active urine sediment with red blood cells and casts will often emerge. Quantitative measurement of urine hemoglobin may rise to 3 g/L during significant hemolysis and in some instances may exceed 10 g/L.

3. Serum bilirubin may show mild to moderate elevations (eg, 2–5 mg/dL) during the first 48 hours, with only a slight rise in liver transaminases.
4. Increases in BUN and serum creatinine will reflect acute renal insufficiency.

V. **Treatment**

A. **Emergency and supportive measures**

1. Provide vigorous **intravenous hydration** and, if needed, **osmotic diuresis with mannitol** (see p 471) to maintain urine output and reduce the risk of acute hemoglobinuric renal failure.
2. Clinical reports indicate that **prompt exchange transfusion with whole blood** is a key therapeutic intervention and should be initiated for plasma or serum hemoglobin levels ≥ 1.5 g/dL and/or signs of renal insufficiency or early acute tubular necrosis. Because of the time delay needed to obtain matched blood, the possible need for exchange transfusion in significantly exposed patients should be anticipated soon after they present.
3. Hemodialysis may be needed to treat progressive renal failure but is not a substitute for exchange transfusion, which, unlike hemodialysis, removes arsenic-hemoprotein complexes thought to contribute to the ongoing hemolytic state.

B. **Specific drugs and antidotes**

1. The scant clinical experience with chelation in acute arsine poisoning is inconclusive, but limited animal and in vitro experimental studies suggest it is reasonable to initiate treatment with **dimercaprol** (BAL, British anti-Lewisite; see p 417), a relatively lipid-soluble chelator, in patients who present within 24 hours of exposure. The dose of dimercaprol during the first 24 hours is 3–5 mg/kg every 4–6 hours by deep intramuscular injection.
2. After 24 hours, consider chelation with the water-soluble dimercapto chelating agents, oral or parenteral **unithiol** (DMPS; see p 515), or oral **succimer** (DMSA, Chemet™; p 510).
3. Note that the recommendation to use dimercaprol rather than unithiol or succimer during the initial phases of poisoning is unique to arsine and differs from the chelation recommendation for poisoning by other inorganic arsenicals, when initial use of unithiol is favored.
4. Chelation is of uncertain efficacy and should not substitute for or delay the vigorous supportive measures outlined above.

C. **Decontamination.** Remove the victim from exposure. First responders should use self-contained breathing apparatus (SCBA) to protect themselves from any arsine remaining in the environment.

D. **Enhanced elimination.** As noted above, **prompt exchange transfusion with whole blood** is useful in patients with evidence of significant active hemolysis or evolving renal insufficiency. Whole donor blood may be infused through a central line at the same rate of blood removal through a peripheral vein, or techniques using modified hemodialysis circuits can be considered.

## ▶ ASBESTOS

*John Balmes, MD*

Asbestos is the name given to a group of naturally occurring silicates, chrysotile, amosite, and crocidolite, as well as the asbestiform types of tremolite, actinolite, and anthophyllite. Exposure to asbestos is a well-documented cause of pulmonary and pleural fibrosis, lung cancer, and mesothelioma, illnesses that may appear many years after exposure.

I. **Mechanism of toxicity.** Inhalation of thin fibers longer than 5 microns produces lung fibrosis and cancer in animals (shorter fibers generally are phagocytosed by macrophages and cleared from the lungs). The exact mechanism of toxicity is unknown. Smoking cigarettes appears to enhance the likelihood of developing lung disease and malignancy.

**II. Toxic dose.** A safe threshold of exposure to asbestos has not been established. Balancing potential health risks against feasibility of workplace control, the current OSHA federal asbestos standard sets a permissible exposure limit (PEL) of 0.1 fiber per cubic centimeter (fibers/cc) as an 8-hour time-weighted average. No worker should be exposed to concentrations in excess of 1 fiber/cc over a 30-minute period.

**III. Clinical presentation.** After a latent period of 15–20 years, the patient may develop one or more of the following clinical syndromes:

- **A. Asbestosis** is a slowly progressive fibrosing disease of the lungs. Pulmonary impairment resulting from lung restriction and decreased gas exchange is common.
- **B. Pleural plaques** typically involve only the parietal pleura and are usually asymptomatic but provide a marker of asbestos exposure. Rarely, significant lung restriction occurs as a result of severe pleural fibrosis involving both parietal and visceral surfaces.
- **C. Pleural effusions** may occur as early as 5–10 years after the onset of exposure and are often not recognized as asbestos-related.
- **D. Lung cancer** is a common cause of death in patients with asbestos exposure, especially in cigarette smokers. **Mesothelioma** is a malignancy that may affect the pleura or the peritoneum. The incidence of **gastrointestinal cancer** may be increased in asbestos-exposed workers.

**IV. Diagnosis** is based on a history of exposure to asbestos (usually at least 15–20 years before the onset of symptoms) and a clinical presentation of one or more of the syndromes described above. Chest x-ray typically shows small, irregular round opacities distributed primarily in the lower lung fields. Pleural plaques, diffuse thickening, or calcification may be present. Pulmonary function tests reveal decreased vital capacity and total lung capacity and impairment of carbon monoxide diffusion.

- **A. Specific tests.** There are no specific blood or urine tests.
- **B. Other useful laboratory studies** include chest x-ray, arterial blood gases, and pulmonary function tests.

**V. Treatment**

- **A. Emergency and supportive measures.** Emphasis should be placed on **prevention** of exposure. All asbestos workers should be encouraged to stop smoking and observe workplace control measures stringently.
- **B. Specific drugs and antidotes.** There are none.
- **C. Decontamination**
  1. **Inhalation.** Persons exposed to asbestos dust and those assisting victims should wear protective equipment, including appropriate respirators and disposable gowns and caps. Watering down any dried material will help prevent its dispersion into the air as dust.
  2. **Skin exposure.** Asbestos is not absorbed through the skin. However, it may be inhaled from skin and clothes, so removal of clothes and washing the skin are recommended.
  3. **Ingestion.** Asbestos is not known to be harmful by ingestion, so no decontamination is necessary.
- **D. Enhanced elimination.** There is no role for these procedures.

## ▶ AZIDE, SODIUM

*Jo Ellen Dyer, PharmD*

**Sodium azide** is a highly toxic white crystalline solid. It has come into widespread use in automobile air bags: its explosive decomposition to nitrogen gas provides rapid inflation of the air bag. In addition, sodium azide is used in the production of metallic azide explosives and as a preservative in laboratories. It has no current medical uses, but because of its potent vasodilatory effects, it has been evaluated as an antihypertensive agent.

**I. Mechanism of toxicity**

**A.** The mechanism of azide toxicity is unclear. Like cyanide and hydrogen sulfide, azide inhibits iron-containing respiratory enzymes such as cytochrome oxidase, resulting in cellular asphyxiation. Azide is also a potent direct-acting vasodilator.

**B.** Although neutral solutions are stable, acidification rapidly converts the azide salt to **hydrazoic acid,** particularly in the presence of solid metals (eg, drain pipes). Hydrazoic acid vapors are pungent and (at high concentrations) explosive. The acute toxicity of hydrazoic acid has been compared with that of hydrogen cyanide and hydrogen sulfide.

**II. Toxic dose.** Although several grams of azide are found in an automobile airbag, it is completely consumed and converted to nitrogen during the explosive inflation process, and toxicity has not been reported from exposure to spent air bags.

**A. Inhalation.** Irritation symptoms or a pungent odor does not give adequate warning of toxicity. The recommended workplace ceiling limit (ACGIH TLV-C) is 0.29 mg/m$^3$ for sodium azide and 0.11 ppm for hydrazoic acid. Air concentrations as low as 0.5 ppm may result in mucous membrane irritation, hypotension, and headache. A chemist who intentionally sniffed the vapor above a 1% hydrazoic acid solution became hypotensive, collapsed, and recovered 15 minutes later with residual headache. Workers in a lead azide plant exposed to air concentrations of 0.3–3.9 ppm experienced symptoms of headache, weakness, palpitations, mild smarting of the eyes and nose, and a drop in blood pressure. Laboratory workers adjacent to a sulfur analyzer that was emitting vapor concentrations of 0.5 ppm experienced symptoms of nasal stuffiness without detecting a pungent odor.

**B. Dermal.** Industrial workers handling bulk sodium azide experienced headache, nausea, faintness, and hypotension, but it is unclear whether the exposure occurred via dermal absorption or inhalation. An explosion of a metal waste drum containing a 1% sodium azide solution caused burns over a 45% body surface area and led to typical azide toxicity with a time course similar to oral ingestion; coma and hypotension developed within 1 hour, followed by refractory metabolic acidosis, shock, and death 14 hours later.

**C. Ingestion.** Several serious or fatal poisonings occurred as a result of drinking large quantities of laboratory saline or distilled water containing 0.1–0.2% sodium azide as a preservative.

1. Ingestion of several grams can cause death within 1–2 hours.
2. Ingestion of 700 mg resulted in myocardial failure after 72 hours. Ingestion of 150 mg produced shortness of breath, tachycardia, restlessness, nausea, vomiting, and diarrhea within 15 minutes. Later, polydipsia, T-wave changes on ECG, leukocytosis, and numbness occurred, lasting 10 days.
3. Doses of 0.65–3.9 mg/day given for up to 2.5 years have been used experimentally as an antihypertensive. The hypotensive effect occurred within 1 minute. Headache was the only complaint noted in these patients.

**III. Clinical presentation**

**A. Irritation.** Exposure to dust or gas may produce reddened conjunctivae and nasal and bronchial irritation that may progress to pulmonary edema.

**B. Systemic toxicity.** Both inhalation and ingestion are associated with a variety of dose-dependent systemic symptoms. Early in the course, hypotension and tachycardia occur that can evolve to bradycardia, ventricular fibrillation, and myocardial failure. Neurologic symptoms include headache, restlessness, facial flushing, loss of vision, faintness, weakness, hyporeflexia, seizures, coma, and respiratory failure. Nausea, vomiting, diarrhea, diaphoresis, and lactic acidosis also appear during the course.

IV. **Diagnosis** is based on the history of exposure and clinical presentation.

A. **Specific levels.** Specific blood or serum levels are not routinely available. A simple qualitative test can be used on powders and solid materials: Azide forms a red precipitate in the presence of ferric chloride (use gloves and respiratory protection when handling the azide).

B. **Other useful laboratory studies** include electrolytes, glucose, arterial blood gases or pulse oximetry, and ECG.

V. **Treatment.** ***Caution:*** Cases involving severe azide ingestion are potentially dangerous to health-care providers. In the acidic environment of the stomach, azide salts are converted to hydrazoic acid, which is highly volatile. Quickly isolate all vomitus or gastric washings and keep the patient in a well-ventilated area. Wear appropriate respiratory protective gear if available; personnel should be trained to use it. Dispose of azide with care. Contact with heavy metals, including copper or lead found in water pipes, forms metal azides that may explode.

A. **Emergency and supportive measures**

1. Protect the airway and assist ventilation (see pp 1–7) if necessary. Insert an intravenous line and monitor the ECG and vital signs.
2. Treat coma (see p 18), hypotension (p 15), seizures (p 22), and arrhythmias (pp 10–15) if they occur.

B. **Specific drugs and antidotes.** There is no specific antidote.

C. **Decontamination** (see p 45)

1. **Inhalation.** Remove the victim from exposure and give supplemental oxygen if available. Rescuers should wear self-contained breathing apparatus and appropriate chemical-protective clothing.
2. **Skin.** Remove and bag contaminated clothing and wash affected areas copiously with soap and water.
3. **Ingestion.** Perform gastric lavage and administer activated charcoal. (The affinity of charcoal for azide is not known.) See the caution statement above; isolate all vomitus or gastric washings to avoid exposure to volatile hydrazoic acid.

D. **Enhanced elimination.** There is no role for dialysis or hemoperfusion in acute azide poisoning.

## ▶ BARBITURATES

*Timothy E. Albertson, MD, PhD*

Barbiturates are used as hypnotic and sedative agents, for the induction of anesthesia, and for the treatment of epilepsy and status epilepticus. They often are divided into four major groups by their pharmacologic activity and clinical use: **ultrashort-acting, short-acting, intermediate-acting,** and **long-acting** (Table II–13). *Common combination products* containing barbiturates include Fiorinal™ (50 mg butalbital) and Donnatal™ (16 mg phenobarbital). Veterinary euthanasia products often contain barbiturates such as pentobarbital.

I. **Mechanism of toxicity**

A. All barbiturates cause generalized **depression of neuronal activity** in the brain. Interaction with a barbiturate receptor leads to enhanced gamma-aminobutyric acid (GABA)-mediated chloride currents and results in synaptic inhibition. Hypotension that occurs with large doses is caused by depression of central sympathetic tone as well as by direct depression of cardiac contractility.

B. **Pharmacokinetics** vary by agent and group (see Tables II–13 and II–59).

1. **Ultrashort-acting** barbiturates are highly lipid soluble and rapidly penetrate the brain to induce anesthesia, then are quickly redistributed to other tissues. For this reason, the clinical duration of effect is much shorter than the elimination half-life for these compounds.

TABLE II–13. BARBITURATES

| Drug | Normal Terminal Elimination Half-Life (h) | Usual Duration of Effect (h) | Usual Hypnotic Dose (Adult) (mg) | Minimum Toxic Level (mg/L) |
|---|---|---|---|---|
| **Ultrashort-acting** | | | | |
| Methohexital | 3–5 | < 0.5 | 50–120 | >5 |
| Thiopental | 8–10 | < 0.5 | 50–75 | >5 |
| **Short-acting** | | | | |
| Pentobarbital | 15–50 | > 3–4 | 50–200 | >10 |
| Secobarbital | 15–40 | > 3–4 | 100–200 | >10 |
| **Intermediate-acting** | | | | |
| Amobarbital | 10–40 | > 4–6 | 65–200 | >10 |
| Aprobarbital | 14–34 | > 4–6 | 40–160 | >10 |
| Butabarbital | 35–50 | > 4–6 | 100–200 | >10 |
| Butalbital | 35 | | 100–200 | >7 |
| **Long-acting** | | | | |
| Mephobarbital | 10–70 | > 6–12 | 50–100 | >30 |
| Phenobarbital | 80–120 | > 6–12 | 100–320 | >30 |

2. **Long-acting barbiturates** are distributed more evenly and have long elimination half-lives, making them useful for once-daily treatment of epilepsy. Primidone (Mysoline) is metabolized to phenobarbital and phenylethylmalonamide (PEMA); although phenobarbital accounts for only about 25% of the metabolites, it has the greatest anticonvulsant activity.

**II. Toxic dose.** The toxic dose of barbiturates varies widely and depends on the drug, the route and rate of administration, and individual patient tolerance. In general, toxicity is likely when the dose exceeds 5–10 times the hypnotic dose. Chronic users or abusers may have striking tolerance to depressant effects.

**A.** The potentially fatal **oral dose** of the shorter-acting agents is 2–3 g, compared with 6–10 g for phenobarbital.

**B.** Several deaths were reported in young women undergoing therapeutic abortion after they received rapid **intravenous injections** of as little as 1–3 mg/kg of methohexital.

**III. Clinical presentation.** The onset of symptoms depends on the drug and the route of administration.

**A.** Lethargy, slurred speech, nystagmus, and ataxia are common with mild to moderate intoxication. With higher doses, hypotension, coma, and respiratory arrest commonly occur. With deep coma, the pupils are usually small or midposition; the patient may lose all reflex activity and appear to be dead.

**B. Hypothermia** is common in patients with deep coma, especially if the victim has suffered exposure to a cool environment. Hypotension and bradycardia commonly accompany hypothermia.

**IV. Diagnosis** is usually based on a history of ingestion and should be suspected in any epileptic patient with stupor or coma. Although skin bullae sometimes are seen with barbiturate overdose, they are not specific for barbiturates. Other causes of coma should also be considered (see p 18).

**A. Specific levels** of phenobarbital are usually readily available from hospital clinical laboratories; concentrations greater than 60–80 mg/L are usually associated with coma, and those greater than 150–200 mg/L with severe hypotension. For short- and intermediate-acting barbiturates, coma is likely when the serum concentration exceeds 20–30 mg/L. Barbiturates are easily detected in routine urine toxicologic screening.

**B. Other useful laboratory studies** include electrolytes, glucose, BUN, creatinine, arterial blood gases or pulse oximetry, and chest x-ray.

**V. Treatment**

**A. Emergency and supportive measures**

1. Protect the airway and assist ventilation (see pp 1–7) if necessary.
2. Treat coma (see p 18), hypothermia (p 19), and hypotension (p 15) if they occur.

**B. Specific drugs and antidotes.** There is no specific antidote.

**C. Decontamination** (see p 45). Administer activated charcoal orally if conditions are appropriate (see Table I–38, p 51). Gastric lavage is not necessary after small to moderate ingestions if activated charcoal can be given promptly.

**D. Enhanced elimination**

1. **Alkalinization** of the urine (see p 54) increases the urinary elimination of phenobarbital but not other barbiturates. Its value in acute overdose is unproved, and it may potentially contribute to fluid overload and pulmonary edema.
2. **Repeat-dose activated charcoal** has been shown to decrease the half-life of phenobarbital, but data are conflicting regarding its effects on the duration of coma, time on mechanical ventilation, and time to extubation.
3. **Hemodialysis** or hemoperfusion may be necessary for severely intoxicated patients who are not responding to supportive care (ie, with intractable hypotension).

## ▶ BARIUM

*Olga F. Woo, PharmD*

Barium poisonings are uncommon and usually result from accidental contamination of food sources, suicidal ingestion, or occupational inhalation exposure.

The water-soluble barium salts (acetate, carbonate, chloride, fluoride, hydroxide, nitrate, and sulfide) are highly toxic, whereas the insoluble salt, barium sulfate, is nontoxic because it is poorly absorbed. Soluble barium salts are found in depilatories, fireworks, ceramic glazes, and rodenticides and are used in the manufacture of glass and in dyeing textiles. Barium sulfide and polysulfide may also produce hydrogen sulfide toxicity (see p 224). Barium may also enter the air during mining and refining processes, from burning coal and gas, and with the production of barium compounds. The oil and gas industries use barium compounds to make drilling mud. Drilling mud lubricates the drill while it is going through rocks.

**I. Mechanism of toxicity**

**A. Systemic barium poisoning** is characterized by profound hypokalemia, leading to respiratory and cardiac arrest. Barium stimulates ATPase and is a selective blocker of passive potassium transport into the extracellular space. The rapid onset of severe hypokalemia most likely is caused by translocation of potassium into cells and blocked cellular potassium channel efflux. Barium ions have a direct action on muscle cell potassium permeability, most notably on striated cardiac muscle. In the gastrointestinal tract, barium stimulates acid and histamine secretion and peristalsis.

**B. Inhalation** of insoluble inorganic barium salts can cause baritosis, a benign pneumoconiosis. One death resulted from barium peroxide inhalation. Detonation of barium styphnate caused severe poisoning from inhalation and dermal absorption.

**C. Pharmacokinetics.** Barium is stored in bone and slowly excreted in feces. Tissue distribution follows a three-compartment model with half-lives of 3.6, 34, and 1033 days.

**II. Toxic dose.** The minimum oral toxic dose of soluble barium salts is undetermined but may be as low as 200 mg. Lethal doses range from 1 to 30 g for various barium salts because absorption is influenced by gastric pH and foods high in sulfate. Patients have survived ingestions of 129 g and 421 g of barium sulfide. The US Environmental Protection agency (EPA) has set an oral reference dose for barium of 0.07 mg/kg/day. A level of 50 $mg/m^3$ may be immediately dangerous to life and health (NIOSH).

**III. Clinical presentation.** Within minutes to a few hours after ingestion, victims develop profound hypokalemia and skeletal muscle weakness that progresses to flaccid paralysis of the limbs and respiratory muscles. Ventricular arrhythmias, hypophosphatemia, rhabdomyolysis, acute renal failure, and coagulopathy may also occur. Gastroenteritis with severe watery diarrhea, mydriasis with impaired visual accommodation, myoclonus, hypertension, profound lactic acidosis, and CNS depression may be present. More often, patients remain conscious even when severely intoxicated.

**IV. Diagnosis** is based on a history of exposure, accompanied by rapidly progressive hypokalemia and muscle weakness.

- **A. Specific levels.** Blood barium levels are not routinely available. One patient survived with a level of 3.7 mg/L, whereas postmortem levels in a fatal poisoning were less than 2 mg/L.
- **B. Other useful laboratory studies** include electrolytes (potassium), BUN, creatinine, phosphorus, arterial blood gases or pulse oximetry, and continuous ECG monitoring. Measure serum potassium levels frequently.

**V. Treatment**

- **A. Emergency and supportive measures**
  1. Maintain an open airway and assist ventilation if necessary (see pp 1–7).
  2. Treat fluid losses from gastroenteritis with intravenous crystalloids.
  3. Attach a cardiac monitor and observe the patient closely for at least 6–8 hours after ingestion.
- **B. Specific drugs and antidotes.** Administer **potassium chloride** (see p 499) to treat symptomatic or severe hypokalemia. Large doses of potassium may be necessary (doses as high as 420 mEq over 24 hours have been given). Use potassium phosphate if the patient has hypophosphatemia.
- **C. Decontamination** (see p 45)
  1. Activated charcoal probably does not adsorb barium and is not recommended unless there are co-ingestants.
  2. Perform gastric lavage for a large recent ingestion.
  3. **Magnesium sulfate or sodium sulfate** (30 g; children 250 mg/kg) should be administered orally to precipitate ingested barium as the insoluble sulfate salt.
- **D. Enhanced elimination**
  1. **Diuresis** with saline and furosemide to obtain a urine flow of 4–6 mL/kg/h may enhance barium elimination.
  2. Hemodialysis and hemoperfusion have not been evaluated in the treatment of serious barium poisoning. Hemodialysis may be helpful in correcting severe electrolyte disturbances.

## ▶ BENZENE

*Chris Camilleri, DO*

Benzene, a clear volatile liquid with an acrid aromatic odor, is one of the most widely used industrial chemicals. It is a constituent by-product in gasoline, and it is used as an industrial solvent and as a chemical intermediate in the synthesis of a variety of materials. Benzene can be found in dyes, plastics, insecticides, and many other materials and products. It is generally not present in household products.

I. **Mechanism of toxicity.** Like other hydrocarbons, benzene can cause a chemical pneumonia if it is aspirated. See p 219 for a general discussion of hydrocarbon toxicity.

   A. Once absorbed, benzene causes CNS depression and may sensitize the myocardium to the arrhythmogenic effects of catecholamines.

   B. Benzene is also known for its chronic effects on the hematopoietic system, which are thought to be mediated by a reactive toxic intermediate metabolite.

   C. Benzene is a known human carcinogen (ACGIH category Al).

II. **Toxic dose.** Benzene is adsorbed rapidly by inhalation and ingestion and, to a limited extent, percutaneously.

   A. Acute ingestion of 2 mL may produce neurotoxicity, and as little as 15 mL has caused death.

   B. The recommended workplace limit (ACGIH TLV-TWA) for benzene **vapor** is 0.5 ppm (1.6 mg/$m^3$) as an 8-hour time-weighted average. The short-term exposure limit (STEL) is 2.5 ppm. The level considered immediately dangerous to life or health (IDLH) is 500 ppm. A single exposure to 7500–20,000 ppm can be fatal. Chronic exposure to air concentrations well below the threshold for smell (2 ppm) is associated with hematopoietic toxicity.

   C. The US Environmental Protection Agency Maximum Contaminant Level (MCL) in water is 5 ppb.

III. **Clinical presentation**

   A. **Acute exposure** may cause immediate CNS effects, including headache, nausea, dizziness, convulsions, and coma. Symptoms of CNS toxicity should be apparent immediately after inhalation or within 30–60 minutes after ingestion. Severe inhalation may result in noncardiogenic pulmonary edema. Ventricular arrhythmias may result from increased sensitivity of the myocardium to catecholamines. Benzene can cause chemical burns to the skin with prolonged or massive exposure.

   B. After **chronic exposure,** hematologic disorders such as pancytopenia, aplastic anemia, and acute myelogenous leukemia and its variants may occur. Causality is suspected for chronic myelogenous leukemia, chronic lymphocytic leukemia, multiple myeloma, Hodgkin's disease, and paroxysmal nocturnal hemoglobinuria. There is an unproven association between benzene exposure and acute lymphoblastic leukemia, myelofibrosis, and lymphomas. Chromosomal abnormalities have been reported, although no effects on fertility have been described in women after occupational exposure.

IV. **Diagnosis** of benzene poisoning is based on a history of exposure and typical clinical findings. With chronic hematologic toxicity, erythrocyte, leukocyte, and thrombocyte counts may first increase and then decrease before the onset of aplastic anemia.

   A. **Specific levels.** ***Note:*** Smoke from one cigarette contains 60–80 mcg of benzene; a typical smoker inhales 1–2 mg of benzene daily. This may confound measurements of low-level benzene exposures.

      1. Urine phenol levels may be useful for monitoring workplace benzene exposure (if diet is carefully controlled for phenol products). A spot urine phenol measurement higher than 50 mg/L suggests excessive occupational exposure. Urinary *trans*-muconic acid and *S*-phenylmercapturic acid (S-PMA) are more sensitive and specific indicators of low-level benzene exposure but are usually not readily available. S-PMA in urine is normally less than 15 mcg/g of creatinine.

      2. Benzene can also be measured in expired air for up to 2 days after exposure.

      3. Blood levels of benzene or metabolites are not clinically useful except after an acute exposure. Normal levels are < 0.5 mcg/L.

   B. **Other useful laboratory studies** include CBC, electrolytes, BUN, creatinine, liver function tests, ECG monitoring, and chest x-ray (if aspiration is suspected).

V. **Treatment**

A. **Emergency and supportive measures**

1. Maintain an open airway and assist ventilation if necessary (see pp 1–7).
2. Treat coma (see p 18), seizures (p 22), arrhythmias (pp 13–15), and other complications if they occur.
3. Be cautious with the use of any adrenergic agents (eg, epinephrine, metoproterenol, albuterol) because of the possibility of myocardial sensitization.
4. Monitor vital signs and ECG for 12–24 hours after significant exposure.

B. **Specific drugs and antidotes.** There is no specific antidote.

C. **Decontamination** (see p 45)

1. **Inhalation.** Immediately move the victim to fresh air and administer oxygen if available.
2. **Skin and eyes.** Remove clothing and wash the skin; irrigate exposed eyes with copious amounts of water or saline.
3. **Ingestion (see p 47).** Administer activated charcoal orally if conditions are appropriate (see Table I–38, p 51). Consider gastric aspiration with a small flexible tube if the ingestion was large (eg, > 150–200 mL) and occurred within the previous 30–60 minutes.

D. **Enhanced elimination.** Dialysis and hemoperfusion are not effective.

## ► BENZODIAZEPINES

*Ben Tsutaoka, PharmD*

The drug class of benzodiazepines includes many compounds that vary widely in potency, duration of effect, presence or absence of active metabolites, and clinical use (Table II–14). Three nonbenzodiazepines—eszopiclone, zolpidem, and zaleplon—have similar effects and are included here. In general, death from benzodiazepine overdose is rare unless the drugs are combined with other CNS-depressant agents such as ethanol, opioids, or barbiturates. Newer potent, short-acting agents have been considered the sole cause of death in recent forensic cases.

I. **Mechanism of toxicity.** Benzodiazepines enhance the action of the inhibitory neurotransmitter GABA. They also inhibit other neuronal systems by poorly defined mechanisms. The result is generalized depression of spinal reflexes and the reticular activating system. This can cause coma and respiratory arrest.

A. Respiratory arrest is more likely with newer short-acting benzodiazepines such as triazolam (Halcion™), alprazolam (Xanax™), and midazolam (Versed™). It has also been reported with zolpidem (Ambien™).

B. Cardiopulmonary arrest has occurred after rapid injection of diazepam, possibly because of CNS-depressant effects or because of the toxic effects of the diluent propylene glycol.

C. **Pharmacokinetics.** Most of these agents are highly protein-bound (80–100%). Time to peak blood level, elimination half-lives, the presence or absence of active metabolites, and other pharmacokinetic values are given in Table II–59, p 382.

II. **Toxic dose.** In general, the toxic:therapeutic ratio for benzodiazepines is very high. For example, oral overdoses of diazepam have been reported in excess of 15–20 times the therapeutic dose without serious depression of consciousness. However, respiratory arrest has been reported after ingestion of 5 mg of triazolam and after rapid intravenous injection of diazepam, midazolam, and many other benzodiazepines. Also, ingestion of another drug with CNS-depressant properties (ethanol, barbiturates, opioids, etc) probably will produce additive effects.

III. **Clinical presentation.** Onset of CNS depression may be observed within 30–120 minutes of ingestion, depending on the compound. Lethargy, slurred speech, ataxia, coma, and respiratory arrest may occur. Generally, patients with benzodiazepine-induced coma have hyporeflexia and midposition or small pupils. Hypo-

**TABLE II–14. BENZODIAZEPINES**

| Drug | Half-Life (h) | Active Metabolite | Oral Adult Dose (mg) |
|---|---|---|---|
| Alprazolam | 6.3–26.9 | No | 0.25–0.5 |
| Chlordiazepoxide | 18–96[a] | Yes | 5–50 |
| Clonazepam | 18–50 | No | 0.5–2 |
| Clorazepate | 40–120[a] | Yes | 3.75–30 |
| Diazepam | 40–120[a] | Yes | 5–20 |
| Estazolam | 8–28 | No | 1–2 |
| Eszopiclone[c] | 6 | No | 2–3 |
| Flunitrazepam | 20 | No | 1–2 |
| Flurazepam | 47–100[a] | Yes | 15–30 |
| Lorazepam | 10–20 | No | 2–4 |
| Midazolam | 2.2–6.8 | Yes | 1–5[b] |
| Oxazepam | 5–20 | No | 15–30 |
| Quazepam | 70–75[a] | Yes | 7.5–15 |
| Temazepam | 3.5–18.4 | No | 15–30 |
| Triazolam | 1.5–5.5 | No | 0.125–0.5 |
| Zaleplon[c] | 1 | No | 5–20 |
| Zolpidem[c] | 1.4–4.5 | No | 5–10 |

[a]Half-life of active metabolite, to which effects can be attributed.
[b]IM or IV.
[c]Not a benzodiazepine, but similar mechanism of action and clinical effects, which may be reversed with flumazenil.

thermia may occur. Serious complications are more likely when newer short-acting agents are involved or when other depressant drugs have been ingested.

**IV. Diagnosis** usually is based on the history of ingestion or recent injection. The differential diagnosis should include other sedative-hypnotic agents, antidepressants, antipsychotics, and narcotics. Coma and small pupils do not respond to naloxone but will reverse with administration of flumazenil (see below).

**A. Specific levels.** Serum drug levels are often available from commercial toxicology laboratories but are rarely of value in emergency management. Urine and blood qualitative screening may provide rapid confirmation of exposure. Certain immunoassays may not detect newer benzodiazepines or those in low concentrations. Triazolam and alprazolam are rarely detectable.

**B. Other useful laboratory studies** include glucose, arterial blood gases, and pulse oximetry.

**V. Treatment**

**A. Emergency and supportive measures**

1. Protect the airway and assist ventilation if necessary (see pp 1–7).
2. Treat coma (see p 18), hypotension (p 15), and hypothermia (p 19) if they occur. Hypotension usually responds promptly to supine position and intravenous fluids.

**B. Specific drugs and antidotes. Flumazenil** (see p 452) is a specific benzodiazepine receptor antagonist that can rapidly reverse coma. However, because benzodiazepine overdose by itself is rarely fatal, the role of flumazenil in routine management has not been established. It is administered intravenously with a starting dose of 0.1–0.2 mg, repeated as needed up to a maximum of 3 mg. It has some important potential drawbacks:

1. It may induce seizures in patients with tricyclic antidepressant overdose.
2. It may induce acute withdrawal, including seizures and autonomic instability, in patients who are addicted to benzodiazepines.
3. Resedation is common when the drug wears off after 1–2 hours, and repeated dosing or a continuous infusion is often required.

**C. Decontamination** (see p 45). Consider activated charcoal if the ingestion occurred within the previous 30 minutes and other conditions are appropriate (see Table I–38, p 51). Gastric lavage is not necessary after small to moderate ingestions if activated charcoal can be given promptly.

**D. Enhanced elimination.** There is no role for diuresis, dialysis, or hemoperfusion. Repeat-dose charcoal has not been studied.

## ► BETA-ADRENERGIC BLOCKERS

*Neal L. Benowitz, MD*

Beta-adrenergic blocking agents are widely used for the treatment of hypertension, arrhythmias, angina pectoris, heart failure, migraine headaches, and glaucoma. Many patients with beta-blocker overdose will have underlying cardiovascular diseases or will be taking other cardioactive medications, both of which may aggravate beta-blocker overdose. Of particular concern are combined ingestions with calcium blockers or tricyclic antidepressants. A variety of beta blockers are available, with various pharmacologic effects and clinical uses (Table II–15).

**I. Mechanism of toxicity.** Excessive beta-adrenergic blockade is common to overdose with all drugs in this category. Although beta-receptor specificity is seen at low doses, it is lost in overdose.

**A. Propranolol, acebutolol,** and other agents with membrane-depressant (quinidine-like) effects further depress myocardial contractility and conduction and may be associated with ventricular tachyarrhythmias. Propranolol is also lipid soluble, which enhances brain penetration and can cause seizures and coma.

**B. Pindolol** and other agents with partial beta-agonist activity may cause tachycardia and hypertension.

**C. Sotalol,** which also has type III antiarrhythmic activity, prolongs the QT interval in a dose-dependent manner and may cause torsade de pointes (see p 14) and ventricular fibrillation.

**D. Labetalol** and **carvedilol** have combined nonselective beta- and alpha-adrenergic blocking actions, both of which can contribute to hypotension in overdose.

**E. Pharmacokinetics.** Peak absorption occurs within 1–4 hours but may be much longer with sustained-release preparations. Volumes of distribution are generally large. Elimination of most agents is by hepatic metabolism, although nadolol is excreted unchanged in the urine and esmolol is rapidly inactivated by red blood cell esterases. (See also Table II–59, p 382.)

**II. Toxic dose.** The response to beta-blocker overdose is highly variable, depending on underlying medical disease or other medications. Susceptible patients may have severe or even fatal reactions to therapeutic doses. There are no clear guidelines, but ingestion of only 2–3 times the therapeutic dose (see Table II–15) should be considered potentially life-threatening in all patients. Atenolol and pindolol appear to be less toxic than other agents.

**III. Clinical presentation.** The pharmacokinetics of beta blockers varies considerably, and duration of poisoning may range from minutes to days.

**A. Cardiac disturbances,** including first-degree heart block, hypotension, and bradycardia, are the most common manifestations of poisoning. Atrioventricu-

**TABLE II–15. BETA-ADRENERGIC BLOCKERS**

| Drug | Usual Daily Adult Dose (mg/24 h) | Cardio-selective | Membrane Depression | Partial Agonist | Normal Half-Life (h) |
|---|---|---|---|---|---|
| Acebutolol | 400–800 | + | + | + | 3–6 |
| Alprenolol | 200–800 | 0 | + | ++ | 2–3 |
| Atenolol | 50–100 | + | 0 | 0 | 4–10 |
| Betaxolol[a] | 10–20 | + | 0 | 0 | 12–22 |
| Bisoprolol | 5–20 | + | 0 | 0 | 8–12 |
| Carteolol | 2.5–10 | 0 | 0 | + | 6 |
| Carvedilol[c] | 6.25–50 | 0 | 0 | 0 | 6–10 |
| Esmolol[b] | | + | 0 | 0 | 9 min |
| Labetalol[c] | 200–800 | 0 | + | 0 | 6–8 |
| Levobunolol[a] | | 0 | 0 | 0 | 5–6 |
| Metoprolol | 100–450 | + | +/– | 0 | 3–7 |
| Nadolol | 80–240 | 0 | 0 | 0 | 10–24 |
| Oxprenolol | 40–480 | 0 | + | ++ | 1–3 |
| Penbutolol | 20–40 | 0 | 0 | + | 17–26 |
| Pindolol | 5–60 | 0 | + | +++ | 3–4 |
| Propranolol | 40–360 | 0 | ++ | 0 | 2–6 |
| Sotalol[d] | 160–480 | 0 | 0 | 0 | 5–15 |
| Timolol[a] | 20–80 | 0 | 0 | +/– | 2–4 |

[a]Also available as ophthalmic preparation.
[b]Intravenous infusion.
[c]Also has alpha-adrenergic blocking activity.
[d]Class III antiarrhythmic activity.

lar block, intraventricular conduction disturbances, cardiogenic shock, and asystole may occur with severe overdose, especially with membrane-depressant drugs such as propranolol. The ECG usually shows a normal QRS duration with increased PR intervals; QRS widening occurs with massive intoxication. QT prolongation and torsade can occur with sotalol.

B. **CNS toxicity,** including convulsions, coma, and respiratory arrest, is commonly seen with propranolol and other membrane-depressant and lipid-soluble drugs.

C. **Bronchospasm** is most common in patients with preexisting asthma or chronic bronchospastic disease.

D. **Hypoglycemia** and **hyperkalemia** may occur.

IV. **Diagnosis** is based on the history of ingestion, accompanied by bradycardia and hypotension. Other drugs that may cause a similar presentation after overdose include sympatholytic and antihypertensive drugs, digitalis, and calcium channel blockers.

A. **Specific levels.** Measurement of beta-blocker serum levels may confirm the diagnosis but does not contribute to emergency management. Metoprolol, labetalol, and propranolol may be detected in comprehensive urine toxicology screening.

**B. Other useful laboratory studies** include electrolytes, glucose, BUN, creatinine, arterial blood gases, and 12-lead ECG and ECG monitoring.

**V. Treatment**

**A. Emergency and supportive measures**

1. Maintain an open airway and assist ventilation if necessary (see pp 1–7).
2. Treat coma (see p 18), seizures (p 22), hypotension (p 15), hyperkalemia (p 37), and hypoglycemia (p 34) if they occur.
3. Treat bradycardia with atropine, 0.01–0.03 mg/kg IV; isoproterenol (start with 4 mcg/min and increase infusion as needed); or cardiac pacing.
4. Treat bronchospasm with nebulized bronchodilators (see p 7).
5. Continuously monitor the vital signs and ECG for at least 6 hours after ingestion.

**B. Specific drugs and antidotes**

1. Bradycardia and hypotension resistant to the measures listed above should be treated with **glucagon,** 5–10 mg IV bolus, repeated as needed and followed by an infusion of 1–5 mg/h (see p 456). **Epinephrine** (intravenous infusion starting at 1–4 mcg/min and titrating to effect; see p 448) may also be useful. **High-dose insulin** plus glucose therapy (see also p 461) has shown benefit in animal studies of beta-blocker poisoning, but clinical studies have not been reported.
2. Wide complex conduction defects caused by membrane-depressant poisoning may respond to **sodium bicarbonate,** 1–2 mEq/kg, as given for tricyclic antidepressant overdose (see p 423).
3. Torsade de pointes polymorphous ventricular tachycardia associated with QT prolongation resulting from sotalol poisoning can be treated with **isoproterenol** infusion, **magnesium,** or **overdrive pacing** (see p 14). Correction of hypokalemia may also be useful.

**C. Decontamination** (see p 45). Administer activated charcoal orally if conditions are appropriate (see Table I–38, p 51). Gastric lavage is not necessary after small to moderate ingestions if activated charcoal can be given promptly. Consider whole-bowel irrigation for large ingestions involving sustained-release formulations.

**D. Enhanced elimination.** Most beta blockers, especially the more toxic drugs such as propranolol, are highly lipophilic and have a large volume of distribution. For those with a relatively small volume of distribution coupled with a long half-life or low intrinsic clearance (eg, acebutolol, atenolol, nadolol, and sotalol), hemoperfusion, hemodialysis, or repeat-dose charcoal may be effective.

## ▶ BETA-2 ADRENERGIC STIMULANTS

*Susan Kim, PharmD*

Beta-adrenergic agonists can be broadly categorized as having beta-1 and beta-2 receptor activity. This section describes the toxicity of beta-2–selective agonists that are commonly available for oral use: albuterol (salbutamol), metaproterenol, and terbutaline (Table II–16).

**I. Mechanism of toxicity**

**A.** Stimulation of beta-2 receptors results in relaxation of smooth muscles in the bronchi, uterus, and skeletal muscle vessels. At high toxic doses, selectivity for beta-2 receptors may be lost, and beta-1 effects may be seen.

**B. Pharmacokinetics.** These agents are readily absorbed orally or by inhalation. Half-lives and other pharmacokinetic parameters are described in Table II–59 (p 382).

**II. Toxic dose.** Generally, a single ingestion of more than the total usual daily dose (see Table II–16) may be expected to produce signs and symptoms of toxicity. Pediatric ingestion of less than 1 mg/kg of albuterol is not likely to cause serious

**TABLE II–16. BETA-2 SELECTIVE AGONISTS**

| Drug | Adult Dose (mg/d) | Pediatric Dose (mg/kg/d) | Duration (h) |
|---|---|---|---|
| Albuterol | 8–16 | 0.3–0.8 | 4–8 |
| Metaproterenol | 60–80 | 0.9–2.0 | 4 |
| Ritodrine[a] | 40–120 | N/A | 4–6 |
| Terbutaline | 7.5–20 | 0.15–0.6 | 4–8 |

[a]No longer available as an oral formulation in the United States.
N/A = dose not available.

toxicity. Dangerously exaggerated responses to therapeutic doses of terbutaline have been reported in pregnant women, presumably as a result of pregnancy-induced hemodynamic changes.

**III. Clinical presentation.** Overdoses of these drugs affect primarily the cardiovascular system. Most overdoses, especially in children, result in only mild toxicity.

- **A. Vasodilation** results in reduced peripheral vascular resistance and can lead to significant hypotension. The diastolic pressure usually is reduced to a greater extent than is the systolic pressure, resulting in a wide pulse pressure and bounding pulse.
- **B. Tachycardia** is a common reflex response to vasodilation and may also be caused by direct stimulation of beta-1 receptors as beta-2 selectivity is lost in high doses. Supraventricular tachycardia or ventricular extrasystoles are reported occasionally.
- **C. Agitation and skeletal muscle tremors** are common. Seizures are rare.
- **D. Metabolic effects** include hypokalemia, hyperglycemia, and lactic acidosis. Delayed hypoglycemia may follow initial hyperglycemia. Hypokalemia is caused by an intracellular shift of potassium rather than true depletion.

**IV. Diagnosis** is based on the history of ingestion. The findings of tachycardia, hypotension with a wide pulse pressure, tremor, and hypokalemia are strongly suggestive. Theophylline overdose (see p 355) may present with similar manifestations.

- **A. Specific levels** are not generally available and do not contribute to emergency management. These drugs are not usually detectable on comprehensive urine toxicology screening.
- **B. Other useful laboratory studies** include electrolytes, glucose, BUN, creatinine, CPK (if excessive muscle activity suggests rhabdomyolysis), and ECG monitoring.

**V. Treatment.** Most overdoses are mild and do not require aggressive treatment.

- **A. Emergency and supportive measures**
  1. Maintain an open airway and assist ventilation if necessary (see pp 1–7).
  2. Monitor the vital signs and ECG for about 4–6 hours after ingestion.
  3. If seizures and/or altered mental status occur, they are most likely caused by cerebral hypoperfusion and should respond to treatment of hypotension (see below).
  4. Treat hypotension initially with boluses of intravenous crystalloid, 10–30 mL/kg. If this fails to improve the blood pressure, use a beta-adrenergic blocker (see B, below).
  5. Sinus tachycardia rarely requires treatment, especially in children, unless accompanied by hypotension or ventricular dysrhythmias. If treatment is necessary, use beta-adrenergic blockers (see B, below).
  6. Hypokalemia does not usually require treatment, since it is transient and does not reflect a total body potassium deficit.

- **B. Specific drugs and antidotes.** Hypotension, tachycardia, and ventricular arrhythmias are caused by excessive beta-adrenergic stimulation, and beta blockers are specific antagonists. Give **propranolol** (see p 504), 0.01–0.02 mg/kg IV, or **esmolol** (see p 449), 0.025–0.1 mg/kg/min IV. Use beta blockers cautiously in patients with a prior history of asthma or wheezing.
- **C. Decontamination** (see p 45). Administer activated charcoal orally if conditions are appropriate (see Table I–38, p 51). Gastric lavage is not necessary after small to moderate ingestions if activated charcoal can be given promptly.
- **D. Enhanced elimination.** There is no role for these procedures.

## ▶ BORIC ACID, BORATES, AND BORON

*Chi-Leung Lai, PharmD*

Boric acid and sodium borate have been used for many years in a variety of products as antiseptics and as fungistatic agents in baby talcum powder. Boric acid powder (99%) is still used as a pesticide against ants and cockroaches. In the past, repeated and indiscriminate application of boric acid to broken or abraded skin resulted in many cases of severe poisoning. Epidemics have also occurred after boric acid was added mistakenly to infant formula or used in food preparation. Although chronic toxicity seldom occurs now, acute ingestion by children at home is common.

Other boron-containing compounds with similar toxicity include boron oxide and orthoboric acid (sassolite).

**I. Mechanism of toxicity**

- **A.** The mechanism of borate poisoning is unknown. Boric acid is not highly corrosive but is irritating to mucous membranes. It probably acts as a general cellular poison. The organ systems most commonly affected are the skin, gastrointestinal tract, brain, liver, and kidneys.
- **B. Pharmacokinetics.** The volume of distribution (Vd) is 0.17–0.50 L/kg. Elimination is mainly through the kidneys, and 85–100% of a dose may be found in the urine over 5–7 days. The elimination half-life is 12–27 hours.

**II. Toxic dose**

- **A.** The **acute** single oral toxic dose is highly variable, but serious poisoning is reported to occur with 1–3 g in newborns, 5 g in infants, and 20 g in adults. A teaspoon of 99% boric acid contains 3–4 g. Most accidental ingestions in children result in minimal or no toxicity.
- **B. Chronic** ingestion or application to abraded skin is much more serious than acute single ingestion. Serious toxicity and death occurred in infants ingesting 5–15 g in formula over several days; serum borate levels were 400–1600 mg/L.

**III. Clinical presentation**

- **A.** After oral or dermal absorption, the earliest symptoms are gastrointestinal, with vomiting and diarrhea. Emesis and diarrhea may have a blue-green color. Significant dehydration and renal failure can occur, with death caused by profound shock.
- **B.** Neurologic symptoms of hyperactivity, agitation, and seizures may occur early.
- **C.** An erythrodermic rash (boiled-lobster appearance) is followed by exfoliation after 2–5 days. Alopecia totalis has been reported.

**IV. Diagnosis** is based on a history of exposure, the presence of gastroenteritis (possibly with blue-green emesis), erythematous rash, acute renal failure, and elevated serum borate levels.

- **A. Specific levels.** Serum or blood borate levels are not generally available and may not correlate accurately with the level of intoxication. Analysis of serum for borates can be obtained from National Medical Services, Inc., telephone (215) 657-4900, or other large regional commercial laboratories. Normal serum or blood levels vary with diet but are usually less than 7 mg/L. The serum boron level can be estimated by dividing the serum borate by 5.72.

**B. Other useful laboratory studies** include electrolytes, glucose, BUN, creatinine, and urinalysis.

**V. Treatment**

**A. Emergency and supportive measures**

1. Maintain an open airway and assist ventilation if necessary (see pp 1–7).
2. Treat coma (see p 18), seizures (p 22), hypotension (p 15), and renal failure (p 38) if they occur.

**B. Specific drugs and antidotes.** There is no specific antidote.

**C. Decontamination** (see p 45). Activated charcoal is not very effective. Consider gastric lavage for very large ingestions.

**D. Enhanced elimination. Hemodialysis** is effective and is indicated after massive ingestions and for supportive care of renal failure. Peritoneal dialysis has not proved effective in enhancing elimination in infants.

## ▶ BOTULISM

*Ilene B. Anderson, PharmD*

German physicians first identified botulism in the late 18th century when patients developed an often fatal disease after eating spoiled sausage. Four distinct clinical syndromes are now recognized: **food-borne botulism, infant botulism, wound botulism,** and adult intestinal colonization (**adult-infant botulism**). Food-borne botulism, the most well-known form, results from ingestion of preformed toxin in improperly preserved home-canned vegetables, fish, or meats. In the last few decades, non-canned foods have also been reported to cause food-borne botulism. Examples include fresh garlic in olive oil, sautéed onions, beef or turkey pot pie, baked potatoes, potato salad, smoked whitefish, turkey loaf, and turkey stuffing.

**I. Mechanism of toxicity**

**A.** Botulism is caused by a heat-labile neurotoxin (botulin) produced by the bacteria *Clostridium botulinum.* Different strains of the bacterium produce seven distinct exotoxins: A, B, C, D, E, F, and G; types A, B, and E are most frequently involved in human disease. Botulin toxin irreversibly binds to cholinergic nerve terminals and prevents acetylcholine release from the axon. Severe muscle weakness results, and death is caused by respiratory failure. The toxin does not cross the blood-brain barrier.

**B.** Botulinum spores are ubiquitous in nature, and except in infants (and, in rare situations, adults), the ingestion of spores is harmless. However, in an anaerobic environment with a pH of 4.6–7 the spores germinate and produce botulinum toxin. The spores are relatively heat stable but can be destroyed by pressure cooking at a temperature of at least 120°C (250°F) for 30 minutes. The toxin can be destroyed by boiling at 100°C (212°F) for 1 minute or heating at 80°C (176°F) for 20 minutes. Nitrites added to meats and canned foods inhibit clostridium growth.

**II. Toxic dose.** Botulin toxin is extremely potent; as little as one taste of botulin-contaminated food (approximately 0.05 mcg of toxin) may be fatal.

**III. Clinical presentation**

**A.** Classic **food-borne botulism** occurs after ingestion of preformed toxin in contaminated food. Initial symptoms are nonspecific and may include nausea, vomiting, sore throat, and abdominal discomfort. The onset of neurologic symptoms is typically delayed 12–36 hours but may vary from a few hours to as long as 8 days. The earlier the onset of symptoms, the more severe the illness. Diplopia, ptosis, sluggishly reactive pupils, dysarthria, dysphagia, dysphonia, and other cranial nerve weaknesses occur, followed by progressive symmetric descending paralysis. The patient's mentation remains clear, and there is no sensory loss. Pupils may be either dilated and unreactive or normal. Constipation and ileus resulting from decreased motility may occur. Profound weakness involving the respiratory muscles may cause respiratory failure and death.

B. **Infant botulism** is caused by ingestion of botulism spores (not preformed toxin) followed by in vivo production of toxin (typically type A or B) in the immature infant gut. Risk factors include age less than 1 year, breast-feeding, and ingestion of honey (which commonly contains botulism spores). The illness is characterized by hypotonia, constipation, tachycardia, difficulty in feeding, poor head control, and diminished gag, sucking, and swallowing reflexes. It is rarely fatal, and infants usually recover strength within 4–6 weeks.

C. **Wound botulism** occurs when the spores contaminate a wound, germinate in the anaerobic environment, and produce toxin in vivo that then is absorbed systemically, resulting in illness. It occurs most commonly in intravenous drug abusers who "skin pop" (inject the drug subcutaneously rather than intravenously), particularly those using "black tar" heroin. It has also been reported rarely with open fractures, dental abscesses, lacerations, puncture wounds, gunshot wounds, and sinusitis. Manifestations of botulism occur after an incubation period of 1–3 weeks.

D. **Adult intestinal colonization (adult-infant) botulism** occurs rarely in adults after ingestion of botulism spores (not preformed toxin). As in infant botulism, spores germinate in the intestinal tract and the toxin is produced in vivo. Conditions predisposing patients to this rare form of botulism include a history of extensive GI surgery, decreased gastric or bile acids, ileus, and prolonged antibiotic therapy resulting in altered GI flora.

IV. **Diagnosis** is based on a high index of suspicion in any patient with a dry sore throat, clinical findings of descending cranial nerve palsies or gastroenteritis, and a history of ingestion of home-canned food. Symptoms may be slow in onset but are sometimes rapidly progressive. Electromyography may reveal normal conduction velocity but decreased motor action potential and no incremental response to repetitive stimulation. The differential diagnosis includes myasthenia gravis, Eaton-Lambert syndrome, the Miller-Fisher variant of Guillain-Barré syndrome, sudden infant death syndrome (SIDS), magnesium intoxication, paralytic shellfish poisoning, and tick-related paralysis (eg, *Dermacentor andersoni*).

A. **Specific levels.** Diagnosis is confirmed by determination of the toxin in serum, stool, gastric aspirate, or a wound; although these tests are useful for public health investigation, they cannot be used to determine initial treatment because the analysis takes more than 24 hours to perform. Obtain serum, stool, wound pus, vomitus, and gastric contents, and suspect food for toxin analysis by the local or state health department. The results may be negative if the samples were collected late or the quantity of toxin is small.

B. **Other useful laboratory studies** include electrolytes, blood sugar, arterial blood gases, electromyography, and cerebrospinal fluid (CSF) if CNS infection is suspected.

V. **Treatment**

A. **Emergency and supportive measures**

1. Maintain an open airway and assist ventilation if necessary (see pp 1–7).
2. Obtain arterial blood gases and observe closely for respiratory weakness; respiratory arrest can occur abruptly.

B. **Specific drugs and antidotes**

1. **Food-borne, wound, and adult intestinal colonization botulism**

a. **Botulinum antitoxin** (see p 424) binds the circulating free toxin and prevents the progression of illness; however, it does not reverse established neurologic manifestations. It is most effective when given within 24 hours of the onset of symptoms.

(1) Contact the local or state health department or the Centers for Disease Control, Atlanta, GA; telephone (404) 639-2888 (24-hour num-

ber) to obtain antitoxin.

(2) Determine sensitivity to horse serum prior to treatment.

(3) The empiric dose for suspected botulism is one to two vials.

b. **Guanidine** increases the release of acetylcholine at the nerve terminal but has not been shown to be clinically effective.

c. For **wound botulism,** antibiotic (eg, penicillin) treatment is indicated, along with wound debridement and irrigation.

2. **Infant botulism**

a. **BabyBIG® (Botulism Immune Globulin Intravenous [Human])** (see page 424) is indicated for the treatment of infant botulism caused by toxin type A or B in patients under 1 year of age. The horse serum-derived antitoxins are not recommended for infant botulism. To inquire about obtaining **BabyBIG®**, contact the Centers for Disease Control, Atlanta, GA; telephone (404) 639-2888. In California, contact the state Department of Health Services, telephone (510) 231-7600.

b. Antibiotics are not recommended except for treatment of secondary infections. Cathartics are not recommended.

C. **Decontamination** (see p 45). Administer activated charcoal orally if conditions are appropriate (see Table I–38, p 51).

D. **Enhanced elimination.** There is no role for enhanced elimination; the toxin binds rapidly to nerve endings, and any free toxin can be readily detoxified with antitoxin.

## ▶ BROMATES

*Thomas R. Sands, PharmD*

Bromate poisoning was most common during the 1940s and 1950s, when bromate was a popular ingredient in home permanent neutralizers. Less toxic substances have been substituted for bromates in kits for home use, but poisonings still occur occasionally from professional products (bromate-containing permanent wave neutralizers have been ingested in suicide attempts by professional hairdressers). Commercial bakeries often use bromate salts to improve bread texture, and bromates are components of the fusing material for some explosives. Bromates previously were used in matchstick heads. Bromate-contaminated sugar was the cause of one reported epidemic of bromate poisoning.

I. **Mechanism of toxicity.** The mechanism is not known. The bromate ion is toxic to the cochlea, causing irreversible hearing loss, and nephrotoxic, causing acute tubular necrosis. Bromates may be converted to hydrobromic acid in the stomach, causing gastritis. Bromates are also strong oxidizing agents that are capable of oxidizing hemoglobin to methemoglobin.

II. **Toxic dose.** The acute ingestion of 200–500 mg/kg of potassium bromate is likely to cause serious poisoning. Ingestion of 2–4 oz of 2% potassium bromate solution caused serious toxicity in children. The sodium salt is believed to be less toxic.

III. **Clinical presentation**

A. Within 2 hours of ingestion, victims develop GI symptoms, including vomiting (occasionally with hematemesis), diarrhea, and epigastric pain. This may be accompanied by restlessness, lethargy, coma, and convulsions.

B. An asymptomatic phase of a few hours may follow before overt renal failure develops. Anuria is usually apparent within 1–2 days of ingestion; renal failure may be irreversible.

C. Tinnitus and irreversible sensorineural deafness occur between 4 and 16 hours after ingestion in adults, but deafness may be delayed for several days in children.

D. Hemolysis and thrombocytopenia have been reported in some pediatric cases.

E. Methemoglobinemia (see p 262) has been reported but is rare.

IV. **Diagnosis** is based on a history of ingestion, especially if accompanied by gastroenteritis, hearing loss, or renal failure.

A. **Specific levels.** Bromates may be reduced to bromide in the serum, but bromide levels do not correlate with the severity of poisoning. There are qualitative tests for bromates, but serum concentrations are not available.

B. **Other useful laboratory studies** include CBC, electrolytes, glucose, BUN, creatinine, urinalysis, audiometry, and methemoglobin.

V. **Treatment**

A. **Emergency and supportive measures**

1. Maintain an open airway and assist ventilation if necessary (see pp 1–7).
2. Treat coma (see p 18) and seizures (p 22) if they occur.
3. Replace fluid losses, treat electrolyte disturbances caused by vomiting and diarrhea, and monitor renal function. Perform hemodialysis as needed for support of renal failure.

B. **Specific drugs and antidotes**

1. **Sodium thiosulfate** (see p 514) theoretically may reduce bromate to the less toxic bromide ion. There are few data to support the use of thiosulfate, but in the recommended dose it is benign. Administer 10% thiosulfate solution, 10–50 mL (0.2–1 mL/kg) IV.
2. Treat methemoglobinemia with **methylene blue** (see p 473).

C. **Decontamination** (see p 45). Sodium bicarbonate (baking soda), 1 tsp in 8 oz of water PO, may prevent formation of hydrobromic acid in the stomach. For large recent ingestions, consider gastric lavage with a 2% sodium bicarbonate solution to prevent formation of hydrobromic acid in the stomach. Activated charcoal may also be administered.

D. **Enhanced elimination.** The bromate ion may be removed by hemodialysis, but this treatment has not been evaluated carefully. Since bromates are primarily excreted renally, initiating hemodialysis early in the course of a documented large ingestion may be prudent therapy to prevent irreversible hearing loss and renal failure.

## ► BROMIDES

*Delia A. Dempsey, MD*

Bromide was once used as a sedative and an effective anticonvulsant, and until 1975 it was a major ingredient in over-the-counter products such as Bromo-Seltzer™ and Dr. Miles' Nervine™. Bromism (chronic bromide intoxication) was once common, accounting for as many as 5–10% of admissions to psychiatric hospitals. Bromism is now rare, although bromides occasionally are used to treat epilepsy. Bromide is still found in photographic chemicals, as the bromide salt or another constituent of numerous medications, in some well water, in bromide-containing hydrocarbons (eg, methyl bromide, ethylene dibromide, halothane), and in some soft drinks containing brominated vegetable oil. Foods fumigated with methyl bromide may contain some residual bromide, but the amounts are too small to cause toxicity.

I. **Mechanism of toxicity**

A. Bromide ions substitute for chloride in various membrane transport systems, particularly within the nervous system. Bromide is preferentially reabsorbed over chloride by the kidney. Up to 30% of chloride may be replaced in the body. With high bromide levels, the membrane-depressant effect progressively impairs neuronal transmission.

B. **Pharmacokinetics.** The volume of distribution of bromide is 0.35–0.48 L/kg. The half-life is 9–12 days, and bioaccumulation occurs with chronic exposure.

Clearance is about 26 mL/kg/day, and elimination is renal. Bromide is excreted in breast milk. It crosses the placenta, and neonatal bromism has been described.

**II. Toxic dose.** The adult therapeutic dose of bromide is 3–5 g. One death has been reported after ingestion of 100 g of sodium bromide. Chronic consumption of 0.5–1 g per day may cause bromism.

**III. Clinical presentation.** Death is rare. Acute oral overdose usually causes nausea and vomiting from gastric irritation. Chronic intoxication can result in a variety of neurologic, psychiatric, gastrointestinal, and dermatologic effects.

**A. Neurologic** and **psychiatric** manifestations are protean and include restlessness, irritability, ataxia, confusion, hallucinations, psychosis, weakness, stupor, and coma. At one time bromism was responsible for 5–10% of admissions to psychiatric facilities.

**B. Gastrointestinal** effects include nausea and vomiting (acute ingestion) and anorexia and constipation (chronic use).

**C. Dermatologic** effects include acneiform, pustular, and erythematous rashes. Up to 25% of patients are affected.

**IV. Diagnosis.** Consider bromism in any confused or psychotic patient with a high serum chloride level and a low or negative anion gap. The serum chloride level is often falsely elevated owing to interference by bromide in the analytic test; the degree of elevation varies with the instrument.

**A. Specific levels.** Endogenous serum bromide does not usually exceed 5 mg/L (0.06 mEq/L). The threshold for detection by usual methods is 50 mg/L. Therapeutic levels are 50–100 mg/L (0.6–1.2 mEq/L); levels above 3000 mg/L (40 mEq/L) may be fatal.

**B. Other useful laboratory studies** include electrolytes, glucose, BUN, creatinine, and abdominal x-ray (bromide is radiopaque).

**V. Treatment**

**A. Emergency and supportive measures**

**1.** Protect the airway and assist ventilation if needed (see pp 1–7).

**2.** Treat coma if it occurs (see p 18).

**B. Specific drugs and antidotes.** There is no specific antidote. However, administering chloride will promote bromide excretion (see below).

**C. Decontamination** (see p 45). After a recent large ingestion, perform gastric lavage. Activated charcoal does not adsorb inorganic bromide ions, but it may adsorb organic bromides.

**D. Enhanced elimination.** Bromide is eliminated entirely by the kidney. The serum half-life can be reduced dramatically with fluids and chloride loading.

**1.** Administer **sodium chloride** intravenously as half-normal saline (D50/0.5 NS) at a rate sufficient to obtain a urine output of 4–6 mL/kg/h. **Furosemide,** 1 mg/kg, may assist urinary excretion.

**2. Hemodialysis** is effective and may be indicated in patients with renal insufficiency or severe toxicity. Hemoperfusion is not effective.

## ► CADMIUM

*Leslie M. Israel, DO, MPH*

Cadmium (Cd) is found in sulfide ores, along with zinc and lead. Exposure is common during the mining and smelting of zinc, copper, and lead. The metallic form of Cd is used in electroplating because of its anticorrosive properties, the metallic salts are used as pigments and stabilizers in plastics, and Cd alloys are used in soldering and welding and in nickel-cadmium batteries. Cd solder in water pipes and Cd pigments in pottery can be sources of contamination of water and acidic foods.

**I. Mechanism of toxicity.** Inhaled Cd is at least 60 times more toxic than the ingested form. Fumes and dust may cause delayed chemical pneumonitis and resultant pulmonary edema and hemorrhage. Cd is a known human carcinogen (IARC Group 1). Ingested Cd is a GI tract irritant. Once absorbed, Cd is bound to metallothionein and filtered by the kidney, where renal tubule damage may occur.

**II. Toxic dose**

**A. Inhalation.** The ACGIH-recommended threshold limit value (TLV-TWA) for air exposure to Cd dusts and fumes, established in 1993, is 0.01 (inhalable fraction) to 0.002 (respirable dusts) mg/m$^3$ as an 8-hour time-weighted average. Exposure to 5 mg/m$^3$ inhaled for 8 hours may be lethal. The level considered immediately hazardous to life or health (IDLH) for Cd dusts or fumes is 9 mg Cd/m$^3$.

**B. Ingestion.** Cd salts in solutions of greater than 15 mg/L may induce vomiting. The lethal oral dose ranges from 350 to 8900 mg.

**C. Water.** The US Environmental Protection Agency has established a safe limit of 0.005 mg/L in drinking water.

**III. Clinical presentation**

**A. Direct contact** may cause local skin or eye irritation. There are no data on dermal absorption of Cd in humans.

**B. Acute inhalation** may cause cough, wheezing, headache, fever, and, if severe, chemical pneumonitis and noncardiogenic pulmonary edema within 12–24 hours after exposure.

**C. Chronic inhalation** at high levels is associated with lung cancer (IARC 2000).

**D. Acute ingestion** of Cd salts causes nausea, vomiting, abdominal cramps, and diarrhea, sometimes bloody, within minutes after exposure. Deaths after oral ingestion result from shock or acute renal failure.

**E. Chronic ingestion** results in accumulation of Cd in bones, causing painful *itai-itai* ("ouch-ouch") disease, and in kidneys, causing renal disease.

**IV. Diagnosis** is based on a history of exposure and the presence of respiratory complaints (after inhalation) or gastroenteritis (after ingestion).

**A. Specific levels.** Whole-blood Cd levels may confirm the exposure; normal levels are less than 1 mcg/L. Very little Cd is excreted in the urine until binding of Cd in the kidney is exceeded and renal damage occurs. Urine Cd values are normally less than 1 mcg/g of creatinine. Measures of tubular microproteinuria (beta-microglobulin, retinol-binding protein, albumin, and metallothionein) are used to monitor the early and toxic effects of Cd on the kidney.

**B. Other useful laboratory studies** include CBC, electrolytes, glucose, BUN, creatinine, arterial blood gases or oximetry, and chest x-ray.

**V. Treatment**

**A. Emergency and supportive measures**

1. **Inhalation.** Monitor arterial blood gases and obtain chest x-ray. Observe for at least 6–8 hours and treat wheezing and pulmonary edema (see pp 7–8) if they occur. After significant exposure, it may be necessary to observe for 1–2 days for delayed-onset noncardiogenic pulmonary edema.
2. **Ingestion.** Treat fluid loss caused by gastroenteritis with intravenous crystalloid fluids (see p 16).

**B. Specific drugs and antidotes.** There is no evidence that chelation therapy (eg, with BAL, EDTA, or penicillamine) is effective, although various chelating agents have been used.

**C. Decontamination**

1. **Inhalation.** Remove the victim from exposure and give supplemental oxygen if available.
2. **Ingestion** (see p 47). Perform gastric lavage after significant ingestion. The effectiveness of activated charcoal is unknown.
3. **Skin and eyes.** Remove contaminated clothing and wash exposed skin with water. Irrigate exposed eyes with copious amounts of tepid water or saline (see p 47).

**D. Enhanced elimination.** There is no role for dialysis, hemoperfusion, or repeat-dose charcoal.

# ▶ CAFFEINE

*Christine A. Haller, MD*

Caffeine is the most widely used psychoactive substance. Besides its well-known presence in coffee, tea, colas, and chocolate, it is available in many over-the-counter and prescription oral medications and as injectable caffeine sodium benzoate (occasionally used for neonatal apnea). Caffeine is widely used as an anorectant, a coanalgesic, a diuretic, and a sleep suppressant. Botanical forms of caffeine, including yerba mate, guarana (*Paullinia cupana*), kola nut (*Cola nitida*), and green tea extract, are common constituents of "thermogenic" dietary supplements that are widely touted for weight loss and athletic enhancement (see also p 215). Although caffeine has a wide therapeutic index and rarely causes serious toxicity, there are many documented cases of accidental, suicidal, and iatrogenic intoxication, some resulting in death.

**I. Mechanism of toxicity**

**A.** Caffeine is a trimethylxanthine that is closely related to theophylline. It acts primarily through nonselective inhibition of adenosine receptors. In addition, with overdose there is considerable beta-1 and beta-2 adrenergic stimulation secondary to release of endogenous catecholamines.

**B. Pharmacokinetics.** Caffeine is rapidly and completely absorbed orally with a volume of distribution of 0.7–0.8 L/kg. Its elimination half-life is approximately 4–6 hours but can range from 3 hours in healthy smokers to 10 hours in nonsmokers; after overdose the half-life may be as long as 15 hours. In infants less than 2–3 months old, metabolism is extremely slow and the half-life may exceed 24 hours. (See also Table II–59.) Caffeine is metabolized in the liver by cytochrome P-450, primarily the CYP 1A2 isoenzyme, and is subject to several potential drug interactions, including inhibition by oral contraceptives, cimetidine, norfloxacin, and alcohol. Tobacco (and marijuana) smoking accelerates caffeine metabolism.

**II. Toxic dose.** The reported lethal oral dose is 10 g (150–200 mg/kg), although one case report documents survival after a 24-g ingestion. In children, ingestion of 35 mg/kg may lead to moderate toxicity. Coffee contains 50–200 mg (tea, 40–100 mg) of caffeine per cup depending on how it is brewed. No-Doz® and other sleep suppressants usually contain about 200 mg each. "Thermogenic" dietary supplements, which are sold as energy beverages (eg, Red Bull), bars, capsules, tablets, or liquid drops, contain the equivalent of 40–200 mg of caffeine per serving as either concentrated plant extracts or synthetic caffeine. As with theophylline, chronic administration of excessive doses may cause serious toxicity with relatively low serum concentrations compared with an acute single ingestion.

**III. Clinical presentation**

**A.** The earliest symptoms of **acute** caffeine poisoning are usually anorexia, tremor, and restlessness, followed by nausea, vomiting, tachycardia, and agitation. With serious intoxication, delirium, seizures, supraventricular and ventricular tachyarrhythmias, hypokalemia, and hyperglycemia may occur. Hypotension is caused by excessive beta-2–mediated vasodilation and is characterized by a low diastolic pressure and a wide pulse pressure.

**B. Chronic** high-dose caffeine intake can lead to "caffeinism" (nervousness, irritability, anxiety, tremulousness, muscle twitching, insomnia, palpitations, and hyperreflexia).

**IV. Diagnosis** is suggested by the history of caffeine exposure or the constellation of nausea, vomiting, tremor, tachycardia, seizures, and hypokalemia (also consider theophylline; see p 355).

**A. Specific levels.** Serum caffeine levels are not routinely available in hospital laboratories but could be determined at reference toxicology laboratories. Toxic concentrations may be detected by cross-reaction with theophylline assays (see Table I–33, p 44). Coffee drinkers have caffeine levels of 1–10 mg/L, and levels exceeding 80 mg/L have been associated with death. The level associated with a high likelihood of seizures is unknown.

B. **Other useful laboratory studies** include electrolytes, glucose, and ECG monitoring.

V. **Treatment**

A. **Emergency and supportive measures**

1. Maintain an open airway and assist ventilation if necessary (see pp 1–7).
2. Treat seizures (see p 22) and hypotension (p 15) if they occur. Extreme anxiety or agitation may respond to benzodiazepines such as IV lorazepam (p 419).
3. Hypokalemia usually resolves without treatment.
4. Monitor ECG and vital signs for at least 6 hours after ingestion.

B. **Specific drugs and antidotes.** Beta blockers effectively reverse cardiotoxic and hypotensive effects mediated by excessive beta-adrenergic stimulation. Treat tachyarrhythmias and hypotension with intravenous **propranolol,** 0.01–0.02 mg/kg (see p 504), or **esmolol,** 0.025–0.1 mg/kg/min (p 449), beginning with low doses and titrating to effect. Because of its short half-life and cardioselectivity, esmolol is preferred for tachyarrhythmias in normotensive patients.

C. **Decontamination** (see p 45). Administer activated charcoal orally if conditions are appropriate (see Table I–38, p 51). Gastric lavage is not necessary after small to moderate ingestions if activated charcoal can be given promptly.

D. **Enhanced elimination.** Repeat-dose activated charcoal (see p 56) may enhance caffeine elimination. Seriously intoxicated patients (with multiple seizures, significant tachyarrhythmias, or intractable hypotension) may require hemodialysis or charcoal hemoperfusion (see p 55).

## ▶ CALCIUM ANTAGONISTS

*Nancy G. Murphy, MD, and Neal L. Benowitz, MD*

Calcium antagonists (also known as calcium channel blockers or calcium blockers) are widely used to treat angina pectoris, coronary spasm, hypertension, hypertrophic cardiomyopathy, supraventricular cardiac arrhythmias, and migraine headache. Toxicity from calcium antagonists may occur with therapeutic use (often owing to drug interactions) or as a result of accidental or intentional overdose. Overdoses of calcium antagonists are frequently life threatening and represent an important source of drug-induced mortality.

I. **Mechanism of toxicity.** Calcium antagonists slow the influx of calcium through cellular calcium channels. Currently marketed agents act primarily on vascular smooth muscle and the heart. They result in coronary and peripheral vasodilation, reduced cardiac contractility, slowed (AV) nodal conduction, and depressed sinus node activity. Lowering of blood pressure through a fall in peripheral vascular resistance may be offset by reflex tachycardia, although this reflex response may be blunted by depressant effects on contractility and sinus node activity. Table II–17 summarizes usual doses, sites of activity, and half-lives of common calcium antagonists.

A. In usual therapeutic doses, amlodipine, felodipine, isradipine, nicardipine, nifedipine, and nitrendipine act primarily on blood vessels, whereas verapamil and diltiazem act on both the heart and blood vessels. In overdose, however, this selectivity may be lost.

B. Bepridil, which is used primarily for refractory angina pectoris, has verapamil-like effects on the heart, inhibits the fast sodium channel, and has type III antiarrhythmic activity. Bepridil also has proarrhythmic effects, especially in the presence of hypokalemia.

C. Nimodipine has a greater action on cerebral arteries and is used to reduce vasospasm after recent subarachnoid hemorrhage.

**TABLE II–17. CALCIUM ANTAGONISTS**

| Drug | Usual Adult Daily Dose (mg) | Elimination Half-Life (h) | Primary Site(s) of Activity[a] |
|---|---|---|---|
| Amlodipine | 2.5–10 | 30–50 | V |
| Bepridil | 200–400 | 24 | M,V |
| Diltiazem | 90–360 (PO)<br>0.25 mg/kg (IV) | 4–6 | M,V |
| Felodipine | 5–30 | 11–16 | V |
| Isradipine | 5–25 | 8 | V |
| Nicardipine | 60–120 | 8 | V |
| Nifedipine | 30–120 | 2–5 | V |
| Nisoldipine | 20–40 | 4 | V |
| Nitrendipine | 40–80 | 2–20 | V |
| Verapamil | 120–480 (PO)<br>0.075–0.15 mg/kg (IV) | 2–8 | M,V |

[a]Major toxicity: M = myocardial (decreased contractility, AV block); V = vascular (vasodilation).

**D.** Important **drug interactions** may result in toxicity. Hypotension is more likely to occur in patients taking beta blockers, nitrates, or both, especially if they are hypovolemic after diuretic therapy. Patients taking disopyramide or other depressant cardioactive drugs and those with severe underlying myocardial disease are also at risk for hypotension. Vasodilatory shock resulting from drug interaction has been described with macrolide antibiotics. Life-threatening bradyarrhythmias, including asystole, may occur when beta blockers and verapamil are given together parenterally. Propranolol also inhibits the metabolism of verapamil. Fatal rhabdomyolysis has occurred with concurrent administration of diltiazem and statins.

**E. Pharmacokinetics.** Absorption may be delayed with sustained-release preparations. Most of these agents are highly protein bound and have large volumes of distribution. They are eliminated mainly via extensive hepatic metabolism. In a report on two patients with verapamil overdoses (serum levels 2200 and 2700 ng/mL), the elimination half-lives were 7.8 and 15.2 hours. (See also Table II–59, p 382.)

**II. Toxic dose.** Usual therapeutic daily doses for each agent are listed in Table II–17. The toxic:therapeutic ratio is relatively small, and serious toxicity may occur with therapeutic doses. For example, severe bradycardia can occur with therapeutic doses of mibefradil. Any dose greater than the usual therapeutic range should be considered potentially life threatening. Note that many of the common agents are available in sustained-release formulations, which can result in delayed onset or sustained toxicity.

**III. Clinical presentation**

**A.** The primary features of calcium antagonist intoxication are **hypotension** and **bradycardia.**

1. Hypotension may be caused by peripheral vasodilation, reduced cardiac contractility, slowed heart rate, or a combination of all three.
2. Bradycardia may result from sinus bradycardia, second- or third-degree AV block, or sinus arrest with junctional rhythm.
3. Most calcium antagonists do not affect intraventricular conduction, so the QRS duration is usually not affected. The PR interval may be prolonged even with therapeutic doses of verapamil. Bepridil prolongs the QT interval

and may cause ventricular arrhythmias, including torsade de pointes (see p 14). Mibefradil also causes QT prolongation and has been associated with ventricular arrhythmias. It has been removed from the US market.

**B. Noncardiac manifestations** of intoxication include nausea and vomiting, abnormal mental status (stupor and confusion), metabolic acidosis (probably resulting from hypotension), and hyperglycemia (owing to blockade of insulin release). Hyperglycemia results in the inability of the myocardium to utilize glucose for fuel, thereby reducing contractility and contributing to hypotension.

**IV. Diagnosis.** The findings of hypotension and bradycardia, particularly with sinus arrest or AV block, in the absence of QRS interval prolongation should suggest calcium antagonist intoxication. The differential diagnosis should include beta blockers and other sympatholytic drugs.

**A. Specific levels.** Serum or blood drug levels are not widely available. Diltiazem and verapamil may be detectable in comprehensive urine toxicology screening.

**B. Other useful laboratory studies** include electrolytes, glucose, BUN, creatinine, arterial blood gases or oximetry, and ECG and ECG monitoring.

**V. Treatment**

**A. Emergency and supportive measures**

1. Maintain an open airway and assist ventilation if necessary (see pp 1–7).
2. Treat coma (see p 18), hypotension (p 15), and bradyarrhythmias (p 10) if they occur. The use of cardiopulmonary bypass to allow time for liver metabolism has been reported in a patient with massive verapamil poisoning. Cardiac pacing should be considered for bradyarrhythmias that are contributing to hypotension.
3. Monitor the vital signs and ECG for at least 6 hours after alleged ingestion of immediate-release compounds. Sustained-release products, especially verapamil, require a longer observation period (24 hours for verapamil, 18 hours for others). Admit symptomatic patients for at least 24 hours.

**B. Specific drugs and antidotes**

1. **Calcium** (see p 428) usually promptly reverses the depression of cardiac contractility, but it does not affect sinus node depression or peripheral vasodilation and has variable effects on AV nodal conduction. Administer **calcium chloride** 10%, 10 mL (0.1–0.2 mL/kg) IV, or **calcium gluconate** 10%, 20 mL (0.3–0.4 mL/kg) IV. Repeat every 5–10 minutes as needed. In case reports, doses as high as 10–15 g over 1–2 hours and 30 g over 12 hours have been administered without apparent calcium toxicity.
2. **Glucagon** (see p 456), **epinephrine** (see p 448), and **inamrinone** (see p 460) have been reported to increase blood pressure in patients with refractory hypotension. Glucagon and epinephrine can also increase the heart rate.
3. **Hyperinsulinemia/euglycemia** (HIE) therapy is effective in animal models of severe intoxication and reportedly has been beneficial in several human case reports. The putative mechanism is correction of calcium antagonist–induced hypoinsulinemia, leading to improved cell carbohydrate metabolism, increased myocardial contractility and peripheral vascular resistance, and correction of acidosis. The treatment is not expected to improve conduction block or bradycardia. A bolus of **insulin** 0.5–1 U/kg (see p 461) is followed by an infusion of 0.5–1 U/kg/h and is accompanied by an initial bolus of **glucose** (25 g or 50 mL of $D_{50}W$; children 0.5 g/kg as $D_{25}W$) followed by additional boluses and infusions to maintain the serum glucose between 100 and 200 mg/dL. Blood sugar levels should be checked every 15–20 minutes, and serum potassium must be followed and corrected as needed.

**C. Decontamination** (see p 45). Administer activated charcoal orally if conditions are appropriate (see Table I–38, p 51). Consider gastric lavage for all but the most trivial ingestions. For large ingestions of a sustained-release preparation, consider whole-bowel irrigation (see p 51) in addition to repeated doses of charcoal (see p 56). Continue charcoal administration for up to 48–72 hours.

**D. Enhanced elimination.** Owing to extensive protein binding, dialysis and hemoperfusion are not effective. Repeat-dose activated charcoal has not been evaluated but may serve as an adjunct to gastrointestinal decontamination after overdose with sustained-release preparations.

## ▶ CAMPHOR AND OTHER ESSENTIAL OILS

*Ilene B. Anderson, PharmD*

Camphor is one of several essential oils (volatile oils) derived from natural plant products that have been used for centuries as topical rubefacients and counterirritant agents for analgesic and antipruritic purposes (Table II–18). Camphor and other essential oils are found in over-the-counter remedies such as BenGay Ultra-Strength™ (4% camphor, 10% menthol, 30% methyl salicylate), Campho-Phenique™ (10.8% camphor, 4.7% phenol), Vicks VapoRub™ (4.7% camphor, 2.6% menthol, 1.2% eucalyptus oil), and camphorated oil (20% camphor). Toxic effects have occurred primarily when essential oils have been intentionally administered orally for purported therapeutic effects and in accidental pediatric ingestions.

**I. Mechanism of toxicity.** After topical application, essential oils produce dermal hyperemia followed by a feeling of comfort, but if ingested, they can cause systemic toxicity. Most essential oils cause CNS stimulation or depression. **Camphor** is a CNS stimulant that causes seizures shortly after ingestion. The underlying mechanism is unknown. Camphor is absorbed rapidly from the GI tract and is metabolized by the liver. It is not known whether metabolites contribute to toxicity.

**II. Toxic dose.** Serious poisonings and death have occurred in children after ingestion of as little as 1 g of camphor. This is equivalent to just 10 mL of Campho-Phenique or 5 mL of camphorated oil. Recovery after ingestion of 42 g in an adult has been reported. The concentrations of other essential oils range from 1 to 20%; doses of 5–15 mL are considered potentially toxic.

**III. Clinical presentation** (see also Table II–18)

**A. Oral.** Manifestations of **acute** oral overdose usually occur within 5–30 minutes after ingestion. Burning in the mouth and throat occurs immediately, followed by nausea and vomiting. Ataxia, drowsiness, confusion, restlessness, delirium, muscle twitching, and coma may occur. Camphor typically causes abrupt onset of seizures about 20–30 minutes after ingestion. Death may result from CNS depression and respiratory arrest or may be secondary to status epilepticus. **Chronic** camphor intoxication may produce symptoms similar to Reye's syndrome.

**B.** Prolonged **skin contact** may result in a burn.

**C. Smoking** (eg, clove cigarettes) or inhaling essential oils may cause tracheobronchitis.

**IV. Diagnosis** usually is based on a history of exposure. The pungent odor of camphor and other volatile oils is usually apparent.

**A. Specific levels** are not available.

**B. Other useful laboratory studies** include electrolytes, glucose, liver transaminases, and arterial blood gases (if the patient is comatose or in status epilepticus).

**V. Treatment**

**A. Emergency and supportive measures**

1. Maintain an open airway and assist ventilation if necessary (see pp 1–7).
2. Treat seizures (see p 22) and coma (p 18) if they occur.

**TABLE II–18. ESSENTIAL OILS**

| Name | Comments |
|---|---|
| Birch oil | Contains 98% methyl salicylate (equivalent to 1.4 g aspirin per mL; see Salicylates, p 333). |
| Camphor | Pediatric toxic dose 1 g (see text). |
| Cinnamon oil | Stomatitis and skin burns can result from prolonged contact. Potent antigen. Smoked as a hallucinogen. |
| Clove oil | Contains 80–90% eugenol. Metabolic acidosis, CNS depression, seizures, coagulopathy, and hepatotoxicity after acute ingestion. Fulminant hepatic failure in a 15-month-old boy after a 10-mL ingestion. *N*-acetylcysteine may be beneficial in preventing or treating the hepatotoxicity. Smoking clove cigarettes may cause irritant tracheobronchitis, hemoptysis. |
| Eucalyptus oil | Contains 70% eucalyptol. Toxic dose is 5 mL. Ingestion causes epigastric burning and may lead to vomiting, seizures, or rapid CNS depression. |
| Guaiacol | Nontoxic. |
| Lavender oil | Used in doses of 0.1 mL as a carminative. Contains trace amounts of coumarin (see p 379). May cause photosensitization. |
| Melaleuca oil | Tea tree oil. Toxic dose in children is 10 mL. Sedation, confusion, ataxia, and coma are reported after ingestion. Onset 30–60 minutes. Contact dermatitis with dermal contact. |
| Menthol | An alcohol derived from various mint oils. Ingestion may cause oral mucosal irritation, vomiting, tremor, ataxia, and CNS depression. Estimated toxic dose in animals is >200 mg/kg. |
| Nutmeg | Myristica oil. A carminative in a dose of 0.03 mL. Used as a hallucinogen and purported to have amphetamine-like effects; 2–4 Tbsp of ground nutmeg can cause psychogenic effects. |
| Pennyroyal oil | Moderate to severe toxicity with ingestion of more than 10 mL. Fatal coma and hepatic necrosis occurred after ingestion of 30 mL by an 18-year-old woman. N-acetylcysteine may be effective in preventing hepatic necrosis. |
| Peppermint oil | Contains 50% menthol. Toxic dose is 5–10 g. Ingestion results in oral mucosal irritation and may lead to vomiting, tremor, CNS depression, bradycardia, and metabolic acidosis. |
| Pine oil | Oral mucosal irritation, CNS depression, bradycardia, hypotension reported after ingestion. |
| Thymol | Used as an antiseptic (see Phenol, p 303). May cause allergic contact dermatitis. |
| Turpentine oils | Toxic dose 15 mL in children; 140 mL in adults may be fatal. |
| Wintergreen oil | Contains methyl salicylate 98% (equivalent to 1.4 g of aspirin per mL; see Salicylates, p 333). |

**B. Specific drugs and antidotes.** There are no specific antidotes for camphor. ***N*-acetylcysteine** (see p 407) may be effective for preventing hepatic injury after pennyroyal and clove oil ingestion.

**C. Decontamination** (see p 45). Administer activated charcoal orally if conditions are appropriate (see Table I–38, p 51). Gastric lavage is not necessary after small to moderate ingestions if activated charcoal can be given promptly.

**D. Enhanced elimination.** The volumes of distribution of camphor and other essential oils are extremely large, and it is unlikely that any enhanced removal procedure will remove significant amounts of camphor. Poorly substantiated case reports have recommended hemoperfusion.

## ► CARBAMAZEPINE AND OXCARBAZEPINE

*Thomas E. Kearney, PharmD*

**Carbamazepine** (Tegretol), an iminostilbene compound, was introduced in the United States in 1974 for the treatment of trigeminal neuralgia. It has become a first-line drug for the treatment of generalized and partial complex seizure disorders and has found expanded use for pain syndromes, psychiatric illnesses, and drug withdrawal reactions. **Oxcarbazepine** (Trileptal) was approved by the US FDA in 2000 and is the 10-keto analog of carbamazepine. It is considered a prodrug with a principal metabolite, 10-hydroxycarbazepine (MHD), that is responsible for its therapeutic effects, which are similar to those of carbamazepine.

**I. Mechanism of toxicity**

**A. Carbamazepine:** Most toxic manifestations appear to be related to its CNS-depressant and anticholinergic effects. It also alters cerebellar-vestibular brainstem function. In addition, presumably because its chemical structure is similar to that of the tricyclic antidepressant imipramine, acute carbamazepine overdose can cause seizures and cardiac conduction disturbances.

**B. Oxcarbazepine** is a CNS depressant and seems to lack the toxicity profile of carbamazepine. This may be attributed to the limited rate of production of the active metabolite and lack of a toxic epoxide metabolite. The exception may be a dose-related nephrogenic dilutional hyponatremia.

**C. Pharmacokinetics.**

1. **Carbamazepine** is slowly and erratically absorbed from the GI tract, and peak levels may be delayed for 6–24 hours, particularly after an overdose (continued absorption for up to 96 hours has been reported with extended-release preparations). The exception may be with oral suspension dosage forms, where absorption may be rapid, with symptoms occurring within 30 minutes of ingestion. It is 75–78% protein bound with a volume of distribution of approximately 1.4 L/kg (up to 3 L/kg after overdose). Up to 28% of a dose is eliminated in the feces, and there is enterohepatic recycling. The parent drug is metabolized by cytochrome P-450, and 40% is converted to its 10,11-epoxide, which is as active as the parent compound. The elimination half-life is variable and is subject to autoinduction of P-450 enzymes; the half-life of carbamazepine is approximately 18–55 hours (initially) to 5–26 hours (with chronic use). The half-life of the epoxide metabolite is approximately 5–10 hours.
2. **Oxcarbazepine** is well absorbed from the GI tract (F >95%) and metabolized rapidly (half-life of 1–5 hours) to its active metabolite, MHD, with peak levels achieved 1–3 hours and 4–12 hours for the parent and the active metabolite, respectively. The active metabolite has 30–40% protein binding, a volume of distribution of 0.8 L/kg, and a half-life of 7–20 hours (average 9 hours). The active metabolite is not subject to autoinduction.

**II. Toxic dose.**

**A. Carbamazepine.** Acute ingestion of more than 10 mg/kg could result in a blood level above the therapeutic range of 4–12 mg/L. The recommended maximum daily dose is 1.6–2.4 g in adults (35 mg/kg/day in children). Death has occurred after adult ingestion of 3.2–60 g, but survival has been reported after an 80-g ingestion. Life-threatening toxicity occurred after ingestion of 5.8–10 g in adults and 2 g (148 mg/kg) in a 23-month-old child.

**B. Oxcarbazepine.** The recommended daily therapeutic dose is 0.6–1.2 g in adults (8–10 mg/kg/day in children up to 600 mg/d) up to a maximum of 2.4 g/day (which is poorly tolerated). Ingestion of 30.6 g by an adult resulted in only mild CNS depression. However, an adult who ingested 3.3 g while on oxcarbazepine therapy developed CNS and cardiovascular symptoms.

**III. Clinical presentation**

**A. Carbamazepine.**

1. Ataxia, nystagmus, ophthalmoplegia, movement disorders (dyskinesia, dys-

tonia), mydriasis, and sinus tachycardia are common with mild to moderate overdose. With more serious intoxication, myoclonus, seizures (including status epilepticus), hyperthermia, coma, and respiratory arrest may occur. Atrioventricular block and bradycardia have been reported, particularly in the elderly. Based on its structural similarity to tricyclic antidepressants, carbamazepine may cause QRS and QT interval prolongation and myocardial depression; however, in case reports of overdose, QRS widening rarely exceeds 100–120 msec and is usually transient.

2. After an acute overdose, manifestations of intoxication may be delayed for several hours because of erratic absorption. Cyclic coma and rebound relapse of symptoms may be caused by continued absorption from a tablet mass as well as enterohepatic circulation of the drug.
3. Chronic use has been associated with bone marrow depression, hepatitis, renal disease, cardiomyopathy, hyponatremia, and exfoliative dermatitis. Carbamazepine also has been implicated in rigidity-hyperthermia syndromes (eg, neuroleptic malignant syndrome and serotonin syndrome) in combination with other drugs.

**B. Oxcarbazepine.** The primary side effects and overdose symptoms are CNS-related (drowsiness, ataxia, diplopia, tinnitus, dizziness, tremor, headache, and fatigue). Status epilepticus was reported in patients with severe mental retardation. There is also a report of a dose-related dystonia (oculogyric crisis). Cardiovascular-related effects (bradycardia and hypotension) were observed after an ingestion of 3.3 g. Significant hyponatremia (most commonly associated with high doses and elderly patients) may be a contributory cause of seizures and coma associated with oxcarbazepine. Hypersensitivity reactions—rash, eosinophilia, and leukopenia—have been reported and have 25–35% cross-reactivity with carbamazepine.

**IV. Diagnosis** is based on a history of exposure and clinical signs such as ataxia and stupor and, in the case of carbamazepine, tachycardia.

**A. Specific levels.** Obtain a stat serum carbamazepine level and repeat levels every 4–6 hours to rule out delayed or prolonged absorption.

1. Serum levels of carbamazepine greater than 10 mg/L are associated with ataxia and nystagmus. Serious intoxication (coma, respiratory depression, seizures) is likely with serum levels greater than 40 mg/L, although there is poor correlation between levels and severity of clinical effects.
2. The epoxide metabolite of carbamazepine may be produced in high concentrations after overdose. It is nearly equipotent and may cross-react with some carbamazepine immunoassays to a variable extent.
3. Carbamazepine can produce a false-positive test for tricyclic antidepressants on drug screening.
4. A 30.6-g ingestion of **oxcarbazepine** resulted in a level of 31.6 mg/L (10-fold above the therapeutic range) for the parent drug and 59 mg/L or two-fold greater than the therapeutic range (10-35 mg/L) for the active metabolite, MHD. A 3.3-g ingestion resulted in an MHD level of 45.6 mg/L.

**B. Other useful laboratory studies** include CBC, electrolytes (in particular sodium), glucose, arterial blood gases or oximetry, and ECG monitoring.

**V. Treatment**

**A. Emergency and supportive measures**

1. Maintain an open airway and assist ventilation if necessary (see pp 1–7). Administer supplemental oxygen.
2. Treat seizures (see p 22), coma (p 18), hyperthermia (p 20), arrhythmias (p 13), hyponatremia (p 36), and dystonias (p 75) if they occur.
3. Asymptomatic patients should be observed for a minimum of 6 hours after ingestion and for at least 12 hours if an extended-release preparation was ingested. Note that CNS depression after oxcarbazepine poisoning may progress over 24 hours owing to prolonged production of the active metabolite.

**B. Specific drugs and antidotes.** There is no specific antidote. Sodium bicarbonate (see p 423) is of unknown value for QRS prolongation. Physostigmine is ***not*** recommended for anticholinergic toxicity.

**C. Decontamination** (see p 45). Administer activated charcoal orally if conditions are appropriate (see Table I–38, p 51). Gastric lavage is not necessary after small to moderate ingestions if activated charcoal can be given promptly. For massive ingestions of carbamazepine, consider additional doses of activated charcoal and possibly whole-bowel irrigation (see p 51).

**D. Enhanced elimination.** In contrast to tricyclic antidepressants, the volumes of distribution of carbamazepine and the active metabolite of oxcarbazepine, MHD, are small, making both accessible to enhanced removal procedures.

1. **Repeat-dose activated charcoal** is effective for carbamazepine and may increase clearance by up to 50%. However, it may be difficult to perform safely in a patient with obtundation and ileus, and there is no demonstrated benefit in terms of morbidity or mortality.
2. **Charcoal hemoperfusion** is highly effective for carbamazepine and may be indicated for severe intoxication (eg, status epilepticus, cardiotoxicity, serum level > 60 mg/L) unresponsive to standard treatment. High-flux (also known as high-efficiency) **hemodialysis** is also reportedly effective.
3. Peritoneal dialysis does not remove carbamazepine effectively.
4. Plasma exchange has been used in children with carbamazepine poisoning.
5. Although no case reports exist utilizing techniques of enhanced elimination for oxcarbazepine poisoning, the pharmacokinetics of its active metabolite, MHD, make it theoretically amenable to dialysis owing to low protein binding and small volume of distribution. However, current case overdose experience suggests that supportive care is sufficient and life-threatening symptoms are unlikely.

# ► CARBON DISULFIDE

*Paul D. Blanc, MD, MSPH*

Carbon disulfide is a volatile organic solvent that is used industrially as a starting material in rayon manufacture in the viscose process. It was important historically in the cold vulcanization of rubber. Although no longer used in this form, carbon disulfide is still a major industrial precursor in rubber industry chemical synthesis and has a number of other industrial applications. Carbon disulfide also is widely used as a solvent in a variety of laboratory settings. It is a metabolite of the drug disulfiram (see p 184) and a spontaneous breakdown by-product of the pesticide metam sodium.

**I. Mechanism of toxicity.** Carbon disulfide toxicity appears to involve disruption of a number of metabolic pathways in various organ systems, including but not limited to the central nervous system. Although key toxic effects have been attributed to the functional disruption of enzymes, especially in dopamine-dependent systems, carbon disulfide is widely reactive with a variety of biologic substrates.

**II. Toxic dose**

**A.** Carbon disulfide is highly volatile (vapor pressure 297 mm Hg), and inhalation is a major route of exposure. The OSHA workplace limit (permissible exposure limit—ceiling; PEL-C) for carbon disulfide is 30 ppm (the PEL is 20 ppm with an allowable 15-minute peak to 100 ppm). The ACGIH-recommended workplace exposure limit (threshold limit value—8-hour time-weighted average) is considerably lower at 1 ppm. The NIOSH recommended exposure limit (REL) is also 1 ppm. Carbon disulfide is also well absorbed through the skin.

**B.** Acute carbon disulfide overexposure via ingestion is unusual, but if ingested, it probably will be very well absorbed. Chronic ingestion of therapeutic doses of disulfiram (200 mg per day) has been suspected to cause carbon disulfide–mediated toxicity, but this has not been firmly established.

**III. Clinical presentation**

**A.** Acute carbon disulfide exposure can cause eye and skin irritation and CNS depression.

**B.** Short-term (days to weeks) high-level exposure to carbon disulfide is associated with psychiatric manifestations ranging from mood change to frank delirium and psychosis.

**C.** Chronic lower-level exposure can cause parkinsonism and other poorly reversible CNS impairments, optic neuritis, peripheral neuropathy, and atherosclerosis. Based on animal data, carbon disulfide exposure is likely to be associated with adverse reproductive outcomes.

**IV. Diagnosis** of carbon disulfide toxicity is based on a history of exposure along with consistent signs and symptoms of one of its toxic manifestations. Industrial hygiene data documenting airborne exposure, if available, are useful diagnostically and in initiating protective measures.

**A. Specific levels.** Biological monitoring for carbon disulfide is not performed routinely.

**B. Other useful laboratory studies** can include nerve conduction studies if neuropathy is suspected and brain magnetic resonance imaging/magnetic resonance angiography (MRI/MRA) to assess the central nervous system.

**V. Treatment**

**A. Emergency and supportive measures.** Severe acute exposure would present as nonspecific CNS depression.

1. Maintain an open airway and assist ventilation if necessary (see pp 1–7). Administer supplemental oxygen.
2. Start an intravenous line and monitor the patient's vital signs and ECG closely.

**B. Specific drugs and antidotes.** There are no specific antidotes for carbon disulfide.

**C. Decontamination** after high-level exposure (see p 45).

1. **Inhalation.** Remove the victim from exposure and give supplemental oxygen if available.
2. **Skin and eyes.** Remove contaminated clothing and wash exposed skin. Irrigate exposed eyes with copious amounts of tepid water or saline (see p 46).
3. **Ingestion.** Administer activated charcoal if it is available and the patient is alert. Consider gastric lavage if the ingestion occurred within 60 minutes of presentation.

**D. Enhanced elimination.** There is no role for these procedures.

## ► CARBON MONOXIDE

*Kent R. Olson, MD*

Carbon monoxide (CO) is a colorless, odorless, tasteless, and nonirritating gas produced by the incomplete combustion of any carbon-containing material. Common sources of human exposure include smoke inhalation in fires; automobile exhaust fumes; faulty or poorly ventilated charcoal, kerosene, or gas stoves; and, to a lesser extent, cigarette smoke and methylene chloride (see p 266). Carbon monoxide poisoning accounts for approximately 40,000 emergency department visits every year in the United States.

**I. Mechanism of toxicity.** Toxicity is a consequence of cellular hypoxia and ischemia.

**A.** CO binds to hemoglobin with an affinity 250 times that of oxygen, resulting in reduced oxyhemoglobin saturation and decreased blood oxygen-carrying capacity. In addition, the oxyhemoglobin dissociation curve is displaced to the left, impairing oxygen delivery at the tissues.

**B.** CO may also directly inhibit cytochrome oxidase, further disrupting cellular function, and it is known to bind to myoglobin, possibly contributing to impaired myocardial contractility.

**C.** In animal models of intoxication, damage is most severe in areas of the brain that are highly sensitive to ischemia and often correlates with the severity of systemic hypotension. Postanoxic injury appears to be complicated by lipid peroxidation, excessive release of excitatory neurotransmitters, and inflammatory changes, including adherence of neutrophils to cerebral vessels.

**D.** Fetal hemoglobin is more sensitive to binding by CO, and fetal or neonatal levels may be higher than maternal levels.

**E. Pharmacokinetics.** The carboxyhemoglobin complex gradually dissociates after removal from exposure. The approximate half-life of elimination of CO-Hgb during treatment with high-flow oxygen by tight-fitting mask or endotracheal tube is 74 minutes (range 24–148). In room air the approximate half-life is as much as 200 minutes, and during hyperbaric oxygen therapy it is as short as 12–20 minutes.

**II. Toxic dose.** The recommended workplace limit (ACGIH TLV-TWA) for carbon monoxide is 25 ppm as an 8-hour time-weighted average. The level considered immediately dangerous to life or health (IDLH) is 1200 ppm (0.12%). However, the *duration* of exposure is very important. Whereas exposure to 1000 ppm (0.1%) eventually will result in 50% saturation of carboxyhemoglobin, it may take several hours to reach that level. In 1895 Haldane experimented on himself by breathing 2100 ppm CO for over an hour, and it was only after 34 minutes, when his level would have been approximately 25%, that he described a throbbing headache. Brief exposure to much higher levels may produce a more rapid rise in CO-Hgb.

**III. Clinical presentation.** Symptoms of intoxication are predominantly in organs with high oxygen consumption such as the brain and heart.

**A.** The majority of patients complain of headache, dizziness, and nausea. Patients with coronary disease may experience angina or myocardial infarction. With more severe exposures, impaired thinking, syncope, coma, convulsions, cardiac arrhythmias, hypotension, and death may occur. Although blood carboxyhemoglobin levels may not correlate reliably with the severity of intoxication, levels greater than 25% are considered significant and levels greater than 40–50% usually are associated with obvious intoxication.

**B.** Survivors of serious poisoning may suffer numerous overt neurologic sequelae consistent with a hypoxic-ischemic insult, ranging from gross deficits such as parkinsonism and a persistent vegetative state to subtler personality and memory disorders. Various studies suggest that the incidence of subtle neuropsychiatric sequelae such as impaired memory and concentration and mood disorders may be as high as 47%.

**C.** Exposure during pregnancy may result in fetal demise.

**IV. Diagnosis** is not difficult if there is a history of exposure (eg, the patient was found in a car in a locked garage) but may be elusive if it is not suspected in less obvious cases. There are no specific reliable clinical findings; cherry-red skin coloration or bright red venous blood is highly suggestive but not frequently noted. The routine arterial blood gas machine measures the partial pressure of oxygen dissolved in plasma ($pO_2$), but oxygen saturation is calculated from the $pO_2$ and is therefore unreliable in patients with CO poisoning. Pulse oximetry also gives falsely normal readings because it is unable to distinguish between oxyhemoglobin and carboxyhemoglobin.

**A. Specific levels.** Obtain a specific carboxyhemoglobin concentration. Persistence of fetal hemoglobin may produce falsely elevated carboxyhemoglobin levels in young infants.

**B. Other useful laboratory studies** include electrolytes, glucose, BUN, creatinine, ECG, and pregnancy tests. Metabolic acidosis suggests more serious poisoning. With smoke inhalation, obtain the blood cyanide level and methemoglobin concentration.

**TABLE II–19. HYPERBARIC OXYGEN: PROPOSED INDICATIONS FOR CO POISONING[a]**

Loss of consciousness
CO Hgb > 25%
Age > 50 years
Metabolic acidosis (base excess less than 2 mEq/L)
Cerebellar dysfunction

[a]From Weaver LK et al: Outcome of acute carbon monoxide poisoning treated with hyperbaric or normobaric oxygen (abstract). *Undersea Hyperb Med* 2001;28(suppl):15, and Weaker LK et al: Hyperbaric oxygen for acute carbon monoxide poisoning. *N Engl J Med* 2002;347:1057–1067.

**V. Treatment**

**A. Emergency and supportive measures**

1. Maintain an open airway and assist ventilation if necessary (see pp 1–7). If smoke inhalation has also occurred, consider early intubation for airway protection.
2. Treat coma (p 18) and seizures (p 22) if they occur.
3. Continuously monitor the ECG for several hours after exposure.
4. Because smoke often contains other toxic gases, consider the possibility of cyanide poisoning (see p 176), methemoglobinemia (p 262), and irritant gas injury (p 212).

**B. Specific drugs and antidotes.** Administer **oxygen** in the highest possible concentration (100%). Breathing 100% oxygen speeds the elimination of CO from hemoglobin to approximately 1 hour, compared with 6 hours in room air. Use a tight-fitting mask and high-flow oxygen with a reservoir (nonrebreather) or administer the oxygen by endotracheal tube. Treat until the carboxyhemoglobin level is less than 5%. Consider **hyperbaric oxygen** in severe cases (see below).

**C. Decontamination.** Remove the patient immediately from exposure and give supplemental oxygen. Rescuers exposed to potentially high concentrations of CO should wear self-contained breathing apparatus.

**D. Enhanced elimination.** Hyperbaric oxygen provides 100% oxygen under 2–3 atmospheres of pressure and can enhance elimination of CO (half-life reduced to 20–30 minutes). In animal models it reduces lipid peroxidation and neutrophil activation, and in a recent randomized controlled trial in humans it reduced the incidence of subtle cognitive sequelae compared with normobaric 100% oxygen, although an earlier similar study found no benefit. Hyperbaric oxygen may be useful in patients with severe intoxication, especially when there is ready access to a chamber. It remains unclear whether its benefits over normobaric oxygen apply to victims who present many hours after exposure or have milder degrees of intoxication. Consult a regional poison control center ([800] 222-1222) for advice and for the location of nearby hyperbaric chambers. See Table II–19 for a list of proposed indications for hyperbaric oxygen.

## ► CARBON TETRACHLORIDE AND CHLOROFORM

*Frederick Fung, MD, MS*

**Carbon tetrachloride** ($CCl_4$, tetrachloromethane) was once used widely as a dry cleaning solvent, degreaser, spot remover, fire extinguisher agent, and antihelminthic. Because of its liver toxicity and known carcinogenicity in animals, its role has become limited; it is now used mainly as an intermediate in chemical manufacturing. **Chloroform** (trichloromethane) is a chlorinated hydrocarbon solvent used as a raw material in the production of freon and as an extractant and solvent in the chemical and pharmaceutical industries. Because of its hepatic toxicity, it is no longer used as a general anesthetic or antihelminthic agent. Chronic low-level exposure may occur in some municipal water supplies owing to chlorination of biologic methanes (trihalomethanes).

I. **Mechanism of toxicity.** Carbon tetrachloride and chloroform are CNS depressants and potent hepatic and renal toxins. They may also increase the sensitivity of the myocardium to arrhythmogenic effects of catecholamines. The mechanism of hepatic and renal toxicity is thought to be a result of a toxic free-radical intermediate (tricholomethyl radical) of cytochrome P-450 metabolism. This radical can bind to cellular molecules (nucleic acid, protein, lipid) and form DNA adducts. Bioactivation of $CCl_4$ has become a model for chemical toxicity induced by free radicals. The toxic reactions are important to elucidate the mechanisms of apoptosis, fibrosis, and carcinogenicity. Chronic use of metabolic enzyme inducers such as phenobarbital and ethanol increases the toxicity of carbon tetrachloride. Carbon tetrachloride is a known animal and a suspected human carcinogen. Chloroform is embryotoxic and is an animal carcinogen.

II. **Toxic dose**

A. Toxicity from **inhalation** is dependent on the concentration in air and the duration of exposure.

1. **Carbon tetrachloride.** Symptoms have occurred after exposure to 160 ppm for 30 minutes. The recommended workplace limit (ACGIH TLV-TWA) is 5 ppm as an 8-hour time-weighted average, and the air level considered immediately dangerous to life or health (IDLH) is 200 ppm.
2. **Chloroform.** The air level considered immediately dangerous to life or health (IDLH) is 500 ppm. The recommended workplace limit (ACGIH TLV-TWA) is 10 ppm as an 8-hour time-weighted average.

B. **Ingestion**

1. **Carbon tetrachloride.** Ingestion of as little as 5 mL has been reported to be fatal.
2. **Chloroform.** The fatal **oral** dose may be as little as 10 mL, although survival after ingestion of more than 100 mL has been reported. The oral $LD_{50}$ in rats is 2000 mg/kg.

III. **Clinical presentation**

A. Persons exposed to carbon tetrachloride or chloroform from **acute inhalation, skin absorption, or ingestion** may present with nausea, vomiting, headache, dizziness, and confusion. Mucous membrane irritation is also seen with ingestion or inhalation. With serious intoxication, respiratory arrest, cardiac arrhythmias, and coma may occur.

B. Severe and sometimes fatal **renal and hepatic damage** may become apparent after 1–3 days.

C. **Skin or eye contact** results in irritation and a defatting type of dermatitis.

IV. **Diagnosis** is based on a history of exposure and the clinical presentation of mucous membrane irritation, CNS depression, arrhythmias, and hepatic necrosis. Carbon tetrachloride is radiopaque and may be visible on abdominal x-ray after acute ingestion.

A. **Specific levels.** Blood, urine, or breath concentrations may document exposure but are rarely available and are not useful for acute management. Qualitative urine screening for chlorinated hydrocarbons (Fujiwara test) may be positive after massive overdose.

B. **Other useful laboratory studies** include electrolytes, glucose, BUN, creatinine, liver transaminases, prothrombin time, and ECG monitoring.

V. **Treatment**

A. **Emergency and supportive measures**

1. Maintain an open airway and assist ventilation if necessary (see pp 1–7).
2. Treat coma (p 18) and arrhythmias (pp 12–15) if they occur. ***Caution:*** Avoid the use of epinephrine or other sympathomimetic amines because

they may induce or aggravate arrhythmias. Tachyarrhythmias caused by increased myocardial sensitivity may be treated with **propranolol,** 1–2 mg IV in adults (see p 504), or **esmolol,** 0.025–0.1 mg/kg/min IV (see p 449). Monitor patients for at least 4–6 hours after exposure and longer if they are symptomatic.

**B. Specific treatment.** ***N*-acetylcysteine** (see p 407) may minimize hepatic and renal toxicity by providing a scavenger for the toxic intermediate. Although its use for carbon tetrachloride or chloroform poisoning has not been studied in humans, acetylcysteine is widely used without serious side effects for treatment of acetaminophen overdose. If possible, it should be given within the first 12 hours after exposure. Animal studies also suggest possible roles for cimetidine, calcium channel blockers, and hyperbaric oxygen in reducing hepatic injury, but there is insufficient human experience with these treatments.

**C. Decontamination** (see p 45)

1. **Inhalation.** Remove from exposure and give supplemental oxygen, if available.
2. **Skin and eyes.** Remove contaminated clothing and wash affected skin with copious soap and water. Irrigate exposed eyes with copious saline or water.
3. **Ingestion.** Administer activated charcoal orally if conditions are appropriate (see Table I–38, p 51). Consider gastric lavage if the ingestion occurred within 60 minutes of presentation.

**D. Enhanced elimination.** There is no role for dialysis, hemoperfusion, or other enhanced removal procedures.

## ► CARDIAC GLYCOSIDES

*Neal L. Benowitz, MD*

Cardiac glycosides are found in several plants, including oleander, foxglove, lily of the valley, red squill, and rhododendron, and in toad venom (*Bufo* spp, which may be found in some Chinese herbal medications and herbal aphrodisiacs). Cardiac glycosides are used therapeutically in tablet form as digoxin and digitoxin. Digoxin is also available in liquid-filled capsules with greater bioavailability.

**I. Mechanism of toxicity**

**A.** Cardiac glycosides inhibit the function of the sodium-potassium-ATPase pump. After acute overdose, this results in hyperkalemia (with chronic intoxication, the serum potassium level is usually normal or low owing to concurrent diuretic therapy).

**B.** Vagal tone is potentiated, and sinus and AV node conduction velocity is decreased.

**C.** Automaticity in Purkinje fibers is increased because of accumulation of intracellular calcium.

**D. Pharmacokinetics.** The bioavailability of digoxin ranges from 60–80%; for digitoxin more than 90% is absorbed. The volume of distribution (Vd) of digoxin is very large (5–10 L/kg), whereas for digitoxin the Vd is small (about 0.5 L/kg). Peak effects occur after a delay of 6–12 hours. The elimination half-life of digoxin is 30–50 hours, and for digitoxin it is 5–8 days (owing to enterohepatic recirculation). (See also Table II–59, p 382.)

**II. Toxic dose.** Acute ingestion of as little as 1 mg of digoxin in a child or 3 mg of digoxin in an adult can result in serum concentrations well above the therapeutic range. More than these amounts of digoxin and other cardiac glycosides may be found in just a few leaves of oleander or foxglove. Generally, children appear to be more resistant than adults to the cardiotoxic effects of cardiac glycosides.

**III. Clinical presentation.** Intoxication may occur after acute accidental or suicidal ingestion or with chronic therapy. Signs and symptoms depend on the chronicity of the intoxication.

**A.** With **acute overdose,** vomiting, hyperkalemia, sinus bradycardia, sinoatrial arrest, and second- or third-degree AV block are common. Ventricular tachycardia or fibrillation may occur.

**B.** With **chronic intoxication,** visual disturbances, weakness, sinus bradycardia, atrial fibrillation with slowed ventricular response rate or junctional escape rhythm, and ventricular arrhythmias (ventricular bigeminy or trigeminy, ventricular tachycardia, bidirectional tachycardia, and ventricular fibrillation) are common. Accelerated junctional tachycardia and paroxysmal atrial tachycardia with block are seen frequently. Hypokalemia and hypomagnesemia from chronic diuretic use may be evident and appear to worsen the tachyarrhythmias.

**IV. Diagnosis** is based on a history of recent overdose or characteristic arrhythmias (eg, bidirectional tachycardia and accelerated junctional rhythm) in a patient receiving chronic therapy. Hyperkalemia suggests acute ingestion but also may be seen with very severe chronic poisoning. Serum potassium levels higher than 5.5 mEq/L are associated with severe poisoning.

**A. Specific levels.** Stat serum digoxin and/or digitoxin levels are recommended, although they may not correlate accurately with the severity of intoxication. This is especially true after acute ingestion, when the serum level is high for 6–12 hours before tissue distribution is complete. After use of digitalis-specific antibodies, the radioimmunoassay digoxin level is falsely markedly elevated. Therapeutic levels of digoxin are 0.5–2 ng/mL; those of digitoxin, 10–30 ng/mL.

**B. Other useful laboratory studies** include electrolytes, BUN, creatinine, serum magnesium, and ECG and ECG monitoring.

**V. Treatment**

**A. Emergency and supportive measures**

1. Maintain an open airway and assist ventilation if necessary (see pp 1–7).
2. Monitor the patient closely for at least 12–24 hours after significant ingestion because of delayed tissue distribution.
3. Treat **hyperkalemia** (see p 37) if it is greater than 5.5 mEq/L with sodium bicarbonate (1 mEq/kg), glucose (0.5 g/kg IV) with insulin (0.1 U/kg IV), or sodium polystyrene sulfonate (Kayexalate, 0.5 g/kg PO). Do ***not*** use calcium; it may worsen ventricular arrhythmias. Mild hyperkalemia may actually protect against tachyarrhythmias.
4. Treat **bradycardia** or **heart block** with atropine, 0.5–2 mg IV (see p 415); a temporary transvenous cardiac pacemaker may be needed for persistent symptomatic bradycardia.
5. **Ventricular tachyarrhythmias** may respond to correction of low potassium or magnesium. Lidocaine (see p 469) and phenytoin (p 304) have been used, but digoxin-specific-antibody is the preferred treatment for life-threatening arrhythmias. Avoid quinidine, procainamide, and other type Ia or type Ic antiarrhythmic drugs.

**B. Specific drugs and antidotes.** Fab fragments of **digoxin-specific antibodies** (Digibind, DigiFab) are indicated for significant poisoning (eg, severe hyperkalemia and symptomatic arrhythmias) and possibly for prophylactic treatment in a massive oral overdose with high serum levels. Antibodies should also be considered for patients with renal insufficiency, which is associated with impaired clearance and a longer anticipated duration of digitalis toxicity. Digibind rapidly binds to digoxin and, to a lesser extent, digitoxin and other cardiac glycosides. The inactive complex that is formed is excreted rapidly in the urine. Details of dose calculation and infusion rate are given on p 441.

**C. Decontamination** (see p 45). Administer activated charcoal orally if conditions are appropriate (see Table I–38, p 51). Gastric lavage is not necessary after small to moderate ingestions if activated charcoal can be given promptly.

**D. Enhanced elimination**

1. Because of its large volume of distribution, **digoxin** is not effectively removed by dialysis or hemoperfusion. Repeat-dose activated charcoal may be useful in patients with severe renal insufficiency, in whom clearance of digoxin is markedly diminished.
2. **Digitoxin** has a small volume of distribution and also undergoes extensive enterohepatic recirculation, and its elimination can be markedly enhanced by repeat-dose charcoal.

# ► CAUSTIC AND CORROSIVE AGENTS

*Walter H. Mullen, PharmD*

A wide variety of chemical and physical agents may cause corrosive injury. They include mineral and organic acids, alkalis, oxidizing agents, denaturants, some hydrocarbons, and agents that cause exothermic reactions. Although the mechanism and the severity of injury may vary, the consequences of mucosal damage and permanent scarring are shared by all these agents.

**Button batteries** are small disk-shaped batteries used in watches, calculators, and cameras. They contain caustic metal salts such as mercuric chloride that may cause corrosive injury.

**I. Mechanism of toxicity**

**A. Acids** cause an immediate coagulation-type necrosis that creates an eschar, which tends to self-limit further damage.

**B.** In contrast, **alkalis** (eg, Drano) cause a liquefactive necrosis with saponification and continued penetration into deeper tissues, resulting in extensive damage.

**C. Other agents** may act by alkylating, oxidizing, reducing, or denaturing cellular proteins or by defatting surface tissues.

**D. Button batteries** cause injury by corrosive effects resulting from leakage of the corrosive metal salts, by direct impaction of the disk-shaped foreign body, and possibly by local discharge of electrical current at the site of impaction.

**II. Toxic dose.** There is no specific toxic dose or level because the concentration of corrosive solutions and the potency of caustic effects vary widely. The concentration or the pH of the solution may indicate the potential for serious injury. For alkalis, the titratable alkalinity (concentration of the base) is a better predictor of corrosive effect than is the pH.

**III. Clinical presentation**

**A. Inhalation** of corrosive gases (eg, chlorine and ammonia) may cause upper respiratory tract injury, with stridor, hoarseness, wheezing, and noncardiogenic pulmonary edema. Pulmonary symptoms may be delayed after exposure to gases with low water solubility (eg, nitrogen dioxide and phosgene; see p 213).

**B. Eye or skin** exposure to corrosive agents usually results in immediate pain and redness, followed by blistering. Conjunctivitis and lacrimation are common. Serious full-thickness burns and blindness can occur.

**C. Ingestion** of corrosives can cause oral pain, dysphagia, drooling, and pain in the throat, chest, or abdomen. Esophageal or gastric perforation may occur, manifested by severe chest or abdominal pain, signs of peritoneal irritation, or pancreatitis. Free air may be visible in the mediastinum or abdomen on x-ray. Hematemesis and shock may occur. Systemic acidosis has been reported after acid ingestion and may be caused partly by absorption of hydrogen ions. Scarring of the esophagus or stomach may result in permanent stricture formation and chronic dysphagia.

**D. Systemic toxicity** can occur after inhalation, skin exposure, or ingestion of a variety of agents (Table II–20).

**TABLE II–20. CORROSIVE AGENTS WITH SYSTEMIC EFFECTS (SELECTED CAUSES)[a]**

| Corrosive Agent | Systemic Symptoms |
|---|---|
| Formaldehyde | Metabolic acidosis; formate poisoning (see p 206) |
| Hydrofluoric acid | Hypocalcemia; hyperkalemia (see p 222) |
| Methylene chloride | CNS depression; cardiac arrhythmias; converted to carbon monoxide (see p 266) |
| Oxalic acid | Hypocalcemia; renal failure (see p 296) |
| Paraquat | Pulmonary fibrosis (see p 297) |
| Permanganate | Methemoglobinemia (see p 262) |
| Phenol | Seizures; coma; hepatic and renal damage (see p 303) |
| Phosphorus | Hepatic and renal injury (see p 308) |
| Picric acid | Renal injury |
| Silver nitrate | Methemoglobinemia (see p 262) |
| Tannic acid | Hepatic injury. |

[a]Reference: Edelman PA: Chemical and electrical burns, pages 183–202. In *Management of the Burned Patient*, Achauer BM (editor). Appleton & Lange, 1987.

E. **Button batteries** usually cause serious injury only if they become impacted in the esophagus, leading to perforation into the aorta or mediastinum. Most cases involve large (25-mm-diameter) batteries. If button batteries reach the stomach without impaction in the esophagus, they nearly always pass uneventfully via the stools within several days.

IV. **Diagnosis** is based on a history of exposure to a corrosive agent and characteristic findings of skin, eye, or mucosal irritation or redness and the presence of injury to the GI tract. Victims with oral or esophageal injury nearly always have drooling or pain on swallowing.

A. **Endoscopy.** Esophageal or gastric injury is unlikely after ingestion if the patient is completely asymptomatic, but studies have shown repeatedly that a small number of patients will have injury in the absence of oral burns or obvious dysphagia. For this reason, many authorities recommend endoscopy for all patients regardless of symptoms.

B. **X-rays** of the chest and abdomen usually reveal impacted button batteries. X-rays may also demonstrate air in the mediastinum from esophageal perforation or free abdominal air from gastric perforation.

C. **Specific levels.** See the specific chemical. Urine mercury levels have been reported to be elevated after button battery ingestion.

D. **Other useful laboratory studies** include CBC, electrolytes, glucose, arterial blood gases, chest x-ray, and upright abdominal x-ray.

V. **Treatment**

A. **Emergency and supportive measures**

1. **Inhalation.** Give supplemental oxygen and observe closely for signs of progressive airway obstruction or noncardiogenic pulmonary edema (see pp 6–7).

2. **Ingestion**

a. Immediately give water or milk to drink.

b. If esophageal or gastric perforation is suspected, obtain immediate surgical or endoscopic consultation.

B. **Specific drugs and antidotes.** For most agents, there is no specific antidote. (See p 222 for hydrofluoric acid burns and p 303 for phenol burns.) In the past, corticosteroids were used by many clinicians in the hope of reducing scarring, but this treatment has been proved ineffective. Moreover, steroids may be harmful in a patient with perforation because they mask early signs of inflammation and inhibit resistance to infection.

**C. Decontamination** (see p 45). ***Caution:*** Rescuers should use appropriate respiratory and skin-protective equipment.

1. **Inhalation.** Remove from exposure; give supplemental oxygen if available.
2. **Skin and eyes.** Remove all clothing; wash skin and irrigate eyes with copious water or saline.
3. **Ingestion**
   a. **Prehospital.** Immediately give water or milk to drink. Do ***not*** induce vomiting or give pH-neutralizing solutions (eg, dilute vinegar or bicarbonate).
   b. **Hospital. Gastric lavage** to remove the corrosive material is controversial but is probably beneficial in acute liquid corrosive ingestion, and it will be required before endoscopy anyway. Use a soft flexible tube and lavage with repeated aliquots of water or saline, frequently checking the pH of the washings.
   c. In general, do ***not*** give activated charcoal, as it may interfere with visibility at endoscopy. Charcoal may be appropriate if the ingested agent can cause significant systemic toxicity.
   d. **Button batteries** lodged in the esophagus must be removed immediately by endoscopy to prevent rapid perforation. Batteries in the stomach or intestine should not be removed unless signs of perforation or obstruction develop.

**D. Enhanced elimination.** In general, there is no role for any of these procedures (see specific chemical).

# ▶ CHLORATES

*Thomas R. Sands, PharmD*

Potassium chlorate is a component of some match heads; barium chlorate (see also p 127) is used in the manufacture of fireworks and explosives; sodium chlorate is still a major ingredient in some weed killers used in commercial agriculture; and other chlorate salts are used in dye production. Safer and more effective compounds have replaced chlorate in toothpaste and antiseptic mouthwashes. Chlorate poisoning is similar to bromate intoxication (see p 138), but chlorates are more likely to cause intravascular hemolysis and methemoglobinemia.

**I. Mechanism of toxicity.** Chlorates are potent oxidizing agents and also attack sulfhydryl groups, particularly in red blood cells and the kidneys. Chlorates cause methemoglobin formation as well as increased fragility of red blood cell membranes, which may result in intravascular hemolysis. Renal failure probably is caused by a combination of direct cellular toxicity and hemolysis.

**II. Toxic dose.** The minimum toxic dose in children is not established but is estimated to range from 1 g in infants to 5 g in older children. Children may ingest up to 1–2 matchbooks without toxic effect (each match head may contain 10–12 mg of chlorate). The adult lethal dose was estimated to be 7.5 g in one case but is probably closer to 20–35 g. A 26-year-old woman survived a 150- to 200-g ingestion.

**III. Clinical presentation.** Within a few minutes to hours after ingestion, abdominal pain, vomiting, and diarrhea may occur. Methemoglobinemia is common (see p 261). Massive hemolysis, hemoglobinuria, and acute tubular necrosis may occur over 1–2 days after ingestion. Coagulopathy and hepatic injury have been described.

**IV. Diagnosis** usually is based on a history of exposure and the presence of methemoglobinemia and hemolysis.

A. **Specific levels.** Blood levels are not available.
B. **Other useful laboratory studies** include CBC, haptoglobin, plasma free hemoglobin, electrolytes, glucose, BUN, creatinine, bilirubin, methemoglobin level, prothrombin time, liver transaminases, and urinalysis.

V. **Treatment**
A. **Emergency and supportive measures**
1. Maintain an open airway and assist ventilation if necessary (see pp 1–7).
2. Treat coma (see p 18), hemolysis, hyperkalemia (p 37), and renal (p 38) or hepatic failure (p 39) if they occur.
3. Massive hemolysis may require blood transfusions. To prevent renal failure resulting from deposition of free hemoglobin in the kidney tubules, administer intravenous fluids and sodium bicarbonate.

B. **Specific drugs and antidotes**
1. Treat methemoglobinemia with **methylene blue** (see p 473), 1–2 mg/kg (0.1–0.2 mL/kg) of 1% solution. Methylene blue is reportedly most effective when used early in mild cases but has poor effectiveness in severe cases in which hemolysis has already occurred.
2. Intravenous **sodium thiosulfate** (see p 514) may inactivate the chlorate ion and has been reported to be successful in anecdotal reports. However, this treatment has not been clinically tested. Administration as a lavage fluid may potentially produce some hydrogen sulfide, and so it is contraindicated.

C. **Decontamination** (see p 45). Administer activated charcoal orally if conditions are appropriate (see Table I–38, p 51). Gastric lavage is not necessary after small to moderate ingestions if activated charcoal can be given promptly. ***Note:*** Spontaneous vomiting is common after significant ingestion.
D. **Enhanced elimination.** Chlorates are eliminated mainly through the kidney; elimination may be hastened by hemodialysis, especially in patients with renal insufficiency. Exchange transfusion and peritoneal dialysis have been used in a few cases.

## ► CHLORINATED HYDROCARBON PESTICIDES

*Darren H. Lew, PharmD*

Chlorinated hydrocarbon pesticides are used widely in agriculture, structural pest control, and malaria control programs around the world. Lindane is used medicinally for the treatment of lice and scabies. Chlorinated hydrocarbons are of major toxicologic concern, and many (eg, DDT and chlordane) have been banned from commercial use because they persist in the environment and accumulate in biologic systems. In 2002, sale of lindane was banned in California.

I. **Mechanism of toxicity**
A. Chlorinated hydrocarbons are neurotoxins that interfere with transmission of nerve impulses, especially in the brain, resulting in behavioral changes, involuntary muscle activity, and depression of the respiratory center. They may also sensitize the myocardium to arrhythmogenic effects of catecholamines, and many can cause liver or renal injury, possibly owing to generation of toxic metabolites. In addition, some chlorinated hydrocarbons may be carcinogenic.
B. **Pharmacokinetics.** Chlorinated hydrocarbons are well absorbed from the GI tract, across the skin, and by inhalation. They are highly lipid soluble and accumulate with repeated exposure. Elimination does not follow first-order kinetics; compounds are released slowly from body stores over days to several months or years.

II. **Toxic dose.** The acute toxic doses of these compounds are highly variable, and reports of acute human poisonings are limited. Table II–21 ranks the relative toxicity of several common compounds.

**TABLE II–21. CHLORINATED HYDROCARBONS**

| Low Toxicity (animal oral $LD_{50}$ > 1 g/kg) | Moderately Toxic (animal oral $LD_{50}$ > 50 mg/kg) | Highly Toxic (animal oral $LD_{50}$ < 50 mg/kg) |
|---|---|---|
| Ethylan (Perthane) | Chlordane | Aldrin |
| Hexachlorobenzene | DDT | Dieldrin |
| Methoxychlor | Heptachlor | Endrin |
| | Kepone | Endosulfan |
| | Lindane | |
| | Mirex | |
| | Toxaphene | |

A. **Ingestion** of as little as 1 g of lindane can produce seizures in a child, and 10–30 g is considered lethal in an adult. The estimated adult lethal oral doses of aldrin and chlordane are 3–7 g each; that of dieldrin, 2–5 g. A 49-year-old man died after ingesting 12 g of endrin. A 20-year-old man survived a 60-g endosulfan ingestion but was left with a chronic seizure disorder.

B. **Skin absorption** is a significant route of exposure, especially with aldrin, dieldrin, and endrin. Extensive or repeated (as little as 2 applications on 2 successive days) whole-body application of lindane to infants has resulted in seizures and death.

III. **Clinical presentation.** Shortly after acute ingestion, nausea and vomiting occur, followed by paresthesias of the tongue, lips, and face; confusion; tremor; obtundation; coma; seizures; and respiratory depression. Because chlorinated hydrocarbons are highly lipid soluble, the duration of toxicity may be prolonged.

A. Recurrent or delayed-onset seizures have been reported.
B. Arrhythmias may occur owing to myocardial sensitivity to catecholamines.
C. Metabolic acidosis may occur.
D. Signs of hepatitis or renal injury may develop.
E. Hematopoietic dyscrasias can develop late.

IV. **Diagnosis** is based on the history of exposure and clinical presentation.

A. **Specific levels.** Chlorinated hydrocarbons can be measured in the serum, but levels are not routinely available.

B. **Other useful laboratory studies** include electrolytes, glucose, BUN, creatinine, hepatic transaminases, prothrombin time, and ECG monitoring.

V. **Treatment**

A. **Emergency and supportive measures**

1. Maintain an open airway and assist ventilation if necessary (see pp 1–7). Administer supplemental oxygen. As most liquid products are formulated in organic solvents, observe for evidence of pulmonary aspiration (see Hydrocarbons, p 219).
2. Treat seizures (p 22), coma (p 18), and respiratory depression (p 5) if they occur. Ventricular arrhythmias may respond to beta-adrenergic blockers such as propranolol (p 504) and esmolol (see p 449).
3. Attach an electrocardiographic monitor and observe the patient for at least 6–8 hours.

B. **Specific drugs and antidotes.** There is no specific antidote.

C. **Decontamination** (see p 45)

1. **Skin and eyes.** Remove contaminated clothing and wash affected skin with copious soap and water, including hair and nails. Irrigate exposed eyes with copious tepid water or saline. Rescuers must take precautions to avoid personal exposure.
2. **Ingestion.** Administer activated charcoal orally if conditions are appropriate (see Table I–38, p 51). Gastric lavage is not necessary after small to moderate ingestions if activated charcoal can be given promptly.

D. **Enhanced elimination** (see p 53)

1. Repeat-dose activated charcoal or cholestyramine resin may be administered to enhance elimination by interrupting enterohepatic circulation.
2. Exchange transfusion, peritoneal dialysis, hemodialysis, and hemoperfusion are not likely to be beneficial because of the large volume of distribution of these chemicals.

## ▶ CHLORINE

*R. Steven Tharratt, MD, MPVM*

Chlorine is a heavier-than-air yellowish-green gas with an irritating odor. It is used widely in chemical manufacturing, in bleaching, and (as hypochlorite) in swimming pool disinfectants and cleaning agents. **Hypochlorite** is an aqueous solution produced by the reaction of chlorine gas with water; most household bleach solutions contain 3–5% hypochlorite; swimming pool disinfectants and industrial-strength cleaners may contain up to 20% hypochlorite. The addition of acid to hypochlorite solution may release chlorine gas. The addition of ammonia to hypochlorite solution may release chloramine, a gas with toxic properties similar to those of chlorine.

I. **Mechanism of toxicity.** Chlorine gas produces a corrosive effect on contact with moist tissues such as the eyes and upper respiratory tract. Exposure to aqueous solutions causes corrosive injury to the eyes, skin, or GI tract (see p 157). Chloramine is less water soluble and may produce more indolent or delayed irritation.

II. **Toxic dose**

A. **Chlorine gas.** The recommended workplace limit (ACGIH TLV-TWA) for chlorine gas is 0.5 ppm (1.5 mg/m$^3$) as an 8-hour time-weighted average. The short-term exposure limit (STEL) is 1 ppm. The level considered immediately dangerous to life or health (IDLH) is 10 ppm.

B. **Aqueous solutions.** Dilute aqueous hypochlorite solutions (3–5%) commonly found in homes rarely cause serious burns but are moderately irritating. However, more concentrated industrial cleaners (20% hypochlorite) are much more likely to cause serious corrosive injury.

III. **Clinical presentation**

A. **Inhalation of chlorine gas.** Symptoms are rapid in onset owing to the relatively high water solubility of chlorine. Immediate burning of the eyes, nose, and throat occurs, accompanied by coughing. Wheezing also may occur, especially in patients with preexisting bronchospastic disease. With serious exposure, upper-airway swelling may rapidly cause airway obstruction, preceded by croupy cough, hoarseness, and stridor. With massive exposure, noncardiogenic pulmonary edema (chemical pneumonitis) may also occur.

B. **Skin or eye contact with gas or concentrated solution.** Serious corrosive burns may occur. Manifestations are similar to those of other corrosive exposures (see p 157).

C. **Ingestion of aqueous solutions.** Immediate burning in the mouth and throat is common, but no further injury is expected after ingestion of 3–5% hypochlorite. With more concentrated solutions, serious esophageal and gastric burns may occur, and victims often have dysphagia, drooling, and severe throat, chest, and abdominal pain. Hematemesis and perforation of the esophagus or stomach may occur.

IV. **Diagnosis** is based on a history of exposure and description of the typical irritating odor, accompanied by irritative or corrosive effects on the eyes, skin, or upper respiratory or GI tract.

A. **Specific levels** are not available.

B. **Other useful laboratory studies** include, with **ingestion,** CBC, electrolytes, and chest and abdominal radiographs; with **inhalation,** arterial blood gases or oximetry and chest radiography.

**V. Treatment**

**A. Emergency and supportive measures**

**1. Inhalation of chlorine gas**

**a.** Immediately give humidified supplemental oxygen. Observe carefully for signs of progressive upper-airway obstruction and intubate the trachea if necessary (see pp 1–7).

**b.** Use bronchodilators for wheezing and treat noncardiogenic pulmonary edema (pp 5–8) if it occurs.

**2. Ingestion of hypochlorite solution.** If a solution of 10% or greater has been ingested or if there are any symptoms of corrosive injury (dysphagia, drooling, or pain), flexible endoscopy is recommended to evaluate for serious esophageal or gastric injury. Obtain chest and abdominal radiographs to look for mediastinal or intra-abdominal air, which suggests perforation.

**B. Specific drugs and antidotes.** There is no proven specific treatment for this or other common caustic burns or inhalations. The inhalation of sodium bicarbonate solutions has not been proved to be beneficial and is not recommended. The administration of corticosteroids is unproven and may be harmful in patients with perforation or serious infection.

**C. Decontamination** (see p 45)

**1. Inhalation.** Remove immediately from exposure and give supplemental oxygen if available. Administer inhaled bronchodilators if wheezing is present.

**2. Skin and eyes.** Remove contaminated clothing and flush exposed skin immediately with copious water. Irrigate exposed eyes with water or saline.

**3. Ingestion of hypochlorite solution.** Immediately give water by mouth. Do ***not*** induce vomiting. Gastric lavage may be useful after concentrated liquid ingestion in order to remove any corrosive material in the stomach and to prepare for endoscopy; use a small flexible tube to avoid injury to damaged mucosa.

**C.** Do ***not*** use activated charcoal; it may obscure the endoscopist's view.

**D. Enhanced elimination.** There is no role for enhanced elimination.

## ▶ CHLOROPHENOXY HERBICIDES

*Michael A. O'Malley, MD, MPH*

Chlorophenoxy compounds have been widely used as herbicides. Agent Orange was a mixture of the chlorophenoxy herbicides 2.4-D (dichlorophenoxyacetic acid) and 2,4,5-T (trichlorophenoxyacetic acid) that also contained small amounts of the highly toxic contaminant TCDD (2,3,7,8-tetrachlorodibenzo-*p*-dioxin; see p 183) derived from the process of manufacturing 2,4,5-T. Manufacture of 2,4-D by chlorination of phenol does not produce TCDD. Populations involved in the manufacture or handling of 2,4,5-T may show elevated levels of TCDD on serum testing and overall increased rates of cancer compared with the general population.

There are numerous formulations available in the United States, including 2,4-D salts (sodium, amine, alkylamine, and alkanolamine) and esters (propanoic acid, butanoic acid, and other alkoxy compounds). Concentrated formulations of 2,4-D esters are likely to contain petroleum solvents (identified on the "first aid" statement on the pesticide label); although these are considered "inert" ingredients because they are not pesticides, they may have their own innate toxicity (see Toluene and Xylene, p 358, and Hydrocarbons, p 219).

**I. Mechanism of toxicity.** In plants, the compounds act as growth hormone stimulators. The mechanism of toxicity is unclear but may involve mitochondrial injury. In animals, cell membrane damage, uncoupling of oxidative phosphorylation, and disruption of acetylcoenzyme A metabolism are found, widespread muscle damage occurs, and the cause of death is usually ventricular fibrillation. Toxicity is markedly increased at doses that exceed the capacity of the renal anion transport mechanism (approximately 50 mg/kg). Massive rhabdomyolysis has been described in human patients, most often in cases involving ingestion of formulations containing more than 10% active ingredient.

**II. Toxic dose.** Doses of 5 mg/kg of 2,4-D are reported to have no effect in human volunteer studies. The minimum toxic dose of 2,4-D in humans is 3–4 g or 40–50 mg/kg, and death has occurred after adult ingestion of 6.5 g. Less than 6% of 2,4-D applied to the skin is absorbed systemically, although dermal exposure may produce skin irritation. The degree of dermal absorption may be less with salt formulations than with 2,4-D esters.

**III. Clinical presentation**

**A. Acute ingestion.** Vomiting, abdominal pain. and diarrhea are common. Tachycardia. muscle weakness, and muscle spasms occur shortly after ingestion and may progress to profound muscle weakness and coma. Massive rhabdomyolysis, metabolic acidosis, and severe and intractable hypotension have been reported, resulting in death within 24 hours. Neurotoxic effects include ataxia, hypertonia, seizures, and coma. Hepatitis and renal failure may occur.

**B. Dermal exposure** to 2,4-D may produce skin irritation. Exposures to formulations containing 2,4,5-T may also produce chloracne. Substantial dermal exposure has been reported to cause a mixed sensory-peripheral neuropathy after a latent period.

**IV. Diagnosis** depends on a history of exposure and the presence of muscle weakness and elevated serum CPK.

**A. Specific levels** of 2,4-D can be measured but may not be available in a timely enough fashion to be of help in establishing the diagnosis. The elimination half-life of 2,4-D is 11.5 hours, and more than 75% is excreted by 96 hours after ingestion. More than 80% is excreted in the urine unchanged.

**B. Other useful laboratory studi**es include electrolytes, glucose, BUN, creatinine, CPK, urinalysis (occult heme test positive in the presence of myoglobin), liver enzymes, 12-lead ECG, and ECG monitoring.

**V. Treatment**

**A. Emergency and supportive measures**

1. Maintain an open airway and assist ventilation if necessary (see pp 1–7).
2. Treat coma (see p 18), hypotension (p 15), and rhabdomyolysis (p 26) if they occur.
3. Monitor the patient closely for at least 6–12 hours after ingestion because of the potential for delayed onset of symptoms.

**B. Specific drugs and antidotes.** There is no specific antidote.

**C. Decontamination (see p 45)**

1. **Skin or eye exposure.** Remove contaminated clothing and wash affected areas.
2. **Ingestion.** Administer activated charcoal orally if conditions are appropriate (see Table I–38, p 51). If a delay of more than 60 minutes is expected before charcoal can be given, consider using ipecac to induce vomiting if it can be administered within a few minutes of exposure and there are no contraindications (see p 51). Consider gastric lavage after a large recent ingestion.

**D. Enhanced elimination.** There is no proven role for these procedures, although alkalinization of the urine may promote excretion of 2,4-D. (As with other weak acids, alkalinization would be expected to promote ionization of thephenoxy acid and decrease reabsorption from the renal tubules.) Hemodialysis has been recommended on the basis of limited clinical data showing clearances similar to alkaline diuresis. Plasmapheresis was reported effective in a pediatric case report involving polyneuropathy associated with 2,4-D ingestion.

## ▶ CHLOROQUINE AND OTHER AMINOQUINOLINES

*Neal L. Benowitz, MD*

Chloroquine and other aminoquinolines are used in the prophylaxis of or therapy for malaria and other parasitic diseases. Chloroquine and hydroxychloroquine also are used in the treatment of rheumatoid arthritis. Drugs in this class include chloroquine phosphate (Aralen™), amodiaquine hydrochloride (Camoquin™), hydroxychloroquine sulfate (Plaquenil™), mefloquine (Lariam™), primaquine phosphate, and quinacrine hydrochloride (Atabrine™). Chloroquine overdose is common, especially in countries where malaria is prevalent, and the mortality rate is 10–30%. Quinine toxicity is described on p 326.

**I. Mechanism of toxicity**

A. **Chloroquine** blocks the synthesis of DNA and RNA and also has some quinidine-like cardiotoxicity. Hydroxychloroquine has similar actions but is considerably less potent.

B. **Primaquine** and **quinacrine** are oxidizing agents and can cause methemoglobinemia or hemolytic anemia (especially in patients with glucose-6-phosphate dehydrogenase [G6PD] deficiency).

C. **Pharmacokinetics.** Chloroquine and related drugs are highly tissue-bound (volume of distribution [Vd] = 150–250 L/kg) and are eliminated very slowly from the body. The terminal half-life of chloroquine is 2 months, and that of hydroxychloroquine is 40 days. Primaquine is extensively metabolized with a half-life of 3–8 hours to an active metabolite that is eliminated much more slowly (half-life 22–30 hours) and can accumulate with chronic dosing. (See also Table II–59.)

**II. Toxic dose.** The therapeutic dose of chloroquine phosphate is 500 mg once a week for malaria prophylaxis or 2.5 g over 2 days for treatment of malaria. Deaths have been reported in children after ingesting one or two tablets—doses as low as 300 mg; the lethal dose of chloroquine for an adult is estimated at 30–50 mg/kg.

**III. Clinical presentation**

A. **Mild to moderate chloroquine overdose** results in dizziness, nausea and vomiting, abdominal pain, headache and visual disturbances (sometimes including irreversible blindness), auditory disturbances (sometimes leading to deafness), agitation, and neuromuscular excitability. The use of chloroquine and proguanil in combination is common and is associated with GI and neuropsychiatric side effects, including acute psychosis.

B. **Severe chloroquine overdose** may cause convulsions, coma, shock, and respiratory or cardiac arrest. Quinidine-like cardiotoxicity may be seen, including sinoatrial arrest, depressed myocardial contractility, QRS and/or QT interval prolongation, heart block, and ventricular arrhythmias. Severe hypokalemia sometimes occurs and may contribute to arrhythmias.

C. **Primaquine** and **quinacrine** intoxication commonly causes GI upset and may also cause severe methemoglobinemia (see p 262) or hemolysis; chronic treatment can cause ototoxicity and retinopathy.

D. **Amodiaquine** in therapeutic doses has caused severe and even fatal neutropenia.

E. **Mefloquine** in therapeutic use or overdose may cause headache, dizziness, vertigo, insomnia, visual and auditory hallucinations, panic attacks, severe depression, psychosis, confusion, and seizures. Neuropsychiatric side effects generally resolve within a few days after withdrawal of mefloquine and with supportive pharmacotherapy, but occasionally symptoms persist for several weeks.

**IV. Diagnosis.** The findings of gastritis, visual disturbances, and neuromuscular excitability, especially if accompanied by hypotension, QRS or QT interval widening, or ventricular arrhythmias, should suggest chloroquine overdose. Hemolysis or methemoglobinemia should suggest primaquine or quinacrine overdose.

A. **Specific levels.** Chloroquine is usually not detected on comprehensive toxicology screening. Quantitative levels can be measured in blood but are not generally available. Because chloroquine is concentrated intracellularly, whole-blood measurements are fivefold higher than serum or plasma levels.
   1. Plasma (trough) concentrations of 10–20 ng/mL (0.01–0.02 mg/L) are effective in the treatment of various types of malaria.
   2. Cardiotoxicity may be seen with serum levels of 1 mg/L (1000 ng/mL); serum levels reported in fatal cases have ranged from 1 to 210 mg/L (average, 60 mg/L).

B. **Other useful laboratory studies** include electrolytes, glucose, BUN, creatinine, and ECG and ECG monitoring. With **primaquine** or **quinacrine,** also include CBC, free plasma hemoglobin, and methemoglobin.

V. **Treatment**

A. **Emergency and supportive measures**
   1. Maintain an open airway and assist ventilation if necessary (see pp 1–7).
   2. Treat seizures (see p 22), coma (p 18), hypotension (p 15), and methemoglobinemia (p 262) if they occur.
   3. Treat massive hemolysis with blood transfusions if needed and prevent hemoglobin deposition in the kidney tubules by alkaline diuresis (as for rhabdomyolysis; see p 26).
   4. Continuously monitor the ECG for at least 6–8 hours or until ECG normalizes.

B. **Specific drugs and antidotes**
   1. Treat cardiotoxicity as for quinidine poisoning (see p 326) with **sodium bicarbonate** (see p 423), 1–2 mEq/kg IV.
   2. Potassium should be administered for severe hypokalemia but should be dosed with caution and with frequent serum potassium measurements, as hyperkalemia may exacerbate quinidine-like cardiotoxicity.
   3. **Epinephrine** infusion (see p 448) may be useful in treating hypotension via combined vasoconstrictor and inotropic actions. Dosing recommendations in one study were 0.25 mcg/kg/min, increasing by increments of 0.25 mcg/kg/min until adequate blood pressure was obtained, along with administration of high-dose diazepam (see below) and mechanical ventilation.
   4. High-dose **diazepam** (2 mg/kg IV given over 30 minutes after endotracheal intubation and mechanical ventilation) has been reported to reduce mortality in animals and to ameliorate cardiotoxicity in human chloroquine poisonings. The mechanism of protection is unknown.

C. **Decontamination** (see p 45). Administer activated charcoal orally if conditions are appropriate (see Table I–38, p 51). Perform gastric lavage for significant ingestions (eg, > 30–50 mg/kg).

D. **Enhanced elimination.** Because of extensive tissue distribution, enhanced removal procedures are ineffective.

## ▶ CHROMIUM

*Thomas J. Ferguson, MD, PhD*

Chromium is a durable metal used in electroplating, paint pigments (chrome yellow), primers and corrosion inhibitors, wood preservatives, textile preservatives, and leather tanning agents. Chromium exposure may occur by inhalation, ingestion, or skin exposure. Although chromium can exist in a variety of oxidation states, most human exposures involve one of two types: trivalent (eg, chromic oxide, chromic sulfate) or hexavalent (eg, chromium trioxide, chromic anhydride, chromic acid, dichromate salts). Toxicity is associated most commonly with hexavalent compounds; however, fatalities have occurred after ingestion of compounds of either type, and chronic skin sensitivity probably is related to the trivalent form. Chromium picolinate is a trivalent chromium compound often promoted as a body-building agent.

**I. Mechanism of toxicity**

**A. Trivalent chromium** compounds are relatively insoluble and noncorrosive and are less likely to be absorbed through intact skin. Biologic toxicity is estimated to be 10- to 100-fold lower than for the hexavalent compounds.

**B. Hexavalent compounds** are powerful oxidizing agents and are corrosive to the airway, skin, mucous membranes, and GI tract. Acute hemolysis and renal tubular necrosis may also occur. Chronic occupational exposure to less soluble hexavalent forms is associated with chronic bronchitis, dermatitis, and lung cancer.

**C. Chromic acid** is a strong acid, whereas some chromate salts are strong bases.

**II. Toxic dose**

**A. Inhalation.** The OSHA workplace permissible exposure limit (PEL, 8-hour time-weighted average) for chromic acid and hexavalent compounds is 0.05 mg/m$^3$ (carcinogen). For bivalent and trivalent chromium the PEL is 0.5 mg/m$^3$.

**B. Skin.** Chromium salts can cause skin burns, which may enhance systemic absorption, and death has occurred after a 10% surface area burn.

**C. Ingestion.** Life-threatening toxicity has occurred from ingestion of as little as 500 mg of hexavalent chromium. The estimated lethal dose of chromic acid is 1–2 g, and of potassium dichromate it is 6–8 g. Drinking water standards are set at 50 mcg/L (1 micromol/L) total chromium.

**III. Clinical presentation**

**A. Inhalation.** Acute inhalation can cause upper respiratory tract irritation, wheezing, and noncardiogenic pulmonary edema (which may be delayed for several hours to days after exposure). Chronic exposure to hexavalent compounds may lead to pulmonary sensitization, asthma, and cancer.

**B. Skin and eyes.** Acute contact may cause severe corneal injury, deep skin burns, and oral or esophageal burns. Hypersensitivity dermatitis may result. It has been estimated that chronic chromium exposure is responsible for about 8% of all cases of contact dermatitis. Nasal ulcers may also occur after chronic exposure.

**C. Ingestion.** Ingestion may cause acute hemorrhagic gastroenteritis; the resulting massive fluid and blood loss may cause shock and oliguric renal failure. Hemolysis, hepatitis, and cerebral edema have been reported. Chromates are capable of oxidizing hemoglobin, but clinically significant methemoglobinemia is relatively uncommon after acute overdose.

**IV. Diagnosis** is based on a history of exposure and clinical manifestations such as skin and mucous membrane burns, gastroenteritis, renal failure, and shock.

**A. Specific levels.** Blood levels are not useful in emergency management and are not widely available. Detection in the urine may confirm exposure; normal urine levels are less than 1 mcg/L.

**B. Other useful laboratory studies** include CBC, plasma free hemoglobin and haptoglobin (if hemolysis is suspected), electrolytes, glucose, BUN, creatinine, liver transaminases, urinalysis (for hemoglobin), arterial blood gas or pulse oximetry, methemoglobin, and chest x-ray.

**V. Treatment**

**A. Emergency and supportive measures**

**1. Inhalation.** Give supplemental oxygen. Treat wheezing (see p 7) and monitor the victim closely for delayed-onset noncardiogenic pulmonary edema (p 6). Delays in the onset of pulmonary edema of up to 72 hours have been reported after inhalation of concentrated solutions of chromic acid.

**2. Ingestion**

**a.** Dilute immediately with water. Treat hemorrhagic gastroenteritis with aggressive fluid and blood replacement (see p 16). Consider early endoscopy to assess the extent of esophageal or gastric injury.

b. Treat hemoglobinuria resulting from hemolysis with alkaline diuresis as for rhabdomyolysis (see p 26). Treat methemoglobinemia (p 262) if it occurs.

B. **Specific drugs and antidotes**

1. Chelation therapy (eg, with BAL) is not effective.
2. After oral ingestion of hexavalent compounds, **ascorbic acid** has been suggested to assist the conversion of hexavalent to less toxic trivalent compounds. Although no definitive studies exist, the treatment is benign and may be helpful. In animal studies the effective dose was 2–4 g of ascorbic acid orally per gram of hexavalent chromium compound ingested.
3. **Acetylcysteine** (see p 407) has been used in several animal studies and one human case of dichromate poisoning.

C. **Decontamination** (see p 45)

1. **Inhalation.** Remove the victim from exposure and give supplemental oxygen if available.
2. **Skin.** Remove contaminated clothing and wash exposed areas immediately with copious soap and water. EDTA (see p 440) 10% ointment may facilitate removal of chromate scabs. A 10% topical solution of ascorbic acid has been advocated to enhance the conversion of hexavalent chromium to the less toxic trivalent state.
3. **Eyes.** Irrigate copiously with tepid water or saline and perform fluorescein examination to rule out corneal injury if pain or irritation persists.
4. **Ingestion.** Give milk or water to dilute corrosive effects. Do ***not*** induce vomiting because of the potential for corrosive injury. For large recent ingestions, perform gastric lavage. Activated charcoal is of uncertain benefit in adsorbing chromium and may obscure the view if endoscopy is performed.

D. **Enhanced elimination.** There is no evidence for the efficacy of enhanced removal procedures such as dialysis and hemoperfusion.

# ▶ CLONIDINE AND RELATED DRUGS

*Cyrus Rangan, MD*

**Clonidine** and the related centrally acting adrenergic inhibitors **guanabenz, guanfacine,** and **methyldopa** are commonly used for the treatment of hypertension. Clonidine also has been used to alleviate opioid and nicotine withdrawal symptoms. Clonidine overdose may occur after ingestion of pills or ingestion of the long-acting skin patches. **Oxymetazoline** and **tetrahydrozoline** are nasal decongestants that may cause toxicity identical to that of clonidine. **Tizanidine** is a chemically related agent used for the treatment of muscle spasticity. **Apraclonidine** and **brimonidine,** ophthalmic preparations for the treatment of glaucoma and ocular hypertension, may cause poisoning from ingestion and from systemic absorption after topical administration.

I. **Mechanism of toxicity.** All these agents decrease central sympathetic outflow by stimulating alpha-2 adrenergic presynaptic (inhibitory) receptors in the brain.

A. **Clonidine, oxymetazoline,** and **tetrahydrozoline** may also stimulate peripheral alpha-1 receptors, resulting in vasoconstriction and transient hypertension.

B. **Guanabenz** is structurally similar to guanethidine, a ganglionic blocker. **Guanfacine** is related closely to guanabenz and has more selective alpha-2–agonist activity than clonidine.

C. **Methyldopa** may further decrease sympathetic outflow by metabolism to a false neurotransmitter (alpha-methylnorepinephrine) or by decreasing plasma renin activity.

D. **Tizanidine** is structurally related to clonidine but has low affinity for alpha-1 receptors.

**E. Pharmacokinetics.** The onset of effects is rapid (30 min) after oral administration of clonidine. Other than methyldopa, these drugs are widely distributed with large volumes of distribution (see also Table II–59).

**II. Toxic dose**

**A. Clonidine.** As little as one tablet of 0.1-mg clonidine has produced toxic effects in children; however, 10 mg shared by twin 34-month-old girls was not lethal. Adults have survived acute ingestions with as much as 100 mg. No fatalities from acute overdoses have been reported, but a child had permanent neurologic damage after a respiratory arrest.

**B. Guanabenz.** Mild toxicity developed in adults who ingested 160–320 mg and in a 3-year-old who ingested 12 mg. Severe toxicity developed in a 19-month-old who ingested 28 mg. A 3-year-old child had moderate symptoms after ingesting 480 mg. All these children recovered by 24 hours.

**C. Guanfacine.** Severe toxicity developed in a 25-year-old woman who ingested 60 mg. A 2-year-old boy ingested 4 mg and became lethargic within 20 minutes, but the peak hypotensive effect occurred 20 hours later.

**D. Methyldopa.** More than 2 g in adults is considered a toxic dose, and death was reported in an adult after an ingestion of 25 g. However, survival was reported after ingestion of 45 g. The therapeutic dose of methyldopa for children is 10–65 mg/kg/day, and the higher dose is expected to cause mild symptoms.

**E. Brimonidine.** Recurrent episodes of unresponsiveness, hypotension, hypotonia, hypothermia, and bradycardia occurred in a 1-month-old infant receiving therapeutic dosing. A 2-week-old infant had severe respiratory depression after one drop was instilled into each eye. Both children recovered with supportive care in less than 24 hours.

**III. Clinical presentation.** Manifestations of intoxication result from generalized sympathetic depression and include pupillary constriction, lethargy, coma, apnea, bradycardia, hypotension, and hypothermia. Paradoxic hypertension caused by stimulation of peripheral alpha-1 receptors may occur with clonidine, oxymetazoline, and tetrahydrozoline (and possibly guanabenz) and is usually transient. The onset of symptoms is usually within 30–60 minutes, although peak effects may occur more than 6–12 hours after ingestion. Full recovery is usual within 24 hours. In an unusual massive overdose, a 28-year-old man who accidentally ingested 100 mg of clonidine powder had a three-phase intoxication over 4 days: initial hypertension, followed by hypotension, and then a withdrawal reaction with hypertension.

**IV. Diagnosis.** Poisoning should be suspected in patients with pinpoint pupils, respiratory depression, hypotension, and bradycardia. Although clonidine overdose may mimic an opioid overdose, it usually does not respond to administration of naloxone.

**A. Specific levels.** Serum drug levels are not routinely available or clinically useful. These drugs are not usually detectable on comprehensive urine toxicology screening.

**B. Other useful laboratory studies** include electrolytes, glucose, and arterial blood gases or oximetry.

**V. Treatment.** Patients usually recover within 24 hours with supportive care.

**A. Emergency and supportive measures**

1. Protect the airway and assist ventilation if necessary (see pp 1–7).
2. Treat coma (see p 18), hypotension (p 15), and bradycardia (p 9) if they occur. They usually resolve with supportive measures such as fluids, atropine, and dopamine. Hypertension is usually transient and does not require treatment.

**B. Specific drugs and antidotes**

1. **Naloxone** (see p 477) has been reported to reverse signs and symptoms of clonidine overdose, but this has not been confirmed. However, because the overdose mimics opioid intoxication, naloxone is indicated because of

the possibility that narcotics may also have been ingested.

2. Tolazoline, a central alpha-2–receptor antagonist, was previously recommended, but the response has been highly variable and it should ***not*** be used.

**C. Decontamination** (see p 45). Administer activated charcoal orally if conditions are appropriate (see Table I–38, p 51). Gastric lavage is not necessary after small to moderate ingestions if activated charcoal can be given promptly. Consider whole-bowel irrigation after ingestion of clonidine skin patches.

**D. Enhanced elimination.** There is no evidence that enhanced removal procedures are effective.

## ► COCAINE

*Nancy G. Murphy, MD, and Neal L. Benowitz, MD*

Cocaine is one of the most popular drugs of abuse. It may be sniffed into the nose (snorted), smoked, or injected intravenously. Occasionally it is combined with heroin and injected (speedball). Cocaine purchased on the street is usually of high purity, but it occasionally may contain substitute drugs such as lidocaine (see p 469) or stimulants such as caffeine (p 142), methamphetamine (p 73), ephedrine (p 322), and phencyclidine (p 301).

The **"free base"** form of cocaine is preferred for smoking because it volatilizes at a lower temperature and is not as easily destroyed by heat as the crystalline hydrochloride salt. Free base is made by dissolving cocaine salt in an aqueous alkaline solution and then extracting the free base form with a solvent such as ether. Heat sometimes is applied to hasten solvent evaporation, creating a fire hazard. **"Crack"** is a free base form of cocaine produced by using sodium bicarbonate to create the alkaline aqueous solution, which is then dried.

**I. Mechanism of toxicity.** The primary actions of cocaine are local anesthetic effects (see p 76), CNS stimulation, and inhibition of neuronal uptake of catecholamines.

**A.** CNS stimulation and inhibition of catecholamine uptake result in a state of generalized sympathetic stimulation very similar to that of amphetamine intoxication (see p 72).

**B.** Cardiovascular effects of high doses of cocaine, presumably related to blockade of cardiac-cell sodium channels, include depression of conduction (QRS prolongation) and contractility. Cocaine-induced QT prolongation also has been described.

**C. Pharmacokinetics.** Cocaine is well absorbed from all routes, and toxicity has been described after mucosal application as a local anesthetic. Smoking and intravenous injection produce maximum effects within 1–2 minutes, whereas oral or mucosal absorption may take up to 20–30 minutes. Once absorbed, cocaine is eliminated by metabolism and hydrolysis, with a half-life of about 60 minutes. In the presence of ethanol, cocaine is transesterified to **cocaethylene,** which has similar pharmacologic effects and a longer half-life than cocaine. (See also Table II–59.)

**II. Toxic dose.** The toxic dose is highly variable and depends on individual tolerance, the route of administration, and the presence of other drugs, as well as other factors. Rapid intravenous injection or smoking may produce transient high brain and heart levels, resulting in convulsions or cardiac arrhythmias, whereas the same dose swallowed or snorted may produce only euphoria.

**A.** The usual maximum recommended dose for intranasal local anesthesia is 100–200 mg (1–2 mL of 10% solution).

**B.** A typical "line" of cocaine to be snorted contains 20–30 mg or more. Crack usually is sold in pellets or "rocks" containing 100–150 mg.

C. Ingestion of 1 g or more of cocaine is very likely to be fatal.

**III. Clinical presentation**

A. **CNS manifestations** of toxicity may occur within minutes after smoking or intravenous injection or may be delayed for 30–60 minutes after snorting, mucosal application, or oral ingestion.

1. Initial euphoria may be followed by anxiety, agitation, delirium, psychosis, tremulousness, muscle rigidity or hyperactivity, and seizures. High doses may cause respiratory arrest.
2. Seizures are usually brief and self-limited; status epilepticus should suggest continued drug absorption (as from ruptured cocaine-filled condoms in the GI tract) or hyperthermia.
3. Coma may be caused by a postictal state, hyperthermia, or intracranial hemorrhage resulting from cocaine-induced hypertension.
4. With chronic cocaine use, insomnia, weight loss, and paranoid psychosis may occur. A "washed-out" syndrome has been observed in cocaine abusers after a prolonged binge, consisting of profound lethargy and deep sleep that may last for several hours to days, followed by spontaneous recovery.

B. **Cardiovascular toxicity** may also occur rapidly after smoking or intravenous injection and is mediated by sympathetic overactivity.

1. Fatal ventricular tachycardia or fibrillation may occur. QRS interval prolongation similar to that with tricyclic antidepressants may occur.
2. Severe hypertension may cause hemorrhagic stroke or aortic dissection.
3. Coronary artery spasm and/or thrombosis may result in myocardial infarction, even in patients with no coronary disease. Diffuse myocardial necrosis similar to catecholamine myocarditis and chronic cardiomyopathy have been described.
4. Shock may be caused by myocardial, intestinal, or brain infarction; hyperthermia; tachyarrhythmias; or hypovolemia produced by extravascular fluid sequestration caused by vasoconstriction.
5. Renal failure may result from shock, renal arterial spasm, or rhabdomyolysis with myoglobinuria.

C. **Death** is usually caused by a sudden fatal arrhythmia, status epilepticus, intracranial hemorrhage, or hyperthermia. Hyperthermia is usually caused by seizures, muscular hyperactivity, or rigidity and typically is associated with rhabdomyolysis, myoglobinuric renal failure, coagulopathy, and multiple organ failure.

D. A variety of **other effects** have occurred after smoking or snorting cocaine.

1. Chest pain without ECG evidence of myocardial ischemia is common. The presumed basis is musculoskeletal, and it may be associated with rhabdomyolysis of chest wall muscle.
2. Pneumothorax and pneumomediastinum cause pleuritic chest pain, and the latter is often recognized by a "crunching" sound ("Hammond's crunch") heard over the anterior chest.
3. Nasal septal perforation may occur after chronic snorting.
4. Accidental subcutaneous injection of cocaine may cause localized necrotic ulcers ("coke burns"), and wound botulism (see p 137) has been reported.

E. **Body "packers"** or **"stuffers."** Persons attempting to smuggle cocaine may swallow large numbers of tightly packed cocaine-filled condoms ("body packers"). Street vendors suddenly surprised by a police raid may quickly swallow their wares, often without carefully wrapping or closing the packets or vials ("body stuffers"). The swallowed condoms, packets, or vials may break open, releasing massive quantities of cocaine. The packages are sometimes, but not always, visible on plain abdominal x-ray.

**IV. Diagnosis** is based on a history of cocaine use or typical features of sympathomimetic intoxication. Skin marks of chronic intravenous drug abuse, especially with scarring from coke burns, and nasal septal perforation after chronic snorting suggest cocaine use. Chest pain with electrocardiographic evidence of ischemia or infarction in a young, otherwise healthy person also suggests cocaine use. Note that young adults, particularly young African-American men, have a high prevalence of normal J-point elevation on ECG, which can be mistaken for acute myocardial infarction.

A. **Specific levels.** Blood cocaine levels are not routinely available and do not assist in emergency management. Cocaine and its metabolite benzoylecgonine are easily detected in the urine and provide qualitative confirmation of cocaine use.

B. **Other useful laboratory studies** include electrolytes, glucose, BUN, creatinine, CPK, urinalysis, urine myoglobin, ECG and ECG monitoring, CT head scan (if hemorrhage is suspected), and abdominal x-ray (if cocaine-filled condom or packet ingestion is suspected).

V. **Treatment**

A. **Emergency and supportive measures**

1. Maintain an open airway and assist ventilation if necessary (see pp 1–7).
2. Treat coma (see p 18), agitation (p 23), seizures (p 22), hyperthermia (p 20), arrhythmias (pp 10–15), and hypotension (p 15) if they occur. Benzodiazepines (p 129) are a good choice for initial management of hypertension and tachycardia associated with agitation.
3. Angina pectoris may be treated with benzodiazepines, aspirin, nitrates, or calcium channel blockers. For acute myocardial infarction, thrombolysis has been recommended but is controversial. Supporting its use is the high prevalence of acute thrombosis, often superimposed on coronary spasm. Against its use are the excellent prognosis for patients with cocaine-induced infarction, even without thrombolysis, and concerns about increased risks of bleeding caused by intracranial hemorrhage or aortic dissection.
4. Monitor vital signs and ECG for several hours. Patients with suspected coronary artery spasm should be admitted to a coronary care unit, and because of reports of persistent or recurrent coronary spasm up to several days after initial exposure, consider the use of an oral calcium antagonist and/or cardiac nitrates for 2–4 weeks after discharge.

B. **Specific drugs and antidotes.** There is no specific antidote.

1. Although propranolol previously was recommended as the drug of choice for treatment of cocaine-induced **tachycardia and hypertension**, it may produce *paradoxic worsening* of hypertension because of blockade of beta-2–mediated vasodilation; if a beta blocker is needed (eg, for tachycardia not responsive to benzodiazepines and IV fluids), administer **esmolol** (a very short-acting beta blocker) (p 449). Esmolol may be also be used **in combination** with a vasodilator such as **phentolamine** (p 495) for management of hypertension.
2. **QRS prolongation** caused by sodium channel blockade can be treated with **sodium bicarbonate** (p 423). Wide complex tachyarrhythmias may also respond to **lidocaine** (p 469).

C. **Decontamination** (see p 46). Decontamination is not necessary after smoking, snorting, or intravenous injection. After **ingestion,** perform the following steps:

1. Administer activated charcoal orally if conditions are appropriate (see Table I–38, p 51).
2. Gastric lavage is not necessary after small to moderate ingestions if activated charcoal can be given promptly.
3. For ingestion of cocaine-filled condoms or packets, give repeated doses of activated charcoal and consider whole-bowel irrigation (see p 51). If large ingested packets (ie, Ziploc™ bags) are not removed by these procedures, laparotomy and surgical removal may be necessary.

D. **Enhanced elimination.** Because cocaine is extensively distributed to tissues and rapidly metabolized, dialysis and hemoperfusion procedures are not effective. Acidification of the urine does not significantly enhance cocaine elimination and may aggravate myoglobinuric renal failure.

## ► COLCHICINE

*David Betten, MD*

Colchicine is marketed as tablets and an injectable solution used for the treatment of gout and familial Mediterranean fever. It is also found in certain plants: autumn crocus or meadow saffron (*Colchicum autumnale*) and glory lily (*Gloriosa superba*). A colchicine overdose is extremely serious, with considerable mortality that is often delayed. Colchicine has been used as a homicidal poison.

I. **Mechanism of toxicity.** Colchicine inhibits mitosis of dividing cells and, in high concentrations, is a general cellular poison. Colchicine is rapidly absorbed and extensively distributed to body tissues (volume of distribution 2–20 L/kg). (See also Table II–59.)

II. **Toxic dose.** The maximum therapeutic dose of oral colchicine is 8–10 mg in 1 day. Tablets contain 0.5–0.6 mg. In a series of 150 cases, doses of 0.5 mg/kg or less were associated with diarrhea and vomiting but not death, doses of 0.5–0.8 mg/kg were associated with marrow aplasia and 10% mortality, and ingestions greater than 0.8 mg/kg uniformly resulted in death. Fatalities, however, have been reported with single ingestions of as little as 7 mg, although other case reports describe survival after ingestions of more than 60 mg. Ingestions of parts of colchicine-containing plants have resulted in severe toxicity and death.

Healthy individuals receiving a cumulative dose of greater than 4 mg of intravenous colchicine per treatment course are also at risk of significant toxicity and death.

III. **Clinical presentation.** Colchicine poisoning affects many organ systems, with toxic effects occurring over days to weeks.

A. After an **acute overdose,** symptoms typically are delayed for 2–12 hours and include nausea, vomiting, abdominal pain, and severe bloody diarrhea. Shock results from depressed cardiac contractility and fluid loss into the GI tract and other tissues. Delirium, seizures, or coma may occur. Lactic acidosis related to shock and inhibition of cellular metabolism is common. Other manifestations of colchicine poisoning include acute myocardial injury, rhabdomyolysis with myoglobinuria, disseminated intravascular coagulation, and acute renal failure.

Chronic colchicine poisoning presents with a more insidious onset. Factors precipitating toxicity from chronic use include renal insufficiency, liver disease, and drug interactions (erythromycin, cimetidine, cyclosporine) that can inhibit colchicine clearance.

B. **Death** usually occurs after 8–36 hours and is caused by respiratory failure, intractable shock, and cardiac arrhythmias or sudden cardiac arrest.

C. **Late complications** include bone marrow suppression, particularly leukopenia and thrombocytopenia (4–5 days) and alopecia (2–3 weeks). Chronic colchicine therapy may produce myopathy (proximal muscle weakness and elevated creatinine kinase levels) and polyneuropathy. This also has occurred after acute poisoning.

IV. **Diagnosis.** A syndrome beginning with severe gastroenteritis, leukocytosis, shock, rhabdomyolysis, and acute renal failure and, several days later, leukopenia and thrombocytopenia should suggest colchicine poisoning. A history of gout or familial Mediterranean fever in the patient or a family member is also suggestive.

A. **Specific levels.** Colchicine levels in blood and urine are not readily available. However, levels may be useful for forensic purposes, especially in cases of unexplained pancytopenia and multiple organ failure. Bone marrow biopsy may reveal metaphase arrest and "pseudo-Pelger-Huet" cells.

**B. Other useful laboratory studies** include CBC, electrolytes, hepatic enzymes, glucose, BUN, creatinine, CPK, troponin I, urinalysis, and ECG monitoring. Elevated serum levels of troponin I suggest greater severity of myocardial necrosis and higher mortality.

**V. Treatment**

**A. Emergency and supportive measures.** Provide aggressive supportive care, with careful monitoring and treatment of fluid and electrolyte disturbances.

1. Anticipate sudden respiratory or cardiac arrest and maintain an open airway and assist ventilation if necessary (see pp 1–7).
2. Treatment of shock (see p 16) may require large amounts of crystalloid fluids, possibly blood (to replace loss from hemorrhagic gastroenteritis), and pressor agents such as dopamine (p 443).
3. Infusion of sodium bicarbonate and mannitol may be considered if there is evidence of rhabdomyolysis (see p 26).
4. Bone marrow depression requires specialized intensive care. Severe neutropenia requires patient isolation and management of febrile episodes as for other neutropenic conditions. Platelet transfusions may be required to control bleeding.

**B. Specific drugs and antidotes.** Colchicine-specific antibodies (Fab fragments) were used successfully in France to treat a 25-year-old woman with severe colchicine overdose. Unfortunately, they are not commercially produced and are unavailable in the United States. Granulocyte colony-stimulating factor (G-CSF) has been used for the treatment of severe leukopenia.

**C. Decontamination** (see p 45). Administer activated charcoal orally if conditions are appropriate (see Table I–38, p 51). If a delay of more than 60 minutes is expected before charcoal can be given, consider using ipecac to induce vomiting if it can be administered within a few minutes of the exposure. Gastric lavage is not necessary after small to moderate ingestions if activated charcoal can be given promptly.

**D. Enhanced elimination.** Because colchicine is highly bound to tissues, with a large volume of distribution, hemodialysis and hemoperfusion are ineffective. Colchicine undergoes enterohepatic recirculation, so **repeat-dose charcoal** might be expected to accelerate elimination, although this has not been documented.

## ▶ COPPER

*Alan Buchwald, MD*

Copper is widely used in its elemental metallic form, in metal alloys, and in the form of copper salts. Elemental metallic copper is used in electrical wiring and plumbing materials and was formerly the main constituent of pennies (now mostly zinc). Copper salts such as copper sulfate, copper oxide, copper chloride, copper nitrate, copper cyanide, and copper acetate are used as pesticides and algaecides and in a variety of industrial processes. Because of its toxicity, copper sulfate is no longer used as an emetic. Copper levels may be elevated in persons who drink from copper containers or use copper plumbing. The increased acidity of beverages stored in copper alloy (eg, brass or bronze) containers enhances leaching of copper into the liquid.

**I. Mechanism of toxicity**

**A. Elemental metallic copper** is poorly absorbed orally and is essentially nontoxic. However, inhalation of copper dust or metallic fumes created when welding or brazing copper alloys may cause chemical pneumonitis or a syndrome similar to metal fume fever (see p 259). Metallic copper dust in the eye (chalcosis) may lead to corneal opacification, uveitis, ocular necrosis, and blindness unless the dust is removed quickly.

**B. Copper sulfate** salt is highly irritating, depending on the concentration, and may produce mucous membrane irritation and severe gastroenteritis.

C. **Systemic absorption** can produce hepatic and renal tubular injury. Hemolysis has been associated with copper exposure from hemodialysis equipment or absorption through burned skin.

II. **Toxic dose.** Copper is an essential trace metal. The daily adult requirement of 2 mg is supplied in a normal diet.

A. **Inhalation.** The recommended workplace limit (ACGIH TLV-TWA) for copper fumes is 0.2 mg/m$^3$; for dusts and mists, it is 1 mg/m$^3$. The air level considered immediately dangerous to life or health for dusts or fumes is 100 mg Cu/m$^3$.

B. **Ingestion** of more than 250 mg of copper sulfate can produce vomiting, and larger ingestions potentially can cause hepatic and renal injury.

C. **Water.** The US Environmental Protection Agency has established a safe limit of 1.3 mg/L in drinking water. The WHO (World Health Organization, 2004) guideline value for drinking water is 2 mg/L.

III. **Clinical presentation**

A. **Inhalation of copper fumes** or **dusts** initially produces a metallic taste and upper respiratory irritation (dry cough, sore throat, and eye irritation). Large exposures may cause severe cough, dyspnea, fever, leukocytosis, and pulmonary infiltrates (see also metal fume fever, p 259).

B. **Ingestion of copper sulfate** or **other salts** causes the rapid onset of nausea and vomiting with characteristic blue-green emesis. Gastrointestinal bleeding may occur. Fluid and blood loss from gastroenteritis may lead to hypotension and oliguria. Intravascular hemolysis can result in acute tubular necrosis. Hepatitis has been reported, caused by centrilobular necrosis. Multisystem failure, shock, and death may occur. Chronic interstitial nephritis has been reported after parenteral copper sulfate poisoning. Methemoglobinemia is uncommon.

C. **Chronic** exposure to Bordeaux mixture (copper sulfate with hydrated lime) may occur in vineyard workers. Pulmonary fibrosis, lung cancer, cirrhosis, angiosarcoma, and portal hypertension have been associated with this occupational exposure.

D. Ingestion of **organocopper** compounds is rare. Suicidal ingestion of an organocopper fungicide containing primarily copper-8-hydroxyquinolate caused lethargy, dyspnea, and cyanosis, with 34% methemoglobinemia.

E. Swimming in water contaminated with copper-based algaecides can cause green discoloration of the hair.

IV. **Diagnosis** is based on a history of acute ingestion or occupational exposure. Occupations at risk include those associated with handling algaecides, herbicides, wood preservatives, pyrotechnics, ceramic glazes, and electrical wiring, as well as welding or brazing copper alloys.

A. **Specific levels.** If copper salt ingestion is suspected, a serum copper level should be obtained. Normal serum copper concentrations average 1 mg/L, and this doubles during pregnancy. Serum copper levels above 5 mg/L are considered very toxic. Whole-blood copper levels may correlate better with acute intoxication because acute excess copper is carried in the red blood cells; however, whole-blood copper levels are not as widely available.

B. **Other useful laboratory studies** include CBC, electrolytes, BUN, creatinine, hepatic transaminases, arterial blood gases or oximetry, and chest x-ray. If hemolysis is suspected, send blood for type and cross-match, plasma free hemoglobin, and haptoglobin and check urinalysis for occult blood (hemoglobinuria).

V. **Treatment**

A. **Emergency and supportive measures**

1. **Inhalation of copper fumes** or **dusts.** Give supplemental oxygen if indicated by arterial blood gases or oximetry and treat bronchospasm (see p 7) and chemical pneumonitis (p 7) if they occur. Symptoms are usually short-lived and resolve without specific treatment.

2. **Ingestion of copper salts**
   a. Treat shock caused by gastroenteritis with aggressive intravenous fluid replacement and, if necessary, pressor drugs (see p 16).
   b. Consider endoscopy to rule out corrosive esophageal or stomach injury, depending on the concentration of the solution and the patient's symptoms.
   c. Blood transfusion may be needed if significant hemolysis or GI bleeding occurs.

B. **Specific drugs and antidotes. BAL** (dimercaprol; see p 417) and **penicillamine** (see p 491) are effective chelating agents and should be used in seriously ill patients with large ingestions. Triethyl tetramine dihydrochloride (Trien or Cuprid) is a specific copper chelator approved for use in Wilson's disease; although it is better tolerated than penicillamine, its role in acute ingestion or chronic environmental exposure has not been established.

C. **Decontamination** (see p 45)
   1. **Inhalation.** Remove the victim from exposure and give supplemental oxygen if available.
   2. **Eyes.** Irrigate copiously and attempt to remove all copper from the surface; perform a careful slit-lamp examination and refer the case to an ophthalmologist urgently if any residual material remains.
   3. **Ingestion.** Perform gastric lavage if there has been a recent ingestion of a large quantity of copper salts. There is no proven benefit for activated charcoal, and its use may obscure the view if endoscopy is performed.

D. **Enhanced elimination.** There is no role for hemodialysis, hemoperfusion, repeat-dose charcoal, or hemodiafiltration. Hemodialysis may be required for supportive care of patients with acute renal failure, and it can marginally increase the elimination of the copper-chelator complex.

## ▶ CYANIDE

*Paul D. Blanc, MD, MSPH*

Cyanide is a highly toxic chemical with a variety of uses, including chemical synthesis, laboratory analysis, and metal plating. Aliphatic nitriles (acrylonitrile and propionitrile) used in plastics manufacturing are metabolized to cyanide. The vasodilator drug nitroprusside releases cyanide upon exposure to light or through metabolism. Natural sources of cyanide (amygdalin and many other cyanogenic glycosides) are found in apricot pits, cassava, and many other plants and seeds, some of which may be important, depending on ethnobotanical practices. Acetonitrile, a component of some artificial nail glue removers, has caused several pediatric deaths.

**Hydrogen cyanide** is a gas easily generated by mixing acid with cyanide salts and is a common combustion by-product of burning plastics, wool, and many other natural and synthetic products. Hydrogen cyanide poisoning is an important cause of death from structural fires, and deliberate cyanide exposure (through cyanide salts) remains an important instrument of homicide and suicide. Hydrogen cyanamide, an agricultural chemical used as a plant regulator, is a potent toxin that inhibits aldehyde dehydrogenase but does not act as a cyanide analog.

I. **Mechanism of toxicity.** Cyanide is a chemical asphyxiant; binding to cellular cytochrome oxidase, it blocks the aerobic utilization of oxygen. Unbound cyanide is detoxified by metabolism to thiocyanate, a much less toxic compound that is excreted in the urine.

II. **Toxic dose**
   A. Exposure to **hydrogen cyanide gas** (HCN) even at low levels (150–200 ppm) can be fatal. The air level considered immediately dangerous to life or health (IDLH) is 50 ppm. The recommended workplace ceiling limit (ACGIH

TLV-C) for HCN is 4.7 ppm (5 mg/m$^3$ for cyanide salts). The OSHA permissible exposure limit (PEL) is 10 ppm. HCN is well absorbed across the skin.

**B.** Adult **ingestion** of as little as 200 mg of the sodium or potassium salt may be fatal. Solutions of cyanide salts can be absorbed through intact skin.

**C.** Acute cyanide poisoning is relatively rare with nitroprusside infusion (at normal infusion rates) or after ingestion of amygdalin-containing seeds (unless they have been pulverized).

**III. Clinical presentation.** Abrupt onset of profound toxic effects shortly after exposure is the hallmark of cyanide poisoning. Symptoms include headache, nausea, dyspnea, and confusion. Syncope, seizures, coma, agonal respirations, and cardiovascular collapse ensue rapidly after heavy exposure.

**A.** A brief delay may occur if the cyanide is ingested as a salt, especially if it is in a capsule or if there is food in the stomach.

**B.** Delayed onset (minutes to hours) also may occur after ingestion of nitriles and plant-derived cyanogenic glycosides, because metabolism to cyanide is required.

**C.** Chronic neurologic sequelae may follow severe cyanide poisoning consistent with anoxic injury.

**IV. Diagnosis** is based on a history of exposure or the presence of rapidly progressive symptoms and signs. Severe lactic acidosis is usually present with significant exposure. The **measured venous oxygen saturation** may be elevated owing to blocked cellular oxygen consumption. The classic "bitter almond" odor of hydrogen cyanide may or may not be noted, in part because of genetic variability in the ability to detect the smell.

**A. Specific levels.** Cyanide determinations are rarely of use in emergency management because they cannot be performed rapidly enough to influence initial treatment. In addition, they must be interpreted with caution because of a variety of complicating technical factors.

1. Whole-blood levels higher than 0.5–1 mg/L are considered toxic.
2. Cigarette smokers may have levels up to 0.1 mg/L.
3. Rapid nitroprusside infusion may produce levels as high as 1 mg/L, accompanied by metabolic acidosis.

**B. Other useful laboratory studies** include electrolytes, glucose, serum lactate, arterial blood gases, mixed venous oxygen saturation, and carboxyhemoglobin (if the patient experienced smoke inhalation exposure).

**V. Treatment**

**A. Emergency and supportive measures.** Treat all cyanide exposures as potentially lethal.

1. Maintain an open airway and assist ventilation if necessary (see pp 1–7). Administer supplemental oxygen.
2. Treat coma (see p 18), hypotension (p 15), and seizures (p 22) if they occur.
3. Start an intravenous line and monitor the patient's vital signs and ECG closely.

**B. Specific drugs and antidotes**

1. The **cyanide antidote package** (Taylor Pharmaceuticals) consists of amyl and sodium **nitrites** (see p 484), which produce cyanide-scavenging methemoglobinemia, and sodium **thiosulfate** (p 514), which accelerates the conversion of cyanide to thiocyanate.
   - **a.** Break a pearl of **amyl nitrite** under the nose of the victim and administer **sodium nitrite,** 300 mg IV (6 mg/kg for children, not to exceed 300 mg). Adjust the dose downward if anemia is present (see p 476). ***Caution***: Nitrite-induced methemoglobinemia can be extremely dangerous and even lethal. Nitrite should not be given if the symptoms are mild or if the diagnosis is uncertain, especially if concomitant carbon monoxide poisoning is suspected.
   - **b.** Administer **sodium thiosulfate,** 12.5 g IV. Thiosulfate is relatively benign and may be given empirically even if the diagnosis is uncertain. It also may be useful in mitigating nitroprusside toxicity (see p 514).

2. The most promising alternative antidote is **hydroxocobalamin** (see p 459). Although available in Europe, it remains an investigational drug in the United States. Dicobalt edentate is also used outside the United States.
3. **Hyperbaric oxygen** has no proven role in cyanide poisoning treatment.

C. **Decontamination** (see p 45). ***Caution***: Avoid contact with cyanide-containing salts or solutions and avoid inhaling vapors from vomitus (which may give off hydrogen cyanide gas).
   1. **Inhalation.** Remove victims from hydrogen cyanide exposure and give supplemental oxygen if available. Each rescuer should wear a positive-pressure, self-contained breathing apparatus and, if possible, chemical-protective clothing.
   2. **Skin.** Remove and isolate all contaminated clothing and wash affected areas with copious soap and water.
   3. **Ingestion** (see p 47). Even though charcoal has a relatively low affinity for cyanide, it will effectively bind the doses typically ingested (eg, 100–500 mg).
      a. **Prehospital.** Immediately administer activated charcoal if it is available and the patient is alert. Do ***not*** induce vomiting unless the victim is more than 30 minutes from a medical facility and charcoal is not available.
      b. **Hospital.** Immediately place a gastric tube and administer activated charcoal, then perform gastric lavage. Give additional activated charcoal and a cathartic after the lavage.

D. **Enhanced elimination.** There is no role for hemodialysis or hemoperfusion in cyanide poisoning treatment. Hemodialysis may be indicated in patients with renal insufficiency who develop high thiocyanate levels while on extended nitroprusside therapy.

## ► DAPSONE

*Kathryn H. Meier, PharmD*

Dapsone is an antibiotic used for treatment of and prophylaxis against various infections, including leprosy, malaria, and *Pneumocystis carinii.* It also has anti-inflammatory actions and is used for some rheumatologic and rare dermatologic disorders.

I. **Mechanism of toxicity.** Acute toxic effects are caused by the P-450 metabolites and include methemoglobinemia, sulfhemoglobinemia, and Heinz-body hemolytic anemia, all of which decrease the oxygen-carrying capacity of the blood.
   A. Dapsone metabolites oxidize the ferrous iron hemoglobin complex to the ferric state, resulting in methemoglobinemia.
   B. Sulfhemoglobinemia occurs when dapsone metabolites irreversibly sulfate the pyrrole hemoglobin ring.
   C. Hemolysis may result from depletion of red blood cell intracellular glutathione by oxidative metabolites.
   D. **Pharmacokinetics.** Absorption of dapsone after overdose is delayed; peak plasma levels occur between 4 and 8 hours after ingestion. The volume of distribution is 1.5 L/kg, and protein binding is 70–90%. Dapsone is metabolized by two primary routes: acetylation and P-450 oxidation. Both dapsone and its acetylated metabolite undergo enterohepatic recirculation. The average elimination half-life is around 30 hours after a therapeutic dose and up to 77 hours after an overdose. (See also Table II–59.)

II. **Toxic dose.** The adult therapeutic dose ranges from 50 to 300 mg/day. Chronic daily dosing of 100 mg can cause methemoglobin levels of 5–12%. Hemolysis has not been reported in adults with doses less than 300 mg/day. Persons with glucose-6-phosphate dehydrogenase (G6PD) deficiency, congenital hemoglobin abnormalities, or underlying hypoxemia may experience greater toxicity at lower doses. Death has occurred with overdoses of 1.4 g and greater, although recovery from severe toxicity has been reported after ingestion of 7.5 g.

**III. Clinical presentation.** Methemoglobinemia and sulfhemoglobinemia usually are observed within a few of hours of the overdose, but intravascular hemolysis may be delayed. The illness lasts several days. Clinical manifestations are more severe in patients with underlying medical conditions that may contribute to hypoxemia.

- **A. Methemoglobinemia** (see p 262) causes cyanosis and dyspnea. Drawn blood may appear "chocolate" brown when the methemoglobin level is greater than 15–20%. Because of the long half-life of dapsone and its metabolites, methemoglobinemia may persist for several days, requiring repeated antidotal treatment.
- **B. Sulfhemoglobinemia** also decreases oxyhemoglobin saturation and is unresponsive to methylene blue. Sulfhemoglobinemia can produce a cyanotic appearance at a lower percentage of total hemoglobin compared with methemoglobin, but the amount of sulfhemoglobin generated is rarely more than 5%.
- **C. Hemolysis** may be delayed in onset 2–3 days after the ingestion.

**IV. Diagnosis**. Overdose should be suspected in cyanotic patients with elevated methemoglobin levels, especially if there is a history of dapsone use or a diagnosis that is likely to be treated with dapsone (eg, HIV/AIDS). Although there are many agents that can cause methemoglobinemia, there are very few that produce both detectable sulfhemoglobin and a prolonged, recurrent methemoglobinemia. Dapsone was the leading cause of methemoglobinemia in one retrospective review of patients in an American hospital.

- **A. Specific levels.** Dapsone levels are not routinely available.
  1. **Methemoglobinemia** (see p 262) is suspected when a cyanotic patient fails to respond to high-flow oxygen or cyanosis persists despite a normal arterial $pO_2$. Pulse oximetry is not a reliable indicator of oxygen saturation in patients with methemoglobinemia. Specific methemoglobin concentrations can be measured by using a multiwave co-oximeter. Qualitatively, a drop of blood on white filter paper will appear brown (when directly compared with normal blood) if the methemoglobin level is greater than 15–20%.
  2. ***Note:*** Administration of the antidote **methylene blue** (see V.B.1. below) can cause transient false elevation of the measured methemoglobin level (up to 15%).
  3. **Sulfhemoglobin** is difficult to detect, in part because its spectrophotometric absorbance is similar to that of methemoglobin on the co-oximeter. A blood sample will turn red if a crystal of potassium cyanide is added but not if significant sulfhemoglobin is present.
  4. The oxygen-carrying capacity of the blood is dependent not only on oxygen saturation but on total hemoglobin concentration. Interpret methemoglobin and sulfhemoglobin levels with reference to the degree of anemia.
- **B. Other useful laboratory studies** include CBC (with differential smear to look for reticulocytes and Heinz bodies), glucose, electrolytes, liver transaminases, bilirubin, and arterial blood gases.

**V. Treatment**

- **A. Emergency and supportive measures**
  1. Maintain an open airway and assist ventilation if needed (pp 1–7). Administer supplemental oxygen.
  2. If hemolysis occurs, administer intravenous fluids and alkalinize the urine, as for rhabdomyolysis (see p 26), to prevent acute renal tubular necrosis. For severe hemolysis, blood transfusions may be required.
  3. Mild symptoms may resolve without intervention, but this may take 2–3 days.

B. **Specific drugs and antidotes**
   1. **Methylene blue** (see p 473) is indicated in a symptomatic patient with a methemoglobin level greater than 20% or with lower levels if even minimal compromise of oxygen-carrying capacity is potentially harmful (eg, severe pneumonia, anemia, or myocardial ischemia).
      a. Give 1–2 mg/kg (0.1–0.2 mL/kg of 1% solution) over several minutes. Therapeutic response may be delayed up to 30 minutes.
      b. Serious overdoses usually require repeated dosing every 6–8 hours for 2–3 days because of the prolonged half-life of dapsone and its metabolites.
      c. Methylene blue is ineffective for sulfhemoglobin and can cause hemolysis in patients with G6PD deficiency. Excessive doses may worsen methemoglobinemia.
   2. Other therapies, such as ascorbic acid, cimetidine, and vitamin E, have been proposed, but their efficacy is unproven.

C. **Decontamination** (see p 45). Administer activated charcoal orally if conditions are appropriate (see Table I–38, p 51). Gastric lavage is not necessary after small to moderate ingestions if activated charcoal can be given promptly, but it may be considered for a very large overdose (more than 75 mg/kg) presenting within 2–3 hours of ingestion.

D. **Enhanced elimination** (see p 53)
   1. **Repeat-dose activated charcoal** interrupts enterohepatic recirculation and can effectively reduce the dapsone half-life (from 77 to 13.5 hours in one report). Continue repeat-dose charcoal for at least 48–72 hours. Do **not** use a charcoal/sorbitol suspension (see p 50).
   2. **Charcoal hemoperfusion** can reduce the dapsone half-life to 1.5 hours and might be considered in a severe intoxication unresponsive to conventional treatment. Hemodialysis is ineffective because dapsone and its metabolites are highly protein bound.

## ▶ DETERGENTS

*Michael J. Walsh, PharmD*

Detergents, familiar and indispensable products in the home, are synthetic surface-active agents that are chemically classified as **anionic, nonionic,** or **cationic** (Table II–22). Most of these products also contain bleaching (chlorine-releasing), bacteriostatic (having a low concentration of quaternary ammonium compound), or enzymatic agents. Accidental ingestion of detergents by children is very common, but severe toxicity rarely occurs.

I. **Mechanism of toxicity.** Detergents may precipitate and denature protein, are irritating to tissues, and have keratolytic and corrosive actions.
   A. **Anionic** and **nonionic** detergents are only mildly irritating, but **cationic** detergents are more hazardous because quaternary ammonium compounds may be caustic (benzalkonium chloride solutions of 10% have been reported to cause corrosive burns).

**TABLE II–22. CATIONIC DETERGENTS**

| Pyridinium compounds | Quaternary ammonium compounds | Quinolinium compounds |
|---|---|---|
| Cetalkonium chloride | Benzalkonium chloride | Dequalinium chloride |
| Cetrimide | Benzethonium chloride | |
| Cetrimonium bromide | | |
| Cetylpyridinium chloride | | |
| Stearalkonium chloride | | |

B. **Low-phosphate** detergents and **electric dishwasher** soaps often contain alkaline corrosive agents such as sodium metasilicate, sodium carbonate, and sodium tripolyphosphate.
C. The **enzyme-containing** detergents may cause skin irritation and have sensitizing properties; they may release bradykinin and histamine, causing bronchospasm.

II. **Toxic dose.** Mortality and serious morbidity are rare, but the nature of the toxic effect varies with the ingredients and concentration of the specific product. Cationic and dishwasher detergents are more dangerous than anionic and nonionic products. For benzalkonium chloride solutions, ingestion of 100–400 mg/kg has been fatal.

III. **Clinical presentation.** Immediate spontaneous vomiting often occurs after oral ingestion. Large ingestions may produce intractable vomiting, diarrhea, and hematemesis. Corrosive injury to the lips mouth, pharynx, and upper GI tract can occur. Exposure to the eye may cause mild to serious corrosive injury, depending on the specific product. Dermal contact generally causes a mild erythema or rash.
A. Phosphate-containing products may produce hypocalcemia, hypomagnesemia, tetany, and respiratory failure.
B. Methemoglobinemia was reported in a 45-year-old woman after copious irrigation of a hydatid cyst with a 0.1% solution of cetrimide, a cationic detergent.

IV. **Diagnosis** is based on a history of exposure and prompt onset of vomiting. A sudsy or foaming mouth may also suggest exposure.
A. **Specific levels.** There are no specific blood or urine levels.
B. **Other useful laboratory studies** include electrolytes, glucose, calcium, magnesium and phosphate (after ingestion of phosphate-containing products), and methemoglobin (cationic detergents).

V. **Treatment**
A. **Emergency and supportive measures**
1. In patients with protracted vomiting or diarrhea, administer intravenous fluids to correct dehydration and electrolyte imbalance (see p 16).
2. If corrosive injury is suspected, consult a gastroenterologist for possible endoscopy. Ingestion of products containing greater than 5–10% cationic detergents is more likely to cause corrosive injury.

B. **Specific drugs and antidotes.** If symptomatic hypocalcemia occurs after ingestion of a phosphate-containing product, administer intravenous **calcium** (see p 428). If methemoglobinemia occurs, administer **methylene blue** (p 473).
C. **Decontamination** (see p 45)
1. **Ingestion.** Dilute orally with small amounts of water or milk. A significant ingestion is unlikely if spontaneous vomiting has not already occurred.
a. Do ***not*** induce vomiting because of the risk for corrosive injury.
b. Consider gentle gastric lavage using a small, flexible tube after very large ingestions of cationic, corrosive, or phosphate-containing detergents.
c. Activated charcoal is not effective. Oral aluminum hydroxide can potentially bind phosphate in the GI tract.
2. **Eyes and skin.** Irrigate with copious amounts of tepid water or saline. Consult an ophthalmologist if eye pain persists or if there is significant corneal injury on fluorescein examination.

D. **Enhanced elimination.** There is no role for these procedures.

## ▶ DEXTROMETHORPHAN

*Timothy E. Albertson, MD, PhD*

Dextromethorphan is a common antitussive agent found in many over-the-counter cough and cold preparations. Many ingestions occur in children, but severe intoxication is rare. Dextromethorphan is often found in combination products containing antihistamines (see p 97), decongestants (p 322), ethanol (p 189), or acetaminophen (p 68). *Common combination products containing dextromethorphan* include Coricidin HBP Cough & Cold Tablets, NyQuil Nighttime Cold Medicine, Triaminic Nite Lite, PediaCare 1, PediaCare 3, Robitussin DM, Robitussin CF, Triaminic DM, and Vicks Pediatric Formula 44. A recent study of dextromethorphan ingestions noted that 71% of cases involved intentional abuse, and 85% of the abusers were 13–17 years old.

I. **Mechanism of toxicity.** Dextromethorphan is the *d*-isomer of 3-methoxy-*N*-methylmorphinan, a synthetic analog of codeine. (The *l*-isomer is the opioid analgesic levorphanol.) Although it has antitussive efficacy approximately equal to that of codeine, dextromethorphan has no apparent analgesic or addictive properties and produces relatively mild opioid effects in overdose.
   A. Both dextromethorphan and its *o*-demethylated metabolite appear to antagonize *N*-methyl-D-aspartate (NMDA) glutamate receptors, which may explain the anticonvulsant properties and protection against hypoxia-ischemia observed in animal models.
   B. Dextromethorphan inhibits reuptake of serotonin and may lead to the **serotonin syndrome** (see p 21) in patients taking monoamine oxidase inhibitors (p 269). Serotoninergic effects, as well as NMDA glutamate receptor inhibition, may explain the acute and chronic abuse potential of dextromethorphan.
   C. Dextromethorphan hydrobromide can cause bromide poisoning (see p 139).
   D. Many of the combination preparations contain acetaminophen, and overdose or abuse may result in hepatotoxicity (see p 68).
   E. **Pharmacokinetics.** Dextromethorphan is well absorbed orally, and effects are often apparent within 15–30 minutes (peak 2.5 hours). The volume of distribution is approximately 5–6 L/kg. The duration of effect is normally 3–6 hours. A genetic polymorphism exists for the debrisoquin hydroxylase enzyme (P-450 2D6). Dextromethorphan is a high-affinity substrate for this enzyme. Rapid metabolizers have a plasma half-life of about 3–4 hours, but in slow metabolizers (about 10% of the population) the half-life may exceed 24 hours. In addition, dextromethorphan competitively inhibits P450 2D6–mediated metabolism, leading to many potential drug interactions. (See also Table II–59.)

II. **Toxic dose.** The toxic dose is highly variable and depends largely on other ingredients in the ingested product. Symptoms usually occur when the amount of dextromethorphan ingested exceeds 10 mg/kg. The usual recommended adult daily dose of dextromethorphan is 60–120 mg/day; in children age 2–5 years, up to 30 mg/day.

III. **Clinical presentation**
   A. **Mild intoxication** produces clumsiness, dizziness, ataxia, nystagmus, mydriasis, and restlessness. Visual and auditory hallucinations have been reported.
   B. With **severe poisoning,** stupor, coma, and respiratory depression may occur, especially if alcohol has been co-ingested. The pupils may be constricted or dilated. A few cases of seizures have been reported after ingestions of more than 20–30 mg/kg.
   C. **Serotonin syndrome** (see p 21). Severe hyperthermia, muscle rigidity, and hypertension may occur with therapeutic doses in patients taking **monoamine oxidase inhibitors** (p 269).

IV. **Diagnosis** should be considered with ingestion of any over-the-counter cough suppressant, especially when there is nystagmus, ataxia, and lethargy. Because dextromethorphan often is combined with other ingredients (eg, antihistamines, phenylpropanolamine, or acetaminophen), suspect mixed ingestion.
   A. **Specific levels.** Assays exist for serum and urine analysis but are not generally available. In seven fatal infant cases, blood levels averaged 0.38 mg/L (range 0.10–0.95). Despite its structural similarity to opioids, dextromethorphan is not likely to produce a false-positive urine opioid immunoassay screen. However, it may produce a false-positive result on methadone and phencyclidine immunoassays. Dextromethorphan is readily detected by comprehensive urine toxicology screening.

B. **Other useful laboratory studies** include electrolytes, glucose, and arterial blood gases (if respiratory depression is suspected). Blood ethanol and acetaminophen levels should be obtained if those drugs are contained in the ingested product.

V. **Treatment**

A. **Emergency and supportive measures.** Most patients with mild symptoms (ie, restlessness, ataxia, or mild drowsiness) can be observed for 4–6 hours and discharged if they are improving.

1. Maintain an open airway and assist ventilation if needed (see pp 1–7).
2. Treat seizures (see p 22) and coma (p 18) if they occur.

B. **Specific drugs and antidotes.** Although **naloxone** (see p 477) has been reported to be effective in doses of 0.06–0.4 mg, other cases have failed to respond to doses up to 2.4 mg.

C. **Decontamination** (see p 45). Administer activated charcoal orally if conditions are appropriate (see Table I–38, p 51). Gastric lavage is not necessary after small to moderate ingestions if activated charcoal can be given promptly.

D. **Enhanced elimination.** The volume of distribution of dextromethorphan is very large, and there is no role for enhanced removal procedures.

## ▶ DIOXINS

*Stephen C. Born, MD, MPH*

Polychlorinated dibenzodioxins (PCDDs) and dibenzofurans (PCDFs) are a group of highly toxic substances commonly known as dioxins. Dioxins are not produced commercially. PCDDs are formed during the production of certain organochlorines (trichlorophenoxyacetic acid [2,4,5-T], hexachlorophene, pentachlorophenol, etc), and PCDDs and PCDFs are formed by the combustion of these and other compounds such as polychlorinated biphenyls (PCBs; see p 321) as well as medical and municipal waste incineration. Agent Orange, a herbicide used by the United States against Vietnam during the Vietnam War, contained dioxins (most importantly 2,3,7,8-tetrachlorodibenzo-*p*-dioxin [TCDD], the most toxic and extensively researched dioxin) as contaminants. Some PCBs have biological activity similar to that of dioxins and are identified as "dioxin-like." The most common route of exposure to dioxins in the United States is through dietary consumption.

I. **Mechanism of toxicity.** Dioxins are highly lipid soluble and are concentrated in fat. Dioxins are known to bind to the aryl hydrocarbon receptor protein (AhR) in cytoplasm and form a heterodimer with nuclear proteins and induce transcription of multiple genes, including cytochrome P-4501A1 (CYP1A1). Dioxins also have endocrine disruptor effects, and exposure may result in reproductive and developmental defects, immunotoxicity, and liver damage. Dioxins are mutagenic and are probable human carcinogens, leading to an overall increase in the rates of all cancers in exposed individuals. TCDD is a known animal carcinogen and is considered a human carcinogen by both the EPA and the IARC.

II. **Toxic dose.** Dioxins are extremely potent animal toxins. With the discovery of significant noncancer developmental abnormalities in environmentally exposed animals, the "no effect" level for exposure to dioxins is under reevaluation and is likely to be within an order of magnitude of current human dietary exposure. The oral 50% lethal dose ($LD_{50}$) in animals varies from 0.0006–0.045 mg/kg. Daily dermal exposure to 10–30 ppm in oil or 100–3000 ppm in soil produces toxicity in animals. Chloracne is likely with daily dermal exposure exceeding 100 ppm. The greatest source of exposure of the general population is food, which is contaminated in minute quantities, usually measured in picograms (trillionths of a gram). Higher exposures have occurred through industrial accidents.

III. **Clinical presentation**

A. **Acute symptoms** after exposure include irritation of the skin, eyes, and mucous membranes and nausea, vomiting, and myalgias.

B. **After a latency period** that may be prolonged (up to several weeks or more), chloracne, porphyria cutanea tarda, hirsutism, or hyperpigmentation may occur. Elevated levels of hepatic transaminases and blood lipids may be found. Polyneuropathies with sensory impairment and lower-extremity motor weakness have been reported.

C. **Death** in laboratory animals occurs a few weeks after a lethal dose and is caused by a "wasting syndrome" characterized by reduced food intake and loss of body weight. Death from acute toxicity in humans is rare, even in cases of intentional poisoning.

IV. **Diagnosis** is difficult and rests mainly on history of exposure; the presence of chloracne (which is considered pathognomonic for exposure to dioxins and related compounds) provides strong supporting evidence. Although many products previously contaminated with dioxins are no longer produced in the United States, exposures to PCDDs and PCDFs occur during many types of chemical fires, and the possibility of exposure can cause considerable public and individual anxiety.

A. **Specific levels.** It is difficult and expensive to detect dioxins in human blood or tissue, and there is no established correlation with symptoms. There are many congeners of PCDDs, PCDFs, and PCBs; the individual contribution of each one to toxicity is assessed by using toxic equivalence factors established by the World Health Organization, based on relative potency estimates for each congener (TCDD by definition has a TEF of 1). As a result of more stringent controls over environmental exposures, the human body burden of dioxins has decreased over the last 30 years. Unexposed persons have a mean of 5.38 pg of 2,3,7,8-TCDD per gram of serum lipid, compared with workers producing trichlorophenols, who had a mean of 220 pg/g. The highest recorded level is 144,000 pg/g blood fat in a patient with few adverse health effects other than chloracne.

B. **Other useful laboratory studies** include glucose, electrolytes, BUN, creatinine, liver transaminases, CBC, and uroporphyrins (if porphyria is suspected).

V. **Treatment**

A. **Emergency and supportive measures.** Treat skin, eye, and respiratory irritation symptomatically.

B. **Specific drugs and antidotes.** There is no specific antidote.

C. **Decontamination** (see p 45)

1. **Inhalation.** Remove victims from exposure and give supplemental oxygen if available.
2. **Eyes and skin.** Remove contaminated clothing and wash affected skin with copious soap and water; irrigate exposed eyes with copious tepid water or saline. Personnel involved in decontamination should wear protective gear appropriate to the suspected level of contamination.
3. **Ingestion.** Administer activated charcoal if conditions are appropriate (see Table I–38, p 51). Gastric emptying is not necessary if activated charcoal can be given promptly.

D. **Enhanced elimination.** Elimination of dioxins may be enhanced by a factor of 4–7 through administration of **olestra,** a nonabsorbable fat substitute that increases fecal excretion. Olestra may decrease the half-life of elimination of TCDD from 7 years to 1–2 years.

## ► DISULFIRAM

*Richard J. Geller, MD, MPH*

Disulfiram (tetraethylthiuram disulfide [CASRN 97-77-8] or Antabuse) is an antioxidant industrial chemical also used as a drug in the treatment of alcoholism. Ingestion of ethanol while a person is taking disulfiram causes a well-defined unpleasant reaction, the fear of which provides a negative incentive to drink. Clinical toxicity is caused by overdose or occurs as a result of a disulfiram-alcohol drug interaction.

**I. Mechanism of toxicity**

**A.** Disulfiram's toxicity is caused by inhibition of two enzymes. Inhibition of aldehyde dehydrogenase leads to accumulation of toxic acetaldehyde after ethanol ingestion. Inhibition of dopamine betahydroxylase (necessary for norepinephrine synthesis) results in norepinephrine depletion at presynaptic sympathetic nerve endings, leading to vasodilation and orthostatic hypotension.

**B.** Disulfiram is metabolized to small amounts of **carbon disulfide** (see also p 150), which may play a role in central and peripheral nervous system toxicity.

**C.** Disulfiram's chemical structure includes sulfur atoms common to chelating agents. Chronic use may increase the elimination of certain essential metals (copper, zinc) by chelation. This may, in part, be the cause of disulfiram's enzyme-inhibiting effects, as both of these enzymes require copper as a cofactor.

**D. Pharmacokinetics.** Disulfiram is absorbed rapidly and completely, but peak effects involve enzyme inhibition and may require 8–12 hours. Although the elimination half-life is 7–8 hours, clinical actions may persist for several days. Disulfiram is metabolized in the liver; it inhibits the metabolism of many other drugs, including isoniazid, phenytoin, theophylline, warfarin, and many benzodiazepines. (See also Table II–59.)

**II. Toxic dose**

**A. Disulfiram overdose.** Ingestion of 2.5 g or more has caused toxicity in children after a delay of 3–12 hours.

**B. Disulfiram-ethanol interaction.** Ingestion of as little as 7 mL of ethanol can cause a severe reaction in patients taking as little as 200 mg/day of disulfiram. Mild reactions have been reported after use of cough syrup, aftershave lotions, and other alcohol-containing products.

**III. Clinical presentation**

**A. Acute disulfiram overdose (without ethanol)** may cause garlic-like breath odor, headache, hypotension, vomiting, ataxia, confusion, lethargy, seizures, and coma. Chronic neuropsychological impairment and fatal hepatic failure have uncommonly followed disulfiram overdose.

**B. Disulfiram-ethanol interaction.** Shortly after ingestion of ethanol, a patient receiving chronic disulfiram therapy develops flushing, throbbing headache, dyspnea, anxiety, vertigo, vomiting, and confusion. Orthostatic hypotension with warm extremities is very common. The severity of the reaction usually depends on the dose of disulfiram and ethanol. Reactions do not usually occur unless the patient has been on oral disulfiram therapy for at least 1 day; the reaction may occur up to several days after the last dose of disulfiram. Disulfiram has been implanted subcutaneously in Europe, leading to reactions after alcohol consumption that are milder but of longer duration.

**IV. Diagnosis** of disulfiram overdose is based on a history of acute ingestion and the presence of CNS symptoms with vomiting. The disulfiram-ethanol interaction is diagnosed in a patient with a history of chronic disulfiram use and possible exposure to ethanol who exhibits a characteristic hypotensive flushing reaction.

**A. Specific levels.** Blood disulfiram levels are not of value in diagnosis or treatment. Blood acetaldehyde levels may be elevated during the disulfiram-ethanol reaction, but this information is of little value in acute management.

**B. Other useful laboratory studies** include electrolytes, glucose, BUN, creatinine, liver transaminases, and ethanol level.

**V. Treatment**

**A. Emergency and supportive measures**

**1. Acute disulfiram overdose**

**a.** Maintain an open airway and assist ventilation if necessary (see pp 1–7).

**b.** Treat coma (see p 18) and seizures (p 22) if they occur.

**2. Disulfiram-ethanol interaction**

**a.** Maintain an open airway and assist ventilation if necessary (see pp 1–7).

**b.** Treat hypotension with supine position and intravenous fluids (eg, saline). If a pressor agent is needed, a direct-acting agent such as norepinephrine (see p 487) is preferred over indirect-acting drugs such as dopamine.

c. Administer benzodiazepine anxiolytics (eg, diazepam or lorazepam, p 419) and reassurance as needed.

d. Treat vomiting with metoclopramide (see p 475) and headache with IV analgesics if needed. Avoid phenothiazine antiemetics (which have an alpha receptor blocking effect) such as prochlorperazine.

**B. Specific drugs and antidotes.** There is no specific antidote.

**C. Decontamination** (see p 45)

1. **Acute disulfiram overdose**. Administer activated charcoal orally if conditions are appropriate (see Table I–38, p 51). Gastric lavage is not necessary after small to moderate ingestions if activated charcoal can be given promptly.

2. **Disulfiram-ethanol interaction.** Decontamination procedures are not likely to be of benefit once the reaction begins.

**D. Enhanced elimination.** Hemodialysis is not indicated for disulfiram overdose, but it may remove ethanol and acetaldehyde and has been reported to be effective in treating the acute disulfiram-ethanol interaction. This is not likely to be necessary in patients receiving adequate fluid and pressor support. There are no data to support the use of repeat-dose activated charcoal for any of the disulfiram syndromes.

# ▶ DIURETICS

*Timothy J. Wiegand M.D.*

Diuretics are prescribed commonly for the management of essential hypertension, congestive heart failure, ascites, and chronic renal insufficiency. Adverse effects from chronic use or misuse (in sports, dieting, and anorexia) are more frequently encountered than those from acute overdose. Overdoses are generally benign, and no serious outcomes have resulted from acute ingestion. Common currently available diuretics are listed in Table II–23.

**I. Mechanism of toxicity**

**A.** The toxicity of these drugs is associated with their pharmacologic effects, which decrease fluid volume and promote electrolyte loss, including dehydra-

**TABLE II–23. DIURETICS**

| Drug | Maximum Adult Daily Dose (mg) | Drug | Maximum Adult Daily Dose (mg) |
|---|---|---|---|
| **Carbonic anhydrase inhibitors** | | **Thiazides** | |
| Acetazolamide | 1000 | Bendroflumethiazide | 20 |
| Dichlorphenamide | 200 | Chlorothiazide | 2000 |
| Methazolamide | 300 | Chlorthalidone | 200 |
| | | Cyclothiazide | 6 |
| **Loop diuretics** | | Flumethiazide | 2000 |
| Bumetanide | 2 | Hydrochlorothiazide | 200 |
| Ethacrynic acid | 200 | Hydroflumethiazide | 200 |
| Furosemide | 600 | Indapamide | 5 |
| Torsemide | 200 | Methyclothiazide | 10 |
| | | Metolazone | 20 |
| **Potassium-sparing** | | Polythiazide | 4 |
| Amiloride | 20 | Quinethazone | 200 |
| Spironolactone | 400 | Trichlormethiazide | 4 |
| Triamterene | 300 | | |

tion, hypokalemia (or hyperkalemia, with spironolactone and triamterene), hypomagnesemia, hyponatremia, and hypochloremic alkalosis. Electrolyte imbalance may lead to cardiac arrhythmias and may enhance digitalis toxicity (see p 155). Diuretics are classified on the basis of the pharmacologic mechanisms by which they affect solute and water loss (see Table II–23).

**B. Pharmacokinetics.** See Table II–59, p 382.

**II. Toxic dose.** Minimum toxic doses have not been established. Significant dehydration or electrolyte imbalance is unlikely if the amount ingested is less than the usual recommended daily dose (see Table II–23). High doses of intravenous ethacrynic acid and furosemide can cause ototoxicity, especially when administered rapidly and in patients with renal failure.

**III. Clinical presentation.** Gastrointestinal symptoms including nausea, vomiting, and diarrhea are common after acute oral overdose. Lethargy, weakness, hyporeflexia, and dehydration (and occasionally hypotension) may be present if volume loss and electrolyte disturbances are present, although the onset of symptoms may be delayed for 2–4 hours or more until diuretic action is obtained. Spironolactone is very slow, with maximal effects after the third day.

**A.** Hypokalemia may cause muscle weakness, cramps, and tetany. Severe hypokalemia may result in flaccid paralysis and rhabdomyolysis. Cardiac rhythm disturbances may also occur.

**B.** Spironolactone and other potassium-sparing agents may cause hyperkalemia.

**C.** Hypocalcemia and hypomagnesemia may also cause tetany.

**D.** Hyperglycemia, hypercalcemia, and hyperuricemia may occur, especially with thiazide diuretics.

**E.** Carbonic anhydrase inhibitors may induce metabolic acidosis.

**IV. Diagnosis** is based on a history of exposure and evidence of dehydration and acid-base or electrolyte imbalance. Note that patients on diuretics may also be taking other cardiac and antihypertensive medications.

**A. Specific levels** are not routinely available or clinically useful.

**B. Other useful laboratory studies** include electrolytes (including calcium and magnesium), glucose, BUN, creatinine, and ECG.

**V. Treatment**

**A. Emergency and supportive measures**

1. Replace fluid loss with intravenous crystalloid solutions and correct electrolyte abnormalities (see p 37). Correction of sodium in patients with diuretic-induced hyponatremia should be limited to 1–2 mEq/hour to avoid central pontine myelinolysis unless seizures or coma is present. In this case 3% hypertonic saline should be used for a more rapid correction.
2. Monitor the ECG until the potassium level is normalized.

**B. Specific drugs and antidotes.** There are no specific antidotes.

**C. Decontamination** (see p 45). Administer activated charcoal orally if conditions are appropriate (see Table I–38, p 51). Gastric lavage is not necessary after small to moderate ingestions if activated charcoal can be given promptly. Cathartics have not been shown to be beneficial in preventing absorption and may worsen dehydration.

**D. Enhanced elimination.** No experience with extracorporeal removal of diuretics has been reported.

## ► ERGOT DERIVATIVES

*Neal L. Benowitz, MD*

Ergot derivatives are used to treat migraine headache and enhance uterine contraction postpartum. Ergots are produced by the fungus *Claviceps purpurea,* which may grow on rye and other grains. Natural or synthetic ergot drugs include ergotamine (Cafergot™, Ergomar™, Gynergen™, and Ergostat™), methysergide (Sansert™), dihydroergotamine (DHE-45™), and ergonovine (Ergotrate™). Some ergoloid derivatives (dihydroergocornine, dihydroergocristine, and dihydroergocryptine) have been used in combination (Hydergine™ and Deapril-ST™) for the treatment of dementia. Bromocriptine (Parlodel™, see p 427) and pergolide (Permax™) are ergot derivatives with dopamine agonist activity that are used to treat Parkinson's disease. Bromocriptine is also used to treat hyperprolactinemic states.

**I. Mechanism of toxicity**

**A.** Ergot derivatives directly stimulate vasoconstriction and uterine contraction, antagonize alpha-adrenergic and serotonin receptors, and may dilate some blood vessels via a CNS sympatholytic action. The relative contribution of each of these mechanisms to toxicity depends on the particular ergot alkaloid and its dose. **Sustained vasoconstriction** causes most of the serious toxicity; reduced blood flow causes local tissue hypoxia and ischemic injury, resulting in tissue edema and local thrombosis, worsening ischemia and causing further injury. At a certain point, reversible vasospasm progresses to irreversible vascular insufficiency and limb gangrene.

**B. Pharmacokinetics.** See Table II–59, p 382.

**II. Toxic dose.** Death has been reported in a 14-month-old child after acute ingestion of 12 mg of ergotamine. However, most cases of severe poisoning occur with chronic overmedication for migraine headaches rather than involving acute single overdoses. Daily doses of 10 mg or more of ergotamine are usually associated with toxicity. There are many case reports of vasospastic complications with normal therapeutic dosing.

**III. Clinical presentation**

**A. Ergotamine and related agents.** Mild intoxication causes nausea and vomiting. Serious poisoning results in vasoconstriction that may involve many parts of the body. Owing to persistence of ergots in tissues, vasospasm may continue for up to 10–14 days.

1. Involvement of the extremities causes paresthesias, pain, pallor, coolness, and loss of peripheral pulses in the hands and feet; gangrene may ensue.
2. Other complications of vasospasm include coronary ischemia and myocardial infarction, abdominal angina and bowel infarction, renal infarction and failure, visual disturbances and blindness, and stroke. Psychosis, seizures, and coma occur rarely.

**B. Bromocriptine** intoxication may present with hallucinations, paranoid behavior, hypertension, and tachycardia. Involuntary movements, hallucinations, and hypotension are reported with **pergolide.**

**C.** Chronic use of **methysergide** occasionally causes retroperitoneal fibrosis.

**IV. Diagnosis** is based on a history of ergot use and clinical findings of vasospasm.

**A. Specific levels.** Ergotamine levels are not widely available, and blood concentrations do not correlate well with toxicity.

**B. Other useful laboratory studies** include CBC, electrolytes, BUN, creatinine, and ECG. Arteriography of the affected vascular bed is indicated occasionally.

**V. Treatment**

**A. Emergency and supportive measures**

1. Maintain an open airway and assist ventilation if necessary (see pp 1–7).
2. Treat coma (see p 18) and convulsions (p 22) if they occur.
3. Immediately discontinue ergot treatment. Hospitalize patients with vasospastic symptoms and treat promptly to prevent complications.

**B. Specific drugs and antidotes**

1. **Peripheral ischemia** requires prompt vasodilator therapy and anticoagulation to prevent local thrombosis.
   a. Administer intravenous **nitroprusside** (see p 485), starting with 1–2 mcg/kg/min, or intravenous **phentolamine** (p 495), starting with 0.5 mg/min, increasing the infusion rate until ischemia is improved or sys-

temic hypotension occurs. Intra-arterial infusion is occasionally required. Nifedipine or other vasodilating calcium antagonists may also enhance peripheral blood flow.

b. Administer **heparin,** 5000 units IV followed by 1000 units/h (in adults), with adjustments in the infusion rate to maintain the activated coagulation time (ACT) or the activated partial thromboplastin time (APTT) at approximately 2 times the baseline.

2. **Coronary spasm.** Administer **nitroglycerin,** 0.15–0.6 mg sublingually or 5–20 mcg/min IV. Intracoronary artery nitroglycerin may be required if there is no response to intravenous infusion. Also consider using a calcium antagonist.

C. **Decontamination** after acute ingestion (see p 45). Administer activated charcoal orally if conditions are appropriate (see Table I–38, p 51). Gastric lavage is not necessary after small to moderate ingestions if activated charcoal can be given promptly.

D. **Enhanced elimination.** Dialysis and hemoperfusion are not effective. Repeat-dose charcoal has not been studied, but because of extensive tissue distribution of ergots it is not likely to be useful.

## ► ETHANOL

*Saralyn R. Williams, MD*

Commercial beer, wine, and liquors contain various amounts of ethanol. Ethanol also is found in a variety of colognes, perfumes, aftershaves, mouthwashes; some rubbing alcohols; many food flavorings (eg, vanilla, almond, and lemon extracts); pharmaceutical preparations (eg, elixirs); and many other products. Ethanol is frequently ingested recreationally and is the most common co-ingestant with other drugs in suicide attempts. Ethanol may also serve as a competitive substrate in the emergency treatment of methanol and ethylene glycol poisonings (see p 193).

I. **Mechanism of toxicity**

A. **CNS depression** is the principal effect of acute ethanol intoxication. Ethanol has additive effects with other CNS depressants such as barbiturates, benzodiazepines, opioids, antidepressants, and antipsychotics.

B. **Hypoglycemia** may be caused by impaired gluconeogenesis in patients with depleted or low glycogen stores (particularly small children and poorly nourished persons).

C. Ethanol intoxication and chronic alcoholism also predispose patients to trauma, exposure-induced hypothermia, injurious effects of alcohol on the GI tract and nervous system, and a number of nutritional disorders and metabolic derangements.

D. **Pharmacokinetics.** Ethanol is readily absorbed (peak 30–120 min) and distributed into the body water (volume of distribution 0.5–0.7 L/kg or about 50 L in the average adult). Elimination is mainly by oxidation in the liver and follows zero-order kinetics. The average adult can metabolize about 7–10 g of alcohol per hour, or about 12–25 mg/dL/h. This rate varies between individuals and is influenced by polymorphisms of the alcohol dehydrogenase enzyme and the activity of the microsomal ethanol-oxidizing systems.

II. **Toxic dose.** Generally, 0.7 g/kg pure ethanol (approximately 3–4 drinks) will produce a blood ethanol concentration of 100 mg/dL (0.1 g/dL). The legal limit for intoxication varies by state, with a range of 0.08 g/dL to 0.1 g/dL.

A. A level of 100 mg/dL decreases reaction time and judgment and may be enough to inhibit gluconeogenesis and cause hypoglycemia in children and patients with liver disease but by itself is not enough to cause coma.

**B.** The level sufficient to cause deep coma or respiratory depression is highly variable, depending on the individual's degree of tolerance to ethanol. Although levels above 300 mg/dL usually cause coma in novice drinkers, chronic alcoholics may be awake with levels of 500–600 mg/dL or higher.

**III. Clinical presentation**

**A. Acute intoxication**

1. With **mild** to moderate intoxication, patients exhibit euphoria, mild incoordination, ataxia, nystagmus, and impaired judgment and reflexes. Social inhibitions are loosened, and boisterous or aggressive behavior is common. Hypoglycemia may occur, especially in children and persons with reduced hepatic glycogen stores.
2. With **deep intoxication,** coma, respiratory depression, and pulmonary aspiration may occur. In these patients, the pupils are usually small and the temperature, blood pressure, and pulse rate are often decreased. Rhabdomyolysis may result from prolonged immobility.

**B. Chronic ethanol abuse** is associated with numerous complications:

1. **Hepatic toxicity** includes fatty infiltration of the liver, alcoholic hepatitis, and eventually cirrhosis. Liver scarring leads to portal hypertension, ascites, and bleeding from esophageal varices and hemorrhoids; hyponatremia from fluid retention; and bacterial peritonitis. Production of clotting factors is impaired, leading to prolonged prothrombin time. Hepatic metabolism of drugs and endogenous toxins is impaired and may contribute to hepatic encephalopathy.
2. **Gastrointestinal** bleeding may result from alcohol-induced gastritis, esophagitis, and duodenitis. Other causes of massive bleeding include Mallory-Weiss tears of the esophagus and esophageal varices. Acute pancreatitis is a common cause of abdominal pain and vomiting.
3. **Cardiac** disorders include various dysrhythmias such as atrial fibrillation that may be associated with potassium and magnesium depletion and poor caloric intake ("holiday heart"). Cardiomyopathy has been associated with long-term alcohol use. (Cardiomyopathy was also historically associated with ingestion of cobalt used to stabilize beer.)
4. **Neurologic** toxicity includes cerebral atrophy, cerebellar degeneration, and peripheral stocking-glove sensory neuropathy. Nutritional disorders such as thiamine (vitamin $B_1$) deficiency can cause Wernicke's encephalopathy or Korsakoff's psychosis.
5. **Alcoholic ketoacidosis** is characterized by anion gap metabolic acidosis and elevated levels of beta-hydroxybutyrate and, to a lesser extent, acetoacetate. The osmolar gap may also be elevated, causing this condition to be mistaken for methanol or ethylene glycol poisoning.

**C. Alcohol withdrawal.** Sudden discontinuation after chronic high-level alcohol use often causes headache, tremulousness, anxiety, palpitations, and insomnia. Brief, generalized seizures may occur, usually within 6–12 hours of decreased ethanol consumption. Sympathetic nervous system overactivity may progress to **delirium tremens,** a life-threatening syndrome characterized by tachycardia, diaphoresis, hyperthermia, and delirium, which usually manifests 48–72 hours after cessation of heavy alcohol use. The "DTs" may cause significant morbidity and mortality if untreated.

**D. Other problems.** Ethanol abusers sometimes intentionally or accidentally ingest ethanol substitutes such as isopropyl alcohol (see p 234), methanol (p 260), and ethylene glycol (p 193). In addition, ethanol may serve as the vehicle for swallowing large numbers of pills in a suicide attempt. Disulfiram (p 184) use can cause a serious acute reaction with ethanol ingestion.

**IV. Diagnosis** of ethanol intoxication is usually simple, based on the history of ingestion, the characteristic smell of fresh alcohol or the fetid odor of acetaldehyde and other metabolic products, and the presence of nystagmus, ataxia, and altered mental status. However, other disorders may accompany or mimic intoxication, such as hypoglycemia, head trauma, hypothermia, meningitis, Wernicke's encephalopathy, and intoxication with other drugs or poisons.

**A. Specific levels.** Serum ethanol levels are usually available at most hospital laboratories and, depending on the method used, are accurate and specific.

1. In general, there is only rough correlation between blood levels and clinical presentation; however, an ethanol level below 300 mg/dL in a comatose patient should initiate a search for alternative causes.
2. If ethanol levels are not readily available, the ethanol concentration may be estimated by calculating the osmolar gap (see p 32).

**B. Suggested laboratory studies** in the acutely intoxicated patient may include glucose, electrolytes, BUN, creatinine, liver transaminases, prothrombin time (PT/INR), magnesium, arterial blood gases or oximetry, and chest x-ray (if pulmonary aspiration is suspected). Consider CT scan of the head if the patient has focal neurologic deficits or altered mental status inconsistent with the degree of blood alcohol elevation.

**V. Treatment**

**A. Emergency and supportive measures**

1. **Acute intoxication.** Treatment is mainly supportive.
   a. Protect the airway to prevent aspiration and intubate and assist ventilation if needed (pp 1–7).
   b. Give glucose and thiamine (see pp 457 and 513), and treat coma (p 18) and seizures (p 22) if they occur. Glucagon is not effective for alcohol-induced hypoglycemia.
   c. Correct hypothermia with gradual rewarming (see p 19).
   d. Most patients will recover within 4–6 hours. Observe children until their blood alcohol level is below 50 mg/dL and there is no evidence of hypoglycemia.
2. **Alcoholic ketoacidosis.** Treat with volume replacement, thiamine (see p 505), and supplemental glucose. Most patients recover rapidly.
3. **Alcohol withdrawal.** Treat with benzodiazepines (eg, diazepam, 2–10 mg IV initially and repeat as needed; see p 419).

**B. Specific drugs and antidotes.** There is no available specific ethanol receptor antagonist despite anecdotal reports of arousal after administration of naloxone.

**C. Decontamination** (see p 45). Because ethanol is rapidly absorbed, gastric decontamination is usually not indicated unless other drug ingestion is suspected. Consider aspirating gastric contents with a small flexible tube if the alcohol ingestion was massive and recent (within 30–45 minutes). Activated charcoal does not effectively adsorb ethanol but may be given if other drugs or toxins were ingested.

**D. Enhanced elimination.** Metabolism of ethanol normally occurs at a fixed rate of approximately 20–30 mg/dL/h. Elimination rates are faster in chronic alcoholics and at serum levels above 300 mg/dL. Hemodialysis efficiently removes ethanol, but enhanced removal is rarely needed because supportive care is usually sufficient. Hemoperfusion and forced diuresis are not effective.

## ▶ ETHYLENE DIBROMIDE

*Janet Weiss, MD*

Ethylene dibromide (EDB, dibromoethane, glycol dibromide, bromofume) is a volatile, nonflammable colorless liquid with a sweet chloroform-like odor produced by the bromination of ethylene. EDB was used as a lead scavenger in leaded gasoline and as a pesticide and fumigant in soil and on grain, fruits, and vegetables, but these uses have almost disappeared in the United States. It is used as a chemical intermediate, as a gauge fluid, and as a nonflammable solvent for resins, gums, and waxes.

Ethylene dibromide's odor is not detectable at a low enough concentration to be considered a good warning of excessive exposure. EDB readily penetrates skin, cloth, and protective clothing made of rubber and leather. Absorption and toxicity can occur by inhalation and by the oral and dermal routes. When heated to decomposition, EDB may release gases and vapors such as hydrogen bromide, bromine, and carbon monoxide. Because EDB has been classified as a suspected human carcinogen and is a male reproductive toxin, its use as a pesticide has been restricted since 1984.

**I. Mechanism of toxicity**

- **A. Liquid EDB is an irritant** capable of causing chemical burns. Inhalation of EDB vapor produces respiratory tract irritation and delayed-onset pulmonary edema.
- **B. Once absorbed systemically,** EDB is converted to 2-bromoacetaldehyde, which becomes irreversibly bound to macromolecules, including DNA, and inhibits enzymes, causing cellular disruption and reduced glutathione levels. Metabolism of EDB involves an oxidative pathway (cytochrome P-450) and a conjugation pathway (glutathione). The liver is a principal target organ for toxicity.

**II. Toxic dose**

- **A. Inhalation.** Because EDB is a suspected carcinogen (ACGIH category A2), no "safe" workplace exposure limit has been determined. Although the current OSHA legal permissible exposure limit (PEL) is 20 ppm as an 8-hour time-weighted average with a ceiling of 30 ppm, the National Institute for Occupational Safety and Health (NIOSH) recommends a ceiling exposure of no more than 0.13 ppm. Exposure to vapor concentrations greater than 200 ppm can produce lung irritation, and 100 ppm is the air level considered immediately dangerous to life or health (IDLH).
- **B. Ingestion** of 4.5 mL of liquid EDB (160 mg/kg) resulted in death.
- **C.** Dermal application of as little as 16 mg/kg caused systemic intoxication.
- **D.** Inhalation. Fatalities have occurred among workers cleaning a tank containing residues of ethylene dibromide.
- **E.** The US Environmental Protection Agency's drinking-water Maximum Contaminant Limit (MCL) for EDB is 0.00005 mg/L.

**III. Clinical presentation**

- **A. Inhalation** of EDB vapor causes irritation of the eyes and upper respiratory tract. Pulmonary edema usually occurs within 1–6 hours but may be delayed as long as 48 hours after exposure.
- **B. Skin exposure** produces painful local inflammation, swelling, and blistering.
- **C. Oral ingestion** causes prompt vomiting and diarrhea.
- **D. Systemic** manifestations of intoxication include CNS depression, delirium, seizures, and metabolic acidosis. Skeletal muscle necrosis, acute renal failure, and hepatic necrosis have also been reported in fatal cases.

**IV. Diagnosis** of EDB poisoning is based on a history of exposure and evidence of upper-airway and eye irritation (in cases of inhalation) or gastroenteritis (after ingestion). EDB vapor has a strong chemical odor.

- **A. Specific levels.** EDB is detectable in expired air, blood, and tissues, although levels are not useful in emergency management. Serum bromide levels may be elevated (> 0.1 mEq/L) in severe cases, because bromide is released from EDB in the body.
- **B. Other useful laboratory studies** include electrolytes, glucose, BUN, creatinine, liver transaminases, CPK, and CBC. In cases of inhalation exposure consider arterial blood gases and chest x-ray.

**V. Treatment**

**A. Emergency and supportive measures**

1. Maintain an open airway and assist ventilation if necessary (see pp 1–7).
2. After inhalation exposure, anticipate and treat wheezing, airway obstruction, and pulmonary edema (pp 7–8). Provide supplemental oxygen if needed, and anticipate possible delayed pulmonary edema.
3. Treat coma (see p 18), seizures (p 22), rhabdomyolysis (p 26), and metabolic acidosis (p 33) if they occur.

**B. Specific drugs and antidotes.** There is no specific antidote. Dimercaprol (BAL) and acetylcysteine (Mucomyst) have been suggested as antidotes on the basis of the postulated mechanism of ethylene dibromide's toxicity. However, no adequate studies have tested the efficacy of these therapies, and they are not recommended for routine use.

**C. Decontamination** (see p 45). ***Caution:*** Victims whose clothing or skin is contaminated with EDB can secondarily contaminate response personnel by direct contact or through off-gassing vapor. Patients do not pose contamination risks after clothing is removed and skin is washed. Rescuers should use self-contained breathing apparatus and wear protective clothing to avoid personal exposure. Patients exposed only to solvent vapor who have no skin or eye irritation do not need decontamination.

1. **Inhalation.** Remove the victim from exposure and provide supplemental oxygen if available.
2. **Skin and eyes.** Remove and safely discard all contaminated clothing and wash exposed skin with copious soap and water. Irrigate exposed eyes with tepid saline or water.
3. **Ingestion.** Administer activated charcoal orally if conditions are appropriate (see Table I–38, p 51). Consider gastric lavage with a small tube if the patient presents within 30 minutes of ingestion or has ingested a large quantity (more than 1–2 oz).

**D. Enhanced elimination.** There is no role for dialysis or hemoperfusion, diuresis, or repeat-dose charcoal.

## ▶ ETHYLENE GLYCOL AND OTHER GLYCOLS

*Ilene B. Anderson, PharmD*

Ethylene glycol is the primary ingredient (up to 95%) in antifreeze. It sometimes is consumed intentionally as an alcohol substitute by alcoholics and is tempting to children because of its sweet taste. Intoxication by ethylene glycol itself causes inebriation and mild gastritis; in addition, its metabolic products cause metabolic acidosis, renal failure, and death. Other glycols may also produce toxicity (Table II–24).

**I. Mechanism of toxicity**

**A. Ethylene glycol** is metabolized by alcohol dehydrogenase to glycoaldehyde, which is then metabolized to glycolic, glyoxylic, and oxalic acids. These acids, along with excess lactic acid, are responsible for the anion gap metabolic acidosis. Oxalate readily precipitates with calcium to form insoluble calcium oxalate crystals. Tissue injury is caused by widespread deposition of oxalate crystals and the toxic effects of glycolic and glyoxylic acids.

**B. Pharmacokinetics.** Ethylene glycol is well absorbed. The volume of distribution is about 0.6–0.8 L/kg. It is not protein bound. Metabolism is by alcohol dehydrogenase, with a half-life of about 3–5 hours. In the presence of ethanol or fomepizole (see below), which block ethylene glycol metabolism, elimination is entirely renal, with a half-life of about 17 hours.

TABLE II–24. OTHER GLYCOLS

| Compounds | Toxicity and Comments | Treatment |
|---|---|---|
| Diethylene glycol (DEG) | Highly nephrotoxic. Renal failure, coma, metabolic acidosis, and death have been reported after ingestion as well as repeated dermal application in patients with extensive burn injuries. Gastritis, hepatitis, pancreatitis, and delayed neurologic sequelae also reported after ingestion. Metabolic acidosis may be delayed > 12 hours after ingestion. Estimated human lethal dose is 0.014–0.170 mg/kg. Calcium oxalate crystal formation documented in animals but not humans after fatal exposure. The metabolism of DEG is unclear; however, a case report documents a good outcome with fomepizole. Molecular weight is 106. | Ethanol and fomepizole may be effective. |
| Dioxane (dimer of ethylene glycol) | May cause coma, liver and kidney damage. The vapor (> 300 ppm) may cause mucous membrane irritation. Dermal exposure to the liquid may have a defatting action. Metabolites unknown. Molecular weight is 88. | Role of ethanol and fomepizole is unknown, but they may be effective. |
| Dipropylene glycol | Relatively low toxicity. Central nervous system depression, hepatic injury, and renal damage have occurred in animal studies after massive exposures. There are no reports of acidosis or lactate elevation. Molecular weight is 134. | Supportive care. There is no role for ethanol therapy. |
| Ethylene glycol mono butyl ether (EGBE, 2-butoxyethanol, butyl Cellosolve). | Clinical toxic effects include lethargy, coma, anion gap metabolic acidosis, hyperchloremia, hypotension, respiratory depression, hemolysis, renal and hepatic dysfunction; rare disseminated intravascular coagulation (DIC) and respiratory distress syndrome (ARDS). Oxalate crystal formation and osmolar gap elevation have been reported, but not in all cases. Serum levels in poisoning cases have ranged from 0.005–432 mg/L. Butoxyethanol is metabolized by alcohol dehydrogenase to butoxyaldehyde and butoxyacetic acid; however, the affinity of alcohol dehydrogenase for butoxyethanol is unknown. Molecular weight is 118. | Ethanol and fomepizole may be effective. |
| Ethylene glycol mono ethyl ether (EGEE, ethyl Cellosolve) | Calcium oxalate crystals have been reported in animals. Animal studies indicate that EGEE is metabolized in part to ethylene glycol; however, the affinity of alcohol dehydrogenase is higher for EGEE than for ethanol. Teratogenic effect has been reported in humans and animals. Molecular weight is 90. | Ethanol and fomepizole may be effective. |
| Ethylene glycol mono methyl ether (EGMe, methyl Cellosolve) | Delayed toxic effects (8 and 18 hours after ingestion) similar to those of ethylene glycol have been reported. Calcium oxalate crystals may or may not occur. Cerebral edema, hemorrhagic gastritis, and degeneration of the liver and kidneys were reported in one autopsy. Animal studies indicate that EGME is metabolized in part to ethylene glycol; however, the affinity of alcohol dehydrogenase is about the same for EGME as for ethanol. Oligospermia has been reported with chronic exposure in humans. Teratogenic effects have been reported in animals. Molecular weight is 76. | Ethanol and fomepizole may be effective. |

| | | |
|---|---|---|
| Polyethylene glycols | Very low toxicity. A group of compounds with molecular weights ranging from 200 to more than 4000. High-molecular-weight compounds (> 500) are poorly absorbed and rapidly excreted by the kidneys. Low-molecular-weight compounds (200–400) may result in metabolic acidosis, renal failure, hypercalcemia after massive oral ingestions or repeated dermal applications in patients with extensive burn injuries. Acute respiratory failure occurred after accidental nasogastric infusion into the lung of a pediatric patient. Alcohol dehydrogenase metabolizes polyethylene glycols. | Supportive care. |
| Propylene glycol (PG) | Relatively low toxicity. Lactic acidosis, central nervous system depression, coma, hypoglycemia, seizures, and hemolysis have been reported rarely after massive exposures or chronic exposures in high-risk patients. Risk factors include renal insufficiency, small infants, epilepsy, and burn patients with extensive dermal application of propylene glycol. Osmolar gap, anion gap, and lactate are commonly elevated. PG levels of 6–42 mg/dL did not result in toxicity after acute infusion. A PG level of 1059 mg/dL was reported in an 8-month-old with extensive burn injuries after repeated dermal application (the child experienced cardiopulmonary arrest). A level of 400 mg/dL was measured in an epileptic patient who experienced status epilepticus, respiratory depression, elevated osmolar gap, and metabolic acidosis. Metabolites are lactate and pyruvate. Molecular weight is 76. | Supportive care, sodium bicarbonate. There is no role for ethanol therapy. Hemodialysis is effective but rarely indicated. |
| Triethylene glycol | Coma, metabolic acidosis with elevated anion gap, osmolar gap of 7 mOsm/L reported 1–1.5 hours after ingestion. Treated with ethanol and recovered by 36 hours. | Ethanol and fomepizole may be effective. |

C. **Other glycols** (see Table II–24). Propylene and dipropylene glycols are of relatively low toxicity. Polypropylene glycol and other high-molecular-weight polyethylene glycols are poorly absorbed and virtually nontoxic. However, diethylene glycol and glycol ethers produce toxic metabolites with toxicity similar to that of ethylene glycol.

II. **Toxic dose.** The approximate lethal oral dose of 95% ethylene glycol (eg, antifreeze) is 1.0–1.5 mL/kg; however, survival has been reported after an ingestion of 2 L in a patient who received treatment within 1 hour of ingestion.

III. **Clinical presentation**

A. **Ethylene glycol**

1. **During the first few hours** after acute ingestion, the victim may appear intoxicated as if by ethanol. The osmolar gap (see p 32) is increased, but there is no initial acidosis. Gastritis with vomiting may also occur.
2. **After a delay of 4–12 hours,** evidence of intoxication by metabolic products occurs, with anion gap acidosis, hyperventilation, convulsions, coma, cardiac conduction disturbances, and arrhythmias. Renal failure is common but usually reversible. Pulmonary edema and cerebral edema may also occur. Hypocalcemia with tetany has been reported.

B. **Other glycols** (see Table II–24). Diethylene glycol and glycol ethers are extremely toxic and may produce acute renal failure and metabolic acidosis. Calcium oxalate crystals may or may not be present.

IV. **Diagnosis** of ethylene glycol poisoning usually is based on the history of antifreeze ingestion, typical symptoms, and elevation of the osmolar and anion gaps. Oxalate or hippurate crystals may be present in the urine (crystals may be cuboidal or elongate in form). Because many antifreeze products contain fluorescein, the urine may fluoresce under a Wood's lamp. However, false-positive and false-negative Wood's lamp results have been reported.

A. **Specific levels.** Tests for ethylene glycol levels are usually available from regional commercial toxicology laboratories but are difficult to obtain quickly.

1. Serum levels higher than 50 mg/dL usually are associated with serious intoxication, although lower levels do not rule out poisoning if the parent compound has already been metabolized (in such a case, the anion gap should be markedly elevated). Calculation of the osmolar gap (see p 32) may be used to estimate the ethylene glycol level.
2. False-positive ethylene glycol levels can be caused by elevated triglycerides (see Table I–33, p 43) or 2,3-butanediol in some assays.
3. Elevated concentrations of the toxic metabolite **glycolic acid** are a better measure of toxicity but are not widely available. Levels less than 10 mmol/L are not toxic.
4. In the absence of a serum ethylene glycol level, if the osmolar and anion gaps are both normal and the patient is asymptomatic, serious ingestion is not likely to have occurred.

B. **Other useful laboratory studies** include electrolytes, lactate, ethanol, glucose, BUN, creatinine, calcium, hepatic transaminases, urinalysis (for crystals and Wood's lamp examination), measured osmolality, arterial blood gases, and ECG monitoring. Serum **beta-hydroxybutyrate** levels may help distinguish ethylene glycol poisoning from **alcoholic ketoacidosis,** which also may cause increased anion and osmolar gaps. (Patients with alcoholic ketoacidosis may not have markedly positive tests for ketones, but the beta-hydroxybutyrate level will usually be elevated.)

V. **Treatment**

A. **Emergency and supportive measures**

1. Maintain an open airway and assist ventilation if necessary (see pp 1–7). Administer supplemental oxygen.

2. Treat coma (see p 18), convulsions (p 22), cardiac arrhythmias (pp 10–15), and metabolic acidosis (p 33) if they occur. Observe the patient for several hours to monitor for development of metabolic acidosis, especially if the patient is symptomatic or there is known co-ingestion of ethanol.
3. Treat hypocalcemia with intravenous calcium gluconate or calcium chloride (see p 428).

**B. Specific drugs and antidotes**

1. Administer **fomepizole** (see p 454) or **ethanol** (p 450) to saturate the enzyme alcohol dehydrogenase and prevent metabolism of ethylene glycol to its toxic metabolites. Indications for therapy include the following:
   a. Ethylene glycol level higher than 20 mg/dL.
   b. History of ethylene glycol ingestion accompanied by two or more of the following:
      (1) Osmolar gap greater than 10 mOsm/L not accounted for by ethanol or other alcohols.
      (2) Serum bicarbonate less than 20 mEq/L.
      (3) Arterial pH less than 7.3.
      (4) Presence of oxalate crystals in the urine.
2. Administer **pyridoxine** (see p 508), **folate** (p 453), and **thiamine** (p 513), cofactors required for the metabolism of ethylene glycol that may alleviate toxicity by enhancing metabolism of glyoxylic acid to nontoxic metabolites.

**C. Decontamination** (see p 45). Perform lavage (or simply aspirate gastric contents with a small flexible tube) if the ingestion was recent (within 30–60 minutes). Activated charcoal is not likely to be of benefit because the required effective dose is large and ethylene glycol is rapidly absorbed, but may be given if other drugs or toxins were ingested.

**D. Enhanced elimination.** The volume of distribution of ethylene glycol is 0.6–0.8 L/kg, making it accessible to enhanced elimination procedures. **Hemodialysis** efficiently removes ethylene glycol and its toxic metabolites and rapidly corrects acidosis and electrolyte and fluid abnormalities.

1. **Indications for hemodialysis** include:
   a. Suspected ethylene glycol poisoning with an osmolar gap greater than 10 mOsm/L not accounted for by ethanol or other alcohols accompanied by metabolic acidosis (pH < 7.25–7.30) unresponsive to therapy.
   b. Ethylene glycol intoxication accompanied by renal failure.
   c. Ethylene glycol serum concentration greater than 50 mg/dL unless the patient is asymptomatic and is receiving fomepizole or ethanol therapy.
   d. Severe metabolic acidosis in a patient with a history of ethylene glycol ingestion, even if the osmolar gap is not elevated (late presenter).
2. **Endpoint of treatment.** The minimum serum concentration of ethylene glycol associated with serious toxicity is not known. In addition, ethylene glycol levels are reported to rebound after dialysis ceases. Therefore, treatment with fomepizole or ethanol should be continued until the osmolar and anion gaps are normalized or (if available) serum ethylene glycol and glycolic acid levels are no longer detectable.

## ▶ ETHYLENE OXIDE

*Stephen C. Born, MD, MPH*

Ethylene oxide is a highly penetrating, chemically reactive flammable gas or liquid that is used widely as a sterilizer of medical equipment and supplies. It is also an important industrial chemical that is used as a chemical intermediate in the production of ethylene glycol, solvents, surfactants, and multiple other industrial chemicals. Ethylene oxide liquid has a boiling point of 10.7°C (760 mm Hg) and is readily miscible with water and organic solvents. Ethylene oxide in air poses a risk of fire/explosion at concentrations greater than 2.6%.

I. **Mechanism of toxicity.** Ethylene oxide is an alkylating agent and reacts directly with proteins and DNA to cause cell death. Direct contact with the gas causes irritation of the eyes, mucous membranes, and lungs. Ethylene oxide is mutagenic, teratogenic, and carcinogenic (regulated as a carcinogen by OSHA; IARC group 1 [carcinogenic to humans]). It may be absorbed through intact skin.

II. **Toxic dose.** Occupational exposure to ethylene oxide is regulated by the Occupational Safety and Health Administration. The OSHA standard and excellent supporting documentation can be found at www.osha.gov. The workplace permissible exposure limit (PEL) in air is 1 ppm (1.8 mg/m$^3$) as an 8-hour time-weighted average (TWA). The air level immediately dangerous to life or health (IDLH) is 800 ppm. Occupational exposure above OSHA-determined trigger levels (0.5 ppm as an 8-hour TWA) requires medical surveillance (29 CFR 1910.1047). The odor threshold is approximately 700 ppm, giving the gas poor warning properties. High levels of ethylene oxide can occur when sterilizers malfunction or during opening or replacing ethylene oxide tanks. Exposure may also occur when fumigated or sterilized materials are inadequately aerated. A minute amount of ethylene oxide is produced endogenously in humans from the metabolism of ethylene.

III. **Clinical presentation**

   A. Ethylene oxide is a potent mucous membrane irritant and can cause eye and oropharyngeal irritation, bronchospasm, and pulmonary edema. Cataract formation has been described after significant eye exposure. Exposure to ethylene oxide in solution can cause vesicant injury to the skin.

   B. Neurotoxicity, including convulsions and delayed peripheral neuropathy, may occur after exposure.

   C. Other systemic effects include cardiac arrhythmias when ethylene oxide is used in combination with freon (see p 208) as a carrier gas.

   D. Leukemia has been described in workers chronically exposed to ethylene oxide.

IV. **Diagnosis** is based on a history of exposure and typical upper-airway irritant effects. Detection of ethylene oxide odor indicates significant exposure. Industrial hygiene sampling is necessary to document air levels of exposure.

   A. **Specific levels.** Blood levels are not available. Ethylene oxide DNA adducts may indicate exposure but are not available for clinical use.

   B. **Other useful laboratory studies** include arterial blood gases or pulse oximetry and chest x-ray.

V. **Treatment**

   A. **Emergency and supportive measures.** Monitor closely for several hours after exposure.

      1. Maintain an open airway and assist ventilation if necessary (see pp 1–7). Treat bronchospasm (p 7) and pulmonary edema (p 7) if they occur.

      2. Treat coma (see p 18), convulsions (p 22), and arrhythmias (pp 10–15) if they occur.

   B. **Specific drugs and antidotes.** There is no specific antidote.

   C. **Decontamination** (see p 45)

      1. Remove the victim from the contaminated environment immediately and administer oxygen. Rescuers should wear self-contained breathing apparatus and chemical-protective clothing.

      2. Remove all contaminated clothing and wash exposed skin. For eye exposures, irrigate copiously with tepid water or saline.

   D. **Enhanced elimination.** There is no role for these procedures.

# ▶ FLUORIDE

*Kathryn H. Meier, PharmD*

Fluoride-liberating chemicals are used in some automobile wheel cleaners, glass etching solutions, insecticides, rodenticides, aluminum production, vitamins and dietary supplements, and products used to prevent dental caries. Most toothpaste contains up to 5 mg fluoride per teaspoon. Fluoride is commonly added to community drinking water. It is also found in hydrofluoric acid (see p 222), which is used for etching glass and silicon chip products. Soluble fluoride salts are rapidly absorbed and are more acutely toxic (Table II–25).

**I. Mechanism of toxicity**

**A.** In addition to its direct cytotoxic and metabolic effects, fluoride binds avidly to calcium and magnesium, causing hypocalcemia and hypomagnesemia. Fluoride disrupts many intracellular mechanisms, including glycolysis, G-protein–mediated signaling, oxidative phosphorylation, adenosine triphosphate (ATP) production, function of Na/K-ATPase, and potassium channels.

**B. Pharmacokinetics.** Fluoride is a weak acid (pKa 3.4) that is passively absorbed from the stomach and small intestine. In an acidic environment more fluoride is present as hydrogen fluoride (HF), which is absorbed more rapidly. Fasting peak absorption occurs in 30–60 minutes. The volume of distribution is 0.5–0.7 L/kg. Fluoride is not protein bound but binds readily to magnesium and calcium in blood, tissues, and bone (most fluoride in the body is bound to bone). The elimination half-life is 2.4–4.3 hours and is prolonged in patients with renal failure.

**II. Toxic dose.** Vomiting and abdominal pain are common with ingestions of 3–5 mg/kg elemental fluoride (see Table II–25); hypocalcemia and muscular symptoms appear with ingestions of 5–10 mg/kg. Death has been reported in a 3-year-old child after ingestion of 16 mg/kg and in adults with doses in excess of 32 mg/kg.

**III. Clinical presentation**

**A. Acute poisoning.** Nausea and vomiting frequently occur within 1 hour of ingestion. Symptoms of serious fluoride intoxication include skeletal muscle weakness, tetanic contractions, respiratory muscle weakness, and respiratory arrest. Serious overdoses are associated with hypocalcemia, hypomagnesemia, and hyperkalemia and with increased QT interval. Death is due to intractable cardiac dysrhythmias and usually occurs within 12 hours.

**B. Chronic effects.** Minor overexposure in children under age 10 can cause tooth mottling. High chronic overexposure (more than 20 mg/day for more than 10 years) can cause skeletal fluorosis (osteosclerosis), ligament calcification, and increased bone density.

**IV. Diagnosis** usually is based on a history of ingestion. Symptoms of GI distress, muscle weakness, hypocalcemia, and hyperkalemia suggest fluoride intoxication.

**TABLE II–25. FLUORIDE-CONTAINING COMPOUNDS**

| Compound | Elemental Fluoride (%) |
|---|---|
| **Soluble salts** | |
| Ammonium bifluoride | 67 |
| Hydrogen fluoride | 95 |
| Sodium fluoride | 45 |
| Sodium fluosilicate | 61 |
| **Less soluble salts** | |
| Cryolite | 54 |
| Sodium monofluorophosphate | 13 |
| Stannous fluoride | 24 |

A. **Specific levels.** The normal serum fluoride concentration is less than 20 mcg/L (ng/mL) but varies considerably with diet and water source. Serum fluoride concentrations are generally difficult to obtain and thus are of limited utility for acute overdose management.

B. **Other useful laboratory studies** include electrolytes, glucose, BUN, creatinine, calcium (and ionized calcium), magnesium, and ECG.

V. **Treatment**

A. **Emergency and supportive measures**

1. Maintain an open airway and assist ventilation if necessary (see pp 1–7).
2. Monitor ECG and serum calcium, magnesium, and potassium for at least 4–6 hours. Admit symptomatic patients with ECG or electrolyte abnormalities to an intensive care setting.

B. **Specific drugs and antidotes.** For hypocalcemia, administer **intravenous calcium gluconate** (see p 428), 10–20 mL (children: 0.2–0.3 mL/kg), monitor ionized calcium levels, and titrate further doses as needed. To date, early IV calcium administration is the only treatment that has increased survival in an animal model. Treat hypomagnesemia with intravenous **magnesium sulfate,** 1–2 g given over 10–15 min (children: 25–50 mg/kg diluted to less than 10 mg/mL). Treat hyperkalemia with intravenous calcium and other usual measures (p 37).

C. **Decontamination** (see p 45)

1. **Prehospital.** Do ***not*** induce vomiting because of the risk of abrupt onset of seizures and arrhythmias. Administer an antacid containing **calcium** (eg, calcium carbonate [Tums, Rolaids]) orally to raise gastric pH and complex free fluoride, reducing absorption. Foods rich in calcium (eg, milk) can also bind fluoride. Magnesium-containing antacids have also been recommended, but there are few data for their effectiveness.
2. **Hospital.** Administer antacids containing **calcium** as described above. Consider gastric lavage for large recent ingestions. Activated charcoal does not adsorb fluoride.

D. **Enhanced elimination.** Because fluoride rapidly binds to free calcium and bone and has a short elimination half-life, hemodialysis is not likely to be effective.

## ▶ FLUOROACETATE

*Steve Offerman, MD*

Fluoroacetate, also known as compound 1080, sodium monofluoroacetate (SMFA), and sodium fluoroacetate, is one of the most toxic substances known. In the past, it was used primarily as a rodenticide by licensed pest control companies, but it largely has been removed from the US market because of its hazardous nature. Compound 1080 use is currently restricted to livestock protection collars designed to protect sheep and cattle from coyotes. Occasionally unlicensed product may be encountered. It is also still used commonly in Australia and New Zealand for vertebrate pest control. It is a tasteless, odorless water-soluble white crystalline powder. Fluoroacetamide (compound 1081) is a similar compound with similar toxicity.

I. **Mechanism of toxicity**

A. Fluoroacetate is metabolized to the toxic compound fluorocitrate, which blocks cellular metabolism by inhibiting the aconitase enzyme within the Krebs cycle. Clinical effects of poisoning are delayed (from 30 minutes to several hours) until fluoroacetate is metabolized to fluorocitrate.

B. **Pharmacokinetics.** The onset of effect is reported to be 30 minutes to several hours after ingestion. The time to peak effect, volume of distribution, duration of action, and elimination half-life in humans are unknown, but there are reports of late-onset coma (36 hours). In rats, only 1% of an oral dose is excreted in the urine and feces within 5 hours, and only 12% by 48 hours.

**II. Toxic dose.** Inhalation or ingestion of as little as 1 mg of fluoroacetate is sufficient to cause serious toxicity. Death is likely after ingestion of more than 5 mg/kg.

**III. Clinical presentation.** After a delay of minutes to several hours (in one report coma was delayed 36 hours), manifestations of diffuse cellular poisoning become apparent; nausea, vomiting, diarrhea, metabolic acidosis (lactic acidosis), shock, renal failure, agitation, confusion, seizures, coma, respiratory arrest, pulmonary edema, and ventricular dysrhythmias may occur. One case series reported a high incidence of hypocalcemia and hypokalemia. Death is usually the result of respiratory failure or ventricular dysrhythmia.

**IV. Diagnosis** is based on a history of ingestion and clinical findings, which may be delayed for several hours. Poisoning with fluoroacetate may mimic poisoning with other cellular toxins such as hydrogen cyanide and hydrogen sulfide, although with these poisons the onset of symptoms is usually more rapid.

- **A. Specific levels.** There is no assay available.
- **B. Other useful laboratory studies** include electrolytes, glucose, BUN, creatinine, calcium, arterial blood gases, ECG, and chest x-ray. Perform continuous ECG monitoring.

**V. Treatment**

- **A. Emergency and supportive measures**
  1. Maintain an open airway and assist ventilation if necessary (see pp 1–7). Administer supplemental oxygen.
  2. Replace fluid losses from gastroenteritis with intravenous saline or other crystalloids.
  3. Treat shock (see p 33), seizures (p 22), and coma (p 18) if they occur. Because of the reported potential delay in the onset of serious symptoms, it is prudent to monitor the patient for at least 36–48 hours.
- **B. Specific drugs and antidotes.** There is no available antidote. Monoacetin (glyceryl monoacetate), which decreases conversion of fluoroacetate to fluorocitrate, has been used experimentally in monkeys but is not available or recommended for human use.
- **C. Decontamination** (see p 45)
  1. **Prehospital.** If it is available and the patient is alert, immediately administer activated charcoal. If a delay of more than 60 minutes is expected before charcoal can be given, consider using ipecac to induce vomiting if it can be administered within a few minutes of exposure and there are no contraindications (see p 51).
  2. **Hospital.** Immediately administer activated charcoal. Consider gastric lavage if it can be performed within 60 minutes of ingestion.
  3. **Skin exposure.** Fluoroacetate is poorly absorbed through intact skin, but a significant exposure could occur through broken skin. Remove contaminated clothing and wash exposed skin thoroughly.
- **D. Enhanced elimination.** There is no role for any enhanced removal procedure.

## ► FOOD POISONING: BACTERIAL

*Susan Kim, PharmD*

Food-borne bacteria and bacterial toxins are a common cause of epidemic gastroenteritis. In general, the illness is relatively mild and self-limited, with recovery within 24 hours. However, severe and even fatal poisoning may occur with listeriosis, salmonellosis, or **botulism** (see p 136) and with certain strains of *Escherichia coli.* Poisoning after the consumption of **fish and shellfish** is discussed on p 204. **Mushroom** poisoning is discussed on p 272. **Viruses** such as the Norwalk virus and Norwalk-like caliciviruses, enteroviruses, and rotaviruses are the causative agent in as many as 80% of food-related illness. Other microbes that can cause food-borne illness include *Cryptosporidium* and *Cyclospora,* which can cause serious illness in immunocompromised patients. However, in over half of reported food-borne outbreaks, no microbiologic pathogens are identified.

I. **Mechanism of toxicity.** Gastroenteritis may be caused by invasive bacterial infection of the intestinal mucosa or by a toxin elaborated by bacteria. Bacterial toxins may be preformed in food that is improperly prepared and improperly stored before use or may be produced in the gut by the bacteria after they are ingested (Table II–26).

II. **Toxic dose.** The toxic dose depends on the type of bacteria or toxin and its concentration in the ingested food, as well as individual susceptibility or resistance. Some of the preformed toxins (eg, staphylococcal toxin) are heat resistant and once in the food are not removed by cooking or boiling.

III. **Clinical presentation.** Commonly, a delay or "incubation period" of 2 hours to 3 days precedes the onset of symptoms (see Table II–26).

   A. **Gastroenteritis** is the most common finding, with nausea, vomiting, abdominal cramps, and diarrhea. Vomiting is more common with preformed toxins. Significant fluid and electrolyte abnormalities may occur, especially in young children or elderly patients.

   B. **Fever, bloody stools,** and **fecal leukocytosis** are common with invasive bacterial infections.

   C. **Systemic infection** can result from *E coli, Salmonella, Shigella, Campylobacter,* or *Listeria.*

      1. **Listeriosis** can cause sepsis and meningitis, particularly in elderly and immunocompromised persons. Infection during pregnancy produces a mild flu-like illness in the mother but serious intrauterine infection resulting in fetal death, neonatal sepsis, or meningitis.

      2. ***Shigella*** and ***E coli*** **0157:H7** strain may cause acute hemorrhagic colitis complicated by hemolytic-uremic syndrome, renal failure, and death, especially in children and immunocompromised adults.

      3. ***Campylobacter*** infections sometimes are followed by Guillain-Barré syndrome or reactive arthritis.

IV. **Diagnosis.** Bacterial food poisoning is often difficult to distinguish from common viral gastroenteritis unless the incubation period is short and there are multiple victims who ate similar foods at one large gathering. The presence of many white blood cells in a stool smear suggests invasive bacterial infection. With any epidemic gastroenteritis, consider other food-borne illnesses, such as those caused by viruses or parasites, illnesses associated with seafood (see p 204), botulism (p 136), and ingestions of certain mushrooms (p 272).

   A. **Specific levels**

      1. **Stool culture** may differentiate *Salmonella, Shigella,* and *Campylobacter* infections. However, culture for *E coli* 0157:H7 must be specifically requested. An enzyme-linked immunosorbent assay (ELISA) test can detect Norwalk virus in stools.

      2. **Blood** and **CSF** may grow invasive organisms, especially *Listeria* (and rarely *Salmonella* or *Shigella*).

      3. **Food samples** should be saved for bacterial culture and toxin analysis, primarily for use by public health investigators.

      4. Antigen testing for *Giardia* can rule out this infection as a cause of diarrhea.

   B. **Other useful laboratory studies** include CBC, electrolytes, glucose, BUN, and creatinine.

V. **Treatment**

   A. **Emergency and supportive measures**

      1. Replace fluid and electrolyte losses with intravenous saline or other crystalloid solutions (patients with mild illness may tolerate oral rehydration).

**TABLE II–26. BACTERIAL FOOD POISONING**

| Organism | Incubation Period | Common Symptoms[a] and Mechanism | Common Foods |
|---|---|---|---|
| *Bacillus cereus* | 1–6 h (emesis) 8–16 h (diarrhea) | V > D. Toxins produced in food and gut. | Reheated fried rice, improperly refrigerated meats. |
| *Campylobacter jejuni* | 1–8 d | D+, F. Invasive and possibly toxin produced in gut. | Poultry; water; milk; direct contact (eg, food handlers). |
| *Clostridium perfringens* | 6–16 h | D > V. Toxin produced in food and gut. | Meats, gravy. |
| *Escherichia coli* "enterotoxigenic" | 12–72 h | D > V. Toxin produced in gut. | "Traveler's diarrhea." Water, various foods; direct contact (eg, food handlers). |
| *Escherichia coli* "enteroinvasive" | 24–72 h | D+. Invasive infection. | Water, various foods; direct contact (eg, food handlers). |
| *Escherichia coli* "enterohemorrhagic" 0157:H7 | 1–8 d | D+, S. Toxin produced in gut. | Water; ground beef, salami and other meats; unpasteurized milk and juice; contaminated lettuce, sprouts; direct contact (eg, food handlers). |
| *Listeria monocytogenes* | 9–32 h | D+, S. Invasive infection. | Milk, soft cheeses. |
| *Salmonella* spp. | 12–36 h | D+. Invasive infection. | Meat; dairy; eggs; water; sprouts; direct contact (eg, food handlers). |
| *Shigella* spp. | 1–7 d | D+. Invasive infection. | Water; fruits, vegetables; direct contact (eg, food handlers). |
| *Staphylococcus aureus* | 1–6 h | V > D. Toxin preformed in food; heat-resistant. | Very common: meats; dairy; bakery foods; direct contact (eg, food handlers). |
| *Vibrio parahemolyticus* | 8–30 h | V, D+. Invasive and toxin produced in gut. | Shellfish; water. |
| *Yersinia enterocolytica* | 3–7 d | D+. Invasive infection. | Water; meats; dairy. |

[a]V = vomiting; D = diarrhea; D+ = diarrhea with blood and/or fecal leukocytes; F = fever; S = systemic manifestations.

Patients with hypotension may require large-volume intravenous fluid resuscitation (see p 15).

2. Antiemetic agents are acceptable for symptomatic treatment, but strong antidiarrheal agents such as Lomotil (diphenoxylate plus atropine) should not be used in patients with suspected invasive bacterial infection (fever and bloody stools).

**B. Specific drugs and antidotes.** There are no specific antidotes.

1. In patients with invasive bacterial infection, antibiotics may be used once the stool culture reveals the specific bacteria responsible, although antibi-

otics do not always shorten the course of illness, and with *E coli* 0157:H7 they may increase the risk of hemolytic-uremic syndrome. Empiric treatment with trimethoprim-sulfamethoxazole or quinolones is often initiated while awaiting culture results.

2. Pregnant women who have eaten *Listeria*-contaminated foods should be treated empirically, even if only mildly symptomatic, to prevent serious intrauterine infection. The antibiotic of choice is intravenous ampicillin, with gentamicin added for severe infection.

C. **Decontamination** (see p 45) procedures are not indicated in most cases. However, consider using activated charcoal if immediately available after ingestion of a highly toxic seafood (eg, fugu fish).

D. **Enhanced elimination.** There is no role for enhanced removal procedures.

http://www.cdc.gov/mmwr/preview/mmwrhtml/rr5002a1.htm (Centers for Disease Control website on food-related illnesses) http://vm.cfsan.fda.gov/~mow/intro.html
(*The Bad Bug Book,* from the FDA, CDC, UDSA, and NIH)

## ▶ FOOD POISONING: FISH AND SHELLFISH

*Susan Kim, PharmD*

A variety of toxins may produce illness after ingestion of fish or shellfish. The most common types of seafood-related toxins include **ciguatera, scombroid, neurotoxic shellfish poisoning, paralytic shellfish poisoning,** and **tetrodotoxin.** Shellfish-induced bacterial diarrhea is described on p 205.

I. **Mechanism of toxicity.** The mechanism varies with each toxin. The toxins are all heat-stable; therefore, cooking the seafood does not prevent illness.

A. **Ciguatera.** The toxin is produced by dinoflagellates, which are then consumed by reef fish. The mechanism of intoxication is uncertain but may involve increased sodium permeability in sodium channels and stimulation of central or ganglionic cholinergic receptors.

B. **Diarrhetic shellfish** poisoning is caused by several identified toxins, all of which appear to be produced by marine dinoflagellates. Suspected toxins include okadaic acid, dinophysistoxins, and azaspiracid.

C. **Domoic acid** is produced by phytoplankton, which are concentrated by filter-feeding fish and shellfish. The toxin is thought to bind to glutamate receptors, causing neuroexcitatory responses.

D. **Neurotoxic shellfish** poisoning is caused by ingestion of brevetoxins, which are produced by "red tide" dinoflagellates. The mechanism appears to involve stimulation of sodium channels, resulting in depolarization of nerve fibers.

E. **Palytoxin** is produced by dinoflagellates. It alters Na and K flux across cell membranes, causing depolarization and contraction of smooth, skeletal, and cardiac muscles. It is also a potent vasoconstrictor.

F. **Paralytic shellfish.** Dinoflagellates ("red tide") produce saxitoxin and related toxins, which are concentrated by filter-feeding clams and mussels. Saxitoxin blocks sodium conductance and neuronal transmission in skeletal muscles.

G. **Scombroid.** Scombrotoxin is a mixture of histamine and histamine-like compounds produced when histidine in fish tissue decomposes.

H. **Tetrodotoxin,** found in puffer fish, California newts, and some South American frogs, blocks the voltage-dependent sodium channel in nerve cell membranes.

II. **Toxic dose.** The concentration of toxin varies widely, depending on geographic and seasonal factors. The amount of toxin necessary to produce symptoms is unknown. Saxitoxin is extremely potent; the estimated lethal dose in humans is 0.3–1 mg, and contaminated mussels may contain 15–20 mg.

III. **Clinical presentation.** The onset of symptoms and clinical manifestations vary with each toxin (Table II–27). In the majority of cases, the seafood appears nor-

**TABLE II–27. FISH AND SHELLFISH INTOXICATIONS**

| Type | Onset | Common Sources | Syndrome |
|---|---|---|---|
| Ciguatera (ciguatoxin) | 1–6 h; milder cases may be delayed | Barracuda, red snapper, grouper | Gastroenteritis, hot and cold reversal (cold allodynia), paresthesias, myalgias, weakness. |
| Diarrhetic shellfish poisoning (various toxins) | 30 min to 2 h | Bivalve mollusks | Nausea, vomiting, diarrhea. |
| Domoic acid (amnestic shellfish poisoning) | Minutes to hours | Mussels, clams, anchovies | Gastroenteritis, headache, myoclonus, seizures, coma. Persistent neuropathy and memory impairment. |
| Neurotoxic shellfish poisoning (brevetoxin) | Minutes to 3 h | Bivalve shellfish, whelks (conchs) | Gastroenteritis, ataxia, paresthesias, seizures. |
| Palytoxin (clupeotoxin) | Hours | Parrotfish, crabs, mackerel, sardines | Gastroenteritis; paresthesias; severe muscle spasms, rhabdomyolysis; seizures; respiratory distress; myocardial damage. |
| Paralytic shellfish poisoning (saxitoxin) | Within 30 min | Bivalve shellfish, "red tide" | Gastroenteritis, paresthesias, ataxia, respiratory paralysis. |
| Scombroid (scombrotoxin) | Minutes to hours | Tuna, mahimahi, bonito, mackerel | Gastroenteritis, flushed skin, hypotension, urticaria, wheezing. |
| Tetrodotoxin | Within 30–40 min | Puffer fish ("fugu"), sun fish, porcupine fish, California newt | Vomiting, paresthesias, muscle twitching, diaphoresis, weakness, respiratory paralysis. |

mal with no adverse smell or taste (scombroid may have a peppery taste; palytoxin may be bitter).

**A. Ciguatera.** Intoxication produces vomiting and watery diarrhea 1–6 hours after ingestion, followed by headache, malaise, myalgias, paresthesias of the mouth and extremities, ataxia, blurred vision, photophobia, cold allodynia ("hot/cold reversal"), extreme pruritus, hypotension, bradycardia, and, rarely, seizures and respiratory arrest.

**B. Diarrhetic shellfish** poisoning causes nausea, vomiting, stomach cramps, and severe diarrhea. In animal studies, azaspiracid toxin caused damage to the liver, spleen, and small intestine.

**C. Domoic acid.** Symptoms begin from 15 minutes to 38 hours after ingestion and consist of gastroenteritis accompanied by unusual neurologic toxicity, including fasciculations, mutism, severe headache, hemiparesis, and myoclonus. Coma, seizures, hypotension, and profuse bronchial secretions have been reported with severe intoxication. Long-term sequelae include persistent severe anterograde memory loss, motor neuropathy, and axonopathy.

**D. Neurotoxic shellfish.** Onset is within a few minutes to 3 hours. Gastroenteritis is accompanied by paresthesias of the mouth, face, and extremities; muscular weakness; seizures; and respiratory arrest. Inhalation of aerosolized brevetoxins may worsen respiratory symptoms in asthmatics.

E. Clinical presentation of **palytoxin** poisoning may initially mimic ciguatera. However, palytoxin produces greater morbidity and mortality as a result of severe muscle spasms, rhabdomyolysis, hypertension, and acute respiratory failure. Clupeotoxism, a highly toxic marine poisoning associated with ingestion of sardines and herring, may be caused by palytoxin.

F. **Paralytic shellfish.** Vomiting, diarrhea, and facial paresthesias usually begin within 30 minutes of ingestion. Headache, myalgias, dysphagia, weakness, and ataxia have been reported. In serious cases respiratory arrest may occur after 1–12 hours.

G. **Scombroid.** Symptoms begin rapidly (minutes to 3 hours) after ingestion. Gastroenteritis, headache, and skin flushing sometimes are accompanied by urticaria, bronchospasm, tachycardia, and hypotension.

H. **Tetrodotoxin.** Symptoms occur within 30–40 minutes after ingestion and include vomiting, paresthesias, salivation, twitching, diaphoresis, weakness, and dysphagia. Hypotension, bradycardia, flaccid paralysis, and respiratory arrest may occur up to 6–24 hours after ingestion.

IV. **Diagnosis** depends on a history of ingestion and is more likely to be recognized when multiple victims present after consumption of a seafood meal. Scombroid may be confused with an allergic reaction because of the histamine-induced urticaria.

A. **Specific levels** are not generally available. However, when epidemic poisoning is suspected, state public health departments or the Centers for Disease Control may be able to analyze suspect food for toxins.

B. **Other useful laboratory studies** include electrolytes, glucose, BUN, creatinine, arterial blood gases, ECG monitoring, and stool for bacterial culture.

V. **Treatment**

A. **Emergency and supportive measures.** Most cases are mild and self-limited and require no specific treatment. However, because of the risk of respiratory arrest, all patients should be observed for several hours (except patients with diarrhetic shellfish poisoning).

1. Maintain an open airway and assist ventilation if necessary (see pp 1–7).
2. Replace fluid and electrolyte losses from gastroenteritis with intravenous crystalloid fluids.

B. **Specific drugs and antidotes**

1. **Scombroid** intoxication can be treated symptomatically with antihistamines, including diphenhydramine (see p 442) and cimetidine, 300 mg IV. Rarely, bronchodilators may also be required.
2. **Ciguatera.** There are anecdotal reports of successful treatment with intravenous mannitol, 0.5–1 g/kg infused IV over 30 minutes (see p 471). However, a recent randomized study showed no difference in outcome between mannitol and saline therapy. Gabapentin (400 mg TID) has also been reported to relieve symptoms.

C. **Decontamination** (see p 45) procedures are not indicated in most cases. However, consider using activated charcoal if immediately available after ingestion of a highly toxic seafood (eg, fugu fish).

D. **Enhanced elimination.** There is no role for these procedures.

## ► FORMALDEHYDE

*John Balmes, MD*

Formaldehyde is a gas with a pungent odor that is used commonly in the processing of paper, fabrics, and wood products and for the production of urea foam insulation. Low-level formaldehyde exposure has been found in stores selling clothing treated with formaldehyde-containing crease-resistant resins, in mobile homes, and in tightly enclosed rooms built with large quantities of formaldehyde-containing products used in construction materials. Formaldehyde aqueous solution (formalin) is used in varying concentrations (usually 37%) as a disinfectant and tissue fixative. Stabilized formalin may also contain 6–15% methanol.

**I. Mechanism of toxicity**

**A.** Formaldehyde causes precipitation of proteins and will cause coagulation necrosis of exposed tissue. The gas is highly water soluble. When inhaled, it produces immediate local irritation of the upper respiratory tract and has been reported to cause spasm and edema of the larynx.

**B.** Metabolism of formaldehyde produces formic acid, which may accumulate and produce metabolic acidosis if sufficient formaldehyde was ingested.

**C.** Formaldehyde is a known animal and a suspected human carcinogen.

**II. Toxic dose**

**A. Inhalation.** The recommended workplace ceiling limit (NIOSH) is 0.016 ppm (8-hour TWA; 0.1 for 15-minute exposure). The air level considered immediately dangerous to life or health (IDLH) is 20 ppm.

**B. Ingestion** of as little as 30 mL of 37% formaldehyde solution has been reported to have caused death in an adult.

**III. Clinical presentation**

**A. Formaldehyde gas** exposure produces irritation of the eyes, and inhalation can produce cough, wheezing, and noncardiogenic pulmonary edema.

**B. Ingestion** of formaldehyde solutions may cause severe corrosive esophageal and gastric injury, depending on the concentration. Lethargy and coma have been reported. Metabolic (anion gap) acidosis may be caused by formic acid accumulation from metabolism of formaldehyde or methanol.

**C.** Hemolysis has occurred when formalin was accidentally introduced into the blood through contaminated hemodialysis equipment.

**IV. Diagnosis** is based on a history of exposure and evidence of mucous membrane, respiratory, or GI tract irritation.

**A. Specific levels**

1. Plasma formaldehyde levels are not useful, but formate levels may indicate the severity of intoxication.
2. Methanol (see p 260) and formate levels may be helpful in cases of intoxication by formalin solutions containing methanol.

**B. Other useful laboratory studies** include electrolytes, glucose, BUN, creatinine, and osmolar gap (see p 32).

**V. Treatment**

**A. Emergency and supportive measures**

1. Maintain an open airway and assist ventilation if necessary (see pp 1–7).
2. **Inhalation.** Treat bronchospasm (see p 7) and pulmonary edema (p 7) if they occur. Administer supplemental oxygen and observe for at least 4–6 hours.
3. **Ingestion**
   - **a.** Treat coma (see p 18) and shock (p 15) if they occur.
   - **b.** Administer intravenous saline or other crystalloids to replace fluid losses caused by gastroenteritis. Avoid fluid overload in patients with inhalation exposure because of the risk of pulmonary edema.
   - **c.** Treat metabolic acidosis with sodium bicarbonate (see p 33).

**B. Specific drugs and antidotes**

1. If a **methanol**-containing solution has been ingested, evaluate and treat with **ethanol** and **folic acid** as for methanol poisoning (see p 260).
2. **Formate** intoxication caused by formaldehyde alone should be treated with **folic acid** (see p 453), but ethanol infusion is not effective.

**C. Decontamination** (see p 45). Rescuers should wear self-contained breathing apparatus and appropriate chemical-protective clothing when handling a heavily contaminated patient.

1. **Inhalation.** Remove victims from exposure and give supplemental oxygen if available.

2. **Skin and eyes.** Remove contaminated clothing and wash exposed skin with soap and water. Irrigate exposed eyes with copious tepid water or saline; perform fluorescein examination to rule out corneal injury if pain and lacrimation persist.
3. **Ingestion.** Give plain water to dilute concentrated solutions of formaldehyde. Perform aspiration of liquid formaldehyde from the stomach if large quantities were swallowed. Depending on the concentration of solution and patient symptoms, consider endoscopy to rule out esophageal or gastric injury. Activated charcoal is of uncertain benefit and may obscure the endoscopist's view.

D. **Enhanced elimination**
1. **Hemodialysis** is effective in removing methanol and formate and in correcting severe metabolic acidosis. Indications for hemodialysis include severe acidosis and an osmolar gap (see p 32) greater than 10 mOsm/L.
2. **Alkalinization** of the urine helps promote excretion of formate.

## ▶ FREONS AND HALONS

*Josef G. Thundiyil, MD, MPH*

**Freons** (fluorocarbons and chlorofluorocarbons [CFCs]) historically have been widely used as aerosol propellants, in refrigeration units, in the manufacture of plastics, in foam blowing, and as degreasing agents. Under provisions of the Montreal Protocol of 1987, the use of CFCs is being phased out to avoid further depletion of stratospheric ozone. Nevertheless, freons remain in older refrigeration and air-conditioning systems, and illicit importation of freons is common. Most freons are gases at room temperature, but some are liquids (freons 11, 21, 113, and 114) and may be ingested. Specialized fire extinguishers contain closely related compounds known as **halons,** which contain bromine, fluorine, and chlorine.

I. **Mechanism of toxicity**

A. Freons are mild CNS depressants and asphyxiants that displace oxygen from the ambient environment. Freons are well absorbed by inhalation or ingestion and are usually rapidly excreted in the breath within 15–60 minutes.

B. As with chlorinated hydrocarbons, freons may potentiate cardiac arrhythmias by sensitizing the myocardium to the effects of catecholamines.

C. Direct freezing of the skin, with frostbite, may occur if the skin is exposed to rapidly expanding gas as it escapes from a pressurized tank.

D. Freons and halons are mild irritants and may produce more potent irritant gases and vapors (eg, phosgene, hydrochloric acid, hydrofluoric acid, and carbonyl fluoride) when heated to high temperatures, as may happen in a fire or if a refrigeration line is cut by a welding torch or electric arc.

E. Some agents are hepatotoxic after large acute or chronic exposure.

II. **Toxic dose**

A. **Inhalation.** The toxic air level is quite variable, depending on the specific agent (see Table IV–4, p 542). Freon 21 (dichlorofluoromethane; TLV 10 ppm [42 mg/m$^3$]) is much more toxic than freon 12 (TLV 2000 ppm). In general, anesthetic or CNS-depressant doses require fairly large air concentrations, which can also displace oxygen, leading to asphyxia. The air level of dichloromonofluoromethane considered immediately dangerous to life or health (IDLH) is 5000 ppm. Other TLV and IDLH values can be found in Table IV–4 (p 542).

B. **Ingestion.** The toxic dose by ingestion is not known.

III. **Clinical presentation**

A. **Skin or mucous membrane** exposure can cause pharyngeal, ocular, and nasal irritation. Dysesthesia of the tongue is commonly reported. Frostbite may occur after contact with rapidly expanding compressed gas. Chronic exposure may result in skin defatting and cracking and erythema.

B. **Respiratory** effects can include cough, dyspnea, bronchospasm, hypoxemia, and pneumonitis.

C. **Systemic effects** of moderate exposure include dizziness, headache, nausea and vomiting, confusion, impaired speech, tinnitus, ataxia, and incoordination. More severe intoxication may result in coma or respiratory arrest. Ventricular arrhythmias may occur even with moderate exposures. A number of deaths, presumably caused by ventricular fibrillation, have been reported after freon abuse by "sniffing" or "huffing" freon products from plastic bags. Hepatic injury may occur.

IV. **Diagnosis** is based on a history of exposure and clinical presentation. Many chlorinated and aromatic hydrocarbon solvents may cause identical symptoms.

A. **Specific levels.** Expired-breath monitoring is possible, and blood levels may be obtained to document exposure, but these procedures are not useful in emergency clinical management.

B. **Other useful laboratory studies** include arterial blood gases or oximetry, ECG monitoring, and liver enzymes.

V. **Treatment**

A. **Emergency and supportive measures**

1. Remove the individual from the contaminated environment.
2. Maintain an open airway and assist ventilation if necessary (see pp 1–7).
3. Treat coma (see p 18) and arrhythmias (pp 10–15) if they occur. Avoid epinephrine or other sympathomimetic amines that may precipitate ventricular arrhythmias. Tachyarrhythmias caused by increased myocardial sensitivity may be treated with **propranolol** (see p 504), 1–2 mg IV, or **esmolol** (see p 449), 0.025–0.1 mg/kg/min IV.
4. Monitor the ECG for 4–6 hours.

B. **Specific drugs and antidotes.** There is no specific antidote.

C. **Decontamination** (see p 45)

1. **Inhalation.** Remove victim from exposure and give supplemental oxygen if available.
2. **Ingestion.** Do ***not*** give charcoal or induce vomiting, because freons are rapidly absorbed and there is a risk of abrupt onset of CNS depression. Consider gastric lavage (or simply aspirate liquid from stomach) if the ingestion was very large and recent (less than 30–45 minutes). The efficacy of activated charcoal is unknown.

D. **Enhanced elimination.** There is no documented efficacy for diuresis, hemodialysis, hemoperfusion, or repeat-dose charcoal.

## ▶ GAMMA-HYDROXYBUTYRATE (GHB)

*Jo Ellen Dyer, PharmD*

**Gamma-hydroxybutyrate (GHB)** originally was investigated as an anesthetic agent during the 1960s but was abandoned because of side effects including myoclonus and emergence delirium. In 2002 it was approved by the FDA as a treatment for cataplexy symptoms in patients with narcolepsy. For abuse purposes GHB is readily available through the illicit drug market and can be made in home labs using recipes posted on the Internet. As a result of increasing abuse, GHB without a legitimate prescription is regulated as a Schedule I substance. Chemical precursors that are converted to GHB in the body, including **gamma-butyrolactone (GBL)** and **1,4-butanediol (1,4-BD),** are also regulated as Schedule I analogs (when intended for human consumption). These chemicals often are sold under constantly changing product names with intentionally obscure chemical synonyms (Table II–28), and to avoid the legal consequences of an analog intended for human consumption, they may be sold as a cleaner, paint stripper, nail polish remover, or solvent, labeled "not for ingestion."

**TABLE II–28. GHB AND RELATED CHEMICALS**

| Chemical | Chemical or Legitimate Names | Slang or Illicit Names |
|---|---|---|
| **Gamma-hydroxybutyric acid**<br>CASRN 591-81-1<br>$C_4H_8O_3$<br>MW 104.11 | Gamma-hydroxybutyric acid; 4-hydroxybutanoic acid; gamma-hydroxybutyrate, sodium; 4-hydroxybutyrate, sodium | Cherry Meth; Easy Lay; Fantasy; G caps; Gamma Hydrate; Georgia Home Boy; GHB; Grievous Bodily Harm; G-riffick; Liquid E; Liquid Ecstasy; Natural Sleep-500; Oxy-sleep; Scoop; Soap; Somatomax PM; Vita G |
| **Gamma-hydroxybutyrate, sodium salt**<br>CASRN 502-85-2<br>$C_4H_7NaO_3$<br>MW 126.09 | *Prescription drug formulations:* sodium oxybate (generic name); Gamma OH (France); Somsanit (Germany); Alcover (Italy); and Xyrem (United States) | |
| **Gamma-butyrolactone**<br>CASRN 96-48-0<br>$C_4H_6O_2$<br>MW 86.09 | 1,2-butanolide; 1,4-butanolide; 3-hydroxybutyric acid lactone; Alpha-butyrolactone; Blon; Butyric acid lactone; Butyric acid; 4-hydroxy-gamma-lactone; Butyrolactone; Butyryl lactone; Dihydro-2(3H)-furanone; Gamma bl; Gamma butanolide; Gamma butyrolactone; Gamma deoxytetronic acid; Gamma hydroxybutanoic acid lactone; Gamma hydroxybutyric acid cyclic ester; Gamma hydroxybutyric acid lactone; Gamma hydroxybutyric acid; gamma-lactone; Gamma hydroxybutyrolactone; Gamma lactone 4-hydroxybutanoic acid; Gamma-6480; Nci-c55875; Tetrahydro-2-furanone | Beta Tech; Blast; BLO; Blow; Blue Moon; Blue Nitro Vitality; Eclipse; Firewater; Furan; Furanone Extreme; Furomax; G3; Gamma G; Gamma Ram; GBL; GenX; GH Gold (GHG); GH Release; GH Relief; GH Revitalizer; Insom-X; Invigorate; Jolt; Nu-Life; Knock out; Liquid Libido; ReActive; Regenerize; Remedy-GH; Remforce; Renewsolvent; RenewTrient; RenewTrient caps; Rest-eze; Revivarant; Revivarant-G; Revitalizer; Thunder; V-3; Verve |
| **1,4-Butanediol**<br>CASRN 110-63-4<br>$C_4H_{10}O_2$<br>MW 90.1 | 1,4-butylene glycol; 1,4-dihydroxybutane; 1,4-tetramethylene glycol; Butane-1,4-diol; Butanediol; BD; BDO; Butylene glycol; Diol 1-4 B; Sucol B; Tetramethylene 1,4-diol; Tetramethylene glycol | AminoFlex; Biocopia PM; BlueRaine; Borametz; BVM; Dormir; Enliven celluplex; FX Cherry Bomb; FX Lemon Drop; FX Orange; FX Rush; GHRE (GH Releasing Extract); Inner G; Liquid Gold; NeuroMod; N-Force; NRG3; Omega-G; Pine Needle Extract; Pro G; Promusol; Rejuv@night; Rest-Q; Revitalize Plus; Serenity; Soma Solutions; SomatoPro caps; Sucol B; Thunder; Thunder Nectar; Ultradiol; Weight belt cleaner; White Magic; X-12; Zen; Ink jet cleaner |

GHB has been promoted as a growth hormone releaser, muscle builder, diet aid, soporific, euphoriant, hallucinogen, antidepressant, alcohol substitute, and enhancer of sexual potency. GHB use in dance clubs and at rave parties commonly involves ingestion along with ethanol and other drugs. GHB has also become known as a "date rape" drug because it can produce a rapid incapacitation or loss of consciousness, facilitating sexual assault.

**I. Mechanism of toxicity**

**A. GHB** is a structural analog of the neurotransmitter gamma-aminobutyric acid (GABA) with agonist activity at both GABA(B) and GHB receptors. It readily crosses the blood-brain barrier, resulting in general anesthesia and respiratory depression. Death results from injury secondary to abrupt loss of consciousness, apnea, pulmonary edema, or pulmonary aspiration of gastric contents. Fatal potentiation of GHB's depressant effects has occurred with ethanol and other depressant drugs.

B. **Gamma-butyrolactone (GBL),** a solvent now regulated by the DEA as a List I Chemical, can be chemically converted by sodium hydroxide to GHB. In addition, GBL is rapidly converted in the body by peripheral lactonases to GHB within minutes.

C. **1,4-Butanediol (1,4-BD),** an intermediate for chemical synthesis, is readily available through chemical suppliers. 1,4-BD is converted in vivo by alcohol dehydrogenase to gamma-hydroxybutyraldehyde, then by aldehyde dehydrogenase to GHB.

D. **Pharmacokinetics.** Onset of CNS depressant effects begins within 10–15 minutes after oral ingestion of GHB and 2–8 minutes after intravenous injection. Peak levels occur within 25–45 minutes, depending on the dose. A recent meal may reduce systemic bioavailability by 37% compared with the fasting state. The duration of effect is 1–2.5 hours after anesthetic doses of 50–60 mg/kg and about 2.5 hours in nonintubated accidental overdoses seen in the emergency department (range 15 minutes–5 hours). The rate of elimination of GHB is saturable. Plasma blood levels of GHB are undetectable within 4–6 hours after therapeutic doses. The volume of distribution is variable owing to saturable absorption and elimination. GHB is not protein bound.

II. **Toxic dose**

A. **GHB.** Response to low oral doses of GHB is unpredictable, with variability between patients and in the same patient. Narcolepsy studies with 30 mg/kg have reported effects including abrupt onset of sleep, enuresis, hallucinations, and myoclonic movements. Anesthetic studies reported unconsciousness with 50 mg/kg and deep coma with 60 mg/kg. Fasting, ethanol, and other depressants enhance the effects of GHB.

B. **GBL,** a nonionized molecule, has greater bioavailability than GHB when given orally in the same doses. A dose of 1.5 g produced sleep lasting 1 hour.

C. **1,4-BD** is equipotent to GHB, although in the presence of ethanol, competition for the metabolic enzyme alcohol dehydrogenase may delay or decrease the peak effect.

III. **Clinical presentation.** Patients with acute GHB overdose commonly present with coma, bradycardia, and myoclonic movements.

A. **Soporific effects and euphoria** usually occur within 15 minutes of an oral dose; unconsciousness and deep coma may follow within 30–40 minutes. When GHB is ingested alone, the duration of coma is usually short, with recovery within 2 to 4 hours and complete resolution of symptoms within 8 hours.

B. **Delirium** and **agitation** are common. **Seizures** occur rarely. Bradypnea with increased tidal volume is seen frequently. Cheyne-Stokes respiration and loss of airway-protective reflexes occur. Vomiting is seen in 30–50% of cases, and incontinence may occur. Stimulation may cause tachycardia and mild hypertension, but bradycardia is more common.

C. **Alkaline corrosive burns** result from misuse of the home manufacture kits: A dangerously basic solution is produced when excess base is added, the reaction is incomplete, or there is inadequate back titration with acid. (The solution can also be acidic from excessive back titration.)

D. Frequent use of GHB in high doses may produce tolerance and dependence. A **withdrawal syndrome** has been reported when chronic use is discontinued. Symptoms include tremor, paranoia, agitation, confusion, delirium, visual and auditory hallucinations, tachycardia, and hypertension. Rhabdomyolysis, myoclonus, and death have occurred.

E. See also the discussion of **drug-facilitated assault,** p 65.

IV. **Diagnosis** is usually suspected clinically in a patient who presents with abrupt onset of coma and recovers rapidly within a few hours.

A. **Specific levels.** Laboratory tests for GHB levels are not readily available but can be obtained from a few national reference laboratories. Serum levels greater than 50 mg/L are associated with loss of consciousness, and levels over 260 mg/L usually produce unresponsive coma. In a small series of accidental overdoses, awakening occurred as levels fell into the range of 75–150 mg/L. GBL and 1,4-BD are rapidly converted in vivo to GHB. The duration of detection of GHB in blood and urine is short (6 and 12 hours, respectively, after therapeutic doses).

B. **Other useful laboratory studies** include glucose, electrolytes, and arterial blood gases or oximetry. Consider urine toxicology screening and blood ethanol to rule out other common drugs of abuse that may enhance or prolong the course of poisoning.

V. **Treatment**

A. **Emergency and supportive measures**

1. Protect the airway and assist ventilation if needed. Note that patients who require intubation are often awake and are extubated within a few hours.
2. Treat coma (see p 18), seizures (p 22), bradycardia (p 9), and corrosive burns (p 157) if they occur.
3. Evaluate for and treat drug-facilitated assault (see p 65).

B. **Specific drugs and antidotes.** There are no specific antidotes available. Flumazenil and naloxone are not clinically effective. GHB withdrawal syndrome is managed with benzodiazepine (see p 419) sedation as in other depressant withdrawal syndromes. Large doses may be needed. Withdrawal refractory to benzodiazepines is not uncommon and may benefit from the addition of barbiturates (pp 493–495) or propofol (p 502).

C. **Decontamination**

1. **Prehospital.** Do ***not*** give charcoal or induce vomiting because of the risk of rapid loss of consciousness and loss of airway-protective reflexes, which may lead to pulmonary aspiration.
2. **Hospital.** The small doses of GHB usually ingested are rapidly absorbed, and gastric lavage and activated charcoal are of doubtful benefit and may increase the risk of pulmonary aspiration. Consider activated charcoal administration for recent, large ingestions or when significant co-ingestion is suspected.

D. **Enhanced elimination.** There is no role for enhanced removal procedures such as dialysis and hemoperfusion.

## ► GASES, IRRITANT

*John Balmes, MD*

A vast number of compounds produce irritant effects when inhaled in the gaseous form. The most common source of exposure to irritant gases is industry, but significant exposures may occur in a variety of circumstances, such as after mixing cleaning agents at home, with smoke inhalation in structural fires, or after highway tanker spills.

I. **Mechanism of toxicity.** Irritant gases often are divided into two major groups on the basis of their water solubility (Table II–29).

A. **Highly soluble gases** (eg, ammonia and chlorine) are readily adsorbed by the upper respiratory tract and rapidly produce their primary effects on moist mucous membranes in the eyes, nose, and throat.

B. **Less soluble gases** (eg, phosgene and nitrogen dioxide) are not rapidly adsorbed by the upper respiratory tract and can be inhaled deeply into the lower respiratory tract to produce delayed-onset pulmonary toxicity.

II. **Toxic dose.** The toxic dose varies with the properties of the gas. Table II–29 illustrates the workplace exposure limits (TLV-TWA) and the levels immediately dangerous to life or health (IDLH) for several common irritant gases.

**TABLE II–29. IRRITANT TOXIC GASES**

| Gas | TLV[a] (ppm) | IDLH[b] (ppm) |
|---|---|---|
| **High water solubility** | | |
| Ammonia | 25 | 300 |
| Formaldehyde | 0.3 (C) | 20 |
| Hydrogen chloride | 2 (C) | 50 |
| Hydrogen fluoride | 3 (C) | 30 |
| Nitric acid | 2 | 25 |
| Sulfur dioxide | 2 | 100 |
| **Moderate water solubility** | | |
| Acrolein | 0.1 | 2 |
| Chlorine | 0.5 | 10 |
| Fluorine | 1 | 25 |
| **Low water solubility** | | |
| Nitric oxide | 25 | 100 |
| Nitrogen dioxide | 3 | 20 |
| Ozone | 0.2[c] | 5 |
| Phosgene | 0.1 | 2 |

[a]TLV = threshold limit value, ACGIH recommended exposure limit as an 8-hour time-weighted average for a 40-hour workweek (TLV-TWA). "(C)" indicates ceiling limit, which should not be exceeded at any time (TLV-C).
[b]IDLH = Air level considered immediately dangerous to life or health, defined as the maximum air concentration from which one could reasonably escape within 30 minutes without any escape-impairing symptoms or any irreversible health effects.
[c]For exposure of no more than 2 hours.

**III. Clinical presentation.** All these gases may produce irritant effects to the upper and/or lower respiratory tract, but warning properties and the onset and location of primary symptoms depend largely on the water solubility of the gas and the concentration of exposure.

**A. Highly soluble gases.** Because of the good warning properties (upper respiratory tract irritation) of highly soluble gases, voluntary prolonged exposure to even low concentrations is unlikely.

1. Low-level exposure causes rapid onset of mucous membrane and upper respiratory tract irritation; conjunctivitis, rhinitis, skin erythema and burns, sore throat, cough, wheezing, and hoarseness are common.
2. With high-level exposure, laryngeal edema, tracheobronchitis, and abrupt airway obstruction may occur. Irritation of the lower respiratory tract and lung parenchyma causes tracheobronchial mucosal sloughing, chemical pneumonitis, and noncardiogenic pulmonary edema.

**B. Less soluble gases.** Because of poor warning properties owing to minimal upper respiratory tract effects, prolonged exposure to moderate levels of these gases often occurs; therefore, chemical pneumonitis and pulmonary edema are more common. The onset of pulmonary edema may be delayed up to 12–24 hours or even longer.

**C. Sequelae.** Although most patients who suffer toxic inhalation injury recover without any permanent impairment, bronchiectasis, bronchiolitis obliterans, persistent asthma, and pulmonary fibrosis can occur.

**IV. Diagnosis** is based on a history of exposure and the presence of typical irritant upper- or lower-respiratory effects. Arterial blood gases and chest x-ray may reveal early evidence of chemical pneumonitis or pulmonary edema. Whereas highly soluble gases have good warning properties and the diagnosis is not difficult, less soluble gases may produce minimal symptoms shortly after exposure; therefore, a high index of suspicion and repeated examinations are required.

- **A. Specific levels.** There are no specific blood or serum levels available.
- **B. Other useful laboratory studies** include arterial blood gases or oximetry, chest x-ray, spirometry, and peak expiratory flow measurement.

**V. Treatment**

- **A. Emergency and supportive measures**
  1. Immediately assess the airway; hoarseness or stridor suggests laryngeal edema, which necessitates direct laryngoscopy and endotracheal intubation if swelling is present (see p 4). Assist ventilation if necessary (p 6).
  2. Give supplemental oxygen, and treat bronchospasm with aerosolized bronchodilators (see p 7).
  3. Monitor arterial blood gases or oximetry, chest x-ray, and pulmonary function. Treat pulmonary edema if it occurs (see p 7).
  4. For victims of smoke inhalation, consider the possibility of concurrent intoxication by carbon monoxide (see p 151) or cyanide (p 176).
- **B. Specific drugs and antidotes.** There is no specific antidote for any of these gases.
- **C. Decontamination** (see p 46). Remove the victim from exposure and give supplemental oxygen if available. Rescuers should take care to avoid personal exposure; in most cases, self-contained breathing apparatus should be worn.
- **D. Enhanced elimination.** There is no role for enhanced elimination.

## ► GLYPHOSATE

*Craig Smollin, MD*

Glyphosate (*N*-[phophonomethyl]glycine) is a herbicide that is used widely in agriculture, forestry, and commercial weed control. Its use is likely to increase, as it is one of the first herbicides against which crops have been genetically modified to increase their tolerance. It functions by inhibiting aromatic amino acid synthesis in plants. Commercial glyphosate-based products (Roundup™, Vantage™, and many others) are marketed in concentrations ranging from 0.5% to 41% or more glyphosate and generally consist of an aqueous mixture of the isopropylamino salt of glyphosate, a surfactant, and various minor components. Concentrated Roundup™, the most commonly used glyphosate preparation in the United States, contains 41% glyphosate and 15% polyoxyethyleneamine (POEA). Accidental exposure has been reported to cause mild skin and eye irritation, whereas suicidal ingestions may lead to mouth and throat irritation, abdominal pain, vomiting, and in some cases death.

**I. Mechanism of toxicity.** The precise mechanisms of toxicity of glyphosate formulations are complicated. There are five different glyphosate salts, and commercial formulations contain surfactants that vary in chemical structure and concentration.

- **A.** It has been hypothesized that toxicity is related to the presence of the surfactant rather than to the glyphosate itself. Surfactants may impair cardiac contractility and increase pulmonary vascular resistance.
- **B.** Some have postulated that glyphosate or the surfactants may uncouple mitochondria oxidative phosphorylation, leading to symptoms of toxicity.
- **C.** Glyphosate is a phosphorus-containing compound, but it does not inhibit acetylcholinesterase.

**II. Toxic dose.** Glyphosate itself has very low toxicity by the oral and dermal routes, with an $LD_{50}$ in animals of > 5000 mg/kg and > 2000 mg/kg, respectively. However, the surfactant (POEA) is more toxick, with an oral $LD_{50}$ of 1200 mg/kg. Ingestion of > 85 mL of a concentrated formulation is likely to cause significant toxicity in adults.

III. **Clinical presentation**

A. **Dermal.** Prolonged exposure to the skin can cause dermal irritation. Severe skin burns are rare. Glyphosate is poorly absorbed across the skin, with only 3% of patients with dermal exposure developing systemic symptoms.

B. **Ocular** exposure can cause a mild conjunctivitis and superficial corneal injury. No serious eye injury occurred among 1513 consecutive ocular exposures reported to a poison control center.

C. **Inhalation** is a minor route of exposure. Aerosolized mist can cause oral or nasal discomfort and throat irritation.

D. **Ingestion**. After acute ingestion of a large amount of a glyphosate/surfactant-containing product, serious GI, cardiopulmonary, and other organ system toxicity may occur.

1. **Gastrointestinal corrosive effects** include mouth, throat, and epigastric pain and dysphagia. Vomiting and diarrhea are common. Esophageal and gastric mucosal injury may occur.
2. **Cardiovascular.** Glyphosate/surfactant-induced myocardial depression can result in cardiogenic shock.
3. **Ventilatory insufficiency** can occur secondary to pulmonary aspiration of the product or noncardiogenic pulmonary edema.
4. **Other.** Renal and hepatic impairment and a diminished level of consciousness may occur secondary to reduced organ perfusion, although a direct toxic effect of glyphosate or surfactant may contribute. Dilated pupils, convulsions, confusion, a neutrophil leukocytosis, fever, and increased serum amylase have also been reported. In a series of 131 cases of glyphosate ingestion, metabolic acidosis was present in 48% of cases and ECG abnormalities (sinus tachycardia and/or nonspecific ST-T wave changes most commonly) occurred in up to 20% of cases.

IV. **Diagnosis** is based on the history of contact with or ingestion of glyphosate-containing products.

A. **Specific levels.** Although unlikely to affect clinical management, serum and urine glyphosate levels may be obtained from a reference laboratory or the manufacturer of Roundup™ (Monsanto, St. Louis, MO).

B. **Other useful laboratory studies** include chest x-ray, electrolytes, renal function studies, and arterial blood gases or pulse oximetry to assess oxygenation.

V. **Treatment**

A. **Emergency and supportive measures**

1. Maintain an open airway and assist ventilation if necessary (see pp 1–7).
2. Treat hypotension (p 15) and coma (p 18) if they occur.
3. If corrosive injury to the GI tract is suspected, consult a gastroenterologist for possible endoscopy.

B. **Specific drugs and antidotes.** No specific antidote is available.

C. **Decontamination** (see p 45)

1. **Skin and eyes.** Remove contaminated clothing and wash exposed skin with water. Flush exposed eyes with copious tepid water or saline.
2. **Ingestion.** For small ingestions of a diluted or low-concentration product, no decontamination is necessary. For larger ingestions, place a flexible nasogastric tube and aspirate gastric contents, then lavage with tepid water or saline. The efficacy of activated charcoal is unknown.

D. **Enhanced elimination.** There is no known role for these procedures.

## ► HERBAL AND ALTERNATIVE PRODUCTS

*Christine A. Haller, MD*

The use of herbal medicines, dietary supplements, and other alternative products has risen sharply since passage of the Dietary Supplement Health and Education Act

(DSHEA) in 1994. In contrast to requirements for prescription or nonprescription drugs, FDA approval is not required prior to the marketing of these products. Premarketing evaluation of safety and efficacy is not mandated, and adherence to good manufacturing practices and quality control standards is not enforced. Consumers often mistakenly believe that these "natural" products are free of harm and may unknowingly be at risk of illness from the products and herb-drug and herb-disease interactions, particularly with "polysupplement" use. Table II–30 lists common uses of selected products that are available as herbal remedies, dietary supplements, or other alternative uses and their potential toxicities.

**I. Mechanism of toxicity**

**A.** A number of poisonings related to herbal preparations are caused by **contaminants** such as cadmium, lead, arsenic, and mercury or pharmaceutical **adulterants** such as diazepam, acetaminophen, phenylbutazone, and prednisone. An epidemic of "eosinophilia-myalgia syndrome" in the late 1980s apparently was caused by contaminants associated with mass production of the amino acid L-tryptophan, and similar contaminants have been identified in some melatonin products.

**B.** Some herbs are intrinsically toxic, and poisoning may occur as a result of **misidentification,** mislabeling, or improper processing of plant materials, as occurred with a Belgian slimming formulation contaminated with the herb *Stephania fangchi* containing the nephrotoxin aristolochic acid.

**C. Herb-drug interactions.** Herbal products may potentiate or diminish the effects of drugs with narrow therapeutic margins. Garlic, ginseng, ginger, and ginkgo biloba appear to have anticoagulant effects and should not be used concomitantly with warfarin, aspirin, or other antiplatelet therapies. St. John's wort has been shown to have several clinically significant pharmacokinetic interactions with substrates for *p*-glycoprotein and the cytochrome P-450 system, resulting in decreased plasma levels of drugs such as indinavir, cyclosporine, digoxin, and oral contraceptives.

**II. Clinical presentation** depends on the toxic constituent of the herbal product and may be acute in onset (eg, with the cardiac stimulant effects of ephedra or guarana) or delayed (as with Chinese herbal nephropathy caused by *Aristolochia*). Allergic reactions to botanical products may manifest with skin rash, including urticaria, bronchospasm, and even anaphylaxis.

**IV. Diagnosis** is based on a history of use of alternative products and exclusion of other medical/toxicologic causes. Identification of an unknown herb may be facilitated by consulting with a local Chinese herbalist, acupuncturist, or naturopathic practitioner. In some cases, chemical analysis of the product may confirm the presence of the suspected causative constituent or contaminant.

**A. Specific levels.** Quantitative levels are not available for most alternative medicine toxins. Ephedrine can be measured in the blood and urine of people taking *Ma huang.*

**B. Laboratory studies.** Serum electrolytes including glucose, BUN, creatinine, liver transaminases, and prothrombin time are useful in cases of suspected organ toxicity resulting from alternative therapies.

**IV. Treatment**

**A. Emergency and supportive measures.** Toxic effects of herbal medicines should be managed with the same approach taken with other ingestions.

1. Replace fluid losses caused by diarrhea or vomiting with intravenous crystalloid (see p 16).
2. Treat hypertension (see p 17), tachycardia (p 12), and arrhythmias (pp 10–15) if they occur.
3. Treat anxiety, agitation, or seizures (see p 22) caused by stimulant herbs with intravenous benzodiazepines (p 419).
4. Maintain an open airway and assist ventilation if necessary in cases of CNS depression or coma related to sedative herb use.

**TABLE II–30. DIETARY SUPPLEMENTS AND ALTERNATIVE REMEDIES**[a]

| Product | Source or Active Ingredient | Common or Purported Use | Clinical Effects and Potential Toxicity |
|---|---|---|---|
| Androstenedione | Sex steroid precursor | Increase muscle size and strength | Virilization in women, increased estrogen in men. |
| Anabolic steroids | Methandrostenolone, oxandrolone, testolactone, many other steroid derivatives | Body building | Virilization; feminization; cholestatic hepatitis; aggressiveness, mania, or psychosis; hypertension; acne; hyperlipidemia; immune suppression. |
| Azarcon (Greta) | Lead salts | Hispanic folk remedy for abdominal pain, colic | Lead poisoning (see p 237). |
| Bitter orange | *Citrus aurantium* (source of synephrine) | Weight loss, athletic enhancement | Synephrine: alpha-adrenergic agonist (see p 322). May cause vasoconstriction, hypertension. |
| Bufotoxin | Bufotenine (toad venom); "love stone"; Chan su | Purported aphrodisiac; hallucinogen | Cardiac glycosides (see p 155). |
| Cascara sagrada | *Rhamnus purshiana* | Cathartic in some diet aids | Abdominal cramps, diarrhea; fluid and electrolyte loss. |
| Chitosan | Derived from marine exoskeletons | Weight loss | Dyspepsia; oily stools; shellfish hypersensitivity reaction. |
| Chondroitin sulfate | Shark or bovine cartilage or synthetic | Osteoarthritis | Possible anticoagulant activity. |
| Chromium | Chromium picolinate | Glucose and cholesterol lowering; athletic performance enhancement | Renal insufficiency; possibly mutagenic in high doses; niacinlike flushing reaction with picolinate salt (see p 166). |
| Comfrey | *Symphytum officinale* | Anti-inflammatory; gastritis; diarrhea | Hepatic veno-occlusive disease; possible teratogen/carcinogen. (Note: many other plants also contain hepatotoxic pyrrolizidine alkaloids; see Table II–46). |
| Creatine | Creatine monohydrate; creatine monophosphate | Athletic performance enhancement | Nausea, diarrhea, muscle cramping, rhabdomyolysis, renal dysfunction |
| DHEA | Dihydroepiandrosterone (an adrenal steroid) | Anticancer; antiaging | Possible androgenic effects. |
| Echinacea | *Echinacea angustifolia; Echinacea pallida; Echinacea purpurea* | Immune stimulation, prevention of colds | Allergic reactions; possible exacerbation of autoimmune diseases. |
| Fenugreek | *Trigonella foenum-graecum* | Increase appetite; promote lactation | Hypoglycemia in large doses; anticoagulant effects possible. |
| Feverfew | *Tanacetum parthenium* | Migraine prophylaxis | Allergic reactions, antiplatelet effects. |
| Garlic | *Allium sativum* | Hyperlipidemia; hypertension | Anticoagulant effect, gastrointestinal irritation, body odor. |
| Ginkgo | Extract of *Ginkgo biloba* | Memory impairment, tinnitus, peripheral vascular disease | Gastrointestinal irritation; antiplatelet effects. |
| Ginseng | *Panex ginseng; Panex quinquefolium* | Fatigue/stress; immune stimulation | Decreases glucose; increases cortisol. *Ginseng abuse syndrome:* nervousness; insomnia; gastrointestinal distress. |

(*continued*)

**TABLE II–30. DIETARY SUPPLEMENTS AND ALTERNATIVE REMEDIES[a] (CONTINUED)**

| Product | Source or Active Ingredient | Common or Purported Use | Clinical Effects and Potential Toxicity |
|---|---|---|---|
| Glucosamine | Marine exoskeletons or synthetic | Osteoarthritis | Possibly decreased insulin production. |
| Goldenseal | *Hydrastis canadensis* | Dyspepsia; postpartum bleeding; drug test adulterant | Nausea; vomiting; diarrhea; paresthesia; seizures; use during pregnancy/lactation can cause kernicteris in infants. |
| Grape seed extract | Procyanidins | Circulatory disorders, antioxidant | None described. |
| Guarana | Caffeine | Athletic performance enhancement; appetite suppressant | Tachycardia, tremor; vomiting (see Caffeine, p 142). |
| Jin bu huan | *l*-Tetrahydropalmatine | Chinese traditional medicine | Acute CNS depression and bradycardia; chronic hepatitis. |
| Kava | *Piper methysticum* | Anxiety, insomnia | Drowsiness; hepatitis, cirrhosis, acute liver failure; habituation, and reversible skin rash. |
| Ma huang | Ephedrine (various *Ephedra* sp.) | Stimulant; athletic performance enhancement; appetite suppressant | Insomnia; hypertension, tachycardia; psychosis, seizures, cardiac dysrhythmias, stroke. |
| Melatonin | Pineal gland | Circadian rhythm sleep disorders | Drowsiness; headache; transient depressive symptoms. |
| Milk thistle | *Silybum marianum* | Toxic hepatitis and other liver diseases | Mild GI distress; possible allergic reaction. |
| SAMe | *S*-adenosyl-L-methionine | Depression | Mild gastrointestinal distress, mania (rare). |
| Saw palmetto | *Serenoa repens* | Benign prostatic hypertrophy | Antiandrogenic, headache. |
| Senna | *Cassia angustifolia; Cassia acutifolia* | Weight loss; laxative | Watery diarrhea; abdominal cramps; fluid and electrolyte loss. |
| Shark cartilage | Pacific Ocean shark *Squalus acanthias* | Cancer, arthritis | Bad taste; hepatitis; hypercalcemia, hyperglycemia. |
| Spirulina | Some blue-green algae | Body building | Niacinlike flushing reaction |
| St. John's wort | *Hypericum perforatum* | Depression | Possible mild MAO inhibition (see p 269); photosensitivity; p-glycoprotein and P450 enzyme induction. |
| Tea tree oil | *Melaleuca alternifolia* | Lice, scabies, ringworm, vaginitis; acne | Sedation and ataxia when taken orally; contact dermatitis, local skin irritation. |
| L-Tryptophan | Essential amino acid | Insomnia, depression | Eosinophilia-myalgia syndrome reported in 1989, due to contaminants in tryptophan. Similar contaminants found in 5-hydroxy-*l*-tryptophan and melatonin. |
| Valerian root | *Valeriana officianalis; Valeriana edulis* | Insomnia | Sedation; vomiting. |
| Vanadium | Vanadyl sulfate | Body building | Greenish discoloration of tongue, intestinal cramps, diarrhea; renal dysfunction. |

(*continued*)

**TABLE II–30. DIETARY SUPPLEMENTS AND ALTERNATIVE REMEDIES[a] (CONTINUED)**

| Product | Source or Active Ingredient | Common or Purported Use | Clinical Effects and Potential Toxicity |
|---|---|---|---|
| Yohimbine | *Corynanthe yohimbe* | Sexual dysfunction | Hallucinations; tachycardia, tremor; hypertension; irritability; gastrointestinal irritation. |
| Zinc | Zinc gluconate lozenges | Flu/cold symptoms | Nausea; mouth/throat irritation. |

[a]Most of these products are legally considered neither food nor drugs and therefore are not regulated by the FDA (Dietary Supplement Health and Education Act, 1994). Toxicity may be related to the active ingredient(s) or to impurities, contaminants, or adulterants in the product. See also caffeine (p 142), essential oils (p 146), salicylates (p 333), and vitamins (p 367).

B. **Specific drugs and antidotes.** There are no specific antidotes for toxicity related to herbal and alternative products.

C. **Decontamination** (see p 45). Administer activated charcoal orally if conditions are appropriate (see Table I–38, p 51). Gastric lavage is not necessary after small to moderate ingestions if activated charcoal can be given promptly.

D. **Enhanced elimination.** The effectiveness of these procedures in removing herbal and alternative medicine toxins has not been studied.

http://www.amfoundation.org/herbmed
(HerbMed: An evidence-based scientific database on herbal medicines supported by the nonprofit Alternative Medicine Foundation.)
http://www.cfsan.fda.gov
(FDA Office of Food Safety and Nutrition: Posts consumer alerts and health professional advisories about safety concerns related to botanical products and other dietary supplements.)

## ▶ HYDROCARBONS

*Collin S. Goto, MD*

Hydrocarbons are used widely as solvents, degreasers, fuels, and lubricants. Hydrocarbons include organic compounds derived from petroleum distillation as well as many other sources, including plant oils, animal fats, and coal. Subcategories of hydrocarbons include aliphatic (saturated carbon structure), aromatic (containing one or more benzene rings), halogenated (containing chlorine, bromine, or fluoride atoms), alcohols and glycols, ethers, ketones, carboxylic acids, and many others. This chapter emphasizes toxicity caused by common household hydrocarbons. See specific chemicals elsewhere in Section II and in Section IV, Table IV–4 (p 542).

I. **Mechanism of toxicity.** Hydrocarbons may cause direct injury to the lung after pulmonary aspiration or systemic intoxication after ingestion, inhalation, or skin absorption (Table II–31). Many hydrocarbons are also irritating to the eyes and skin.

A. **Pulmonary aspiration.** Chemical pneumonitis is caused by direct tissue damage and disruption of surfactant. Aspiration risk is greatest for hydrocarbons with low viscosity and low surface tension (eg, petroleum naphtha, gasoline, turpentine).

B. **Ingestion**

1. **Aliphatic hydrocarbons** and **simple petroleum distillates** such as lighter fluid, kerosene, furniture polish, and gasoline are poorly absorbed from the GI tract and do not pose a significant risk of systemic toxicity after ingestion as long as they are not aspirated.

**TABLE II–31. HYDROCARBON INGESTION**

| Common Compounds | Risk of Systemic Toxicity After Ingestion | Risk of Chemical Aspiration Pneumonia | Treatment |
|---|---|---|---|
| **No systemic toxicity, high viscosity**<br>Petrolatum jelly, motor oil | Low | Low | Supportive. |
| **No systemic toxicity, low viscosity**<br>Gasoline, kerosene, petroleum naphtha, mineral seal oil, petroleum ether | Low | High | Observe for pneumonia; do ***not*** empty stomach. |
| **Unknown or uncertain systemic toxicity**<br>Turpentine, pine oil | Uncertain | High | Observe for pneumonia; consider removal by nasogastric suction and/or administration of activated charcoal if ingestion is > 2 mL/kg. |
| **Systemic toxins**<br>Camphor, phenol, halogenated or aromatic compounds | High | High | Observe for pneumonia; consider removal by nasogastric suction and/or administration of activated charcoal. |

2. In contrast, many **aromatic** and **halogenated hydrocarbons, alcohols, ethers, ketones,** and other **substituted or complex hydrocarbons** are capable of causing serious systemic toxicity, such as coma, seizures, and cardiac arrhythmias.

C. **Inhalation** of hydrocarbon vapors in an enclosed space may cause intoxication as a result of systemic absorption or by displacing oxygen from the atmosphere.

D. **Injection** of hydrocarbons into skin, subcutaneous tissue, or muscle may cause a severe local inflammatory reaction and liquefaction necrosis.

E. **Skin and eye contact** can cause local irritation. **Dermal** absorption can be significant for some agents but is insignificant for most of the simple aliphatic compounds.

II. **Toxic dose.** The toxic dose is variable, depending on the agent involved and whether it is aspirated, ingested, injected, or inhaled.

A. **Pulmonary aspiration** of as little as a few milliliters may produce chemical pneumonitis.

B. **Ingestion** of as little as 10–20 mL of some systemic toxins, such as camphor and carbon tetrachloride, may cause serious or fatal poisoning.

C. For recommended **inhalation** exposure limits for common hydrocarbons, see Table IV–4, p 542.

D. **Injection** of less than 1 mL can cause significant local tissue inflammation.

E. **Dermal** absorption is insignificant for most simple aliphatic compounds but may occur with other agents.

III. **Clinical presentation**

A. **Pulmonary aspiration** usually causes immediate onset of coughing or choking. This may progress within minutes or hours to a chemical pneumonitis characterized by respiratory distress, including tachypnea, retractions, grunting, wheezing, rales, hypoxia, and hypercarbia. Death may ensue from respiratory failure, secondary bacterial infection, and other respiratory complications.

B. **Ingestion** often causes abrupt nausea and vomiting, occasionally with hemorrhagic gastroenteritis. Some compounds may be absorbed and produce systemic toxicity.

C. **Systemic toxicity** caused by hydrocarbon ingestion, inhalation, intravenous injection, or dermal absorption is highly variable, depending on the compound, but often includes confusion, ataxia, lethargy, and headache. With significant exposure, syncope, coma, and respiratory arrest may occur. Cardiac arrhythmias may occur as a result of myocardial sensitization, especially with halogenated and aromatic compounds. With many agents, hepatic and renal injury may occur.

D. **Injection** of hydrocarbons can cause local tissue inflammation, pain, and necrosis. Severe scarring and loss of function have occurred after injection into a finger with a paint gun or another high-pressure spray device containing a hydrocarbon solvent. Often the puncture wound and local swelling appear minor, but tracking of hydrocarbon solvent down fascial planes into the palm and forearm may cause widespread inflammation and injury.

E. **Skin or eye contact** may cause local irritation, burns, or corneal injury. Chronic skin exposure often causes a defatting dermatitis (resulting from removal of oils from the skin). Some agents are absorbed through the skin and can produce systemic effects.

**IV. Diagnosis**

A. **Aspiration pneumonitis.** Diagnosis is based on a history of exposure and the presence of respiratory symptoms such as coughing, tachypnea, and wheezing. If these symptoms are not present within 6 hours of exposure, it is very unlikely that chemical pneumonitis will occur. Chest x-ray and arterial blood gases or oximetry may assist in the diagnosis of chemical pneumonitis, although chest x-ray findings may be delayed for more than 12–24 hours.

B. **Systemic intoxication.** Diagnosis is based on a history of ingestion or inhalation, accompanied by the appropriate systemic clinical manifestations.

C. **Specific levels.** Specific levels are generally not available or useful.

D. **Other useful laboratory studies.** For suspected aspiration pneumonitis, obtain arterial blood gases or oximetry and a chest x-ray; for suspected systemic toxicity, obtain electrolytes, glucose, BUN, creatinine, and liver transaminases and perform ECG monitoring.

**V. Treatment**

**A. Emergency and supportive measures**

1. **General.** Provide basic supportive care for all symptomatic patients.
   a. Maintain an open airway and assist ventilation if necessary (see pp 1–7). Administer supplemental oxygen.
   b. Monitor arterial blood gases or oximetry, chest x-ray, and ECG and admit symptomatic patients to an intensive care setting.
   c. Use epinephrine and other sympathomimetic amines with caution in patients with significant hydrocarbon intoxication, because arrhythmias may be induced.
2. **Pulmonary aspiration.** Patients who remain completely asymptomatic after 4–6 hours of observation may be discharged. In contrast, if the patient is coughing on arrival, aspiration probably has occurred.
   a. Administer supplemental oxygen and treat bronchospasm (see p 7) and hypoxia (p 7) if they occur.
   b. Do ***not*** use steroids or prophylactic antibiotics.
3. **Ingestion.** In the vast majority of accidental childhood ingestions, less than 5–10 mL is actually swallowed and systemic toxicity is rare. Treatment is primarily supportive.
4. **Injection.** For injections into the fingertip or hand, especially those involving a high-pressure paint gun, consult with a plastic or hand surgeon immediately, as prompt wide exposure, irrigation, and debridement are often required.

**B. Specific drugs and antidotes**

1. There is no specific antidote for aspiration pneumonitis; corticosteroids are of no proven value.
2. Specific drugs or antidotes may be available for systemic toxicity of some hydrocarbons (eg, acetylcysteine for carbon tetrachloride and methylene

blue for methemoglobin formers) or their solutes (eg, chelation therapy for leaded gasoline and antidotes for pesticides, etc).

**C. Decontamination**

1. **Inhalation.** Move the victim to fresh air and administer oxygen if available.
2. **Skin and eyes.** Remove contaminated clothing and wash exposed skin with water and soap. Irrigate exposed eyes with copious water or saline and perform fluorescein examination for corneal injury.
3. **Ingestion** (see p 45). For agents with no known systemic toxicity, gut decontamination is neither necessary nor desirable because any gut-emptying procedure increases the risk of aspiration. For systemic toxins, consider aspiration of the liquid via nasogastric tube and administration of activated charcoal. Take precautions to prevent pulmonary aspiration if the patient is obtunded.
4. **Injection.** See A.4, above.

**D. Enhanced elimination.** There is no known role for any of these procedures.

## ▶ HYDROGEN FLUORIDE AND HYDROFLUORIC ACID

*Jennifer Hannum, MD, and Binh T. Ly, MD*

Hydrogen fluoride (HF) is an irritant gas that liquefies at 19.5°C; in an aqueous solution it produces hydrofluoric acid. HF gas is used in chemical manufacturing. In addition, it may be released from fluorosilicates, fluorocarbons, or Teflon when heated to over 350°C. Hydrofluoric acid (aqueous HF solution) is widely used as a rust remover, in glass etching, and in the manufacture of silicon semiconductor chips. Hydrofluoric acid events at the workplace were shown to be two times more likely to involve injuries compared with other acids. Poisoning usually occurs after dermal exposure, although ingestions occasionally occur. Similar toxicity can result from exposure to ammonium bifluoride.

**I. Mechanism of toxicity.** HF is a dermal and respiratory irritant. Hydrofluoric acid is a relatively weak acid (the dissociation constant is about 1000 times less than that of hydrochloric acid), and toxic effects result primarily from the highly reactive fluoride ion.

**A.** HF is able to penetrate tissues deeply, where the highly cytotoxic fluoride ion is released and cellular destruction occurs.

**B.** In addition, fluoride readily precipitates with divalent cations; this may cause systemic hypocalcemia, hypomagnesemia, and local bone demineralization.

**II. Toxic dose.** Toxicity depends on the air levels and duration of exposure to HF gas or the concentration and extent of exposure to aqueous HF solutions.

**A. Hydrogen fluoride gas.** The recommended workplace ceiling limit (ACGIH TLV-C) for HF gas is 3 ppm (2.6 mg/m$^3$); 30 ppm is considered immediately dangerous to life or health (IDLH). A 5-minute exposure to air concentrations of 50–250 ppm is likely to be lethal.

**B. Aqueous solutions.** Solutions of 50–70% are highly toxic and produce immediate pain; concomitant inhalation exposure may occur with exposure to higher concentrations caused by the release of HF gas. Intermediate concentrations (20–40%) may cause little pain initially but result in deep injury after a delay of 1–8 hours; weak solutions (5–15%) cause almost no pain on contact but may cause serious delayed injury after 12–24 hours. Most household products containing aqueous HF contain 5–8% or less.

**III. Clinical presentation.** Symptoms and signs depend on the type of exposure (gas or liquid), concentration, duration, and extent of exposure.

**A. Inhalation** of HF gas produces ocular and nasopharyngeal irritation, coughing, and bronchospasm. After a delay of up to several hours, chemical pneumonitis and noncardiogenic pulmonary edema may occur. Corneal injury may result from ocular exposure.

B. **Skin exposure.** After acute exposure to weak (5–15%) or intermediate (20–40%) solutions, there may be no symptoms because the pH effect is not pronounced. Concentrated (50–70%) solutions have better warning properties because of immediate pain. After a delay of 1–12 hours, progressive redness, swelling, skin blanching, and pain occur owing to penetration to deeper tissues by the fluoride ion. The exposure is typically through a pinhole-size defect in a rubber glove, and the fingertip is the most common site of injury. The pain is progressive and unrelenting. Severe deep-tissue destruction may occur, including full-thickness skin loss and destruction of underlying bone.

C. **Ingestion** of HF may cause corrosive injury to the mouth, esophagus, and stomach.

D. **Systemic hypocalcemia, hypomagnesemia,** and **hyperkalemia** may occur after ingestion or skin burns involving a large body surface area or highly concentrated solutions (can occur with exposure to > 2.5% body surface area and a highly concentrated solution). These electrolyte imbalances, either alone or in combination, can lead to cardiac dysrhythmias, the primary cause of death in HF injuries. Prolonged QT interval may be the initial manifestation of hypocalcemia or hypomagnesemia.

IV. **Diagnosis** is based on a history of exposure and typical findings. Immediately after exposure to weak or intermediate solutions, there may be few or no symptoms even though potentially severe injury may develop later.

A. **Specific levels.** Serum fluoride concentrations are not useful after acute exposure but may be used in evaluating chronic occupational exposure. Normal serum fluoride is less than 20 mcg/L but varies considerably with dietary and environmental intake. In workers, preshift urine excretion of fluoride should not exceed 3 mg/g of creatinine.

B. **Other useful laboratory studies** include electrolytes, BUN, creatinine, calcium, magnesium, and continuous ECG monitoring.

V. **Treatment**

A. **Emergency and supportive measures**

1. Maintain an open airway and assist ventilation if necessary (see pp 1–7). Administer supplemental oxygen. Treat pulmonary edema (pp 1–7) if it occurs.
2. Patients with HF ingestion should be evaluated for corrosive injury, with consultation by a gastroenterologist for consideration of endoscopic evaluation (p 157). All HF ingestions should be considered potentially life threatening.
3. Monitor the ECG and serum calcium, magnesium, and potassium concentrations; give intravenous calcium (p 428; also see below) if there is evidence of hypocalcemia or severe hyperkalemia; replace magnesium as indicated.

B. **Specific drugs and antidotes. Calcium** (see p 428) rapidly precipitates fluoride ions and is an effective antidote for dermal exposures and systemic hypocalcemia resulting from absorbed fluoride. In addition, serum magnesium should be monitored and replaced as appropriate.

1. **Skin burns.** For exposures involving the hands or fingers, immediately consult an experienced hand surgeon, medical toxicologist, or Poison Control Center ([800] 222-1222). Historically, fingernail removal was utilized, but this can result in disfiguring morbidity. Occasionally calcium will have to be given by the intra-arterial route or by intravenous Bier block technique. ***Caution:*** Do ***not*** use calcium ***chloride*** salt for subcutaneous or intra-arterial injections; this form contains a larger proportion of calcium ion compared with the gluconate salt and may cause vasospasm and tissue necrosis.

   a. **Topical.** Apply a gel containing calcium gluconate or carbonate (see p 424), using an occlusive dressing or a rubber glove to enhance skin penetration. Alternately, soak in a quaternary ammonium solution such as Zephiran (1.3 g/L of water) or an Epsom salt solution. If pain is not significantly improved within 30–60 minutes, consider subcutaneous or intra-arterial injection.

b. **Subcutaneous.** Inject calcium gluconate 5–10% subcutaneously in affected areas, using a 27- or 30-gauge needle and no more than 0.5 mL per digit or 1 mL/cm2 in other regions.

c. **Intra-arterial.** Injection of calcium by the intra-arterial route (see p 428) may be necessary for burns involving several digits or subungual areas.

d. **Bier block.** This intravenous regional perfusion technique has been reported to be useful (see Calcium chapter).

2. **Systemic hypocalcemia or hyperkalemia.** Administer calcium gluconate 10%, 0.2–0.4 mL/kg IV, or calcium chloride 10%, 0.1–0.2 mL/kg IV.

C. **Decontamination** (see p 45). Rescuers entering a contaminated area should wear self-contained breathing apparatus and appropriate personal protective equipment to avoid exposure.

1. **Inhalation.** Immediately remove victims from exposure and give supplemental oxygen if available. The use of 2.5% calcium gluconate by nebulization is recommended by some authorities.

2. **Skin.** Immediately remove contaminated clothing and flood exposed areas with copious amounts of water. Then soak in a solution of Epsom salts (magnesium sulfate) or calcium; immediate topical use of calcium or magnesium may help prevent deep burns. Some facilities that frequently manage HF cases purchase or prepare a 2.5% calcium gluconate gel (in water-based jelly). This intervention can be highly effective if applied immediately. Soaking in a dilute benzalkonium chloride (Zephiran) solution has been advocated as an alternative to calcium.

3. **Eyes.** Flush with copious amounts of water or saline. The effectiveness of a weak (1–2%) calcium gluconate solution is not established. Consult with an ophthalmologist if there is evidence or suspicion of ocular exposure.

4. **Ingestion**

a. **Prehospital.** Immediately give any available calcium-containing (calcium carbonate or milk) or magnesium-containing (Epsom salts, magnesium hydroxide, etc) substance by mouth. Do ***not*** induce vomiting because of the risk of corrosive injury. Activated charcoal is not effective.

b. **Hospital.** Consider gastric suctioning with a nasogastric tube. Administer magnesium- or calcium-containing substance as in **4.a** above.

D. **Enhanced elimination.** There is no role for enhanced elimination procedures.

## ► HYDROGEN SULFIDE

*Stephen W. Munday, MD, MPH, MS*

Hydrogen sulfide is a highly toxic, flammable, colorless gas that is heavier than air. It is produced naturally by decaying organic matter and is also a by-product of many industrial processes. Hazardous levels may be found in petroleum refineries, tanneries, mines, pulp-making factories, sulfur hot springs, carbon disulfide production, commercial fishing holds, hot asphalt fumes, and pools of sewage sludge or liquid manure. It sometimes is referred to as "pit gas."

I. **Mechanism of toxicity.** Hydrogen sulfide causes cellular asphyxia by inhibition of the cytochrome oxidase system, similar to the action of cyanide. Because it is absorbed rapidly by inhalation, symptoms occur nearly immediately after exposure, leading to rapid unconsciousness or "knockdown." Hydrogen sulfide is also a mucous membrane irritant.

II. **Toxic dose.** The characteristic rotten egg odor of hydrogen sulfide is detectable at concentrations as low as 0.025 ppm. The recommended workplace limit (ACGIH TLV-TWA) is 10 ppm (14 mg/m$^3$) as an 8-hour time-weighted average, with a short-term exposure limit (STEL) of 15 ppm (21 mg/m$^3$). The federal OSHA permissible exposure limit (PEL) is 20 ppm as a 15-minute ceiling during an 8-hour workday. Marked respiratory tract irritation occurs with levels of 50–100 ppm. Olfactory nerve paralysis occurs with levels of 100–150 ppm. The level considered immediately dangerous to life or health (IDLH) is 100 ppm. Pulmonary edema occurs at levels of 300–500 ppm. Levels of 600–800 ppm are rapidly fatal.

**III. Clinical presentation**

A. **Irritant effects.** Upper-airway irritation, burning eyes, and blepharospasm may occur at relatively low levels. Skin exposure can cause painful dermatitis. Chemical pneumonitis and noncardiogenic pulmonary edema may occur after a delay of several hours.

B. **Acute systemic effects** include headache, nausea and vomiting, dizziness, confusion, seizures, and coma. Massive exposure may cause immediate cardiovascular collapse, respiratory arrest, and death. Survivors may be left with serious neurologic impairment.

**IV. Diagnosis** is based on a history of exposure and rapidly progressive manifestations of airway irritation and cellular asphyxia, with sudden collapse. The victim or coworkers may describe the smell of rotten eggs, but because of olfactory nerve paralysis, the absence of this smell does not rule out exposure. Silver coins in the pockets of victims have been blackened (by conversion to silver sulfide).

A. **Specific levels** are not available (sulfide is unstable in vitro). Sulfhemoglobin is not thought to be produced after hydrogen sulfide exposure.

B. **Other useful laboratory studies** include electrolytes, glucose, arterial blood gases, and chest x-ray.

**V. Treatment**

A. **Emergency and supportive measures.** ***Note:*** Rescuers should use self-contained breathing apparatus to prevent personal exposure.

1. Maintain an open airway and assist ventilation if necessary (see pp 1–7). Administer high-flow humidified supplemental oxygen. Observe for several hours for delayed-onset chemical pneumonia or pulmonary edema (p 7).
2. Treat coma (see p 18), seizures (p 22), and hypotension (p 15) if they occur.

B. **Specific drugs and antidotes.** Theoretically, administration of nitrites (see p 476) to produce methemoglobinemia may promote conversion of sulfide ions to sulfmethemoglobin, which is far less toxic. However, there is limited evidence for the effectiveness of nitrites, and they can cause hypotension and impaired oxygen delivery. Animal data and limited human case reports have suggested that hyperbaric oxygen (HBO, see p 490) may be helpful if it is provided early after exposure, but this therapy remains unproven.

C. **Decontamination** (see p 45). Remove the victim from exposure and give supplemental oxygen if available.

D. **Enhanced elimination.** There is no role for enhanced elimination procedures. Although hyperbaric oxygen therapy has been promoted for treatment of hydrogen sulfide poisoning, this is based on anecdotal cases and there is no convincing rationale or scientific evidence for its effectiveness.

## ▶ HYMENOPTERA

*Richard F. Clark, MD*

Venomous insects are grouped into four families of the order Hymenoptera: Apidae (honeybees), Bombidae (bumblebees), Vespidae (wasps, hornets, and yellow jackets), and Formicidae (ants). With the exception of Vespidae, most Hymenoptera sting only when disturbed or when the hive is threatened. Yellow jackets may attack without provocation and are the most common cause of insect-induced anaphylactic reactions.

I. **Mechanism of toxicity.** The venoms of Hymenoptera are complex mixtures of enzymes and are delivered by various methods. The venom apparatus is located in the posterior abdomen of the females.
   A. The terminal end of the stinger of the **Apidae** (honeybee) is barbed, so the stinger remains in the victim and some or all of the venom apparatus is torn from the body of the bee, resulting in its death as it flies away. The musculature surrounding the venom sac continues to contract for several minutes after evisceration, causing venom to be ejected persistently. The **Bombidae** and **Vespidae** have stingers that remain functionally intact after a sting, resulting in their ability to inflict multiple stings.
   B. The envenomating **Formicidae** have secretory venom glands in the posterior abdomen and envenomate either by injecting venom through a stinger or by spraying venom from the posterior abdomen into a bite wound produced by their mandibles.

II. **Toxic dose.** The dose of venom delivered per sting may vary from none to the entire contents of the venom gland. The toxic response is highly variable, depending on individual sensitivity. Some Hymenoptera, such as wasps, have the ability to sting several times, increasing the venom load. Disturbing a fire ant nest may result in as many as 3000–5000 stings within seconds.

III. **Clinical presentation.** The patient may present with local or systemic signs of envenomation or an allergic reaction.
   A. **Envenomation.** Once venom is injected, there is usually immediate onset of severe pain followed by a local inflammatory reaction that may include erythema, wheal formation, ecchymosis, edema, vesiculation and blisters, itching, and a sensation of warmth. Multiple stings, and very rarely severe single stings, may also produce vomiting, diarrhea, hypotension, syncope, cyanosis, dyspnea, rhabdomyolysis, coagulopathy, and death.
   B. **Allergic reactions.** Numerous deaths occur annually in the United States from immediate hypersensitivity (anaphylactic) reactions characterized by urticaria, angioedema, bronchospasm, and shock. Most anaphylactic reactions occur within 15 minutes of envenomation. Rarely, delayed-onset reactions may occur, including Arthus reactions (arthralgias and fever), nephritis, transverse myelitis, and Guillain-Barré syndrome. Cross-sensitivity to fire ant venom can exist in some patients with apid or vespid allergies.

IV. **Diagnosis** is usually obvious from the history of exposure and typical findings.
   A. **Specific levels.** Not relevant.
   B. **Other useful laboratory studies.** CPK and renal function should be checked in severe cases of multiple stings.

V. **Treatment**
   A. **Emergency and supportive measures**
      1. Monitor the victim closely for at least 30–60 minutes.
      2. Treat anaphylaxis (see p 27), if it occurs, with epinephrine (p 448) and diphenhydramine (p 442) or hydroxyzine. Persistent urticaria may respond to the addition of cimetidine, 300 mg PO or IV, or another H2 receptor antagonist. Persons known to be sensitive to Hymenoptera venom should wear medical alert jewelry and carry an epinephrine emergency kit at all times.
      3. In most cases the painful localized tissue response will resolve in a few hours without therapy. Some symptomatic relief may be obtained by topical application of ice, papain (meat tenderizer), or creams containing corticosteroids or antihistamines.
      4. Provide tetanus prophylaxis if appropriate.
   B. **Specific drugs and antidotes.** There is no available antidote.

C. **Decontamination.** Examine the sting site carefully for any retained stingers; stingers can be removed by gentle scraping with a sharp edge (eg, a knife blade) or with tweezers (venom gland contents have almost always been quickly and completely expelled). Wash the area with soap and water.

D. **Enhanced elimination.** These procedures are not applicable.

## ▶ IODINE

*Walter H. Mullen, PharmD*

The chief use of iodine is for its antiseptic property. It is bactericidal, sporicidal, protozoacidal, cysticidal, and virucidal. Because it is poorly soluble in water, liquid formulations usually are prepared as a tincture in ethanol (50% or higher). Iodoform, iodochlorhydroxyquin, iodophors (povidone-iodine), and sodium and potassium iodides also exert their bactericidal effect by liberating iodine. Lugol's solution (5% iodine and 10% potassium iodide) is used in the treatment of hyperthyroidism and for the prevention of radioactive iodine absorption after nuclear accidents. The antiarrhythmic drug amiodarone releases iodine and may cause thyrotoxicosis after prolonged use. Iodine also is used in the manufacture of dyes and photographic reagents.

I. **Mechanism of toxicity.** Iodine is corrosive because of its oxidizing properties. When ingested, iodine is poorly absorbed but may cause severe gastroenteritis. Iodine is readily inactivated by starch to convert it to iodide, which is nontoxic. In the body, iodine is converted rapidly to iodide and stored in the thyroid gland.

II. **The toxic dose** depends on the product and the route of exposure. Iodophors and iodoform liberate only small amounts of iodine and are generally nontoxic and noncaustic.

   A. **Iodine vapor.** The ACGIH-recommended workplace ceiling limit (TLV-C) for iodine vapor is 0.1 ppm (1 mg/m$^3$). The air level considered immediately dangerous to life or health (IDLH) is 2 ppm.

   B. **Skin and mucous membranes.** Strong iodine tincture (7% iodine and 5% potassium iodide in 83% ethanol) may cause burns, but USP iodine tincture (2% iodine and 2% sodium iodide in 50% ethanol) is not likely to produce corrosive damage. Systemic absorption of iodine may occur after an acute application of strong iodine tincture or after chronic applications of less concentrated products.

   C. **Ingestion.** Reported fatal doses vary from 200 mg to more than 20 g of iodine; an estimated mean lethal dose is approximately 2–4 g of free iodine. USP iodine tincture contains 100 mg iodine per 5 mL, and strong iodine tincture contains 350 mg of iodine per 5 mL. Iodine ointment contains 4% iodine. Consider ethanol toxicity with large exposures (see p 190).

III. **Clinical presentation.** The manifestations of iodine poisoning are related largely to the corrosive effect on mucous membranes.

   A. **Inhalation** of iodine vapor can cause severe pulmonary irritation that leads to pulmonary edema.

   B. **Skin** and eye exposures may result in severe corrosive burns.

   C. **Ingestion** can cause corrosive gastroenteritis with vomiting, hematemesis, and diarrhea, which can result in significant volume loss and circulatory collapse. Pharyngeal swelling and glottic edema have been reported. Mucous membranes are usually stained brown, and the vomitus may be blue if starchy foods are already present in the stomach.

   D. **Chronic** ingestions or absorption may result in hypothyroidism and goiter. Iodides cross the placenta, and neonatal hypothyroidism and death from respiratory distress secondary to goiter have been reported.

IV. **Diagnosis** is based on a history of exposure and evidence of corrosive injury. Mucous membranes are usually stained brown, and vomitus may be blue.

A. **Specific levels.** Blood levels are not clinically useful but may confirm exposure.

B. **Other useful laboratory studies** include, for serious corrosive injury, CBC, electrolytes, BUN, and creatinine. For serious inhalation, arterial blood gases or oximetry and chest x-ray are useful.

V. **Treatment**

A. **Emergency and supportive measures**

1. Maintain an open airway and perform endotracheal intubation if airway edema is progressive (see pp 1–7). Treat bronchospasm (see p 7) and pulmonary edema (p 7) if they occur.
2. Treat fluid loss from gastroenteritis aggressively with intravenous crystalloid solutions.
3. If corrosive injury to the esophagus or stomach is suspected, consult a gastroenterologist to perform endoscopy.

B. **Specific drugs and antidotes.** Sodium thiosulfate may convert iodine to iodide and tetrathionate but is not recommended for intravenous use because iodine is converted rapidly to iodide in the body.

C. **Decontamination** (see p 45)

1. **Inhalation.** Remove the victim from exposure.
2. **Skin and eyes.** Remove contaminated clothing and flush exposed skin with water. Irrigate exposed eyes copiously with tepid water or saline for at least 15 minutes.
3. **Ingestion.** Do ***not*** induce vomiting because of the corrosive effects of iodine. Administer a starchy food (potato, flour, or cornstarch) or milk to lessen GI irritation. For large exposures, consider gastric lavage, using milk, cornstarch, or sodium thiosulfate. Activated charcoal is of unknown efficacy.

D. **Enhanced elimination.** Once absorbed into the circulation, iodine is converted rapidly to the far less toxic iodide. Therefore, there is no need for enhanced drug removal.

## ► IPECAC SYRUP

*Jon Lorett, PharmD*

Ipecac syrup is an alkaloid derivative of the ipecacuanha plant (*Cephaline ipecacuanha*). The principal alkaloids, emetine and cephaeline, both have emetogenic properties. The emetine extract has been used for the treatment of amebiasis. Syrup of ipecac is widely available over the counter as an effective, rapidly acting emetic agent. Currently, the major source of poisoning is chronic intoxication resulting from intentional misuse by patients with eating disorders. Cases of "Munchausen's syndrome by proxy," in which a parent repeatedly administers ipecac to a child, have also been reported.

I. **Mechanism of toxicity**

A. **Mechanism of action.** Ipecac causes vomiting in two phases: by direct irritation of the gastric mucosa and by systemic absorption and stimulation of the central chemoreceptor trigger zone.

B. **Acute ingestion** can cause profuse vomiting and diarrhea, especially with ingestion of the more concentrated fluid extract (no longer available in the United States).

C. **Chronic repeated dosing.** The emetine component causes inhibition of protein synthesis that is particularly demonstrated in human myocytes and skeletal muscle cells after overdose or prolonged use. Another proposed mechanism for cellular toxicity is blockade of sodium and calcium channels.

II. **Toxic dose.** Toxicity depends on the formulation and whether the exposure is acute or chronic.

A. **Acute ingestion** of 60–120 mL of **syrup of ipecac** is not likely to cause serious poisoning. However, the **fluid extract,** which is approximately 14 times more potent than syrup of ipecac, has caused death after ingestion of as little as 10 mL.

B. **Chronic dosing** results in cumulative toxicity because of the slow elimination of emetine. Repeated ingestion over time, as in cases of Munchausen by proxy or eating disorders, has been reported to cause myotoxicity with total accumulated doses of 600–1250 mg. Daily ingestion of 90–120 mL of syrup of ipecac for 3 months caused death from cardiomyopathy.

III. **Clinical presentation**

A. **Acute ingestion** of ipecac causes nausea and vomiting. In patients with depressed airway-protective reflexes, pulmonary aspiration of gastric contents may occur. Prolonged or forceful vomiting may cause gastritis, gastric rupture, pneumomediastinum, retropneumoperitoneum, or Mallory-Weiss tears of the cardioesophageal junction. One fatal case of intracerebral hemorrhage was reported in an elderly patient after a single therapeutic dose of ipecac syrup.

B. **Chronic intoxication.** In patients with chronic misuse, dehydration and electrolyte abnormalities (eg, hypokalemia) occur as a result of frequent vomiting and diarrhea, and myopathy or cardiomyopathy may develop. Symptoms of myopathy include muscle weakness and tenderness, hyporeflexia, and elevated serum CPK. Cardiomyopathy, with congestive heart failure and arrhythmias, may be fatal.

1. **Munchausen by proxy.** Children intentionally poisoned with ipecac typically have a history of recurrent hospitalizations for vomiting that seems refractory to outpatient medical treatment. The symptoms usually improve in the hospital but worsen when the child returns home. Progressive weight loss and loss of developmental milestones are common. Physical examination reveals muscle weakness and other signs of chronic myopathy. Some children have been reported to develop a secondary eating disorder, such as rumination, as a result of their recurrent vomiting.
2. **Adults with an eating disorder** and frequent use of ipecac often present with a history of recent weight loss. Malnutrition and chronic vomiting may cause electrolyte disturbances, dental changes, and skin changes associated with various vitamin deficiencies.

IV. **Diagnosis** is based on a careful history of ingestion. Chronic ipecac poisoning should be suspected in any patient with an eating disorder and evidence of dehydration, electrolyte imbalance, or myopathy or in a young child with repeated unexplained episodes of vomiting, diarrhea, and failure to thrive. The electrocardiogram may show prolonged QRS and QT intervals, flat or inverted T waves, and supraventricular and ventricular arrhythmias.

A. **Specific levels.** Emetine may be detected in the urine for up to several weeks after ingestion, and its presence may provide qualitative confirmation of ipecac exposure but does not correlate with the degree of effect. It is not part of a routine comprehensive toxicology screen and must be requested specifically. Levels as low as 95 ng/mL in urine and 21 ng/mL in blood have been found in cases of confirmed Munchausen by proxy. A urinary level of 1700 ng/mL was found in a 4-year-old child who died after chronic vomiting, diarrhea, and failure to thrive. Pathologic findings of the heart muscle included marked autolytic changes with swollen mitochondria and fragmented irregular alignment of Z bands.

B. **Other useful laboratory studies** include electrolytes, BUN, creatinine, CPK, LDH, and ECG.

V. **Treatment**

A. **Emergency and supportive measures**

1. Correct fluid and electrolyte abnormalities with intravenous fluids and potassium as needed.

2. Diuretics and pressor support may be required in patients with congestive cardiomyopathy.
3. Monitor the ECG for 6–8 hours and admit patients with evidence of myopathy or cardiomyopathy. Treat arrhythmias with standard drugs (see pp 10–15).

B. **Specific drugs and antidotes.** There is no specific antidote.

C. **Decontamination** (acute ingestions only; see p 45). Consider using activated charcoal orally, but only if it can be given within a few minutes after a large ipecac ingestion.

D. **Enhanced elimination.** There is no known role for enhanced elimination. The alkaloids are highly bound to tissue.

## ▶ IRON

*Anthony S. Manoguerra, PharmD*

Iron is widely used for treatment of anemia, for prenatal supplementation, and as a common daily mineral supplement. Because of its wide availability and presumed harmlessness as a common over-the-counter nutritional supplement, it remains a common childhood ingestion and is one of the leading causes of fatal poisonings in children. There are many different iron preparations that contain various amounts of iron salts. Most children's preparations contain 12–18 mg of elemental iron per dose, and most adult preparations contain 60–90 mg of elemental iron per dose.

I. **Mechanism of toxicity.** Toxicity results from direct corrosive effects and cellular toxicity.

A. Iron has a direct corrosive effect on mucosal tissue and may cause hemorrhagic necrosis and perforation. Fluid loss from the GI tract results in severe hypovolemia.

B. Absorbed iron, in excess of protein binding capacity, causes cellular dysfunction and death, resulting in lactic acidosis and organ failure. The exact mechanism for cellular toxicity is not known, but iron ligands can cause oxidative and free-radical injury.

II. **Toxic dose.** The acute lethal dose in animal studies is 150–200 mg/kg of elemental iron. The lowest reported lethal dose in a child was 600 mg. Symptoms are unlikely if less than 20 mg/kg of elemental iron has been ingested. Doses of 20–30 mg/kg may produce self-limited vomiting, abdominal pain, and diarrhea. Ingestion of more than 40 mg/kg is considered potentially serious, and more than 60 mg/kg potentially lethal.

III. **Clinical presentation.** Iron poisoning is usually described in four stages, although the clinical manifestations may overlap.

A. Shortly after ingestion, the corrosive effects of iron cause vomiting and diarrhea, often bloody. Massive fluid or blood loss into the GI tract may result in shock, renal failure, and death.

B. Victims who survive this phase may experience a latent period of apparent improvement over 12 hours.

C. This may be followed by an abrupt relapse with coma, shock, seizures, metabolic acidosis, coagulopathy, hepatic failure, and death. *Yersinia enterocolitica* sepsis may occur.

D. If the victim survives, scarring from the initial corrosive injury may result in pyloric stricture or other intestinal obstructions.

IV. **Diagnosis** is based on a history of exposure and the presence of vomiting, diarrhea, hypotension, and other clinical signs. Elevation of the white blood count (> 15,000) or blood glucose (> 150 mg/dL) or visible radiopaque pills on abdominal x-ray also suggest significant ingestion. Serious toxicity is very unlikely if the white count, glucose, and x-ray are normal and there is no spontaneous vomiting or diarrhea.

A. **Specific levels.** If the total serum iron level is higher than 450–500 mcg/dL, toxicity is more likely to be present. Serum levels higher than 800–1000 mcg/

dL are associated with severe poisoning. Determine the serum iron level at 4–6 hours after ingestion and repeat determinations after 8–12 hours to rule out delayed absorption (eg, from a sustained-release tablet or a tablet bezoar). The total iron-binding capacity (TIBC) is unreliable in iron overdose and should not be used to estimate free iron levels.

B. **Other useful laboratory studies** include CBC, electrolytes, glucose, BUN, creatinine, liver function tests, coagulation studies, and abdominal x-ray.

V. **Treatment.** Patients who have self-limited mild GI symptoms or who remain asymptomatic for 6 hours are unlikely to develop serious intoxication. In contrast, those few with serious ingestion must be managed promptly and aggressively.

A. **Emergency and supportive measures**
   1. Maintain an open airway and assist ventilation if necessary (see pp 1–7).
   2. Treat shock caused by hemorrhagic gastroenteritis aggressively with intravenous crystalloid fluids (see p 16) and replace blood if needed. Patients are often markedly hypovolemic owing to GI losses and third-spacing of fluids into the intestinal wall and interstitial space.
   3. Treat coma (see p 18), seizures (p 22), and metabolic acidosis (p 33) if they occur.

B. **Specific treatment.** For seriously intoxicated victims (eg, shock, severe acidosis, and/or serum iron > 500–600 mcg/dL), administer **deferoxamine** (see p 437). Monitor the urine for the characteristic orange or pink-red ("vin rosé") color of the chelated deferoxamine-iron complex, although this may not always be seen. Therapy may be stopped when the urine color returns to normal or when the serum iron level decreases to the normal range. Prolonged deferoxamine therapy (longer than 36–72 hours) has been associated with adult respiratory distress syndrome (ARDS) and *Yersinia* sepsis.
   1. The intravenous route is preferred: Give 10–15 mg/kg/h by constant infusion; faster rates (up to 45 mg/kg/h) reportedly have been well tolerated in single cases, but rapid boluses usually cause hypotension. The manufacturer's recommended maximum daily dose is 6 g, but larger amounts have been given safely in massive iron overdoses.
   2. Deferoxamine has also been given intramuscularly (eg, as a test dose in suspected poisonings while awaiting laboratory confirmation); the usual dose is 50 mg/kg, with a maximum of 1 g. However, in severe poisonings, absorption of the drug by this route is unreliable and is not recommended.

C. **Decontamination** (see p 45). Activated charcoal is not effective. Ipecac is not recommended, because it can aggravate iron-induced GI irritation and interfere with whole-bowel irrigation (see below).
   1. Consider gastric lavage only if the product was a liquid formulation or tablets were chewed. (Intact tablets are not likely to pass through a lavage tube.) Do ***not*** use phosphate-containing solutions for lavage; they may result in life-threatening hypernatremia, hyperphosphatemia, and hypocalcemia. Deferoxamine lavage is not effective and may enhance iron absorption.
   2. **Whole-bowel irrigation** (see p 51) is very effective for ingested tablets and may be considered first-line treatment, especially if large numbers of tablets are visible on plain abdominal x-ray.
   3. **Activated charcoal does not adsorb iron** and is not recommended unless other drugs have been ingested.
      a. Massive ingestions may result in tablet concretions or bezoars. Repeated or prolonged whole-bowel irrigation may be considered (44.3 L over 5 days in one reported case). Endoscopy or surgical gastrotomy is rarely required but has been used.

D. **Enhanced elimination**
   1. Hemodialysis and hemoperfusion are not effective at removing iron but may be necessary to remove deferoxamine-iron complex in patients with renal failure.

2. **Exchange transfusion** is used occasionally for massive pediatric ingestion but is of questionable efficacy.

## ▶ ISOCYANATES

*Paul D. Blanc, MD, MSPH*

**Toluene diisocyanate (TDI), methylene diisocyanate (MDI),** and related chemicals are industrial components in the polymerization of urethane coatings and insulation materials. Most two-part urethane products contain some amount of one of these chemicals, and lesser amounts may contaminate one-part systems. **Methyl isocyanate** (the toxin released in the disaster in Bhopal, India) is a carbamate insecticide precursor; it is not used in urethanes, has actions different from those of the TDI group of chemicals, and is not discussed here (see Table IV–4, p 542).

I. **Mechanism of toxicity.** Toluene diisocyanate and related isocyanates act as irritants and sensitizers at very low concentrations. The mechanism is poorly understood. They may act as haptens or act through cell-mediated immune pathways. Once a person is sensitized to one isocyanate, cross-reactivity to others often occurs.

II. **Toxic dose.** The ACGIH-recommended workplace limit (threshold limit value—short-term exposure limit; TLV-STEL) and the OSHA limit (permissible exposure limit-ceiling; PEL-C) for TDI are both 0.02 ppm (0.14 mg/m$^3$). The ACGIH recommended 8-hour TLV-time weighted average (TWA) is considerable lower at 0.005 ppm (0.036 mg/m$^3$). These exposure limits prevent acute irritant effects. In individuals with prior TDI sensitivity, however, even this level may induce asthma responses. The level considered immediately dangerous to life or health (IDLH) is 2.5 ppm. Other isocyanates (eg, MDI, hexamethylene diisocyanate [HDI]) are less volatile, but overexposure can occur from inhalation of spray aerosols and, potentially, through direct skin contact. The ACGIH TLV-TWA values for MDI and HDI are the same as those for TDI.

III. **Clinical presentation**

A. **Acute exposure** to irritant levels causes skin and upper respiratory tract toxicity. Burning eyes and skin, cough, and wheezing are common. Noncardiogenic pulmonary edema may occur with severe exposure. Symptoms may occur immediately with exposure or may occasionally be delayed several hours.

B. **Low-level chronic exposure** may produce dyspnea, wheezing, and other signs and symptoms consistent with asthma. Interstitial lung responses, with radiographic infiltrates and hypoxemia, may occur less commonly.

IV. **Diagnosis** requires a careful occupational history. Pulmonary function testing may document an obstructive deficit or may be normal. Variable airflow or changing measures of airway reactivity (methacholine or histamine challenge) temporally linked to exposure strongly support the diagnosis of isocyanate-induced asthma.

A. **Specific levels.** There are no clinical blood or urine tests for isocyanates.

1. Test inhalation challenge to isocyanate is not advised except in experienced laboratories owing to the danger of severe asthma attack.
2. Isocyanate antibody testing, although used in research, is difficult to interpret in an individual patient and may not correlate with non-IgE responses.

B. **Other useful laboratory studies** include arterial blood gases or oximetry, chest x-ray, and pulmonary function tests.

V. **Treatment**

A. **Emergency and supportive measures**

1. After acute high-intensity inhalational exposure, maintain an open airway (see pp 1–4), give bronchodilators as needed for wheezing (p 7), and observe for 8–12 hours for pulmonary edema (p 7).

2. Once airway hyperreactivity has been documented, further exposure to isocyanate is contraindicated. Involve public health or OSHA agencies to determine whether other workers are at increased risk through improper workplace controls.

B. **Specific drugs and antidotes.** There is no specific antidote.

C. **Decontamination** after high-level exposure (see p 45)

1. **Inhalation.** Remove the victim from exposure and give supplemental oxygen if available.
2. **Skin and eyes.** Remove contaminated clothing (liquid or heavy vapor exposure) and wash exposed skin with copious soap and water. Irrigate exposed eyes with saline or tepid water.

D. **Enhanced elimination.** There is no role for these procedures.

## ▶ ISONIAZID (INH)

*Andrew Erdman, MD*

Isoniazid (INH), a hydrazide derivative of isonicotinic acid, is the bactericidal drug of choice for tuberculosis. INH is well known for its propensity to cause hepatitis with chronic use. Acute isoniazid overdose is a common cause of drug-induced seizures and metabolic acidosis.

I. **Mechanism of toxicity**

A. **Acute overdose.** Isoniazid produces acute toxic effects by reducing brain pyridoxal 5-phosphate, which is the active form of vitamin $B_6$ and is an essential cofactor for the enzyme glutamic acid decarboxylase. This results in lower CNS levels of gamma-aminobutyric acid (GABA), an inhibitory neurotransmitter, which leads to uninhibited electrical activity manifested as seizures. INH may also inhibit the hepatic conversion of lactate to pyruvate, exacerbating the lactic acidosis from seizures.

B. **Chronic toxicity.** Peripheral neuritis with chronic use is thought to be related to competition with pyridoxine. The mechanism of chronic hepatic injury and INH-induced systemic lupus erythematosus (SLE) is not discussed here.

C. **Pharmacokinetics.** Peak absorption occurs in 1–2 hours. The volume of distribution is 0.6–0.7 L/kg. Elimination is by hepatic metabolism; the half-life is 0.5–1.6 hours in fast acetylators and 2–5 hours in slow acetylators. See also Table II–59.

II. **Toxic dose**

A. **Acute ingestion** of as little as 15–40 mg/kg can produce toxicity. Severe toxicity is common after ingestion of 80–150 mg/kg.

B. With **chronic use,** 10–20% of patients will develop hepatic toxicity when the dose is 10 mg/kg/day, but less than 2% will develop this toxicity if the dose is 3–5 mg/kg/day. Older persons are more susceptible to chronic toxicity.

III. **Clinical presentation**

A. After **acute overdose,** nausea, vomiting, slurred speech, ataxia, depressed sensorium, coma, respiratory depression, and seizures may occur rapidly (usually within 30–120 minutes). Profound anion gap metabolic acidosis (pH 6.8–6.9) often occurs after only one or two seizures, probably owing to muscle release of lactic acid. This usually clears slowly even after the seizure activity is controlled. Liver injury may occur after an acute overdose and may be delayed up to several days. Hemolysis may occur in patients with G6PD deficiency. Rhabdomyolysis can be a complication of recurrent seizures.

B. **Chronic therapeutic** INH use may cause peripheral neuritis, hepatitis, hypersensitivity reactions including drug-induced lupus erythematosus, and pyridoxine deficiency.

IV. **Diagnosis** usually is made by history and clinical presentation. INH toxicity should be considered in any patient with acute-onset seizures, especially if they are unresponsive to routine anticonvulsant medications and if accompanied by profound metabolic acidosis.

**A. Specific levels.** Isoniazid usually is not detected in routine toxicology screening. Specific levels may be obtained but are rarely available or helpful for management of acute overdoses. A 5 mg/kg dose produces a peak INH concentration of 3 mg/L at 1 hour (1–7 mg/L is considered antitubercular). Serum levels higher than 30 mg/L are associated with acute toxicity.

**B. Other useful laboratory studies** include electrolytes, glucose, BUN, creatinine, liver function tests, creatine phosphokinase, and arterial blood gases.

**V. Treatment**

**A. Emergency and supportive measures**

1. Maintain an open airway and assist ventilation if necessary (see pp 1–7).
2. Treat coma (see p 18), seizures (p 22), and metabolic acidosis (p 33) if they occur. Administer diazepam, 0.1–0.2 mg/kg IV, for treatment of seizures.

**B. Specific drugs and antidotes. Pyridoxine** (vitamin $B_6$) is a specific antidote and usually terminates diazepam-resistant seizures and results in improved mental status. Administer at least 5 g IV (see p 508) if the amount of INH ingested is not known; if the amount is known, give an equivalent amount in grams of pyridoxine to grams of ingested INH. Concomitant treatment with diazepam may improve the outcome. If no pyridoxine is available, high-dose diazepam (0.3–0.4 mg/kg) may be effective for status epilepticus. Pyridoxine treatment may also hasten the resolution of metabolic acidosis.

**C. Decontamination** (see p 45). Administer activated charcoal orally if conditions are appropriate (see Table I–38, p 51). Consider gastric lavage for massive ingestions.

**D. Enhanced elimination.** Forced diuresis and hemodialysis have been reported to be successful but are unnecessary for most cases, because the half-life of INH is relatively short (1–5 hours, depending on acetylator status), and toxicity usually can be easily managed with pyridoxine and diazepam. Symptoms generally resolve over a course of 8–24 hours.

## ► ISOPROPYL ALCOHOL

*Michael J. Matteucci, MD*

Isopropyl alcohol is used widely as a solvent, an antiseptic, and a disinfectant and is commonly available in the home as a 70% solution (rubbing alcohol). It is often ingested by alcoholics as a cheap substitute for liquor. Unlike the other common alcohol substitutes methanol and ethylene glycol, isopropyl alcohol is not metabolized to highly toxic organic acids and therefore does not produce a profound anion gap acidosis. Hospitals sometimes color isopropyl alcohol with blue dye to distinguish it from other clear liquids; this has led abusers to refer to it as "blue heaven."

**I. Mechanism of toxicity**

**A.** Isopropyl alcohol is a potent depressant of the CNS, and intoxication by ingestion or inhalation may result in coma and respiratory arrest. It is metabolized to acetone (dimethyl ketone), which may contribute to and prolong CNS depression.

**B.** Very large doses of isopropyl alcohol may cause hypotension secondary to vasodilation and possibly myocardial depression.

**C.** Isopropyl alcohol is irritating to the GI tract and commonly causes gastritis.

**D. Pharmacokinetics.** Isopropyl alcohol is well absorbed within 2 hours and quickly distributes into body water (volume of distribution 0.6 L/kg). It is metabolized (half-life 3-7 hours) by alcohol dehydrogenase to acetone.

**II. Toxic dose.** Isopropyl alcohol is an approximately two- to threefold more potent CNS depressant than ethanol.

A. **Ingestion.** The toxic oral dose is about 0.5–1 mL/kg of rubbing alcohol (70% isopropyl alcohol) but varies depending on individual tolerance and whether any other depressants were ingested. Fatalities have occurred after adult ingestion of 240 mL, but patients with up to 1-L ingestions have recovered with supportive care.

B. **Inhalation.** The odor of isopropyl alcohol can be detected at an air level of 40–200 ppm. The recommended workplace limit (ACGIH TLV-TWA) is 400 ppm (983 mg/$m^3$) as an 8-hour time-weighted average. The air level considered immediately dangerous to life or health (IDLH) is 2000 ppm. Toxicity has been reported in children after isopropyl alcohol sponge baths, probably as a result of inhalation rather than skin absorption.

III. **Clinical presentation.** Intoxication mimics drunkenness from ethanol, with slurred speech, ataxia, and stupor followed in large ingestions by coma, hypotension, and respiratory arrest.

A. Because of the gastric irritant properties of isopropyl alcohol, abdominal pain and vomiting are common, and hematemesis occasionally occurs.

B. Metabolic acidosis may occur but is usually mild. The osmolar gap is usually elevated (see p 33).

C. Isopropyl alcohol is metabolized to **acetone,** which contributes to CNS depression and gives a distinct odor to the breath (in contrast, methanol and ethylene glycol and their toxic metabolites are odorless). Acetone is also found in nail polish remover and is used widely as a solvent in industry and chemical laboratories.

IV. **Diagnosis** usually is based on a history of ingestion and the presence of an elevated osmolar gap, the absence of severe acidosis, and the characteristic smell of isopropyl alcohol or its metabolite, acetone. Ketonemia and ketonuria may be present within 1–3 hours of ingestion.

A. **Specific levels.** Serum isopropyl alcohol and acetone levels are usually available from commercial toxicology laboratories. The serum level may also be estimated by calculating the osmolar gap (see Table I–22, p 32). Isopropyl alcohol levels higher than 150 mg/dL usually cause coma, but patients with levels up to 560 mg/dL have survived with supportive care and dialysis. Serum acetone concentrations may be elevated.

B. **Other useful laboratory studies** include electrolytes, glucose, BUN, creatinine, serum osmolality and osmolar gap, and arterial blood gases or oximetry.

V. **Treatment**

A. **Emergency and supportive measures**

1. Maintain an open airway and assist ventilation if necessary (see pp 1–4). Administer supplemental oxygen.
2. Treat coma (see p 18), hypotension (p 15), and hypoglycemia (p 34) if they occur.
3. Admit and observe symptomatic patients for at least 6–12 hours.

B. **Specific drugs and antidotes.** There is no specific antidote. Ethanol therapy is ***not*** indicated because isopropyl alcohol does not produce a toxic organic acid metabolite.

C. **Decontamination** (see p 45). Because isopropyl alcohol is absorbed rapidly after ingestion, gastric emptying procedures are not likely to be useful if the ingestion is small (a swallow or two) or if more than 30 minutes has passed. For large, recent ingestion, consider performing aspiration of gastric contents with a small flexible tube.

D. **Enhanced elimination**

1. **Hemodialysis** effectively removes isopropyl alcohol and acetone but is rarely indicated because the majority of patients can be managed with supportive care alone. Dialysis should be considered when levels are extremely high (eg, > 500–600 mg/dL), if hypotension does not respond to fluids and vasopressors, and in acute renal failure.
2. Hemoperfusion, repeat-dose charcoal, and forced diuresis are not effective.

# ▶ JELLYFISH AND OTHER CNIDARIA

*Susan Kim, PharmD*

The large phylum Cnidaria (coelenterates), numbering about 5000 species, includes **fire coral, Portuguese man-o-war, box jellyfish, sea nettle,** and **anemones.** Despite considerable morphologic variation, all these organisms have venom contained in microscopic structures like water balloons, called nematocysts.

I. **Mechanism of toxicity.** Each nematocyst contains a small ejectable thread soaking in viscous venom. The thread has a barb on the tip and is fired from the nematocyst with enough velocity to pierce human skin. The nematocysts are contained in outer sacs (cnidoblasts) arranged along the tentacles of jellyfish or along the surface of fire coral and the finger-like projections of sea anemones. When the cnidoblasts are opened by hydrostatic pressure, physical contact, changes in osmolarity, or chemical stimulants that have not been identified, they release their nematocysts, which eject the thread and spread venom into the skin of the victim. The venom contains numerous chemical components, including neuromuscular toxins, cardiotoxins, hemolysins, dermonecrotoxins, and histamine-like compounds.

II. **Toxic dose.** Each time a nematocyst is opened, all the contained venom is released. The degree of effect depends on the particular species, the number of nematocysts that successfully discharge venom, the envenomation site, contact time, and individual patient sensitivity (especially in children). Hundreds of thousands of nematocysts may be discharged with a single exposure.

   A. Deaths from jellyfish stings in the Northern Hemisphere are rare and almost always are due to the **Portuguese man-o-war** (*Physalia* sp), though *Chiropsalmus quadrumanus* (a type of box jellyfish) was implicated in the death of a child off the coast of Texas.

   B. The **Australian box jellyfish** (*Chironex fleckeri,* "sea wasp") is the most venomous marine animal and is responsible for numerous fatalities. It should not be confused with the Hawaiian box jellyfish (*Carybdea alata*).

III. **Clinical presentation**

   A. **Acute effects**

      1. Stinging produces immediate burning pain, pruritis, papular lesions, and local tissue inflammation, which may progress to pustules and desquamation.
      2. Nausea, vertigo, dizziness, muscle cramping, myalgia, arthralgia, anaphylactoid reaction, and transient elevation in liver transaminases may follow.
      3. Severe envenomation may result in respiratory distress, severe muscle cramping with hypotension, arrhythmias, shock, and pulmonary edema. Lethal outcomes are associated with rapid onset of cardiovascular collapse. Fulminant hepatic failure and renal failure have been reported after sea anemone stings.
      4. "Irukandji syndrome," which is associated with *Carukia barnesi* jellyfish from Australia and Hawaii, has been reported to cause pulmonary edema and fatal cardiac injury.

   B. **Potential sequelae** include skin necrosis, infections, cosmetic tissue damage (fat atrophy and hyperpigmentation), contractures, paresthesias, neuritis, recurrent cutaneous eruptions, paralysis, and regional vasospasm with vascular insufficiency.

   C. **Corneal stings** from the sea nettle are usually painful but resolve within 1–2 days. However, there are reports of prolonged iritis, elevated intraocular pressure, mydriasis, and decreased visual acuity lasting months to years.

IV. **Diagnosis** is based on the history and observation of characteristic lines of inflammation along the sites of exposure ("tentacle tracks").

   A. **Specific levels.** Specific toxin levels are not available.

   B. **Other useful laboratory studies** include CBC, electrolytes, glucose, BUN, creatinine, CPK, liver transaminases, and urinalysis for hemoglobin.

**V. Treatment.** Symptomatic care is sufficient for the majority of envenomations, even that of the box jellyfish.

**A. Emergency and supportive measures**

1. Maintain an open airway and assist ventilation if necessary (see pp 1–7). Administer supplemental oxygen.
2. Treat hypotension (see p 15), arrhythmias (pp 10–15), coma (p 18), and seizures (p 22) if they occur.

**B. Specific drugs and antidotes.** Box jellyfish *(Chironex fleckeri)* antivenin from Australia terminates acute pain and cardiovascular symptoms, prevents tissue effects, and may be located by a regional poison control center (in the United States, [800] 222-1222) for use in severe cases. Local marine biologists can help identify indigenous species for the planning of specific therapy.

**C. Decontamination.** Avoid thrashing about, scratching, scraping, or other mechanical maneuvers that may break open the nematocysts. Without touching the affected areas, wash them with cold sea or salt water. ***Do not use fresh water*** because it may cause nematocysts to discharge.

1. **For most cnidarian envenomations** (including the box jellyfish), experts recommend spraying, soaking, or flooding the affected area with **vinegar** for 30 minutes to disarm nematocysts. Other remedies for neutralizing nematocysts include rubbing alcohol, household ammonia (diluted 1:10), and a slurry of meat tenderizer or baking soda. (One report even recommended urinating on the area if these agents are not available.) ***Note:*** None of these remedies relieves the pain of already discharged nematocysts and may actually worsen it.
2. However, for *Chrysaora quinquecirrha* (American sea nettle), *Pelagia noctiluca* (little mauve stinger jellyfish), and *Cyanea captillata* (hair or "lion's mane" jellyfish), ***do not apply vinegar*** because it may precipitate firing in these species.
3. To remove nematocysts, apply a slurry of baking soda or flour and then shave the area with the dull edge of a knife or remove the nematocyst manually, using doubled-gloved hands or forceps. Afterward, cool compresses may be applied for pain relief.

**D. Enhanced elimination.** These procedures are not applicable.

## ▶ LEAD

*Michael J. Kosnett, MD, MPH*

Lead is a soft, malleable metal that is obtained chiefly by the primary smelting and refining of natural ores or by the widespread practice of recycling and secondary smelting of scrap lead products. Recycling accounts for nearly 85% of domestic lead consumption, approximately 85% of which is used in the manufacture of lead acid batteries. Lead is used for weights and radiation shielding, and lead alloys are used in the manufacture of pipes; cable sheathing; brass, bronze, and steel; ammunition; and solder (predominantly electrical devices and automotive radiators). Lead compounds are added as pigments, stabilizers, or binders in paints, ceramics, glass, and plastic.

Although the use of lead in house paint has been curtailed since the 1970s, industrial use of corrosion-resistant lead-based paint continues, and high-level exposure may result from renovation, sandblasting, torching, or demolition. Young children are particularly at risk from repeated ingestion of lead-contaminated house dust, yard soil, or paint chips or from mouthing toy jewelry or other decorative items containing lead. Children may also be exposed to lead carried into the home on contaminated work clothes worn by adults.

Lead exposure may occur from the use of lead-glazed ceramics or containers for food or beverage preparation or storage. Certain folk medicines (eg, the Mexican remedies *azarcon* and *greta,* the Dominican remedy *litargirio*, and some Indian Ayurvedic preparations) may contain high amounts of lead salts.

**I. Mechanism of toxicity**

**A.** The multisystem toxicity of lead is mediated by several mechanisms, including inactivation or alteration of enzymes and other macromolecules by binding to sulfhydryl, phosphate, or carboxyl ligands and interaction with essential cations, most notably calcium, zinc, and iron. Pathologic alterations in cellular and mitochondrial membranes, neurotransmitter synthesis and function, heme synthesis, cellular redox status, and nucleotide metabolism may occur. Adverse impacts on the nervous, renal, GI, hematopoietic, reproductive, and cardiovascular systems can result.

**B. Pharmacokinetics.** Inhalation of lead fume or other fine, soluble particulate results in rapid and extensive pulmonary absorption, the major though not exclusive route of exposure in industry. Nonindustrial exposure occurs predominantly by ingestion, particularly in children, who absorb 45–50% of soluble lead compared with approximately 10–15% in adults. After absorption, lead is distributed via the blood (where 99% is bound to the erythrocyte) to multiple tissues, including transplacental transport to the fetus, and CNS transport across the blood-brain barrier. Clearance of lead from the body follows a multicompartment kinetic model, consisting of "fast" compartments in the blood and soft tissues (half-life of 1 to 2 months) and slow compartments in the bone (half-life of years to decades). Approximately 70% of lead excretion occurs via the urine, with smaller amounts eliminated via the feces and scant amounts via the hair, nails, and sweat. Greater than 90% of the lead burden in adults and more than two-thirds of the burden in young children occur in the skeleton. Slow redistribution of lead from bone to soft tissues may elevate blood lead concentrations for months to years after a patient with chronic high-dose exposure has been removed from external sources. In patients with high bone lead burden, pathologic states associated with rapid bone turnover or demineralization, such as hyperthyroidism and immobilization osteoporosis, have resulted in symptomatic lead intoxication.

**II. Toxic dose**

**A. Dermal** absorption is minimal with inorganic lead but may be substantial with organic lead compounds, which may also cause skin irritation.

**B. Ingestion.** In general, absorption of lead compounds is directly proportional to solubility and inversely proportional to particle size. Gastrointestinal lead absorption is increased by iron deficiency and low dietary calcium and decreased by co-ingestion with food.

1. Acute symptomatic intoxication is rare after a single exposure but may occur within hours after ingestion of gram quantities of soluble lead compounds or days after GI retention of swallowed lead objects, such as fishing weights and curtain weights.
2. Studies have not established a low-dose threshold for adverse subclinical effects of lead. Recent epidemiologic studies in children have observed effects of lead on cognitive function at blood lead concentrations less than 5 mcg/dL, and other studies suggest that background levels of lead exposure in recent decades may have been associated with hypertension in some adults. The geometric mean blood lead concentration in the United States during 2001–2002 was estimated to be 1.45 mcg/dL; background dietary lead intake may be in the range of 1–4 mcg per day.
3. The US Environmental Protection Agency action level for lead in drinking water is 15 ppb (parts per billion). However, the Maximum Contaminant Level (MCL) goal for drinking water is zero ppb, and EPA has set no "reference dose" for lead because of the lack of a recognized low-dose threshold for adverse effects.

**C. Inhalation.** Unprotected exposure to the massive airborne lead levels (> 2500 mcg/m$^3$) encountered during abrasive blasting, welding, or torch cutting metal surfaces coated with lead-based paint poses an acute hazard and has resulted in symptomatic lead intoxication from within a day to a few weeks. The OSHA workplace permissible exposure limit (PEL) for inorganic lead dusts and fumes is 50 mcg/$m^3$ as an 8-hour time-weighted average. The level considered immediately dangerous to life or health (IDLH) is 100 mg/$m^3$.

**III. Clinical presentation.** The multisystem toxicity of lead presents a spectrum of clinical findings ranging from overt, life-threatening intoxication to subtle, subclinical effects.

**A. Acute ingestion** of very large amounts of lead (gram quantities) may cause abdominal pain, anemia (usually hemolytic), toxic hepatitis, and encephalopathy.

**B. Subacute or chronic exposure** is more common than acute poisoning.

1. **Constitutional** effects include fatigue, malaise, irritability, anorexia, insomnia, weight loss, decreased libido, arthralgias, and myalgias. Hypertension may be associated with lead exposure in susceptible populations.
2. **Gastrointestinal** effects include crampy abdominal pain (lead colic), nausea, constipation, or (less commonly) diarrhea.
3. **Central nervous system** manifestations range from impaired concentration, headache, diminished visual-motor coordination, and tremor to overt encephalopathy (a life-threatening emergency characterized by agitated delirium or lethargy, ataxia, convulsions, and coma). Chronic low-level exposure in infants and children may lead to decreased intelligence and impaired neurobehavioral development, stunted growth, and diminished auditory acuity. Recent studies in adults suggest that lead may accentuate age-related decline in cognitive function.
4. **Peripheral motor neuropathy,** affecting mainly the upper extremities, can cause severe extensor muscle weakness ("wrist drop").
5. **Hematologic** effects include normochromic or microcytic anemia, which may be accompanied by basophilic stippling. Hemolysis may occur after acute or subacute high-dose exposure.
6. **Nephrotoxic** effects include reversible acute tubular dysfunction (including Fanconi-like aminoaciduria in children) and chronic interstitial fibrosis. Hyperuricemia and gout may occur.
7. **Adverse reproductive outcomes** may include diminished or aberrant sperm production, increased rate of miscarriage, preterm delivery, decreased gestational age, low birth weight, and impaired neurologic development.

**C. Repeated, intentional inhalation of leaded gasoline** has resulted in ataxia, myoclonic jerking, hyperreflexia, delirium, and convulsions.

**IV. Diagnosis.** Although overt encephalopathy or abdominal colic associated with a suspect activity may readily suggest the diagnosis of severe lead poisoning, the nonspecific symptoms and multisystem signs associated with mild or moderate intoxication may be mistaken for a viral illness or another disorder. Consider lead poisoning in any patient with multisystem findings including abdominal pain, headache, and anemia and, less commonly, motor neuropathy, gout, and renal insufficiency. Consider lead encephalopathy in any child or adult with delirium or convulsions (especially with coexistent anemia) and chronic lead poisoning in any child with neurobehavioral deficits or developmental delays.

**A. Specific levels.** The **whole-blood lead** level is the most useful indicator of lead exposure. Relationships between blood lead levels and clinical findings generally have been based on subacute or chronic exposure and not on transiently high values that may result immediately after acute exposure. In addition, there may be considerable interindividual variability. ***Note:*** *Blood lead samples must be drawn and stored in lead-free syringes and tubes* ("trace metals" tube or royal blue stopper tube containing heparin or EDTA).

1. Blood lead levels are less than 5 mcg/dL in populations without occupational or specific environmental exposure. Levels between 5 (or lower)

and 25 mcg/dL have been associated with subclinical decreases in intelligence and impaired neurobehavioral development in children exposed in utero or in early childhood. Studies in adults suggest that long-term blood lead concentrations in the range of 10–25 mcg/dL may pose a risk for hypertension and might possibly contribute to age-related decline in cognitive function.

2. Blood lead levels of 25–60 mcg/dL may be associated with headache, irritability, difficulty concentrating, slowed reaction time, and other neuropsychiatric effects. Anemia may occur, and subclinical slowing of motor nerve conduction may be detectable.
3. Blood levels of 60–80 mcg/dL may be associated with GI symptoms and subclinical renal effects.
4. With blood levels in excess of 80 mcg/dL, serious overt intoxication may occur, including abdominal pain (lead colic) and nephropathy. Encephalopathy and neuropathy usually are associated with levels over 100 mcg/dL.

B. Elevations in **free erythrocyte protoporphyrin (FEP) or zinc protoporphyrin (ZPP)** (> 35 mcg/dL) reflect lead-induced inhibition of heme synthesis. Because only actively forming and not mature erythrocytes are affected, elevations typically lag lead exposure by a few weeks. High blood lead in the presence of a normal FEP or ZPP therefore suggests very recent exposure. Protoporphyrin elevation is not specific for lead and may also occur with iron deficiency. Protoporphyrin levels are not sensitive for low-level exposure (blood lead < 30 mcg/dL).

C. **Urinary lead excretion** increases and decreases more rapidly than blood lead. In the CDC's Third National Report on Human Exposure to Environmental Chemicals, the geometric mean urinary lead concentration of subjects age 6 and older was 0.7 mcg/L. Normal, baseline urinary lead excretion for the general population is less than 10 mcg/day. Several empiric protocols that measure 6- or 24-hour urinary lead excretion after calcium EDTA challenge have been developed to identify persons with elevated body lead burdens. However, since chelatable lead predominantly reflects lead in soft tissues, which in most cases already correlates satisfactorily with blood lead, chelation challenges are seldom indicated in clinical practice.

D. Noninvasive in vivo **x-ray fluorescence measurement of lead in bone,** a test predominantly available in research settings, may provide the best index of long-term cumulative lead exposure and total body lead burden.

E. **Other tests.** Nonspecific laboratory findings that support the diagnosis of lead poisoning include anemia (normocytic or microcytic) and basophilic stippling of erythrocytes, a useful but insensitive clue. Acute high-dose exposure sometimes may be associated with transient azotemia (elevated BUN and serum creatinine) and mild to moderate elevation in serum transaminases. Recently ingested lead paint, glazes, chips, or solid lead objects may be visible on abdominal x-rays. CT or MRI of the brain often reveals cerebral edema in patients with lead encephalopathy. Because iron deficiency increases lead absorption, iron status should be evaluated.

**V. Treatment**

**A. Emergency and supportive measures**

1. Treat seizures (see p 22) and coma (p 18) if they occur. Provide adequate fluids to maintain urine flow (optimally 1–2 mL/kg/h) but avoid overhydration, which may aggravate cerebral edema. Avoid phenothiazines for delirium, as they may lower the seizure threshold.
2. Patients with increased intracranial pressure may benefit from corticosteroids (eg, dexamethasone, 10 mg IV) and mannitol (0.25–1.0 g/kg IV as a 20–25% solution).

B. **Specific drugs and antidotes.** Treatment with chelating agents decreases blood lead concentrations and increases urinary lead excretion. Although chelation has been associated with improvement in symptoms and decreased mortality, controlled clinical trials demonstrating efficacy are lacking, and *treatment recommendations have been largely empiric.*

1. **Encephalopathy.** Administer intravenous **calcium EDTA** (see p 446). Some clinicians initiate treatment with a single dose of **BAL** (p 417), followed 4 hours later by concomitant administration of calcium EDTA and BAL.
2. **Symptomatic without encephalopathy.** Administer oral **succimer** (DMSA, p 510) or parenteral **calcium EDTA** (p 446). Calcium EDTA is preferred as initial treatment if the patient has severe GI toxicity (eg, lead colic) or if the blood lead concentration is extremely elevated (eg, > 150 mcg/dL). **Unithiol** (p 515) may be considered as an alternative to DMSA.
3. **Asymptomatic children with elevated blood lead levels.** The Centers for Disease Control and Prevention (CDC) recommend treatment of children with levels of 45 mcg/dL or higher. Use oral **succimer** (DMSA, p 510). A large randomized, double-blind, placebo-controlled trial of DMSA in children with blood lead concentrations between 25 and 44 mcg/dL found no evidence of clinical benefit.
4. **Asymptomatic adults.** The usual treatment is removal from exposure and observation. Consider oral **succimer** (DMSA, p 510) for patients with markedly elevated levels (eg, > 80–100 mcg/dL).
5. Although **D-penicillamine** (see p 491) is an alternative oral treatment, it may be associated with more side effects and less efficient lead diuresis.
6. **Blood lead monitoring during chelation.** Obtain a blood lead measurement immediately prior to chelation and recheck the measurement within 24–48 hours after starting chelation to confirm that levels are declining. Recheck measurements 1 and 7 to 21 days after chelation to assess the extent of rebound in blood lead level associated with redistribution of lead from high bone stores and/or the possibility of reexposure. Additional courses of treatment and further investigation of exposure sources may be warranted.

**C. Decontamination** (see p 45)

1. **Acute ingestion.** Because even small items (eg, a paint chip or a sip of lead-containing glaze) may contain tens to hundreds of milligrams of lead, gut decontamination is indicated after acute ingestion of virtually any lead-containing substance.
   - **a.** Administer activated charcoal (although efficacy is unknown).
   - **b.** If lead-containing material is still visible on abdominal x-ray after initial treatment, consider whole-bowel irrigation (see p 51).
   - **c.** Consider endoscopic or surgical removal of lead foreign bodies that exhibit prolonged GI retention.
2. **Lead-containing buckshot, shrapnel, or bullets** in or adjacent to synovial spaces or fluid-filled spaces such as a paravertebral pseudocyst or a subscapular bursa should be surgically removed if possible, particularly if associated with evidence of systemic lead absorption.

**D. Enhanced elimination.** There is no role for dialysis, hemoperfusion, or repeat-dose charcoal. However, in anuric patients with chronic renal failure, limited study suggests that calcium EDTA combined with hemofiltration may increase lead clearance.

**E. Other required measures.** Remove the patient from the source of exposure and institute control measures to prevent repeated intoxication. Other possibly exposed persons (eg, coworkers or siblings or playmates of young children) should be evaluated promptly.

1. **Infants and children.** The CDC has recommended universal blood lead screening of children at 12 and 24 months of age in communities where > 27% of dwellings were constructed prior to 1950. For other communities, screening targeted to children from families with low income or other se-

lected risk factors is recommended. General management guidelines are based on the results of the blood lead test:

**a.** 10–14 mcg/dL: repeat screening; educate parents about risk factors.

**b.** 15–19 mcg/dL: repeat screening, and if elevated, refer for public health case management to investigate and abate sources.

**c.** 20–44 mcg/dL: perform complete medical evaluation; refer for case management.

**d.** 45–69 mcg/dL: perform complete medical evaluation; chelate with oral succimer; refer for case management.

**e.** 70 mcg/dL or higher: hospitalize child for immediate chelation; refer for case management.

**f.** Detailed guidelines for case management of children with elevated blood lead levels are found at the CDC website: www.cdc.gov/nceh/lead/CaseManagement/caseManage_main.htm.

**2. Adults with occupational exposure**

**a.** Federal OSHA standards for workers exposed to lead provide specific guidelines for periodic blood lead monitoring and medical surveillance (see www.osha-slc.gov/OshStd_toc/OSHA_Std_toc_1910.html). Under the general industry standard, workers must be removed from exposure if a single blood lead level exceeds 60 mcg/dL or if the average of three successive levels exceeds 50 mcg/dL. In construction workers, removal is required if a single blood lead level exceeds 50 mcg/dL. Workers may not return to work until the blood lead level is below 40 mcg/dL and any clinical manifestations of toxicity have resolved. Prophylactic chelation is prohibited. OSHA standards mandate that workers removed from work because of elevated blood lead levels retain full pay and benefits.

**b.** Medical removal parameters in the OSHA standards summarized above were established in the late 1970s and are outdated based on current background blood levels and recent concern about the hazards of lower-level exposure. The standards explicitly empower physicians to order medical removal at lower blood lead levels. It may now be prudent and feasible for employers to maintain workers' blood lead levels below 20 mcg/dL and possibly below 10 mcg/dL. In 2005, the Association of Occupational and Environmental Clinics (www.aoec.org) approved "Medical Management Guidelines for Lead-Exposed Adults" that call for worker protection more stringent than current OSHA standards.

Centers for Disease Control and Prevention. Preventing Lead Poisoning in Young Children. Atlanta: CDC, 2005. [www.cdc.gov/nceh/lead/Publications/PrevLeadPoisoning.pdf] (The latest statement by the CDC maintains 10 mcg/dL as a blood lead level of concern but acknowledges impacts at lower levels and calls for primary prevention).

## ▶ LIONFISH AND OTHER SCORPAENIDAE

*Richard F. Clark, MD*

The family Scorpaenidae are saltwater fish that are mostly bottom dwellers that are noted for their ability to camouflage themselves and disappear into the environment. There are 30 genera and about 300 species, some 30 of which can envenomate humans. Although they once were considered an occupational hazard only of commercial fishing, increasing contact with these fish by scuba divers and home aquarists has increased the frequency of envenomations.

**I. Mechanism of toxicity.** Envenomation usually occurs when the fish is being handled or stepped on or when the aquarist has hands in the tank. The dorsal, anal, and pectoral fins are supported by spines that are connected to venom glands. The fish will erect its spines and jab the victim, causing release of venom (and often sloughing of the integumentary sheath of the spine into the wound). The venom of all these organisms is a heat-labile mixture that is not completely characterized.

**II. Toxic dose.** The dose of venom involved in any sting is variable. Interspecies difference in the severity of envenomation is generally the result of the relation between the venom gland and the spines.

- **A.** ***Synanceja*** (Australian stonefish) have short, strong spines with the venom gland located near the tip; therefore, large doses of venom are delivered, and severe envenomation results.
- **B. Pterois** (lionfish, turkeyfish) have long delicate spines with poorly developed venom glands near the base of the spine and therefore are usually capable of delivering only small doses of venom.

**III. Clinical presentation.** Envenomation typically produces immediate onset of excruciating, sharp, throbbing, intense pain. In untreated cases, the intensity of pain peaks at 60–90 minutes and the pain may last for 1–2 days.

- **A. Systemic intoxication** associated with stonefish envenomation can include the rapid onset of hypotension, tachycardia, cardiac arrhythmias, myocardial ischemia, syncope, diaphoresis, nausea, vomiting, abdominal cramping, dyspnea, pulmonary edema, cyanosis, headache, muscular weakness, and spasticity.
- **B. Local tissue effects** include erythema, ecchymosis, and swelling. Infection may occur owing to retained portions of integumentary sheath. Hyperalgesia, anesthesia, or paresthesias of the affected extremity may occur, and persistent neuropathy has been reported.

**IV. Diagnosis** usually is based on a history of exposure, and the severity of envenomation is usually readily apparent.

- **A. Specific levels.** There are no specific toxin levels available.
- **B. Other useful laboratory studies** for severe intoxication include electrolytes, glucose, BUN, creatinine, CPK, urinalysis, ECG monitoring, and chest x-ray.

**V. Treatment**

- **A. Emergency and supportive measures**
  - **1.** After severe stonefish envenomation:
    - **a.** Maintain an open airway and assist ventilation if needed (see pp 1–7). Administer supplemental oxygen.
    - **b.** Treat hypotension (see p 15) and arrhythmias (pp 10–15) if they occur.
  - **2.** General wound care:
    - **a.** Clean the wound carefully and remove any visible integumentary sheath. Monitor wounds for development of infection.
    - **b.** Give tetanus prophylaxis if needed.
- **B. Specific drugs and antidotes.** Immediately immerse the extremity in **hot water** (45°C [113°F]) for 30–60 minutes. This should result in prompt relief of pain within several minutes. For stonefish envenomations, a specific antivenin can be located by a regional poison control center (in the United States, [800] 222-1222), but most of these cases can be managed successfully with hot water immersion and supportive symptomatic care.
- **C. Decontamination** procedures are not applicable.
- **D. Enhanced elimination.** There is no role for these procedures.

## ► LITHIUM

*Timothy J. Wiegand, MD, and Neal L. Benowitz, MD*

Lithium is used for the treatment of bipolar depression and other psychiatric disorders and occasionally to raise the white blood cell count in patients with leukopenia. Serious toxicity is caused most commonly by chronic overmedication in patients with renal impairment. Acute overdose, in contrast, is generally less severe.

**I. Mechanism of toxicity**

**A.** Lithium is a cation that enters cells and substitutes for sodium or potassium. Lithium is thought to stabilize cell membranes. With excessive levels, it depresses neural excitation and synaptic transmission.

**B. Pharmacokinetics.** Lithium is completely absorbed within 6–8 hours of ingestion. The initial volume of distribution (Vd) is about 0.5 L/kg, with slow entry into tissues and a final Vd of 0.7–1.4 L/kg. Entry into the brain is slow; this explains the delay between peak blood levels and CNS effects after an acute overdose. Elimination is virtually entirely by the kidney, with a half-life of 14–30 hours.

**II. Toxic dose.** The usual daily dose of lithium ranges from 300 to 2400 mg (8–64 mEq/day), and the therapeutic serum lithium level is 0.6–1.2 mEq/L. The toxicity of lithium depends on whether the overdose is acute or chronic.

**A. Acute ingestion** of 1 mEq/kg (40 mg/kg) will produce a blood level after tissue equilibration of approximately 1.2 mEq/L. Acute ingestion of more than 20–30 tablets by an adult potentially could cause serious toxicity.

**B. Chronic intoxication** may occur in patients on stable therapeutic doses. Lithium is excreted by the kidney, where it is handled like sodium; any state that causes dehydration, sodium depletion, or excessive sodium reabsorption may lead to increased lithium reabsorption, accumulation, and possibly intoxication. Common states causing lithium retention include acute gastroenteritis, diuretic use (particularly thiazides), use of nonsteroidal anti-inflammatory drugs or ACE inhibitors, and lithium-induced nephrogenic diabetes insipidus.

**III. Clinical presentation.** Mild to moderate intoxication results in lethargy, muscular weakness, slurred speech, ataxia, tremor, and myoclonic jerks. Rigidity and extrapyramidal effects may be seen. Severe intoxication may result in agitated delirium, coma, convulsions, and hyperthermia. Recovery is often very slow, and patients may remain confused or obtunded for several days to weeks. Rarely, cerebellar and cognitive dysfunction is persistent. Cases of rapidly progressive dementia, similar to Jakob-Creutzfeldt disease, have occurred and are usually reversible. The ECG commonly shows T-wave flattening or inversions and depressed ST segments in the lateral leads; less commonly, bradycardia and sinus node arrest may occur. The white cell count often is elevated (15–20,000/mm$^3$).

**A. Acute ingestion** may cause initial mild nausea and vomiting, but systemic signs of intoxication are minimal and usually are delayed for several hours while lithium distributes into tissues. Initially high serum levels fall by 50–70% or more with tissue equilibration.

**B.** In contrast, patients with **chronic intoxication** usually already have systemic manifestations on admission, and toxicity may be severe with levels only slightly above therapeutic levels. Typically, patients with chronic intoxication have elevated BUN and creatinine levels and other evidence of dehydration or renal insufficiency.

**C. Nephrogenic diabetes insipidus** (see p 35) is a recognized complication of chronic lithium therapy and may lead to dehydration and hypernatremia.

**IV. Diagnosis.** Lithium intoxication should be suspected in any patient with a known psychiatric history who is confused, ataxic, or tremulous.

**A. Specific levels.** The diagnosis is supported by an elevated **lithium** level.

1. Most hospital clinical laboratories can perform a stat serum lithium concentration. However, the serum lithium level is not an accurate predictor of toxicity.
   - **a.** With chronic poisoning, toxicity may be associated with levels only slightly above the therapeutic range.
   - **b.** In contrast, peak levels as high as 9.3 mEq/L have been reported early after acute ingestion without signs of intoxication owing to measurement before final tissue distribution.
   - **c.** ***Note:*** Specimens obtained in a green-top tube (lithium heparin) will give a markedly false elevation of the serum lithium level.

2. Cerebrospinal fluid lithium levels higher than 0.4 mEq/L were associated in one case report with CNS toxicity. However, CSF lithium levels generally do not generally with toxicity and are not clinically useful.

B. **Other useful laboratory studies** include electrolytes (the anion gap may be narrowed owing to elevated chloride or bicarbonate), glucose, BUN, creatinine, and ECG monitoring.

V. **Treatment**

A. **Emergency and supportive measures**

1. In obtunded patients, maintain an open airway and assist ventilation if necessary (see pp 1–7). Administer supplemental oxygen.
2. Treat coma (see p 18), seizures (p 22), and hyperthermia (p 20) if they occur.
3. In dehydrated patients, replace fluid deficits with intravenous crystalloid solutions. Initial treatment should include repletion of sodium and water with 1–2 L of normal saline (children: 10–20 mL/kg). Once fluid deficits are replaced, give hypotonic (eg, half-normal saline) solutions because continued administration of normal saline often leads to hypernatremia, especially in patients with lithium-induced nephrogenic diabetes insipidus.

B. **Specific drugs and antidotes.** There is no specific antidote. Thiazides and indomethacin have been used for treatment of nephrogenic diabetes insipidus (see p 35).

C. **Decontamination** (see p 45) measures are appropriate after acute ingestion but not chronic intoxication.

1. Consider gastric lavage for a large recent ingestion. Activated charcoal does not adsorb lithium but may be useful if other drug ingestion is suspected.
2. Whole-bowel irrigation (see p 51) may enhance gut decontamination, especially in cases involving sustained-release preparations that are not likely to dissolve readily during the lavage procedure.
3. Oral administration of sodium polystyrene sulfonate (SPS, Kayexalate) has been advocated for attempts to reduce lithium absorption, but there is insufficient evidence of safety or effectiveness.

D. **Enhanced elimination** (see p 53). Lithium is excreted exclusively by the kidneys. The clearance is about 25% of the glomerular filtration rate and is reduced by sodium depletion or dehydration.

1. **Hemodialysis** removes lithium effectively and is indicated for intoxicated patients with seizures or severely abnormal mental status and for patients unable to excrete lithium renally (ie, anephric or anuric patients). Repeated and prolonged dialysis may be necessary because of slow movement of lithium out of the CNS. There is no consensus on the level of lithium at which one must dialyze for lithium toxicity.
2. **Continuous venovenous hemodiafiltration** (CVVHD) has been shown to be effective in removing lithium in several human cases. The clearance of lithium via CVVHD is 28–62 mL/min compared with a normal renal clearance of 20–25 mL/min. (The clearance of lithium during hemodialysis is 60–170 mL/min.) Advantages of CVVDH over hemodialysis include its wide availability in many intensive care units, reduced risk in patients with hemodynamic instability, and no postdialysis rebound in lithium concentrations as equilibration between the tissue and vascular compartments occurs between runs of dialysis.
3. Forced diuresis only slightly increases lithium excretion compared with normal hydration and is not recommended. However, establishing normal urine output may bring the urinary lithium clearance to 25–30 mL/min.
4. Oral sodium polystyrene sulfonate (SPS, Kayexalate) enhances elimination of lithium in animal models, but there is insufficient experience in humans.
5. Hemoperfusion and repeat-dose charcoal are not effective.

# ▶ LOMOTIL AND OTHER ANTIDIARRHEALS

*Ilene B. Anderson, PharmD*

**Lomotil** is a combination product containing diphenoxylate and atropine that is prescribed commonly for symptomatic treatment of diarrhea. Children are especially sensitive to small doses of Lomotil and may develop delayed toxicity after accidental ingestion. **Motofen** is a similar drug that contains difenoxin and atropine. **Loperamide** (Imodium™) is a nonprescription drug with similar properties.

I. **Mechanism of toxicity**
   A. **Diphenoxylate** is an opioid analog of meperidine. It is metabolized to **difenoxin,** which has fivefold the antidiarrheal activity of diphenoxylate. Both agents have opioid effects (see p 288) in overdose.
   B. **Atropine** is an anticholinergic agent (see p 85) that may contribute to lethargy and coma. It also slows drug absorption and may delay the onset of symptoms.
   C. **Loperamide** is a synthetic piperidine derivative that is structurally similar to diphenoxylate and haloperidol. It may produce opioid-like toxicity in overdose.

II. **Toxic dose**
   A. **Lomotil™.** The toxic dose is difficult to predict because of wide individual variability in response to drug effects and promptness of treatment. The lethal dose is unknown, but death in children has been reported after ingestion of **fewer than five tablets.**
   B. **Loperamide.** A single acute ingestion of less than 0.4 mg/kg is not likely to cause serious toxicity in children over 1 year of age. Fatalities, abdominal distension, and paralytic ileus have been reported in children less than 1 year of age after ingestion of 0.6–3 mg per day.

III. **Clinical presentation.** Depending on the individual and the time since ingestion, manifestations may be those of primarily anticholinergic or opioid intoxication.
   A. **Atropine** intoxication may occur before, during, or after opioid effects. Anticholinergic effects include lethargy or agitation, flushed face, dry mucous membranes, mydriasis (dilated pupils), ileus, hyperpyrexia, and tachycardia.
   B. **Opioid intoxication** produces small pupils, coma, and respiratory arrest, and the onset of these effects often is delayed for several hours after ingestion.
   C. All the antidiarrheals may cause vomiting, abdominal distention, and paralytic ileus.

IV. **Diagnosis** is based on the history and signs of anticholinergic or opioid intoxication.
   A. **Specific levels.** Specific serum levels are not available.
   B. **Other useful laboratory studies** include electrolytes, glucose, and arterial blood gases (if respiratory insufficiency is suspected).

V. **Treatment**
   A. **Emergency and supportive measures**
      1. Maintain an open airway and assist ventilation if necessary (see pp 1–7).
      2. Treat coma (see p 18) and hypotension (p 15) if they occur.
      3. Because of the danger of abrupt respiratory arrest, observe all children with Lomotil™ or Motofen™ ingestion in an intensive care unit for 18–24 hours. Similar precautions should be taken for patients with very large ingestions of loperamide.
   B. **Specific drugs and antidotes**
      1. Administer **naloxone,** 1–2 mg IV (see p 477), to patients with lethargy, apnea, or coma. Repeated doses of naloxone may be required, because its duration of effect (1–2 hours or less) is much shorter than that of the opioids in these products.
      2. There is no evidence that **physostigmine** (see p 497) is beneficial for this overdose, although it may reverse signs of anticholinergic poisoning.
   C. **Decontamination** (see p 45). Administer activated charcoal orally if conditions are appropriate (see Table I–38, p 51). Gastric lavage is not necessary

after small to moderate ingestions if activated charcoal can be given promptly.

**D. Enhanced elimination.** There is no role for these procedures.

## ▶ LYSERGIC ACID DIETHYLAMIDE (LSD) AND OTHER HALLUCINOGENS

*Lisa Wu, MD*

Patients who seek medical care after self-administering mind-altering substances may have used any of a large variety of chemicals. Several of these agents are discussed elsewhere in this manual (eg, amphetamines [p 73], cocaine [p 170], marijuana [p 252], phencyclidine [p 301], and toluene [p 358]). The drugs discussed in this section, LSD and other hallucinogens, have become known in some circles as *entactogens* ("to touch within"), and several have been used widely for personal experimentation as well as clinically to facilitate psychotherapeutic interviews. Table II–32 lists some common and uncommon hallucinogens.

**I. Mechanism of toxicity.** Despite many intriguing theories and much current research, the biochemical mechanism of hallucinations is not known. LSD stimulates 5-HT2 receptors, and many other agents are thought to alter the activity of serotonin and dopamine in the brain. Central and peripheral sympathetic stimulation may account for some of the side effects, such as anxiety, psychosis, dilated pupils, and hyperthermia. Some agents (eg, MDMA) are directly neurotoxic.

**II. Toxic dose.** The toxic dose is highly variable, depending on the agent and the circumstances (see Table II–32). In general, entactogenic effects do not appear to be dose-related; therefore, increasing the dose does not intensify the desired effects. Likewise, paranoia or panic attacks may occur with any dose and depend on the surroundings and the patient's current emotional state. In contrast, hallucinations, visual illusions, and sympathomimetic side effects are dose-related. The toxic dose may be only slightly greater than the recreational dose. In human volunteers receiving recreational doses of MDMA, elimination was nonlinear, implying that small increases in dosing may increase the risk of toxicity.

**III. Clinical presentation**

**A. Mild to moderate intoxication**

1. A person experiencing a "bad trip" is conscious, coherent, and oriented but is anxious and fearful and may display paranoid or bizarre reasoning. The patient may also be tearful, combative, or self-destructive. Delayed intermittent "flashbacks" may occur after the acute effects have worn off and are usually precipitated by use of another mind-altering drug.
2. A person with dose-related sympathomimetic side effects may also exhibit tachycardia, mydriasis (dilated pupils), diaphoresis, bruxism, short attention span, tremor, hyperreflexia, hypertension, and fever.

**B. Life-threatening toxicity**

1. Intense sympathomimetic stimulation can cause seizures, severe hyperthermia, hypertension, intracranial hemorrhage, and cardiac arrhythmias. Hyperthermic patients are usually obtunded, agitated or thrashing about, diaphoretic, and hyperreflexic. Untreated, hyperthermia may result in hypotension, coagulopathy, rhabdomyolysis, and hepatic and other organ failure (see p 20). Hyperthermia has been associated with LSD, methylene dioxyamphetamine (MDA), MDMA, and paramethoxyamphetamine (PMA).
2. Severe hyponatremia has been reported after use of MDMA and may result from both excess water intake and inappropriate secretion of antidiuretic hormone.
3. The use of 2,5-dimethoxy-4-bromoamphetamine (DOB) has resulted in ergot-like vascular spasm, circulatory insufficiency, and gangrene (see p 187).

TABLE II–32. HALLUCINOGENS

| Drug or Compound | Common Name | Comments |
|---|---|---|
| 5-Hydroxy-*N,N*-dimethyltryptamine | Bufotenine | From skin secretions of the toad *Bufo vulgaris.* |
| *N,N*-dimethyltryptamine | DMT, "Businessman's trip" | Slang term refers to short duration (30–60 minutes). Found in plants and ayahuasca brews of South America. |
| 2,5-Dimethoxy-4-bromo-amphetamine[a] | DOB | Potent ergot-like vascular spasm may result in ischemia, gangrene. |
| 2,5-Dimethoxy-4-methyl-amphetamine[a] | DOM, STP (Serenity, Tranquility Peace) | Potent sympathomimetic. |
| 4,9-Dihydro-7-methoxy-1-methyl-3-pyrido(3,4)-indole | Harmaline | South American religious and cultural drink called yage or ayahuasca. |
| Lysergic acid diethylamide | LSD, acid | Potent hallucinogen. Average dose 50–150 mcg in tablets, papers. |
| *n*-Methyl-1-(1,3-benzodioxol-5-yl)-2-butanamine | MBDB | Nearly pure entactogen without hallucinosis or sympathomimetic stimulation. |
| 3,4-Methylenedioxy-amphetamine[a] | MDA, "Love drug" | Potent sympathomimetic. Several hyperthermic deaths reported. MDMA analog but reportedly more hallucinogenic. Sometimes found in "Ecstasy" tablets. |
| 3,4-Methylenedioxy-methamphetamine[a] | MDMA, "Ecstasy," "Adam" | Sympathomimetic: hyperthermia, seizures, cerebral hemorrhage, and arrhythmias reported; hyponatremia. |
| 3,4-Methylenedioxy-*n*-ethylamphetamine[a] | MDE, "Eve" | MDMA analog but reportedly less pronounced empathogen. Sometimes found in "Ecstasy" tablets. |
| 3,4,5-Trimethoxyphenethylamine | Mescaline | Derived from peyote cactus. Commonly used by some Native Americans. |
| 3-Methoxy-4,5-methylene-dioxyallylbenzene | Myristicin, nutmeg | Anticholinergic presentation. Used as aphrodisiac and antidiarrheal. |
| *p*-Methoxyamphetamine[a] | PMA, "Death," "Doctor Death" | Contaminant or adulterant in some pills sold as MDMA; very potent sympathomimetic. High morbidity and mortalitiy associated with overdose. |
| 4-Phosphoryloxy-*N-N*-dimethyltryptamine | Psilocybin | From *Psilocybe* mushrooms. |

[a]Amphetamine derivatives. See also p 73.

IV. **Diagnosis** is based on a history of use and the presence of signs of sympathetic stimulation. Diagnosis of hyperthermia requires a high level of suspicion and use of a thermometer that accurately measures core temperature (eg, rectal probe).

A. **Specific levels.** Serum drug levels are neither widely available nor clinically useful in emergency management. The amphetamine derivatives (DOB, STP, MDA, MDMA, etc) cross-react in many of the available screening procedures for amphetamine-class drugs. However, LSD and the other nonamphetamine hallucinogens listed in Table II–32 are not identified on routine toxicology screening. Recently, several LSD screening immunoassays have become available, although they are of limited use because of false-positive and false-negative results and a short window of detection (4–12 hours).

B. **Other useful laboratory studies** include electrolytes, glucose, BUN, and creatinine. In hyperthermic patients, obtain prothrombin time, CPK, and urinalysis for occult blood (myoglobinuria will be present).

V. **Treatment**

A. For a patient with a "bad trip" or panic reaction, provide gentle reassurance and relaxation techniques in a quiet environment.

1. Treat agitation (see p 23) or severe anxiety states with diazepam or midazolam (p 419). Butyrophenones such as haloperidol (p 458) are useful despite a small theoretic risk of lowering the seizure threshold.
2. Treat seizures (see p 22), hyperthermia (p 20), rhabdomyolysis (p 26), hypertension (p 17), and cardiac arrhythmias (p 13) if they occur.

B. **Specific drugs and antidotes.** There is no specific antidote. Sedating doses of diazepam (2–10 mg) may alleviate anxiety, and hypnotic doses (10–20 mg) can induce sleep for the duration of the "trip."

C. **Decontamination** (see p 45). Most of these drugs are taken orally in small doses, and decontamination procedures are relatively ineffective and likely to aggravate psychological distress. Consider the use of activated charcoal or gastric lavage only after recent (within 30-60 minutes) large ingestions.

D. **Enhanced elimination.** These procedures are not useful. Although urinary acidification may increase the urine concentration of some agents, it does not significantly enhance total-body elimination and may aggravate myoglobinuric renal failure.

## ► MAGNESIUM

*Kathryn H. Meier, PharmD*

Magnesium (Mg) is a divalent cation that is required for a variety of enzymatic reactions involving protein synthesis and carbohydrate metabolism. It is also an essential ion for proper neuromuscular functioning. Oral magnesium is widely available in over-the-counter antacids (eg, Maalox and Mylanta) and cathartics (milk of magnesia and magnesium citrate and sulfate). Intravenous magnesium is used to treat toxemia of pregnancy, polymorphous ventricular tachycardia, refractory ventricular arrhythmias, and severe bronchospasm.

I. **Mechanism of toxicity**

A. Elevated serum magnesium concentrations act as a CNS depressant and block neuromuscular transmission by inhibiting acetylcholine release at the motor endplate. Hypermagnesemia amplifies the response to neuromuscular blockers.

B. Magnesium also competitively antagonizes calcium at calcium channels, thus impeding calcium flux and impairing both muscle contraction and electrical conduction.

C. **Pharmacokinetics.** The usual body content of Mg is approximately 1700–2200 mEq in a 70-kg person; it is stored primarily in bone and intracellular fluids. The oral bioavailability ranges from 20–40% depending on the salt form. Although best modeled with two-compartment pharmacokinetics, the average volume of distribution is around 0.5 L/Kg, and the elimination half-life averages 4–5 hours in healthy adults. Normal kidney function is essential for clearance because 97% of ingested Mg is eliminated in the urine.

**II. Toxic dose.** Although most acute or chronic overexposures do not result in hypermagnesemia, poisoning has been reported after intravenous overdose or massive oral or rectal overdose. Patients with renal insuffiency (creatinine clearance < 30 mL/min) are at higher risk with standard doses because of impaired clearance.

**A.** Commonly available antacids (Maalox, Mylanta, and others) contain 12.5–37.5 mEq of magnesium per 15 mL (one tablespoon), milk of magnesia contains about 40 mEq per 15 mL, and magnesium sulfate contains 8 mEq per g.

**B.** Ingestion of 200 g of magnesium sulfate caused coma in a young woman with normal renal function. Pediatric deaths have been reported after the use of Epsom salt enemas.

**III. Clinical presentation.** Orally administered magnesium causes diarrhea, usually within 3 hours. Repeated or excessive doses of magnesium-containing cathartics can cause serious fluid and electrolyte abnormalities. Moderate toxicity may cause nausea, vomiting, muscle weakness, and cutaneous flushing. Higher levels can cause cardiac conduction abnormalities, hypotension, and severe muscle weakness and lethargy. Very high levels can cause coma, respiratory arrest, and asystole (see Table II–33).

**IV. Diagnosis** should be suspected in a patient who presents with hypotonia, hypotension, and CNS depression, especially if there is a history of using magnesium-containing antacids or cathartics or renal insufficiency.

**A. Specific levels.** Determination of serum magnesium concentration is usually rapidly available. The normal range is 1.8–3.0 mg/dL (0.75–1.25 mmol/L, or 1.5–2.5 mEq/L) total Mg. Therapeutic levels for treatment of toxemia of pregnancy (eclampsia) are 5–7.4 mg/dL (2–3 mmol/L, or 4–6 mEq/L) total Mg. Ionized levels correlate with total Mg levels and are not needed to assess overdose.

**B. Other useful laboratory studies** include electrolytes, calcium, BUN, creatinine, serum osmolality and osmolar gap (magnesium may elevate the osmolar gap), calcium, arterial blood gases (if respiratory depression is suspected), and ECG.

**V. Treatment**

**A. Emergency and supportive measures**

1. Maintain an open airway and assist ventilation if necessary (see pp 1–7).
2. Replace fluid and electrolyte losses caused by excessive catharsis.
3. Treat hypotension with intravenous fluids and dopamine (see p 15).

**B. Specific drugs and antidotes.** There is no specific antidote. However, administration of intravenous **calcium** (see p 428) may temporarily alleviate respiratory depression, hypotension, and arrhythmias.

**TABLE II–33. MAGNESIUM POISONING**

| Magnesium (mg/dL) | Magnesium (mEq/L) | Magnesium (mmol/L) | Possible clinical effects |
|---|---|---|---|
| > 3.5 | > 3 | > 1.5 | Nausea, vomiting, weakness, cutaneous flushing |
| > 6 | > 5 | > 2.5 | ECG changes: prolonged PR, QRS, QT intervals |
| 8–12 | 7–10 | 3.5–5 | Hypotension, loss of deep tendon reflexes, sedation |
| > 12 | > 10 | > 5 | Muscle paralysis, respiratory arrest , hypotension, arrhythmias |
| > 17 | > 14 | > 7 | Death from respiratory arrest or asystole |

C. **Decontamination** (see p 45). Activated charcoal is not effective. Consider gastric emptying with a nasogastric tube for large recent ingestions. Do ***not*** administer a cathartic.

D. **Enhanced elimination**
   1. **Hemodialysis** rapidly removes magnesium and is the only route of elimination in anuric patients.
   2. Hemoperfusion and repeat-dose charcoal are not effective.
   3. Forced diuresis using intravenous furosemide and normal saline may enhance Mg elimination, but there are insufficient human data to recommend it.

## ► MANGANESE

*Paul D. Blanc, MD, MSPH*

Manganese intoxication generally is caused by chronic exposure. Sources of inorganic manganese exposure include mining, metal working, smelting, foundries, and welding. Recent studies also suggest a possible link between an organic manganese fungicide (Maneb) and chronic neurologic toxicity. A gasoline additive, methylcyclopentadienyl manganese tricarbonyl (MMT), has been promoted for combustion efficiency but creates potential health concerns as a source of manganese.

I. **Mechanism of toxicity.** The precise mechanism is not known. The CNS is the target organ.

II. **Toxic dose.** The primary route of exposure is inhalation, but there is evidence that absorption to the CNS through the olfactory system may play a role in toxicity Inorganic manganese is poorly absorbed from the GI tract. The OSHA workplace limit (permissible exposure limit—ceiling; PEL-C) for inorganic manganese is 5 mg/m$^3$; The ACGIH-recommended workplace exposure limit (threshold limit value—8-hour time-weighted average; TLV-TWA) is considerably lower at 0.2 mg/m$^3$. The AGGIH TLV-TWA for MMT is 0.1 mg/m$^3$. The air level considered immediately dangerous to life or health (IDLH) is 10,000 ppm.

III. **Clinical presentation.** Acute high-level manganese inhalation can produce an irritant-type pneumonitis, but this is rare (see p 212). More typically, toxicity occurs after chronic exposure to low levels over months or years. The patient may present with a psychiatric disorder that can be misdiagnosed as schizophrenia or atypical psychosis. Organic signs of neurologic toxicity, such as parkinsonism and other extrapyramidal movement disorders, usually appear later, up to years after any primarily psychiatric presentation.

IV. **Diagnosis** depends on a thorough occupational and psychiatric history.

A. **Specific levels.** Testing of whole blood, serum, or urine may be performed, but the results should be interpreted with caution, as they may not correlate with clinical effects. Whole-blood levels are 20 times greater than levels in serum or plasma, and red blood cell contamination can falsely elevate serum or plasma levels.
   1. Normal serum manganese concentrations are usually less than 1.2 mcg/L.
   2. Elevated urine manganese concentrations (> 2 mcg/L) may confirm recent acute exposure. Exposures at the OSHA PEL usually do not raise urinary levels above 8 mcg/L. Chelation challenge does not have a role in diagnosis.
   3. Hair and nail levels are not useful.

B. **Other useful laboratory studies** include arterial blood gases or oximetry and chest x-ray (after acute, heavy symptomatic inhalation exposure if acute lung injury is suspected). MRI of the brain may show findings suggestive of manganese deposition.

V. **Treatment**

A. **Emergency and supportive measures**
   1. **Acute inhalation.** Administer supplemental oxygen. Treat bronchospasm (see p 7) and noncardiogenic pulmonary edema (p 7) if they occur.

2. **Chronic intoxication.** Psychiatric and neurologic effects are treated with the usual psychiatric and antiparkinsonian drugs but often respond poorly.

B. **Specific drugs and antidotes.** Calcium EDTA and other chelators have ***not*** been proved effective after chronic neurologic damage has occurred. The efficacy of chelators early after acute exposure has not been studied.

C. **Decontamination** (see p 45)

1. **Acute inhalation.** Remove the victim from exposure and give supplemental oxygen if available.
2. **Ingestion.** Because inorganic manganese is so poorly absorbed from the GI tract, gut decontamination is probably not necessary. For massive ingestions, particularly of organic compounds (eg, Maneb and MMT), gastric lavage and activated charcoal may be appropriate but have not been studied.

D. **Enhanced elimination.** There is no known role for dialysis or hemoperfusion.

## ▶ MARIJUANA

*Neal L. Benowitz, MD*

Marijuana consists of the leaves and flowering parts of the plant *Cannabis sativa* and usually is smoked in cigarettes ("joints" or "reefers") or pipes or added to food (usually cookies or brownies). Resin from the plant may be dried and compressed into blocks called hashish. Marijuana contains a number of cannabinoids; the primary psychoactive one is delta-9-tetrahydrocannabinol (THC). THC is also available in capsule form (dronabinol or Marinol) as an appetite stimulant used primarily for AIDS-related anorexia and as treatment for vomiting associated with cancer chemotherapy.

I. **Mechanism of toxicity**

A. THC, which binds to anandamide receptors in the brain, may have stimulant, sedative, or hallucinogenic actions, depending on the dose and time after consumption. Both catecholamine release (resulting in tachycardia) and inhibition of sympathetic reflexes (resulting in orthostatic hypotension) may be observed.

B. **Pharmacokinetics.** Only about 10–20% of ingested dronabinol is absorbed, with onset of effects within 30–60 minutes and peak absorption at 2–4 hours. It is metabolized by hydroxylation to active and inactive metabolites. Elimination half-life is 20–30 hours but may be longer in chronic users.

II. **Toxic dose.** Typical marijuana cigarettes contain 1–3% THC, but more potent varieties may contain up to 15% THC. Hashish contains 3–6% and hashish oil 30–50% THC. Dronabinol is available in 2.5-, 5-, and 10-mg capsules. Toxicity is dose-related, but there is much individual variability, influenced in part by prior experience and degree of tolerance.

III. **Clinical presentation**

A. **Subjective effects** after smoking a marijuana cigarette include euphoria, palpitations, heightened sensory awareness, and altered time perception followed after about 30 minutes by sedation. More severe intoxication may result in impaired short-term memory, depersonalization, visual hallucinations, and acute paranoid psychosis. Cannabis use may precipitate or exacerbate psychosis in schizophrenic individuals. Occasionally, even with low doses of THC, subjective effects may precipitate a panic reaction. Acute cannabis intoxication may result in impaired driving and motor vehicle accidents. Cannabis dependence, both behavioral and physical, occurs in 7–10% of users.

B. **Physical findings** may include tachycardia, orthostatic hypotension, conjunctival injection, incoordination, slurred speech, and ataxia. Stupor with pallor, conjunctival injection, fine tremor, and ataxia has been observed in children after they have eaten marijuana cookies.

- **C. Other health problems** include salmonellosis and pulmonary aspergillosis from use of contaminated marijuana. Marijuana may be contaminated by paraquat, but paraquat is destroyed by pyrolysis and there have been no reports of paraquat toxicity from smoking marijuana.
- **D. Intravenous use** of marijuana extract or hash oil may cause dyspnea, abdominal pain, fever, shock, disseminated intravascular coagulation, acute renal failure, and death.

**IV. Diagnosis** usually is based on the history and typical findings such as tachycardia and conjunctival injection combined with evidence of altered mood or cognitive function.

- **A. Specific levels.** Blood levels are not commonly available. Cannabinoid metabolites may be detected in the urine by enzyme immunoassay up to several days after a single acute exposure or weeks after chronic THC exposure. Urine levels do not correlate with the degree of intoxication or functional impairment. Hemp and hemp seed products (eg, hemp seed nutrition bars) may provide alternative explanations for positive urine testing. Although barely capable of causing a true positive for THC metabolite, they have no pharmacologic effect.
- **B. Other useful laboratory studies** include electrolytes and glucose.

**V. Treatment**

- **A. Emergency and supportive measures**
  1. Most psychological disturbances can be managed by simple reassurance, possibly with adjunctive use of lorazepam, diazepam, or midazolam (see p 415).
  2. Sinus tachycardia usually does not require treatment but, if necessary, may be controlled with beta blockers.
  3. Orthostatic hypotension responds to head-down position and intravenous fluids.
- **B. Specific drugs and antidotes.** There is no specific antidote.
- **C. Decontamination** after ingestion (see p 47). Administer activated charcoal orally if conditions are appropriate (see Table I–38, p 51). Gastric lavage is not necessary if activated charcoal can be given promptly.
- **D. Enhanced elimination.** These procedures are not effective owing to the large volume of distribution of cannabinoids.

## ▶ MERCURY

*Michael J. Kosnett, MD, MPH*

Mercury (Hg) is a naturally occurring metal that is mined chiefly as HgS in cinnabar ore. It is converted to three primary forms, each with a distinct toxicology: elemental (metallic) mercury ($Hg^0$), inorganic mercury salts (eg, mercuric chloride [$HgCl_2$]), and organic (alkyl and aryl) mercury (eg, methylmercury). Approximately one-half to one-third of commercial mercury use is in the manufacture of chlorine and caustic soda, one-half to one third in electrical equipment, and the remainder in various applications, such as dental amalgam, fluorescent lamps, switches, thermostats, and artisanal gold production. In the United States, mercury use in batteries and paints has been discontinued. Previous use in pharmaceuticals and biocides has declined sharply, although mercuric chloride is still used as a stool fixative, and some organomercury compounds (such as mercurochrome, phenylmercuric acetate, and thimerosal) are still used as topical antiseptics or preservatives. Some folk medicines contain inorganic mercury compounds, and some Latin American and Caribbean communities have used elemental mercury in religious or cultural rituals. Aquatic organisms can convert inorganic mercury into methylmercury, with resulting bioaccumulation in large carnivorous fish such as swordfish.

**TABLE II–34. MERCURY COMPOUNDS**

| Form | Absorption | | Toxicity | |
|---|---|---|---|---|
| | Oral | Inhalation | Neurologic | Renal |
| **Elemental (metallic) mercury** | | | | |
| $Hg^{0}$ liquid | Poor | NA* | Rare | Rare |
| $Hg^{0}$ vapor | NA* | Good | Likely | Possible |
| **Inorganic mercuric salts** | | | | |
| $Hg^{2+}$ | Good | Rare but possible | Rare | Likely |
| **Organic (alkyl) mercury** | | | | |
| $RHg^{+}$ | Good | Rare but possible | Likely | Possible |

*NA = Not applicable.

I. **Mechanism of toxicity.** Mercury reacts with sulfhydryl (SH) groups, resulting in enzyme inhibition and pathologic alteration of cellular membranes.
   A. Elemental mercury and methylmercury are particularly toxic to the CNS. Metallic mercury vapor is also a pulmonary irritant. Methylmercury is associated with neurodevelopmental disorders.
   B. Inorganic mercuric salts are corrosive to the skin, eyes, and GI tract and are nephrotoxic.
   C. Inorganic and organic mercury compounds may cause contact dermatitis.

II. **Toxic dose.** The pattern and severity of toxicity are highly dependent on the form of mercury and the route of exposure, mostly because of different pharmacokinetic profiles. Chronic exposure to any form may result in toxicity. See Table II–34 for a summary of absorption and toxicity.
   A. **Elemental (metallic) mercury** is a volatile liquid at room temperature.
      1. **$Hg^{0}$ vapor** is absorbed rapidly by the lungs and distributed to the CNS. Airborne exposure to 10 $mg/m^3$ is considered immediately dangerous to life or health (IDLH), and chemical pneumonitis may occur at levels in excess of 1 $mg/m^3$. In occupational settings, overt signs and symptoms of elemental mercury intoxication generally have required months to years of sustained daily exposure to airborne mercury levels of 0.05–0.2 $mg/m^3$. The recommended workplace limit (ACGIH TLV-TWA) is 0.025 $mg/m^3$ as an 8-hour time-weighted average; however, some studies suggest that subclinical effects on the CNS and kidneys may occur below this level.
      2. **Liquid metallic mercury** is poorly absorbed from the GI tract, and acute ingestion has been associated with poisoning only in the presence of abnormal gut motility that markedly delays normal fecal elimination or after peritoneal contamination.
   B. **Inorganic mercuric salts.** The acute lethal oral dose of mercuric chloride is approximately 1–4 g. Severe toxicity and death have been reported after use of peritoneal lavage solutions containing mercuric chloride concentrations of 0.2–0.8%.
   C. **Organic mercury**
      1. **Mercury-containing antiseptics** such as mercurochrome have limited skin penetration; however, in rare cases, such as topical application to an infected omphalocele, intoxication has resulted. Oral absorption is significant and may also pose a hazard.
      2. **Methylmercury** is well absorbed after inhalation, ingestion, and probably dermal exposure. Ingestion of 10–60 mg/kg may be lethal, and chronic daily ingestion of 10 mcg/kg may be associated with adverse neurologic

and reproductive effects. The US Environmental Protection Agency reference dose (RfD), the daily lifetime dose believed to be without potential hazard, is 0.1 mcg/kg/day. The RfD was derived from studies of neuropsychologic deficits arising from in utero exposure in humans. To minimize neurodevelopmental risk, the US EPA and FDA have advised pregnant women, women who might become pregnant, nursing mothers, and young children to avoid consumption of fish with high levels of mercury (such as swordfish) and to limit consumption of fish and shellfish with lower mercury levels to no more than 12 ounces (two average meals) per week (www.epa.gov/waterscience/fishadvice/advice.html).

3. **Dimethylmercury,** a highly toxic synthetic liquid used in analytic chemistry, is well absorbed through the skin, and cutaneous exposure to only a few drops has resulted in a delayed but fatal encephalopathy.

**III. Clinical presentation**

A. **Acute inhalation of high concentrations of metallic mercury vapor** may cause severe chemical pneumonitis and noncardiogenic pulmonary edema. Acute gingivostomatitis may also occur.

B. **Chronic intoxication from inhalation of mercury vapor** produces a classic triad of tremor, neuropsychiatric disturbances, and gingivostomatitis.

1. Early stages feature a fine intention tremor of the fingers, but involvement of the face and progression to choreiform movements of the limbs may occur.
2. **Neuropsychiatric manifestations** include fatigue, insomnia, anorexia, and memory loss. There may be an insidious change in mood to shyness, withdrawal, and depression, combined with explosive irritability and frequent blushing ("erethism").
3. Subclinical changes in peripheral nerve function and renal function have been reported, but frank neuropathy and nephropathy are rare.
4. **Acrodynia,** a rare idiosyncratic reaction to chronic mercury exposure, occurs mainly in children and has the following features: pain in the extremities, often accompanied by pinkish discoloration and desquamation ("pink disease"); hypertension; profuse sweating; anorexia, insomnia, irritability, and/or apathy; and a miliarial rash.

C. **Acute ingestion of inorganic mercuric salts,** particularly mercuric chloride, causes an abrupt onset of hemorrhagic gastroenteritis and abdominal pain. Intestinal necrosis, shock, and death may ensue. Acute oliguric renal failure from acute tubular necrosis may occur within days. Chronic exposure may result in CNS toxicity.

D. **Organic mercury compounds,** particularly short-chain alkyl compounds such as methylmercury, primarily affect the CNS, causing paresthesias, ataxia, dysarthria, hearing impairment, and progressive constriction of the visual fields. Symptoms first become apparent after a latent interval of several weeks or months.

1. **Ethylmercury** undergoes less CNS penetration than does methylmercury and has faster total body clearance. In addition to neurotoxicity, symptoms of acute poisoning may include gastroenteritis and nephrotoxicity. Thimerosal (ethylmercury thiosalicylate), a preservative that undergoes metabolism to ethylmercury, was removed from most childhood vaccines in the United States on a precautionary basis. No causal link between thimerosal-containing vaccines and neurodevelopmental disorders has been established. A 2004 Institute of Medicine report concluded that evidence favors *rejection* of a causal relationship between thimerosal-containing vaccines and autism.
2. **Phenylmercury** compounds, which undergo deacylation in vivo, produce a pattern of toxicity intermediate between alkyl mercury and inorganic mercury.
3. **Methylmercury** is a potent reproductive toxin, and perinatal exposure has caused mental retardation and a cerebral palsy–type syndrome in offspring.

**IV. Diagnosis** depends on integration of characteristic findings with a history of known or potential exposure and the presence of elevated mercury blood levels or urinary excretion.

**A. Specific levels.** Elemental and inorganic mercury follow a biphasic elimination rate (initially rapid, then slow), and both urinary and fecal excretion occur. The urinary elimination half-life is approximately 40 days. ***Note:*** Urine mercury may be reported as the mass of the metal per volume of urine (ie, mcg/L) or as the mass of the metal per gram of creatinine (ie, mcg/g creatinine). Adjustment for creatinine, which reduces the impact of variation in urine flow rate, can be of value in comparing serial measurements obtained in the same individual (eg, workplace biomonitoring) or in evaluating dose-response trends in small population studies. However, when one is assessing a "creatinine-corrected" result, the urine concentration of the metal (Hg/L) and of creatinine (g creatinine/L) should also be reviewed individually. Specimens in which the creatinine concentration is very low (eg, < 0.5 g/L) or very high (> 3 g/L) may be unreliable and should be interpreted cautiously. The urine creatinine concentration of adults is on average close to 1 g/L, and therefore urine mercury values expressed as mcg/g creatinine will often be similar to values expressed as mcg/L. In infants, creatinine-corrected values may appear anomalously elevated owing to infants' relatively low rate of creatinine excretion.

1. **Metallic and inorganic mercury.** Whole-blood and urine mercury levels are useful in confirming exposure. Shortly after acute exposures, whole-blood mercury values may rise faster than urine mercury levels. Urine mercury levels, reflecting the mercury content of the kidney, are in general a better biomarker of chronic exposure. In most people without occupational exposure, whole-blood Hg is less than 10 mcg/L and urine Hg is less than 10 mcg/L. Based on the ACGIH Biological Exposure Index for workers exposed to elemental or inorganic mercury, it has been recommended that end of workweek blood Hg remain less than 15 mcg/L and that the urine mercury level remain less than 35 mcg/g creatinine. Recent studies have noted a small, reversible increase in urinary *N*-acetyl-glucosaminidase, a biomarker of perturbation in renal tubular function, in workers with urinary mercury levels 25–35 mcg/L. Overt neurologic effects have occurred in persons with chronic urine Hg levels greater than 100–200 mcg/L, although lower levels have been reported in some pediatric cases of acrodynia. In patients with acute inorganic mercury poisoning resulting in gastroenteritis and acute tubular necrosis, blood Hg levels are often greater than 500 mcg/L.
2. **Organic mercury.** Methylmercury undergoes biliary excretion and enterohepatic recirculation, with 90% eventually excreted in the feces; as a result, urine levels are not useful. The blood mercury half-life is variable but averages 50 days. Whole-blood Hg levels greater than 200 mcg/L have been associated with symptoms. In a 2001 analysis, the US EPA considered umbilical cord blood mercury levels of 46–79 mcg/L to represent lower-bound estimates of levels associated with a significant increase in adverse neurodevelopmental effects in children. Among US women age 16–49 studied in the 1999–2002 National Health and Nutrition Examination Survey (NHANES), the geometric mean whole-blood mercury level was 0.92 mcg/L, and the 95th percentile level was 6.04 mcg/L (greater than 90% present as methylmercury). Among a subset of women consuming fish and/or shellfish 2 times per week, the 95th percentile whole-blood mercury level was 12.1 mcg/L. Because methylmercury undergoes bioconcentration across the placenta, umbilical cord blood mercury levels are on average 1.7 times higher than maternal whole-blood mercury levels.

   Hair levels have been used to document remote or chronic exposure to methylmercury. In US females age 16–49 (NHANES 1999–2000) the geometric mean hair mercury concentration was 0.20 mcg/g and the 95th percentile was 1.73 mcg/g.

**B. Other useful laboratory studies** include electrolytes, glucose, BUN, creatinine, liver transaminases, urinalysis, chest x-ray, and arterial blood gases (if pneumonitis is suspected). Urinary markers of early nephrotoxicity (microalbuminuria, retinol binding protein, beta-2 microglobulin, and *N*-acetylglucosaminidase) may aid in the detection of early adverse effects. Formal visual field examination may be useful for organic mercury exposure. ***Note:*** Empiric protocols that measure urine mercury concentration after administration of a single dose of a chelating agent such as unithiol (DMPS) have been described, but their diagnostic or prognostic utility has not been established. After administration of a dose of unithiol, urine mercury concentration may transiently increase on the order of 10-fold regardless of whether basal (prechallenge) levels are low or high.

**V. Treatment**

**A. Emergency and supportive measures**

1. **Inhalation.** Observe closely for several hours for development of acute pneumonitis and pulmonary edema (see p 7) and give supplemental oxygen if indicated.
2. **Mercuric salt ingestion.** Anticipate severe gastroenteritis and treat shock aggressively with intravenous fluid replacement (see p 15). Vigorous hydration may also help maintain urine output. Acute renal failure is usually reversible, but hemodialysis may be required for 1–2 weeks.
3. **Organic mercury ingestion.** Provide symptomatic supportive care.

**B. Specific drugs and antidotes**

1. **Metallic (elemental) mercury.** In acute or chronic poisoning, oral **succimer** (DMSA, p 510) or oral **unithiol** (DMPS, p 515) may enhance urinary Hg excretion (although its effect on clinical outcome has not been fully studied). Although **penicillamine** (p 491) is an alternative oral treatment, it may be associated with more side effects and less efficient Hg excretion.
2. **Inorganic mercury salts.** Treatment with intravenous **unithiol** (DMPS, p 515) or intramuscular **BAL** (p 417), if begun within minutes to a few hours after ingestion, may reduce or avert severe renal injury. Because prompt intervention is necessary, do not delay treatment while waiting for specific laboratory confirmation. Oral **succimer** (DMSA, p 510) is also effective, but its absorption may be limited by gastroenteritis and shock, and it is more appropriately used as a follow-up to DMPS or BAL treatment.
3. **Organic mercury.** In methylmercury intoxication, limited data suggest that oral **succimer** (DMSA, p 510) and oral ***N*-acetylcysteine** (NAC, p 407) may be effective in decreasing Hg levels in tissues, including the brain.
4. Because BAL may redistribute mercury to the brain from other tissue sites, it should not be used in poisoning by metallic or organic mercury, because the brain is a key target organ.

**C. Decontamination** (see p 45)

1. **Inhalation**
   a. Immediately remove the victim from exposure and give supplemental oxygen if needed.
   b. Even minute indoor spills (eg, 1 mL) of metallic mercury can result in hazardous chronic airborne levels. Cover the spill with powdered sulfur and carefully clean up and discard all residue and contaminated carpeting, porous furniture, and permeable floor covering. Do ***not*** use a home vacuum cleaner, as this may disperse the liquid mercury, increasing its airborne concentration. For large spills, professional cleanup with self-contained vacuum systems is recommended. Instruments that provide instantaneous (real-time) measurement of mercury vapor concentration are available for monitoring contamination and cleanup. Guidance on the management of mercury spills is available from the US EPA at www.epa.gov/epaoswer/hazwaste/mercury/spills.htm.

2. **Ingestion of metallic mercury.** In healthy persons, metallic mercury passes through the intestinal tract with minimal absorption, and there is no need for gut decontamination after minor ingestions. With large ingestions or in patients with abnormally diminished bowel motility or intestinal perforation, there is a risk of chronic intoxication. Multiple-dose cathartics, whole-bowel irrigation (see p 51), or even surgical removal may be necessary, depending on x-ray evidence of mercury retention or elevated blood or urine Hg levels.
3. **Ingestion of inorganic mercuric salts**
   a. **Prehospital.** Administer activated charcoal if available. Do ***not*** induce vomiting because of the risk of serious corrosive injury.
   b. **Hospital.** Perform gastric lavage. Administer activated charcoal, although it is of uncertain benefit.
   c. Arrange for endoscopic examination if corrosive injury is suspected.
4. **Ingestion of organic mercury.** After acute ingestion, perform gastric lavage and administer activated charcoal. Immediately stop breast-feeding but continue to express and discard milk, as some data suggest this may accelerate reduction of blood Hg levels.

D. **Enhanced elimination**
1. There is no role for dialysis, hemoperfusion, or repeat-dose charcoal in removing metallic or inorganic mercury. However, dialysis may be required for supportive treatment of renal failure, and it may slightly enhance removal of the mercury-chelator complex in patients with renal failure (hemodialysis clearance of the mercury-BAL complex is about 5 mL/min). Somewhat higher mercury clearance (10 mL/min) was described when high-flux continuous venovenous hemodiafiltration was combined with unithiol in the treatment of mercuric sulfate–induced acute renal failure.
2. In patients with chronic methylmercury intoxication, repeated oral administration of an experimental polythiol resin was effective in enhancing Hg elimination by interrupting enterohepatic recirculation.

## ▶ METALDEHYDE

*Winnie W. Tai, PharmD*

Metaldehyde is used widely in the United States as a snail and slug poison. In Europe, it is also used as a solid fuel for small heaters. In Japan, tablets containing up to 90% metaldehyde are used for producing colored flames for entertaining. The pellets often are mistaken for cereal or candy. Common commercial products containing metaldehyde (2–4%) include Cory's Slug and Snail Death, Deadline for Slugs and Snails, and Bug-Geta Snail and Slug Pellets.

I. **Mechanism of toxicity**
   A. The mechanism of toxicity is not well understood. Metaldehyde, like paraldehyde, is a polymer of acetaldehyde, and depolymerization to form acetaldehyde may account for some of its toxic effects. Further metabolism to acetone bodies may contribute to metabolic acidosis.
   B. **Pharmacokinetics.** Metaldehyde is readily absorbed, with onset of effects in 1–3 hours. Volume of distribution and protein binding are not known. The elimination half-life is approximately 27 hours.

II. **Toxic dose.** Ingestion of 100–150 mg/kg may cause myoclonus and convulsions, and ingestion of more than 400 mg/kg is potentially lethal. Death occurred in a child after ingestion of 3 g.

III. **Clinical presentation.** Symptoms usually begin within 1–3 hours after ingestion.
   A. Small ingestions (5–10 mg/kg) cause salivation, facial flushing, vomiting, abdominal cramps, diarrhea, and fever.

**B.** Larger doses may produce irritability, ataxia, drowsiness, myoclonus, opisthotonus, convulsions, and coma. Rhabdomyolysis and hyperthermia may result from seizures or excessive muscle activity. Liver and kidney damage has been reported.

**C.** Metabolic acidosis and an elevated osmolar gap have been reported.

**IV. Diagnosis** is based on a history of ingestion and clinical presentation. Ask about containers in the garage or planting shed; metaldehyde frequently is packaged in brightly colored cardboard boxes similar to cereal containers.

**A. Specific levels.** Serum levels are not generally available.

**B. Other useful laboratory studies** include electrolytes, glucose, BUN, creatinine, osmolar gap (may be elevated), and liver enzymes. If rhabdomyolysis is suspected, also perform a urine dipstick for occult blood (myoglobin is positive) and obtain a serum CPK.

**V. Treatment**

**A. Emergency and supportive measures**

1. Maintain an open airway and assist ventilation if necessary (see pp 1–7).
2. Treat coma (see p 18) and seizures (p 22) if they occur. Paraldehyde should ***not*** be used to treat seizures because of its chemical similarity to metaldehyde.
3. Treat fluid loss from vomiting or diarrhea with intravenous crystalloid fluids (p 15).
4. Monitor asymptomatic patients for at least 4–6 hours after ingestion.

**B. Specific drugs and antidotes.** There is no specific antidote.

**C. Decontamination** (see p 45). Administer activated charcoal orally if conditions are appropriate (see Table I–38, p 51). Do ***not*** induce vomiting because of the risk of abrupt onset of seizures. Gastric lavage is not necessary after small to moderate ingestions if activated charcoal can be given promptly.

**D. Enhanced elimination.** There is no apparent benefit from dialysis, hemoperfusion, or forced diuresis. Repeat-dose charcoal has not been studied.

# ▶ METAL FUME FEVER

*Paul D. Blanc, MD, MSPH*

Metal fume fever is an acute febrile illness associated with the inhalation of respirable particles (fume) of zinc oxide. Although metal fume fever has also been invoked as a generic effect of exposure to numerous other metal oxides (copper, cadmium, iron, magnesium, and manganese), there is little evidence to support this. Metal fume fever usually occurs in workplace settings involving welding, melting, or flame-cutting galvanized metal (zinc-coated steel) or in brass foundry operations. Zinc chloride exposure may occur from smoke bombs; although it can cause severe lung injury, it does not cause metal fume fever.

**I. Mechanism of toxicity.** Metal fume fever results from inhalation of zinc oxide (neither ingestion nor parenteral administration induces this syndrome). The mechanism is uncertain but may be cytokine-mediated. It does not involve sensitization (it is not an allergy) and can occur with the first exposure.

**II. Toxic dose.** The toxic dose is variable. Resistance to the condition develops after repeated days of exposure but wears off rapidly when exposure ceases. The ACGIH recommended workplace exposure limit (TLV-TWA) for zinc oxide fumes is 5 $mg/m^3$ as an 8-hour time-weighted average, which is intended to prevent metal fume fever in most exposed workers. The air level considered immediately dangerous to life or health (IDLH) is 500 $mg/m^3$.

**III. Clinical presentation**

**A.** Symptoms typically begin 4–8 hours after exposure with fever, malaise, myalgia, and headache. The white blood cell count may be elevated (12,000–

16,000/mm$^3$). The chest x-ray is usually normal. Typically, all symptoms resolve on their own within 24–36 hours.

- **B.** Rare asthmatic or allergic responses to zinc oxide fume have been reported. These responses are not part of the metal fume fever syndrome.
- **C.** Pulmonary infiltrates and hypoxemia are not consistent with pure metal fume fever. If present, this suggests possible heavy metal pneumonitis resulting from cadmium or other toxic inhalations (eg, phosgene and nitrogen oxides) associated with metal working, foundry operations, or welding.

**IV. Diagnosis.** A history of welding, especially with galvanized metal, and typical symptoms and signs are sufficient to make the diagnosis.

- **A. Specific levels.** There are no specific tests to diagnose or exclude metal fume fever. Blood or urine zinc determinations do not have a role in clinical diagnosis of the syndrome.
- **B. Other useful laboratory studies** include CBC. Oximetry or arterial blood gases and chest x-ray are used to exclude other disorders involving acute lung injury.

**V. Treatment**

- **A. Emergency and supportive measures**
  1. Administer supplemental oxygen and give bronchodilators if there is wheezing and consider other diagnoses such as an allergic response (see pp 7–8). If hypoxemia or wheezing is present, consider other toxic inhalations (see p 212).
  2. Provide symptomatic care (eg, acetaminophen or another antipyretic) as needed; symptoms are self-limited.
- **B. Specific drugs and antidotes.** There is no specific antidote.
- **C. Decontamination** is not necessary; by the time symptoms develop, the exposure has usually been over for several hours.
- **D. Enhanced elimination.** There is no role for these procedures.

## ▶ METHANOL

*Ilene B. Anderson, PharmD*

Methanol (wood alcohol) is a common ingredient in many solvents, windshield-washing solutions, duplicating fluids, and paint removers. It sometimes is used as an ethanol substitute by alcoholics. Although methanol produces mainly inebriation, its metabolic products may cause metabolic acidosis, blindness, and death after a characteristic latent period of 6–30 hours.

**I. Mechanism of toxicity**

- **A.** Methanol is slowly metabolized by alcohol dehydrogenase to formaldehyde and subsequently by aldehyde dehydrogenase to formic acid (formate). Systemic acidosis is caused by both formate and lactate, whereas blindness is caused primarily by formate. Both ethanol and methanol compete for the enzyme alcohol dehydrogenase and block the metabolism of methanol to its toxic metabolites.
- **B. Pharmacokinetics.** Methanol is readily absorbed and quickly distributed to the body water (Vd = 0.6–0.77 L/kg). It is not protein bound. It is metabolized slowly by alcohol dehydrogenase via zero-order kinetics at a rate about one-tenth that of ethanol. The reported "half-life" ranges from 1 to 24 hours, depending on whether metabolism is blocked (eg, by ethanol or fomepizole). Only about 3% is excreted unchanged by the kidneys, and less than 10–20% through the breath. Formate half-life ranges from 3–20 hours; during dialysis the half-life decreases to 1–2.6 hours.

**II. Toxic dose.** The fatal oral dose of methanol is estimated to be 30–240 mL (20–150 g). The minimum toxic dose is approximately 100 mg/kg. Elevated serum methanol levels have been reported after extensive dermal exposure and concentrated inhalation. The ACGIH recommended workplace exposure limit (TLV-TWA) for inhalation is 200 ppm as an 8-hour time-weighted average, and the level considered immediately dangerous to life or health (IDLH) is 6000 ppm.

**III. Clinical presentation**

**A. In the first few hours** after ingestion, methanol-intoxicated patients present with inebriation and gastritis. Acidosis is not usually present because metabolism to toxic products has not yet occurred. There may be a noticeable elevation in the osmolar gap (see p 32); an osmolar gap as low as 10 mOsm/L is consistent with toxic concentrations of methanol.

**B. After a latent period** of up to 30 hours, severe anion gap metabolic acidosis, visual disturbances, blindness, seizures, coma, acute renal failure with myoglobinuria, and death may occur. Patients describe the visual disturbance as blurred vision, haziness, or "like standing in a snowfield." Fundoscopic examination may reveal optic disc hyperemia, venous engorgement, peripapilledema, and retinal or optic disc edema. The latent period is longer when ethanol has been ingested concurrently with methanol. Visual disturbances may occur within 6 hours in patients with a clear sensorium.

**IV. Diagnosis** usually is based on the history, symptoms, and laboratory findings because stat methanol levels are rarely available. Calculation of the osmolar and anion gaps (see p 32) can be used to estimate the methanol level and predict the severity of the ingestion. A large anion gap not accounted for by elevated lactate suggests possible methanol (or ethylene glycol) poisoning, because the anion gap in these cases is mostly nonlactate.

**A. Specific levels**

1. **Serum methanol** levels higher than 20 mg/dL should be considered toxic, and levels higher than 40 mg/dL should be considered very serious. After the latent period, a low or nondetectable methanol level does not rule out serious intoxication in a symptomatic patient because all the methanol may already have been metabolized to formate.
2. Elevated **serum formate** concentrations may confirm the diagnosis and are a better measure of toxicity, but formate levels are not widely available.

**B. Other useful laboratory studies** include electrolytes (and anion gap), glucose, BUN, creatinine, serum osmolality and osmolar gap, arterial blood gases, ethanol level, and lactate level.

**V. Treatment**

**A. Emergency and supportive measures**

1. Maintain an open airway and assist ventilation if necessary (see pp 1–7).
2. Treat coma (see p 18) and seizures (p 22) if they occur.
3. Treat metabolic acidosis with intravenous sodium bicarbonate (see p 423). Correction of acidosis should be guided by arterial blood gases.

**B. Specific drugs and antidotes**

1. Administer **fomepizole** (see p 454) or **ethanol** (p 450) to saturate the enzyme alcohol dehydrogenase and prevent the formation of methanol's toxic metabolites. Therapy is indicated in patients with the following:
   - **a.** A history of significant methanol ingestion when methanol serum levels are not immediately available and the osmolar gap is greater than 10 mOsm/L.
   - **b.** Metabolic acidosis (arterial pH $< 7.3$, serum bicarbonate $< 20$ mEq/L) and an osmolar gap greater than 10 mOsm/L not accounted for by ethanol.
   - **c.** A methanol blood concentration greater than 20 mg/dL.
2. **Folic or folinic acid** (see p 453) may enhance the conversion of formate to carbon dioxide and water. A suggested dose of folinic or folic acid is 1 mg/kg (up to 50 mg) IV every 4 hours.

**C. Decontamination** (see p 45). Aspirate gastric contents if this can be performed within 30–60 minutes of ingestion. Activated charcoal is not likely to be useful because the effective dose is very large and methanol is absorbed rapidly from the GI tract.

**D. Enhanced elimination.** Hemodialysis rapidly removes both methanol (half-life reduced to 3–6 hours) and formate.

1. The indications for dialysis include.
   a. Suspected methanol poisoning with significant metabolic acidosis.
   b. Visual abnormalities.
   c. Renal failure.
   d. An osmolar gap greater than 10 mOsm/L or a measured serum methanol concentration greater than 50 mg/dL.
2. Endpoint of treatment. Dialysis, fomepizole, or ethanol should be continued until the methanol concentration is less than 20 mg/dL and the osmolar and anion gaps are normalized.

## ▶ METHEMOGLOBINEMIA

*Paul D. Blanc, MD, MSPH*

Methemoglobin is an oxidized form of hemoglobin. Many oxidant chemicals and drugs are capable of inducing methemoglobinemia. Selected agents include nitrites and nitrates, bromates and chlorates, aniline derivatives, antimalarial agents, dapsone, propanil (a herbicide), sulfonamides, and local anesthetics (Table II–35). High-risk occupations include chemical and munitions work. An important environmental source for methemoglobinemia in infants is nitrate-contaminated well water. Amyl nitrite and butyl nitrite are abused for their alleged sexual enhancement properties. Oxides of nitrogen and other oxidant combustion products make smoke inhalation an important potential cause of methemoglobinemia.

**I. Mechanism of toxicity**

**A.** Methemoglobin inducers act by oxidizing ferrous ($Fe^{2+}$) to ferric ($Fe^{3+}$) hemoglobin. This abnormal hemoglobin is incapable of carrying oxygen, inducing a functional anemia. In addition, the shape of the oxygen-hemoglobin dissociation curve is altered, aggravating cellular hypoxia.

**B.** Methemoglobinemia does not cause hemolysis directly; however, many oxidizing agents that induce methemoglobinemia may also cause hemolysis through either hemoglobin (Heinz body) or cell membrane effects, particularly in patients with low tolerance for oxidative stress (eg, those with G6PD deficiency).

**II. Toxic dose.** The ingested dose or inhaled air level of toxin required to induce methemoglobinemia is highly variable. Neonates and persons with congenital methemoglobin reductase deficiency or G6PD deficiency have an impaired ability

**TABLE II–35. METHEMOGLOBINEMIA (SELECTED CAUSES)**

| Local anesthetics | Analgesics | Miscellaneous |
|---|---|---|
| Benzocaine | Phenazopyridine | Aminophenol |
| Lidocaine | Phenacetin | Aniline dyes |
| Prilocaine | **Nitrites and nitrates** | Bromates |
| **Antimicrobials** | Ammonium nitrate | Chlorates |
| Chloroquine | Amyl nitrite | 4-Dimethyl amino phenolate (4-DMAP) |
| Dapsone | Butyl nitrite | Metoclopramide |
| Primaquine | Isobutyl nitrite | Nitrobenzene |
| Sulfonamides | Potassium nitrate | Nitroethane |
| Trimethoprim | Sodium nitrate | Nitrogen oxides |
| | | Nitroglycerin |
| | | Propanil |

**TABLE II–36. METHEMOGLOBIN LEVELS**

| Methemoglobin Level[a] | Typical Symptoms |
|---|---|
| < 15% | Usually asymptomatic |
| 15–20% | Cyanosis, mild symptoms |
| 20–45% | Marked cyanosis, moderate symptoms |
| 45–70% | Severe cyanosis, severe symptoms |
| > 70% | Usually lethal |

[a]These percentages assume normal range total hemoglobin concentrations. Concomitant anemia may lead to more severe symptoms at lower proportional methemoglobinemia.

to regenerate normal hemoglobin and are therefore more likely to accumulate methemoglobin after oxidant exposure. Concomitant hemolysis suggests either heavy oxidant exposure or increased cell vulnerability.

**III. Clinical presentation.** The severity of symptoms usually correlates with measured methemoglobin levels (Table II–36).

**A.** Symptoms and signs are caused by decreased blood oxygen content and cellular hypoxia and include headache, dizziness, and nausea, progressing to dyspnea, confusion, seizures, and coma. Even at low levels, skin discoloration ("chocolate cyanosis"), especially of the nails, lips, and ears, can be striking.

**B.** Usually, mild methemoglobinemia (less than 15–20%) is well tolerated and will resolve spontaneously. This presumes that preexisting anemia has not already compromised the patient, thus making a smaller proportional impairment more clinically relevant. Continued metabolism of oxidant compounds from a long-acting parent compound (eg, dapsone) may lead to prolonged effects (2–3 days).

**IV. Diagnosis.** A patient with mild to moderate methemoglobinemia appears markedly cyanotic yet may be relatively asymptomatic. The arterial oxygen partial pressure ($pO_2$) is normal. The diagnosis is suggested by the finding of "chocolate brown" blood (dry a drop of blood on filter paper and compare with normal blood), which is usually apparent when the methemoglobin level exceeds 15%. Differential diagnosis includes other causes of cellular hypoxia (eg, carbon monoxide, cyanide, and hydrogen sulfide) and sulfhemoglobinemia.

**A. Specific levels.** The co-oximeter type of arterial blood gas analyzer directly measures oxygen saturation and methemoglobin percentages (measure as soon as possible, because levels fall rapidly in vitro).

1. ***Note:*** Sulfhemoglobin and the antidote methylene blue both produce erroneously high levels on the co-oximeter: A dose of 2 mL/kg methylene blue can lead to a false-positive methemoglobin reading of approximately 15%.
2. The routine arterial blood gas machine measures the serum $pO_2$ (which is normal) and calculates a falsely normal oxygen saturation in the face of methemoglobinemia.
3. Pulse oximetry is ***not*** reliable; it does not accurately reflect the degree of hypoxemia in a patient with severe methemoglobinemia and may appear falsely abnormal in a patient who has been given methylene blue.

**B. Other useful laboratory studies** include electrolytes and glucose. If hemolysis is suspected, add CBC, haptoglobin, peripheral smear, and urinalysis dipstick for occult blood (free hemoglobin is positive).

**V. Treatment**

**A. Emergency and supportive measures**

1. Maintain an open airway and assist ventilation if necessary (see pp 1–7). Administer supplemental oxygen.
2. Usually, mild methemoglobinemia (<15–20%) will resolve spontaneously and requires no intervention.

B. **Specific drugs and antidotes**
   1. **Methylene blue** (see p 473) is indicated in a symptomatic patient with methemoglobin levels higher than 20% or when even minimal compromise of oxygen-carrying capacity is potentially harmful (preexisting anemia, congestive heart failure, pneumocystis pneumonia, angina pectoris, etc). Give methylene blue, 1–2 mg/kg (0.1–0.2 mL/kg of 1% solution), over several minutes. ***Caution:*** Methylene blue can slightly worsen methemoglobinemia when given in excessive amounts; in patients with G6PD deficiency, it may aggravate methemoglobinemia and cause hemolysis.
   2. **Ascorbic acid,** which can reverse methemoglobin by an alternate metabolic pathway, is of minimal use acutely because of its slow action.

C. **Decontamination** (see p 45) depends on the specific agent involved.

D. **Enhanced elimination** (see p 53)
   1. If methylene blue is contraindicated (eg, G6PD deficiency) or has not been effective, **exchange transfusion** may rarely be necessary in patients with severe methemoglobinemia.
   2. **Hyperbaric oxygen** is theoretically capable of supplying sufficient oxygen independent of hemoglobin and may be useful in extremely serious cases that do not respond rapidly to antidotal treatment.

## ▶ METHYL BROMIDE

*Delia A. Dempsey, MS, MD*

Methyl bromide, a potent alkylating agent, is an odorless, colorless extremely toxic gas used as a fumigant in soil, perishable foods, and buildings. It is also used in the chemical industry. Fields or buildings to be fumigated are evacuated and covered with a giant tarp, and the gas is introduced. After 12–24 hours, the tarp is removed, and the area ventilated and then tested for residual methyl bromide before reoccupation. Methyl bromide is a major source of ozone-destroying bromine in the stratosphere, and most production and use was scheduled to be phased out by 2005 in developed countries and by 2015 in developing countries.

I. **Mechanism of toxicity**

A. Methyl bromide is a potent nonspecific alkylating agent with a special affinity for sulfhydryl and amino groups. Limited data indicate that toxicity is the result of direct alkylation of cellular components (eg, glutathione, proteins, or DNA) or formation of toxic metabolites from methylated glutathione. Animal data clearly indicate that its toxicity does not result from the bromide ion.

B. **Pharmacokinetics.** Inhaled methyl bromide is distributed rapidly to all tissues and metabolized. In sublethal animal studies, approximately 50% is eliminated as exhaled carbon dioxide, 25% is excreted in urine and feces, and 25% is bound to tissues as a methyl group. The elimination half-life of the bromide ion is 9–15 days.

II. **Toxic dose.** Methyl bromide is threefold heavier than air and may accumulate in low-lying areas, and it may seep via piping or conduits from fumigated buildings into adjacent structures. It may condense to a liquid at cold temperatures (3.6°C [38.5°F]) and then vaporize when temperatures rise. Methyl bromide gas lacks warning properties, so the lacrimator chloropicrin (2%) usually is added. However, chloropicrin has a different vapor pressure and may dissipate at a different rate, limiting its warning properties.

A. **Inhalation** is the most important route of exposure. The ACGIH recommended workplace exposure limit (TLV-TWA) in air is 1 ppm (3.9 mg/m$^3$) as an 8-hour time-weighted average. Toxic effects generally are seen at levels of 200 ppm, and the air level considered immediately dangerous to life or health (IDLH) is 250 ppm. NIOSH considers methyl bromide a potential occupational carcinogen.

B. **Skin** irritation and absorption may occur, causing burns and systemic toxicity. Methyl bromide may penetrate clothing and some protective gear. Retention of the gas in clothing and rubber boots can be a source of prolonged dermal exposure.

**III. Clinical presentation**

A. **Acute irritant effects** on the eyes, mucous membranes, and upper respiratory tract are attributed to the added lacrimator chloropicrin. (Lethal exposures can occur without warning if chloropicrin has not been added.) Moderate skin exposure can result in dermatitis and, in severe cases, chemical burns.

B. **Acute systemic effects** usually are delayed by 2–24 hours. Initial toxicity may include malaise, visual disturbances, headache, nausea, vomiting, and tremor, which may advance to intractable seizures and coma. Death may be caused by fulminant respiratory failure with noncardiogenic pulmonary edema or complications of status epilepticus. Sublethal exposure may result in flu-like symptoms, respiratory complaints, or chronic effects.

C. **Chronic neurologic sequelae** can result from chronic exposure or a sublethal acute exposure. A wide spectrum of neurologic and psychiatric problems may occur that may be reversible (months to years) or irreversible. They include agitation, delirium, dementia, psychoneurotic symptoms, psychosis, visual disturbances, vertigo, aphasia, ataxia, peripheral neuropathies, myoclonic jerking, tremors, and seizures.

**IV. Diagnosis** is based on a history of exposure to the compound and on clinical presentation.

A. **Specific levels.** Bromide levels in patients with acute methyl bromide exposure are usually well below the toxic range for bromism and may be only mildly elevated compared with levels in unexposed persons (see Bromides, p 140). Nontoxic bromide levels do not rule out methyl bromide poisoning. Levels of methylated proteins or DNA are being investigated as possible biomarkers for methyl bromide exposure.

B. **Other useful laboratory studies** include electrolytes, glucose, BUN, and creatinine. If there is respiratory distress, also perform arterial blood gases or oximetry and chest x-ray.

**V. Treatment**

A. **Emergency and supportive measures**

1. Administer supplemental oxygen and treat bronchospasm (see p 7), pulmonary edema (p 7), seizures (p 22), and coma (p 18) if they occur. Intractable seizures usually predict a fatal outcome. Consider induction of barbiturate coma with a short-acting agent such as pentobarbital (p 493) and consult a neurologist as soon as possible.
2. Monitor patients for a minimum of 6–12 hours to detect development of delayed symptoms, including seizures and noncardiogenic pulmonary edema.

B. **Specific drugs and antidotes.** Theoretically, *N*-acetylcysteine (NAC, p 407) or dimercaprol (BAL, p 417) can offer a reactive sulfhydryl group to bind free methyl bromide, although neither agent has been critically tested. There were strikingly different outcomes for two patients with the same exposure but different glutathione transferase activity, suggesting that NAC could possibly exacerbate toxicity. Neither agent can be recommended at this time.

C. **Decontamination** (see p 45). Properly trained personnel should use self-contained breathing apparatus and chemical-protective clothing before entering contaminated areas. The absence of irritant effects from chloropicrin does not guarantee that it is safe to enter without protection.

1. Remove victims from exposure and administer supplemental oxygen if available.
2. If exposure is to liquid methyl bromide, remove contaminated clothing and wash affected skin with soap and water. Irrigate exposed eyes with copious water or saline.

D. **Enhanced elimination.** There is no role for these procedures.

# ► METHYLENE CHLORIDE

*Binh T. Ly, MD, and Jennifer Hannum, MD*

Methylene chloride (dichloromethane, DCM) is a volatile colorless liquid with a chloroform-like odor. It has a wide variety of industrial uses, many of which are based on its solvent properties, including paint stripping, pharmaceutical manufacturing, metal cleaning and degreasing, film base production, agricultural fumigation, and plastics manufacturing. It is not known to occur naturally. Methylene chloride is metabolized to carbon monoxide in vivo and may produce phosgene, chlorine, or hydrogen chloride upon combustion.

**I. Mechanism of toxicity**

**A. Solvent effects.** Similar to other hydrocarbons, DCM is an irritant to mucous membranes, defats the skin epithelium, and may sensitize the myocardium to the dysrhythmogenic effects of catecholamines.

**B. Anesthetic effects.** Like other halogenated hydrocarbons, DCM can cause CNS depression and general anesthesia.

**C. Carbon monoxide** (CO) is generated in vivo during metabolism by the mixed-function oxidases (P-450 2E1) in the liver. Elevated carboxyhemoglobin (CO Hgb) levels may be delayed and prolonged, with CO Hgb levels as high as 50% reported. (See also Carbon Monoxide, p 151.)

**D.** Methylene chloride is a **suspected human carcinogen** (IARC 2B, see p 537).

**II. Toxic dose.** Toxicity may occur after inhalation or ingestion.

**A. Inhalation.** The permissible exposure limit (PEL) is 25 ppm as an 8-hour time-weighted average. The ACGIH workplace threshold limit value (TLV-TWA) is 50 ppm (174 mg/m$^3$) for an 8-hour shift, which may result in a CO Hgb level of 3–4%. The air level considered immediately dangerous to life or health (IDLH) is 2300 ppm. The odor threshold is about 100–200 ppm.

**B. Ingestion.** The acute oral toxic dose is approximately 0.5–5 mL/kg.

**III. Clinical presentation**

**A. Inhalation** is the most common route of exposure and may cause mucous membrane and skin irritation, nausea, vomiting, and headache. Ocular exposure can cause conjunctival irritation. Severe exposure may lead to pulmonary edema or hemorrhage, cardiac dysrhythmias, and CNS depression with respiratory arrest.

**B. Ingestion** can cause corrosive injury to the GI tract and systemic intoxication. Renal and hepatic injury and pancreatitis have been reported.

**C. Dermal exposure** can cause dermatitis or chemical burns, and systemic symptoms can result from skin absorption.

**D. Chronic exposure** can cause bone marrow, hepatic, and renal toxicity. Methylene chloride is a known animal and a suspected human carcinogen (IARC 2B).

**IV. Diagnosis** is based on a history of exposure and clinical presentation.

**A. Specific levels**

1. **Carboxyhemoglobin** levels should be obtained serially as peak CO Hgb levels may be delayed.
2. Expired air and blood or urine levels of **methylene chloride** may be obtained to assess workplace exposure but are not useful in clinical management.

**B. Other useful laboratory studies** include CBC, electrolytes, glucose, BUN, creatinine, liver transaminases, and ECG monitoring.

**V. Treatment**

**A. Emergency and supportive measures**

1. Maintain an open airway and assist ventilation if necessary (see pp 1–7).
2. Administer supplemental oxygen treat coma (see p 18) and pulmonary edema (p 7) if they occur.
3. Monitor the ECG for at least 4–6 hours and treat dysrhythmias (pp 10–15)

if they occur. Avoid the use of catecholamines (eg, epinephrine, dopamine), which may precipitate cardiac dysrhythmias. Tachydysrhythmias caused by myocardial sensitization may be treated with **esmolol** (see p 449), 0.025–0.1 mg/kg/min IV, or **propranolol** (p 504), 1–2 mg IV.

4. If corrosive injury is suspected after ingestion, consult a gastroenterologist regarding possible endoscopic evaluation.

B. **Specific drugs and antidotes.** Administer 100% **oxygen** by tight-fitting mask or endotracheal tube if the CO Hgb level is elevated. Consider hyperbaric oxygen (HBO) if the CO Hgb level is elevated and the patient has findings of CNS toxicity.

C. **Decontamination** (see p 45)

1. **Inhalation.** Remove the victim from exposure and give supplemental oxygen, if available.
2. **Skin and eyes.** Remove contaminated clothing and wash exposed skin with soap and water. Irrigate exposed eyes with copious saline or water.
3. **Ingestion.** Activated charcoal is of limited value and may make endoscopic evaluation difficult if corrosive injury is suspected. Perform nasogastric suction (if there has been a large, recent ingestion).

D. **Enhanced elimination.** There is no documented efficacy for repeat-dose activated charcoal, hemodialysis, or hemoperfusion. Although treatment with HBO may enhance elimination of carbon monoxide, its efficacy for patients with acute methylene chloride poisoning remains unproven.

## ► MOLDS

*John R. Balmes, MD*

Fungi are ubiquitous in all environments and play a critical ecologic role by decomposing organic matter. "Mold" is the common term for multicellular fungi that grow as a mat of intertwined microscopic filaments (hyphae). Molds are pervasive in the outdoor environment but may also be present indoors under certain conditions, primarily in the presence of excessive moisture from leaks in roofs or walls, plant pots, or pet urine. The most common indoor molds are *Cladosporium, Penicillium, Aspergillus,* and *Alternaria.* Other molds that can grow indoors include *Fusarium, Trichoderma,* and *Stachybotrys;* the presence of these molds often indicates a long-standing problem with water leakage or damage.

I. **Mechanism of toxicity.** Molds and other fungi may affect human health adversely through three processes: allergy, infection, and toxicity.

A. **Allergy.** Outdoor molds are generally more abundant and important in allergic disease than indoor molds. The most important indoor allergenic molds are *Penicillium* and *Aspergillus* species. Outdoor molds, such as *Cladosporium* and *Alternaria,* often can be found at high levels indoors if there is abundant access for outdoor air (eg, open windows). Homes and buildings that have excessive moisture or water damage can lead to enhanced growth of allergenic fungi.

B. **Infection.** Several fungi cause superficial infections involving the skin or nails. A very limited number of pathogenic fungi (eg, *Blastomyces, Coccidioides, Cryptococcus,* and *Histoplasma*) can infect nonimmunocompromised individuals. In contrast, persons with severe immune dysfunction (eg, cancer patients on chemotherapy, organ transplant patients on immunosuppressive drugs, patients with HIV infection) are at significant risk for more severe opportunistic fungal infection (eg, *Candida* and *Aspergillus*).

C. **Mycotoxins and glucans.** Some species of fungi are capable of producing mycotoxins, whereas most molds have one of a group of substances known as glucans in their cell walls. Serious veterinary and human mycotoxicoses have been documented after ingestion of foods heavily overgrown with toxigenic mold species. Inhalational exposure to high concentrations of mixed organic dusts (often in occupational settings) is associated with **organic dust toxic syndrome** (ODTS), an acute febrile illness. This self-limited condition generally is attributed to bacterial endotoxins and potentially to mold glucans rather than to mycotoxins. Currently there is insufficient evidence to confirm that indoor environmental exposures to mycotoxins from toxigenic mold species result in disease. In 1994 the CDC reported that a cluster of cases of acute idiopathic pulmonary hemorrhage (AIPH) in infants from Cleveland was associated with home contamination by *Stachybotrys chartarum.* However, a subsequent detailed reevaluation of the original data led the CDC to conclude that there was insufficient evidence to link the Cleveland cluster of AIPH causally to *S chartarum* exposure.

**D. Volatile organic compounds (VOCs),** including low-molecular-weight alcohols, aldehydes, and ketones, are generated by molds and are often responsible for the musty, disagreeable odor associated with indoor molds. A role for these VOCs in some building-related symptoms is possible.

**II. Toxic dose.** Because mycotoxins are not volatile, exposure would require inhalation of aerosolized spores, mycelial fragments, or contaminated substrates. The toxic inhaled dose of mycotoxin for humans is not known. Based on experimental data from single-dose in vivo studies, *Stachybotrys chartarum* spores (intranasally in mice or intratracheally in rats) in high doses (more than 30 million spores/kg) can produce pulmonary inflammation and hemorrhage. The no-effect dose in rats (3 million spores/kg) corresponds to a continuous 24-hour exposure to 2.1 million spores/$m^3$ for infants, 6.6 million spores/$m^3$ for a school-age child, or 15.3 million spores/$m^3$ for an adult. These spore concentrations are much higher than those measured in building surveys.

**III. Clinical presentation**

**A. Mold allergy** occurs in atopic individuals who develop IgE antibodies to a wide range of indoor and outdoor allergens, including animal dander, dust mites, and weed, tree, and grass pollens. Allergic responses are most commonly experienced as asthma or allergic rhinitis ("hay fever"). A much less common but more serious immunologic condition, **hypersensitivity pneumonitis** (HP), may follow exposure (often occupational) to relatively high concentrations of fungal (and other microbial) proteins.

**B. Infection** caused by pathogenic fungi is generally unrelated to exposure to molds from identifiable point sources and is beyond the scope of this chapter.

**C. Organic dust toxic syndrome** presents as a flu-like illness with an onset 4 to 8 hours after a heavy exposure (such as shoveling compost). Symptoms resolve without treatment over 24 hours.

**D.** "**Sick building syndrome,**" or "nonspecific building-related illness," represents a poorly defined set of symptoms that are attributed to a building's indoor environment and can include neurologic, GI, dermatologic, and respiratory complaints. The potential role of building-associated exposure to molds in some of these cases is suspected, but the mechanism is not clear. Existing data do not support a specific role for mycotoxins in this syndrome.

**IV. Diagnosis.** A history of recurrent respiratory symptoms associated with a specific building environment is consistent with either asthma or HP. Inquire about home, school, or work building conditions. If the conditions suggest the likelihood of mold contamination, consult with a specialist trained in the evaluation of building environments (eg, an industrial hygienist or a structural engineer). Mold risk is increased with a history of prior water damage or leak even when not ongoing, especially in the context of damaged drywall or carpeting on concrete.

**A. Specific tests.** Allergen skin prick testing or radioallergosorbent (RAST) testing can confirm the presence of specific IgE-mediated allergy to common fungi. Testing for the presence of IgG precipitating antibodies can confirm exposure to HP-inducing fungi, but a positive test does not confirm the diagnosis of HP. There are no specific blood or urine tests for mycotoxin exposure.

B. **Other useful laboratory studies.** Pulmonary function testing is helpful in distinguishing asthma (obstructive pattern with a normal diffusing capacity) from HP (restrictive pattern with a low diffusing capacity). Chest x-ray or high-resolution chest CT scanning may suggest the presence of interstitial lung disease consistent with HP or active or past fungal infection. Histologic examination of lung tissue obtained from transbronchial or open-lung biopsy may be necessary to confirm the diagnosis of HP.

C. **Environmental evaluation.** Indoor air samples with contemporaneous outdoor air samples can assist in evaluating whether there is mold growth indoors; air samples may also assist in evaluating the extent of potential indoor exposure. Bulk, wipe, and wall cavity samples may indicate the presence of mold but do not adequately characterize inhalational exposures of building occupants.

V. **Treatment**

A. **Emergency and supportive measures.** Treat bronchospasm (see p 7) and hypoxemia (p 7) if they are present.

B. **Specific drugs and antidotes.** None.

C. **Decontamination of the environment (remediation).** Mold overgrowth in indoor environments should be remediated not only because it may produce offensive odors and adverse health effects but because mold physically destroys the building materials on which it grows. A patient with HP caused by sensitization to a specific fungus present in a building environment is not likely to improve until excess exposure is eliminated. Once the source of moisture that supports mold growth has been eliminated, active mold growth can be halted. Colonized porous materials such as clothing and upholstery can be cleaned, using washing or dry cleaning as appropriate, and need not be discarded unless cleaning fails to restore an acceptable appearance and odor. Carpeting, drywall, and other structural materials, once contaminated, may present a greater remediation challenge.

D. **Enhanced elimination.** Not relevant.

See also the American College of Occupational and Environmental Medicine Position Statement/ Guideline: "Adverse Human Health Effects Associated with Molds in the Indoor Environment" http://www.acoem.org/position/statements.asp?CATA_ID=52.

## ▶ MONOAMINE OXIDASE INHIBITORS

*Lada Kokan, MD, and Neal L. Benowitz, MD*

Most monoamine oxidase (MAO) inhibitors are used primarily to treat severe depression but are also used occasionally to treat phobias and anxiety disorders. First-generation MAO inhibitors include **isocarboxazid** (Marplan™), **phenelzine** (Nardil™), and **tranylcypromine** (Parnate™). Newer-generation MAO inhibitors with reputed lower toxicity include **selegiline** (Eldepryl™), used in the treatment of Parkinson's disease, and **moclobemide** (Aurorix™), a much less toxic antidepressant that is available in many countries but not in the United States. Serious toxicity from MAO inhibitors occurs with overdose or owing to interactions with certain other drugs or foods (Table II–37).

A few drugs of other classes have some MAO-inhibiting activity. **Procarbazine** (Matulane™) is a cancer chemotherapeutic drug. **Linezolid** (Zyvox™) is increasingly important as one of the few antibiotics available to treat methicillin-resistant *Staphylococcus aureus* (MRSA) infections. The recreational drug paramethoxyamphetamine (PMA), which is often mistaken for ecstasy (MDMA, see p 73), also is also a potent MAO inhibitor. Both drugs increase serotonin levels, but PMA is reported to be more toxic. The popular herbal product used for depression **St. John's Wort** (*Hypericum perforatum*) appears to act in part as an MAO inhibitor. A number of other

TABLE II–37. MONOAMINE OXIDASE INHIBITOR INTERACTIONS[a]

| Drugs | | Foods |
|---|---|---|
| Amphetamines | Metaraminol | Beer |
| Buspirone | Methyldopa | Broad bean pods and fava beans |
| Clomipramine | Methylphenidate | Cheese (natural or aged) |
| Cocaine | Paroxetine | Chicken liver |
| Dextromethorphan | Phenylephrine | Pickled herring |
| Ephedrine | Phenylpropanolamine | Smoked, pickled, or aged meats |
| Fluvoxamine | Reserpine | Snails |
| Fluoxetine | Sertraline | Spoiled or bacterially contaminated foods |
| Guanethidine | Tramadol | Summer sausage |
| L-Dopa | Trazodone | Wine (red) |
| LSD (lysergic acid diethylamide) | Tryptophan | Yeast (dietary supplement and Marmite) |
| MDMA | Venlafaxine | |
| Meperidine (Demerol) | | |

[a]Possible interactions based on case reports or pharmacologic considerations.

plant products containing tryptamines, harmines, hydroxoindole, and other extracts have also been shown to have MAO-inhibiting activity.

I. **Mechanism of toxicity.** MAO inhibitors inactivate MAO, an enzyme responsible for degradation of catecholamines within neurons in the CNS. MAO is an enzyme with two major subtypes, MAO-A and MAO-B. MAO-A is also found in the liver and the intestinal wall, where it metabolizes tyramine and therefore limits its entry into the systemic circulation.

A. Toxicity results from the release of excessive neuronal stores of vasoactive amines, inhibition of metabolism of catecholamines, or absorption of large amounts of dietary tyramine (which in turn releases catecholamines from neurons).

1. **Selegiline** was developed as a *selective* MAO-B inhibitor that does not require a restrictive diet. (MAO-B selectivity is lost above doses of 20 g/day; thus, overdose with selegiline resembles that of the older MAO inhibitors.)

2. Older MAO inhibitors and selegiline are *irreversible* inhibitors of the enzyme. Since effects can last up to 2 weeks, drug and food interactions are common and potentially fatal with the first-generation drugs. However, **moclobemide** is a *reversible* competitive MAO inhibitor. As a result, it does not require food restrictions, has much less potential for drug interactions, and is much safer in overdose than are the older MAO inhibitors.

B. Toxic reactions to MAO inhibitors can be classified into four distinct types: food interactions, interactions with **certain drugs, serotonin syndrome, and acute overdose.**

1. **Food interactions**. Tyramine is a dietary monoamine that normally is degraded by GI MAO-A. MAO inhibition allows excessive absorption of tyramine, which acts indirectly to release norepinephrine, causing a hyperadrenergic syndrome. Patients taking therapeutic doses of the MAO-B-specific selegiline or the reversible inhibitor moclobemide (up to 900 mg/day) are not prone to this interaction and can eat a nonrestrictive diet.

2. **Interactions with indirect-acting monoamine drugs**. MAO inhibits degradation of presynaptic norepinephrine so that increased amounts are stored in the nerve endings. Drugs that act indirectly to release norepinephrine, such as pseudoephedrine and phenylephrine, can cause marked hypertension and tachycardia. Selegiline is not likely to cause this reaction because MAO-B has a much greater effect on brain dopamine than on norepinephrine levels.

3. **Serotonin syndrome**. Severe muscle hyperactivity, clonus, and hyperthermia may occur when patients receiving MAO inhibitors use even thera-

peutic doses of meperidine (Demerol), dextromethorphan, tricyclic antidepressants, SSRIs, or tryptophan; the mechanism is unknown but may be related to inhibition of serotonin metabolism in the CNS.

4. **Acute overdose** involving any MAO inhibitor is very serious and can be fatal. Selectivity for MAO-B is lost in selegiline overdose. In addition, selegiline is metabolized to amphetamine, which can contribute to hyperadrenergic symptoms in overdose.

C. ***Note:*** Because of irreversible MAO inhibition, adverse drug interactions may occur for up to 2 weeks after discontinuation of older MAO inhibitors. Interactions may also occur when MAO inhibitors are started within 10 days of stopping fluoxetine, owing to the long half-life of fluoxetine.

II. **Toxic dose.** First-generation MAO inhibitors have a low therapeutic index; acute ingestion of 2–3 mg/kg or more of tranylcypromine, isocarboxazid, or phenelzine should be considered potentially life threatening. In contrast, overdoses of up to 13 times the daily starting dose of moclobemide alone (about 28 mg/kg) typically result in mild or no symptoms. (However, overdose of moclobemide along with SSRIs can result in life-threatening toxicity with lower doses of moclobemide.)

III. **Clinical presentation.** Symptoms may be delayed 6–24 hours after acute overdose but occur rapidly after ingestion of interacting drugs or foods in a patient on chronic MAO inhibitor therapy. Because of irreversible inactivation of MAO, toxic effects (and the potential for drug or food interactions) may persist for several days when first-generation drugs are involved.

A. **Drug or food interactions** typically cause tachycardia, hypertension, anxiety, flushing, diaphoresis, and headache. Hypertensive crisis can lead to ischemia and end-organ damage such as intracranial hemorrhage, myocardial infarction, or renal failure.

B. With the **serotonin syndrome,** signs of both neuromuscular and autonomic instability such as hyperthermia, tremor, myoclonic jerking, hyperreflexia, and shivering may develop. Lower-extremity clonus is often reported, and patients are usually agitated and/or delirious. Severe hyperthermia can lead to acute cardiovascular collapse and multiorgan failure (see p 21).

C. **Acute overdose** can cause a clinical syndrome characterized by elements of both adrenergic hyperactivity and excessive serotonin activity, including severe hypertension, delirium, hyperthermia, dysrhythmias, seizures, obtundation, and eventually hypotension and cardiovascular collapse with multisystem failure. Other findings may include mydriasis, nystagmus, hallucinations, and tachypnea.

D. **Hypotension,** particularly when upright (orthostatic hypotension), is seen with therapeutic dosing and also may occur with overdose.

IV. **Diagnosis** is based on clinical features of sympathomimetic drug intoxication with a history of MAO inhibitor use, particularly with the use of drugs or foods known to interact. Serotonin syndrome (see p 21) is suspected when the patient has myoclonic jerking, hyperreflexia, diaphoresis, and hyperthermia.

A. **Specific levels.** Drug levels are not generally available. Most agents are not detectable on comprehensive urine toxicology screening. Selegiline is metabolized to amphetamine, which may be detected on urine toxicology screening tests.

B. Other useful laboratory studies include electrolytes, glucose, BUN, creatinine, CPK, troponin, 12-lead ECG, and ECG monitoring. If intracranial hemorrhage is suspected, perform a CT head scan.

V. **Treatment**

A. **Emergency and supportive measures**

1. Maintain an open airway and assist ventilation if necessary (see pp 1–7). Administer supplemental oxygen.
2. Treat hypertension (p 17), coma (p 18), seizures (p 22), and hyperthermia (p 20) if they occur.
   a. Use titratable intravenous antihypertensives such as nitroprusside (see p 485) and phentolamine (see p 495) because of the potential for rapid changes in hemodynamics.

   b. If hypotension occurs, it may reflect depletion of neuronal catecholamine stores, and in this case the direct-acting agent norepinephrine is preferred over the indirect-acting drug dopamine.
  3. Continuously monitor temperature, other vital signs, and ECG for a minimum of 6 hours in asymptomatic patients and admit all symptomatic patients for continuous monitoring for 24 hours.

**B. Specific drugs and antidotes**

1. Since the hypertension is catecholamine-mediated, alpha-adrenergic blockers (eg, phentolamine, p 495) or combined alpha- and beta-adrenergic blockers (eg, labetalol, p 466) are particularly useful. ***Note:*** Use of nonselective beta blockers without a vasodilator may cause paradoxic worsening of hypertension owing to unopposed alpha-adrenergic effects.
2. **Serotonin syndrome** should be treated with sedation and cooling. Anecdotal reports suggest possible benefit with the serotonin antagonists cyproheptadine (Periactin™), 4 mg PO or per nasogastric (NG) tube every hour for 3 doses), and methysergide (Sansert™), 2 mg PO or per NG tube every 6 hours for 3 doses.

**C. Decontamination.** Administer activated charcoal orally if conditions are appropriate (see Table I–38, p 51). Consider gastric lavage if the patient presents early after a very large ingestion of a first-generation drug or selegiline.

**D. Enhanced elimination.** Dialysis and hemoperfusion are not effective. Repeat-dose activated charcoal has not been studied.

## ▶ MUSHROOMS, AMATOXIN-TYPE

*Kathy Marquardt, PharmD*

Amatoxins are a group of highly toxic peptides found in several species of mushrooms, including *Amanita phalloides, Amanita virosa, Amanita bisporigera, Amanita ocreata, Amanita verna, Galerina autumnalis, Galerina marginata,* and some species of *Lepiota* and *Conocybe.* This category of mushrooms is responsible for more than 90% of mushroom deaths worldwide.

This group is also referred to as cyclopeptide-containing mushrooms. The three cyclopeptides are amatoxin, phallotoxin, and virotoxin. Amatoxins, principally alpha amanitin, are the most toxic and are responsible for the hepatic and renal toxicity. Phallotoxins are not well absorbed and cause GI symptoms. Virotoxins are not implicated in human poisoning.

**I. Mechanism of toxicity.** Amatoxins are highly stable and resistant to heat and are not removed by any form of cooking. They bind to DNA-dependent RNA polymerase II and inhibit the elongation essential to transcription. The result is a decrease in mRNA that causes an arrest of protein synthesis and cell death. Metabolically active tissue dependent on high rates of protein synthesis, such as cells of the GI tract, hepatocytes, and the proximal convoluted tubules of the kidney, are disproportionately affected. Cellular damage has also been found in the pancreas, adrenal glands, and testes.

**A. Pharmacokinetics.** Amatoxins are readily absorbed from the intestine and are transported across the hepatocyte by bile transport carriers. About 60% undergo enterohepatic recirculation. They have limited protein binding and are eliminated in urine, vomitus, and feces. Toxins are detectable in urine within 90–120 minutes after ingestion. No metabolites of amatoxin have been detected. The half-life in humans is unknown, but there is a rapid decrease in serum levels, with detection of toxin unlikely after 36 hours.

**II. Toxic dose.** Amatoxins are among the most potent toxins known; the minimum lethal dose is about 0.1 mg/kg. One *Amanita phalloides* cap may contain 10–15 mg. In contrast, *Galerina* species contain far less toxin; 15–20 caps would be a fatal dose for an adult.

**III. Clinical presentation.** Amatoxin poisoning can be divided into three phases. There is an initial phase of delayed GI toxicity followed by a false recovery period and then late-onset hepatic failure. This triphasic syndrome is pathognomic for amatoxin mushroom poisoning.

**A. Phase 1.** Onset of symptoms is 6–24 hours after ingestion. Symptoms consist of vomiting, severe abdominal cramps, and explosive watery diarrhea, which may become grossly bloody. This GI phase may be severe enough to cause acid-base disturbances, electrolyte abnormalities, hypoglycemia, dehydration, and hypotension. Death may occur within the first 24 hours from massive fluid loss.

**B. Phase 2** occurs 18–36 hours after ingestion. There is a period of transient clinical improvement in the gastroenteritis but rising liver enzymes. During this phase, patients may be discharged home only to return in 1–2 days with hepatic and renal failure.

**C. Phase 3** begins 2–4 days after ingestion and is characterized by markedly elevated transaminases, hyperbilirubinemia, coagulopathy, hypoglycemia, acidosis, hepatic encephalopathy, hepatorenal syndrome, multiorgan failure, disseminated intravascular coagulation, and convulsions. Death usually occurs 6–16 days after ingestion. Encephalopathy, metabolic acidosis, severe coagulopathy, and hypoglycemia are grave prognostic signs and usually predict a fatal outcome.

**IV. Diagnosis** is usually based on a history of wild mushroom ingestion and a delay of 6–24 hours before onset of severe gastroenteritis (see also monomethylhydrazine-type mushrooms, Table II–38, p 274). However, if a variety of mushrooms have been eaten, stomach upset may occur much earlier owing to a different toxic species, making diagnosis of amatoxin poisoning more difficult.

Any available mushroom specimens that may have been ingested should be examined by a mycologist. Pieces of mushroom retrieved from the emesis or even mushroom spores found on microscopic examination may provide clues to the ingested species.

**A. Specific levels**

1. Amatoxin can be detected in serum, urine, and gastric fluids by radioimmunoassay or high-performance liquid chromatography (HPLC), but these methods are not readily available. Using HPLC, amatoxin has been detected in serum for up to 36 hours and urine for up to 4 days. Radioimmunoassay has detected amatoxins in urine in 100% of cases tested within 24 hours and in 80% of cases tested within 48 hours.
2. A qualitative test (the Meixner test) may determine the presence of amatoxins in mushroom specimens. Juice from the mushroom is dripped onto newspaper or other high-lignin-content paper and allowed to dry. A single drop of concentrated hydrochloric acid is then added; a blue color suggests the presence of amatoxins. ***Caution:*** This test has unknown reliability and can be misinterpreted or poorly performed; it should not be used to determine the edibility of mushroom specimens. In addition, false-positive reactions can be caused by drying at a temperature greater than 63°C, exposure of the test paper to sunlight, or the presence of psilocybin, bufotenin, or certain terpenes.

**B. Other useful laboratory studies** include electrolytes, glucose, BUN, creatinine, liver transaminases, bilirubin, and prothrombin time (PT/INR). Transaminases usually peak 60–72 hours after ingestion. Measures of liver function such as the INR are more useful in evaluating the severity of hepatic failure.

**V. Treatment.** The mortality rate is approximately 10–15% with intensive supportive care.

**A. Emergency and supportive measures**

1. Maintain an open airway and assist ventilation if necessary (see pp 1–7). Administer supplemental oxygen.

TABLE I–38. MUSHROOM TOXICITY

| Syndrome | Toxin(s) | Causative Mushrooms | Symptoms and Signs |
|---|---|---|---|
| Delayed gastroenteritis and liver failure | Amatoxins (See p 272) | *Amanita phalloides, A ocreata, A verna, A virosa, A bisporigera, Galerina autumnalis, G marginata,* and some *Lepiota* and *Conocybe* species. | Delayed onset 6–24 h: vomiting, diarrhea, abdominal cramps, followed by fulminant hepatic failure after 2–3 days. |
| Delayed gastroenteritis, CNS abnormalities, hemolysis, hepatitis | Monomethylhydrazine | *Gyrometra (Helvella) esculenta*, others. | Delayed onset 6–12 h: vomiting, diarrhea, dizziness, weakness, headache, delirium, seizures, coma; hemolysis, methemoglobinemia, hepatic and renal injury may also occur. |
| Cholinergic syndrome | Muscarine | *Clitocybe dealbata, C cerusata, Inocybe, Omphalotus olearius.* | Onset 30 min–2 h: diaphoresis, bradycardia, bronchospasm, lacrimation, salivation, sweating, vomiting, diarrhea, miosis. Treat with atropine (p 415). |
| Disulfiram-like reaction with alcohol | Coprine | *Coprinus atramentarius, Clitocybe clavipes.* | Within 30 min after ingestion of alcohol: nausea, vomiting, flushing, tachycardia, hypotension; risk of reaction for up to 5 days after ingesting fungi. (See Disulfiram, p 184.) |
| Isoxazole syndrome | Ibotenic acid, muscimol | *Amanita muscaria, A pantherina,* others. | Onset 30 min–2 h: vomiting, followed by drowsiness, muscular jerking, hallucinations, delirium, psychosis. |
| Gastritis and renal failure | Allenic norleucine | *Amanita smithiana, Amanita proxima.* | Abdominal pain, vomiting within 30 min to 12 hours, followed by progressive acute renal failure within 2–3 days. |
| Delayed onset gastritis and renal failure | Orellanine | *Cortinarius orellanus,* other *Cortinarius* spp. | Abdominal pain, anorexia, vomiting starting after 24–36 hours, followed by progressive acute renal failure (tubulointerstitial nephritis) 3–14 days later. |
| Hallucinogenic | Psilocybin, psilocyn | *Psilocybe cubensis, panaeolina foenisecii,* others. | Onset 30 min–2 h: visual hallucinations, sensory distortion, tachycardia, mydriasis, occasionally seizures. |
| Gastrointestinal irritants | Unidentified | *Chlorophyllum molybdites, Boletus satanas,* many others. | Vomiting, diarrhea within 30 min–2 h of ingestion. |
| Immunohemolytic anemia | Unidentified | *Paxillus involutus.* | GI irritant for most, but a few people develop immune-mediated hemolysis within 2 h of ingestion. |
| Allergic pneumonitis (inhaled spores) | Lycoperdon spores | *Lycoperdon* species | Inhalation of dry spores can cause acute nausea, vomiting, and nasopharyngitis, followed within days by fever, malaise, dyspnea, and inflammatory pneumonitis |
| Erythromelalgia | Acromelic acids | *Clitocybe acromelalga, Clitocybe amoenolens* | Onset 6–24 hours. Symptoms of numbness, burning pain, paresthesias, reddish edema in fingers and toes. |
| Rhabdomyolysis | Unidentified | *Tricholoma equestre, Russula subnigricans* | Onset 24–72 hours. Fatigue, muscle weakness, rhabdomyolysis, renal insufficiency, and myocarditis. |
| Delayed CNS toxicity | Polyporic acid | *Hapalopilus rutilans* | Onset after 24 hours. Decreased visual acuity, somnolence, reduced motor tone and activity, electrolyte disturbances, and hepatorenal failure. |

2. Treat fluid and electrolyte losses aggressively, because massive fluid losses may cause circulatory collapse. Administer normal saline or another crystalloid solution, 10- to 20-mL/kg boluses, with monitoring of central venous pressure or even pulmonary artery pressure to guide fluid therapy.
3. Provide vigorous supportive care for hepatic failure (p 39); orthotopic **liver transplantation** may be lifesaving in patients who develop fulminant hepatic failure. Contact a liver transplantation service for assistance.

**B. Specific drugs and antidotes.** No antidote has been proved effective for amatoxin poisoning, although over the years many therapies have been promoted. Animal studies and retrospective comparisons in human cases suggest that early treatment with **silibinin** (an extract of milk thistle that is used in Europe intravenously in a dose of 20–50 mg/kg/day but is not available as a pharmaceutical preparation in the United States; see p 500) may be effective in reducing hepatocyte uptake of amatoxin. High doses of penicillin showed some hepatoprotective effects in dog and rat studies, but controlled human studies are lacking. A retrospective analysis of 20 years of amatoxin treatment found that high-dose penicillin was the most frequently utilized chemotherapy but showed little efficacy. The therapies thought most effective based on this review were silibinin, *N*-acetylcysteine, and detoxication procedures. There are no data to support the use of cimetidine or steroids, and thioctic acid causes a severe hypoglycemia. Amatoxin-specific FAB fragments enhanced the activity of amatoxins. Consult a medical toxicologist or a regional poison control center ([800] 222-1222 in the United States) for further information.

**C. Decontamination** (see p 45). Administer activated charcoal orally. Gastric lavage may not remove mushroom pieces.

**D. Enhanced elimination.** There is no proven role for forced diuresis, hemoperfusion, hemofiltration, or hemodialysis in the removal of amatoxins.

1. Repeat-dose activated charcoal may trap small quantities of amatoxin undergoing enterohepatic recirculation and should be continued for the first 48 hours.
2. Cannulation of the bile duct and removal of bile have been effective in dog studies.

## ► MUSHROOMS

*Kathy Marquardt, PharmD*

There are more than 5000 varieties of mushrooms, of which about 50–100 are known to be toxic and only 200–300 are known to be safely edible. The majority of toxic mushrooms cause mild to moderate self-limited gastroenteritis. A few species may cause severe or even fatal reactions. The major categories of poisonous mushrooms are described in Table II–38. *Amanita phalloides* and other amatoxin-containing mushrooms are discussed on p 272.

**I. Mechanism of toxicity.** The various mechanisms thought responsible for poisoning are listed in Table II–38. The majority of toxic incidents are caused by GI irritants that produce vomiting and diarrhea shortly after ingestion.

**II. Toxic dose.** This is not known. The amount of toxin varies considerably among members of the same species, depending on local geography and weather conditions. In most cases, the exact amount of toxic mushroom ingested is unknown because the victim has unwittingly added a toxic species to a meal of edible fungi.

**III. Clinical presentation.** The various clinical presentations are described in Table II–38. These presentations often can be recognized by onset of action. If symptom onset is within 6 hours, the likely categories will be GI irritants, cholinergic syndrome, hallucinogenic, the isoxazole syndrome, immunohemolytic, allergic pneumonitis, or allenic norleucine class.

Mushrooms that cause symptoms from 6–24 hours after ingestion include those containing amatoxins or monomethylhydrazine and those causing erythromelalgia.

Onset of symptoms more than 24 hours after ingestion suggests poisoning by the orellanines that cause kidney damage, mushrooms causing rhabdomyolysis, and mushrooms causing delayed CNS toxicity. Mushrooms in the coprine category do not cause symptoms unless the patient ingests alcohol. This disulfiram-like effect can occur from 2 hours to as long as 5 days after ingestion.

**IV. Diagnosis** may be difficult because the victim may not realize that the illness was caused by mushrooms, especially if symptoms are delayed 12 or more hours after ingestion. If leftover mushrooms are available, obtain assistance from a mycologist through a local university or mycologic society. However, note that the mushrooms brought for identification may not be the same ones that were eaten.

History is key to determining the category of toxic mushroom. It is important to get a description of the mushroom and the environment from which it was obtained. Was the mushroom dish cooked or eaten raw? Were several types of mushrooms ingested? What was the time of ingestion in relation to the onset of symptoms? Was alcohol ingested since the mushrooms were eaten? Is everyone who ate the mushroom ill? Are those who did not eat the mushroom also ill? Were the mushrooms eaten several times? Were they stored properly?

**A. Specific levels.** Qualitative detection of the toxins of several mushroom species has been reported, but these tests are not routinely available.

**B. Other useful laboratory studies** include CBC, electrolytes, glucose, BUN, creatinine, liver transaminases, and prothrombin time (PT/INR). Obtain a methemoglobin level if gyromitrin-containing mushrooms are suspected or the patient is cyanotic. Obtain a chest x-ray if allergic pneumonitis syndrome is suspected and serial creatinine phosphokinase (CPK) levels for suspected rhabdomyolysis.

**V. Treatment**

**A. Emergency and supportive measures**

1. Treat hypotension from gastroenteritis with intravenous crystalloid solutions (see p 15) and supine positioning. Treat agitation (p 23), hyperthermia (p 20), rhabdomyolysis (p 26), and seizures (p 22) if they occur.
2. Monitor patients for 12–24 hours for delayed-onset gastroenteritis associated with amatoxin or monomethylhydrazine poisoning.
3. Monitor renal function for 1–2 weeks after suspected *Cortinarius* spp ingestion, or 2–3 days after *Amanita smithiana* ingestion. Provide supportive care, including hemodialysis if needed, for renal dysfunction.

**B. Specific drugs and antidotes**

1. For **monomethylhydrazine** poisoning, give pyridoxine, 20–30 mg/kg IV (see p 508), for seizures; treat methemoglobinemia with methylene blue, 1 mg/kg IV (p 473).
2. For **muscarine** intoxication, atropine, 0.01–0.03 mg/kg IV (see p 415), may alleviate cholinergic symptoms.
3. **Allergic pneumonitis** may benefit from steroid administration.
4. Treat **amatoxin-type** poisoning as described on p 272.

**C. Decontamination** (see p 45). Administer activated charcoal orally if conditions are appropriate (see Table I–38, p 51).

1. Charcoal is probably not warranted after a trivial ingestion (eg, a lick or a nibble) of an unknown mushroom by a toddler.
2. Repeat-dose activated charcoal (see p 50) may be helpful after amatoxin ingestion (see p 272).

**D. Enhanced elimination.** There is no accepted role for these procedures.

## ▶ NAPHTHALENE AND PARADICHLOROBENZENE

*Mark J. Galbo, MS*

Naphthalene and paradichlorobenzene are common ingredients in diaper pail and toilet bowl deodorizers and moth repellents. Both compounds have a similar pungent odor and are clear to white crystalline substances; therefore, they are difficult to distinguish visually. Naphthalene 10% in oil was used as a scabicide in the past. Naphthalene is no longer commonly used because it largely has been replaced by the far less toxic paradichlorobenzene.

I. **Mechanism of toxicity.** Both compounds cause GI upset, and both may cause CNS stimulation. In addition, naphthalene may produce hemolysis, especially in patients with glucose-6-phosphate dehydrogenase (G6PD) deficiency.

II. **Toxic dose**

A. **Naphthalene.** As little as one mothball containing naphthalene (250–500 mg) may produce hemolysis in a patient with G6PD deficiency. The amount necessary to produce lethargy or seizures is not known but may be as little as 1–2 g (4–8 mothballs). Several infants developed serious poisoning from clothes and bedding that had been stored in naphthalene mothballs.

B. **Paradichlorobenzene** is much less toxic than naphthalene; up to 20-g ingestions have been well tolerated in adults. The oral LD50 for paradichlorobenzene in rats is 2.5–3.2 g/kg.

C. **Pharmacokinetics.** Both compounds are rapidly absorbed orally or by inhalation.

III. **Clinical presentation.** Acute ingestion usually causes prompt nausea and vomiting. Both compounds are volatile, and inhalation of vapors may cause eye, nose, and throat irritation.

A. **Naphthalene.** Agitation, lethargy, and seizures may occur with naphthalene ingestion. Acute hemolysis may occur, especially in patients with G6PD deficiency. Chronic inhalation has also caused hemolytic anemia.

B. **Paradichlorobenzene** ingestions are virtually always innocuous. Serious poisoning in animals is reported to cause tremors and hepatic necrosis. Paradichlorobenzene decomposes to hydrochloric acid; this may explain some of its irritant effects.

IV. **Diagnosis** usually is based on a history of ingestion and the characteristic "mothball" smell around the mouth and in the vomitus. Differentiation between naphthalene and paradichlorobenzene by odor or color is difficult. In an in vitro x-ray study, paradichlorobenzene was radiopaque but naphthalene was not visible. In a saturated salt solution (about 1 tablespoon of salt in 4 ounces of water), naphthalene will float and paradichlorobenzene will sink.

A. **Specific levels.** Serum levels are not available.

B. **Other useful laboratory studies** include CBC and, if hemolysis is suspected, haptoglobin, free hemoglobin, and urine dipstick for occult blood (positive with hemoglobinuria).

V. **Treatment**

A. **Emergency and supportive measures**

1. Maintain an open airway and assist ventilation if necessary (see pp 1–7).
2. Treat coma (see p 18) and seizures (p 22) if they occur.
3. Treat hemolysis and resulting hemoglobinuria, if they occur, by intravenous hydration and urinary alkalinization (see Rhabdomyolysis, p 26).

B. **Specific drugs and antidotes.** There is no specific antidote.

C. **Decontamination** (see p 45)

1. **Naphthalene.** Administer activated charcoal orally if conditions are appropriate (see Table I–38, p 51). Gastric lavage is not necessary after small to moderate ingestions if activated charcoal can be given
2. **Paradichlorobenzene.** Gut emptying and charcoal are not necessary unless a massive dose has been ingested. Do not administer milk, fats, or oils, which may enhance absorption.
3. **Inhalation.** Either agent: Remove the victim from exposure; fresh air is all that is required.

D. **Enhanced elimination.** There is no role for these procedures.

# ▶ NICOTINE

*Neal L. Benowitz, MD*

Nicotine poisoning may occur in children after they ingest tobacco or drink saliva expectorated by a tobacco chewer (which is often collected in a can or other containers), in children or adults after accidental or suicidal ingestion of nicotine-containing pesticides (such as Black Leaf 40, which contains 40% nicotine sulfate), and occasionally after cutaneous exposure to nicotine, such as among tobacco harvesters ("green tobacco sickness"). Nicotine chewing gum (Nicorette), transdermal delivery formulations (Habitrol, Nicoderm, Nicotrol, Prostep, and generics), and nicotine nasal spray, inhalers, and lozenges are widely available as adjunctive therapy for smoking cessation. Alkaloids similar to nicotine (anabasine, cytisine, coniine, and lobeline) are found in several plant species (see Plants, p 309).

**I. Mechanism of toxicity**

- **A.** Nicotine binds to nicotinic cholinergic receptors, resulting initially, via actions on ganglia, in predominantly sympathetic nervous stimulation. With higher doses, parasympathetic stimulation and then ganglionic and neuromuscular blockage may occur. Direct effects on the brain may also result in vomiting and seizures.
- **B. Pharmacokinetics.** Nicotine is absorbed rapidly by all routes. The apparent volume of distribution is 3 L/kg. It is rapidly metabolized and to a lesser extent excreted in the urine, with a half-life of 120 minutes.

**II. Toxic dose.** Owing to presystemic metabolism and spontaneous vomiting, which limit absorption, the bioavailability of nicotine that is swallowed is about 30–40%. Rapid absorption of 2–5 mg can cause nausea and vomiting, particularly in a person who does not use tobacco habitually. Absorption of 40–60 mg in an adult is said to be lethal, although this dose spread throughout the day is not unusual in a cigarette smoker.

- **A. Tobacco.** Cigarette tobacco contains about 1.5% nicotine, or 10–15 mg of nicotine per cigarette. Moist snuff is also about 1.5% nicotine; most containers hold 30 g of tobacco. Chewing tobacco contains 2.5–8% nicotine. In a child, ingestion of one cigarette or three cigarette butts should be considered potentially toxic, although serious poisoning from ingestion of cigarettes is very uncommon.
- **B. Nicotine gum** contains 2 or 4 mg per piece, but owing to its slow absorption and high degree of presystemic metabolism, nicotine intoxication from these products is uncommon.
- **C. Transdermal nicotine patches** deliver an average of 5–22 mg of nicotine over the 16–24 hours of intended application, depending on the brand and size. Transdermal patches may produce intoxication in light smokers or in nonsmokers, particularly children to whom a used patch inadvertently sticks. Ingestion of a discarded patch may also potentially produce poisoning.
- **D. Nicotine nasal spray** delivers about 1 mg (a single dose is one spray in each nostril).
- **E. Nicotine inhaler systems** consist of a plastic mouthpiece and replaceable cartridges containing 10 mg of nicotine. If accidentally ingested, the cartridge would release the nicotine slowly, and no serious intoxication has been reported.
- **F. Nicotine lozenges** contain 2–4 mg nicotine, and ingestion could cause serious toxicity in a child.

**III. Clinical presentation.** Nicotine intoxication commonly causes dizziness, nausea, vomiting, pallor, and diaphoresis. Abdominal pain, salivation, lacrimation, and diarrhea may be noted. Pupils may be dilated or constricted. Confusion, agitation, lethargy, and convulsions are seen with severe poisonings. Initial tachycardia and hypertension may be followed by bradycardia and hypotension. Respiratory muscle weakness with respiratory arrest is the most likely cause of death. Symptoms usually begin within 15 minutes after acute liquid nicotine exposure and resolve in 1 or 2 hours, although more prolonged symptoms may be seen with higher doses or cutaneous exposure, with the latter resulting from continued absorption from the skin. Delayed onset and prolonged symptoms may also be seen with nicotine gum or transdermal patches.

IV. **Diagnosis** is suggested by vomiting, pallor, and diaphoresis, although these symptoms are nonspecific. The diagnosis usually is made by a history of tobacco, insecticide, or therapeutic nicotine product exposure. Nicotine poisoning should be considered in a small child with unexplained vomiting whose parents consume tobacco.

A. **Specific levels.** Nicotine and its metabolite cotinine are detected in comprehensive urine toxicology screens, but because they are so commonly present, they will not usually be reported unless a specific request is made. Serum levels can be performed but are not useful in acute management.

B. **Other useful laboratory studies** include electrolytes, glucose, and arterial blood gases or oximetry.

V. **Treatment**

A. **Emergency and supportive measures**

1. Maintain an open airway and assist ventilation if necessary (see pp 1–7). Administer supplemental oxygen.
2. Treat seizures (see p 22), coma (p 18), hypotension (p 15), hypertension (p 17), and arrhythmias (pp 10–15) if they occur.
3. Observe for at least 4–6 hours to rule out delayed toxicity, especially after skin exposure. For ingestion of intact gum tablets or transdermal patches, observe for a longer period (up to 12–24 hours).

B. **Specific drugs and antidotes**

1. **Mecamylamine** (Inversine) is a specific antagonist of nicotine actions; however, it is available only in tablets, a form not suitable for a patient who is vomiting, convulsing, or hypotensive.
2. Signs of muscarinic stimulation (bradycardia, salivation, wheezing, etc), if they occur, may respond to **atropine** (see p 415).

C. **Decontamination** (see p 45). ***Caution:*** Rescuers should wear appropriate skin-protective gear when treating patients with oral or skin exposure to liquid nicotine.

1. **Skin and eyes.** Remove all contaminated clothing and wash exposed skin with copious soap and water. Irrigate exposed eyes with copious saline or water.
2. **Ingestion.** Administer activated charcoal orally if conditions are appropriate (see Table I–38, p 51). Gastric lavage is not necessary after tobacco ingestions if activated charcoal can be given promptly. Consider gastric lavage for large recent ingestions of liquid nicotine.
   a. For asymptomatic small-quantity cigarette ingestions, no gut decontamination is necessary.
   b. For ingestion of transdermal patches or large amounts of gum, consider repeated doses of charcoal and whole-bowel irrigation (see p 51).

D. **Enhanced elimination.** These procedures are not likely to be useful because the endogenous clearance of nicotine is high, its half-life is relatively short (2 hours), and the volume of distribution is large.

## ► NITRATES AND NITRITES

*Neal L. Benowitz, MD*

Organic nitrates (eg, nitroglycerin, isosorbide dinitrate, and isosorbide mononitrate) are widely used as vasodilators for the treatment of ischemic heart disease and heart failure. Organic nitrates such as nitroglycerin also are used in explosives. Bismuth subnitrate, ammonium nitrate, and silver nitrate are used in antidiarrheal drugs, cold packs, and topical burn medications, respectively. Sodium and potassium nitrate and nitrite are used in preserving cured foods and may also occur in high concentrations in some well water. Butyl, amyl, ethyl, and isobutyl nitrites often are sold as "room deodorizers" or "liquid incense" and sometimes are inhaled for abuse purposes.

**I. Mechanism of toxicity.** Nitrates and nitrites both cause vasodilation, which can result in hypotension.

- **A. Nitrates** relax veins at lower doses and arteries at higher doses. Nitrates may be converted into nitrites in the GI tract, especially in infants.
- **B. Nitrites** are potent oxidizing agents. Oxidation of hemoglobin by nitrites may result in methemoglobinemia (see p 262), which hinders oxygen-carrying capacity and oxygen delivery. Many organic nitrites (eg, amyl nitrite and butyl nitrite) are volatile and may be inhaled.

**II. Toxic dose.** In the quantities found in food, nitrates and nitrites are generally not toxic; however, infants may develop methemoglobinemia after ingestion of sausages or well water because they readily convert nitrate to nitrite and because their hemoglobin is more susceptible to oxidation than is that of adults.

- **A. Nitrates.** The estimated adult lethal oral dose of nitroglycerin is 200–1200 mg. Hypotension occurs at low doses, but massive doses are required to produce methemoglobinemia.
- **B. Nitrites.** Ingestion of as little as 15 mL of butyl nitrite produced 40% methemoglobinemia in an adult. The estimated adult lethal oral dose of sodium nitrite is 1 g.

**III. Clinical presentation.** Headache, skin flushing, and orthostatic hypotension with reflex tachycardia are the most common adverse effects of nitrates and nitrites and occur commonly even with therapeutic doses of organic nitrates.

- **A. Hypotension** may aggravate or produce symptoms of cardiac ischemia or cerebrovascular disease and may even cause seizures. However, fatalities from hypotension are rare.
- **B.** Workers or patients regularly exposed to nitrates may develop tolerance and may suffer **angina** or **myocardial infarction** owing to rebound coronary vasoconstriction upon sudden withdrawal of the drug.
- **C. Methemoglobinemia** (see p 262) is most common after nitrite exposure; the skin is cyanotic even at levels low enough to be otherwise asymptomatic (eg, 15%).
- **D.** Use of **sildenafil** (Viagra™) and other selective phosphodiesterase inhibitors (tadalafil [Cialis™], vardenafil [Levitra™]) used to treat erectile dysfunction can prolong and intensify the vasodilating effects of nitrates, causing severe hypotension.

**IV. Diagnosis** is suggested by hypotension with reflex tachycardia and headache. Methemoglobinemia of 15% or more may be diagnosed by noting a chocolate brown coloration of the blood when it is dried on filter paper.

- **A. Specific levels.** Blood levels are not commercially available. With the use of a nitrite dipstick (normally used to detect bacteria in urine), nitrite can be detected in the serum of patients intoxicated by alkyl nitrites.
- **B. Other useful laboratory studies** include electrolytes, glucose, arterial blood gases or oximetry, methemoglobin concentration, and ECG monitoring.

**V. Treatment**

- **A. Emergency and supportive measures**
  1. Maintain an open airway and assist ventilation if necessary (see pp 1–7). Administer supplemental oxygen.
  2. Treat hypotension with supine positioning, intravenous crystalloid fluids, and low-dose pressors if needed (see p 15).
  3. Monitor vital signs and ECG for 4–6 hours.
- **B. Specific drugs and antidotes.** Symptomatic methemoglobinemia may be treated with **methylene blue** (see p 473).
- **C. Decontamination** (see p 45)

1. **Inhalation.** Remove victims from exposure and administer supplemental oxygen if available.
2. **Skin and eyes.** Remove contaminated clothing and wash with copious soap and water. Irrigate exposed eyes with water or saline.
3. **Ingestion.** Administer activated charcoal orally if conditions are appropriate (see Table I–38, p 51). Gastric lavage is not necessary after small to moderate ingestions if activated charcoal can be given promptly.

**D. Enhanced elimination.** Hemodialysis and hemoperfusion are not effective. Severe methemoglobinemia in infants not responsive to methylene blue therapy may require **exchange transfusion.**

# ► NITROGEN OXIDES

*Paul D. Blanc, MD, MSPH*

Nitrogen oxides (nitric oxide and nitrogen dioxide; *not* nitrous oxide [p 282]) are gases commonly released from nitrous or nitric acid, from reactions between nitric acid and organic materials, from burning of nitrocellulose and many other products, and as a by-product of explosions. Exposure to nitrogen oxides occurs in electric arc welding, electroplating, and engraving. Nitrogen oxides are found in engine exhaust, and they are produced when stored grain with a high nitrite content ferments in storage silos. Nitric oxide used as a therapeutic agent reacts with oxygen to form nitrogen dioxide.

**I. Mechanism of toxicity.** Nitrogen oxides are irritant gases with relatively low water solubility. Nitrogen oxides cause delayed-onset chemical pneumonitis. In addition, they can oxidize hemoglobin to methemoglobin.

**II. Toxic dose.** The ACGIH-recommended workplace exposure limit (threshold limit value—8-hour time-weighted average; TLV-TWA) for nitric oxide is 25 ppm (31 $mg/m^3$), and for nitrogen dioxide it is 3 ppm (5.6 $mg/m^3$). The air levels considered immediately dangerous to life or health (IDLH) are 100 and 20 ppm, respectively. The OSHA exposure limit (permissible exposure limit-ceiling; PEL-C) is higher for nitrogen dioxide at 5.0 ppm.

**III. Clinical presentation.** Because of the poor water solubility of nitrogen oxides, there is very little mucous membrane or upper respiratory irritation at low levels (< 10 ppm nitrogen dioxide). This allows prolonged exposure with few warning symptoms other than mild cough or nausea. With more concentrated exposures, upper respiratory symptoms such as burning eyes, sore throat, and cough may occur.

**A.** After a delay of up to 24 hours, chemical pneumonitis may develop, with progressive hypoxemia and pulmonary edema. The onset may be more rapid after exposure to higher concentrations. Some cases may evolve to bronchiolitis obliterans in the days after an initial improvement.

**B.** After recovery from acute chemical pneumonitis and after chronic low-level exposure to nitrogen oxides, permanent lung disease from bronchiolar damage may become evident.

**C.** Methemoglobinemia (see p 262) has been described in victims exposed to nitrogen oxides in smoke during major structural fires.

**D.** Inhaled nitric oxide (eg, used for therapeutic purposes as a pulmonary vasodilator, especially in neonates) can have extrapulmonary effects, including reduced platelet aggregation, methemoglobinemia, and systemic vasodilation.

**IV. Diagnosis** is based on a history of exposure, if known. Because of the potential for delayed effects, all patients with significant smoke inhalation should be observed for several hours.

**A. Specific levels.** There are no specific blood levels.

**B. Other useful laboratory studies** include arterial blood gases with co-oximetry to assess concomitant methemoglobinemia, chest x-ray, and pulmonary function tests.

**V. Treatment**

**A. Emergency and supportive measures**

1. Observe closely for signs of upper-airway obstruction and intubate the trachea and assist ventilation if necessary (see pp 1–7). Administer humidified supplemental oxygen.
2. Observe symptomatic victims for a minimum of 24 hours after exposure and treat chemical pneumonia and noncardiogenic pulmonary edema (see p 7) if they occur.

**B. Specific drugs and antidotes**

1. The role of corticosteroids is most clearly indicated for later onset of bronchiolitis obliterans. In acute lung injury from chemical inhalation, including nitrogen oxide, a beneficial role of steroids has not been established.
2. Treat methemoglobinemia with **methylene blue** (see p 473).

**C. Decontamination** (see p 45). Rescuers should wear self-contained breathing apparatus and, if there is the potential for high-level gas exposure or exposure to liquid nitric acid, chemical-protective clothing.

1. **Inhalation.** Remove victims from exposure immediately and give supplemental oxygen, if available.
2. **Skin and eyes.** Remove any wet clothing and flush exposed skin with water. Irrigate exposed eyes with copious water or saline.

**D. Enhanced elimination.** There is no role for enhanced elimination procedures.

## ▶ NITROPRUSSIDE

*Neal L. Benowitz, MD*

Sodium nitroprusside is a short-acting parenterally administered vasodilator that is used to treat severe hypertension and cardiac failure. It also is used to induce hypotension for certain surgical procedures. Toxicity may occur with acute high-dose nitroprusside treatment or with prolonged infusions.

**I. Mechanism of toxicity.** Nitroprusside is rapidly hydrolyzed (half-life 11 minutes) and releases free cyanide, which normally is converted quickly to thiocyanate by rhodanase enzymes in the liver and blood vessels.

**A. Acute cyanide poisoning** (see p 176) may occur with short-term high-dose nitroprusside infusions (eg, > 10–15 mcg/kg/min for 1 hour or longer).

**B. Thiocyanate** is eliminated by the kidney and may accumulate in patients with renal insufficiency, especially after prolonged infusions.

**II. Toxic dose.** The toxic dose depends on renal function and the rate of infusion.

**A. Cyanide** poisoning is uncommon at nitroprusside infusion rates less than 8–10 mcg/kg/min but has been reported after infusion of 4 mcg/kg/min for 3 hours.

**B. Thiocyanate** toxicity does not occur with acute brief use in persons with normal renal function but may result from prolonged infusions (eg, > 3 mcg/kg/min for 48 hours or longer), especially in persons with renal insufficiency (with rates as low as 1 mcg/kg/min).

**III. Clinical presentation.** The most common adverse effect of nitroprusside is hypotension, which often is accompanied by reflex tachycardia. Peripheral and cerebral hypoperfusion can lead to lactic acidosis and altered mental status.

**A. Cyanide** poisoning is accompanied by headache, hyperventilation, anxiety, agitation, seizures, and metabolic acidosis. ECG may reveal ischemic patterns.

**B. Thiocyanate** accumulation causes somnolence, confusion, delirium, tremor, and hyperreflexia. Seizures and coma may rarely occur with severe toxicity.

C. Methemoglobinemia occurs rarely and is usually mild.

IV. **Diagnosis.** Lactic acidosis, coma, or seizures after short-term high-dose nitroprusside infusion should suggest cyanide poisoning, whereas confusion or delirium developing gradually after several days of continuous use should suggest thiocyanate poisoning.

A. **Specific levels.** Cyanide levels may be obtained but are not usually available rapidly enough to guide treatment when cyanide poisoning is suspected. Cyanide levels may not reflect toxicity accurately because of simultaneous production of methemoglobin, which binds some of the cyanide. Cyanide levels higher than 1 mg/L usually produce a demonstrable lactic acidosis. **Thiocyanate** levels higher than 50–100 mg/L may cause delirium and somnolence.

B. **Other useful laboratory studies** include electrolytes, glucose, BUN, creatinine, serum lactate, ECG, arterial blood gases and measured arterial and venous oxygen saturation (see Cyanide, p 176), and methemoglobin level.

V. **Treatment**

A. **Emergency and supportive measures**

1. Maintain an open airway and assist ventilation if necessary (see pp 1–7). Administer supplemental oxygen.
2. For hypotension, stop the infusion immediately and administer intravenous fluids or even pressors if necessary (see p 15).

B. **Specific drugs and antidotes.** If cyanide poisoning is suspected, administer **sodium thiosulfate** (see p 514). Sodium nitrite treatment may aggravate hypotension and should not be used. **Hydroxocobalamin** (p 459), 25 mg/h IV infusion, sometimes is co-administered with high-dose nitroprusside as prophylaxis against cyanide toxicity.

C. **Decontamination.** These procedures are not relevant because the drug is administered only parenterally.

D. **Enhanced elimination.** Nitroprusside and cyanide are both metabolized rapidly, so there is no need to consider enhanced elimination for them. Hemodialysis may accelerate **thiocyanate** elimination and is especially useful in patients with renal failure.

## ▶ NITROUS OXIDE

*Aaron Schneir, MD*

Nitrous oxide, or laughing gas, is used as an adjuvant for general anesthesia, an anesthetic and analgesic agent for minor procedures, and a propellant in many commercial products, such as whipped cream and cooking oil spray. ("Whippets" are small cartridges of nitrous oxide that can be purchased at restaurant supply stores, grocery convenience stores, and "head shops.") Nitrous oxide is used by many US dentists, in some cases without adequate scavenging equipment. Abuse of nitrous oxide is not uncommon in the medical and dental professions.

I. **Mechanism of toxicity**

A. **Acute toxicity** after exposure to nitrous oxide is caused mainly by asphyxia if adequate oxygen is not supplied with the gas.

B. **Chronic toxicity** to the hematologic and nervous systems results from inactivation of vitamin $B_{12}$ after irreversible oxidation of its cobalt atom. Vitamin $B_{12}$ is required for the synthesis of methionine from homocysteine and for the production of tetrahydrofolate. Methionine is essential for myelin production, and tetrahydrofolate is essential for DNA synthesis. Use of nitrous oxide can precipitate neurologic symptoms in patients with subclinical $B_{12}$ or folic acid deficiency.

C. **Adverse reproductive** outcomes have been reported in workers chronically exposed to nitrous oxide.

II. **Toxic dose.** The toxic dose is not established. Chronic occupational exposure to 2000 ppm nitrous oxide produced asymptomatic but measurable depression of vitamin $B_{12}$ in dentists. The ACGIH-recommended workplace exposure limit (TLV-TWA) is 50 ppm (90 mg/$m^3$) as an 8-hour time-weighted average.

**III. Clinical presentation**

**A.** Signs of **acute toxicity** are related to **asphyxia,** and include headache, dizziness, confusion, syncope, seizures, and cardiac arrhythmias. Interstitial emphysema and pneumomediastinum have been reported after forceful inhalation from a pressurized whipped cream dispenser.

**B. Chronic nitrous oxide abuse** may produce megaloblastic anemia, thrombocytopenia, leukopenia, peripheral neuropathy (especially posterior column findings), and myelopathy, similar to the effects of vitamin $B_{12}$ deficiency.

**IV. Diagnosis** is based on a history of exposure and clinical presentation (eg, evidence of asphyxia and an empty can or tank). It also should be considered in a patient with manifestations suggesting chronic vitamin $B_{12}$ deficiency but with normal vitamin $B_{12}$ levels.

**A. Specific levels.** Specific levels are not generally available and are unreliable owing to off-gassing.

**B. Other useful laboratory studies** include CBC with manual differential, vitamin $B_{12}$, folic acid, nerve conduction studies, and MRI if the patient has neuropathy. Elevated homocysteine and methylmalonic acid levels have been documented in nitrous oxide abusers who had normal vitamin $B_{12}$ levels.

**V. Treatment**

**A. Emergency and supportive measures**

**1.** Maintain an open airway and assist ventilation if necessary (see pp 1–7). Administer high-flow supplemental oxygen.

**2.** After significant asphyxia, anticipate and treat coma (see p 18), seizures (p 22), and cardiac arrhythmias (pp 10–15).

**B. Specific drugs and antidotes.** Chronic effects may resolve over 2–3 months after discontinuation of exposure. Vitamin $B_{12}$ and folinic acid supplementation is indicated to correct underlying deficiencies. Successful treatment with methionine has been reported.

**C. Decontamination.** Remove victims from exposure and give supplemental oxygen if available.

**D. Enhanced elimination.** These procedures are not effective.

## ▶ NONSTEROIDAL ANTI-INFLAMMATORY DRUGS

*Winnie W. Tai, PharmD*

The nonsteroidal anti-inflammatory drugs (NSAIDs) are a chemically diverse group of agents that have similar pharmacologic properties and are widely used for control of pain and inflammation (Table II–39). Overdose by most of the agents in this group usually produces only mild GI upset. However, toxicity may be more severe after overdose with **oxyphenbutazone, phenylbutazone, mefenamic acid, piroxicam,** or **diflunisal.**

**I. Mechanism of toxicity**

**A.** NSAIDs produce their pharmacologic and most toxicologic effects by inhibiting the enzyme cyclooxygenase (isoforms COX-1 and COX-2); this results in decreased production of prostaglandins and decreased pain and inflammation. CNS, hemodynamic, pulmonary, and hepatic dysfunction also occurs with some agents, but the relationship to prostaglandin production remains uncertain. Prostaglandins are also involved in maintaining the integrity of the gastric mucosa and regulating renal blood flow; thus, acute or chronic intoxication may affect these organs.

**B.** The newest generation of NSAIDs, known as the COX-2 inhibitors (rofecoxib, or Vioxx™; celecoxib, or Celebrex™, valdecoxib, or Bextra™), selectively in-

**TABLE II–39. NSAIDS**

| Drug | Maximum Daily Adult Dose (mg) | Half-Life (h) | Comments |
|---|---|---|---|
| **Carboxylic acids** | | | |
| Bromfenac sodium | 150 | 1–2 | Chronic use associated with severe liver injury. |
| Carprofen | 4 mg/kg (PO or SC) | 4–10 (PO) 12 (IV) | Approved for use in dogs only. |
| Diclofenac | 200 | 2 | |
| Diflunisal | 1500 | 8–12 | |
| Etodolac | 1000 | 7 | |
| Fenoprofen | 3200 | 3 | Acute renal failure. |
| Ibuprofen[a] | 3200 | 2–4 | Massive overdose may cause coma, renal failure, metabolic acidosis, and cardiorespiratory depression. |
| Indomethacin | 200 | 3–11 | |
| Ketoprofen[a] | 300 | 2–4 | Large overdoses may cause respiratory depression, coma, seizures. |
| Ketorolac | 40 (PO) 60–120 (IV) | 4–6 | High risk of renal failure. |
| Meclofenamate | 400 | 1–3 | |
| Mefenamic acid | 1000 | 2 | Seizures, twitching. |
| Naproxen[a] | 1500 | 12–17 | Seizures, acidosis. |
| Oxaprozin | 1800 | 42–50 | |
| Sulindac | 400 | 7–16 | Extensive enterohepatic recirculation. |
| Tolmetin | 1800 | 1 | |
| **Enolic acids** | | | |
| Nabumetone | 2000 | 24 | |
| Oxyphenbutazone | 600 | 27–64 | Seizures, acidosis. |
| Phenylbutazone | 600 | 50–100 | Seizures, acidosis. |
| Piroxicam | 20 | 45–50 | Seizures, coma. |
| Meloxicam | 15 | 15–20 | |
| **Cox-2 inhibitors** | | | |
| Celecoxib | 400 | 11 | |
| Rofecoxib | 50 | 17 | Removed from US market due to concern for increased risk of cardiovascular events. |
| Parecoxib | | | Prodrug for valdecoxib; IM/IV use only; investigational in United States. |
| Valdecoxib | 40 | 8–11 | Removed from US market in 2005 due to concern for increased risk of cardiovascular events and serious skin reactions. |

[a]Currently available in the United States as nonprescription formulations.

hibit the cyclooxygenase-2 isoform with no COX-1 inhibition at therapeutic doses. Since COX-1 is involved in GI mucosal protection, these drugs reduce the likelihood of GI bleeding compared with conventional NSAIDs.

**C. Pharmacokinetics.** NSAIDs are generally well absorbed, and volumes of distribution are relatively small (eg, 0.15 L/kg for ibuprofen). COX-2 inhibitors have larger volumes of distribution (86–91 L in adults for rofecoxib, 400 L for celecoxib). Most of these agents are highly protein bound, and most are eliminated through hepatic metabolism and renal excretion, with variable half-lives (eg, 1.5–2.5 hours for ibuprofen and 12–17 hours for naproxen). (See also Table II–59.)

**II. Toxic dose.** Human data are insufficient to establish a reliable correlation between amount ingested, plasma concentrations, and clinical toxic effects. Generally, significant symptoms occur after ingestion of more than 5–10 times the usual therapeutic dose.

**III. Clinical presentation.** In general, patients with NSAID overdose are asymptomatic or have mild GI upset (nausea, vomiting, abdominal pain, sometimes hematemesis). Occasionally patients exhibit drowsiness, lethargy, ataxia, nystagmus, tinnitus, and disorientation.

**A.** With the more toxic agents **oxyphenbutazone, phenylbutazone, mefenamic acid,** and **piroxicam** and with massive **ibuprofen** or **fenoprofen** overdose, seizures, coma, renal failure, and cardiorespiratory arrest may occur. Hepatic dysfunction, hypoprothrombinemia, and metabolic acidosis are also reported.

**B. Diflunisal** overdose produces toxicity resembling salicylate poisoning (see p 331).

**C.** Chronic use of **bromfenac** for more than 10 days has resulted in fatal hepatotoxicity.

**D. Phenylbutazone** and **antipyrine** use has been associated with agranulocytosis and other blood dyscrasias.

**E.** There is limited information regarding overdoses of COX-2 inhibitors. The manufacturers of rofecoxib and celecoxib speculate that hypertension, acute renal failure, respiratory depression, and coma may occur in overdose. Rofecoxib and valdecoxib have been removed from the US market because of concerns about increased risk of cardiovascular events (including myocardial infarctions and strokes). There is also an increased risk for serious skin reactions with valdecoxib.

**IV. Diagnosis** usually is based primarily on a history of ingestion of NSAIDs, because symptoms are mild and nonspecific and quantitative levels are not usually available.

**A. Specific levels** are not usually readily available and do not contribute to clinical management.

**B. Other useful laboratory studies** include CBC, electrolytes, glucose, BUN, creatinine, liver transaminases, prothrombin time (PT/INR), and urinalysis.

**V. Treatment**

**A. Emergency and supportive measures**

1. Maintain an open airway and assist ventilation if necessary (see pp 1–7). Administer supplemental oxygen.
2. Treat seizures (see p 22), coma (p 18), and hypotension (p 15) if they occur.
3. Antacids may be used for mild GI upset. Replace fluid losses with intravenous crystalloid solutions.

**B. Specific drugs and antidotes.** There is no antidote. Vitamin K (see p 508) may be used for patients with elevated prothrombin time caused by hypoprothrombinemia.

**C. Decontamination** (see p 45). Administer activated charcoal orally if conditions are appropriate (see Table I–38, p 51). Gastric lavage is not necessary after small to moderate ingestions if activated charcoal can be given promptly.

**D. Enhanced elimination.** NSAIDs are highly protein bound and extensively metabolized. Thus, hemodialysis, peritoneal dialysis, and forced diuresis are not likely to be effective.

1. **Charcoal hemoperfusion** may be effective for **phenylbutazone** overdose, although there are limited clinical data to support its use.
2. Repeat-dose activated charcoal therapy may enhance the elimination of meloxicam, oxyphenbutazone, phenylbutazone, and piroxicam.
3. Repeated oral doses of cholestyramine have been reported to increase the clearance of meloxicam and piroxicam.

## ► NONTOXIC OR MINIMALLY TOXIC HOUSEHOLD PRODUCTS

*Eileen Morentz and Jay Schrader*

A variety of products commonly found around the home are completely nontoxic or have little or no toxicity after typical accidental exposures. Treatment is rarely required because the ingredients are not toxic, the concentrations of potentially toxic ingredients are minimal, or the construction or packaging of the product is such that a significant dose of a harmful ingredient is extremely unlikely.

Table II–40 lists a number of products considered nontoxic. However, the taste or texture of the product may be disagreeable or cause mild stomach upset. Also, some

**TABLE II–40. NONTOXIC OR MINIMALLY TOXIC PRODUCTS[a]**

| | | |
|---|---|---|
| Air fresheners | Diapers, disposable | Plastic |
| Aluminum foil | Erasers | Playdoh |
| Antiperspirants | Eye makeup | Putty |
| Ashes, wood/fireplace | Felt-tip markers and pens | Rouge |
| Aspartame | Fingernail polish (dry) | Rust |
| Baby lotion (Note: baby oil can cause aspiration pneumonitis; see p 146) | Glitter | Saccharin |
| | Glow stick/jewelry | Shellac (dry) |
| | Gum | Sheetrock |
| Baby powder (without talc) | Gypsum | Shoe polish |
| Baby wipes | Incense | Silica gel |
| Ball-point pen ink | Indelible markers | Silly putty |
| Calamine lotion | Ink (w/out aniline dyes) | Soil |
| Candles | Kitty litter | Stamp pad ink |
| Chalk[b] | Lip balm | Starch |
| Charcoal | Lipstick | Styrofoam |
| Charcoal briquettes | Magic markers | Superglue |
| Cigarette ashes | Makeup | Teething rings |
| Cigarette filter tips (unsmoked) | Mascara | Thermometers (phthalates/alcohol, gallium) |
| Clay | Matches (< 3 paper books) | |
| Cold packs (for large ingestions, see Nitrates, p 279) | Mylar balloons | Wall board |
| | Newspaper | Watercolor paints |
| Crayons | Paraffin | Wax |
| Cyanoacrylate glues | Pencils (contain graphite, not lead) | Zinc oxide ointment |
| Deodorants | Photographs | |
| Desiccants | Plaster | |

[a]These items are virtually nontoxic in small to moderate exposures. However, the taste or texture of the product may result in mild stomach upset. In addition, some of the products may cause a foreign body effect or choking hazard, depending on the size of the product and the age of the child.

[b]Plain drawing chalk. (Old pool-cue chalk may contain lead. "Chinese chalk" contains pyrethrins.)

**TABLE II–41. MILD GASTROINTESTINAL IRRITANTS[a]**

| | | |
|---|---|---|
| A & D Ointment | Corticosteroids | Lanolin |
| Antacids | Dishwashing liquid soaps (not electric dishwashing type) | Latex paint |
| Antibiotic ointments | Fabric softeners | Liquid soaps |
| Baby bath | Fertilizers (nitrogen, phosphoric acid, and potash) | Miconazole |
| Baby shampoo | Glycerin | Petroleum jelly |
| Bar soap | Guaifenesin | Plant food |
| Bath oil beads | Hair conditioners | Prednisone |
| Bleach (household, less than 6% hypochlorite) | Hair shampoos | Shaving cream |
| Body lotions and creams | Hand soaps | Simethicone |
| Bubble bath | Hydrocortisone cream | Spermicides (nonoxynol-9 < 10%) |
| Bubbles | Hydrogen peroxide 3% | Steroid creams |
| Carbamide peroxide 6.5% | Kaolin | Sunscreen/suntan lotions (allergic reactions possible) |
| Chalk (calcium carbonate) | Lactase | Toothpaste (without fluoride) |
| Clotrimazole cream | | |

[a]The items in this list usually have little or no effect in small ingestions. In moderate to large ingestions, gastrointestinal effects such as diarrhea, constipation, stomach cramps, and vomiting may occur. The effects are usually mild and rarely require medical intervention.

of the products listed can create a foreign body effect or a choking hazard, depending on the formulation and the age of the child. Table II–41 provides examples of products that may cause mild GI upset but are generally not considered toxic after small ingestions. Stomach cramps, vomiting, or diarrhea may occur but each one is usually mild and self-limited. Table II–42 lists several other products that often are ingested by small children with minimal effect. Although they may contain potentially toxic ingredients, the concentration or packaging makes it very unlikely that symptoms will occur after a small exposure.

In all cases involving exposures to these substances, attempt to confirm the identity and/or ingredients of the product and assure that no other more toxic products were involved. Determine whether there are any unexpected symptoms or evidence of choking or foreign body effect. Advise the parent that mild GI upset may occur. Water or another liquid may be given to reduce the taste or texture of the product. For symptomatic eye exposures, follow the instructions for ocular decontamination (see p 47).

## ► OPIATES AND OPIOIDS

*Timothy E. Albertson, MD, PhD*

Opiates are a group of naturally occurring compounds derived from the juice of the poppy *Papaver somniferum.* Morphine is the classic opiate derivative used widely in medicine; heroin (diacetylmorphine) is a well-known, highly addictive street narcotic. The term *opioids* refers to these and other derivatives of naturally occurring opium (eg, morphine, heroin, codeine, and hydrocodone) as well as new, totally synthetic opiate analogs (eg, fentanyl, butorphanol, meperidine, and methadone; Table II–43). A wide variety of prescription medications contain opioids, often in combination with aspirin or acetaminophen. **Dextromethorphan** (see p 181) is an opioid derivative with potent antitussive but no analgesic or addictive properties. **Tramadol** (Ultram™) is a newer analgesic that is unrelated chemically to the opiates but acts on *mu* opioid receptors and blocks serotonin reuptake. **Butorphanol** is available as a nasal spray with rapid absorption. **Buprenorphine** is a partial opioid agonist that recently has been approved for treatment of opioid addiction.

**TABLE II–42. OTHER LOW-TOXICITY PRODUCTS[a]**

| Products | Comments |
|---|---|
| **Holiday hazards** | |
| Angel hair | Finely spun glass. Dermal or ocular irritation or corneal abrasion is possible. |
| Bubble lights | May contain a tiny amount of methylene chloride. |
| Christmas tree ornaments | Can cause foreign body effect or choking hazard. Antique or foreign-made ornaments may be decorated with lead-based paint. |
| Christmas tree preservatives | Homemade solutions may contain aspirin, bleach, or sugar. Commercial products usually contain only concentrated sugar solution. |
| Easter egg dyes | Most of these contain nontoxic dyes and sodium bicarbonate. Older formulations may contain sodium chloride, which can cause hypernatremia if a large amount is ingested (see p 35). |
| Fireplace crystals | May contain salts of copper, selenium, arsenic, and antimony. Small amounts can cause irritation to the mouth or stomach. (Larger ingestions could conceivably result in heavy metal poisoning; see specific heavy metal.) |
| Halloween candy | Tampering rarely occurs. X-ray of candy provides a false sense of security; although it may reveal radiopaque glass or metallic objects, most poisons are radiolucent. Prudent approach is to discard candy or food items that are not commercially packaged or if the package is damaged. |
| Snow scenes | The "snow" is composed of insoluble particles of calcium carbonate that are not toxic. The fluid may have bacterial growth. |
| Snow sprays | Sprays may contain hydrocarbon solvent or methylene chloride (see pp 219 and 266) vehicle. Inhalation may cause headache and nausea. Once dried, the snow is not toxic. |
| **Miscellaneous** | |
| Capsaicin sprays | These products contain capsaicin, the main ingredient in chili peppers. Exposure causes intense mucous membrane irritation and burning sensation. Treat with topical liquid antacids. |
| Cyanoacrylate glues | Ingestion is harmless. Cyanide is not released. Corneal abrasions may occur after ocular exposure. Adhesion of skin and eyelids is possible after dermal exposure. Treat adhesions with petrolatum-based ointment. |
| Fire extinguishers | The two common types contain sodium bicarbonate (white powder) or monoammonium phosphate (yellow powder). Small ingestions result in little to no effect. Mucous membrane irritation is common. Major risk is pneumonitis after extensive inhalation. |
| Fluorescent light bulbs | Contain inert gases and nontoxic powder that may be irritating to mucous membranes. |
| Oral contraceptives | Birth control pills contain varying amounts of estrogens and progesterones. In excessive amounts these may cause stomach upset and in females (even prepubertal) may cause transient vaginal spotting. Some formulations may contain iron. |
| Thermometers (mercury) | Household fever thermometers contain less than 0.5 mL liquid mercury, which is harmless if swallowed. Clean up cautiously to avoid dispersing Hg as mist or vapor (ie, do not vacuum). |
| **Household pesticides** | Numerous formulations. Some contain hydrocarbon solvents; others are water-based. Pesticides used may include pyrethrins, organophosphates, or carbamates, but generally low potency and in concentrations less than 1.5%. The risk of pesticide poisoning is very low unless intentional massive exposure. Symptoms after exposure are due mainly to inhalation of the hydrocarbon solvent. |
| Topical monthly flea control products | Formulations include fipronil, imidacloprid. Low oral toxicity after ingestion of less than 2–3 mL. Dermal and ocular irritation may occur. |
| **Respiratory irritants** | |
| Baby powders (talc-containing), spray starch | These products have little or no toxicity when ingested. However, if aspirated into the lungs, they can cause an inflammatory pneumonitis. |

[a]These products may contain small amounts of potentially toxic ingredients but rarely cause problems because of the small concentrations or conditions of exposure.

**TABLE II–43. OPIATES AND OPIOIDS[a]**

| Drug | Type of Activity | Usual Adult Dose[a] (mg) | Elimination Half-Life (h) | Duration of Analgesia (h) |
|---|---|---|---|---|
| Butorphanol | Mixed | 2 | 5-6 | 3–4 |
| Codeine | Agonist | 60 | 2–4 | 4–6 |
| Fentanyl | Agonist | 0.2 | 1–5 | 0.5–2 |
| Heroin[b] | Agonist | 4 | (b) | 3–4 |
| Hydrocodone | Agonist | 5 | 3–4 | 4–8 |
| Hydromorphone | Agonist | 1.5 | 1–4 | 4–5 |
| Meperidine | Agonist[c] | 100 | 2–5 | 2–4 |
| Methadone | Agonist | 10 | 20–30 | 4–8[d] |
| Morphine | Agonist | 10 | 2–4 | 3–6 |
| Nalbuphine | Mixed | 10 | 5 | 3–6 |
| Oxycodone | Agonist | 4.5 | 2–5 | 4–6 |
| Pentazocine | Mixed | 50 | 2–3 | 2–3 |
| Propoxyphene | Agonist | 100 | 6–12 | 4–6 |
| Tramadol | Agonist[c] | 50–100 | 6–7.5 | 4–6 |

[a]Usual dose: dose equivalent to 10 mg of morphine.
[b]Rapidly hydrolyzed to morphine.
[c]Also inhibits serotonin reuptake.
[d]Sedation and coma may last 2–3 days.

**I. Mechanism of toxicity**

**A.** In general, opioids share the ability to stimulate a number of specific opiate receptors in the CNS, causing sedation and respiratory depression. Death results from respiratory failure, usually as a result of apnea or pulmonary aspiration of gastric contents. In addition, acute noncardiogenic pulmonary edema may occur by unknown mechanisms.

**B. Pharmacokinetics.** Usually, peak effects occur within 2–3 hours, but absorption may be slowed by their pharmacologic effects on GI motility. Slow-release preparations of morphine (eg, MS-Contin) or oxycodone (eg, OxyContin) may have a delayed onset and prolonged effects. Fentanyl patches can cause continued dermal absorption even after removal. Smoking or ingesting fentanyl patches can result in rapid and high levels. Most of these drugs have large volumes of distribution (3–5 L/kg). The rate of elimination is highly variable, from 1–2 hours for fentanyl derivatives to 15–30 hours for methadone. See also Tables II–43 and II–59.

**II. Toxic dose.** The toxic dose varies widely, depending on the specific compound, the route and rate of administration, and tolerance to the effects of the drug as a result of chronic use. Some newer fentanyl derivatives have potency up to 2000 times that of morphine.

**III. Clinical presentation**

**A. With mild or moderate overdose,** lethargy is common. The pupils are usually small, often "pinpoint" size. Blood pressure and pulse rate are decreased, bowel sounds are diminished, and the muscles are usually flaccid.

**B. With higher doses,** coma is accompanied by respiratory depression, and apnea often results in sudden death. Noncardiogenic pulmonary edema may occur, often after resuscitation and administration of the opiate antagonist naloxone.

C. **Seizures** are not common after opioid overdose but occur occasionally with certain compounds (eg, codeine, dextromethorphan, meperidine, propoxyphene, and tramadol). Seizures may occur in patients with renal compromise who receive repeated doses of meperidine owing to accumulation of the metabolite normeperidine.

D. **Cardiotoxicity** similar to that seen with tricyclic antidepressants (see p 91) and quinidine (p 324) can occur in patients with severe **propoxyphene** intoxication.

E. Some newer synthetic opioids have mixed agonist and antagonist effects, with unpredictable results in overdose. **Buprenorphine** causes less maximal opioid effect than morphine does, and because of strong binding to opioid receptors it can cause acute withdrawal symptoms in persons on high doses of conventional opioids.

F. Opioid **withdrawal syndrome** can cause anxiety, piloerection (goosebumps), abdominal cramps and diarrhea, and insomnia.

IV. **Diagnosis** is simple when typical manifestations of opiate intoxication are present (pinpoint pupils and respiratory and CNS depression), and the patient quickly awakens after administration of naloxone. Signs of intravenous drug abuse (eg, needle track marks) may be present.

A. **Specific levels** are not usually performed because of poor correlation with clinical effects. Qualitative screening of the urine is an effective way to confirm recent use. Fentanyl derivatives, tramadol, and some other synthetic opioids may not be detected by routine toxicologic screens (see Table I–31, p 42).

B. **Other useful laboratory studies** include electrolytes, glucose, arterial blood gases or oximetry, chest x-ray, and stat serum acetaminophen or salicylate levels (if the ingested overdose was of a combination product).

V. **Treatment**

A. **Emergency and supportive measures**

1. Maintain an open airway and assist ventilation if necessary (see pp 1–7). Administer supplemental oxygen.
2. Treat coma (see p 18), seizures (p 22), hypotension (p 15), and noncardiogenic pulmonary edema (p 7) if they occur.

B. **Specific drugs and antidotes**

1. **Naloxone** (see p 477) is a specific opioid antagonist with no agonist properties of its own; large doses may be given safely.
   a. Administer naloxone, 0.4–2 mg IV. As little as 0.2–0.4 mg is usually effective for heroin overdose. Repeat doses every 2–3 minutes if there is no response, up to a total dose of 10–20 mg if an opioid overdose is strongly suspected. Intranasal naloxone is effective but is not as effective as intramuscular naloxone in the prehospital setting.
   b. ***Caution:*** The duration of effect of naloxone (1–2 hours) is shorter than that of many opioids. Therefore, do not release a patient who has awakened after naloxone treatment until at least 3–4 hours has passed since the last dose of naloxone. In general, if naloxone was required to reverse opioid-induced coma, it is safer to admit the patient for at least 6–12 hours of observation.
2. **Nalmefene** (see p 477) is an opioid antagonist with a longer duration of effect (3–5 hours).
   a. Nalmefene may be given in doses of 0.1–2 mg IV, with repeated doses up to 10–20 mg if an opioid overdose is strongly suspected.
   b. ***Caution:*** Although nalmefene's duration of effect is longer than that of naloxone, it is still much shorter than that of methadone. If a methadone overdose is suspected, the patient should be observed for at least 8–12 hours after the last dose of nalmefene.

3. **Sodium bicarbonate** (see p 423) may be effective for QRS interval prolongation or hypotension associated with propoxyphene poisoning.

C. **Decontamination** (see p 45). Administer activated charcoal orally if conditions are appropriate (see Table I–38, p 51). Gastric lavage is not necessary after small to moderate ingestions if activated charcoal can be given promptly. Consider whole-bowel irrigation after ingestion of sustained-release products (eg, MS-Contin, OxyContin).

D. **Enhanced elimination.** Because of the very large volumes of distribution of the opioids and the availability of an effective antidotal treatment, there is no role for enhanced elimination procedures.

## ▶ ORGANOPHOSPHORUS AND CARBAMATE INSECTICIDES

*David A. Tanen, MD*

Organophosphorus compounds and carbamates, also known more generally as *cholinesterase inhibitors,* are widely used pesticides that may cause poisonings after accidental or suicidal exposure. Poisonings are particularly common in rural areas and third-world countries where more potent agents are widely available, and it has been estimated by the World Health Organization that millions of people are affected yearly. During the 1930s, pesticide research in Germany led to the synthesis of numerous organophosphorus compounds including parathion along with several **chemical warfare agents** (eg, GA [Tabun], GB [Sarin], and GD [Soman]; see p 373 and Table II–57). Household exposures usually do not cause a significant problem because insect sprays often contain low-potency cholinesterase inhibitors.

I. **Mechanism of toxicity**

A. **Organophosphorus (OP) compounds** inhibit the enzyme acetylcholinesterase (AChE) found in synaptic junctions, red blood cells (RBCs), and butyrylcholinesterase (also known as pseudocholinesterase or plasma cholinesterase) in the blood. Blockade of AChE leads to the accumulation of excessive acetylcholine at muscarinic receptors (cholinergic effector cells), at nicotinic receptors (skeletal neuromuscular junctions and autonomic ganglia), and in the CNS.

Permanent inhibition of acetylcholinesterase may occur through covalent binding by the OP to the enzyme. This is known as "aging," and its rate of development is variable and depends on the specific OP. Dimethyl compounds (eg, dimethoate) generally age more quickly than diethyl agents (eg, chlorpyrifos). Antidotal treatment with an oxime (see Pralidoxime, p 500) may delay the onset of aging; early administration of oximes is therefore recommended.

B. **Carbamates** also inhibit the acetylcholinesterases and lead to accumulation of acetylcholine, similar to the effects of OPs. CNS effects are often less pronounced than in OP poisoning because they have more difficulty crossing the blood-brain barrier. Carbamates also do not "age," leading to faster reactivation of the AChE. Toxicity is therefore usually brief and self-limited. **Aldicarb** is an important carbamate because it is relatively more potent and is translocated systemically by certain plants (eg, melons) and concentrated in their fruit. An acute outbreak of aldicarb poisoning occurred in California in 1985 after ingestion of watermelons that had been grown in a field previously sprayed with aldicarb. The use of the imported rodenticide "Tres Pasitos" led to an epidemic of aldicarb poisoning in New York in 1994–1997.

C. Most OPs and carbamates can be absorbed by any route: inhalation, ingestion, and absorption through the skin. **Highly lipophilic organophosphates** (disulfoton, fenthion, and others) are stored in fat tissue, and this may lead to persistent toxicity lasting several days after exposure.

**II. Toxic dose.** There is a wide spectrum of relative potency of the organophosphorus and carbamate compounds (Table II–44). The severity and tempo of intoxication are also affected by the rate of exposure (acute versus chronic), the ongoing metabolic degradation and elimination of the agent, and, for some organophosphorus compounds (indirect inhibitors), the rate of metabolism to their toxic "-oxone" derivatives.

**TABLE II–44. ORGANOPHOSPHORUS AND CARBAMATE COMPOUNDS[a]**

| ORGANOPHOSPHATES | | |
|---|---|---|
| **Low toxicity ($LD_{50}$ > 1000 mg/kg)** | **Moderate toxicity ($LD_{50}$ 50–1000 mg/kg)** | **High Toxicity ($LD_{50}$ < 50 mg/kg)** |
| Bromophos | Acephate | Azinphos-methyl |
| Etrimfos | Bensulide | Bomyl |
| Iodofenphos (jodfenphos) | Chlorpyrifos | Carbophenothion |
| Malathion | Crotoxyphos | Chlorfenvinphos |
| Phoxim | Cyanophos | Chlormephos |
| Primiphos-methyl | Cythioate | Coumaphos |
| Propylthiopyrophosphate | DEF | Cyanofenphos |
| Temephos | Demeton-S-methyl | Demeton |
| Tetrachlorvinphos | Diazinon | Dialifor |
| | Dichlofenthion | Dicrotophos |
| | Dichlorvos (DDVP) | Disulfoton |
| | Dimethoate | EPN |
| | Edifenphos | Famphur |
| | EPBP | Fenamiphos |
| | Ethion | Fenophosphon |
| | Ethoprop | Fensulfothion |
| | Fenthion | Fonofos |
| | Fenitrothion | Isofenphos |
| | Formothion | Isofluorphate |
| | Heptenophos | Mephosfolan |
| | IBP (Kitacin) | Methamidophos |
| | Isoxathion | Methidathion |
| | Leptophos | Mevinphos |
| | Methyl trithion | Monocrotophos |
| | Naled | Parathion |
| | Oxydemeton-methyl | Phorate |
| | Oxydeprofos | Phosfolan |
| | Phencapton | Phosphamidon |
| | Phenthoate | Prothoate |
| | Phosalone | Schradan |
| | Phosmet | Sulfotep |
| | Pirimiphos-ethyl | Terbufos |
| | Profenofos | Tetraethylpyrophosphate |
| | Propetamphos | Triorthocresylphosphate |
| | Pyrazophos | |
| | Pyridaphenthion | |
| | Quinalphos | |
| | Sulprofos | |
| | Thiometon | |
| | Triazophos | |
| | Tribufos | |
| | Trichlorfon | |

*(continued)*

**TABLE II–44. ORGANOPHOSPHORUS AND CARBAMATE COMPOUNDS[a] (CONTINUED)**

| CARBAMATES | | |
|---|---|---|
| **Low toxicity ($LD_{50}$ > 200 mg/kg)** | **Moderate Toxicity ($LD_{50}$ 50–200 mg/kg)** | **High Toxicity ($LD_{50}$ < 50 mg/kg)** |
| BPMC (Fenocarb) | Benfuracarb | Aldicarb |
| Carbaryl | Bufencarb | Aldoxycarb |
| Ethiofencarb | Carbosulfan | Aminocarb |
| Isoprocarb | Dioxacarb | Bendiocarb |
| MPMC (Meobal) | Propoxur | Carbofuran |
| MTMC (Metacrate) | Pirimicarb | Dimetilan |
| XMC (Cosban) | Promecarb | Formetanate |
| | Thiodicarb | Isolan |
| | Trimethacarb | Mecarbam |
| | | Methiocarb |
| | | Methomyl |
| | | Mexacarbate |
| | | Oxamyl |

[a]Based on oral $LD_{50}$ values in the rat. **Note:** The likelihood of serious toxicity depends not only on the dose of the pesticide but also on the route of exposure, circumstances of the exposure, and preexisting cholinesterase activity. Moreover, agents that are highly lipid soluble, such as fenthion and sulfoton, may cause prolonged intoxication.

**III. Clinical presentation.** Signs and symptoms of acute organophosphate poisoning may occur almost immediately or be delayed several hours, depending on the route and the degree of exposure. Delayed onset may result from dermal exposures or indirect agents such as malathion and fenthion that require metabolism to the active form. Clinical manifestations may be classified into muscarinic, nicotinic, and CNS effects. In addition, chemical pneumonitis (see p 219) may occur if a product containing a hydrocarbon solvent is aspirated into the lungs.

**A. Muscarinic** manifestations include vomiting, diarrhea, abdominal cramping, bronchospasm, miosis, bradycardia, and excessive salivation and sweating. Fluid losses can lead to systemic hypovolemia, resulting in shock.

**B. Nicotinic** effects include muscle fasciculations, tremor, and weakness. Respiratory muscle weakness complicated by bronchorrhea may lead to respiratory arrest and death.

**C. Central nervous system** poisoning may cause agitation, seizures, and coma.

**D. Intermediate syndrome.** Patients may develop proximal muscle weakness 2–4 days after the resolution of the acute cholinergic crisis. This is often first noted as neck weakness, progressing to proximal limb weakness and cranial nerve palsies. Respiratory muscle weakness and respiratory arrest may occur abruptly. The intermediate syndrome is thought to be caused by a redistribution of lipophilic pesticides or result from inadequate oxime therapy. Symptoms may last 1–2 weeks and do not usually respond to additional treatment with oximes or atropine.

**E.** In addition to CNS sequelae, some cholinesterase inhibitors may cause a delayed, often permanent **peripheral neuropathy.** The mechanism appears to be the result of inhibition of neuropathy target esterase (NTE). Notably, the outbreak of "Jamaican ginger paralysis" in the 1930s was due to drinking rum contaminated with triorthocresyl phosphate.

**IV. Diagnosis** is based on the history of exposure and the presence of characteristic muscarinic, nicotinic, and CNS manifestations of acetylcholine excess. There may be a solvent odor, and some agents have a strong garlicky odor.

**A. Specific levels**

1. **Organophosphorus compounds.** Laboratory evidence of poisoning may be obtained by measuring decreases in the plasma pseudocholinesterase (PChE) and red blood cell acetylcholinesterase (RBC AChE) activities. However, because of wide interindividual variability, significant depression of enzyme activity may occur but still fall within the "normal" range. It is most helpful if the patient had a preexposure baseline measurement for comparison (eg, as part of a workplace health surveillance program).
   a. The RBC AChE activity provides a more reliable measure of the toxic effect; a 50% or greater depression in activity from baseline generally indicates a true exposure effect.
   b. PChE activity is a sensitive indicator of exposure but is not as specific as AChE activity (PChE may be depressed owing to genetic deficiency, medical illness, or chronic organophosphorus exposure). PChE activity usually falls before AChE and recovers faster than AChE.
2. **Carbamate** poisoning produces reversible acetylcholinesterase inhibition, and spontaneous recovery of enzyme activity may occur within several hours, making these tests less useful.
3. Assay of blood, urine, gastric lavage fluid, and excrement for specific agents and their metabolites may also provide evidence of exposure, but these tests are not widely available.

**B. Other useful laboratory studies** include electrolytes, glucose, BUN, creatinine, liver transaminases, arterial blood gases or oximetry, ECG monitoring, and chest x-ray (if pulmonary edema or aspiration of hydrocarbon solvent is suspected).

**V. Treatment**

**A. Emergency and supportive measures.** ***Caution:*** Rescuers and health-care providers must take measures to prevent direct contact with the skin or clothing of contaminated victims, because secondary contamination and serious illness may result, especially with potent pesticides or nerve agents (see Section IV, p 520.)

1. Maintain an open airway and assist ventilation if necessary (see pp 1–7). Pay careful attention to respiratory muscle weakness because sudden respiratory arrest may occur. This is often preceded by increasing weakness of neck flexion muscles. If intubation is required, a nondepolarizing agent (see p 480) should be used because the effect of succinylcholine will be extended secondary to the inhibition of PChE. Administer supplemental oxygen.
2. Treat hydrocarbon pneumonitis (see p 219), seizures (p 22), and coma (p 18) if they occur. Seizures should be treated with benzodiazepines such as diazepam (see p 419).
3. Observe asymptomatic patients for at least 8–12 hours to rule out delayed-onset symptoms, especially after extensive skin exposure or ingestion of a highly fat-soluble agent.

**B. Specific drugs and antidotes.** Specific treatment includes the antimuscarinic agent **atropine** and the enzyme reactivator **pralidoxime.**

1. Give **atropine,** 0.5–2 mg IV initially (see p 417), then double the dose every 5 minutes until signs of atropinization are present (decreased secretions and wheezing, increased heart rate). The most clinically important indication for continued atropine administration is persistent wheezing or bronchorrhea. Tachycardia is not a contraindication to more atropine. ***Note:*** Atropine will reverse muscarinic but not nicotinic effects.
2. **Pralidoxime** (2-PAM, Protopam; see p 500) is a specific antidote that acts to regenerate the enzyme activity at all affected sites prior to aging. Other oximes include obidoxime and HI-6. Oximes may be less effective against dimethyl compounds compared with diethyl agents.
   a. Pralidoxime should be given immediately to reverse muscular weak-

ness and fasciculations: 1–2 g initial bolus dose (20–40 mg/kg in children) IV over 5–10 minutes, followed by a continuous infusion (see p 492). It is most effective if started early, before irreversible phosphorylation of the enzyme, but may still be effective if given later, particularly after exposure to highly lipid-soluble compounds. It is unclear how long oxime therapy should be continued, but it seems reasonable to continue it for 24 h after the patient becomes asymptomatic.

**b.** Pralidoxime generally is not recommended for carbamate intoxication, because in such cases the cholinesterase inhibition is spontaneously reversible and short-lived. However, if the exact agent is not identified and the patient has significant toxicity, pralidoxime should be given empirically.

**C. Decontamination** (see p 46). ***Note:*** Rescuers should wear chemical-protective clothing and gloves when handling a grossly contaminated victim. If there is heavy liquid contamination with a solvent such as xylene or toluene, clothing removal and victim decontamination should be carried out outdoors or in a room with high-flow ventilation.

1. **Skin.** Remove all contaminated clothing and wash exposed areas with soap and water, including the hair and under the nails. Irrigate exposed eyes with copious tepid water or saline.
2. **Ingestion.** Administer activated charcoal orally if conditions are appropriate (see Table I–38, p 51). Gastric lavage may be appropriate soon after moderate to large ingestions, but because of the possibility of seizures or rapidly changing mental status, lavage should be done only after intubation.

**D. Enhanced elimination.** Dialysis and hemoperfusion generally are not indicated because of the large volume of distribution of organophosphates.

# ► OXALIC ACID

*Kent R. Olson, MD*

Oxalic acid and oxalates are used as bleaches, metal cleaners, and rust removers and in chemical synthesis and leather tanning. Soluble and insoluble oxalate salts are found in several species of plants.

**I. Mechanism of toxicity**

**A. Oxalic acid solutions** are highly irritating and corrosive. Ingestion and absorption of oxalate cause acute hypocalcemia resulting from precipitation of the insoluble calcium oxalate salt. Calcium oxalate crystals may then deposit in the brain, heart, kidneys, and other sites, causing serious systemic damage.

**B. Insoluble calcium oxalate** salt found in dieffenbachia and similar plants is not absorbed but causes local mucous membrane irritation.

**II. Toxic dose.** Ingestion of 5–15 g of oxalic acid has caused death. The recommended workplace limit (ACGIH TLV-TWA) for oxalic acid vapor is 1 mg/m$^3$ as an 8-hour time-weighted average. The level considered immediately dangerous to life or health (IDLH) is 500 mg/m$^3$.

**III. Clinical presentation.** Toxicity may occur as a result of skin or eye contact, inhalation, or ingestion.

**A. Acute skin or eye contact** causes irritation and burning, which may lead to serious corrosive injury if the exposure and concentration are high.

**B. Inhalation** may cause sore throat, cough, and wheezing. Large exposures may lead to chemical pneumonitis or pulmonary edema.

**C. Ingestion** of soluble oxalates may result in weakness, tetany, convulsions, and cardiac arrest owing to profound hypocalcemia. The QT interval may be prolonged, and variable conduction defects may occur. Oxalate crystals may be found on urinalysis. Insoluble oxalate crystals are not absorbed but can cause irritation and swelling in the oropharynx and esophagus.

**IV. Diagnosis** is based on a history of exposure and evidence of local or systemic effects or oxalate crystalluria.

**A. Specific levels.** Serum oxalate levels are not available.

**B. Other useful laboratory studies** include electrolytes, glucose, BUN, creatinine, calcium, ECG monitoring, and urinalysis.

**V. Treatment**

**A. Emergency and supportive measures**

1. Protect the airway (see p 1), which may become acutely swollen and obstructed after a significant ingestion or inhalation. Administer supplemental oxygen and assist ventilation if necessary (pp 1–7).
2. Treat coma (see p 18), seizures (p 22), and arrhythmias (pp 10–15) if they occur.
3. Monitor the ECG and vital signs for at least 6 hours after significant exposure and admit symptomatic patients to an intensive care unit.

**B. Specific drugs and antidotes.** Administer 10% **calcium solution** (chloride or gluconate) to counteract symptomatic hypocalcemia (see p 428).

**C. Decontamination** (see p 45)

1. **Insoluble oxalates** in plants. Flush exposed areas. For ingestions, dilute with plain water; do not induce vomiting or give charcoal.
2. **Oxalic acid or strong commercial oxalate solutions.** Immediately flush with copious water. Do ***not*** induce vomiting because of the risk of aggravating corrosive injury; instead, give water to dilute, and on arrival in the hospital perform gastric lavage.
3. **Plants containing soluble oxalates.** Attempt to precipitate ingested oxalate in the stomach by administering calcium (calcium chloride or gluconate, 1–2 g, or calcium carbonate [Tums], several tablets) orally or via a gastric tube. The effectiveness of activated charcoal is unknown.

**D. Enhanced elimination.** Maintain high-volume urine flow (3–5 mL/kg/h) to help prevent calcium oxalate precipitation in the tubules. Oxalate is removed by hemodialysis, but the indications for this treatment are not established.

## ► PARAQUAT AND DIQUAT

*Richard J. Geller, MD, MPH*

Paraquat dichloride (CAS # 1910-42-5) and diquat dibromide (CAS # 85-00-7) are dipyridyl herbicides used for weed control and as preharvest (desiccant) defoliants. Dipyridyl product formulations differ by country. In the United States, paraquat has been available as a concentrated (29–44%) liquid. Diquat is found in aqueous concentrates containing 8–37.3% of the herbicide. Granular formulations that contain a 2.5% mixture of paraquat and diquat salts are also available. Recently a formulation containing diquat 0.73% and glyphosate 18% was marketed (Roundup Grass and Weed Killer).

**I. Mechanism of toxicity**

**A. Paraquat and diquat** are strong cations in aqueous solution, and concentrated solutions (eg, > 20%) may cause severe corrosive injury when ingested, injected, or applied to the skin, eyes, or mucous membranes. The dipyridyl herbicides are extremely potent systemic toxins when absorbed and can cause multiple system organ damage. Reaction of these dicationic compounds with nicotinamide adenosine dinucleotide phosphate (NADPH) produces highly reactive free radicals, including superoxide anions, leading to cell death and tissue destruction through lipid peroxidation.

1. **Paraquat** is selectively taken up and concentrated by pulmonary alveolar cells, leading to cell necrosis followed by connective tissue proliferation and pulmonary fibrosis.

2. **Diquat** is not taken up by pulmonary alveolar cells and does not cause pulmonary fibrosis, but it accumulates in the kidney, causing renal failure. It is also associated with GI fluid sequestration and cerebral and brainstem hemorrhagic infarctions.

**B. Pharmacokinetics**

1. **Absorption.** Paraquat and diquat are rapidly absorbed from the GI tract, and peak serum levels are reached within 2 hours of ingestion. The presence of food may reduce absorption significantly. Although absorption is poor through intact skin, the dipyridyl herbicides can be taken up through abraded skin or after prolonged contact with concentrated solutions. Fatalities usually result from ingestion but have been reported after intramuscular injection, after vaginal and percutaneous exposure, and rarely after inhalation.
2. **Distribution.** Paraquat has an apparent volume of distribution of 1.2–1.6 L/kg. It is distributed most avidly to lung, kidney, liver, and muscle tissue; in the lungs, paraquat is actively taken up against a concentration gradient.
3. **Elimination.** Paraquat is eliminated renally, with more than 90% excreted unchanged within 12–24 hours if renal function is normal. Diquat is eliminated renally and via the GI tract.

**II. Toxic dose.** Diquat is slightly less toxic than paraquat. However, this distinction may be of little comfort, as both compounds are extremely poisonous.

**A. Paraquat.** Ingestion of as little as 2–4 g, or 10–20 mL, of concentrated 20% paraquat solution has resulted in death. The estimated lethal dose of 20% paraquat is 10–20 mL for adults and 4–5 mL for children. The mean oral $LD_{50}$ in monkeys is approximately 50 mg/kg.

1. If food is present in the stomach, it may bind paraquat, preventing its absorption and reducing its toxicity.
2. Once applied to plants or soil, paraquat is rapidly bound and is not likely to be toxic. When burned, it is combusted and does not produce poisoning. Paraquat is not systemically incorporated by plants.

**B. Diquat.** The estimated lethal dose for adults is 30–60 mL of 20% diquat. The oral LD50 in monkeys is approximately 100–300 mg/kg.

**III. Clinical presentation**

**A. Paraquat.** After ingestion of concentrated solutions, there is pain and swelling in the mouth and throat and oral ulcerations may be visible. Nausea, vomiting, and abdominal pain are common. The severity and tempo of illness depend on the dose. Ingestion of more than 40 mg/kg (about 14 mL of a 20% solution in an adult) leads to corrosive GI injury, rapid onset of renal failure, myonecrosis, shock, and death within hours to a few days. Ingestion of 20–40 mg/kg causes a more indolent course evolving over several days, with most patients dying from pulmonary fibrosis after days to weeks. Patients with ingestions of less than 20 mg/kg usually recover fully.

**B. Diquat** causes similar initial symptoms but does not cause pulmonary fibrosis. Severe gastroenteritis and GI fluid sequestration may cause massive fluid and electrolyte loss that contributes to renal failure. Agitation, seizures, and coma have been described. Cerebral and brainstem hemorrhagic infarctions may occur.

**IV. Diagnosis** is based on a history of ingestion and the presence of gastroenteritis and oral burns. The oral mucosal burns may have the appearance of a pseudomembrane on the soft palate that sometimes is confused with diphtheria. Rapidly progressive pulmonary fibrosis suggests paraquat poisoning.

**A. Specific levels.** The prognosis may be correlated with specific serum levels, but these levels are not likely to be available in a time frame useful for emergency management. Assistance in obtaining and interpreting plasma and urine paraquat and diquat levels can be obtained through Syngenta ([800] 327-8633). Plasma paraquat levels associated with a high likelihood of death are 2 mg/L at 4 hours, 0.9 mg/L at 6 hours, and 0.1 mg/L at 24 hours after ingestion.

**B. Other useful laboratory studies** include electrolytes, glucose, BUN, creatinine, liver transaminases, urinalysis, arterial blood gases or oximetry, and chest x-ray. Rapid rise of creatinine (out of proportion to the BUN) has been seen.

**V. Treatment**

**A. Emergency and supportive measures.** Assistance in managing paraquat and diquat exposure can be obtained 24 hours a day by contacting the **Syngenta Agricultural Products Emergency Information Network ([800] 327-8633).**

1. Maintain an open airway and assist ventilation if necessary (see pp 1–7).
2. Treat fluid and electrolyte imbalance caused by gastroenteritis with intravenous crystalloid solutions.
3. Avoid excessive oxygen administration in patients with **paraquat** poisoning, as this may aggravate lipid peroxidation reactions in the lungs. Treat significant hypoxemia with supplemental oxygen, but use only the lowest oxygen concentration necessary to achieve a $pO_2$ of about 60 mm.

**B. Specific drugs and antidotes.** There is no specific antidote.

**C. Decontamination** (see p 45)

1. **Skin and eyes.** Remove all contaminated clothing and wash exposed skin with soap and water. Irrigate exposed eyes with copious saline or water.
2. **Ingestion.** Immediate and aggressive GI decontamination is probably the only treatment that may affect the outcome significantly after paraquat or diquat ingestion.
   a. **Prehospital.** Prompt ingestion of *any* food may afford some protection if charcoal is not immediately available. Do ***not*** administer ipecac.
   b. **Hospital.** Immediately administer 100 g of activated charcoal and repeat the dose in 1–2 hours. Gastric lavage may be helpful if performed within an hour of the ingestion but should be preceded by a dose of activated charcoal. Various clays, such as bentonite and fuller's earth, also adsorb paraquat and diquat but are probably no more effective than charcoal.

**D. Enhanced elimination** (see p 53). Although charcoal hemoperfusion has been advocated and early animal studies and human case reports suggested benefits, no controlled study has demonstrated improved outcome, and the current consensus is that the procedure is not indicated. Hemodialysis and forced diuresis do not enhance elimination, though renal failure may necessitate hemodialysis.

## ▶ PENTACHLOROPHENOL AND DINITROPHENOL

*Delia A. Dempsey, MS, MD*

**Pentachlorophenol** (Penchloro, Penta, PCP, others) is a chlorinated aromatic hydrocarbon that is used as a fungicide to preserve wood (eg, telephone poles). Since 1984 its use in the United States has been restricted to industrial uses by certified applicators. It is a ubiquitous environmental contaminant detectable in the general population. It appears to be a thyroid hormone and immune disrupter. It is a probable carcinogen (EPA).

**Dinitrophenols** (Dinosam, Dnoc, DNP, and analogs) have been used as insecticides, herbicides, fungicides, and chemical intermediaries and are used in some explosives, dyes, and photographic chemicals. Dinitrophenol has also been taken orally for weight reduction. The use of dinitrophenol as a pesticide or as a weight-reducing agent is banned in the United States, although the chemical appears to be available over the Internet.

**I. Mechanism of toxicity**

**A.** Pentachlorophenol and dinitrophenols uncouple oxidative phosphorylation in the mitochondria. Substrates are metabolized, but the energy produced is dissipated as heat instead of producing adenosine triphosphate (ATP). The basal metabolic rate increases, placing increased demands on the cardiorespiratory system. Excess lactic acid results from anaerobic glycolysis.

**B.** Dinitrophenols may oxidize hemoglobin to methemoglobin (see p 262).

**C.** In animal studies, pentachlorophenol is mutagenic, teratogenic, and carcinogenic. DNP is teratogenic and may be weakly carcinogenic.

**II. Toxic dose.** These agents are readily absorbed through the skin, lungs, and GI tract.

**A. Inhalation.** The air level of pentachlorophenol considered immediately dangerous to life or health (IDLH) is 2.5 mg/m$^3$. The ACGIH recommended workplace air exposure limit (TLV-TWA) is 0.5 mg/m$^3$ as an 8-hour time-weighted average.

**B. Skin.** This is the main route associated with accidental poisoning. An epidemic of intoxication occurred in a neonatal nursery after diapers were inadvertently washed in 23% sodium pentachlorophenate.

**C. Ingestion.** The minimum lethal oral dose of pentachlorophenol for humans is not known, but death occurred after ingestion of 2 g. Ingestion of 1–3 g of dinitrophenol is considered lethal.

**III. Clinical presentation.** The toxic manifestations of pentachlorophenol and dinitrophenol are nearly identical. Profuse sweating, fever, tachypnea, and tachycardia are universally reported in serious poisonings.

**A. Acute exposure** causes irritation of the skin, eyes, and upper respiratory tract. Systemic absorption may cause headache, vomiting, weakness, and lethargy. Profound sweating, hyperthermia, tachycardia, tachypnea, convulsions, and coma are associated with severe or fatal poisonings. Pulmonary edema may occur. Death usually is caused by cardiovascular collapse or hyperthermia. After death an extremely rapid onset of rigor mortis is reported frequently. Dinitrophenol may also induce methemoglobinemia, liver and kidney failure, and yellow-stained skin.

**B. Chronic exposure** may present in a similar manner and in addition may cause weight loss, GI disturbances, fevers and night sweats, weakness, flu-like symptoms, contact dermatitis, and aplastic anemia (rare). Cataracts and glaucoma have been associated with DNP.

**IV. Diagnosis** is based on history of exposure and clinical findings and should be suspected in patients with fever, metabolic acidosis, diaphoresis, and tachypnea.

**A. Specific levels.** Blood levels are not readily available or useful for emergency management.

**B. Other useful laboratory studies** include CBC, electrolytes, glucose, BUN, creatinine, CPK, liver transaminases, amylase, urine dipstick for occult blood (positive with hemolysis or rhabdomyolysis), arterial blood gases, methemoglobin level, and chest x-ray.

**V. Treatment**

**A. Emergency and supportive measures**

1. Maintain an open airway and assist ventilation if necessary (see pp 1–7).
2. Treat coma (see p 18), seizures (p 22), hypotension (p 15), and hyperthermia (p 20) if they occur. Dehydration from tachypnea, fever, and sweating is common and may require large-volume fluid replacement.
3. Monitor asymptomatic patients for at least 6 hours after exposure.
4. Do ***not*** use salicylates or anticholinergic agents, as they may worsen hyperthermia. Paralysis with neuromuscular blockers may not be helpful because of the intracellular mechanism for hyperthermia. Barbiturates (see pp 493, 494) may be of some value.

**B. Specific drugs and antidotes.** There is no specific antidote. Treat methemoglobinemia with methylene blue (see p 473).

**C. Decontamination** (see p 45)

1. **Inhalation.** Remove the victim from exposure and administer supplemental oxygen if available.
2. **Skin and eyes.** Remove contaminated clothing and store in a plastic bag; wash exposed areas thoroughly with soap and copious water. Irrigate exposed eyes with copious saline or tepid water. Rescuers should wear appropriate protective clothing and respirators to avoid exposure.
3. **Ingestion.** Administer activated charcoal orally if conditions are appropriate (see Table I–38, p 51). Gastric lavage is not necessary after small to moderate ingestions if activated charcoal can be given promptly.

**D. Enhanced elimination.** There is no evidence that enhanced elimination procedures are effective.

## ▶ PHENCYCLIDINE (PCP) AND KETAMINE

*Timothy J. Wiegand, MD, and Neal L. Benowitz, MD*

**Phencyclidine** [PCP, 1-(1-phenylcyclohexyl)-piperidine] is a dissociative anesthetic agent with properties similar to those of ketamine. It previously was marketed for veterinary use, and it became popular as an inexpensive street drug in the late 1960s. PCP is most commonly smoked but may also be snorted, ingested, or injected, and it is frequently substituted for or added to illicit psychoactive drugs such as THC (tetrahydrocannabinol or marijuana), mescaline, and LSD. PCP is known by a variety of street names, including “Peace pill,” “Angel dust,” “Hog,” “Goon,” “Animal tranquilizer,” and “Krystal.” “Sherms” is slang for Sherman cigarettes laced with PCP. Various chemical analogs of PCP have been synthesized, including PCC (1-piperidonocyclohexanecarbinol), PCE (1-phenyl-cyclohexylethylamine), PHP (phenylcyclohexylpyrrolidine), and TCP (1[1-cyclohexyl]piperidine).

**Ketamine** [2-(2-chlorophenyl)-2-(methylamino)cyclohexanone] shares many pharmacologic and clinical characteristics with PCP. Although currently used as an anesthetic agent and for procedural sedation, ketamine is a popular drug of abuse. Although the effects differ, it sometimes is misrepresented as MDMA (methylenedioxymethamphetamine). Street names for ketamine include “Jet,” “Kit-kat,” “Special K,” “Special LA Coke,” “Super C,” and “Vitamin K.”

**I. Mechanism of toxicity**

**A.** PCP and ketamine are dissociative anesthetics that produce generalized loss of pain perception with little or no depression of airway reflexes or ventilation. Psychotropic effects are mediated through several mechanisms, including stimulation of sigma opioid receptors; inhibition of reuptake of dopamine, norepinephrine, and serotonin; and blocking of potassium conductance. PCP also binds to a site within the L-type calcium channel, thus attenuating the influx of calcium when excitatory neurotransmitters bind to this receptor.

**B. Pharmacokinetics.** PCP is absorbed rapidly by inhalation or ingestion. PCP is highly lipophilic and has a large volume of distribution (Vd) of about 6 L/kg. The duration of clinical effects after an overdose is highly variable and ranges from 11–14 hours in one report to 1–4 days in another. PCP is eliminated mainly by hepatic metabolism, although renal and gastric excretion accounts for a small fraction and is pH dependent. (See also Table II–59.) Ketamine is well absorbed after snorting, ingestion, rectal administration, or injection. Effects last 30 minutes to 2 hours, depending on the route of administration. It is metabolized by the liver. Renal elimination is an important route of elimination for norketamine, the active metabolite of ketamine. The volume of distribution of ketamine is approximately 2–4 L/kg.

**II. Toxic dose**

**A. PCP.** In tablet form the usual street dose is 1–6 mg, which results in hallucinations, euphoria, and disinhibition. Ingestion of 6–10 mg causes toxic psychosis and signs of sympathomimetic stimulation. Acute ingestion of 150–200 mg has resulted in death. Smoking PCP produces rapid onset of effects and thus may be an easier route for users to titrate to the desired level of intoxication.

B. **Ketamine.** Usual therapeutic anesthetic doses are 1–5 mg/kg IV or 5–10 mg/kg IM. Recreational doses range from 10 to 250 mg nasally, 40 to 450 mg orally or rectally, and 10 to 100 mg IM. The higher recreational doses are purported to lead to a psychic state called "the K-hole."

III. **Clinical presentation.** Clinical effects may be seen within minutes of smoking PCP and can last 24 hours or longer, depending on the dose. Because users of PCP and ketamine often present having co-ingested multiple drugs of abuse (cocaine, THC, alcohol, MDMA, etc), the initial presentation may be difficult to discern from other toxidromes. Although the clinical effects of PCP and ketamine are similar, reports of ketamine causing similar degrees of agitation and violent behavior to PCP are lacking.

A. **Mild intoxication** causes lethargy, euphoria, hallucinations, and occasionally bizarre or violent behavior. Hypersalivation and lacrimation may occur. Patients may abruptly swing between quiet catatonia and loud or agitated behavior. Vertical and horizontal nystagmus may be prominent with PCP intoxication.

B. **Severe PCP intoxication** produces signs of adrenergic hyperactivity, including hypertension, rigidity, localized dystonic reactions, hyperthermia, tachycardia, diaphoresis, pulmonary edema, convulsions, and coma. The pupils are sometimes paradoxically small. Death may occur as a result of self-destructive behavior or as a complication of hyperthermia and subsequent multiorgan system dysfunction (eg, rhabdomyolysis, renal failure, coagulopathy, or brain damage). Sudden death, probably from ventricular arrhythmia, has occurred during restraint for agitated delirium (such as in police custody).

C. Chronic ketamine abuse may cause memory impairment.

IV. **Diagnosis** is suggested by the presence of rapidly fluctuating behavior, vertical nystagmus, and sympathomimetic signs.

A. **Specific levels**

1. Specific serum PCP levels are not readily available and do not correlate reliably with the degree of intoxication. Levels of 30–100 ng/mL have been associated with toxic psychosis.
2. Qualitative urine screening for PCP is widely available. PCP analogs may not be detected on routine screening, although they can cross-react in some immunologic assays (see Table I–33, p 44). Ketamine is not detected on routine screening.

B. **Other useful laboratory studies** include electrolytes, glucose, BUN, creatinine, CPK, and urinalysis dipstick for occult blood (positive with myoglobinuria).

V. **Treatment**

A. **Emergency and supportive measures**

1. Maintain an open airway and assist ventilation if necessary (see pp 1–7).
2. Treat coma (p 18), seizures (p 22), hypertension (p 17), hyperthermia (p 20), and rhabdomyolysis (p 26) if they occur.
3. Agitated behavior (p 23) may respond to limiting sensory stimulation but may require sedation with haloperidol (see p 458), midazolam, or diazepam (see p 419). Do ***not*** use physostigmine. In the initial management of an extremely agitated patient, midazolam or haloperidol may be given intramuscularly if IV access is absent.
4. Monitor temperature and other vital signs for a minimum of 6 hours and admit all patients with hyperthermia or other evidence of significant intoxication.

B. **Specific drugs and antidotes.** There is no specific antidote. Clonidine at a dose of 2.5–5 mcg/kg orally has been used to attenuate the sympathomimetic effects of ketamine seen during anesthesia.

**C. Decontamination.** No decontamination measures are necessary after snorting, smoking, or injecting PCP or ketamine. For ingestion, administer activated charcoal if conditions are appropriate (see Table I–38, p 51). Gastric lavage is not necessary after small to moderate ingestions if activated charcoal can be given promptly.

**D. Enhanced elimination.** Because of its large volume of distribution, PCP is not effectively removed by dialysis, hemoperfusion, or other enhanced removal procedures.

1. Repeat-dose activated charcoal has not been studied but might marginally increase elimination by adsorbing PCP partitioned into the acidic stomach fluid. Continuous nasogastric suction has also been proposed for removal of gastric-partitioned PCP.
2. Although urinary acidification increases the urinary concentration of PCP, there is no evidence that this significantly enhances systemic elimination, and it may be dangerous because urinary acidification can aggravate myoglobinuric renal failure.

## ► PHENOL AND RELATED COMPOUNDS

*Gary W. Everson, PharmD*

**Phenol** (carbolic acid) was introduced into household use as a potent germicidal agent but has limited use today because less toxic compounds have replaced it. Now phenol is most commonly found in topical skin products (eg, Campho-phenique contains 4.7% phenol) and is also used cosmetically as a skin-peeling agent. **Hexachlorophene** is a chlorinated biphenol that was used widely as a topical antiseptic and preoperative scrub until its adverse neurologic effects were recognized. Other phenolic compounds include **creosote, creosol, cresol, cresylic acid, hydroquinone, eugenol,** and **phenylphenol** (bisphenol, the active ingredient in Lysol). **Pentachlorophenol** and **dinitrophenols** are discussed on p 299.

I. **Mechanism of toxicity.** Phenol denatures protein, disrupts the cell wall, and produces a coagulative tissue necrosis. It may cause corrosive injury to the eyes, skin, and respiratory tract. Systemic absorption may result in cardiac arrhythmias and CNS stimulation, but the mechanisms of these effects are not known. Some phenolic compounds (eg, dinitrophenol and hydroquinone) may induce hemolysis and **methemoglobinemia** (see p 262).

II. **Toxic dose.** The minimum toxic and lethal doses have not been well established. Phenol is well absorbed via inhalation, skin application, and ingestion.

**A. Inhalation.** The ACGIH-recommended workplace exposure limit (TLV-TWA) for pure phenol is 5 ppm (19 mg/m$^3$) as an 8-hour time-weighted average. The level considered immediately dangerous to life or health (IDLH) is 250 ppm.

**B. Skin application.** Death has occurred in infants from repeated dermal applications of small doses (one infant died after a 2% solution of phenol was applied for 11 hours on the umbilicus under a closed bandage). Cardiac arrhythmias occurred after dermal application of 3 mL of an 88% phenol solution. Solutions of > 5% are corrosive.

**C. Ingestion.** Deaths have occurred after adult ingestions of 1–32 g of phenol; however, survival after ingestion of 45–65 g has been reported. As little as 50–500 mg has been reported as fatal in infants.

**D. Pharmacokinetics.** Phenol is rapidly absorbed by all routes. Its elimination half-life is 0.5–4.5 hours.

III. **Clinical presentation.** Toxicity may result from inhalation, skin or eye exposure, or ingestion.

**A. Inhalation.** Vapors of phenol may cause respiratory tract irritation and chemical pneumonia. Smoking of clove cigarettes (clove oil contains the phenol derivative eugenol) may cause severe tracheobronchitis.

B. **Skin and eyes.** Topical exposure to the skin may produce a deep white patch that turns red and then stains the skin brown. This lesion is often relatively painless. Irritation and severe corneal damage may occur if concentrated phenolic compounds come in contact with eyes.

C. **Ingestion** usually causes vomiting and diarrhea, and diffuse corrosive GI tract injury may occur. Systemic absorption may cause agitation, confusion, seizures, coma, hypotension, arrhythmias, and respiratory arrest.

IV. **Diagnosis** is based on a history of exposure, the presence of a characteristic odor, and painless skin burns with white discoloration.

A. **Specific levels.** Normal urine phenol levels are less than 20 mg/L. Urine phenol levels may be elevated in workers exposed to benzene and after the use of phenol-containing throat lozenges and mouthwashes.

B. **Other useful laboratory studies** include CBC, electrolytes, glucose, BUN, creatinine, and ECG. Obtain a methemoglobin level after hydroquinone exposures.

V. **Treatment**

A. **Emergency and supportive measures**

1. Maintain an open airway and assist ventilation if necessary (see pp 1–7).
2. Treat coma (see p 18), seizures (p 22), hypotension (p 15), and arrhythmias (pp 10–15) if they occur.
3. If corrosive injury to the GI tract is suspected, consult a gastroenterologist for possible endoscopy.

B. **Specific drugs and antidotes.** No specific antidote is available. If **methemoglobinemia** occurs, administer methylene blue (see p 473).

C. **Decontamination** (see p 45)

1. **Inhalation.** Remove victims from exposure and administer supplemental oxygen if available.
2. **Skin and eyes.** Remove contaminated clothing and wash exposed skin with soapy water or, if available, Polyethylene Glycol 300, mineral oil, olive oil, or petroleum jelly. Immediately flush exposed eyes with copious tepid water or saline.
3. **Ingestion.** Administer activated charcoal orally if conditions are appropriate (see Table I–38, p 51). Use caution because phenol can cause convulsions, increasing the risk of pulmonary aspiration. Gastric lavage is not necessary after small to moderate ingestions if activated charcoal can be given promptly.

D. **Enhanced elimination.** Enhanced removal methods are generally not effective because of the large volume of distribution of these lipid-soluble compounds. Hexachlorophene is excreted in the bile, and repeat-dose activated charcoal (see p 50) may possibly be effective in increasing its clearance from the gut.

## ▶ PHENYTOIN

*Craig Smollin, MD*

Phenytoin is used orally for the prevention of generalized (grand mal) and partial complex seizures. Intravenous phenytoin is used to treat status epilepticus and occasionally as an antiarrhythmic agent. Oral formulations include suspensions, capsules, and tablet preparations. The brand Dilantin Kapseals exhibits delayed absorption characteristics not usually shared by generic products.

I. **Mechanism of toxicity.** Toxicity may be caused by the phenytoin itself or by the propylene glycol diluent used in parenteral preparations. To make it available for intravenous use, phenytoin must be dissolved in 40% propylene glycol and 10% ethanol at pH 12.

A. **Phenytoin** suppresses high-frequency neuronal firing, primarily by increasing the refractory period of voltage-dependent sodium channels. Toxic levels usually cause CNS depression.

**B.** The **propylene glycol** diluent in parenteral preparations may cause myocardial depression and cardiac arrest when infused rapidly (> 40–50 mg/min [0.5–1 mg/kg/min]). The mechanism is not known. The injectable form of phenytoin also is highly alkaline and can cause tissue necrosis if it infiltrates ("purple glove syndrome").

**C. Fosphenytoin,** a water-soluble prodrug, does not contain the propylene glycol diluent and does not cause these toxic effects. As a result, it can be given at rates twice as fast as those for phenytoin. It does not appear to provide faster times to peak plasma phenytoin concentration or to result in fewer adverse effects compared with phenytoin.

**D. Pharmacokinetics.** Absorption may be slow and unpredictable. The time to peak plasma levels varies with the dosage. The volume of distribution is about 0.5–0.8 L/kg. Protein binding is about 90% at therapeutic levels. Hepatic elimination is saturable (zero-order kinetics) at levels near the therapeutic range, so the apparent "half-life" increases as levels rise (26 hours at 10 mg/L, 40 hours at 20 mg/L, and 60 hours at 40 mg/L). See also Table II–59 (p 382).

**II. Toxic dose.** The minimum acute toxic oral overdose is approximately 20 mg/kg. Because phenytoin exhibits dose-dependent elimination kinetics, accidental intoxication can easily occur in patients on chronic therapy owing to drug interactions or slight dosage adjustments.

**III. Clinical presentation.** Toxicity caused by phenytoin may be associated with acute oral overdose or chronic accidental overmedication. In acute oral overdose, absorption and peak effects may be delayed.

**A. Mild to moderate intoxication** commonly causes nystagmus, ataxia, and dysarthria. Nausea, vomiting, diplopia, hyperglycemia, agitation, and irritability have also been reported.

**B. Severe intoxication** can cause stupor, coma, and respiratory arrest. Although seizures have been reported, seizures in a phenytoin-intoxicated patient should prompt a search for other causes (eg, anoxia, hyperthermia, or an overdose of another drug). Death from isolated oral phenytoin overdose is extremely rare.

**C. Rapid intravenous injection,** usually at rates exceeding 50 mg/min, can cause profound hypotension, bradycardia, and cardiac arrest. These effects are attributed to the propylene glycol diluent. Cardiac toxicity does not occur with an oral overdose or with fosphenytoin.

**IV. Diagnosis** is based on a history of ingestion or is suspected in any epileptic patient with altered mental status or ataxia.

**A. Specific levels.** Serum phenytoin concentrations are generally available in all hospital clinical laboratories. Obtain repeated blood samples because slow absorption may result in delayed peak levels. The therapeutic concentration range is 10–20 mg/L.

1. Above 20 mg/L, nystagmus is common. Above 30 mg/L, ataxia, slurred speech, and tremor are common. With levels higher than 40 mg/L, lethargy, confusion, and stupor ensue. Survival has been reported in three patients with levels above 100 mg/L.
2. Because phenytoin is protein bound, patients with renal failure or hypoalbuminemia may experience toxicity at lower serum levels. Free (unbound) serum phenytoin levels are not routinely available.

**B. Other useful laboratory studies** include electrolytes, glucose, BUN, creatinine, serum albumin, and ECG monitoring (during intravenous infusion).

**V. Treatment**

**A. Emergency and supportive measures**

1. Maintain an open airway and assist ventilation if necessary (see pp 1–7). Administer supplemental oxygen.
2. Treat stupor and coma (see p 15) if they occur. Protect the patient from self-injury caused by ataxia.

3. If seizures occur, consider an alternative diagnosis and treat with other usual anticonvulsants (see p 22).
4. If hypotension occurs with intravenous phenytoin administration, immediately stop the infusion and administer intravenous fluids and pressors (see p 15) if necessary.

B. **Specific drugs and antidotes.** There is no specific antidote.
C. **Decontamination** (see p 45). Administer activated charcoal orally if conditions are appropriate (see Table I–38, p 51). Gastric lavage is not necessary after small to moderate ingestions if activated charcoal can be given promptly.
D. **Enhanced elimination.** Repeat-dose activated charcoal (see p 50) may enhance phenytoin elimination but is not necessary and may increase the risk of aspiration pneumonitis in drowsy patients. There is no role for diuresis, dialysis, or hemoperfusion.

## ▶ PHOSGENE

*John Balmes, MD*

Phosgene originally was manufactured as a war gas. It is now used in the manufacture of dyes, resins, and pesticides. It is also commonly produced when chlorinated compounds are burned, such as in a fire, or in the process of welding metal that has been cleaned with chlorinated solvents.

I. **Mechanism of toxicity.** Phosgene is an irritant. However, because it is poorly water soluble, in lower concentrations it does not cause immediate upper-airway or skin irritation. Thus, an exposed individual may inhale phosgene for prolonged periods deeply into the lungs, where it is slowly hydrolyzed to hydrochloric acid. This results in necrosis and inflammation of the small airways and alveoli, which may lead to noncardiogenic pulmonary edema.

II. **Toxic dose.** The ACGIH-recommended workplace exposure limit (TLV-TWA) is 0.1 ppm (0.4 mg/m$^3$) as an 8-hour time-weighted average. The level considered immediately dangerous to life or health (IDLH) is 2 ppm. Exposure to 50 ppm may be rapidly fatal.

III. **Clinical presentation.** Exposure to moderate concentrations of phosgene causes mild cough and minimal mucous membrane irritation. After an asymptomatic interval of 30 minutes to 8 hours (depending on the duration and concentration of exposure), the victim develops dyspnea and hypoxemia. Pulmonary edema may be delayed up to 24 hours. Permanent pulmonary impairment may be a sequela of serious exposure.

IV. **Diagnosis** is based on a history of exposure and the clinical presentation. Many other toxic gases may cause delayed-onset pulmonary edema (see p 7).
   A. **Specific levels.** There are no specific blood or urine levels.
   B. **Other useful laboratory studies** include chest x-ray and arterial blood gases or oximetry.

V. **Treatment**
   A. **Emergency and supportive measures**
      1. Maintain an open airway and assist ventilation if necessary (see pp 1–7). Administer supplemental oxygen, and treat noncardiogenic pulmonary edema (see p 7) if it occurs.
      2. Monitor the patient for at least 12–24 hours after exposure because of the potential for delayed-onset pulmonary edema.
   B. **Specific drugs and antidotes.** There is no specific antidote.
   C. **Decontamination.** Remove the victim from exposure and give supplemental oxygen if available. Rescuers should wear self-contained breathing apparatus.
   D. **Enhanced elimination.** These procedures are not effective.

## ► PHOSPHINE AND PHOSPHIDES

*Kent R. Olson, MD*

**Phosphine** is a colorless gas that is heavier than air. It is odorless in its pure form, but impurities give it a characteristic fishy or garlic-like odor. It has been used for fumigation, and it is a serious potential hazard in operations producing metal phosphides, in which phosphine can be released in the chemical reaction of water and metal alloys. Workers at risk include metal refiners, acetylene workers, fire fighters, pest-control operators, and those in the semiconductor industry. **Magnesium phosphide** and **aluminum phosphide** are available in pellets or tablets and are used as fumigants and rodenticides. **Zinc phosphide** is a crystalline dark gray powder mixed into food as rodent bait. Phosphides are a leading cause of fatal suicides and accidental ingestions in India and many developing countries.

**I. Mechanism of toxicity.** Phosphine is a highly toxic gas, especially to the lungs, brain, kidneys, heart, and liver. The pathophysiologic action of phosphine is not clearly understood but may be related to inhibition of electron transport in mitochondria. Phosphides liberate phosphine gas upon contact with moisture, and this reaction is enhanced in the acidity of the stomach. Phosphine is then absorbed through the GI and respiratory tracts.

**II. Toxic dose**

**A. Phosphine gas.** The ACGIH-recommended workplace exposure limit (TLV-TWA) is 0.3 ppm (0.42 mg/$m^3$), which is much lower than the minimal detectable (fishy odor) concentration of 1–3 ppm. Hence, the odor threshold does not provide sufficient warning of dangerous concentrations. An air level of 50 ppm is considered immediately dangerous to life or health (IDLH). Chronic exposure to sublethal concentrations for extended periods may produce toxic symptoms.

**B. Phosphides.** Ingestion of as little as 500 mg of **aluminum phosphide** has caused death in an adult. In a reported case series, survivors ingested about 1.5 g (range 1.5–18), whereas fatal cases had ingested an average of 2.3 g (range 1.5–36). The $LD_{50}$ for **zinc phosphide** in rats is 40 mg/kg; the lowest reported lethal dose in humans is 4 g. A 36-year-old man who ingested 6 mg/kg of zinc phosphide and was treated with ipecac and activated charcoal remained asymptomatic.

**III. Clinical presentation.** Inhalation of phosphine gas is associated with cough, dyspnea, headache, dizziness, and vomiting. Phosphide ingestion may cause nausea, vomiting, diarrhea, hypotension unresponsive to pressors, and a rotten fish or garlicky odor. Adult respiratory distress syndrome (ARDS), acute renal failure, hepatitis, seizures, and coma may occur. Myocardial injury manifested by elevated cardiac enzymes, ST-T wave changes, global hypokinesia, and various atrial and ventricular arrhythmias have been reported, as well as pericardial and pleural effusions, adrenal necrosis, and pancreatitis. Methemoglobinemia has also been reported. The onset of symptoms is usually rapid, although delayed onset of pulmonary edema has been described.

**IV. Diagnosis** is based on a history of exposure to the agent. ***Caution:*** Pulmonary edema may have a delayed onset, and initial respiratory symptoms may be mild or absent.

**A. Specific levels.** Body fluid phosphine levels are not clinically useful.

**B. Other useful laboratory studies** include BUN, creatinine, electrolytes, liver transaminases, arterial blood gases or oximetry, and chest x-ray.

**V. Treatment**

**A. Emergency and supportive measures**

1. Maintain an open airway and assist ventilation if necessary (see pp 1–7). Administer supplemental oxygen and treat noncardiogenic pulmonary edema (p 7) if it occurs.
2. Treat seizures (see p 22) and hypotension (p 15) if they occur.
3. Patients with a history of significant phosphine inhalation or phosphide in-

gestion should be admitted and observed for 48–72 hours for delayed onset of pulmonary edema.

4. Intravenous **magnesium** has been used to treat cardiac arrhythmias otherwise unresponsive to treatment.
5. In severe poisoning, adrenal function may be compromised and intravenous **hydrocortisone** should be considered, especially if hypotension does not respond to IV fluids and vasopressors.

B. **Specific drugs and antidotes.** There is no specific antidote.

C. **Decontamination**

1. Caregivers are at a low risk for secondary contamination, but off-gassing of phosphine may occur if the patient vomits or if gastric lavage fluid is not isolated.
2. Administer activated charcoal orally if conditions are appropriate (see Table I–38, p 51), although studies have not determined its binding affinity for phosphides. Consider gastric lavage for large recent ingestion. Use of 3–5% sodium bicarbonate in the lavage has been proposed (to reduce stomach acid and resulting production of phosphine) but is not of proven benefit.

D. **Enhanced elimination.** Dialysis and hemoperfusion have not been shown to be useful in hastening elimination of phosphine.

## ▶ PHOSPHORUS

*Matthew D. Cook, DO*

There are two naturally occurring types of elemental phosphorus: red and yellow. **Red phosphorus** is not absorbed and is essentially nontoxic. In contrast, **yellow phosphorus** (also called **white phosphorus**) is a highly toxic cellular poison. Yellow/white phosphorus is a colorless or yellow wax-like crystalline solid with a garlic-like odor and is almost insoluble in water. Although no longer a component of matches, yellow/white phosphorus is still used in the manufacture of fireworks, fertilizer, and methamphetamine. It is also used as a rodenticide and as an incendiary in military ammunition.

I. **Mechanism of toxicity**

A. Phosphorus is highly corrosive and is also a general cellular poison. Cardiovascular collapse occurring after ingestion probably results not only from fluid loss caused by vomiting and diarrhea but also from direct toxicity on the heart and vascular tone.

B. Yellow/white phosphorus spontaneously combusts in air at room temperature to yield phosphorus oxide, a highly irritating fume.

II. **Toxic dose**

A. **Ingestion.** The fatal oral dose of yellow/white phosphorus is approximately 1 mg/kg. Deaths have been reported after ingestion of as little as 3 mg in a 2-year-old child.

B. **Inhalation.** The recommended workplace limit (ACGIH TLV-TWA) for yellow or white phosphorus is 0.1 mg/m$^3$ (0.02 ppm) as an 8-hour time-weighted average. The air level considered immediately dangerous to life or health (IDLH) is 5 mg/m$^3$.

III. **Clinical presentation**

A. **Acute inhalation** may cause mucous membrane irritation, cough, wheezing, chemical pneumonitis, and noncardiogenic pulmonary edema. **Chronic inhalation** of phosphorus (over at least 10 months) may result in mandibular necrosis (“phossy jaw”).

B. **Skin or eye contact** may cause conjunctivitis or severe dermal or ocular burns.

C. **Acute ingestion** may cause GI burns, severe vomiting and abdominal pain, and diarrhea with “smoking” stools. Systemic effects include headache, delirium, shock, seizures, coma, and arrhythmias (atrial fibrillation, QRS and QT prolongation, ventricular tachycardia, and fibrillation). Metabolic derangements, including hypocalcemia and hyperphosphatemia (or hypophosphatemia), may occur. Fulminant hepatic or renal failure may occur after 2–3 days. Reversible bone marrow toxicity with neutropenia has been described.

**IV. Diagnosis** is based on a history of exposure and the clinical presentation. Cutaneous burns, a garlic odor of the vomitus, and "smoking" or luminescent stools and vomitus caused by spontaneous combustion of elemental phosphorus suggest ingestion. Wood's lamp examination of the skin will cause embedded phosphorus particles to fluoresce.

- **A. Specific levels.** Because serum phosphorus may be elevated, depressed, or normal, it is not a useful test for diagnosis or estimation of severity.
- **B. Other useful laboratory studies** include BUN, creatinine, calcium, liver transaminases, urinalysis, arterial blood gases or oximetry, ECG, and chest x-ray (after acute inhalation).

**V. Treatment**

- **A. Emergency and supportive measures**
  1. Observe a victim of inhalation closely for signs of upper-airway injury and perform endotracheal intubation and assist ventilation if necessary (see p 4). Administer supplemental oxygen. Treat bronchospasm (p 7) and pulmonary edema (p 7) if they occur.
  2. Treat fluid losses from gastroenteritis with aggressive intravenous crystalloid fluid replacement.
  3. Consider endoscopy if oral, esophageal, or gastric burns are suspected (see p 157).
- **B. Specific drugs and antidotes.** There is no specific antidote.
- **C. Decontamination** (see p 45). Rescuers should wear appropriate protective gear to prevent accidental skin or inhalation exposure. If solid phosphorus is brought into the emergency department, immediately cover it with water or wet sand.
  1. **Inhalation.** Remove the victim from exposure and give supplemental oxygen, if available.
  2. **Skin and eyes.** Remove contaminated clothing and wash exposed areas with soap and water. Irrigate exposed eyes with copious tepid water or saline. Covering exposed areas may help prevent spontaneous combustion of yellow/white phosphorus.
  3. **Ingestion.** Perform gastric lavage if the ingestion occurred within the previous 60 minutes. Activated charcoal is of unknown benefit. Do ***not*** induce vomiting because of the risk of corrosive injury.
- **D. Enhanced elimination.** There is no effective method of enhanced elimination.

## ► PLANTS

*Judith A. Alsop, PharmD*

Ingestion of plants and berries by children is one of the top five reasons for calls to poison control centers. Decorative plants are found in many homes, and landscaped yards provide access to a variety of attractive and potentially toxic plants. Fortunately, serious poisoning from plants is rare in children because the quantity of plant material required to cause serious poisoning is greater than what a small child ingests. Serious toxicity or death from plant ingestion is usually a result of intentional abuse (eg, jimson weed), misuse (eg, various teas steeped from plants), or suicide attempts (eg, oleander).

**I. Mechanism of toxicity.** Plants can be categorized by their potential toxicity. Table II–45 describes the effects of various plant toxins. Table II–46 provides an alphabetical list of potentially toxic plants and herbs.

**TABLE II–45. PLANTS: SOME TOXIC COMPONENTS**

| Toxin | Clinical Effects |
|---|---|
| Aconitum | Tingling in digits followed by paresthesias, feeling of intense cold, gastroenteritis, skeletal muscle paralysis, ventricular arrhythmias, respiratory paralysis, death. |
| Aesculin | Single seed can cause gastroenteritis. Larger amounts can cause ataxia, gastroenteritis, CNS depression, and paralysis. |
| Anthraquinone | Severe diarrhea with GI bleeding, renal damage, dyspnea, and seizures. |
| Chinaberry | Tetranortriterpene neurotoxin: gastroenteritis, lethargy, coma, respiratory failure, seizures, paralysis. |
| Coniine | Salivation, vomiting, seizures followed by CNS depression and respiratory depression, rhabdomyolysis, renal failure, muscle paralysis, rapid death secondary to respiratory paralysis. |
| Cyanogenic glycosides | Dyspnea, cyanosis, weakness, seizures, coma, cardiovascular collapse. Symptoms may be delayed for 3-4 hours or more as glycoside is hydrolyzed to cyanide in the gut. |
| Cytisine | Vomiting, hypotension, tachycardia, paralysis, seizures, respiratory depression. |
| Euphorbiaceae | Oral irritation, gastroenteritis. Erythema, edema, followed by vesicle and blister formation. Eye exposure may result in corneal ulceration, iritis, conjunctivitis, and temporary blindness. Systemic symptoms: seizures, coma, and death. |
| Gelsemium indole-alkaloids | Headache, sweating, muscular weakness or rigidity, seizures, dyspnea, bradycardia, respiratory arrest. |
| Grayanotoxin | Burning, numbness, tingling of mouth, vomiting, hypotension, bradycardia, coma, seizures. |
| Hydroquinone | Vomiting, jaundice, dizziness, headache, delirium, pallor, anoxia, seizures, respiratory failure, cyanosis, cardiovascular collapse. Allergic contact dermatitis. |
| Lantadene | Anticholinergic effects with gastroenteritis, respiratory distress, ataxia, coma, depressed deep tendon reflexes, weakness, cyanosis, death. |
| Lobeline | Vomiting, bradycardia, hypertension, tachypnea, tremors, seizures, paralysis. |
| Nicotine alkaloids | Salivation, gastroenteritis, agitation followed by seizures and coma. Hypertension, tachycardia, tachypnea followed by hypotension, bradycardia and bradypnea. |
| Protoanemonin | Acrid taste, burning in mouth and throat, oral ulceration, gastroenteritis, hematemesis. |
| Pyrrolizidine alkaloids | Gastroenteritis, hepatic veno-occlusive disease. |
| Quinolizidine | Vomiting, hypotension, tachycardia, seizures, paralysis, respiratory depression. |
| Sanguinaria | Gastroenteritis, CNS depression, ataxia, dyspnea, respiratory paralysis. |
| Saponin | Gastroenteritis, dermatitis, mydriasis, hyperthermia, ataxia, muscle weakness, dyspnea, coma. |
| Solanine | Salivation, gastroenteritis, coma, hypotension, bradycardia, cramping, paresthesias. |
| Tannin | Abdominal pain, extreme thirst, frequent urination, bloody diarrhea, rapid but weak pulse. Liver and kidney damage may occur several weeks later. |
| Toxalbumin | Severe gastroenteritis, sloughing of the GI tract followed by toxicity to the liver, CNS, kidney and adrenals. |
| Veratrum alkaloids | Gastroenteritis, bradycardia, syncope, paresthesias, hypotension. |

**TABLE II–46. PLANTS: ALPHABETICAL LIST**

| Common Name | Botanical Name | Toxic Group | Remarks (see text and Table II–45) |
|---|---|---|---|
| Acacia, black | *Robinia pseudoacacia* | 1 | Toxalbumin |
| Aconite | *Aconitum* spp | 1 | Nausea, vomiting, arrhythmias, shock |
| Acorn | *Quercus* spp | 3 | Tannin; dermatitis |
| Agapanthus | *Agapanthus* spp | 3 | Dermatitis |
| Akee | *Blighia sapida* | 1 | Hypoglycemia and hepatotoxicity |
| Alder, American | *Alnus crispus* | 3 | Dermatitis |
| Alder buckthorn | *Rhamnus frangula* | 1 | Anthraquinone |
| Almond, bitter | *Prunus* spp | 1 | Cyanogenic glycosides (see p 176) |
| Aloe vera | *Aloe vera* | 3 | GI upset; skin irritant |
| Amaryllis | *Amaryllidaceae* | 3 | GI upset |
| Amaryllis | *Hippeastrum equestre* | 3 | GI upset |
| American bittersweet | *Celastrus scandens* | 3 | GI upset |
| American ivy | *Parthenocissus* spp | 2b | Soluble oxalates |
| Anemone | *Anemone* spp | 1, 3 | Protoanemonin, dermatitis |
| Angelica | *Angelica archangelica* | 3 | Dermatitis |
| Angel's trumpet | *Brugmansia arborea, Datura* spp | 1, 3 | Anticholinergic alkaloids (see p 85) |
| Anthurium | *Anthurium* spp | 2a | Calcium oxalate crystals |
| Apple (chewed seeds) | *Malus domestica* | 1 | Cyanogenic glycosides (see p 176) |
| Apricot (chewed pits) | *Prunus* spp | 1 | Cyanogenic glycosides (see p 176) |
| Arrowhead vine | *Syngonium podophyllum* | 2a | Calcium oxalate crystals |
| Arum | *Arum* spp | 2a | Calcium oxalate crystals |
| Ash tree | *Fraxinus* spp | 3 | Dermatitis |
| Aspen tree | *Populus tremuloides* | 3 | Dermatitis |
| Autumn crocus | *Colchicum autumnale* | 1 | Colchicine (see p 173) |
| Avocado (leaves and seeds) | *Persea americana* | 1 | Unknown toxin causing hepatitis, myocarditis in animals |
| Azalea | *Rhododendron* genus | 1 | Grayanotoxin |
| Bahia | *Bahia oppositifolia* | 1 | Cyanogenic glycosides (see p 176) |
| Baneberry | *Actaea* spp | 1, 3 | Irritant oil protoanemonin: severe gastroenteritis |
| Barbados nut; purging nut | *Jatropha* spp | 1 | Toxalbumin, Euphorbiaceae |
| Barberry | *Berberis* spp | 1, 3 | GI upset, hypotension, seizures |
| Beech, European | *Fagus sylvatica* | 3 | Saponins |
| Beech, Japanese | *Fagus crenta* | 3 | Saponins |
| Begonia | *Begonia rex* | 2a | Calcium oxalate crystals |
| Belladonna | *Atropa belladonna* | 1 | Atropine (see p 415) |
| Bellyache bush | *Jatropha* spp | 1 | Euphorbiaceae |
| Be-still tree | *Thevetia peruviana* | 1 | Cardiac glycosides (see p 155) |
| Birch (bark, leaves) | *Betula* spp | 1, 3 | Methyl salicylate (see p 333), irritant oils causing GI upset |
| Bird of paradise | *Poinciana gillesi* | 3 | GI upset |
| Bird of paradise flower | *Streelizia reginae* | 3 | GI upset |
| Black cohosh | *Cimicifuga* spp | 3 | GI upset |
| Black-eyed Susan | *Rudbeckia hirta* | 3 | Dermatitis |
| Black henbane | *Hyoscyamus niger* | 1 | Anticholinergic alkaloids (see p 84) |
| Black lily | *Dracunculus vulgaris* | 2a | Calcium oxalate crystals |
| Black locust | *Robinia pseudoacacia* | 1 | Toxalbumin |
| Black nightshade | *Hyoscyamus* spp, *Solanum nigrum* | 1 | Solanine |
| Black snakeroot | *Cimicifuga racemosa* | 3 | GI upset |
| Black snakeroot | *Zigadenus* spp | 1 | Veratrum alkaloids |

*(continued)*

**TABLE II–46. PLANTS: ALPHABETICAL LIST (CONTINUED)**

| Common Name | Botanical Name | Toxic Group | Remarks (see text and Table II–45) |
|---|---|---|---|
| Bleeding heart | *Dicentra* | 3 | Dermatitis |
| Bloodroot | *Sanguinaria canadensis* | 3 | Sanguinaria |
| Blue cohosh | *Caulophyllum thalictroides* | 1, 3 | Cytisine; dermatitis |
| Boston ivy | *Parthenocissus* spp | 2b | Soluble oxalates |
| Bougainvillea | *Bougainvillea glabra* | 3 | Dermatitis |
| Box elder | *Acer negundo* | 3 | Dermatitis |
| Boxwood; box plant | *Buxus* spp | 3 | GI upset, dermatitis |
| Bracken fern | *Pteridium aquilinum* | 1 | Potential carcinogen |
| Bradford pear | *Pyrus calleryana* | 3 | Dermatitis |
| Broom | *Cytisus* spp | 1, 3 | Cytisine; dermatitis |
| Buckeye | *Aesculus* spp | 1, 3 | Aesculin |
| Buckthorn | *Karwinskia humboltiana* | 1 | Chronic ingestion may cause ascending paralysis |
| Buckthorn | *Rhamnus* spp | 3 | Anthraquinone |
| Bunchberry | *Cornus canadensis* | 3 | Dermatitis |
| Burdock root | *Arctium lappa* | 1,3 | Anticholinergic alkaloids (see p 85) |
| Burning bush | *Dictamnus albus* | 3 | Dermatitis |
| Burning bush | *Euonymus* spp | 3 | GI upset |
| Burning bush | *Kochia* spp | 2a, 2b, 3 | Soluble and insoluble oxalates, dermatitis |
| Buttercups | *Ranunculus* spp | 3 | Irritant oil protoanemonin |
| Cactus (thorn) | *Cactus* | 3 | Dermatitis, cellulitis (abscess may result) |
| Caladium | *Caladium* spp; *Xanthosoma* spp | 2a | Calcium oxalate crystals |
| California geranium | *Senecio* spp | 1 | Hepatotoxic pyrrolizidine alkaloids |
| California poppy | *Eschscholzia californica* | 3 | Potentially mildly narcotic; sanguinaria |
| California privet | *Ligustrum* spp | 3 | GI upset |
| Calla lily | *Zantedeschia* spp | 2a | Calcium oxalate crystals |
| Cannabis | *Cannabis sativa* | 1 | Mild hallucinogen (see Marijuana, p 252) |
| Caraway | *Carum carvi* | 3 | Dermatitis |
| Cardinal flower | *Lobelia* spp | 1 | Lobeline: nicotinelike alkaloid (see p 278) |
| Carnation | *Dianthus caryophyllus* | 3 | Dermatitis |
| Carolina allspice | *Calycanthus* spp | 1 | Strychnine-like alkaloid (see p 350) |
| Cascara | *Rhamnus* spp | 3 | Anthraquinone cathartic |
| Cassava | *Manihot esculenta* | 1 | Cyanogenic glycosides (see p 176); Euphorbiaceae |
| Castor bean | *Ricinus communis* | 1 | Toxalbumin (ricin) |
| Catnip | *Nepeta cataria* | 1, 3 | Mild hallucinogen |
| Cedar | *Thuja* spp | 3 | Dermatitis |
| Century plant | *Agave americana* | 3 | Thorns can cause cellulitis |
| Chamomile | *Anthemis cotula* | 3 | Dermatitis |
| Chamomile | *Chamomilla recucita* | 3 | GI upset, dermatitis |
| Cherry (chewed pits) | *Prunus* spp | 1 | Cyanogenic glycosides (see p 176) |
| Chili pepper | *Capsicum* spp | 3 | Irritant to skin, eyes, mucous membranes |
| Chinaberry | *Melia azedarach* | 1, 3 | Chinaberry: severe GI upset, seizures |
| Chokecherry | *Prunus virginiana* | 1 | Cyanogenic glycosides (see p 176) |
| Christmas rose | *Helleborus niger* | 1, 3 | Protoanemonin |
| Chrysanthemum; mum | *Chrysanthemum* spp | 3 | Dermatitis, GI upset |
| Clematis | *Clematis* spp | 3 | Protoanemonin |
| Clover | *Trifolium* spp | 1 | Cyanogenic glycosides (see p 176) |
| Clover, sweet | *Melilotus alba* | 1 | Coumarin (see p 379) |
| Coffeeberry | *Rhamnus* spp | 3 | Anthraquinone cathartic |

(*continued*)

**TABLE II–46. PLANTS: ALPHABETICAL LIST (CONTINUED)**

| Common Name | Botanical Name | Toxic Group | Remarks (see text and Table II–45) |
|---|---|---|---|
| Cola nut | *Cola nitida* | 1 | Caffeine (see p 142) |
| Comfrey | *Symphytum officinale* | 1, 3 | Irritant tannin and hepatotoxic pyrrolizidine alkaloids |
| Conquerer root | *Exogonium purga* | 3 | GI upset |
| Coral bean | *Erythrina* spp | 1 | Cyanogenic glycosides (see p 155) |
| Coral berry | *Symphoricarpos* spp | 3 | GI upset |
| Coriaria | *Coriaria* spp | 1 | Contains convulsant agent |
| Cotoneaster | *Cotoneaster* | 1,3 | Cyanogenic glycosides (see p 155) |
| Cottonwood | *Populus deltoides* | 3 | Dermatitis |
| Coyotillo | *Karwinskia humboldtiana* | 1 | Chronic ingestion may cause ascending paralysis |
| Crab apples | *Malus* spp | 1 | Cyanogenic glycosides (chewed seeds) |
| Creeping charlie | *Glecoma hederacea* | 3 | GI upset |
| Crocus, wild or prairie | *Anemone* spp | 3 | Protoanemonin |
| Croton | *Codiaeum* spp | 3 | GI upset, dermatitis |
| Crowfoot | *Ranunculus repens* | 1 | Protoanemonin |
| Crown of thorns | *Euphorbia* spp | 1,3 | Euphorbiaceae |
| Cyclamen | *Cyclamen* | 3 | GI upset |
| Daffodil (bulb) | *Narcissus* spp | 2a,3 | Calcium oxalate crystals, GI upset |
| Dagga | *Cannabis sativa* | 1 | Mild hallucinogen |
| Daisy | *Chrysanthemum* spp | 3 | GI upset, dermatitis |
| Daisy, butter | *Ranunculus repens* | 1 | Protoanemonin |
| Daisy, seaside | *Erigeron karvinskianus* | 3 | Dermatitis |
| Daphne | *Daphne* spp | 1, 3 | GI upset, dermatitis. Bark contains coumarin glycosides (see p 155) |
| Datura | *Datura* spp | 1 | Anticholinergic alkaloids (see p 85) |
| Deadly nightshade | *Atropa belladonna* | 1 | Atropine (see p 85) |
| Deadly nightshade | *Solanum* spp | 1 | Solanine |
| Death camas | *Zigadenus* spp | 1 | Veratrum alkaloids |
| Devils ivy | *Scindapsus aureus, Epipremnum aureum* | 2a | Calcium oxalate crystals |
| Dieffenbachia | *Dieffenbachia* spp | 2a | Calcium oxalate crystal |
| Dogbane | *Apocynum* spp | 1 | Cardiac glycosides (see p 155) |
| Dogwood, bloodtwig | *Cornus sanguinea* | 3 | Dermatitis |
| Dolls-eyes | *Actaea* spp | 3 | Irritant oil protoanemonin: severe gastroenteritis |
| Dragon root | *Arisaema* spp | 2a | Calcium oxalate crystals |
| Dumbcane | *Dieffenbachia* spp | 2a | Calcium oxalate crystals |
| Dusty miller | *Senecio* spp | 1 | Hepatotoxic pyrrolizidine alkaloids |
| Eggplant (green parts) | *Solanum melongena* | 1 | Solanine |
| Elderberry | *Sambucus* | 1 | Unripe berries contain cyanogenic glycosides (see p 155) |
| Elephant's ear; taro | *Alacasia* spp; *Colocasia* spp; *Philodendron* spp | 2a | Calcium oxalate crystals |
| Elm, Chinese | *Ulmus parvifolia* | 3 | Dermatitis |
| English ivy; heart ivy | *Hedera helix* | 3 | Saponins; dermatitis |
| English laurel | *Prunus laurocerasus* | 1 | Cyanogenic glycosides (see p 155) |
| Eucalyptus | *Eucalyptus* | 3 | GI upset |
| False hellebore | *Veratrum* spp | 1, 3 | Veratrum alkaloids |
| False parsley | *Cicuta maculata* | 1 | Water hemlock: cicutoxin causes seizures |
| False parsley | *Aethusa cynapium* | 1 | Poison hemlock: coniine (similar to nicotine, see p 278) |

(*continued*)

**TABLE II–46. PLANTS: ALPHABETICAL LIST (CONTINUED)**

| Common Name | Botanical Name | Toxic Group | Remarks (see text and Table II–45) |
|---|---|---|---|
| Fava bean | *Vicia faba* | 1 | Hemolytic anemia in G6PD-deficient persons |
| Ficus (sap) | *Ficus* spp | 3 | Dermatitis |
| Firethorn | *Pyracantha* | 3 | GI upset |
| Flag | *Iris* spp | 3 | GI upset, dermatitis |
| Fleabane | *Erigeron* spp | 3 | Dermatitis |
| Fool's parsley | *Conium maculatum* | 1 | Conine: nicotinelike alkaloid (see p 278) |
| Four o'clock | *Mirabilis jalapa* | 3 | Seeds have hallucinogenic effects |
| Foxglove | *Digitalis purpurea* | 1 | Cardiac glycosides (see p 155) |
| Garden sorrel | *Rumex* spp | 2b | Soluble oxalates |
| Geranium | *Pelargonium* spp | 3 | Dermatitis |
| Geranium, California | *Senecio* spp | 3 | Hepatotoxic pyrrolizidine alkaloids |
| Ginkgo | *Ginkgo biloba* | 1, 3 | Dermatitis; chronic: increased bleeding time |
| Glory pea | *Sesbania* spp | 1 | Saponins, pyrrolizidine alkaloids |
| Goldenrod; rayless | *Haplopappus heterophyllus* | 1 | CNS depression in animals |
| Golden chain | *Labumum anagyroides* | 1 | Cytisine |
| Golden seal | *Hydrastis* spp | 1, 3 | GI upset; possible systemic toxicity |
| Gordoloba | *Achillea millefolium* | 3 | GI upset, dermatitis |
| Gotu kola | *Hydrocotyle asiatica* | 1, 3 | CNS depression, dermatitis |
| Groundsel | *Senecio* spp | 1 | Hepatotoxic pyrrolizidine alkaloids |
| Guaiac | *Guaiacum officinale* | 3 | GI upset |
| Harmaline | *Banisteriopsis* spp | 1 | Harmaline: hallucinogen (see p 247) |
| Harmel; Syrian rue | *Peganum harmala* | 1 | Harmaline: hallucinogen (see p 247) |
| Hawaiian woodrose | *Merremia tuberosa* | 1 | Hallucinogen |
| Hawaiian baby woodrose | *Argyreia nervosa* | 1 | Hallucinogen |
| Heart leaf philodendron | *Philodendron* spp | 2a | Calcium oxalate crystals |
| Heath | *Calluna vulggaris* | 1 | Grayanotoxin |
| Heliotrope | *Heliotropium* spp | 1 | Pyrrolizidine alkaloids: hepatotoxicity |
| Hells bells | *Datura stramonium* | 1 | Anticholinergic |
| Hemlock (poison hemlock) | *Conium maculatum* | 1 | Coniine: nicotinelike alkaloid (see p 278) |
| Hemlock (water hemlock) | *Cicuta maculata* | 1 | Cicutoxin: seizures |
| Henbane; black henbane | *Hyoscyamus* spp | 1 | Anticholinergic alkaloids (see p 85) |
| Holly (berry) | *Ilex aquifolium* | 3 | GI upset |
| Hops, European | *Humulus lupulus* | 3 | Dermatitis |
| Hops, wild | *Bryonia* spp | 3 | GI upset, dermatitis |
| Horse chestnut | *Aesculus* spp | 1, 3 | Aesculin |
| Hyacinth | *Hyacinthus* | 3 | GI upset, dermatitis |
| Hydrangea | *Hydrangea* spp | 1, 3 | Cyanogenic glycosides (see p 155) |
| Indian currant | *Symphoricarpos* spp | 3 | GI upset |
| Indian tobacco | *Lobelia* spp | 1 | Lobeline: nicotine-like alkaloid (see p 278) |
| Inkberry | *Ilex glabra* | 3 | GI upset |
| Inkberry (pokeweed) | *Phytolacca americana* | 3 | Saponin |
| Iris | *Iris* | 3 | GI upset, dermatitis |
| Ithang | *Miragyna* spp | 1 | Sedative and hallucinogen |
| I-thien-hung | *Emilia sonchifolia* | 1 | Pyrrolizidine alkaloids |
| Ivy | *Hedera* spp | 3 | GI upset, dermatitis |
| Ivy bush | *Kalmia* spp | 1 | Grayanotoxin |
| Jack-in-the-pulpit | *Arisaema* spp | 2a | Calcium oxalate crystals |
| Jaggery palm | *Caryota urens* | 2a | Calcium oxalate crystals |

(*continued*)

**TABLE II–46. PLANTS: ALPHABETICAL LIST (CONTINUED)**

| Common Name | Botanical Name | Toxic Group | Remarks (see text and Table II–45) |
|---|---|---|---|
| Jalap root | *Exogonium purga* | 3 | GI upset |
| Jasmine, Carolina | *Gelsemium sempervirens* | 1 | Gelsemium |
| Jequirity bean | *Abrus precatorius* | 1 | Toxalbumin (abrin): severe fatal gastroenteritis reported |
| Jerusalem cherry | *Solanum pseudocapsicum* | 1, 3 | Unripe berry contains solanine and anticholinergic alkaloids (see p 85) |
| Jessamine, Carolina or yellow | *Gelsemium sempervirens* | 1 | Gelsemium |
| Jessamine, day or night | *Cestrum* spp | 1, 3 | Solanine and anticholinergic alkaloids (see p 85) |
| Jessamine, poet's | *Jasminum officianale* | 3 | Dermatitis |
| Jimmyweed | *Haplopappus heterophyllus* | 1 | High alcohol tremetol: CNS depression |
| Jimsonweed | *Brugmansia arborea, Datura stramonium* | 1 | Anticholinergic alkaloids (see p 85) |
| Juniper | *Juniperus* spp | 1,3 | GI upset, dermatitis; chronic: renal toxicity |
| Kanna | *Sceletium tortuosum* | 1 | Mild hallucinogen |
| Kava-kava | *Piper methysticum* | 1 | Acute: sedation, ataxia. Chronic: dermatitis and hepatotoxicity |
| Kentucky coffee tree | *Gymaocladus dioica* | 1 | Cytisine: similar to nicotine (see p 278) |
| Khat; chat | *Catha edulis* | 1 | Mild hallucinogen and stimulant |
| Kratom | *Mitragynas* spp | 1 | Sedative and hallucinogen |
| Lady's slipper | *Cypripedium* spp | 3 | Dermatitis |
| Lady's slipper | *Pedilanthus tithymaloides* | 1 | Euphorbiaceae |
| Lantana | *Lantana camara* | 1 | Lantadene |
| Larkspur | *Delphinium* | 1 | Aconitum-like |
| Laurel | *Laurus nobilis* | 3 | Dermatitis, GI upset |
| Licorice root | *Glycyrrhiza lepidata* | 1, 3 | Hypokalemia after chronic use |
| Licorice, wild | *Abrus precatorius* | 1 | Toxalbumin |
| Lily of the Nile | *Agapanthus* | 3 | GI upset, dermatitis |
| Lily-of-the-valley | *Convallaria majalis* | 1 | Cardiac glycosides (see p 155) |
| Lily-of-the-valley bush | *Pieris japonica* | 1 | Grayanotoxin |
| Lion's ear | *Leonotis leonurus* | 1 | Mild hallucinogen |
| Lobelia | *Lobelia berlandieri* | 1 | Lobeline |
| Locoweed | *Astragalus* spp | 1 | Pyrrolizidine alkaloids |
| Locoweed | *Datura stramonium* | 1 | Anticholinergic alkaloids (see p 85) |
| Locoweed | *Cannabis sativa* | 1 | Mild hallucinogen (see p 247) |
| Lupine | *Lupinus* spp | 1 | Quinolizidine |
| Mandrake root | *Mandragora officinarum* | 1 | Anticholinergic alkaloids (see p 85) |
| Mandrake | *Podophyllum peltatum* | 1, 3 | Oil is keratolytic, irritant; hypotension, seizures reported after ingestion of resin |
| Marble queen | *Scindapsus aureus* | 2a | Calcium oxalate crystals |
| Marijuana | *Cannabis sativa* | 1 | Mild hallucinogen |
| Marsh marigold | *Caltha palustris* | 3 | Protoanemonin |
| Mate | *Ilex paraguayensis* | 1 | Caffeine |
| Mayapple | *Podophyllum peltatum* | 1, 3 | Oil is keratolytic, irritant; hypotension, seizures reported |
| Meadow crocus | *Colchicum autumnale* | 1 | Colchicine (see p 173) |
| Mescal bean | *Sophora secundiflora* | 1 | Cytisine: similar to nicotine (see p 278) |
| Mescal button | *Lophophora williamsii* | 1 | Mescaline: hallucinogen (see p 247) |

(*continued*)

**TABLE II–46. PLANTS: ALPHABETICAL LIST (CONTINUED)**

| Common Name | Botanical Name | Toxic Group | Remarks (see text and Table II–45) |
|---|---|---|---|
| Milkweed | *Asclepias* spp | 3 | Cardiac glycosides (see p 155), myocarditis and neuropathy in animals |
| Mistletoe, American | *Phoradendron flavescens* | 3 | GI upset |
| Mistletoe, European | *Viscum album* | 1, 3 | Hemoagglutination, seizures, GI upset |
| Mock azalea | *Menziesia ferruginea* | 1 | Cardiac glycosides (see p 155) |
| Monkshood | *Aconitum napellus* | 1 | Aconite: hypotension, AV block, arrhythmias; seizures |
| Moonflower | *Ipomoea alba* | 3 | Dermatitis |
| Moonflower | *Datura inoxia* | 1.3 | Anticholinergic alkaloids, dermatitis |
| Moonseed | *Menispermaceae* | 1 | Picrotoxin-like seizures |
| Moonseed, Carolina | *Cocculus carolinus* | 1 | Seizures possible |
| Mormon tea | *Ephedra viridis* | 1 | Ephedra: tachycardia, hypertension (see p 322) |
| Morning glory | *Ipomoea violacea* | 1 | Seeds are hallucinogenic |
| Mountain laurel | *Kalmia* spp | 1 | Grayanotoxin |
| Naked lady | *Amaryllis belladonna* | 3 | GI upset |
| Narcissus | *Narcissus* spp | 2a, 3 | GI upset, possibly calcium oxalates |
| Nectarine (chewed pits) | *Prunus* spp | 1 | Cyanogenic glycosides (see p 176) |
| Nephthytis | *Syngonium podophyllum* | 2a | Calcium oxalate crystals |
| Nightshade | *Solanum* spp | 1 | Solanine and anticholinergic alkaloids (see p 85) |
| Nightshade, black | *Solanum nigrum, Hyoscyamus* spp | 1 | Solanine; anticholinergic alkaloids (see p 85) |
| Nightshade, deadly | *Atropa belladonna* | 1 | Atropine (see p 415) |
| Nutmeg | *Myristica fragrans* | 1 | Hallucinogen (see p 247) |
| Oak | *Quercus* spp | 1 | Tannin |
| Oakleaf ivy | *Hedera helix* | 3 | GI upset, dermatitis |
| Oakleaf ivy | *Toxicodendron* spp | 3 | Urushiol oleoresin: contact dermatitis |
| Oleander | *Nerium oleander* | 1 | Cardiac glycosides (see p 155) |
| Oleander, yellow | *Thevetia peruviana* | 1 | Cardiac glycosides (see p 155); more toxic than *Nerium* |
| Olive | *Olea europaea* | 3 | Dermatitis |
| Ornamental cherry | *Prunus* spp | 1 | Cyanogenic glycosides (see p 176) |
| Ornamental pear | *Pyrus calleryana* | 3 | Dermatitis |
| Ornamental plum (chewed seeds) | *Prunus* spp | 1 | Cyanogenic glycosides (see p 176) |
| Ornamental pepper | *Capsicum annuum* | 3 | GI upset, dermatitis |
| Ornamental pepper | *Solanum pseudocapsicum* | 1 | Solanine |
| Palm (thorns or spines) | Various | 3 | Cellulitis, synovitis |
| Paper white narcissus | *Narcissus* spp | 2a, 3 | GI upset, may contain calcium oxalates |
| Paradise tree | *Melia azedarach* | 1, 3 | Chinaberry; severe GI upset; seizures |
| Paraguay tea | *Ilex paraguayensis* | 1 | Caffeine (see p 142) |
| Pasque flower | *Anemone* spp | 1 | Protoanemonin |
| Peach (chewed pits) | *Prunus* spp | 1 | Cyanogenic glycosides (see p 176) |
| Pear (chewed seeds) | *Pyrus* spp | 1 | Cyanogenic glycosides (see p 176) |
| Pecan | *Carya illinonensis* | 3 | Dermatitis |
| Pennyroyal (oil) | *Mentha pulegium* | 1 | Hepatotoxic, seizures, multi-system failure (see p 146) |
| Periwinkle | *Vinca* | 1 | Vinca alkaloids |
| Periwinkle, rose | *Catharanthus roseus* | 1 | Vinca alkaloids, possible hallucinogen |
| Peyote; mescal | *Lophophora williamsii* | 1 | Mescaline: hallucinogen (see p 247) |

(*continued*)

**TABLE II–46. PLANTS: ALPHABETICAL LIST (CONTINUED)**

| Common Name | Botanical Name | Toxic Group | Remarks (see text and Table II–45) |
|---|---|---|---|
| Pheasant's-eye | *Adonis* spp | 1 | Cardiac glycosides (see p 155) |
| Photinia | *Photinia arbutifolia* | 1 | Cyanogenic glycosides |
| Pigeonberry | *Duranta repens* | 3 | Saponins |
| Pigeonberry | *Cornus canadensis* | 3 | Dermatitis |
| Pigeonberry | *Rivina humilis* | 3 | GI upset |
| Pigeonberry | *Phytolacca americana* | 3 | Saponin |
| Pinks | *Dianthus caryophyllus* | 3 | GI upset, dermatitis |
| Plum (chewed pits) | *Prunus* spp | 1 | Cyanogenic glycosides (see p 176) |
| Poinsettia | *Euphorbia* spp | 3 | Possible GI upset |
| Poison ivy; poison oak; poison sumac; poison vine | *Toxicodendron* spp | 3 | Urushiol oleoresin contact dermatitis (*Rhus* dermatitis) |
| Pokeweed (unripe berries) | *Phytolacca americana* | 3 | Saponin |
| Poplar | *Populus* spp | 3 | Dermatitis |
| Poppy, common | *Papaver somniferum* | 1 | Opiates (see p 288) |
| Potato (unripe, leaves) | *Solanum* spp | 1, 3 | Solanine and anticholinergic alkaloids (see p 85) |
| Pothos | *Scindapsus aureus* | 2a | Calcium oxalate crystals |
| Pothos | *Epipremnum aureum* | 2a | Calcium oxalate crystals |
| Prayer bean | *Arbus prectorius* | 1 | Toxalbumin |
| Prickly pear (thorn) | *Opuntia* spp | 3 | Dermatitis, cellulitis |
| Prickly poppy | *Argemone mexicana* | 1 | Sanguinaria. Narcotic-analgesic, smoked as euphoriant |
| Pride of China, Pride of India | *Melia azedarach* | 1 | Chinaberry: severe GI upset, seizures |
| Pride-of-Madeira | *Echium* spp | 1 | Pyrrolizidine alkaloids: hepatotoxicity |
| Primrose | *Primula vulgaris* | 3 | Dermatitis |
| Privet; common privet | *Ligustrum* spp | 3 | GI upset |
| Purge nut | *Jatropha curcas* | 1 | Toxalbumin, Euphorbiaceae |
| Purslane, milk | *Euphorbia* spp | 3 | Dermatitis |
| Pussy willow | *Salix caprea* | 3 | Dermatitis |
| Pyracantha | *Pyracantha* | 3 | GI upset, thorn stab wounds can cause cellulitis |
| Queen Anne's Lace | *Daucus carota* | 3 | Dermatitis |
| Ragweed | *Ambrosia artemisiifolia* | 3 | Dermatitis |
| Ragwort, tansy | *Senecio* spp | 1 | Hepatotoxic pyrrolizidine alkaloids |
| Ranunculus | *Ranunculus* spp | 1 | Protoanemonin |
| Rattlebox | *Crotalaria* spp | 1 | Hepatotoxic pyrrolizidine alkaloids |
| Rattlebox, purple | *Daubentonia* spp | 3 | Hepatotoxic pyrrolizidine alkaloids |
| Rattlebush | *Baptista tinctoria* | 1 | Cytisine |
| Redwood tree | *Sequoia sempervirens* | 3 | Dermatitis |
| Rhododendron | *Rhododendron genus* | 1 | Grayanotoxin |
| Rhubarb (leaves) | *Rheum rhaponticum* | 2b | Soluble oxalates |
| Rosary pea; rosary bean | *Abrus precatorius* | 1 | Toxalbumin (abrin): severe fatal gastroenteritis reported |
| Rose (thorn) | *Rosa* spp | 3 | Cellulitis |
| Rose periwinkle | *Catharanthus roseus* | 1 | Vincristine, vinblastine (see p 100) |
| Rue | *Ruta graveolens* | 3 | Dermatitis |
| Rustyleaf | *Menziesia ferruginea* | 1 | Grayanotoxins |
| Sagebrush | *Artemsia* spp | 1, 3 | GI upset; CNS stimulant |
| Salvia | *Salvia divinorum* | 1 | Mild hallucinogen |
| Sassafras | *Sassafras* spp | 1 | Abortifacient, narcotic |
| Scotch broom | *Cytisus scoparius* | 1, 3 | Cytisine; GI upset |

(*continued*)

**TABLE II–46. PLANTS: ALPHABETICAL LIST (CONTINUED)**

| Common Name | Botanical Name | Toxic Group | Remarks (see text and Table II–45) |
|---|---|---|---|
| Shamrock | *Oxalis* spp | 2b | Soluble oxalates |
| Skunk cabbage | *Symplocarpus foetidus* | 2a | Calcium oxalate crystals |
| Skunk cabbage | *Veratrum* spp | 1, 3 | Veratrum alkaloids |
| Sky-flower | *Duranta repens* | 3 | Saponins |
| Snakeroot | *Eupatorium rugosum* | 1 | Hepatotoxic pyrrolizidine alkaloids |
| Snakeroot | *Cicuta maculata* | 1 | Water hemlock: seizures |
| Snakeroot | *Aristolochia serpentina* | 1 | Acute: cardiac effect; Chronic: nephropathy |
| Snowberry | *Symphoricarpos* spp | 3 | GI upset |
| Sorrel | *Oxalis* spp, *Rhumex* spp | 2b | Soluble oxalate |
| Soursob | *Oxalis* spp | 2b | Soluble oxalates |
| Spathiphyllum | *Spathiphyllum* | 2a | Calcium oxalate crystals |
| Spindle tree | *Euonymous* spp | 3 | GI upset |
| Split leaf philodendron | *Philodendron* spp | 2a | Calcium oxalate crystals |
| Squill | *Scilla; Urginea maritima* | 1 | Cardiac glycosides (see p 155) |
| Star-of-Bethlehem | *Ornithogalum* spp | 1 | Cardiac glycosides (see p 155) |
| Star-of-Bethlehem | *Hippobroma longiflora* | 1 | Lobeline |
| St. John's wort | *Hypericum perforatum* | 1 | Mild GI upset, dermatitis; mild serotonin enhancer (see p 215) |
| String of pearls/beads | *Senecio* spp | 1 | Hepatotoxic pyrrolizidine alkaloids |
| Strychnine | *Strychnos nux-vomica* | 1 | Strychnine: seizures (see p 350) |
| Sweet clover | *Melilotus* spp | 1 | Coumarin glycosides (see p 155) |
| Sweet pea | *Lathyrus odoratus* | 1 | Neuropathy (lathyrism) after chronic use |
| Sweet William | *Dianthus barbatus* | 3 | GI upset, dermatitis |
| Swiss cheese plant | *Monstera friedrichsthali* | 2a | Calcium oxalate crystals |
| Tansy | *Tanacetum* spp | 3 | Dermatitis |
| Taro | *Alocasia macrorrhia* | 2a | Calcium oxalate crystals |
| Taro | *Colocasia esculenta* | 2a | Calcium oxalate crystals |
| Texas umbrella tree | *Melia azedarach* | 1 | Chinaberry: severe GI upset; seizures |
| Thornapple | *Datura stramonium and inoxia* | 1 | Anticholinergic (see p 85) |
| Thornapple | *Argemone mexicana* | 1 | Sanguinaria, cardiomyopathy, edema |
| Tobacco | *Nicotiana* spp | 1 | Nicotine (see p 278) |
| Tobacco, wild | *Lobelia inflata* | 1 | Lobeline |
| Tomato (leaves) | *Lycopersicon esculentum* | 1 | Solanine |
| Tonka bean | *Dipteryx odorata* | 1 | Coumarin glycosides (see p 379) |
| Toyon (leaves) | *Heteromeles arbutifolia, Photinia arbutifolia* | 1 | Cyanogenic glycosides (see p 176) |
| Tulip (bulb) | *Tulipa* | 3 | Dermatitis |
| Tung nut, tung tree; candle nut | *Aleurites* spp | 1, 3 | Euphorbiaceae |
| T'u-san-chi | *Gynura segetum* | 1 | Hepatotoxic pyrrolizidine alkaloids |
| Umbrella plant | *Cyperus alternifolius* | 1 | Acute: gastrointestinal. Chronic: renal toxicity, seizures |
| Uva-ursi | *Arctostaphylos uvo-ursi* | 1, 3 | Hydroquinone: berries edible |
| Valerian | *Valeriana officinalis* | 1 | Valerine alkaloids: used as mild tranquilizer |
| Verbena | *Verbena officinalis and hastata* | 3 | Dermatitis |
| Virginia creeper | *Parthenocissus* spp | 2b | Soluble oxalates |
| Walnut (green shells) | *Juglans* | 3 | Dermatitis |
| Water hemlock | *Cicuta maculata* | 1 | Cicutoxin: seizures |
| Weeping fig (sap) | *Ficus benjamina* | 3 | Dermatitis |

(*continued*)

**TABLE II–46. PLANTS: ALPHABETICAL LIST (CONTINUED)**

| Common Name | Botanical Name | Toxic Group | Remarks (see text and Table II–45) |
|---|---|---|---|
| Weeping pagoda tree | *Saphora japonica* | 1 | Cytisine |
| Weeping tea tree | *Melaleuca leucadendron* | 3 | Dermatitis |
| Weeping willow | *Salix babylonica* | 3 | Dermatitis |
| White cedar | *Melia azedarach* | 1 | Chinaberry: severe GI upset; seizures |
| White cedar | *Hura crepitans* | 3 | GI upset, dermatitis |
| White cedar | *Thuja occidentalis* | 1 | Abortifacient, stimulant |
| Wild calla | *Calla palustris* | 2a | Calcium oxalates |
| Wild carrot | *Daucus carota* | 3 | Dermatitis |
| Wild carrot | *Cicuta maculata* | 1 | Cicutoxin, seizures |
| Wild cassada | *Jatropha gossypifolia* | 1 | Euphorbiaceae |
| Wild cherry | *Prunus* spp | 1 | Cyanogenic glycosides (chewed seeds) |
| Wild coffee | *Polyscias guilfoyei* | 3 | Saponin |
| Wild cotton | *Asclepias syriaca* | 1 | Cardiac glycosides (see p 155) |
| Wild dagga | *Leonotis leonurus* | 1 | Mild hallucinogen |
| Wild fennel | *Nigella damascena* | 3 | Irritant, possible protoanemonin |
| Wild garlic | *Allium canadense* | 3 | GI upset, dermatitis |
| Wild hops | *Bryonia* spp | 3 | GI upset, dermatitis |
| Wild iris | *Iris versicolor* | 3 | GI upset, dermatitis |
| Wild lemon | *Podophyllum pelatum* | 1, 3 | Oil is keratolytic, irritant; CNS depressant |
| Wild marjoram | *Origanum vulgare* | 3 | GI upset |
| Wild oats | *Arena fatua* | 3 | GI upset |
| Wild onion | *Allium* spp | 3 | GI upset |
| Wild onion | *Zigadenus* spp | 3 | GI upset, dermatitis |
| Wild passion flower | *Passiflora incarnata* | 1, 3 | CNS depressant, dermatitis |
| Wild parsnip | *Pastinaca sativa* | 3 | Dermatitis |
| Wild parsnip | *Cicuta maculata* | 1 | Cicutoxin, seizures |
| Wild parsnip | *Heracleum mantegazzianum* | 3 | Dermatitis |
| Wild parsnip | *Angelica archangelica* | 3 | Dermatitis |
| Wild pepper | *Daphne mezereum* | 3 | Dermatitis |
| Wild rock rose | *Cistus incanus* | 3 | Dermatitis |
| Windflower | *Anemone* | 1, 3 | Protoanemonin, dermatitis |
| Wisteria | *Wisteria* | 3 | GI upset |
| Woodbind | *Parthenocissus* spp | 2b | Soluble oxalates |
| Wood rose | *Ipomoea violacea; Merremia tuberosa* | 1 | Seeds are hallucinogenic |
| Wormwood | *Artemesia absinthium* | 1 | Absinthe: possible CNS effects, porphyria with chronic use |
| Yarrow | *Achillea millefolium* | 3 | GI upset, dermatitis |
| Yellow oleander | *Thevetia peruviana* | 1 | Cardiac glycosides (see p 155) |
| Yerba buena | *Poliomintha incana* | 1 | Hepatotoxic, seizures, multisystem failure |
| Yerba lechera | *Euphorbia* spp | 1 | Euphorbiaceae |
| Yerba mala | *Euphorbia* spp | 1 | Euphorbiaceae |
| Yerba mate | *Ilex paraguariensis* | 1 | Caffeine |
| Yew | *Taxus* spp | 1 | Taxine; similar to cardiac glycosides (see p 155); seizures |
| Yew, Japanese | *Podocarpus macrophylla* | 3 | Dermatitis |
| Yohimbine | *Corynanthe yohimbe* | 1 | Purported aphrodisiac; mild hallucinogen; alpha-2-blocker |

A. **Group 1** plants contain systemically active poisons that may cause serious poisoning.
B. **Group 2a** plants contain insoluble calcium oxalate crystals that may cause burning pain and swelling of mucous membranes. Many houseplants are found in this category.
C. **Group 2b** plants contain soluble oxalate salts (sodium or potassium) that can produce acute hypocalcemia, renal injury, and other organ damage secondary to precipitation of calcium oxalate crystals in various organs (see p 296). Mucous membrane irritation is rare, allowing patients to ingest sufficient quantities to cause systemic toxicity. Gastroenteritis also may occur.
D. **Group 3** plants contain various toxins that generally produce mild to moderate GI irritation after ingestion or dermatitis after skin contact.

II. **Toxic dose.** The amount of toxin ingested is usually unknown. Concentrations of the toxic agent may vary depending on the plant part, the season, and soil conditions. In general, childhood ingestions of a single leaf or a few petals, even of group 1 plants, results in little or no toxicity because of the small amount of toxin absorbed. Steeping the plant in hot water (eg, an "herbal" tea) may allow very large amounts of toxin to be absorbed.

III. **Clinical presentation** depends on the active toxic agent (see Table II–45), although even nontoxic plants can cause coughing, choking, and gagging if a large piece is swallowed.

A. **Group 1.** In most cases, vomiting, abdominal pain, and diarrhea occur within 60–90 minutes of a significant ingestion, but systemic symptoms may be delayed a few hours while toxins are activated in the gut (eg, cyanogenic glycosides) or distributed to tissues (eg, cardiac glycosides). With some toxins, (eg, ricin), severe gastroenteritis may result in massive fluid and electrolyte loss and GI sloughing.
B. **Group 2a.** Insoluble calcium oxalate crystals cause immediate oral burning, pain, and stinging upon contact with mucous membranes. Swelling of the lips, tongue, and pharynx may occur. In rare cases, glottic edema may result in airway obstruction. Symptoms usually resolve within a few hours.
C. **Group 2b.** Soluble oxalates may be absorbed into the circulation, where they precipitate with calcium. Acute hypocalcemia and multiple-organ injury, including renal tubular necrosis, may result (see Oxalates, p 296).
D. **Group 3.** Skin or mucous membrane irritation may occur, although it is less severe than with group 2 plants. Vomiting and diarrhea are common but are usually mild to moderate and are self-limited. Fluid and electrolyte imbalances caused by severe gastroenteritis are rare.

IV. **Diagnosis** usually is based on a history of exposure and the presence of plant material in vomitus. Identification of the plant is often difficult. Because common names sometimes refer to more than one plant, it is preferable to confirm the botanical name. If in doubt about the plant identification, take a cutting of the plant (not just a leaf or a berry) to a local nursery, florist, or college botany department.

A. **Specific levels.** Serum toxin levels are not available for most plant toxins. In selected cases, laboratory analyses for therapeutic drugs may be used (eg, digoxin assay for oleander glycosides, cyanide level for cyanogenic glycosides).
B. **Other useful laboratory studies** for patients with gastroenteritis include CBC, electrolytes, glucose, BUN, creatinine, and urinalysis. If hepatotoxicity is suspected, obtain liver transaminases and prothrombin time (PT/INR).

V. **Treatment.** Most ingestions cause no symptoms or only mild gastroenteritis. Patients recover quickly with supportive care.

A. **Emergency and supportive measures**
1. Maintain an open airway and assist ventilation if necessary (see pp 1–7). Administer supplemental oxygen.
2. Treat coma (see p 18), seizures (p 22), arrhythmias (pp 10–15), and hypotension (p 15) if they occur.

3. Replace fluid losses caused by gastroenteritis with intravenous crystalloid solutions.

B. **Specific drugs and antidotes.** There are few effective antidotes. Refer to discussions elsewhere in Section II for further details.

C. **Decontamination** (see page 45)

1. **Group 1 and group 2b plants.** Administer activated charcoal orally if conditions are appropriate (see Table I–38, p 51). Gastric lavage is not necessary after small to moderate ingestions if activated charcoal can be given promptly.

2. **Group 2a and group 3 plants**

a. Wash the affected areas with soap and water and give sips of water to drink.

b. Administer ice cream, juice bars, pudding, or cold milk to soothe irritated oral mucous membranes after exposure to insoluble oxalate plants.

c. Do ***not*** induce vomiting because of potential aggravation or irritant effects. Activated charcoal is not necessary.

D. **Enhanced elimination.** These procedures are generally not effective.

## ▶ POLYCHLORINATED BIPHENYLS (PCBs)

*Robert L. Goldberg, MD*

Polychlorinated biphenyls (PCBs) are a group of chlorinated hydrocarbon compounds that once were used widely as high-temperature insulators for transformers and other electrical equipment and were also found in carbonless copy papers and some inks and paints. Since 1974, all uses in the United States have been confined to closed systems. Most PCB poisonings are chronic occupational exposures, with delayed-onset symptoms being the first indication that an exposure has occurred. In 1977, the US Environmental Protection Agency (EPA) banned further manufacturing of PCBs because they are suspected carcinogens and are highly persistent in the environment. The primary exposures occur from leaking transformers and other electrical equipment, hazardous waste sites, and environmental exposure from ingestion of contaminated water, fish, or wildlife.

I. **Mechanism of toxicity.** PCBs are irritating to mucous membranes. When burned, PCBs may produce the more highly toxic polychlorinated dibenzodioxins (PCDDs) and polychlorinated dibenzofurans (PCDFs; see p 183). It is difficult to establish the specific effects of PCB intoxication because PCBs are nearly always contaminated with small amounts of these compounds. PCBs, and particularly the PCDD and PCDF contaminants, are mutagenic and teratogenic and are considered probable human carcinogens.

II. **Toxic dose.** PCBs are well absorbed by all routes (skin, inhalation, and ingestion) and are widely distributed in fat; bioaccumulation occurs even with low-level exposure.

A. **Inhalation.** PCBs are mildly irritating to the skin at airborne levels of 0.1 $mg/m^3$ and very irritating at 10 $mg/m^3$. The recommended workplace limits (ACGIH TLV-TWA) are 0.5 $mg/m^3$ (for PCBs with 54% chlorine) and 1 $mg/m^3$ (for PCBs with 42% chlorine) as 8-hour time-weighted averages. The air level considered immediately dangerous to life or health (IDLH) for either type is 5 $mg/m^3$.

B. **Ingestion.** Acute toxicity after ingestion is unlikely; the oral LD50 is 1–10 g/kg.

III. **Clinical presentation**

A. **Acute PCB exposure** may cause skin, eye, nose, and throat irritation.

B. **Chronic exposure** may cause **chloracne** (cystic acneiform lesions predominantly found on the posterior neck, axillae, and upper back); the onset usually occurs 6 weeks or longer after exposure. Skin pigmentation and porphyria may occur. Elevation of hepatic transaminases may occur.

**C.** Epidemiologic studies suggest that PCB exposure can be associated with neurobehavioral effects in newborns and children. Other effects include decreased birth weight and immune system effects in babies as a result of transplacental transmission or breast-feeding by mothers exposed to elevated levels of PCBs. There is evidence that PCBs cause adverse estrogen activity in male neonates.

**IV. Diagnosis** usually is based on a history of exposure and the presence of chloracne or elevated hepatic transaminases.

**A. Specific levels.** PCB serum and fat levels are poorly correlated with health effects. Serum PCB concentrations are usually less than 20 mcg/L; higher levels may indicate exposure but not necessarily toxicity.

**B. Other useful laboratory studies** include BUN, creatinine, and liver enzymes.

**V. Treatment**

**A. Emergency and supportive measures**

1. Treat bronchospasm (see p 7) if it occurs.
2. Monitor for elevated hepatic enzymes, chloracne, and nonspecific eye, GI, and neurologic symptoms.

**B. Specific drugs and antidotes.** There is no specific antidote.

**C. Decontamination** (see p 45)

1. **Inhalation.** Remove the victim from exposure and give supplemental oxygen if available.
2. **Skin and eyes.** Remove contaminated clothing and wash exposed skin with soap and water. Irrigate exposed eyes with copious tepid water or saline.
3. **Ingestion.** Administer activated charcoal orally if conditions are appropriate (see Table I–38, p 51). Gastric lavage is not necessary after small to moderate ingestions if activated charcoal can be given promptly.

**D. Enhanced elimination.** There is no role for dialysis, hemoperfusion, or repeat-dose charcoal. Lipid-clearing drugs (eg, clofibrate and resins) have been suggested, but insufficient data exist to recommend them.

## ▶ PSEUDOEPHEDRINE, PHENYLEPHRINE, AND OTHER DECONGESTANTS

*Neal L. Benowitz, MD*

Pseudoephedrine and phenylephrine are sympathomimetic drugs that are widely available in nonprescription nasal decongestants and cold preparations. These remedies usually also contain antihistamines and cough suppressants. Nonprescription ephedrine-containing cough and cold preparations as well as ephedrine-containing dietary supplements were widely consumed until 2004, when their use was banned by the FDA because of the unacceptable risk of toxicity. **Ephedrine** and ephedra-containing herbal preparations (eg, *Ma huang* and "Herbal Ecstasy"), often in combination with caffeine, were also used as alternatives to the amphetamine derivative Ecstasy (see p 73) or as adjuncts to body-building or weight-loss programs. **Phenylpropanolamine** (PPA) had been marketed as a nonprescription decongestant and appetite suppressant for many years but was removed from the US market in 2000 because of an association with hemorrhagic stroke in women.

**I. Mechanism of toxicity.** All these agents stimulate the adrenergic system, with variable effects on alpha- and beta-adrenergic receptors, depending on the compound. Generally, these agents stimulate the CNS much less than do other phenylethylamines (see amphetamines, p 73).

**A. PPA and phenylephrine** are direct alpha-adrenergic agonists. In addition, PPA produces mild beta-1 adrenergic stimulation and acts in part indirectly by enhancing norepinephrine release.

**B. Ephedrine and pseudoephedrine** have both direct and indirect alpha- and beta-adrenergic activity but clinically produce more beta-adrenergic stimulation than does PPA or phenylephrine.

**TABLE II–47. EPHEDRINE AND OTHER OTC DECONGESTANTS**

| Drug | Major Effects[a] | Usual Daily Adult Dose (mg) | Usual Daily Pediatric Dose (mg/kg) |
|---|---|---|---|
| Ephedrine | Beta, alpha | 100–200 | 2–3 |
| Phenylephrine | Alpha | 40–60 | 0.5–1 |
| Phenylpropanolamine[b] | Alpha | 100–150 | 1–2 |
| Pseudoephedrine | Beta, alpha | 180–360 | 3–5 |

[a]Alpha = alpha-adrenergic receptor agonist; beta = beta-adrenergic receptor agonist.
[b]Removed from US market.

**C. Pharmacokinetics.** Peak effects occur within 1–3 hours, although absorption may be delayed with sustained-release products. These drugs have large volumes of distribution (eg, the Vd for PPA is 2.5–5 L/kg). Elimination half-lives are 3–7 hours. See also Table II–59, p 382.

**II. Toxic dose.** Table II–47 lists the usual therapeutic doses of each agent. Patients with autonomic insufficiency and those taking MAO inhibitors (see p 269) may be extraordinarily sensitive to these and other sympathomimetic drugs, developing severe hypertension after ingestion of even subtherapeutic doses.

**A.** PPA, phenylephrine, and ephedrine have low toxic:therapeutic ratios. Toxicity often occurs after ingestion of just 2–3 times the therapeutic dose. Strokes and cardiac toxicity have been reported after therapeutic doses of ephedra and PPA.

**B.** Pseudoephedrine is less toxic, with symptoms occurring after four- to fivefold the usual therapeutic dose.

**III. Clinical presentation.** The time course of intoxication by these drugs is usually brief, with resolution within 4–6 hours (unless sustained-release preparations are involved). The major toxic effect of these drugs is **hypertension,** which may lead to headache, confusion, seizures, and intracranial hemorrhage.

**A. Intracranial hemorrhage** may occur in normal, healthy young persons after what might appear to be only modest elevation of blood pressure (ie, 170/110 mm Hg) and is often associated with focal neurologic deficits, coma, or seizures.

**B. Bradycardia or atrioventricular block** is common in patients with moderate to severe hypertension associated with PPA and phenylephrine owing to the baroreceptor reflex response to hypertension. The presence of drugs such as antihistamines and caffeine prevents reflex bradycardia and may enhance the hypertensive effects of PPA and phenylephrine.

**C. Myocardial infarction** and diffuse myocardial necrosis have been associated with ephedra use and PPA intoxication.

**IV. Diagnosis** usually is based on a history of ingestion of diet pills or decongestant medications and the presence of hypertension. Bradycardia or AV block suggests PPA or phenylephrine. Severe headache, focal neurologic deficits, or coma should raise the possibility of intracerebral hemorrhage.

**A. Specific levels.** Serum drug levels are not generally available and do not alter treatment. In high doses, these agents may produce positive results for amphetamines on urine testing (see Table I–33, p 43) but can be distinguished on confirmatory testing.

**B. Other useful laboratory studies** include electrolytes, glucose, BUN, creatinine, CPK with MB isoenzymes, 12-lead ECG and ECG monitoring, and CT head scan if intracranial hemorrhage is suspected.

**V. Treatment**

**A. Emergency and supportive measures**

1. Maintain an open airway and assist ventilation if necessary (see pp 1–7). Administer supplemental oxygen.

2. Treat hypertension aggressively (see p 17 and **B**, below). Treat seizures (p 22) and ventricular tachyarrhythmias (p 12) if they occur. Do ***not*** treat reflex bradycardia except indirectly by lowering blood pressure.
3. Monitor the vital signs and ECG for a minimum of 4–6 hours after exposure and longer if a sustained-release preparation has been ingested.

**B. Specific drugs and antidotes**

1. **Hypertension.** Treat hypertension if the diastolic pressure is higher than 100–105 mm Hg, especially in a patient with no prior history of hypertension. If there is CT or obvious clinical evidence of intracranial hemorrhage, lower the diastolic pressure cautiously to no lower than 90 mm Hg and consult a neurosurgeon immediately.
   a. Use a vasodilator such as **phentolamine** (see p 495) or **nitroprusside** (p 485).
   b. ***Caution:*** Do not use beta blockers to treat hypertension without first giving a vasodilator; otherwise, paradoxic worsening of the hypertension may result.
   c. Many patients have moderate orthostatic variation in blood pressure; therefore, for immediate partial relief of severe hypertension, try placing the patient in an upright position.
2. **Arrhythmias**
   a. Tachyarrhythmias usually respond to low-dose **esmolol** (see p 449) or **metoprolol.**
   b. Caution: Do ***not*** treat AV block or sinus bradycardia associated with hypertension; increasing the heart rate with atropine may abolish this reflex response that serves to limit hypertension, resulting in worsening elevation of the blood pressure.

**C. Decontamination** (see p 45). Administer activated charcoal orally if conditions are appropriate (see Table I–38, p 51). Gastric lavage is not necessary after small to moderate ingestions if activated charcoal can be given promptly.

**D. Enhanced elimination.** Dialysis and hemoperfusion are not effective. Urinary acidification may enhance elimination of PPA, ephedrine, and pseudoephedrine but may also aggravate myoglobin deposition in the kidney if the patient has rhabdomyolysis.

## ▶ PYRETHRINS AND PYRETHROIDS

*John P. Lamb, PharmD*

Pyrethrins are naturally occurring insecticides derived from the chrysanthemum plant. Pyrethroids (Table II–48) are synthetically derived compounds. Acute human poisoning from exposure to these insecticides is rare; however, they can cause skin and upper-airway irritation and hypersensitivity reactions. Piperonyl butoxide is added to these compounds to prolong their activity by inhibiting mixed oxidase enzymes in the liver that metabolize the pyrethrins. Common pyrethrin-containing pediculicides include A-200, Triple-X, and RID.

**I. Mechanism of toxicity.** In insects, pyrethrins and pyrethroids rapidly cause death by paralyzing the nervous system through disruption of the membrane ion

**TABLE II–48. PYRETHROIDS**

| | | |
|---|---|---|
| Allethrin | Cypermethrin | Furamethrin |
| Barthrin | Decamethrin | Permethrin |
| Bioallethrin | Deltamethrin | Phenothrin |
| Bioresmethrin | Dimethrin | Phthalthrin |
| Cismethrin | Fenothrin | Resmethrin |
| Cyhalothrin | Fenvalerate | Supermethrin |
| Cymethrin | | Tetramethrin |

transport system in nerve axons, and pyrethroids prolong sodium influx and also may block inhibitory pathways. Mammals are generally able to metabolize these compounds rapidly and thereby render them harmless.

**II. Toxic dose.** The toxic oral dose in mammals is greater than 100–1000 mg/kg, and the potentially lethal acute oral dose is 10–100 g. Pyrethrins are not well absorbed across the skin or from the GI tract. They have been used for many years as oral anthelminthic agents with minimum adverse effects other than mild GI upset.

- **A. Deltamethrin.** There is one report of seizures in a young woman who ingested 30 mL of 2.5% deltamethrin (750 mg). **Miraculous Insecticide Chalk™** (from China) contains up to 37.6 mg of deltamethrin per stick of chalk. Ingestion of a single chalk is generally considered nontoxic.
- **B. Cypermethrin.** A 45-year-old man died after ingesting beans cooked in 10% cypermethrin.

**III. Clinical presentation.** Toxicity to humans is associated primarily with hypersensitivity reactions and direct irritant effects rather than with any pharmacologic property.

- **A. Anaphylactic** reactions including bronchospasm, oropharyngeal edema, and shock may occur in hypersensitive individuals.
- **B. Inhalation** of these compounds may precipitate wheezing in asthmatics. An 11-year-old girl had a fatal asthma attack after applying a pyrethrin-containing shampoo to her dog. Inhalation or pulmonary aspiration may also cause a hypersensitivity pneumonitis.
- **C. Skin** exposure may cause burning, tingling, numbness, and erythema. The paresthesias are believed to result from a direct effect on cutaneous nerve endings.
- **D. Eyes.** Accidental eye exposure during scalp application of A-200 Pyrinate has caused corneal injury including keratitis and denudation. The cause is uncertain but may be related to the surfactant (Triton-X) contained in the product.
- **E. Ingestion.** With large ingestions (200–500 mL of concentrated solution), the CNS may be affected, resulting in seizures, coma, or respiratory arrest.

**IV. Diagnosis** is based on a history of exposure. No characteristic clinical symptoms or laboratory tests are specific for identifying these compounds.

- **A. Specific levels.** These compounds are metabolized rapidly in the body, and methods for determining the parent compound are not routinely available.
- **B. Other useful laboratory studies** include electrolytes, glucose, and arterial blood gases or oximetry.

**V. Treatment**

- **A. Emergency and supportive measures**
  1. Treat bronchospasm (see p 7) and anaphylaxis (p 27) if they occur.
  2. Observe patients with a history of large ingestions for at least 4–6 hours for any signs of CNS depression or seizures.
- **B. Specific drugs and antidotes.** There is no specific antidote.
- **C. Decontamination** (see p 45)
  1. **Inhalation.** Remove victims from exposure and give supplemental oxygen if needed.
  2. **Skin.** Wash with copious soap and water. Topical application of vitamin E in vegetable oil was reported anecdotally to relieve paresthesias.
  3. **Eyes.** Irrigate with copious water. After irrigation, perform a fluorescein examination and refer the victim to an ophthalmologist if there is evidence of corneal injury.
  4. **Ingestion.** In the majority of cases, a subtoxic dose has been ingested and no decontamination is necessary. However, after a large ingestion of Chinese chalk or a concentrated solution, administer activated charcoal orally if conditions are appropriate (see Table I–38, p 51). Gastric lavage is not necessary after small to moderate ingestions if activated charcoal can be given promptly.
- **D. Enhanced elimination.** These compounds are metabolized rapidly by the body, and extracorporeal methods of elimination would not be expected to enhance their elimination.

## ▶ QUINIDINE AND OTHER TYPE IA ANTIARRHYTHMIC DRUGS

*Neal L. Benowitz, MD*

Quinidine, procainamide (Pronestyl™), and disopyramide (Norpace™) are type Ia antiarrhythmic agents. Quinidine and procainamide are used commonly for suppression of supraventricular and ventricular arrhythmias. Disopyramide is used for ventricular arrhythmias. All three agents have a low toxic:therapeutic ratio and may produce fatal intoxication (Table II–49). See the description of other antiarrhythmic agents on p 79.

**I. Mechanism of toxicity**

**A.** Type Ia agents depress the fast sodium-dependent channel, slowing phase zero of the cardiac action potential. At high concentrations, this results in reduced myocardial contractility and excitability and severe depression of cardiac conduction velocity. Repolarization is also delayed, resulting in a prolonged QT interval that may be associated with polymorphic ventricular tachycardia (torsade de pointes).

**B.** Quinidine and disopyramide also have anticholinergic activity; quinidine has alpha-adrenergic receptor-blocking activity, and procainamide has ganglionic- and neuromuscular-blocking activity.

**C. Pharmacokinetics.** See Table II–59, p 382.

**II. Toxic dose.** Acute adult ingestion of 1 g of quinidine, 5 g of procainamide, or 1 g of disopyramide and any ingestion in children should be considered potentially lethal.

**III. Clinical presentation.** The primary manifestations of toxicity involve the cardiovascular and central nervous systems.

**A. Cardiotoxic effects** of the type Ia agents include sinus bradycardia; sinus node arrest or asystole; PR, QRS, or QT interval prolongation; sinus tachycardia (caused by anticholinergic effects); polymorphous ventricular tachycardia (torsade de pointes); and depressed myocardial contractility, which, along with alpha-adrenergic or ganglionic blockade, may result in hypotension and occasionally pulmonary edema.

**B. Central nervous system toxicity.** Quinidine and disopyramide can cause anticholinergic effects such as dry mouth, dilated pupils, and delirium. All type Ia agents can produce seizures, coma, and respiratory arrest.

**C. Other effects.** Quinidine commonly causes nausea, vomiting, and diarrhea after acute ingestion and, especially with chronic doses, cinchonism (tinnitus, vertigo, deafness, and visual disturbances). Procainamide may cause GI upset and, with chronic therapy, a lupus-like syndrome.

**IV. Diagnosis** is based on a history of exposure and typical cardiotoxic features such as QRS and QT interval prolongation, AV block, and polymorphous ventricular tachycardia.

**TABLE II-49. QUINIDINE AND TYPE IA ANTIARRHYTHMIC DRUGS**

| Drug | Serum Half-Life (h) | Usual Adult Daily Dose (mg) | Therapeutic Serum Levels (mg/L) | Major Toxicity[a] |
|---|---|---|---|---|
| Quinidine | 6–8 | 1000–2000 | 2–4 | S, B, V, H |
| Disopyramide | 4–10 | 400–800 | 2–4 | B, V, H |
| Procainamide | 4 | 1000–4000 | 4–10 | B, V, H |
| NAPA[b] | 5–7 | N/A | 15–25 | H |

[a]S = seizures; B = bradycardia; V = ventricular tachycardia; H = hypotension.
[b]NAPA = *N*-acetylprocainamide, an active metabolite of procainamide.

A. **Specific levels.** Serum levels for each agent are generally available. Serious toxicity with these drugs usually occurs only with levels above the therapeutic range; however, some complications, such as QT prolongation and polymorphous ventricular tachycardia, may occur at therapeutic levels.
   1. Methods for detecting quinidine may vary in specificity, with some also measuring metabolites and contaminants.
   2. Procainamide has an active metabolite, *N*-acetylprocainamide (NAPA); with therapeutic procainamide dosing, NAPA levels can range from 15 to 25 mg/L.

B. **Other useful laboratory studies** include electrolytes, glucose, BUN, creatinine, arterial blood gases or oximetry, and ECG monitoring.

V. **Treatment**

A. **Emergency and supportive measures**
   1. Maintain an open airway and assist ventilation if necessary (see pp 1–7).
   2. Treat hypotension (see p 15), arrhythmias (pp 13–15), coma (p 18), and seizures (p 22) if they occur.
   3. Treat recurrent ventricular tachycardia with lidocaine, phenytoin, or overdrive pacing (p 13). Do ***not*** use other type Ia or Ic agents, because they may worsen cardiac toxicity.
   4. Continuously monitor vital signs and ECG for a minimum of 6 hours and admit symptomatic patients until the ECG returns to normal.

B. **Specific drugs and antidotes.** Treat cardiotoxic effects such as wide QRS intervals and hypotension with **sodium bicarbonate** (see p 423), 1–2 mEq/kg rapid IV bolus, repeated every 5–10 minutes and as needed. Markedly impaired conduction or high-degree AV block unresponsive to bicarbonate therapy is an indication for insertion of a cardiac pacemaker.

C. **Decontamination** (see p 45). Administer activated charcoal orally if conditions are appropriate (see Table I–38, p 51). Gastric lavage is not necessary after small to moderate ingestions if activated charcoal can be given promptly.

D. **Enhanced elimination** (see p 53)
   1. **Quinidine** has a very large volume of distribution, and therefore it is not effectively removed by dialysis. Acidification of the urine may enhance excretion, but this is not recommended because it may aggravate cardiac toxicity.
   2. **Disopyramide, procainamide,** and ***N*-acetylprocainamide** have smaller volumes of distribution and are effectively removed by hemoperfusion or dialysis.
   3. The efficacy of repeat-dose activated charcoal has not been studied for the type Ia agents.

## ► QUININE

*Neal L. Benowitz, MD*

Quinine is an optical isomer of quinidine. Quinine was once widely used for treatment of malaria and is still occasionally used for chloroquine-resistant cases, but it is now prescribed primarily for the treatment of nocturnal muscle cramps. Quinine is found in tonic water and has been used to cut street heroin. It has also been used as an abortifacient.

I. **Mechanism of toxicity.** The mechanism of quinine toxicity is believed to be similar to that of quinidine (see p 326); however, quinine is a much less potent cardiotoxin. Quinine also has toxic effects on the retina that can result in blindness. At one time, vasoconstriction of retinal arterioles resulting in retinal ischemia was thought to be the cause of blindness; however, recent evidence indicates a direct toxic effect on photoreceptor and ganglion cells.

II. **Toxic dose.** Quinine sulfate is available in capsules and tablets containing 130–325 mg. The minimum toxic dose is approximately 3–4 g in adults; 1 g has been fatal in a child.

**III. Clinical presentation.** Toxic effects involve the cardiovascular and central nervous systems, the eyes, and other organ systems.

**A. Mild intoxication** produces nausea, vomiting, and cinchonism (tinnitus, deafness, vertigo, headache, and visual disturbances).

**B. Severe intoxication** may cause ataxia, obtundation, convulsions, coma, and respiratory arrest. With massive intoxication, quinidine-like cardiotoxicity (hypotension, QRS and QT interval prolongation, AV block, and ventricular arrhythmias) may be fatal.

**C. Retinal toxicity** occurs 9–10 hours after ingestion and includes blurred vision, impaired color perception, constriction of visual fields, and blindness. The pupils are often fixed and dilated. Fundoscopy may reveal retinal artery spasm, disk pallor, and macular edema. Although gradual recovery occurs, many patients are left with permanent visual impairment.

**D. Other toxic effects** of quinine include hypokalemia, hypoglycemia, hemolysis (in patients with glucose-6-phosphate dehydrogenase [G6PD] deficiency), and congenital malformations when used in pregnancy.

**IV. Diagnosis** is based on a history of ingestion and the presence of cinchonism and visual disturbances. Quinidine-like cardiotoxic effects may or may not be present.

**A. Specific levels.** Serum quinine levels can be measured by the same assay as for quinidine, as long as quinidine is not present. Plasma quinine levels above 10 mg/L have been associated with visual impairment; 87% of patients with levels above 20 mg/L reported blindness. Levels above 16 mg/L have been associated with cardiac toxicity.

**B. Other useful laboratory studies** include CBC, electrolytes, glucose, BUN, creatinine, arterial blood gases or oximetry, and ECG monitoring.

**V. Treatment**

**A. Emergency and supportive measures**

1. Maintain an open airway and assist ventilation if necessary (see pp 1–7).
2. Treat coma (see p 18), seizures (p 22), hypotension (p 15), and arrhythmias (pp 10–15) if they occur.
3. Avoid types Ia and Ic antiarrhythmic drugs; they may worsen cardiotoxicity.
4. Continuously monitor vital signs and the ECG for at least 6 hours after ingestion, and admit symptomatic patients to an intensive care unit.

**B. Specific drugs and antidotes**

1. Treat cardiotoxicity with **sodium bicarbonate** (see p 423), 1–2 mEq/kg by rapid IV bolus.
2. Stellate ganglion block has previously been recommended for quinine-induced blindness, the rationale being to increase retinal blood flow. However, recent evidence indicates that this treatment is not effective, and the procedure may have serious complications.

**C. Decontamination** (see p 45). Administer activated charcoal orally, if conditions are appropriate (see Table I–38, p 51). Gastric lavage is not necessary after small to moderate ingestions if activated charcoal can be given promptly.

**D. Enhanced elimination.** Because of extensive tissue distribution (volume of distribution is 3 L/kg), dialysis and hemoperfusion procedures are ineffective. Acidification of the urine may slightly increase renal excretion but does not significantly alter the overall elimination rate and may aggravate cardiotoxicity.

## ▶ RADIATION (IONIZING)

*Evan T. Wythe, MD*

Radiation poisoning is a rare but potentially challenging complication of the nuclear age. Dependence on nuclear energy and the expanded use of radioactive isotopes in industry and medicine have increased the possibility of accidental exposures. Ionizing radiation may be generated from a variety of sources. **Particle-emitting** sources may produce beta and alpha particles and neutrons. **Ionizing electromagnetic** radiation includes gamma rays and x-rays. In contrast, magnetic fields, microwaves, radio waves, and ultrasound are examples of **nonionizing** electromagnetic radiation.

Management of a radiation accident depends on whether the victim has been contaminated or only irradiated. **Irradiated** victims pose no threat to health-care providers and can be managed with no special precautions. In contrast, **contaminated** victims must be decontaminated to prevent spread of radioactive materials to others and the environment.

A terrorist **"dirty bomb"** (dispersion bomb) probably would contain commonly acquired radioactive materials such as americium (alpha emitter: found in smoke detectors and oil exploration equipment), cobalt (gamma emitter: used in food and mail irradiation), iridium (gamma emitter: used in cancer therapy), strontium (gamma emitter: used in medical treatment and power generation), and cesium (gamma emitter: used to sterilize medical equipment and for medical and industrial uses). Psychological effects (ie, panic) probably would overshadow medical concerns, as medically significant acute radiation exposure by contamination would be confined only to the immediate blast area. Long-term exposure could increase cancer rates significantly; adequate decontamination of blast areas may be problematic, potentially making them uninhabitable.

**I. Mechanism of toxicity**

**A.** Radiation impairs biologic function by ionizing atoms and breaking chemical bonds, leading to the formation of highly reactive free radicals that can damage cell walls, organelles, and DNA. Affected cells are either killed or inhibited in division. Cells with a high turnover rate (eg, bone marrow and epithelial coverings such as skin, GI tract, and pulmonary system) are more sensitive to radiation. Lymphocytes are particularly sensitive.

**B.** Radiation also causes a poorly understood inflammatory response and microvascular effects after moderately high doses (eg, 600 rad).

**C.** Radiation effects may be deterministic or stochastic. Deterministic effects are associated with a threshold dose and usually occur within an acute time frame (within a year). Stochastic effects have no known threshold and may occur after a latency period of years (eg, cancer).

**II. Toxic dose.** Various terms are used to describe radiation exposure and dose: **R** (roentgen) is a measure of exposure, whereas **rad** (radiation absorbed dose) and **rem** (radiation equivalent, man) are measures of dose. In the United States, rad is the unit of radiation dose commonly referred to in exposures, whereas rem is useful in describing dose-equivalent biologic damage. For most exposures, these units can be considered interchangeable. The exception is alpha particle exposure (eg, plutonium), which causes greater double-stranded DNA damage and a higher rem compared with rad. The International System of Units (SI) is replacing the rad and rem nomenclature; 1 grey (Gy) = 100 rad and 1 sievert (Sv) = 100 rem.

**A. Toxicity thresholds**

1. **Acute effects.** Exposure to more than 75 rad causes nausea and vomiting. Exposure to more than 400 rad is potentially lethal without medical intervention. Vomiting within 1–5 hours of exposure suggests an exposure of at least 600 rad. Brief exposure to 5000 rad or more usually causes death within minutes to hours.
2. **Carcinogenesis.** Radiation protection organizations have not agreed on a threshold dose for stochastic effects such as cancer.

**B. Recommended exposure limits**

1. **Exposure to the general population.** The National Council on Radiation Protection (NCRP) recommends a maximum of 0.5 rem per person per year. The background radiation level at sea level is about 35 millirem (0.035 rem) per year.
2. **Occupational exposure to x-rays.** The federal government has set standards for such exposures: 5 rem/year to the total body, gonads, or blood-

forming organs; 75 rem/year to the hands or feet. A single chest x-ray results in a radiation exposure of about 15 millirem (mrem) to the patient and about 0.006 mrem to nearby health-care personnel (at a distance of 160 cm). A head CT scan gives about 1 rad to the head; an abdominal CT scan may give as much as 2–5 rad to the area of concern.

3. **Radiation during pregnancy.** Established guidelines vary but generally recommend a maximum exposure of no more than 50 mrem per month (NCRP). Exposure to the ovaries and fetus from a routine abdominal (KUB) film may be as high as 146 mrem; from a chest x-ray, the dose is about 15 mrem.
4. **Exposure guidelines for emergency health-care personnel.** To save a life, the NCRP-recommended maximum exposure for a rescuer is 50–75 rem whole-body exposure.

**III. Clinical presentation**

**A. Acute radiation syndrome** (ARS) consists of a constellation of symptoms and signs indicative of systemic radiation injury. It often is described in four stages (prodrome, latency, manifest illness, and recovery). The onset and severity of each stage of radiation poisoning are determined largely by the dose.

1. The *prodromal* stage, from 0–48 hours, may include nausea, vomiting, abdominal cramps, and diarrhea. Severe exposures are associated with diaphoresis, disorientation, fever, ataxia, coma, shock, and death.
2. During the *latent* stage, there may be an improvement in symptoms. The duration of this stage is usually hours to days, but it may be shorter or absent with massive exposures.
3. The *manifest illness* stage, from 1–60 days, is characterized by multiple organ system involvement, particularly bone marrow suppression, which may lead to sepsis and death.
4. The *recovery* phase may be accompanied by hair loss, disfiguring burns, and scars.

**B. Gastrointestinal system.** Exposure to 100 R or more usually produces nausea, vomiting, abdominal cramps, and diarrhea within a few hours. After exposure to 600 rad or more, loss of integrity of the GI mucosal layer results in denudation and severe necrotic gastroenteritis, which may lead to marked dehydration, GI bleeding, and death within a few days. Doses of 1500 rad are thought to destroy GI stem cells completely.

**C. Central nervous system.** With acute exposures of several thousand rad, confusion and stupor may occur, followed within minutes to hours by ataxia, convulsions, coma, and death. In animal models of massive exposure, a phenomenon known as "early transient incapacitation" occurs.

**D. Bone marrow depression** may be subclinical but apparent on a CBC after exposure to as little as 25 rad. Immunocompromise usually follows exposure to more than 100 rad.

1. Early neutropenia is caused by margination; the true nadir occurs at about 30 days or as soon as 14 days after severe exposure. Neutropenia is the most significant factor in septicemia.
2. Thrombocytopenia is usually not evident for 2 weeks or more after exposure.
3. The lymphocyte count is of great prognostic importance and usually reaches a nadir within 48 hours of serious exposure; a count of less than 300–500 lymphocytes/mm$^3$ during this period indicates a poor prognosis, whereas 1200/mm$^3$ or more suggests likely survival.

**E. Other complications** of high-dose acute radiation syndrome include multisystem organ failure, veno-occlusive disease of the liver, interstitial pneumonitis, renal failure, tissue fibrosis, skin burns, and hair loss.

**IV. Diagnosis** depends on the history of exposure. The potential for contamination should be assessed by determining the type of radionuclide involved and the potential route(s) of exposure.

A. **Specific levels**
   1. **Detection.** Depending on the circumstances, the presence of radionuclides may be verified by one or more of the following devices: survey meters with pancake or alpha probes, whole-body counts, chest counts, and nuclear medicine cameras.
   2. **Biologic specimens.** Nasopharyngeal and wound swabs, sputum, vomitus, skin wipes, wound bandages, and clothing articles (particularly shoes) may be collected for radionuclide analysis and counts. Collection of urine and feces for 24–72 hours may assist in the estimation of an internal dose. Serum levels of radioactive materials are not generally available or clinically useful.
   3. **Other methods.** Chromosomal changes in lymphocytes are the most sensitive indication of exposures to as little as 10 rad; DNA fragments, dicentric rings, and deletions may be present. Exposure to 15 rad may cause oligospermia first seen about 45 days after the exposure.

B. **Other useful laboratory studies** include CBC (repeat every 6 hours), electrolytes, glucose, BUN, creatinine, and urinalysis. Immediately draw lymphocytes for human leukocyte antigen (HLA) typing in case bone marrow transplant is required later.

V. **Treatment.** For expert assistance in evaluation and treatment of victims and in on-scene management, immediately contact the **Radiation Emergency Assistance Center and Training Site (REAC/TS)** at **www.orau.gov/reacts**: **telephone 865-576-3131 or 865-576-1005.** REAC/TS is operated for the US Department of Energy (DOE) by the Oak Ridge Associated Universities, and assistance is available 24 hours a day. Also contact the local state agency responsible for radiation safety.

A. **Emergency and supportive measures.** Depending on the risk to rescuers, treatment of serious medical problems takes precedence over radiologic concerns. If there is a potential for contamination of rescuers and equipment, appropriate radiation response protocols should be implemented, and rescuers should wear protective clothing and respirators. ***Note:*** If the exposure was to electromagnetic radiation only, the victim is not contaminating and does not pose a risk to downstream personnel.
   1. Maintain an open airway and assist ventilation if necessary (see pp 1–7).
   2. Treat coma (see p 18) and seizures (p 22) if they occur.
   3. Replace fluid losses from gastroenteritis with intravenous crystalloid solutions (see p 15).
   4. Treat leukopenia and resulting infections as needed. Immunosuppressed patients require reverse isolation and appropriate broad-spectrum antibiotic therapy. Bone marrow stimulants may help selected patients.

B. **Specific drugs and antidotes.** Chelating agents or pharmacologic blocking drugs may be useful in some cases of ingestion or inhalation of certain biologically active radioactive materials if they are given before or shortly after exposure (Table II–50). Contact REAC/TS (see above) for specific advice on the use of these agents.

C. Decontamination (p 45)
   1. **Exposure to particle-emitting solids or liquids.** *The victim is potentially highly contaminating to rescuers, transport vehicles, and attending health personnel.*
      a. Remove victims from exposure, and if their conditions permit, remove all contaminated clothing and wash the victims with soap and water.
      b. All clothing and cleansing water must be saved, evaluated for radioactivity, and disposed of properly.
      c. Rescuers should wear protective clothing and respiratory gear to avoid contamination. At the hospital, measures must be taken to prevent contamination of facilities and personnel (see Section IV, p 520).

**TABLE II–50. CHELATING AGENTS FOR SOME RADIATION EXPOSURES[a]**

| Radionuclide | Chelating or Blocking Agents |
|---|---|
| Americium-241 | Ca-DTPA or Zn-DTPA (see p 444): chelator. Dose: 1 g in 250 mL $D_5W$ IV over 30–60 min daily. Wounds: Irrigate with 1 g DTPA in 250 mL water.<br>EDTA (see p 446) may also be effective if DTPA is not immediately available. |
| Cesium-137 | Prussian blue (ferric hexacyanoferrate) adsorbs cesium in the GI tract and may also enhance elimination. Exposure burden establishes dose, at low exposure burden 500 mg PO 6 times daily in 100–200 mL of water. |
| Cobalt-60 | Limited evidence suggests possible use of Ca-DTPA or Zn DTPA (see p 444): chelator. Dose: 1 g in 250 mL $D_5W$ IV over 30–60 min daily. Wounds: Irrigate with 1 g DTPA in 250 mL water.<br>EDTA (see p 446) may also be tried if DTPA is not immediately available. |
| Iodine-131 | Potassium iodide dilutes radioactive iodine and blocks thyroid iodine uptake. Adult dose: 300 mg PO immediately, then 130 mg PO daily. See p 499.<br>Perchlorate, 200 mg PO, then 100 mg every 5 h, has also been recommended. |
| Plutonium-239 | Ca-DTPA or Zn DTPA (see p 444): chelator. Dose: 1 g in 250 mL $D_5W$ IV over 30–60 min daily. Wounds: Irrigate with 1 g DTPA in 250 mL water.<br>EDTA (see p 446) may also be effective if DTPA is not immediately available.<br>Aluminum-containing antacids may bind plutonium in GI tract. |
| Strontium-90 | Alginate or aluminum hydroxide-containing antacids may reduce intestinal absorption of strontium. Dose: 10 g, then 1 g 4 times daily.<br>Barium sulfate may also reduce strontium absorption. Dose: 100 g in 250 mL water PO.<br>Calcium gluconate may dilute the effect of strontium. Dose: 2 g in 500 mL PO or IV.<br>Ammonium chloride is a demineralizing agent. Dose: 3 g PO 3 times daily |
| Tritium | Forced fluids, diuretics, (?) hemodialysis. Water dilutes tritium, enhances urinary excretion. |
| Uranium-233, -235, -238 | Sodium bicarbonate forms a carbonate complex with uranyl ion, which is then eliminated in the urine. Dose: 100 mEq in 500 mL $D_5W$ by slow constant IV infusion.<br>Aluminum-containing antacids may help prevent uranium absorption. |

[a]References: Bhattacharyya ANL et al: Methods of treatment. Pages 27–36 in: *Radiation Protection Dosimetr.* Gerber GB, Thomas RG (editors). Vol. 41, No. 1 (1992); and Ricks RC; *Hospital Emergency Department Management of Radiation Accidents.* Oak Ridge Associated Universities, 1984.

**d.** Induce vomiting or perform gastric lavage (see p 48) if radioactive material has been ingested. Administer activated charcoal (see p 50), although its effectiveness is unknown. Certain other adsorbent materials may also be effective (see Table II–50).

**e.** Contact REAC/TS (see above) and the state radiologic health department for further advice. In some exposures, unusually aggressive steps may be needed (eg, lung lavage for significant inhalation of plutonium).

**2. Electromagnetic radiation exposure.** *The patient is not radioactive and does not pose a contamination threat.* There is no need for decontamination once the patient has been removed from the source of exposure unless electromagnetic radiation emitter fragments are embedded in body tissues.

**D. Enhanced elimination.** Chelating agents and forced diuresis may be useful for certain exposures (see Table II–50).

## ► SALICYLATES

*Susan Kim, PharmD*

Salicylates are used widely for their analgesic and anti-inflammatory properties. They are found in a variety of prescription and over-the-counter analgesics, cold preparations, topical keratolytic products (methyl salicylate), and even Pepto-Bismol (bismuth subsalicylate). Before the introduction of child-resistant containers, aspirin overdose was one of the leading causes of accidental death in children. Two distinct syndromes of intoxication may occur, depending on whether the exposure is **acute** or **chronic.**

**I. Mechanism of toxicity.** Salicylates have a variety of toxic effects.

**A.** Central stimulation of the respiratory center results in hyperventilation, leading to respiratory alkalosis. Secondary consequences from hyperventilation include dehydration and compensatory metabolic acidosis.

**B.** Intracellular effects include uncoupling of oxidative phosphorylation and interruption of glucose and fatty acid metabolism, which contribute to metabolic acidosis.

**C.** The mechanism by which cerebral and pulmonary edema occurs is not known but may be related to an alteration in capillary integrity.

**D.** Salicylates alter platelet function and may also prolong the prothrombin time.

**E. Pharmacokinetics.** Acetylsalicylic acid is well absorbed from the stomach and small intestine. Large tablet masses and enteric-coated products may dramatically delay absorption (hours to days). The volume of distribution of salicylate is about 0.1–0.3 L/kg, but this can be increased by acidemia, which enhances movement of the drug into cells. Elimination is mostly by hepatic metabolism at therapeutic doses, but renal excretion becomes important with overdose. The elimination half-life is normally 2–4.5 hours but can be as long as 18–36 hours after overdose. Renal elimination is dependent on urine pH. See also Table II–59 (p 382).

**II. Toxic dose.** The average therapeutic single dose is 10 mg/kg, and the usual daily therapeutic dose is 40–60 mg/kg/day. Each tablet of aspirin contains 325–650 mg of acetylsalicylic acid. One teaspoon of concentrated **oil of wintergreen** contains 5 g of methyl salicylate, equivalent to about 7.5 g of aspirin.

**A. Acute ingestion** of 150–200 mg/kg will produce mild intoxication; severe intoxication is likely after acute ingestion of 300–500 mg/kg.

**B. Chronic intoxication** may occur with ingestion of more than 100 mg/kg/day for 2 or more days.

**III. Clinical presentation.** Patients may become intoxicated after an acute accidental or suicidal overdose or as a result of chronic repeated overmedication for several days.

**A. Acute ingestion.** Vomiting occurs shortly after ingestion, followed by hyperpnea, tinnitus, and lethargy. Mixed respiratory alkalemia and metabolic acidosis are apparent when arterial blood gases are determined. With severe intoxication, coma, seizures, hypoglycemia, hyperthermia, and pulmonary edema may occur. Death is caused by CNS failure and cardiovascular collapse.

**B. Chronic intoxication.** Victims are usually confused elderly persons who are taking salicylates therapeutically. The diagnosis is often overlooked because the presentation is nonspecific; confusion, dehydration, and metabolic acidosis are often attributed to sepsis, pneumonia, or gastroenteritis. However, morbidity and mortality rates are much higher than they are after acute overdose. Cerebral and pulmonary edema is more common than with acute intoxication, and severe poisoning occurs at lower salicylate levels.

**IV. Diagnosis** is not difficult if there is a history of acute ingestion accompanied by typical signs and symptoms. In the absence of a history of overdose, diagnosis is suggested by the characteristic arterial blood gases, which reveal a mixed respiratory alkalemia and metabolic acidosis.

**A. Specific levels.** Obtain stat and serial serum salicylate concentrations. Systemic acidemia increases brain salicylate concentrations, worsening toxicity.

1. **Acute ingestion.** Serum levels greater than 90–100 mg/dL (900–1000 mg/L, or 6.6–7.3 mmol/L) usually are associated with severe toxicity. Single determinations are ***not*** sufficient because of the possibility of prolonged or delayed absorption from sustained-release tablets or a tablet mass or bezoar (especially after massive ingestion). Most toxicologists no longer use the Done nomogram to estimate toxicity.
2. **Chronic intoxication.** Symptoms correlate poorly with serum levels, and the Done nomogram cannot be used to predict toxicity. Chronic therapeutic concentrations in arthritis patients range from 100–300 mg/L (10–30 mg/dL). A level greater than 600 mg/L (60 mg/dL) accompanied by acidosis and altered mental status is considered very serious.

**B. Other useful laboratory studies** include electrolytes (anion gap calculation), glucose, BUN, creatinine, prothrombin time, arterial blood gases, and chest x-ray.

**V. Treatment**

**A. Emergency and supportive measures**

1. Maintain an open airway and assist ventilation if necessary (see pp 1–7). ***Warning:*** Ensure adequate ventilation to prevent respiratory acidosis and do not allow controlled mechanical ventilation to interfere with the patient's need for compensatory efforts to maintain the serum pH. Administer supplemental oxygen. Obtain serial arterial blood gases and chest x-rays to observe for pulmonary edema (more common with chronic or severe intoxication).
2. Treat coma (see p 18), seizures (p 22), pulmonary edema (p 7), and hyperthermia (p 20) if they occur.
3. Treat metabolic acidosis with intravenous sodium bicarbonate (see p 423). Do ***not*** allow the serum pH to fall below 7.4.
4. Replace fluid and electrolyte deficits caused by vomiting and hyperventilation with intravenous crystalloid solutions. Be cautious with fluid therapy, because excessive fluid administration may contribute to pulmonary edema.
5. Administer supplemental glucose, and treat hypoglycemia (see p 34) if it occurs.
6. Monitor asymptomatic patients for a minimum of 6 hours (longer if an enteric-coated preparation or a massive overdose has been ingested and there is suspicion of a tablet bezoar). Admit symptomatic patients to an intensive care unit.

**B. Specific drugs and antidotes.** There is no specific antidote for salicylate intoxication. **Sodium bicarbonate** is given frequently both to prevent acidemia and to promote salicylate elimination by the kidneys (see **D**, below).

**C. Decontamination** (see p 45). Decontamination is not necessary for patients with *chronic* intoxication.

1. Administer activated charcoal orally if conditions are appropriate (see Table I–38, p 51). Gastric lavage is not necessary after small to moderate ingestions if activated charcoal can be given promptly.
2. ***Note:*** With large ingestions of salicylate (eg, 30–60 g), very large doses of activated charcoal (300–600 g) are theoretically necessary to adsorb all the salicylate. In such cases, the charcoal can be given in several 25- to 50-g doses at 3- to 5-hour intervals. Whole bowel irrigation (see p 52) is recommended to help move the pills and charcoal through the intestinal tract.

**D. Enhanced elimination** (see p 53)

1. **Urinary alkalinization** is effective in enhancing urinary excretion of salicylate, although it is often difficult to achieve in dehydrated or critically ill patients. The goal is to maintain urine pH of ≥ 7.5.
   a. Add 100 mEq of sodium bicarbonate to 1 L of 5% dextrose in quarter normal saline and infuse intravenously at 200 mL/h (3–4 mL/kg/h). If the patient is dehydrated, start with a bolus of 10–20 mL/kg. Fluid and bicarbonate administration is potentially dangerous in patients at high risk for pulmonary edema (eg, chronic intoxication).
   b. Unless renal failure is present, also add potassium, 30–40 mEq, to each liter of intravenous fluids (potassium depletion inhibits alkalinization).
   c. Alkalemia is not a contraindication to bicarbonate therapy in light of the fact that patients often have a significant base deficit in spite of the elevated serum pH.
2. **Hemodialysis** is very effective in rapidly removing salicylate and correcting acid-base and fluid abnormalities. Indications for urgent hemodialysis are as follows:
   a. Patients with acute ingestion and serum levels higher than 1000 mg/L (100 mg/dL) with severe acidosis and other manifestations of intoxication.
   b. Patients with chronic intoxication with serum levels higher than 600 mg/L (60 mg/dL) accompanied by acidosis, confusion, or lethargy, especially if the patient is elderly or debilitated.
   c. Any patient with severe manifestations of intoxication.
3. **Hemoperfusion** is also very effective but does not correct acid-base or fluid disturbances.
4. **Repeat-dose activated charcoal** therapy effectively reduces the serum salicylate half-life, but it is not as rapidly effective as dialysis, and frequent stooling may contribute to dehydration and electrolyte disturbances.
5. **Continuous venovenous hemodiafiltration** was reported to be effective in two cases, but there is insufficient information about clearance rates to recommend this procedure.

## ► SCORPIONS

*Richard F. Clark, MD*

The order Scorpionida contains several families, genera, and species of scorpions. All have paired venom glands in a bulbous segment called the telson that is situated just anterior to a stinger on the end of the six terminal segments of the abdomen (often called a tail). The only systemically poisonous species in the United States is *Centruroides exilicauda* (formerly *C sculpturatus*), also known as the bark scorpion. The most serious envenomations usually are reported in children under age 10 years. This scorpion is found primarily in the arid southwestern United States but has been found as a stowaway in cargo as far north as Michigan. Other dangerous scorpions are found in Mexico (*Centruroides* spp), Brazil (*Tityus* spp), India (*Buthus* spp), the Middle East, and north Africa and the eastern Mediterranean (*Leiurus* and *Androctonus* spp).

I. **Mechanism of toxicity.** The scorpion grasps its prey with its anterior pincers, arches its pseudoabdomen, and stabs with the stinger. Stings also result from stepping on the stinger. The venom of *C exilicauda* contains numerous digestive enzymes (eg, hyaluronidase and phospholipase) and several neurotoxins. These neurotoxins can cause alterations in sodium channel flow, resulting in excessive stimulation at neuromuscular junctions and the autonomic nervous system.

II. **Toxic dose.** Variable amounts of venom from none to the complete contents of the telson may be ejected through the stinger.

**III. Clinical presentation**

**A. Common scorpion stings.** Most stings result only in local, immediate burning pain. Some local tissue inflammation and occasionally local paresthesias may occur. Symptoms usually resolve within several hours. This represents the typical scorpion sting most often seen in the United States.

**B. Dangerous scorpion stings.** In some victims, especially children under age 10 years, systemic symptoms can occur after stings by *Centruroides* species, including weakness, restlessness, diaphoresis, diplopia, nystagmus, roving eye movements, hyperexcitability, muscle fasciculations, opisthotonus, priapism, salivation, slurred speech, hypertension, tachycardia, and, rarely, convulsions, paralysis, and respiratory arrest. Envenomations by *Tityus, Buthus, Androctonus,* and *Leiurus* species have caused pulmonary edema, cardiovascular collapse, and death, as well as coagulopathies, disseminated intravascular coagulation, pancreatitis, and renal failure with hemoglobinuria and jaundice. In nonfatal cases, recovery usually occurs within 12–36 hours.

**IV. Diagnosis.** Either the patient saw the scorpion or the clinician must recognize the symptoms. In the case of *Centruroides* stings, tapping on the sting site usually produces severe pain ("tap test").

**A. Specific levels.** Body fluid toxin levels are not available.

**B.** No other useful laboratory studies are needed for minor envenomations. For severe envenomations, obtain CBC, electrolytes, glucose, BUN, creatinine, coagulation profile, and arterial blood gases.

**V. Treatment.** The majority of scorpion stings in the United States, including those by *Centruroides,* can be managed with symptomatic home care consisting of oral analgesics and cool compresses or intermittent ice packs.

**A. Emergency and supportive measures**

1. For severe envenomations, maintain an open airway and assist ventilation if necessary (see pp 1–7). Administer supplemental oxygen. Atropine has been used successfully in some cases to dry mouth and airway secretions.
2. Treat hypertension (see p 17), tachycardia (p 12), and convulsions (p 22) if they occur.
3. Do ***not*** overtreat with excessive sedation. One study reported benefit with a continuous infusion of midazolam in patients with severe *Centruroides* stings.
4. Clean the wound and provide tetanus prophylaxis if indicated.
5. Do ***not*** immerse the injured extremity in ice or perform local incision or suction.

**B. Specific drugs and antidotes.** An antivenom effective against severe *Centruroides* envenomations was available at one time in Arizona. However, production of this antivenom has ceased, and supplies may be depleted. Specific antivenoms against other species may be available in other parts of the world but are not approved in the United States.

**C. Decontamination.** These procedures are not applicable.

**D. Enhanced elimination.** These procedures are not applicable.

## ► SEDATIVE-HYPNOTIC AGENTS

*Ben T. Tsutaoka, PharmD*

Sedative-hypnotic agents are used widely for the treatment of anxiety and insomnia. As a group they are one of the most frequently prescribed medications. Barbiturates (see p 124), benzodiazepines (p 129), antihistamines (p 97), skeletal muscle relaxants (p 341), antidepressants (pp 89 and 91), and anticholinergic agents (p 85) are discussed elsewhere in this book. This section and Table II–51 list some of the less commonly used hypnotic agents.

TABLE II–51. SEDATIVE-HYPNOTIC AGENTS[a]

| Drug | Usual Adult Oral Hypnotic Dose (mg) | Approximate Lethal Dose (g) | Toxic Concentration (mg/L) | Usual Half-Life[b] (h) |
|---|---|---|---|---|
| Buspirone | 5–20 | Unknown | — | 2–4 |
| Chloral hydrate | 500–1000 | 5–10 | > 20[c] | 8–11[d] |
| Ethchlorvynol | 500–1000 | 5–10 | > 10 | 10–20 |
| Glutethimide | 250–500 | 10–20 | > 10 | 10–12 |
| Meprobamate | 600–1200 | 10–20 | > 60 | 10–11 |
| Methaqualone | 150–250 | 3–8 | > 5 | 20–60 |
| Methyprylon | 200–400 | 5–10 | > 10 | 7–11 |
| Paraldehyde | 5–10 mL | 25 mL | > 200 | 6–7 |

[a]See also anticholinergic agents (p 85), antihistamines (p 97), barbiturates (pp 493–494), benzodiazepines (p 419), and skeletal muscle relaxants (p 341).
[b]Half-life in overdose may be considerably longer.
[c]Toxic concentration is measured as the metabolite trichloroethanol.
[d]Half-life of the metabolite trichloroethanol.

**I. Mechanism of toxicity.** The exact mechanism of action and the pharmacokinetics (see Table II–59, p 382) vary for each agent. The major toxic effect that causes serious poisoning or death is CNS depression resulting in coma, respiratory arrest, and pulmonary aspiration of gastric contents.

**II. Toxic dose.** The toxic dose varies considerably between drugs and also depends largely on individual tolerance and the presence of other drugs, such as alcohol. For most of these drugs, ingestion of 3–5 times the usual hypnotic dose results in coma. However, co-ingestion of alcohol or other drugs may cause coma after smaller ingestions, whereas individuals who chronically use large doses of these drugs may tolerate much higher acute doses.

**III. Clinical presentation.** Overdose with any of these drugs may cause drowsiness, ataxia, nystagmus, stupor, coma, and respiratory arrest. Deep coma may result in absent reflexes, fixed pupils, and depressed or absent EEG activity. Hypothermia is common. Most of these agents also slow gastric motility and decrease muscle tone. Hypotension with a large overdose is caused primarily by depression of cardiac contractility and, to a lesser extent, loss of venous tone.

**A. Chloral hydrate** is metabolized to trichloroethanol, which also has CNS-depressant activity. Trichloroethanol may also sensitize the myocardium to the effects of catecholamines, resulting in cardiac arrhythmias.

**B. Buspirone** may cause nausea, vomiting, drowsiness, and miosis. There have been no reported deaths.

**C. Ethchlorvynol** has a pungent odor sometimes described as pear-like, and gastric fluid often has a pink or green color, depending on the capsule form (200- and 500-mg capsules are red; 750-mg capsules are green).

**D. Glutethimide** often produces mydriasis (dilated pupils) and other anticholinergic side effects, and patients may exhibit prolonged and cyclic or fluctuating coma. It sometimes is taken in combination with codeine (“loads”), which may produce opioid effects.

**E. Meprobamate** has been reported to form tablet concretions in large overdoses, occasionally requiring surgical removal. Hypotension is more common with this agent than with other sedative-hypnotics. Meprobamate is the metabolite of the skeletal muscle relaxant carisoprodol (see p 341).

F. **Methaqualone** is unusual among sedative-hypnotic agents in that it frequently causes muscular hypertonicity, clonus, and hyperreflexia.

IV. **Diagnosis** usually is based on a history of ingestion, because clinical manifestations are fairly nonspecific. Hypothermia and deep coma may cause the patient to appear dead; thus, careful evaluation should precede the diagnosis of brain death. Chloral hydrate is radiopaque and may be visible on plain abdominal x-rays.

A. **Specific levels** and qualitative urine screening are usually available through commercial toxicology laboratories but are rarely of value in emergency management.

1. Drug levels do not always correlate with severity of intoxication, especially in patients who have tolerance to the drug or have also ingested other drugs or alcohol. In addition, early after ingestion blood levels may not reflect brain concentrations.
2. Some agents (ie, chloral hydrate) have active metabolites whose levels may correlate better with the state of intoxication.

B. **Other useful laboratory studies** include electrolytes, glucose, serum ethanol, BUN, creatinine, arterial blood gases, ECG, and chest x-ray.

V. **Treatment**

A. **Emergency and supportive measures**

1. Maintain an open airway and assist ventilation if necessary (see pp 1–7). Administer supplemental oxygen.
2. Treat coma (see p 18), hypothermia (p 19), hypotension (p 15), and pulmonary edema (p 7) if they occur.
3. Monitor patients for at least 6 hours after ingestion, because delayed absorption may occur. Patients with **chloral hydrate** ingestion should be monitored for at least 18–24 hours because of the risk of cardiac arrhythmias. Tachyarrhythmias caused by myocardial sensitization may be treated with **propranolol** (see p 504), 1–2 mg IV, or **esmolol** (see p 449), 0.025–0.1 mg/kg/min IV.

B. **Specific drugs and antidotes.** Flumazenil (see p 452) is a specific antagonist of benzodiazepine receptors. It does not appear to cross-react with other sedative agents.

C. **Decontamination** (see p 45). Administer activated charcoal orally if conditions are appropriate (see Table I–38, p 51). Gastric lavage is not necessary after small to moderate ingestions if activated charcoal can be given promptly.

D. **Enhanced elimination.** Because of extensive tissue distribution, dialysis and hemoperfusion are not very effective for most of the drugs in this group.

1. Repeat-dose charcoal may enhance elimination of glutethimide (which undergoes enterohepatic recirculation) and meprobamate, although no studies have been performed to document clinical effectiveness.
2. Meprobamate has a relatively small volume of distribution (0.7 L/kg), and hemoperfusion may be useful for deep coma complicated by intractable hypotension.
3. Resin hemoperfusion has been reported to be partially effective for ethchlorvynol overdose.

## ▶ SELENIUM

*Richard J. Geller, MD, MPH*

Selenium (element 34) belongs to column VIa of the periodic table of the elements and shares chemical properties with sulfur and tellurium. It exists in four natural oxidation states and is found in a variety of compounds capable of causing human poisoning. Table II–52 describes the chemistry of selenium compounds. Selenium is an essential trace element in the human diet, and exposures may occur through the use

**TABLE II–52. SELENIUM COMPOUNDS**

| Compound (Synonyms) | Physical Properties | Toxic Dose or Air Concentration[a] |
|---|---|---|
| Elemental selenium<br>CASRN 7782-49-2 (Se) | Amorphous or crystalline, red to gray solid | PEL 0.2 mg/$m^3$<br>IDLH 1 mg/$m^3$ |
| Hydrogen selenide<br>(Selenium hydride)<br>CASRN 7783-07-5 ($H_2Se$) | Odiferous colorless gas | PEL 0.05 ppm<br>IDLH 1 ppm |
| Sodium selenide<br>CASRN 1313-85-5 ($Na_2Se$) | Red to white powder | PEL 0.2 mg/$m^3$ (as Se) |
| Selenious acid<br>(Hydrogen selenite)<br>CASRN 7783-00-8<br>($H_2Se^o{}_3$) | White powder encountered as 2% solution in gun blueing | Ingestion of as little as 15 mL of a 2% solution was reported fatal in a child. |
| Sodium selenite<br>(Selenium trioxide)<br>CASRN 10102-18-8<br>($O_3Se.2Na$) | White powder | Mean lethal dose of selenite salts in dogs 4 mg/kg. Human ingestion of 1-5 mg/kg sodium selenite caused moderate toxicity. |
| Selenium oxide<br>(Selenium dioxide)<br>CASRN 7446-08-4 ($O_2Se$) | White crystal or powder | PEL 0.2 mg/$m^3$ (as Se) |
| Sodium selenate<br>CASRN 13410-01-0<br>($O_4Se.2Na$) | White crystals | PEL 0.2 mg/$m^3$ (as Se) |
| Selenic acid<br>CASRN 7783-08-6 ($H_2SeO_4$) | White solid | PEL 0.2 mg/$m^3$ (as Se) |
| Selenium hexafluoride<br>(Selenium fluoride)<br>CASRN 7783-79-1 ($F_6Se$) | Colorless gas | PEL 0.05 ppm<br>IDLH 2 ppm |

[a]PEL = OSHA-regulated permissible exposure limit for occupational exposure as an 8-hour time-weighted average (TWA); IDLH = level considered immediately dangerous to life or health (NIOSH).

of dietary supplements as well as via exposure to industrial compounds. Serious acute poisoning is reported most commonly from ingestion of selenious acid in gun bluing (coating) solutions. Illness caused by chronic exposure to selenium is uncommon but is seen in regions with high selenium content in food. Industries using selenium compounds include ceramics, electronics, glass, rubber, and metallurgy. Selenium dioxide is the most commonly used compound industrially. Selenium is produced largely as a by-product of copper refining.

**I. Mechanism of toxicity.** Precise cellular toxopathology is poorly understood. Animal studies implicate mechanisms involving the formation of superoxide and hydroxyl anions as well as hydrogen peroxide. Mechanistic knowledge makes no contribution to treatment currently. A garlic breath odor observed in various selenium poisonings is due to in vivo creation of dimethyl selenium.

**II. Toxic dose**

**A. Ingestion.** Little is known about the oral toxic dose because there are few reports of poisoning.

**1. Acute overdose.** The most commonly reported fatal selenium ingestion involves selenious acid. Ingestion of as little as 15 mL of gun bluing solution (2% selenious acid) has been fatal. The oral mean lethal dose (MLD) of selenite salts in the dog is about 4 mg/kg. Ingestion of 1–5 mg/kg sodium selenite in five adults caused moderate reversible toxicity. Survival after ingestion of 2000 mg of selenium dioxide has been reported.

2. **Chronic ingestion.** The recommended nutritional daily intake is 50–200 mcg. The drinking water maximum contaminant level (MCL) is 10 mcg/L. Chronic ingestion of 850 mcg/day has been associated with toxicity.

B. **Inhalation.** The ACGIH recommended threshold limit value (TLV) for occupational exposure to elemental selenium, as well as selenium compounds in general, has been set at 0.2 mg/m$^3$. The exposure levels considered immediately dangerous to life or health (IDLH) are listed in Table II–52.

III. **Clinical presentation**

A. **Acute ingestion** of **selenious acid** causes upper GI corrosive injury, vomiting and diarrhea, hypersalivation, and a garlic odor on the breath, with rapid deterioration of mental status and restlessness progressing to coma, hypotension from myocardial depression and decreased vascular resistance, respiratory insufficiency, and death. Suicidal ingestion of an unknown amount of **selenium dioxide** has been fatal. Ingestions of **sodium selenate** have produced gastroenteritis with garlic breath and T-wave inversion on the ECG. Five patients who ingested large amounts of **sodium selenite** developed vomiting, diarrhea, chills, and tremor but survived.

B. **Chronic ingestion** of **elemental selenium, sodium selenite, sodium selenate,** or **selenium dioxide** may cause pallor, stomach disorders, nervousness, metallic taste, and garlic breath.

C. **Acute inhalation** of **hydrogen selenide** produces dyspnea, abdominal cramps, and diarrhea. Inhalation of **selenium hexafluoride** produces severe corrosive injury and systemic toxicity from acids of selenium plus fluoride ion toxicity. **Selenium salt** inhalation causes dyspnea and skin and mucous membrane irritation.

IV. **Diagnosis** is difficult without a history of exposure. Acute severe gastroenteritis with garlic breath odor and hypotension may suggest selenious acid poisoning, but these findings are not specific.

A. **Specific levels** are not generally available. Selenium can be measured in the blood, hair, and urine. Whole-blood levels remain elevated longer than do serum levels (which are typically 40–60% lower) and may reflect long-term exposure.

1. On a normal diet, whole-blood selenium levels range from 0.1–0.2 mg/L. One patient with chronic intoxication after ingestion of 31 mg/day had a whole-blood selenium level of 0.53 mg/L.
2. Average hair levels are up to 0.5 ppm. The relationship between hair and tissue concentrations is not well understood. The utility of hair testing is complicated by the widespread use of selenium in shampoos.
3. Both whole-blood and urinary concentrations reflect dietary intake. Overexposure should be considered when blood selenium levels exceed 0.4 mg/L or urinary excretion exceeds 600–1000 mcg/day.

B. **Other useful laboratory studies** include electrolytes, glucose, BUN, creatinine, liver transaminases, and ECG. After inhalation exposure, obtain arterial blood gases or oximetry and chest x-ray.

V. **Treatment**

A. **Emergency and supportive measures**

1. Maintain an open airway and assist ventilation if necessary (see pp 1–7). Administer supplemental oxygen.
2. Treat coma (see p 18), convulsions (p 22), bronchospasm (p 7), hypotension (p 15), and pulmonary edema (p 7) if they occur. Since hypotension is often multifactorial, evaluate and optimize volume status, peripheral vascular resistance, and myocardial contractility.
3. Observe for at least 6 hours after exposure.
4. After ingestion of selenious acid, consider endoscopy to rule out esophageal or gastric corrosive injury.

**B. Specific drugs and antidotes.** There is no specific antidote. The value of suggested therapies such as chelation, vitamin C, and *N*-acetylcysteine is not established.

**C. Decontamination** (see p 45)

1. **Inhalation.** Immediately remove the victim from exposure and give supplemental oxygen if available.
2. **Skin and eyes.** Remove contaminated clothing and wash exposed skin with soap and copious water. Irrigate exposed eyes with copious tepid water or saline.
3. **Ingestion**
   a. Ingestion of elemental selenium or selenium salts does not usually benefit from GI decontamination. In light of the risk of severe corrosive GI injury, gastric lavage plus activated charcoal may be of value for ingestions of selenious acid seen within 1 hour.
   b. In vitro experiments indicate that **vitamin C** can reduce selenium salts to elemental selenium, which is poorly absorbed. Its use has not been studied in vivo, but oral or nasogastric administration of several grams of ascorbic acid has been recommended.

**D. Enhanced elimination.** There is no known role for any enhanced removal procedure.

## ▶ SKELETAL MUSCLE RELAXANTS

*Susan Kim, PharmD*

Most compounds in this group act as simple sedative-hypnotic agents that provide skeletal muscle relaxation indirectly. The drugs commonly used as skeletal muscle relaxants are listed in Table II–53. Carisoprodol (Soma™) and baclofen have been abused as recreational drugs.

**I. Mechanism of toxicity**

**A. Central nervous system.** Most of these drugs cause generalized CNS depression.

1. **Baclofen** is an agonist at the GABA(B) receptor and can produce profound CNS and respiratory depression as well as paradoxic muscle hyper-

**TABLE II–53. SKELETAL MUSCLE RELAXANTS**

| Drug | Usual Half-Life (hours) | Usual Daily Adult Dose (mg) |
|---|---|---|
| Baclofen | 2.5–4 | 40–80 |
| Carisoprodol[a] | 1.5–8 | 800–1600 |
| Chlorphenesin carbamate | 3.5 | 1600–2400 |
| Chlorzoxazone | 1 | 1500–3000 |
| Cyclobenzaprine | 24–72 | 30–60 |
| Metaxalone | 2–3 | 2400–3200 |
| Methocarbamol | 1–2 | 4000–4500 |
| Orphenadrine | 14–16 | 200 |
| Tizanidine | 2.5 | 12–36 |

[a]Metabolized to meprobamate (see p 336).

tonicity and seizure-like activity. Hallucinations, seizures, and hyperthermia have occurred after abrupt withdrawal from baclofen.

2. Spastic encephalopathy is also common with **carisoprodol** overdose.
3. Tizanidine, a centrally acting alpha-2 agonist, has effects similar to those of clonidine (see p 168)

**B. Cardiovascular effects.** Hypotension may occur after overdose. **Baclofen** has caused bradycardia in up to 30% of ingestions. Massive **orphenadrine** ingestions have caused supraventricular and ventricular tachycardia.

**C. Pharmacokinetics** varies with the drug. Absorption may be delayed because of anticholinergic effects. See also Table II–59, p 382.

**II. Toxic dose.** The toxic dose varies considerably among drugs, depends largely on individual tolerance, and can be influenced by the presence of other drugs, such as ethanol. For most of these drugs, ingestion of more than 3–5 times the usual therapeutic dose may cause stupor or coma. Death was reported in a 4-year-old who ingested approximately 3500 mg of carisoprodol, and a 2-year-old who ingested two tablets (350 mg each) required intubation. A 2-year-old developed seizures and ventricular tachycardia after ingesting 400 mg of orphenadrine.

**III. Clinical presentation.** Onset of CNS depression usually is seen within 30–120 minutes of ingestion. Lethargy, slurred speech, ataxia, coma, and respiratory arrest may occur. Larger ingestions, especially when combined with alcohol, can produce unresponsive coma.

**A. Carisoprodol** may cause hyperreflexia, opisthotonus, and increased muscle tone.

**B. Cyclobenzaprine** and **orphenadrine** can produce anticholinergic findings such as tachycardia, dilated pupils, and delirium. Despite its structural similarity to tricyclic antidepressants, cyclobenzaprine has not been reported to cause quinidine-like cardiotoxicity. Status epilepticus, ventricular tachycardia, and asystolic arrest have been reported after **orphenadrine** overdose.

**C. Baclofen** overdose causes coma, respiratory depression, bradycardia, and paradoxic seizure-like activity. Onset is rapid but may last 12–48 hours.

**D. Tizanidine** is similar to clonidine and can cause coma, profound hypotension, and bradycardia (see p 168); in addition, sinoatrial (SA) and AV nodal dysfunction was reported after an overdose.

**IV. Diagnosis** usually is based on the history of ingestion and findings of CNS depression, often accompanied by muscle twitching or hyperreflexia. The differential diagnosis should include other sedative-hypnotic agents (see p 336).

**A. Specific levels.** Many of these drugs can be detected on comprehensive urine toxicology screening. Quantitative drug levels do not always correlate with severity of intoxication, especially in patients who have tolerance to the drug or have also ingested other drugs or alcohol.

**B. Other useful laboratory studies** include electrolytes, glucose, serum ethanol, BUN, creatinine, arterial blood gases, and chest x-ray.

**V. Treatment**

**A. Emergency and supportive measures**

1. Maintain an open airway and assist ventilation if necessary (see pp 1–7). Administer supplemental oxygen.
2. Treat coma (see p 18), hypothermia (p 19), hypotension (p 15), and pulmonary edema (p 7) if they occur. Hypotension usually responds promptly to supine position and intravenous fluids.
3. Monitor patients for at least 6 hours after ingestion, because delayed absorption may occur.

**B. Specific drugs and antidotes.** There are no specific antidotes. Flumazenil (see p 446) is a specific antagonist of benzodiazepine receptors and would not be expected to be beneficial for skeletal muscle relaxants, but it reportedly has been used successfully for chlorzoxazone and carisoprodol overdose. Although physostigmine may reverse the anticholinergic symptoms associated with cyclobenzaprine and orphenadrine overdose, it is not generally needed and may potentially cause seizures.

C. **Decontamination** (see p 45). Administer activated charcoal orally if conditions are appropriate (see Table I–38, p 51). Gastric lavage is not necessary after small to moderate ingestions if activated charcoal can be given promptly.

D. **Enhanced elimination.** Because of extensive tissue distribution, dialysis and hemoperfusion are not very effective for most of the drugs in this group. Repeat-dose charcoal may enhance elimination of meprobamate, although no studies have been performed to document this.

## ▶ SMOKE INHALATION

*Kent R. Olson, MD*

Smoke inhalation commonly occurs in fire victims and is associated with high morbidity and mortality. In addition to thermal injury, burning organic and inorganic materials can produce a very large number of different toxins, leading to chemical injury to the respiratory tract as well as systemic effects from absorption of poisons through the lungs. "Smoke bombs" do not release true smoke but can be hazardous because of irritant components, particularly zinc chloride.

I. **Mechanism of toxicity.** Smoke is a complex mixture of gases, fumes, and suspended particles. Injury may result from:

   A. **Thermal damage** to the airway and tracheobronchial passages.

   B. **Irritant gases, vapors, and fumes** that can damage the upper and lower respiratory tract (see p 212). Many common irritant substances are produced by thermal breakdown and combustion, including acrolein, hydrogen chloride, phosgene, and nitrogen oxides.

   C. **Asphyxia** due to consumption of oxygen by the fire and production of carbon dioxide and other gases.

   D. **Toxic systemic effects** of inhaled carbon monoxide, cyanide, and other systemic poisons. Cyanide is a common product of combustion of plastics, wool, and many other natural and synthetic polymers.

II. **Toxic dose.** The toxic dose varies depending on the intensity and duration of the exposure. Inhalation in a confined space with limited egress is typically associated with delivery of a greater toxic dose.

III. **Clinical presentation**

   A. **Thermal and irritant effects** include singed nasal hairs, carbonaceous material in the nose and pharynx, cough, wheezing, and dyspnea. Stridor is an ominous finding that suggests imminent airway compromise due to swelling in and around the larynx. Pulmonary edema, pneumonitis, and adult respiratory distress syndrome (ARDS) may occur. Inhalation of steam is strongly associated with deep thermal injury but is not complicated by systemic toxicity.

   B. **Asphyxia and systemic intoxicants** may cause dizziness, confusion, syncope, seizures and coma. In addition, carbon monoxide (see p 151), cyanide poisoning (p 176), and methemoglobinemia (p 262) have been documented in victims of smoke inhalation.

IV. **Diagnosis** should be suspected in any patient brought from a fire, especially with facial burns, singed nasal hairs, carbonaceous deposits in the upper airways or in the sputum, or dyspnea.

   A. **Specific levels.** Carboxyhemoglobin, methemoglobin, and blood cyanide levels can be performed. Unfortunately, cyanide levels are not readily available with short turnaround time in most hospitals. Thus, the diagnosis may be empiric.

   B. **Other useful laboratory studies** include arterial blood gases or oximetry, chest x-ray, spirometry, or peak expiratory flow measurement. Arterial blood gases, pulse oximetry, and chest x-ray may reveal early evidence of chemical pneumonitis or pulmonary edema. However, arterial blood gases and pulse oximetry are *not* reliable in patients with carbon monoxide poisoning or methemoglobinemia.

**V. Treatment**

**A. Emergency and supportive measures**

1. Immediately assess the airway; hoarseness or stridor suggests laryngeal edema, which may necessitate direct laryngoscopy and endotracheal intubation if sufficient swelling is present (see p 4). Assist ventilation if necessary (p 5).
2. Administer high-flow supplemental oxygen by tight-fitting nonrebreather mask (see p 490).
3. Treat bronchospasm with aerosolized bronchodilators (see p 7).
4. Treat pulmonary edema if it occurs (see p 7).

**B. Specific drugs and antidotes**

1. **Carbon monoxide** poisoning. Provide 100% oxygen by mask or endotracheal tube. Consider hyperbaric oxygen (see p 490).
2. **Cyanide** poisoning. Empiric antidotal therapy with **sodium thiosulfate** (see p 514) and (if available) **hydroxocobalamin** (p 459) is recommended for patients with altered mental status, hypotension, or acidosis. Use of sodium nitrite is discouraged because it may cause hypotension and aggravate methemoglobinemia.
3. Treat **methemoglobinemia** with **methylene blue** (see p 473).

**C. Decontamination** (see p 47). Once the victim is removed from the smoke environment, further decontamination is not needed.

**D. Enhanced elimination.** Consider hyperbaric oxygen (see p 490) for carbon monoxide poisoning.

## ▶ SNAKEBITE

*Richard F. Clark, MD*

Among the 14 families of snakes, 5 are poisonous (Table II–54). The annual incidence of snakebite in the United States is three to four bites per 100,000 population. Clinically significant morbidity occurs in less than 60%, and only a few deaths are reported each year. Rattlesnake bite is the most common snake envenomation in the United States, and the victim is often a young intoxicated male who was teasing or trying to capture the snake. Snakes strike accurately to about one-third of their body length, with a maximum striking distance of a few feet.

**I. Mechanism of toxicity.** Snake venoms are complex mixtures of 50 or more components that function to immobilize, kill, and predigest prey. In human victims, these substances produce local "digestive" or cytotoxic effects on tissues as well as hemotoxic, neurotoxic, and other systemic effects. The relative predominance of cytotoxic, hemotoxic, and neurotoxic venom components depends on the species of the snake and geographic and seasonal variables.

**II. Toxic dose.** The potency of the venom and the amount of venom injected vary considerably. About 20% of all snake strikes are "dry" bites in which no venom is injected.

**III. Clinical presentation.** The most common snake envenomations in the United States are from rattlesnakes (Viperidae, subfamily Crotalinae). Bites from common North American Elapidae (eg, coral snakes) and Colubridae (eg, king snakes) are also discussed here. For information about bites from other exotic snakes, contact a regional poison control center ([800] 222-1222) for a specific consultation.

**A. Crotalinae.** Fang marks may look like puncture wounds or lacerations, with the latter resulting from a glancing blow by the snake or a sudden movement

**TABLE II–54. POISONOUS SNAKES (SELECTED)**

| Family and Genera | Common Name | Comments |
|---|---|---|
| **Colubridae** | | |
| *Lampropeltis* | King snake | Human envenomation difficult because of small mouth and small fixed fangs in the rear of mouth. Larger African species may cause severe systemic coagulopathy. |
| *Heterodon* | Hognose | |
| *Coluber* | Racer | |
| *Dispholidus* | Boomslang | |
| **Elapidae** | | |
| *Micrurus* | Coral snake | Human envenomation difficult because of small mouth and small fixed fangs in rear of mouth. Neurotoxicity usually predominates. |
| *Naja* | Cobra | |
| *Bungarus* | Krait | |
| *Dendroaspis* | Mamba | |
| **Hydrophidae** | Sea snakes | Also have small rear-located fangs. |
| **Viperidae, subfamily Crotalinae** | | |
| *Crotalus* | Rattlesnake | Most common envenomation in United States. Long rotating fangs in the front of the mouth. Heat-sensing facial pits (hence the name "pit vipers"). |
| *Agkistrodon* | Copperhead, cottonmouth | |
| *Bothrops* | Fer-de-lance | |
| **Viperidae, subfamily Viperinae** | | |
| *Bitis* | Puff adder, gaboon viper | Long rotating fangs in the front of the mouth but no heat-sensing facial pits. |
| *Cerastes* | Cleopatra's asp | |
| *Echis* | Saw-scaled viper | |

by the victim. The fangs often penetrate only a few millimeters but occasionally enter deeper tissue spaces or blood vessels. Signs and symptoms of toxicity are almost always apparent within 8–12 hours of envenomation.

1. **Local effects.** Within minutes of envenomation, stinging, burning pain begins. Progressive swelling, erythema, petechiae, ecchymosis, and hemorrhagic blebs may develop over the next several hours. The limb may swell to twice its normal size within the first few hours. Hypovolemic shock and local compartment syndrome may occur secondary to fluid and blood sequestration in injured areas.
2. **Systemic effects** may include nausea and vomiting, weakness, muscle fasciculations, diaphoresis, perioral and peripheral paresthesias, a metallic taste, thrombocytopenia, and coagulopathy. Circulating vasodilatory compounds may contribute to hypotension. Pulmonary edema and cardiovascular collapse have been reported.
3. **Mojave rattlesnake** (*Crotalus scutulatus*) bites merit special consideration and caution, because neurologic signs and symptoms of envenomation may be delayed and there is often little swelling or evidence of tissue damage. The onset of muscle weakness, ptosis, and respiratory arrest may occur several hours after envenomation. Facial and laryngeal edema has also been reported.

**B. Elapidae.** Coral snake envenomation is rare because of the snake's small mouth and fangs. The snake must hold on and "chew" the extremity for several seconds or more to work its fangs into the skin. The largest and most venomous coral snakes reside in the southeastern United States, where bites are more often severe when they occur.

1. **Local effects.** There is usually minimal swelling and inflammation around the fang marks. Local paresthesias may occur.
2. **Systemic effects.** Systemic symptoms usually occur within a few hours but may rarely be delayed 12 hours or more. Nausea and vomiting, confu-

sion, diplopia, dysarthria, muscle fasciculations, generalized muscle weakness, and respiratory arrest may occur.

C. **Colubridae.** These small-mouthed rear-fanged snakes must also hang on to their victims and "chew" the venom into the skin before significant envenomation can occur.

1. **Local effects.** There is usually little local reaction other than mild pain and paresthesias, although swelling of the extremity may occur.
2. **Systemic effects.** The most serious effect of envenomation is systemic coagulopathy, which can be fatal but is rare in all but a few African colubrids.

D. **Exotic species.** "Collectors" are increasingly importing exotic snake species into the United States. In some states, such as Florida, laws in the past permitted this practice. The most commonly found exotic species, such as cobras and mambas, are also elapids, but their bites probably will result in much larger venom injection than is the case with coral snakes. Symptoms may occur more rapidly and be more severe than those seen in coral snakebites, but the spectrum of toxicity may be similar. Neurologic signs and symptoms, progressing to respiratory arrest, may occur.

IV. **Diagnosis.** Correct diagnosis and treatment depend on proper identification of the offending snake, especially if more than one indigenous poisonous species or an exotic snake is involved.

A. Determine whether the bite was by an indigenous (wild) species or an exotic zoo animal or illegally imported pet. (The owner of an illegal pet snake may be reluctant to admit this for fear of fines or confiscation.) Envenomation occurring during the fall and winter months (October–March), when snakes usually hibernate, is not likely to be caused by a wild species.

B. If the snake is available, attempt to have it identified by a herpetologist. ***Caution:*** Accidental envenomation may occur even after the snake is dead.

C. **Specific levels.** These tests are not applicable.

D. **Other useful laboratory studies** include CBC, platelet count, prothrombin time (PT/INR), fibrin split products, fibrinogen, CPK, and urine dipstick for occult blood (positive with free myoglobin or hemoglobin). For severe envenomations with frank bleeding, hemolysis, or anticipated bleeding problems, obtain a blood type and screen early. If compromised respiratory function is suspected, closely monitor oximetry and arterial blood gases.

V. **Treatment**

A. **Emergency and supportive measures.** Regardless of the species, prepare for both local and systemic manifestations. Monitor patients closely for at least 6–8 hours after a typical crotaline bite and for at least 12–24 hours after a *C scutulatus* or an elapid bite.

1. **Local effects**
   a. **Monitor local swelling** at least hourly with measurements of limb girth, the presence and extent of local ecchymosis, and assessment of circulation.
   b. When indicated, obtain consultation with an experienced surgeon for management of serious wound complications. Do not perform fasciotomy unless compartment syndrome is documented with tissue compartment pressure monitoring.
   c. Provide tetanus prophylaxis if needed.
   d. Administer broad-spectrum antibiotics only if there are signs of infection.
2. **Systemic effects**
   a. **Monitor the victim for respiratory muscle weakness.** Maintain an open airway and assist ventilation if necessary (see pp 1–7). Administer supplemental oxygen.
   b. Treat bleeding complications with fresh-frozen plasma (and antivenom; see below). Treat hypotension with intravenous crystalloid fluids (see p 15) and rhabdomyolysis (p 26) with fluids and sodium bicarbonate.

B. **Specific drugs and antidotes.** For patients with documented envenomation, be prepared to administer specific **antivenom.** Virtually all local and systemic manifestations of envenomation improve after antivenom administration. ***Caution:*** Life-threatening anaphylactic reactions may occur with antivenom administration, even after a negative skin test.

1. For **rattlesnake** and other **Crotalinae** envenomations, fang marks, limb swelling, ecchymosis, and severe pain at the bite site are considered minimal indications for **antivenom** (see p 410). Progressive systemic manifestations such as generalized fasciculations, coagulopathy, and muscle weakness are indications for prompt and aggressive treatment. For a Mojave rattlesnake bite, the decision to administer antivenom is more difficult because there are few local signs of toxicity.
2. For **coral snake** envenomation, consult a regional poison control center ([800] 222-1222) or an experienced medical toxicologist to determine the advisability of ***Micrurus fulvius*** **antivenin** (see p 413). In general, if there is evidence of coagulopathy or neurologic toxicity, administer antivenom.
3. For **Colubridae** envenomations, there is no antivenom available.
4. For **other exotic snakes,** consult a regional poison control center ([800] 222-1222) for assistance in diagnosis, location of specific antivenom, and indications for administration. Many herpetologists in areas where exotic species are common may have private supplies of antivenom. Even if this supply is older than the expiration date on the package, it may be usable in severe cases.

C. **Decontamination.** First-aid measures are generally ineffective and may cause additional tissue damage.

1. Remain calm, remove the victim to at least 20 feet from the snake, wash the area with soap and water, and remove any constricting clothing or jewelry. Apply ice sparingly to the site (excessive ice application or immersion in ice water can lead to frostbite and aggravate tissue damage).
2. Loosely splint or immobilize the extremity near heart level. *Do **not** apply a tourniquet.*
3. Do ***not*** make cuts over the bite site.
4. If performed within 15 minutes, **suction** over the fang marks (ie, with a Sawyer extractor) may remove some venom, but this should not delay transport to a hospital. Suction devices have not been demonstrated to improve outcome, and studies suggest this therapy may increase tissue damage. Mouth suction of the wound is not advised.

D. **Enhanced elimination.** Dialysis, hemoperfusion, and charcoal administration are not applicable.

## ▶ SPIDERS

*Jeffrey R. Suchard, MD*

Many thousands of spider species are found worldwide, and nearly all possess poison glands connected to fangs in the large, paired jaw-like structures known as chelicerae. Fortunately, only a very few spiders have fangs long and tough enough to pierce human skin. In the United States, these spiders include ***Latrodectus*** (black widow) and ***Loxosceles*** (brown spider) species, **tarantulas** (a common name given to several large spider species), and a few others.

Patient complaints of "spider bites" occur much more commonly than do actual spider bites. Unexplained skin lesions, especially those with a necrotic component, often areascribed to spiders, especially the brown recluse spider. Health-care providers should consider alternative etiologies in the absence of a convincing clinical history and presentation. Many alleged "spider bites" are actually infections, with community-acquired methicillin-resistant *Staphylococcus aureus* (MRSA) being a common etiology.

***Latrodectus*** species (black widow spiders) are ubiquitous in the continental United States, and the female can cause serious envenomations with rare fatalities. Black widows construct their chaotic webs in dark places, often near human habitation in garages, wood piles, outdoor toilets, and patio furniture. The spider has a body size of 1–2 cm and is characteristically shiny black with a red hourglass shape on the ventral abdomen. Related species or immature specimens may have brown, red, or orange markings or have irregular markings on a black body.

***Loxosceles reclusa*** (the brown recluse spider) is found only in the central and southeastern United States (eg, Missouri, Kansas, Arkansas, and Tennessee). Rare individual specimens have been found in other areas, but they represent stowaways on shipments from endemic areas. Other *Loxosceles* species may be found in the desert southwest, although they tend to cause less serious envenomations. The spider's nocturnal hunting habits and reclusive temperament result in infrequent contact with humans, and bites are generally defensive in nature. The spider is 1–3 cm in length and light to dark brown in color, with a characteristic violin- or fiddle-shaped marking on the dorsum of the cephalothorax.

**Tarantulas** rarely cause significant envenomation but can produce a painful bite because of their large size. Tarantulas also bear urticating hairs that they can flick at predators and that cause intense mucosal irritation. People who keep pet tarantulas have developed ophthalmia nodosa when these hairs embed in their corneas, usually while they are cleaning their spiders' cages.

**I. Mechanism of toxicity.** Spiders use their hollow fangs (chelicerae) to inject their venoms, which contain various protein and polypeptide toxins that are poorly characterized but appear to be designed to induce rapid paralysis of the insect victim and aid in digestion.

**A. *Latrodectus*** (black widow) spider venom contains *alpha-latrotoxin,* which causes opening of nonspecific cation channels, leading to an increased influx of calcium and indiscriminate release of acetylcholine (at the motor endplate) and norepinephrine.

**B. *Loxosceles*** (brown spiders) venom contains a variety of digestive enzymes and sphingomyelinase D, which is cytotoxic and chemotactically attracts white blood cells to the bite site and also has a role in producing systemic symptoms such as hemolysis.

**II. Toxic dose.** Spider venoms are generally extremely potent toxins (far more potent than most snake venoms), but the delivered dose is extremely small. The size of the victim may be an important variable.

**III. Clinical presentation.** Manifestations of envenomation are quite different depending on the species.

**A. *Latrodectus*** (black widow) bites may produce local signs ranging from mild erythema to a target lesion with a central punctate site, central blanching, and an outer erythematous ring.

1. The bite is often initially painful but may go unnoticed. It almost always becomes painful within 30–120 minutes. By 3–4 hours, painful cramping and muscle fasciculations occur in the involved extremity. This cramping progresses centripetally toward the chest, back, or abdomen and can produce board-like rigidity, weakness, dyspnea, headache, and paresthesias. Black widow envenomation may mimic myocardial infarction or an acute surgical abdomen. Symptoms often persist for 1–2 days.
2. Additional common symptoms may include hypertension, regional diaphoresis, restlessness, nausea, vomiting, and tachycardia.
3. Other, less common symptoms include leukocytosis, fever, delirium, arrhythmias, and paresthesias. Rarely, hypertensive crisis or respiratory arrest may occur after severe envenomation, mainly in very young or very old victims.

**B. *Loxosceles*** bites are best known for causing slowly healing skin ulcers, a syndrome often called "necrotic arachnidism."

1. Envenomation usually produces a painful burning sensation at the bite site within 10 minutes but can be delayed. Over the next 1–12 hours, a "bull's-

eye" lesion forms, consisting of a blanched ring enclosed by a ring of ecchymosis. The entire lesion can range from 1–5 cm in diameter. Over the next 24–72 hours, an indolent necrotic ulcer develops that may take a month or more to heal. However, in most cases, necrosis is limited and healing occurs rapidly.

2. Systemic illness may occur in the first 24–48 hours and does not necessarily correlate with the severity of the ulcer. Systemic manifestations include fever, chills, malaise, nausea, and myalgias. Rarely, intravascular hemolysis and disseminated intravascular coagulopathy may occur.

C. **Other spiders.** Bites from most other spider species are of minimal clinical consequence. As with many arthropod bites, a self-limited local inflammatory reaction may occur, and any break in the skin may become secondarily infected. Bites from a few species can cause systemic symptoms (myalgias, arthralgias, headache, nausea, vomiting) or have been reported to cause necrotic ulcers (eg, *Phidippus* spp and *Tegenaria agrestis*).

IV. **Diagnosis** most commonly is based on the characteristic clinical presentation. Bite marks of all spiders but the tarantulas are usually too small to be easily visualized, and victims may not recall feeling the bite or seeing the spider. Spiders (especially the brown recluse) have bad reputations that far exceed their actual danger to humans, and patients may ascribe a wide variety of skin lesions and other problems to spider bites. Many other arthropods and insects also produce small puncture wounds, pain, itching, redness, swelling, and even necrotic ulcers. Arthropods that seek blood meals from mammals are more likely to bite humans than are spiders. Several other medical conditions can cause necrotic skin ulcers, including bacterial, viral, and fungal infections and vascular, dermatologic, and even factitious disorders. Thus, any prospective diagnosis of "brown recluse spider bite" requires careful scrutiny. Unless the patient gives a reliable eyewitness history, brings the offending animal for identification (not just any spider found around the home), or exhibits systemic manifestations clearly demonstrating spider envenomation, the evidence is circumstantial at best.

A. **Specific levels.** Serum toxin detection is used experimentally but is not commercially available.

B. **Other useful laboratory studies**

1. ***Latrodectus.*** Electrolytes, calcium, glucose, CPK, and ECG (for chest pain).

2. ***Loxosceles.*** CBC, BUN, and creatinine. If hemolysis is suspected, haptoglobin and urine dipstick for occult blood (positive with free hemoglobin) are useful; repeat daily for 1–2 days.

V. **Treatment**

A. **Emergency and supportive measures**

1. **General**

a. Cleanse the wound and apply cool compresses or intermittent ice packs. Treat infection if it occurs.

b. Give tetanus prophylaxis if indicated.

2. ***Latrodectus* envenomation**

a. Monitor victims for at least 6–8 hours. Because symptoms typically wax and wane, patients may appear to benefit from any therapy offered.

b. Maintain an open airway and assist ventilation if necessary (see pp 1–7), and treat severe hypertension (p 17) if it occurs.

3. ***Loxosceles* envenomation**

a. Admit patients with systemic symptoms and monitor for hemolysis, renal failure, and other complications.

b. The usual approach to wound care in cases of necrotic arachnidism is watchful waiting. The majority of these lesions will heal with minimal intervention over the course of a few weeks. Standard wound care measures are indicated, and secondary infections should be treated with antibiotics if they occur. Surgical debridement and skin grafting may be indicated for large and/or very slowly healing wounds; however, prophylactic early surgical excision of the bite site is not recommended.

**B. Specific drugs and antidotes**

1. ***Latrodectus***
   - **a.** Most patients will benefit from opiate analgesics such as **morphine** (see p 476) and often are admitted for 24–48 hours for pain control in serious cases.
   - **b.** Muscle cramping has been treated with **intravenous calcium** (see p 428) or muscle relaxants such as **methocarbamol** (p 472). However, these therapies are often ineffective when used alone.
   - **c.** Equine-derived antivenin (**antivenin *Latrodectus mactans;*** see p 412) is rapidly effective but infrequently used because symptomatic therapy is often adequate and because of the small risk of anaphylaxis. It may still be indicated for seriously ill, elderly, or pediatric patients who do not respond to conventional therapy for hypertension, muscle cramping, or respiratory distress and for pregnant victims threatening premature labor.
2. ***Loxosceles.*** Therapy for necrotic arachnidism has been difficult to evaluate because of the inherent difficulty of accurate diagnosis.
   - **a.** Dapsone has shown some promise in reducing the severity of necrotic ulcers in anecdotal case reports but has not been effective in controlled animal models.
   - **b.** Steroids usually are not recommended.
   - **c.** A goat-derived antivenin has been studied but is not FDA-approved or commercially available.
   - **d.** Hyperbaric oxygen has been proposed for significant necrotic ulcers, but results from animal studies are equivocal, and insufficient data exist to recommend its use.

**C. Decontamination.** These measures are not applicable. There is no proven value in the sometimes popular early excision of *Loxosceles* bites to prevent necrotic ulcer formation.

**D. Enhanced elimination.** These procedures are not applicable.

## ▶ STRYCHNINE

*Saralyn R. Williams, MD*

Strychnine is an alkaloid derived from the seeds of a tree, *Strychnos nux-vomica.* At one time strychnine was an ingredient in a variety of over-the-counter tonics and laxatives. Strychnine no longer is used in pharmaceuticals; however, it is still available as a rodenticide and sometimes is found as an adulterant in illicit drugs such as cocaine and heroin.

**I. Mechanism of toxicity**

**A.** Strychnine competitively antagonizes the binding of glycine, an inhibitory neurotransmitter released by postsynaptic inhibitory neurons in the spinal cord. This causes increased neuronal excitability and exaggerated reflex arcs, resulting in generalized seizure-like contraction of skeletal muscles. Simultaneous contraction of opposing flexor and extensor muscles causes severe muscle injury, with rhabdomyolysis, myoglobinuria, and, in some cases, acute renal failure.

**B. Pharmacokinetics.** Strychnine is absorbed rapidly after ingestion or nasal inhalation and distributed rapidly into the tissues. The volume of distribution is very large (Vd = 13 L/kg). Elimination is by hepatic metabolism via first-order kinetics, with a half-life of about 10–16 hours after overdose.

**II. Toxic dose.** A toxic threshold dose is difficult to establish, although 16 mg was fatal in an adult in one case. Manifestations of toxicity can occur rapidly, and since management decisions are based on clinical findings rather than on a history of ingested amounts, any dose of strychnine should be considered life threatening.

**III. Clinical presentation.** Symptoms and signs usually develop within 15–30 minutes of ingestion and may last several hours.

**A.** Muscular stiffness and painful cramps precede generalized muscle contractions, extensor muscle spasms, and opisthotonus. The face may be drawn into a forced grimace ("sardonic grin," or *risus sardonicus*). Muscle contractions are intermittent and are easily triggered by emotional or minimal physical stimuli. Repeated and prolonged muscle contractions often result in hyperthermia, rhabdomyolysis, myoglobinuria, and renal failure.

**B.** Muscle spasms may resemble the tonic phase of a grand mal seizure, but strychnine does not cause true convulsions, as its target area is the spinal cord, not the brain. The patient is usually awake and painfully aware of the contractions.

**C.** Victims may also experience hyperacusis, hyperalgesia, and increased visual stimulation. Sudden noises or other sensory input may trigger muscle contractions.

**D.** Death usually is caused by respiratory arrest that results from intense contraction of the respiratory muscles. Death may also be secondary to hyperthermia or rhabdomyolysis and renal failure.

**IV. Diagnosis** is based on a history of ingestion of a rodenticide or recent intravenous drug abuse and the presence of seizure-like generalized muscle contractions, often accompanied by hyperthermia, lactic acidosis, and rhabdomyolysis (with myoglobinuria and elevated CPK). In the differential diagnosis (see Table I–16, p 26), one should consider other causes of generalized muscle rigidity such as a black widow spider bite (p 347), neuroleptic malignant syndrome (p 21), and tetanus (see p 353).

**A. Specific levels.** Strychnine can be measured in the gastric fluid, urine, or blood. The toxic serum concentration is reported to be 1 mg/L, although in general, blood levels do not correlate well with the severity of toxicity.

**B. Other useful laboratory studies** include electrolytes, BUN, creatinine, CPK, arterial blood gases or oximetry, and urine test for occult blood (positive in the presence of urine myoglobinuria).

**V. Treatment**

**A. Emergency and supportive measures**

1. Maintain an open airway and assist ventilation if necessary (see pp 1–7).
2. Treat hyperthermia (see p 20), metabolic acidosis (p 33), and rhabdomyolysis (p 26) if they occur.
3. Limit external stimuli such as noise, light, and touch.
4. **Treat muscle spasms** aggressively.
   a. Administer **diazepam** (see p 419), 0.1–0.2 mg/kg IV, or **midazolam,** 0.05–0.1 mg/kg IV, to patients with mild muscle contractions. Give **morphine** (p 476) for pain relief. ***Note:*** These agents may impair respiratory drive.
   b. In more severe cases, use **pancuronium,** 0.06–0.1 mg/kg IV, or another nondepolarizing neuromuscular blocker (see p 480) to produce complete neuromuscular paralysis. ***Caution:*** Neuromuscular paralysis will cause respiratory arrest; patients will need endotracheal intubation and assisted ventilation.

**B. Specific drugs and antidotes.** There is no specific antidote.

**C. Decontamination** (see p 45). Administer activated charcoal orally if conditions are appropriate (see Table I–38, p 51). Do ***not*** induce vomiting because of the risk of aggravating muscle spasms. Gastric lavage is not necessary after small to moderate ingestions if activated charcoal can be given promptly.

**D. Enhanced elimination.** Symptoms usually abate within several hours and can be managed effectively with intensive supportive care. Hemodialysis and hemoperfusion have not been beneficial for enhancing the clearance of strychnine. The use of repeat-dose activated charcoal has not been studied.

## ▶ SULFUR DIOXIDE

*John Balmes, MD*

Sulfur dioxide is a colorless nonflammable gas formed by the burning of materials that contain sulfur. It is a major air pollutant from automobiles, smelters, and plants that burn soft coal or oils with a high sulfur content. It is soluble in water to form sulfurous acid, which may be oxidized to sulfuric acid; both are components of acid rain. Occupational exposures to sulfur dioxide occur in ore and metal refining, chemical manufacturing, and wood pulp treatment and in its use as a disinfectant, refrigerant, and dried-food preservative.

I. **Mechanism of toxicity.** Sulfur dioxide is an irritant because it rapidly forms sulfurous acid on contact with moist mucous membranes. Most effects occur in the upper respiratory tract because 90% of inhaled sulfur dioxide is deposited rapidly there, but with very large exposures sufficient gas reaches the lower airways to cause chemical pneumonitis and pulmonary edema.

II. **Toxic dose.** The sharp odor or taste of sulfur dioxide is noticed at 1–5 ppm. Throat and conjunctival irritation begins at 8–12 ppm and is severe at 50 ppm. The ACGIH-recommended workplace permissible limit (TLV-TWA) is 2 ppm (5.2 mg/m$^3$) as an 8-hour time-weighted average, the short-term exposure limit (STEL) is 5 ppm (13 mg/m$^3$), and the air level considered immediately dangerous to life or health (IDLH) is 100 ppm. Persons with asthma may experience bronchospasm with brief exposure to 0.5–1 ppm.

III. **Clinical presentation**
   - A. **Acute exposure** causes burning of the eyes, nose, and throat; lacrimation; and cough. Laryngospasm may occur. Wheezing may be seen in normal subjects as well as asthmatics. Chemical bronchitis is not uncommon. With a very high-level exposure, chemical pneumonitis and noncardiogenic pulmonary edema may occur.
   - B. **Asthma and chronic bronchitis** may be exacerbated.
   - C. **Sulfhemoglobinemia** resulting from absorption of sulfur has been reported.
   - D. **Frostbite** injury to the skin may occur from exposure to liquid sulfur dioxide.

IV. **Diagnosis** is based on a history of exposure and the presence of airway and mucous membrane irritation. Symptoms usually occur rapidly after exposure.
   - A. **Specific levels.** Blood levels are not available.
   - B. **Other useful laboratory studies** include arterial blood gases or oximetry, chest x-ray, and spirometry or peak expiratory flow rate.

V. **Treatment**
   - A. **Emergency and supportive measures**
     1. Remain alert for progressive upper-airway edema or obstruction and be prepared to intubate the trachea and assist ventilation if necessary (see pp 1–7).
     2. Administer humidified oxygen, treat wheezing with bronchodilators (see p 7), and observe the victim for at least 4–6 hours for development of pulmonary edema (p 7).
   - B. **Specific drugs and antidotes.** There is no specific antidote.
   - C. **Decontamination**
     1. **Inhalation.** Remove the victim from exposure and give supplemental oxygen if available.
     2. **Skin and eyes.** Wash exposed skin and eyes with copious tepid water or saline. Treat frostbite injury as for thermal burns.
   - D. **Enhanced elimination.** There is no role for these procedures.

# ▶ TETANUS

*Karl A. Sporer, MD*

Tetanus is a rare disease in the United States. In 2002, only 2 cases were reported in the United States, none in Canada, and 101 in Mexico. It is caused by an exotoxin produced by *Clostridium tetani,* an anaerobic, spore-forming, gram-positive rod found widely in soil and in the GI tract. Tetanus typically is seen in older persons (especially older women), recent immigrants, and intravenous drug users who have not maintained adequate tetanus immunization.

**I. Mechanism of toxicity.** The growth of *C tetani* in a wound under anaerobic conditions produces the toxin tetanospasmin. The toxin enters the myoneural junction of alpha motor neurons and travels by retrograde axonal transport to the synapse. There it blocks the release of the presynaptic inhibitory neurotransmitters GABA and glycine, causing intense muscular spasms.

**II. Toxic dose.** Tetanospasmin is an extremely potent toxin. Fatal tetanus can result from a minor puncture wound in a susceptible individual.

**III. Clinical presentation.** The incubation period between the initial wound and the development of symptoms averages 1–2 weeks (range 2–56 days). The wound is not apparent in about 5% of cases. Wound cultures are positive for *C tetani* only about one-third of the time.

- **A.** The most common initial complaint is pain and stiffness of the jaw, progressing to trismus, *risus sardonicus,* and opisthotonus over several days. Uncontrollable and painful reflex spasms involving all muscle groups are precipitated by minimal stimuli and can result in fractures, rhabdomyolysis, hyperpyrexia, and asphyxia. The patient remains awake during the spasms. In survivors, the spasms may persist for days or weeks.
- **B.** A syndrome of sympathetic hyperactivity often accompanies the muscular manifestations, with hypertension, tachycardia, arrhythmias, and diaphoresis that in some reports alternate with hypotension and bradycardia.
- **C.** Neonatal tetanus occurs frequently in developing countries as a result of inadequate maternal immunity and poor hygiene, especially around the necrotic umbilical stump. Localized tetanus has been reported, involving rigidity and spasm only in the affected limb. Cephalic tetanus is uncommonly associated with head wounds and involves primarily the cranial nerves.

**IV. Diagnosis** is based on the finding of characteristic muscle spasms in an awake person with a wound and an inadequate immunization history. Strychnine poisoning (see p 348) produces identical muscle spasms and should be considered in the differential diagnosis. Other considerations include hypocalcemia and dystonic reactions.

- **A. Specific levels.** There are no specific toxin assays. A serum antibody level of 0.01 IU/mL or greater suggests prior immunity and makes the diagnosis less likely.
- **B. Other useful laboratory studies** include electrolytes, glucose, calcium, BUN, creatinine, CPK, arterial blood gases, and urine dipstick for occult blood (positive with myoglobinuria).

**V. Treatment**

- **A. Emergency and supportive measures**
  1. Maintain an open airway and assist ventilation if necessary (see pp 1–7).
  2. Treat hyperthermia (see p 20), arrhythmias (pp 10–15), metabolic acidosis (p 33), and rhabdomyolysis (p 26) if they occur.
  3. Limit external stimuli such as noise, light, and touch.
  4. **Treat muscle spasms** aggressively:
     - **a.** Administer **diazepam** (see p 419), 0.1–0.2 mg/kg IV, or **midazolam,** 0.05–0.1 mg/kg IV, to patients with mild muscle contractions. Give **morphine** (see p 476) for pain relief. ***Note:*** These agents may impair respiratory drive.

b. In more severe cases, use **pancuronium,** 0.06–0.1 mg/kg IV, or another neuromuscular blocker (see p 480) to produce complete neuromuscular paralysis. ***Caution:*** Neuromuscular paralysis will cause respiratory arrest; patients will need endotracheal intubation and assisted ventilation.

**B. Specific drugs and antidotes**

1. **Human tetanus immune globulin** (TIG), 3000–5000 IU administered IM, will neutralize circulating toxin but has no effect on toxin that already is fixed to neurons. TIG should be given as early as possible to a patient with suspected tetanus and to persons with a fresh wound but possibly inadequate prior immunization. Use of TIG has not decreased mortality but may decrease the severity and duration of disease.
2. **Prevention** can be ensured by an adequate immunization series with tetanus toxoid in childhood and repeated boosters at 10-year intervals. Survival of tetanus may not protect against future exposures, because the small amount of toxin required to cause disease is inadequate to confer immunity.

**C. Decontamination.** Thoroughly debride and irrigate the wound and administer appropriate antibiotics (penicillin is adequate for *C tetani*).

**D. Enhanced elimination.** There is no role for these procedures.

# ▶ THALLIUM

*Thomas J. Ferguson, MD, PhD*

Thallium is a soft metal that quickly oxidizes upon exposure to air. It is a minor constituent in a variety of ores. Thallium salts are used in the manufacture of jewelry, semiconductors, and optical devices. Thallium no longer is used in the United States as a depilatory or a rodenticide because of its high human toxicity.

**I. Mechanism of toxicity.** The mechanism of thallium toxicity is not known. It appears to affect a variety of enzyme systems, resulting in generalized cellular poisoning. Thallium metabolism has some similarities to that of potassium, and it may inhibit potassium flux across biologic membranes by binding to Na-K ATP transport enzymes.

**II. Toxic dose.** The minimum lethal dose of thallium salts is probably 12–15 mg/kg, although toxicity varies widely with the compound, and there have been reports of death after adult ingestion of as little as 200 mg. The more water-soluble salts (eg, thallous acetate and thallic chloride) are slightly more toxic than the less soluble forms (thallic oxide and thallous iodide). Some thallium salts are well absorbed across intact skin.

**III. Clinical presentation.** Symptoms do not occur immediately but are typically delayed 12–14 hours after ingestion.

**A. Acute effects** include abdominal pain, nausea, vomiting, and diarrhea (sometimes with hemorrhage). Shock may result from massive fluid or blood loss. Within 2–3 days, delirium, seizures, respiratory failure, and death may occur.

**B. Chronic effects** include painful peripheral neuropathy, myopathy, chorea, stomatitis, and ophthalmoplegia. Hair loss and nail dystrophy (Mees' lines) may appear after 2–4 weeks.

**IV. Diagnosis.** Thallotoxicosis should be considered when gastroenteritis and painful paresthesia are followed by alopecia.

**A. Specific levels.** Urinary thallium is normally less than 0.8 mcg/L. Concentrations higher than 20 mcg/L provide evidence of excessive exposure and may be associated with subclinical toxicity during workplace exposures. Blood thallium levels are not considered reliable measures of exposure except after large exposures. Hair levels are of limited value, used mainly in documenting past exposure and in forensic cases.

B. **Other useful laboratory studies** include CBC, electrolytes, glucose, BUN, creatinine, and hepatic transaminases. Since thallium is radiopaque, plain abdominal x-rays may be useful after acute ingestion.

V. **Treatment**

A. **Emergency and supportive measures**

1. Maintain an open airway and assist ventilation if necessary (see pp 1–7).
2. Treat seizures (see p 22) and coma (p 18) if they occur.
3. Treat gastroenteritis with aggressive intravenous replacement of fluids (and blood if needed). Use pressors only if shock does not respond to fluid therapy (see p 15).

B. **Specific drugs and antidotes.** There is currently no recommended specific treatment in the United States.

1. **Prussian blue** (ferric ferrocyanide) is the mainstay of therapy in Europe and received FDA approval for use in the United States in 2003. This compound has a crystal lattice structure that binds thallium ions and interrupts enterohepatic recycling. Insoluble Prussian blue (Radiogardase) is available as 500-mg tablets, and the recommended adult dose is 3 g orally three times per day. Prussian blue appears to be nontoxic at these doses. In the United States, Prussian blue should be available through pharmaceutical suppliers, and an emergency supply may be available through Oak Ridge Associated Universities ([865] 576-3131 or [865] 576-1005, the Operation Center Oak Ridge/REACTS 24-hour phone line). Radiogardase is manufactured by HEYL Chemisch-pharmazeutische Fabrik GmbH & Co. KG in Berlin, Germany.
2. **Activated charcoal** is readily available and has been shown to bind thallium in vitro. Multiple-dose charcoal is recommended because thallium apparently undergoes enterohepatic recirculation. In one study, charcoal was shown to be superior to Prussian blue in eliminating thallium.
3. **BAL** (see p 417) and other chelators have been tried with varying success. Penicillamine and diethyldithiocarbamate should be avoided because of studies suggesting that they contribute to redistribution of thallium to the brain.

C. **Decontamination** (see p 45). Administer activated charcoal orally if conditions are appropriate (see Table I–38, p 51). Ipecac-induced vomiting may be useful for initial treatment at the scene (eg, children at home) if it can be given within a few minutes of exposure. Consider gastric lavage for large recent ingestions.

D. **Enhanced elimination.** Repeat-dose activated charcoal may enhance fecal elimination by binding thallium secreted into the gut lumen or via the biliary system, interrupting enterohepatic or enteroenteric recirculation. Forced diuresis, dialysis, and hemoperfusion are of no proven benefit.

## ▶ THEOPHYLLINE

*Kent R. Olson, MD*

Theophylline is a methylxanthine that once was used widely for the treatment of asthma. Intravenous infusions of aminophylline, the ethylenediamine salt of theophylline, are used to treat bronchospasm, congestive heart failure, and neonatal apnea. Theophylline most commonly is used orally in sustained-release preparations (Theo-Dur™, Slo-Phyllin™, Theo-24™, and many others).

I. **Mechanism of toxicity**

A. The exact mechanism of toxicity is not known. Theophylline is an antagonist of adenosine receptors, and it inhibits phosphodiesterase at high levels, increasing intracellular cyclic adenosine monophosphate (cAMP). It also is known to release endogenous catecholamines at therapeutic concentrations and may stimulate beta-adrenergic receptors.

B. **Pharmacokinetics.** Absorption may be delayed with sustained-release preparations. The volume of distribution is approximately 0.5 L/kg. The normal elimination half-life is 4–6 hours; this may be doubled by illnesses or interacting drugs that slow hepatic metabolism, such as liver disease, congestive heart failure, influenza, erythromycin, and cimetidine, and may increase to as much as 20 hours after overdose. (See also Table II–59, p 382.)

II. **Toxic dose.** An acute single dose of 8–10 mg/kg could raise the serum level by up to 15–20 mg/L, depending on the rate of absorption. Acute oral overdose of more than 50 mg/kg may potentially result in a level above 100 mg/L and severe toxicity.

III. **Clinical presentation.** Two distinct syndromes of intoxication may occur, depending on whether the exposure is **acute** or **chronic.**

A. **Acute single overdose** is usually a result of a suicide attempt or accidental childhood ingestion but also may be caused by accidental or iatrogenic misuse (therapeutic overdose).

1. Usual manifestations include vomiting (sometimes with hematemesis), tremor, anxiety, and tachycardia. Metabolic effects include pronounced hypokalemia, hypophosphatemia, hyperglycemia, and metabolic acidosis.
2. With serum levels above 90–100 mg/L, hypotension, ventricular arrhythmias, and seizures are common; status epilepticus is frequently resistant to anticonvulsant drugs.
3. Seizures and other manifestations of severe toxicity may be delayed 12–16 hours or more after ingestion, in part owing to delayed absorption of drug from sustained-release preparations.

B. **Chronic intoxication** occurs when excessive doses are administered repeatedly over 24 hours or longer or when intercurrent illness or an interacting drug interferes with the hepatic metabolism of theophylline. The usual victims are very young infants and elderly patients, especially those with chronic obstructive lung disease.

1. Vomiting may occur but is not as common as in acute overdose. Tachycardia is common, but hypotension is rare. Metabolic effects such as hypokalemia and hyperglycemia do not occur.
2. Seizures may occur with lower serum levels (eg, 40–60 mg/L) and have been reported with levels as low as 20 mg/L.

IV. **Diagnosis** is based on a history of ingestion or the presence of tremor, tachycardia, and other manifestations in a patient known to be on theophylline. Hypokalemia strongly suggests an acute overdose rather than chronic intoxication.

A. **Specific levels.** Serum theophylline levels are essential for diagnosis and determination of emergency treatment. After acute oral overdose, obtain repeated levels every 2–4 hours; single determinations are not sufficient, because continued absorption from sustained-release preparations may result in peak levels 12–16 hours or longer after ingestion.

1. Levels less than 90–100 mg/L after acute overdose usually are not associated with severe symptoms such as seizures and ventricular arrhythmias.
2. However, with chronic intoxication, severe toxicity may occur with levels of 40–60 mg/L. ***Note:*** Acute caffeine overdose (see p 142) will cause a similar clinical picture and produce falsely elevated theophylline concentrations with most commercial immunoassays.

B. **Other useful laboratory studies** include electrolytes, glucose, BUN, creatinine, hepatic function tests, and ECG monitoring.

V. **Treatment**

A. **Emergency and supportive measures**

1. Maintain an open airway and assist ventilation if necessary (see pp 1–7).
2. Treat seizures (see p 22), arrhythmias (pp 12–15), and hypotension (p 15) if they occur. Tachyarrhythmias and hypotension are best treated with a beta-adrenergic agent (see B, below).

3. Hypokalemia is caused by intracellular movement of potassium and does not reflect a significant total body deficit; it usually resolves spontaneously without aggressive treatment.
4. Monitor vital signs, ECG, and serial theophylline levels for at least 16–18 hours after a significant oral overdose.

B. **Specific drugs and antidotes.** Hypotension, tachycardia, and ventricular arrhythmias are caused primarily by excessive beta-adrenergic stimulation. Treat with low-dose **propranolol** (see p 504), 0.01–0.03 mg/kg IV, or **esmolol** (see p 449), 0.025–0.05 mg/kg/min. Use beta blockers cautiously in patients with a prior history of asthma or wheezing.

C. **Decontamination** (see p 45). Administer activated charcoal orally if conditions are appropriate (see Table I–38, p 51). Gastric lavage is not necessary after small to moderate ingestions if activated charcoal can be given promptly. Consider the use of repeated doses of activated charcoal and whole-bowel irrigation after a large ingestion of a sustained-released formulation.

D. **Enhanced elimination** (see p 53). Theophylline has a small volume of distribution (0.5 L/kg) and is efficiently removed by hemodialysis, charcoal hemoperfusion, or repeat-dose activated charcoal.
1. **Hemodialysis** or **hemoperfusion** should be performed if the patient is in status epilepticus or if the serum theophylline concentration is greater than 100 mg/L.
2. **Repeat-dose activated charcoal** (see p 50) is not as effective but may be used for stable patients with levels below 100 mg/L.

# ▶ THYROID HORMONE

*F. Lee Cantrell, PharmD*

Thyroid hormone is available in the synthetic forms triiodothyronine ($T_3$, or liothyronine), tetraiodothyronine ($T_4$, levothyroxine), and liotrix (both $T_3$ and $T_4$) and as natural desiccated animal thyroid (both $T_3$ and $T_4$; Table II–55). Despite concern about the potentially life-threatening manifestations of thyrotoxicosis, serious toxicity rarely occurs after acute thyroid hormone ingestion.

I. **Mechanism of toxicity.** Excessive thyroid hormone potentiates adrenergic activity in the cardiovascular, GI, and neurologic systems. The effects of $T_3$ overdose are manifested within the first 6 hours after ingestion. In contrast, symptoms of $T_4$ overdose may be delayed 2–5 days after ingestion while metabolic conversion to $T_3$ occurs.

II. **Toxic dose**

A. An acute ingestion of more than 5 mg of **levothyroxine** ($T_4$) or 0.75 mg of **triiodothyronine** ($T_3$) is considered potentially toxic. An adult has survived an ingestion of 48 g of unspecified thyroid tablets; a 15-month-old child had moderate symptoms after ingesting 1.5 g of desiccated thyroid.

B. Euthyroid adults and children appear to have a high tolerance to the effects of an acute overdose. Patients with preexisting cardiac disease and those with chronic overmedication have a lower threshold of toxicity. Sudden deaths have been reported after chronic thyroid hormone abuse in healthy adults.

**TABLE II–55. THYROID HORMONE: DOSAGE EQUIVALENTS**

| | |
|---|---|
| Dessicated animal thyroid | 65 mg (1 grain) |
| Thyroxine ($T_4$, levothyroxine) | 0.1 mg (100 mcg) |
| Triiodothyronine ($T_3$) | 0.025 mg (25 mcg) |

**III. Clinical presentation.** The effects of an acute $T_4$ overdose may not be evident for several days because of a delay in the metabolism of $T_4$ to the more active $T_3$.

**A. Mild to moderate intoxication** may cause sinus tachycardia, elevated temperature, flushing, diarrhea, vomiting, headache, anxiety, agitation, psychosis, and confusion.

**B. Severe toxicity** may include supraventricular tachycardia, hyperthermia, and hypotension. There is one case report of a seizure after an acute overdose.

**IV. Diagnosis** is based on a history of ingestion and signs and symptoms of increased sympathetic activity.

**A. Specific levels.** Elevated $T_4$ and $T_3$ concentrations do not correlate well with the risk of developing clinical symptoms and are therefore of minimal use in the overdose setting.

**B. Other useful laboratory studies** include electrolytes, glucose, BUN, creatinine, and ECG monitoring.

**V. Treatment**

**A. Emergency and supportive measures**

1. Maintain an open airway and assist ventilation if necessary (see pp 1–7).
2. Treat seizures (see p 22), hyperthermia (p 20), hypotension (p 15), and arrhythmias (pp 10–15) if they occur.
3. Repeated evaluation over several days is recommended after large $T_4$ or combined ingestions, because serious symptoms may be delayed.
4. Most patients will suffer no serious toxicity or will recover with simple supportive care.

**B. Specific drugs and antidotes**

1. Treat serious tachyarrhythmias with **propranolol** (see p 504), 0.01–0.1 mg/kg IV repeated every 2–5 minutes to the desired effect, or **esmolol** (see p 449), 0.025–0.1 mg/kg/min IV. Simple sinus tachycardia may be treated with oral propranolol, 0.1–0.5 mg/kg every 4–6 hours.
2. In cases of massive $T_4$ ingestion, peripheral metabolic conversion of $T_4$ to $T_3$ can be inhibited by **propylthiouracil,** 6–10 mg/kg/day (maximum 1 g) divided into three oral doses for 5–7 days, or **iopanoic acid,** 125 mg/day orally for up to 6 days.

**C. Decontamination** (see p 45). Administer activated charcoal orally if conditions are appropriate (see Table I–38, p 51). Gastric lavage is not necessary after small to moderate ingestions if activated charcoal can be given promptly.

**D. Enhanced elimination.** Diuresis and hemodialysis are not useful because thyroid hormones are extensively protein bound. Treatment with charcoal hemoperfusion, plasmapheresis, and exchange transfusion has been employed but did not appear to influence clinical outcome.

## ▶ TOLUENE AND XYLENE

*Janet Weiss, MD*

Toluene (methylbenzene, methyl benzol, phenyl methane, toluol) and xylene (dimethylbenzene, methyl toluene, and xylol) are very common aromatic solvents that are used widely in glues, inks, dyes, lacquers, varnishes, paints, paint removers, pesticides, cleaners, and degreasers. The largest source of exposure is the production and use of gasoline. They are clear, colorless volatile liquids with a sweet, pungent odor. They have good warning properties in that the odor threshold of xylene is about 1 ppm, which is 100 times less than the OSHA PEL, and the odor threshold of toluene is 8 ppm, which is 25 times less than the OSHA PEL. They are less dense than water and readily produce flammable and toxic concentrations at room temperature. The vapor is heavier than air and may accumulate in low-lying areas. Toluene frequently is abused intentionally by inhaling lacquer thinner and paints containing toluene to induce a "sniffer's high."

**I. Mechanism of toxicity**

**A.** Toluene and xylene cause generalized CNS depression. Like other aromatic hydrocarbons, they may sensitize the myocardium to the arrhythmogenic effects of catecholamines. They are mild mucous membrane irritants that affect the eyes and the respiratory and GI tracts.

**B.** Pulmonary aspiration can cause a hydrocarbon pneumonitis (see p 219).

**C.** Chronic abuse of toluene can cause diffuse CNS demyelination, renal tubular damage, and myopathy.

**D. Kinetics.** Symptoms of CNS toxicity are apparent immediately after inhalation of high concentrations and 30 to 60 minutes after ingestion. Pulmonary effects may not appear for up to 6 hours after exposure. Toluene is metabolized by alcohol dehydrogenase, and the presence of ethanol can inhibit toluene metabolism and prolong systemic toxicity.

**II. Toxic dose**

**A. Ingestion.** As little as 15–20 mL of toluene is reported to cause serious toxicity. A 60-mL dose was fatal in an adult male, with death occurring within 30 minutes.

**B. Inhalation.** The recommended workplace limits are 50 ppm (188 $mg/m^3$) (ACGIH TLV-TWA) and 200 ppm (OSHA PEL) for toluene and 100 ppm (434 $mg/m^3$) (ACGIH TLV-TWA and OSHA PEL) for xylene as 8-hour time-weighted averages, with a "skin" notation indicating the potential for appreciable skin absorption. The air levels considered immediately dangerous to life or health (IDLH) are 500 ppm for toluene and 900 ppm for xylene. Death has been reported after exposure to 1800–2000 ppm toluene for 1 hour.

**C.** Prolonged **dermal** exposure may cause chemical burns; both toluene and xylene are well absorbed across the skin.

**III. Clinical presentation.** Toxicity may be a result of ingestion, pulmonary aspiration, or inhalation.

**A. Inhalation** produces euphoria, dizziness, headache, nausea, and weakness. Exposure to high concentrations may rapidly cause delirium, coma, pulmonary edema, respiratory arrest, and death, although most victims regain consciousness rapidly after they are removed from exposure. Arrhythmias may result from cardiac sensitization. Acute exposure to vapor can irritate the mucous membranes of the respiratory tract, leading to reactive airway dysfunction syndrome (RADS). Massive exposures can lead to pulmonary edema and respiratory arrest.

**B. Ingestion** of toluene or xylene may cause vomiting and diarrhea, and if pulmonary aspiration occurs, chemical pneumonitis may result. Systemic absorption may lead to CNS depression.

**C. Chronic exposure** to toluene may cause permanent CNS impairment, including tremors; ataxia; brainstem, cerebellar, and cerebral atrophy; and cognitive and neurobehavioral abnormalities. Myopathy, hypokalemia, electrolyte and acid-base imbalance and renal tubular acidosis are also common. Workers repeatedly exposed to toluene at 200–500 ppm have reported loss of coordination, memory loss, and loss of appetite.

**D.** Toluene and xylene are not confirmed human reproductive hazards, but animal studies suggest that toluene may cause adverse reproductive effects, and both solvents cross the placenta and are excreted in breast milk. Microcephaly has been reported in the offspring of mothers who regularly used toluene recreationally while pregnant.

**IV. Diagnosis** is based on a history of exposure and typical manifestations of acute CNS effects such as euphoria and "drunkenness." After acute ingestion, pulmonary aspiration is suggested by coughing, choking, tachypnea, or wheezing and is confirmed by chest x-ray.

**A. Specific levels.** In acute symptomatic exposures, toluene or xylene may be detectable in blood drawn with a gas-tight syringe, but usually only for a few hours. The metabolites hippuric acid, ortho-cresol (toluene), and methylhippuric acid (xylene) are excreted in the urine and can be used to document exposure, but urine levels do not correlate with systemic effects.

**B. Other useful laboratory studies** include CBC, electrolytes, glucose, BUN, creatinine, liver transaminases, CPK, and urinalysis. Chest radiography and pulse oximetry (or arterial blood gas measurements) are recommended for severe inhalation or if pulmonary aspiration is suspected.

**V. Treatment**

**A. Emergency and supportive measures**

1. **Inhalational exposure.** Maintain an open airway and assist ventilation if necessary (see pp 1–7). Administer supplemental oxygen and monitor arterial blood gases and chest x-rays.
   - **a.** If the patient is coughing or dyspneic, aspiration pneumonia is likely. Treat as for hydrocarbon pneumonia (see p 219).
   - **b.** If the patient remains asymptomatic after a 6-hour observation period, chemical pneumonia is unlikely and further observation or chest x-ray is not needed.
2. Treat coma (see p 18), arrhythmias (pp 13–15), and bronchospasm (p 7) if they occur. ***Caution:*** Epinephrine and other sympathomimetic amines can provoke or aggravate cardiac arrhythmias. Tachyarrhythmias may be treated with **propranolol** (p 504), 1–2 mg IV, or **esmolol** (p 449), 0.025–0.1 mg/kg/min IV.

**B. Specific drugs and antidotes.** There is no specific antidote.

**C. Decontamination.** Patients exposed only to solvent vapor who have no skin or eye irritation do not need decontamination. However, victims whose clothing or skin is contaminated with liquid solvent can secondarily contaminate response personnel by direct contact or through off-gassing vapor.

1. **Inhalation.** Remove the victim from exposure and give supplemental oxygen if available.
2. **Skin and eyes.** Remove contaminated clothing and wash exposed skin with soap and water. Flush exposed or irritated eyes with plain water or saline.
3. **Ingestion.** Administer activated charcoal orally if conditions are appropriate (see Table I–38, p 51). Consider gastric lavage for large ingestions (> 1–2 oz) if it can be performed within 30 minutes of ingestion.

**D. Enhanced elimination.** There is no role for enhanced elimination.

## ▶ TRICHLOROETHANE, TRICHLOROETHYLENE, AND TETRACHLOROETHYLENE

*Josef G. Thundiyil, MD, MPH*

Trichloroethane and trichloroethylene are widely used solvents that are ingredients in many products, including typewriter correction fluid (“white-out”), color film cleaners, insecticides, spot removers, fabric-cleaning solutions, adhesives, and paint removers. They are used extensively in industry as degreasers. Trichloroethane is available in two isomeric forms, 1,1,2- and 1,1,1-, with the latter (also known as methyl chloroform) being the more common. Tetrachloroethylene (perchloroethylene) is another related solvent that is used widely in the dry cleaning industry.

**I. Mechanism of toxicity**

**A.** These solvents act as respiratory and CNS depressants and skin and mucous membrane irritants. As a result of their high lipid solubility and CNS penetration, they have rapid anesthetic action, and both tricholorethylene and trichloroethane were used for this purpose medically until the advent of safer agents. Peak blood levels occur within minutes of inhalation exposure or 1–2 hours after ingestion. Their proposed mechanism of action includes neuronal calcium channel blockade and GABA stimulation.

**B.** Trichloroethane, trichloroethylene, their metabolite trichloroethanol, and tetrachloroethylene may sensitize the myocardium to the arrhythmogenic effects of catecholamines.

**C.** Trichloroethylene or a metabolite may act to inhibit acetaldehyde dehydrogenase, blocking the metabolism of ethanol and causing "degreaser's flush."

**D. Carcinogenicity.** The National Institute of Occupational Safety and Health (NIOSH) and the International Agency for Research on Cancer (IARC) consider tetrachloroethylene and trichloroethylene probable carcinogens (Class 2A). Although 1,1,2-trichloroethane is a NIOSH-suspected carcinogen, there is insufficient evidence to label 1,1,1-trichloroethane a carcinogen.

**II. Toxic dose**

**A. Trichloroethane.** The acute lethal oral dose to humans is reportedly between 0.5–5 mL/kg. The recommended workplace limits (ACGIH TLV-TWA) in air for the 1,1,1- and 1,1,2-isomers are 350 and 10 ppm, respectively, and the air levels considered immediately dangerous to life or health (IDLH) are 700 and 100 ppm, respectively. Anesthetic levels are in the range of 10,000–26,000 ppm. The odor is detectable by a majority of people at 500 ppm, but olfactory fatigue commonly occurs.

**B. Trichloroethylene.** The acute lethal oral dose is reported to be approximately 3–5 mL/kg. The recommended workplace limit (ACGIH TLV-TWA) is 50 ppm (269 mg/m$^3$), and the air level considered immediately dangerous to life or health (IDLH) is 1000 ppm.

**C. Tetrachloroethylene.** The recommended workplace limit (ACGIH TLV-TWA) is 25 ppm (170 mg/m$^3$), and the air level considered immediately dangerous to life or health (IDLH) is 150 ppm.

**III. Clinical presentation.** Toxicity may be a result of inhalation, skin contact, or ingestion.

**A. Inhalation or ingestion** may cause nausea, euphoria, headache, ataxia, dizziness, agitation, confusion, and lethargy and, if intoxication is significant, respiratory arrest, seizures, and coma. Hypotension and cardiac arrhythmias may occur. Inhalational exposure may result in cough, dyspnea, and bronchospasm. With severe overdose, renal and hepatic injury may be apparent 1–2 days after exposure.

**B. Local effects** of exposure to liquid or vapors include irritation of the eyes, nose, and throat. Prolonged skin contact can cause defatting, dermatitis and, in the case of trichloroethane and tetrachloroethylene, scleroderma-like skin changes.

**C. Ingestion** can produce GI irritation associated with nausea, vomiting, and abdominal pain. Aspiration into the tracheobronchial tree may result in hydrocarbon pneumonia (see p 219).

**D. Degreaser's flush.** Workers exposed to these vapors may have a transient flushing and orthostatic hypotension if they ingest alcohol, owing to a disulfiram-like effect (see Disulfiram, p 184).

**E. Other.** Severe exposures have caused development of cranial nerve neuropathies, optic neuritis, and skeletal muscle toxicity. Trichloroethylene has been shown to cross the placenta and is associated with preeclampsia and spontaneous abortion. Tetrachloroethylene is present in breast milk.

**IV. Diagnosis** is based on a history of exposure and typical symptoms. Addictive inhalational abuse of typewriter correction fluid suggests trichloroethylene poisoning.

**A. Specific levels**

1. Although all three solvents can be measured in expired air, blood, and urine, levels are not routinely rapidly available and are not needed for emergency evaluation or treatment. Confirmation of exposure to trichloroethane may be possible by detecting the metabolite trichloroethanol in the blood or urine. Hospital laboratory methods are not usually sensitive to these amounts.

2. Breath analysis is becoming more widely used for workplace exposure control, and serial measurements may allow for estimation of the amount absorbed.

B. **Other useful laboratory studies** include electrolytes, glucose, BUN, creatinine, liver transaminases, arterial blood gases, chest radiography, and ECG monitoring.

V. **Treatment**

A. **Emergency and supportive measures**

1. Maintain an open airway and assist ventilation if necessary (see pp 1–7). Administer supplemental oxygen and treat hydrocarbon aspiration pneumonitis (p 219) if it occurs.
2. Treat seizures (see p 22), coma (p 18), and arrhythmias (pp 12–15) if they occur. ***Caution:*** Avoid the use of epinephrine or other sympathomimetic amines because of the risk of inducing or aggravating cardiac arrhythmias. Tachyarrhythmias caused by myocardial sensitization may be treated with **propranolol** (p 504), 1–2 mg IV, or **esmolol** (p 449), 0.025–0.1 mg/kg/min IV.
3. Monitor for a minimum of 4–6 hours after significant exposure.

B. **Specific drugs and antidotes.** There is no specific antidote.

C. **Decontamination** (see p 45)

1. **Inhalation.** Remove the victim from exposure and administer supplemental oxygen, if available.
2. **Skin and eyes.** Remove contaminated clothing and wash exposed skin with soap and water. Irrigate exposed eyes with copious tepid water or saline.
3. **Ingestion.** Do ***not*** give activated charcoal or induce vomiting because of the danger of rapid absorption and abrupt onset of seizures or coma. Perform gastric lavage only if the ingestion was very large and recent (less than 30 minutes). The efficacy of activated charcoal is unknown.

D. **Enhanced elimination.** These procedures are not effective or necessary.

## ▶ VACOR (PNU)

*Neal L. Benowitz, MD*

Vacor rat killer (2% *N*-3-pyridylmethyl-*N*'-*p*-nitrophenylurea; PNU) is a unique rodenticide that causes irreversible insulin-dependent diabetes and autonomic nervous system injury. It was removed from general sale in the United States in 1979 but is still available in some homes and for use by licensed exterminators. The product was sold in 39-g packets of cornmeal-like material containing 2% PNU.

I. **Mechanism of toxicity.** PNU is believed to antagonize the actions of nicotinamide and, in a manner similar to that of alloxan and streptozocin, injure pancreatic beta cells. The mechanisms of autonomic neuropathy and CNS effects are unknown. Adrenergic neurons acting on blood vessels but not the heart are affected. As a result, orthostatic hypotension associated with an intact reflex tachycardia is the usual picture.

II. **Toxic dose.** Acute toxicity usually has occurred after ingestion of one 39-g packet of Vacor (approximately 8 g of PNU). The smallest dose reported to cause toxicity was 390 mg.

III. **Clinical presentation.** Initial symptoms include nausea and vomiting. Occasionally, confusion, stupor, and coma occur after several hours. After a delay of several hours to days, irreversible autonomic neuropathy, peripheral neuropathy, and diabetes may occur.

A. **Autonomic dysfunction.** Dizziness or syncope or both caused by severe orthostatic hypotension occur with an onset from 6 hours to 2 days after ingestion. Orthostatic hypotension usually is accompanied by intact reflex tachycardia. Other manifestations of autonomic neuropathy include dysphagia, recurrent vomiting, and constipation.

**B. Insulin-dependent diabetes mellitus,** with polyuria, polydipsia, hyperglycemia, and ketoacidosis, occurs after a few days. Hypoglycemia, resulting from insulin release, occasionally precedes hyperglycemia.

**C. Peripheral neuropathy** may cause paresthesias and muscle weakness.

**IV. Diagnosis.** A sudden onset of orthostatic hypotension or diabetes mellitus should suggest the possibility of Vacor ingestion. A careful investigation should be performed to determine what rat-killing chemicals may be present in the home.

**A. Specific levels.** PNU levels are not available.

**B. Other useful laboratory studies** include electrolytes, glucose, BUN, and creatinine.

**V. Treatment**

**A. Emergency and supportive measures**

1. Maintain an open airway and assist ventilation if necessary (see pp 1–7).
2. Orthostatic hypotension usually responds to supine positioning and intravenous fluids. Chronic therapy includes a high-salt diet and fludrocortisone (0.1–1 mg/day).
3. Treat diabetes in the usual manner with fluids and insulin.

**B. Specific drugs and antidotes.** Immediately administer **nicotinamide** (see p 483). Although its efficacy in humans is not proven, nicotinamide can prevent PNU-induced diabetes in rats.

**C. Decontamination** (see p 45). Administer activated charcoal orally if conditions are appropriate (see Table I–38, p 51). If a delay of more than 60 minutes is expected before charcoal can be given, consider using ipecac to induce vomiting if it can be administered within a few minutes of exposure and there are no contraindications (see p 464). Gastric lavage is not necessary after small to moderate ingestions if activated charcoal can be given promptly. For large ingestions (eg, more than one packet), consider gastric lavage and extra doses of charcoal (ie, to maintain a 10:1 ratio of charcoal to PNU).

**D. Enhanced elimination.** Forced diuresis, dialysis, and hemoperfusion are not effective. Repeat-dose charcoal treatment has not been studied.

## ► VALPROIC ACID

*Thomas E. Kearney, PharmD*

Valproic acid (Depakene or Depakote [divalproex sodium]) is a structurally unique anticonvulsant. It is used for the treatment of absence seizures, partial complex seizures, and generalized seizure disorders and is a secondary agent for refractory status epilepticus. It also is used commonly for the prophylaxis and treatment of acute manic episodes and other affective disorders, migraine prophylaxis, and chronic pain syndromes.

**I. Mechanism of toxicity**

**A.** Valproic acid is a low-molecular-weight (144.21) branched-chain carboxylic acid (pKa = 4.8) that increases levels of the inhibitory neurotransmitter gamma-aminobutyric acid (GABA) and prolongs the recovery of inactivated sodium channels. These properties may be responsible for its action as a general CNS depressant. Valproic acid also alters fatty acid metabolism with impaired mitochondrial beta-oxidation and disruption of the urea cycle and can cause hyperammonemia, hepatotoxicity, metabolic perturbations, pancreatitis, cerebral edema, and bone marrow depression. Some of these effects may be associated with carnitine deficiency.

**B. Pharmacokinetics**

1. Valproic acid is absorbed rapidly and completely absorbed from the GI tract. There is a delay in the absorption with the preparation Depakote (di-

valproex sodium) because of its delayed-release formulation as well as the intestinal conversion of divalproex to two molecules of valproic acid.

2. At therapeutic levels, valproic acid is highly protein bound (80–95%) and primarily confined to the extracellular space with a small (0.1–0.5 L/kg) volume of distribution (Vd). In overdose and at levels exceeding 90 mg/L, saturation of protein-binding sites occurs, resulting in a greater circulating free fraction of valproic acid and a larger Vd.
3. Valproic acid is metabolized predominantly by the liver and may undergo some degree of enterohepatic recirculation. The elimination half-life is 5–20 hours (average 10.6 hours). In overdose, the half-life may be prolonged to as long as 30 hours (there are case reports of up to 60 hours, but this may have been due to delayed absorption). A level exceeding 1000 mg/L may not drop into the therapeutic range for at least 3 days. In addition, active metabolites (eg, the neurotoxic 2-en-valproic acid, hepatotoxic 4-en-valproic acid) produced via beta-oxidation and omega-oxidation pathways may contribute to prolonged or delayed toxicity.

II. **Toxic dose.** The usual daily dose for adults is 1.2–1.5 g to achieve therapeutic serum levels of 50–150 mg/L, and the suggested maximum daily dose is 60 mg/kg. Acute ingestions exceeding 200 mg/kg are associated with a high risk for significant CNS depression. The lowest published fatal dose is 15 g (750 mg/kg) in a 20-month-old child, but adult patients have survived after ingestions of 75 g.

III. **Clinical presentation**

A. **Acute overdose**

1. Acute ingestion commonly causes GI upset, variable CNS depression (confusion, disorientation, obtundation, and coma with respiratory failure), and occasionally hypotension with tachycardia and a prolonged QT interval. The pupils may be miotic, and the presentation may mimic an opiate poisoning. Cardiorespiratory arrest has been associated with severe intoxication, and the morbidity and mortality from valproic acid poisoning seem to be related primarily to hypoxia and refractory hypotension.
2. Paradoxic seizures may occur in patients with a preexisting seizure disorder.
3. Transient rises of transaminase levels have been observed without evidence of liver toxicity. Hyperammonemia with encephalopathy has been observed with therapeutic levels and in overdose and without other evidence of hepatic dysfunction. It may also be associated with a higher risk of cerebral edema.
4. At very high serum levels (> 1000 mg/L) after large ingestions, other metabolic and electrolyte abnormalities may be observed, including an increased anion gap acidosis, hypocalcemia, and hypernatremia.
5. Other complications or late sequelae (days after ingestion) associated with severe intoxication may include optic nerve atrophy, cerebral edema, noncardiogenic pulmonary edema, anuria, and hemorrhagic pancreatitis.

B. **Adverse effects of chronic valproic acid therapy** include hepatic failure (high-risk patients are less than 2 years of age, are receiving multiple anticonvulsants, or have other long-term neurologic complications) and weight gain. Hepatitis is not dose related and usually is not seen after an acute overdose. Pancreatitis usually is considered a non–dose-related effect but has been reported with acute fatal overdoses. Alopecia, red cell aplasia, thrombocytopenia, and neutropenia have been associated with both acute and chronic valproic acid intoxication.

C. Valproic acid is a known **human teratogen.**

IV. **Diagnosis** is based on the history of exposure and typical findings of CNS depression and metabolic disturbances. The differential diagnosis is broad and includes most CNS depressants. Encephalopathy and hyperammonemia may mimic Reye's syndrome.

A. **Specific levels.** Obtain a stat serum valproic acid level. Serial valproic acid level determinations should be obtained, particularly after ingestion of divalproex-containing preparations (Depakote), because of the potential for delayed absorption. Peak levels have been reported up to 18 hours after Depakote overdose and could be reached even later after ingestion of the extended-release formulation, Depakote ER.

1. In general, serum levels exceeding 450 mg/L are associated with drowsiness or obtundation, and levels greater than 850 mg/L are associated with coma, respiratory depression, and metabolic perturbations. However, there appears to be poor correlation of serum levels with outcome. Moreover, assays may or may not include metabolites.
2. Death from acute valproic acid poisoning has been associated with peak levels ranging from 106–2728 mg/L, but survival was reported in a patient with a peak level of 2120 mg/L.

**B. Other useful laboratory studies** include electrolytes, glucose, BUN, creatinine, calcium, ammonia, liver transaminases, bilirubin, prothrombin time, lipase, amylase, serum osmolality and osmolar gap (see p 32; serum levels > 1500 mg/L may increase the osmolar gap by 10 mOsm/L or more), arterial blood gases or oximetry, ECG monitoring, and CBC. Valproic acid may cause a false-positive urine ketone determination.

**V. Treatment**

**A. Emergency and supportive measures**

1. Maintain an open airway and assist ventilation if needed (see pp 4–5). Administer supplemental oxygen.
2. Treat coma (see p 18), hypotension (p 15), and seizures (p 22) if they occur. There are anecdotal reports of the use of corticosteroids, hyperventilation, barbiturates, and osmotic agents to treat cerebral edema.
3. Treat acidosis, hypocalcemia, and hypernatremia if they are severe and symptomatic.
4. Monitor patients for at least 6 hours after ingestion and for up to 12 hours after ingestion of Depakote (divalproex sodium) because of the potential for delayed absorption.

**B. Specific drugs and antidotes.** There is no specific antidote. Naloxone (see p 477) has been reported to increase arousal, but inconsistently, with the greatest success in patients with serum valproic acid levels of 185–190 mg/L. L-Carnitine (p 431) has been used to treat valproic acid–induced hyperammonemia and hepatotoxicity. Although data are lacking on clinical outcomes, it appears to have a safe adverse reaction profile.

**C. Decontamination** (see p 51)

1. Administer activated charcoal orally if conditions are appropriate (see Table I–38, p 51). Gastric lavage is not necessary after small to moderate ingestions if activated charcoal can be given promptly.
2. Moderately large ingestions (eg, > 10 g) theoretically require extra doses of activated charcoal to maintain the desired charcoal:drug ratio of 10:1. The charcoal is given not all at once but in repeated 25- to 50-g quantities over the first 12–24 hours.
3. The addition of **whole-bowel irrigation** (see p 51) may be helpful in large ingestions of sustained-release products such as divalproex (Depakote or Depakote ER).

**D. Enhanced elimination** (see p 53). Although valproic acid is highly protein bound at therapeutic serum levels, saturation of protein binding in overdose (binding decreases to 35% at 300 mg/L) makes valproic acid favorably disposed to enhanced removal methods.

1. **Hemodialysis and hemoperfusion.** Hemodialysis may result in a fourfold to 10-fold decrease in elimination half-life in overdose patients. Dialysis also corrects metabolic disturbances, removes valproic acid metabolites and ammonia, and is associated with a rise in free carnitine levels. Consider dialysis in patients with serum valproic acid levels that exceed 850 mg/L, since these cases are associated with higher morbidity and mortality. Charcoal

hemoperfusion (alone and in series with hemodialysis) has also been utilized with clearances similar to those observed with hemodialysis.

2. **Continuous renal replacement therapy** (CVVH, CAVH) has also been used, but with lower reported clearances.
3. **Repeat-dose activated charcoal.** Theoretically, repeated doses of charcoal may enhance clearance by interrupting enterohepatic recirculation, but no controlled data exist to confirm or quantify this benefit. Another benefit is enhanced GI decontamination after a large or massive ingestion, since single doses of charcoal are inadequate to adsorb all ingested drug.

## ▶ VASODILATORS

*Jeffrey Fay, PharmD*

A variety of vasodilators and alpha-receptor blockers are used in clinical medicine. Nonselective alpha-adrenergic blocking agents (eg, phenoxybenzamine, phentolamine, and tolazoline) have been used in clinical practice since the 1940s. The first selective alpha-1 blocker, prazosin, was introduced in the early 1970s; doxazosin, indoramin, terazosin, trimazosin, urapidil, and tamsulosin (approved for benign prostatic hypertrophy) are newer alpha-1–selective agents. Minoxidil, hydralazine, and diazoxide are direct-acting peripheral vasodilators. Fenoldopam is a dopamine-1 receptor agonist that has been approved by the FDA for in-hospital, short-term management of severe hypertension. Nesiritide is a recombinant human B-type natriuretic peptide that is used for the intravenous treatment of acutely decompensated congestive heart failure. Sildenafil is one of a class of agents used in the treatment of male erectile dysfunction. Nitroprusside (see p 485) and nitrates (p 279) are discussed elsewhere.

I. **Mechanism of toxicity.** All these drugs dilate peripheral arterioles to lower blood pressure. A reflex sympathetic response results in tachycardia and occasionally cardiac arrhythmias. Prazosin and other newer alpha-1–specific agents are associated with little or no reflex tachycardia; however, postural hypotension is common, especially in patients with hypovolemia.

II. **Toxic dose.** The minimum toxic or lethal doses of these drugs have not been established. Fatalities have been reported with indoramin overdose and excessive intravenous doses of phentolamine.

   A. **Indoramin.** A 43-year-old woman died 6 hours after ingesting 2.5 g; CNS stimulation and seizures were also reported.
   B. **Prazosin.** A young man developed priapism 24 hours after an overdose of 150 mg. A 19-year-old man became hypotensive after taking 200 mg and recovered within 36 hours. Two elderly men who ingested 40–120 mg were found comatose with Cheyne-Stokes breathing and recovered after 15–18 hours.
   C. **Minoxidil.** Two adults developed profound hypotension (with tachycardia) that required pressor support after 1.3-g and 3-g ingestions of topical minoxidil solutions.
   D. **Sildenafil** is generally well tolerated in accidental pediatric ingestions.
   E. **Pharmacokinetics.** See Table II–59, p 382.

III. **Clinical presentation.** Acute overdose may cause headache, nausea, dizziness, weakness, syncope, orthostatic hypotension, warm flushed skin, and palpitations. Lethargy and ataxia may occur in children. Severe hypotension may result in cerebral and myocardial ischemia and acute renal failure. First-time users of alpha-1 blockers may experience syncope after therapeutic dosing.

IV. **Diagnosis** is based on a history of exposure and the presence of orthostatic hypotension, which may or may not be accompanied by reflex tachycardia.

   A. **Specific levels.** Blood levels of these drugs are not routinely available or clinically useful.

B. **Other useful laboratory studies** include electrolytes, glucose, BUN, creatinine, and ECG monitoring.

V. **Treatment**

A. **Emergency and supportive measures**

1. Maintain an open airway and assist ventilation if necessary (see pp 1–7).
2. Hypotension usually responds to supine positioning and intravenous crystalloid fluids. Occasionally, pressor therapy is needed (p 16).

B. **Specific drugs and antidotes.** There is no specific antidote.

C. **Decontamination** (see p 45). Administer activated charcoal orally if conditions are appropriate (see Table I–38, p 51). Gastric lavage is not necessary after small to moderate ingestions if activated charcoal can be given promptly.

D. **Enhanced elimination.** There is no clinical experience with extracorporeal drug removal for these agents. Terazosin and doxazosin are long-acting and are eliminated 60% in feces; thus, repeat-dose activated charcoal may enhance their elimination.

## ▶ VITAMINS

*David L. Irons, PharmD*

Acute toxicity is unlikely after ingestion of vitamin products that do not contain iron (for situations in which iron is present, see p 230). Vitamins A and D may cause toxicity, but usually only after chronic use.

I. **Mechanism of toxicity**

A. **Vitamin A.** The mechanism by which excessive amounts of vitamin A produce increased intracranial pressure is not known.

B. **Vitamin C.** Chronic excessive use and large IV doses can produce increased levels of the metabolite oxalic acid. Urinary acidification promotes calcium oxalate crystal formation, which can result in nephropathy or acute renal failure.

C. **Vitamin D.** Chronic ingestion of excessive amounts of vitamin D enhances calcium absorption and produces hypercalcemia.

D. **Niacin.** Histamine release results in cutaneous flushing and pruritus.

E. **Pyridoxine.** Chronic overdose may alter neuronal conduction, resulting in paresthesias and muscular incoordination.

II. **Toxic dose**

A. **Vitamin A.** Acute ingestion of more than 12,000 IU/kg is considered toxic. Chronic ingestion of more than 25,000 IU/day for 2–3 weeks may produce toxicity.

B. **Vitamin C.** Acute intravenous doses of more than 1.5 g and chronic ingestion of more than 4 g/day have produced nephropathy.

C. **Vitamin D.** Acute ingestion is highly unlikely to produce toxicity. In children, chronic ingestion of more than 5000 IU/day for several weeks may result in toxicity (adults > 25,000 IU/day).

D. **Niacin.** Acute ingestion of more than 100 mg may cause a dermal flushing reaction.

E. **Pyridoxine.** Chronic ingestion of 2–5 g/day for several months has resulted in neuropathy.

III. **Clinical presentation.** Most acute overdoses of multivitamins are associated with nausea, vomiting, and diarrhea.

A. Chronic **vitamin A** toxicity is characterized by dry, peeling skin, alopecia, and signs of increased intracranial pressure (headache, altered mental status, and blurred vision; pseudotumor cerebri). Bulging fontanelles have been described in infants. Liver injury may cause jaundice and ascites.

B. **Vitamin C.** Calcium oxalate crystals may cause acute renal failure or chronic nephropathy.

C. Chronic excessive use of **vitamin D** is associated with hypercalcemia, producing weakness, altered mental status, GI upset, renal tubular injury, and occasionally cardiac arrhythmias.

D. Chronic excessive use of **vitamin E** can cause nausea, headaches, and weakness.

E. **Vitamin K** can cause hemolysis in newborns (particularly if they are G6PD deficient).

F. Acute ingestion of **niacin** but not niacinamide (nicotinamide) may produce unpleasant dramatic cutaneous flushing and pruritus that may last for a few hours. Chronic excessive use (particularly of the sustained-release form) has been associated with hepatitis.

G. Chronic excessive **pyridoxine** use may result in peripheral neuropathy.

H. Large doses of **B vitamins** may intensify the yellow color of urine, and **riboflavin** may produce yellow perspiration.

IV. **Diagnosis** of vitamin overdose usually is based on a history of ingestion. Cutaneous flushing and pruritus suggest a niacin reaction but may be caused by other histaminergic agents.

A. **Specific levels.** Serum vitamin A (retinol) or carotenoid assays may assist in the diagnosis of hypervitaminosis A. Levels of 25-hydroxy vitamin D are useful in assessing excessive intake. Other serum vitamin concentration measurements are not useful.

B. **Other useful laboratory studies** include CBC, electrolytes, glucose, BUN, calcium, creatinine, liver transaminases, and urinalysis.

V. **Treatment**

A. **Emergency and supportive measures**

1. Treat fluid losses caused by gastroenteritis with intravenous crystalloid solutions (see p 16).
2. Treat vitamin A–induced elevated intracranial pressure and vitamin D–induced hypercalcemia if they occur.
3. Antihistamines may alleviate niacin-induced histamine release.

B. **Specific drugs and antidotes.** There is no specific antidote.

C. **Decontamination** (see p 45). Usually, gut decontamination is unnecessary unless a toxic dose of vitamin A or D has been ingested or the product contains a toxic amount of iron.

D. **Enhanced elimination.** Forced diuresis, dialysis, and hemoperfusion are of no clinical benefit.

## ▶ WARFARE AGENTS—BIOLOGICAL

*David Tanen, MD*

Biological weapons have been used since antiquity, with documented cases dating back to the 6th century BC, when the Assyrians poisoned wells with ergots. In the late 1930s and early 1940s, the Japanese Army (Unit 731) experimented on prisoners of war in Manchuria with biological agents that are thought to have resulted in at least 10,000 deaths. Although in 1972 over 100 nations signed the Biological Weapons Convention (BWC), both the Soviet Union and Iraq have admitted to the production of biological weapons and many other countries are suspected of continuing their programs. Today, bioweapons are considered the cheapest and easiest weapons of mass destruction to produce. Some agents (see Table II–56) that are thought to be likely to be used include *Bacillus anthracis* (anthrax), *Yersinia pestis* (plague), *Clostridium botulinum* toxin (botulism), *Variola major* (smallpox), and *Francisella tularensis* (tularemia). All these agents can be weaponized easily for aerial dispersion.

The effect of a biological weapon on a population can be seen in the terrorist attack on the east coast of the United States in September 2001. Anthrax spores were delivered through the mail and resulted in 11 cases of inhalational anthrax and 12

**TABLE II–56. BIOLOGICAL WARFARE AGENTS (SELECTED)**

| Agent | Mode of Transmission | Latency Period | Clinical Effects |
|---|---|---|---|
| Anthrax | Spores can be inhaled or ingested or cross the skin. No person-to-person transmission, so patient isolation not required. Lethal dose estimated 2500–50,000 spores. | Typically 1–7 days but can be as long as 60 days | *Inhaled:* fever; malaise; dyspnea; nonproductive cough; hemorrhagic mediastinitis; shock.<br>*Ingested:* nausea, vomiting, abdominal pain, hematemesis or hematochezia; sepsis.<br>*Cutaneous:* painless red macule or papule enlarges over days into ulcer, leading to eschar; adenopathy; untreated may lead to sepsis.<br>*Treatment:* ciprofloxacin, other antibiotics (see text). Anthrax vaccine. |
| Plague | Inhalation of aerosolized bacteria or inoculation via flea bite or wound. Victims are contagious via respiratory droplets. Toxic dose 100–500 organisms. | 1–6 days | After aerosol attack, most victims would develop pulmonary form: malaise, high fever, chills, headache; nausea, vomiting, abdominal pain; dyspnea; pneumonia; respiratory failure; sepsis and multiorgan failure. Black necrotic skin lesions can result from hematogenous spread. Skin buboes otherwise unlikely unless bacteria inoculated through skin (eg, flea bite, wound).<br>*Treatment:* tetracyclines, aminoglycosides, other antibiotics (see text). Vaccine not available. |
| Smallpox | Virus transmitted in clothing, on exposed skin, as aerosol. Victims most contagious from start of exanthem. Toxic dose 100–500 organisms. | 7–17 days | Fever, chills, malaise, headache, vomiting, followed 23 days later by maculopapular rash starting on the face and oral mucosa and spreading to trunk and legs. Pustular vesicles are usually in the same stage of development (unlike chickenpox). Death in about 30% from generalized toxemia.<br>*Treatment:* vaccinia vaccine; immune globulin (see text). |
| Tularemia | Inhalation of aerosolized bacteria, ingestion, or inoculation via tick or mosquito bite. Skin and clothing contaminated. Person-to-person transmission not reported. Toxic dose 10–50 organisms if inhaled. | 3–5 days (range 1–14) | *Inhalation:* fever, chills, sore throat, fatigue, myalgias, nonproductive cough, hilar lymphadenopathy, pneumonia with hemoptysis and respiratory failure.<br>*Skin:* ulcer, painful regional adenopathy, fever, chills, headache, malaise.<br>*Treatment:* doxycycline, aminoglycosides, fluoroquinolones (see text). Investigational vaccine. |
| Viral hemorrhagic fevers | Variety of routes, including insect or arthropod bites, handling contaminated tissues, and person-to-person transmission. | Variable (up to 2–3 weeks) | Includes *Ebola, Marburg, Arenaviruses, Hantavirus*, several others. Severe multisystem febrile illness with shock, delirium, seizures, and coma and diffuse bleeding into skin, internal organs, and body orifices.<br>*Treatment:* none. Isolate victims, provide supportive care. |
| Botulinum toxins | Toxin aerosolized or added to food or water. Exposed surfaces may be contaminated with toxin. Toxic dose 0.01 mcg/kg for inhalation and 70 mcg for ingestion. | Hours to a few days | See p 136. Symmetric, descending flaccid paralysis with initial bulbar palsies (ptosis, diplopia, dysarthria, dysphagia) progressing to diaphragmatic muscle weakness and respiratory arrest. Dry mouth and blurred vision due to toxin blockade of muscarinic receptors. Toxin cannot penetrate intact skin but is absorbed across mucous membranes or wounds.<br>*Treatment:* botulinum antitoxin (see p 424). |

(*continued*)

**TABLE II–56. BIOLOGICAL WARFARE AGENTS (SELECTED) (CONTINUED)**

| | | | |
|---|---|---|---|
| Ricin | Derived from castor bean (*Ricinus communis*); may be delivered as a powder or dissolved in water and may be inhaled, ingested, or injected. | Onset within 4–6 hours; death usually within 3–4 days. | Nausea, vomiting, abdominal pain, diarrhea, often bloody. Not well absorbed orally. Severe toxicity such as cardiovascular collapse, rhabdomyolysis, renal failure and death more likely after injection. Lethal dose by injection estimated to be 5-20 mcg/kg. Inhalation might cause congestion, wheezing, pneumonitis.<br>*Treatment:* supportive. Not contagious, no need to isolate victims. Prophylactic immunization with ricin toxoid and passive postexposure treatment with antiricin antibody have been reported in animals. |
| Staphylococcal enterotoxin B | Enterotoxin produced by *Staphylococcus aureus;* may be inhaled or ingested | Onset as early as 3–4 hours, duration 3–4 days. | Fever, chills, myalgia, cough, dyspnea, headache, nausea, vomiting; symptoms usual onset 8–12 hours after exposure.<br>*Treatment:* supportive. Victims are not contagious, do not need isolation. Vaccine and immunotherapy effective in animals. |
| T-2 mycotoxin | Yellow sticky liquid aerosol or dust (alleged "Yellow Rain" in 1970s), poorly soluble in water | Minutes to hours | Highly toxic tricothecene toxin can cause burning skin discomfort; nausea, vomiting, and diarrhea, sometimes bloody; weakness, dizziness and difficulty walking; chest pain and cough; gingival bleeding and hematemesis; hypotension; skin vesicles and bullae, ecchymosis, and necrosis. Eye exposure causes pain, tearing, redness. Leukopenia, granulocytopenia, and thrombocytopenia reported.<br>*Treatment:* supportive. Rapid skin decontamination with copious water, soap; consider using military skin decontamination kit. |

cases of the cutaneous form of the disease. Even on that small scale, the effect on the public health system was enormous, and an estimated 32,000 people received prophylactic antibiotic therapy.

**I. Mechanism of toxicity**

A. **Anthrax** spores penetrate the body's defenses by inhalation into terminal alveoli, through exposed skin, or by penetration of the GI mucosa. They then are ingested by macrophages and transported to lymph nodes, where germination occurs (this may take up to 60 days). The bacteria multiply and produce two toxins: "lethal factor" and "edema factor." Lethal factor produces local necrosis and toxemia by stimulating the release of tumor necrosis factor and interleukin-1-beta from macrophages.

B. **Plague** bacteria (*Yersinia pestis*) penetrate the body's defenses either by inhalation into terminal alveoli or by the bite of an infected flea. Dissemination occurs through lymphatics where the bacteria multiply, leading to lymph node necrosis. Bacteremia, septicemia, and endotoxemia result in shock, coagulopathy, and coma. Historically, plague is famous as the "Black Death" of the 14th and 15th centuries, which killed 20–30 million people in Europe.

C. **Botulinum toxins** cannot penetrate intact skin but can be absorbed through wounds or across mucosal surfaces. Once absorbed, the toxins are carried to presynaptic nerve endings at neuromuscular junctions and cholinergic synapses, where they bind irreversibly, impairing the release of acetylcholine.

D. **Smallpox** virus particles reach the lower respiratory tract, cross the mucosa, and travel to lymph nodes, where they replicate and cause a viremia that leads to further spread and multiplication in the spleen, bone marrow, and lymph nodes. A secondary viremia occurs, and the virus spreads to the dermis and oral mucosa. Death results from the toxemia associated with circulating immune complexes and soluble variola antigens.

E. **Tularemia.** *Francisella tularensis* bacteria usually cause infection by exposure to bodily fluids of infected animals or through the bites of ticks or mosquitoes. Aerosolized bacteria can also be inhaled. An initial focal, suppurative necrosis is followed by bacterial multiplication within macrophages and dissemination to lymph nodes, lungs, spleen, liver, and kidneys. In the lungs, the lesions progress to pneumonic consolidation and granuloma formation and can result in chronic interstitial fibrosis.

**II. Toxic doses** are variable but generally extremely small. As few as 10–50 *Francisella tularensis* organisms may cause tularemia, and less than 100 mcg of botulinum toxin can result in botulism.

**III. Clinical presentation.** See Table II–56 and the Centers for Disease Control (CDC) website on biological and chemical terrorism: http://www.bt.cdc.gov.

A. **Anthrax** may present in three different forms: inhalational, cutaneous, and GI. Inhalational is extremely rare, and any case should raise the suspicion of a biological attack. Cutaneous typically follows exposure to infected animals and is the most common form, with over 2000 cases reported annually. GI is rare and follows the ingestion of contaminated meat.

B. **Plague.** Although plague traditionally is spread through infected fleas, biological weapons programs have attempted to increase its potential by developing techniques to aerosolize it. Depending on the mode of transmission, there are two forms of plague: bubonic and pneumonic. The *bubonic* form would be seen after the dissemination of the bacteria through infected fleas into a population (this was investigated by the Japanese in the 1930s in Manchuria). After an aerosolized release, the predominant form would be *pneumonic.*

C. **Botulism** poisoning is described in more detail on p 136. Patients may present with blurred vision, ptosis, difficulty swallowing or speaking, and dry mouth, with progressive muscle weakness leading to flaccid paralysis and respiratory arrest within 24 hours. Since the toxins act irreversibly, recovery may take months.

D. **Smallpox** infection causes generalized malaise and fever owing to viremia, followed by a characteristic diffuse pustular rash with most of the lesions in the same stage of development.

E. **Tularemia.** After inhalation, victims may develop nonspecific symptoms resembling those of any respiratory illness, including fever, nonproductive cough, headache, myalgias, sore throat, fatigue, and weight loss. Skin inoculation causes an ulcer, painful regional lymphadenopathy, fever, chills, headache, and malaise.

IV. **Diagnosis.** Recognition of a bioweapon attack most likely will be made retrospectively, based on epidemiologic investigations. Specific indicators might include patients presenting with exotic or nonendemic infections, clusters of a particular disease, and infected animals in the region where an outbreak is occurring. A historical example was the downwind pattern of disease and proximity of animal deaths that helped prove that the anthrax outbreak in Sverdlovsk (in the former Soviet Union) in 1979 was caused by the release of anthrax spores from a biological weapons plant.

A. **Anthrax**

1. Obtain a Gram stain and culture of vesicle fluid and blood. Rapid diagnostic tests (ELISA, polymerase chain reaction [PCR]) are available at national reference labs.
2. Chest x-ray may reveal widened mediastinum and pleural effusions. Chest CT may reveal mediastinal lymphadenopathy.

B. **Plague**

1. Obtain a Gram stain of blood, CSF, lymph node aspirate, or sputum. Other diagnostic tests include direct fluorescent antibody testing and PCR for antigen detection.
2. Chest x-ray may reveal patchy or consolidated bilateral opacities.

C. **Botulism** (see also p 136)

1. The toxin may be present on nasal mucous membranes and be detected by ELISA for 24 hours after inhalation. Refrigerated samples of serum, stool, or gastric aspirate can be sent to the CDC or specialized public health labs that can run a mouse bioassay.
2. Electromyography (EMG) may reveal normal nerve conduction velocity, normal sensory nerve function, a pattern of brief, small-amplitude motor potentials, and, most distinctively, an incremental response to repetitive stimulation often seen only at 50 Hz.

D. **Smallpox** virus can be isolated from the blood and scabs and can be seen under light microscopy as Guarnieri bodies or by electron microscopy. Cell culture and PCR may also be employed.

E. **Tularemia**

1. Obtain blood and sputum cultures. *F tularensis* may be identified by direct examination of secretions, exudates, or biopsy specimens, using direct fluorescent antibody or immunohistochemical stains. Serology may confirm the diagnosis retrospectively.
2. Chest x-ray may reveal evidence of opacities with pleural effusions that are consistent with pneumonia.

V. **Treatment.** Contact the **Centers for Disease Control and Prevention (CDC) 24-hour Emergency Response Hotline at (770) 488-7100** for assistance with diagnosis and management.

A. **Emergency and supportive measures**

1. Provide aggressive supportive care. Treat hypotension (see p 15) with intravenous fluids and vasopressors and respiratory failure (p 5) with assisted ventilation.
2. **Isolate** patients with suspected plague, smallpox, or viral hemorrhagic fevers, who may be highly contagious. Patient isolation is not needed for suspected anthrax, botulism, or tularemia since person-to-person transmission is not likely. However, health-care workers should always use universal precautions.

**B. Specific drugs and antidotes**

1. **Antibiotics** are indicated for suspected anthrax, plague, or tularemia. All three bacteria are generally susceptible to fluoroquinolones, tetracyclines, and aminoglycosides. The following drugs and doses often are recommended as *initial empiric treatment,* pending results of culture and sensitivity testing (see also *MMWR* 2001 Oct 26;50(42):909–919, which is available on the Internet at http://www.cdc.gov/mmwr/preview/mmwrhtml/mm5042a1.htm).
   a. **Ciprofloxacin,** 400 mg IV every 12 h (children: 20–30 mg/kg/day up to 1 g/day).
   b. **Doxycycline,** 100 mg PO or IV every 12 h (children 45 kg: 2.2 mg/kg). ***Note:*** May discolor teeth in children under 8 years old.
   c. **Gentamicin,** 5 mg/kg IM or IV once daily, or streptomycin.
   d. Antibiotics should be continued for 60 days in patients with anthrax infection. **Postexposure antibiotic prophylaxis** is recommended after exposure to anthrax, plague, and tularemia.
   e. Antibiotics are ***not*** indicated for ingested or inhaled botulism; aminoglycosides can make muscle weakness worse (see p 136). Treat with **botulinum antitoxin** (p 424).
2. **Vaccines.** Anthrax and smallpox vaccines can be used before exposure and also for postexposure prophylaxis. A pentavalent (ABCDE) botulinum toxoid currently is used for laboratory workers at high risk of exposure. It is ***not*** effective for postexposure prophylaxis. Vaccines are not currently available for plague, tularemia, and viral hemorrhagic fevers.

**C. Decontamination. *Note:*** The clothing and skin of exposed individuals may be contaminated with spores, toxin, or bacteria. Rescuers and health-care providers should take precautions to avoid secondary contamination.

1. Remove all potentially contaminated clothing and wash the patient thoroughly with soap and water.
2. Dilute bleach (0.5%) and ammonia are effective for cleaning surfaces possibly contaminated with viruses and bacteria.
3. All clothing should be cleaned with hot water and bleach.

**D. Enhanced elimination.** These procedures are not relevant.

## ► WARFARE AGENTS—CHEMICAL

*Mark Galbo, MS, and David A. Tanen, MD*

Chemical warfare has a long history that may have reached its zenith during World War I with the battlefield use of chlorine, phosgene, and mustard gases. More recently, Iraq used chemical agents in its war with Iran and against its own Kurdish population. In 1995 Aum Shinrikyo, a terrorist cult, released the nerve agent Sarin in the Tokyo subway system during rush hour.

Chemical warfare agents are divided into groups largely on the basis of their mechanism of toxicity (Table II–57): nerve agents, vesicants or blister agents, blood agents or cyanides, choking agents, and incapacitating agents. Presenting symptoms as well as the clinical circumstances may help identify the agent and lead to effective treatment as well as proper decontamination.

**I. Mechanism of toxicity**

**A. Nerve agents** include GA (Tabun), GB (Sarin), GD (Soman), GF, and VX. These potent organophosphorus agents cause inhibition of acetylcholinesterase and subsequent excessive muscarinic and nicotinic stimulation (see p 291).

**B. Vesicants (blister agents).** Nitrogen and sulfur mustards are hypothesized to act by alkylating cellular DNA and depleting glutathione, leading to lipid peroxidation by oxygen free radicals; Lewisite combines with thiol moieties in

TABLE II–57. CHEMICAL WARFARE AGENTS (SELECTED)

| | Appearance | Vapor Pressure and Saturated Air Concentration (at 25°C) | Persistence in Soil | Toxic Doses (for 70-kg man) | Comments (see text for additional clinical description) |
|---|---|---|---|---|---|
| **Nerve agents (cholinesterase inhibitors; see text and p 373)** | | | | | |
| Tabun (GA) | Colorless to brown liquid with fairly fruity odor | 0.07 mm Hg<br>610 $mg/m^3$<br>Low volatility | 1–1.5 days | $LC_{50}$ 400 mg-min/$m^3$<br>$LD_{50}$ skin 1 g | Rapid onset; aging half-time 13–14 hrs. |
| Sarin (GB) | Colorless, odorless liquid | 2.9 mm Hg<br>22,000 $mg/m^3$<br>Highly volatile | 2–24 hrs | $LC_{50}$ 100 mg-min/$m^3$<br>$LD_{50}$ skin 1.7 g | Rapid onset; aging half-time 3–5 hrs. |
| Soman (GD) | Colorless liquid with fruity or camphor odor | 0.4 mm Hg<br>3,060 $mg/m^3$<br>Mod. volatile | Relatively persistent | $LC_{50}$ 50 mg-min/$m^3$<br>$LD_{50}$ skin 350 mg | Rapid onset; aging half-time 2–6 min. |
| VX | Colorless to straw-colored odorless liquid | 0.0007 mm Hg<br>10.5 $mg/m^3$<br>Very low volatility | 2–6 days | $LC_{50}$ 10 mg-min/$m^3$<br>$LD_{50}$ skin 10 mg | Rapid onset; aging half-time 48 hrs. |
| **Vesicants** | | | | | |
| Sulfur mustard (HD) | Pale yellow to dark brown liquid | 0.011 mm Hg<br>600 $mg/m^3$<br>Low volatility | 2 weeks – 3 years | $LC_{50}$ 1500 mg-min/$m^3$<br>$LD_{50}$ 100 mg/kg | Pain onset hours after exposure; fluid-filled blisters. |
| Phosgene oxime (CX) | Colorless crystalline solid or liquid with intense irritating odor | 11.2 mm Hg<br>1,800 $mg/m^3$<br>Moderately volatile | 2 hrs | $LC_{50}$ 3200 mg-min/$m^3$<br>$LD_{50}$ unknown | Immediate pain, tissue damage within seconds, solid wheal formation. |
| Lewisite (L) | Colorless to amber or brown oily liquid with geranium odor | 0.58 mm Hg<br>4,480 $mg/m^3$<br>Volatile | Days | $LC_{50}$ 1200 mg-min/$m^3$<br>$LD_{50}$ 40-50 mg/kg | Immediate pain, tissue damage in seconds to minutes; fluid-filled blisters. |

| | | | | | |
|---|---|---|---|---|---|
| **Riot control agents (Lacrimators)** | | | | | |
| CS<br>Chlorobenzylidene-malonitrile | White crystalline powder with pungent pepper odor | 0.00034 mm Hg<br>0.71 mg/$m^3$<br>Very low volatility | Variable | $LC_{50}$ 60,000 mg-min/$m^3$<br>Incapacitating dose:<br>$IC_{50}$ 3–5 mg-min/$m^3$ | Rapid severe eye pain and blepharospasm; skin tingling or burning sensation; duration 30–60 min after leaving exposure. |
| CN (mace)<br>chloroacetophenone | Solid or powder with fragrant apple-blossom odor | 0.0054 mm Hg<br>34.3 mg/$m^3$<br>Low volatility | Short | $LC_{50}$ 7–14,000 mg-min/$m^3$<br>Incapacitating dose:<br>$IC_{50}$ 20–40 mg-min/$m^3$ | |
| DM (diphenyl-aminearsine) | Yellow-green odorless crystalline substance | $4.5 \times 10^{-11}$ mm Hg<br>Insignificant<br>Virtually nonvolatile | Persistent | $LC_{50}$ 11–35,000 mg-min/$m^3$<br>Incapacitating dose:<br>$IC_{50}$ 22–150 mg-min/$m^3$<br>Nausea and vomiting: 370 mg-min/$m^3$ | Delayed onset (minutes) irritation, uncontrollable coughing and sneezing. Vomiting and diarrhea can last hours. |
| **Cyanides (see p 176)** | | | | | |
| Hydrogen cyanide (AC) | Gas with odor of bitter almonds or peach kernels | 630 mm Hg<br>1,100,000 mg/$m^3$<br>Gas lighter than air | Less than 1 hr | LC50 2500–5,000 mg-min/$m^3$<br>$LD_{50}$ skin 100 mg/kg | Rapidly acting gaseous cyanide. |
| Cyanogen chloride (CK) | Colorless gas or liquid | 1,230 mm Hg<br>2,600,000 mg/$m^3$<br>Gas density heavier than air | Nonpersistent | $LC_{50}$ 11,000 mg-min/$m^3$ | Irritating to eyes and lungs, can cause delayed pulmonary edema. |
| **Incapacitating agents (see text)** | | | | | |

Sources: *Medical Management of Chemical Casualties Handbook*, Chemical Casualty Care Office, Medical Research Institute of Chemical Defense, Aberdeen Proving Ground, MD 21010, 1995; and *Textbook of Military Medicine: Medical Aspects of Chemical and Biological Warfare*. U.S. Army, 1997. Available free on the internet after registration at https://ccc.apgea.army.mil/products/handbooks/books.htm.

many enzymes and also contains trivalent arsenic.

**C. Choking agents** include chlorine and lacrimator agents. These gases and mists are highly irritating to mucous membranes. In addition, some may combine with the moisture in the respiratory tract to form free radicals that lead to lipid peroxidation of cell walls. Phosgene causes less acute irritation but may lead to delayed pulmonary injury (see also p 306).

**D. Cyanides (blood agents)** include cyanide, hydrogen cyanide, and cyanogen chloride. These compounds have high affinity for metalloenzymes such as cytochrome aa3, thus derailing cellular respiration and leading to the development of a metabolic acidosis.

**E. Incapacitating agents.** A variety of agents have been considered, including strong anticholinergic agents such as BZ and scopolamine (see Anticholinergics, p 85), stimulants such as amphetamines and cocaine, hallucinogens such as LSD (p 247), and CNS depressants such as opioids (p 288). A form of fentanyl gas mixed with an inhalational anesthetic may have been used by Russian authorities in 2002 in an attempt to free hostages being held in a Moscow theater.

**II. Toxic doses** vary widely and also depend on the physical properties of the agents as well as the route and duration of exposure. Apart from the mechanism of toxicity of the chemical weapon, the following are important for consideration:

**A. Physical state of the chemical.** Agents delivered as aerosols and in large droplets generally have more persistence and can accumulate on surfaces. Gases tend to disperse, whereas vaporized forms of liquids may reliquefy in a cooler environment, leading to the potential for delayed dermal exposure. The use of high-molecular-weight thickeners to decrease evaporation of substances has been shown to increase agent persistence.

**B. Volatility.** Highly volatile agents (eg, hydrogen cyanide) vaporize rapidly and can be easily inhaled, while chemicals with low volatility (eg, VX) can remain in the environment for long periods.

**C. Environmental factors.** The presence of wind and rain can reduce the effectiveness of chemical weapon delivery by increasing dispersion and dilutional effects. Cold weather may reduce vapor formation but increase the persistence of the liquid form of some agents. Gases and vapors heavier than air may accumulate in low-lying areas.

**D. Agent decomposition** (see also Table II–57). Some warfare agents produce toxic by-products when exposed to acidic environments. GA may produce hydrogen cyanide and carbon monoxide. GB and GD produce hydrogen fluoride under acidic conditions. Lewisite is corrosive to steel and in nonalkaline conditions may decompose to trisodium arsenate. VX forms the toxic product EA2192 when it undergoes alkaline hydrolysis.

**III. Clinical presentation**

**A. Nerve agents** are potent cholinesterase-inhibiting organophosphorus compounds (see also p 292). Symptoms of muscarinic and nicotinic overstimulation include abdominal pain, vomiting, diarrhea, excessive salivation and sweating, bronchospasm, copious pulmonary secretions, muscle fasciculations and weakness, and respiratory arrest. Seizures, bradycardia, or tachycardia may be present. Severe dehydration can result from volume loss caused by sweating, vomiting, and diarrhea.

**B. Vesicants (blister agents).** The timing of onset of symptoms depends on the agent, route, and degree of exposure.

1. Skin blistering is the major cause of morbidity and can lead to severe tissue damage.
2. Ocular exposure causes tearing, itching, and burning and can lead to severe corneal damage, chronic conjunctivitis, and keratitis. Permanent blindness usually does not occur.
3. Pulmonary effects include cough and dyspnea, chemical pneumonitis, and chronic bronchitis.

C. **Choking agents** can cause varying degrees of mucous membrane irritation, cough, wheezing, and chemical pneumonitis. Phosgene exposure may also present with delayed pulmonary edema that can be severe and sometimes lethal.

D. **Cyanides** cause dizziness, dyspnea, confusion, agitation, and weakness, with progressive obtundation and even coma. Seizures and hypotension followed by cardiovascular collapse may occur rapidly. The effects tend to be all or nothing in a gas exposure, so if patients survive the initial insult, they can be expected to recover.

E. **Incapacitating agents.** The clinical features depend on the agent (see **I.E**, p 376).

1. **Anticholinergics.** As little as 1.5 mg of scopolamine can cause delirium, poor coordination, stupor, tachycardia, and blurred vision. BZ (3-quinuclidinyl benzilate, or QNB) is about 3 times more potent than scopolamine. Other signs include dry mouth, flushed skin, and dilated pupils.
2. **LSD** and similar hallucinogens cause dilated pupils, tachycardia, CNS stimulation, and varying degrees of emotional and perceptual distortion.
3. **CNS stimulants** can cause acute psychosis, paranoia, tachycardia, sweating, and seizures.
4. **CNS depressants** generally cause somnolence and depressed respiratory drive (with apnea a serious risk).

IV. **Diagnosis** is based mainly on symptoms as well as the setting in which the exposure occurred.

A. **Specific levels**

1. **Nerve agents.** Plasma and RBC cholinesterase activity is depressed, but interpretation may be difficult because of the wide interindividual variability and broad normal range (see also p 292).
2. **Pulmonary agents and vesicants.** There are no specific blood or urine levels that will assist in diagnosis or management.
3. **Cyanides.** Cyanide levels will be elevated, but rapid testing is not widely available. Suspect cyanide poisoning if a patient has severe metabolic acidosis, especially if mixed venous oxygen saturation is greater than 90%.

B. **Other laboratory tests** include CBC, electrolytes, glucose, BUN, creatinine, arterial blood gases, amylase/lipase and liver transaminases, chest x-ray, and ECG monitoring. In addition, obtain serum lactate and mixed venous oxygen saturation if cyanide poisoning is suspected (see p 176).

C. **Methods of detection** The military has developed various devices to detect commonly known chemical warfare agents encountered in liquid or vapor forms. These devices include individual soldier detection systems such as **M8 paper and M9 tape** that identify persistent and nonpersistent nerve or blister agents. These tests are sensitive but not specific. More sophisticated chemical agent detector kits such as the **M256** and **M256A1 kits,** which can identify a larger number of liquids or vapors, are also available. Systems that monitor air concentrations of various agents also have been used, such as the US military's CAM and ICAM (chemical agent monitors) and ACADA (automatic chemical agent detection alarm). Complexity and portability vary widely among detection methods: M9 paper may simply iindicate that an agent is present, whereas the Chemical Biological Mass Spectrometer Block II analyzes air samples by using a mass spectrometer. Further development of such systems is under way in both the private and governmental/military sectors.

V. **Treatment.** For expert assistance in management of chemical agent exposures and to access pharmaceutical antidote stockpiles that may be needed, contact your local or state health agency or local Poison Control Center (1-800-222-1222). In addition, if an act of terrorism is suspected, contact the Federal Bureau of Investigation (FBI).

A. **Emergency and supportive measures.** ***Caution:*** Rescuers and health-care providers should take measures to prevent direct contact with the skin or clothing of contaminated victims, because secondary contamination and serious illness may result. (See Section IV, pp 524 and 525.)

1. Maintain an open airway and assist ventilation if necessary (see pp 1–7). Administer supplemental oxygen. Monitor patients closely; airway injury may result in abrupt obstruction and asphyxia. Muscle weakness caused by nerve agents may cause abrupt respiratory arrest. Delayed pulmonary edema may follow exposure to less soluble gases such as phosgene (p 306).
2. Treat hypotension (see p 15), seizures (p 22), and coma (p 18) if they occur.

**B. Specific drugs and antidotes**

1. **Nerve agents** (see also p 292)
   a. **Atropine.** Give 0.5–2 mg IV initially (see p 415) and repeat the dose as needed. Initial doses may be given intramuscularly. The most clinically important indication for continued atropine administration is persistent wheezing or bronchorrhea. ***Note:*** Atropine will reverse muscarinic but not nicotinic (muscle weakness) effects.
   b. **Pralidoxime** (2-PAM, Protopam; see p 500) is a specific antidote for organophosphorus agents. It should be given immediately to reverse muscular weakness and fasciculations: 1–2 g initial bolus dose (20–40 mg/kg in children) IV over 5–10 minutes, followed by a continuous infusion (p 500). It is most effective if started early, before irreversible phosphorylation of the enzyme, but may still be effective if given later. Initial doses can be given by the intramuscular route if IV access is not immediately available. ***Note:*** Oximes such as HI-6, Obidoxime, and P2S offer promise for better reactivation of cholinesterases in the setting of nerve agent exposure. The availability of these agents in the United States is currently very limited.
   c. Valium anticonvulsant therapy may be beneficial even before the onset of seizures and should be administered as soon as exposure is recognized. The initial dose is 10 mg IM or IV in adult patients (0.1–0.3 mg/kg in children).
2. **Vesicants.** Treat primarily as a chemical burn (see p 157).
   a. British anti-Lewisite (BAL, see p 417), a chelating agent used in the treatment of arsenic, mercury, and lead poisoning, originally was developed for treatment of Lewisite exposures. Topical BAL has been recommended for eye and skin exposure to Lewisite; however, preparations for ocular and dermal use are not widely available.
   b. Sulfur donors such as sodium thiosulfate have shown promise in animal models of mustard exposures when given before or just after an exposure. The role of this antidote in human exposures is not clear.
3. **Choking agents.** Treatment is mainly symptomatic with the use of bronchodilators as needed for wheezing. Hypoxia should be treated with humidified oxygen, but caution should be exercised in treating severe chlorine or phosgene exposure because excessive oxygen administration may worsen the lipid peroxidation caused by oxygen free radicals. Steroids are indicated for patients with underlying reactive airways disease.
4. **Cyanides** (see p 176). The **cyanide antidote package** (Taylor Pharmaceuticals) consists of amyl and sodium **nitrites** (p 484), which produce cyanide-scavenging methemoglobinemia, and sodium **thiosulfate** (p 514), which accelerates the conversion of cyanide to thiocyanate.
5. **Incapacitating agents**
   a. Anticholinergic delirium may respond to physostigmine (see p 497).
   b. Stimulant toxicity and bad reactions to hallucinogens may respond to lorazepam, diazepam, and other benzodiazepines (see p 410).
   c. Treat suspected opioid overdose with naloxone (p 477).

**C. Decontamination.** ***Note:*** Rescuers should wear appropriate chemical protective clothing, as some agents can penetrate clothing and latex gloves. Butyl chemical protective gloves should be worn, especially in the presence of mustard agents. Preferably, a well-trained hazardous materials team should perform initial decontamination prior to transport to a health-care facility (see Section IV, pp 525–526). Decontamination of exposed equipment and materials may also be necessary but can be difficult because agents may persist or even polymerize on surfaces. Currently, the primary methods of decontamination are physical removal and chemical deactivation of the agent. Gases and vapors in general do not require any further decontamination other than simple physical removal of the victim from the toxic environment. Off-gassing is unlikely to cause a problem unless the victim was thoroughly soaked with a volatile liquid.

1. **Physical removal** involves removal of clothing, dry removal of gross contamination, and flushing of exposed skin and eyes with copious amounts of water. The **M291 kit** employed by the US military for individual decontamination on the battlefield uses ion-exchange resins and adsorbents to enhance physical removal of chemical agents prior to dilution and chemical deactivation. It consists of a carrying pouch that contains six individual pads impregnated with a resin-based powder. The **M258A1 kit** contains two types of packets for removal of liquid chemical agents, one for the G-type nerve agents (Packet 1) and the other for nerve agent VX and liquid mustard (Packet 2).
2. **Chemical deactivation of chemical agents.** Nerve agents typically contain phosphorus groups and are subject to deactivation by hydrolysis, whereas mustard and VX contain sulfur moieties subject to deactivation via oxidation reactions. Various chemical means of promoting these reactions have been utilized.
   a. **Oxidation.** Dilute sodium or calcium hypochlorite (0.5%) can oxidize susceptible chemicals. This alkaline solution is useful for both organophosphorus compounds and mustard agents. ***Caution:*** *Dilute hypochlorite solutions should NOT be used for ocular decontamination or for irrigation of wounds involving the peritoneal cavity, brain, or spinal cord.* A 5% hypochlorite solution is used for equipment.
   b. **Hydrolysis.** Alkaline hydrolysis of phosphorus-containing nerve agents is an effective means of decontamination of personnel exposed to these agents (VX, Tabun, Sarin, Soman). Dilute hypochlorite is slightly alkaline. The simple use of water with soap to wash an area may also cause slow hydrolysis.

D. **Enhanced elimination.** There is no role for these procedures in managing illness caused by chemical warfare agents.

## ▶ WARFARIN AND RELATED RODENTICIDES

*Ilene B. Anderson, PharmD*

Dicumarol and other natural anticoagulants are found in sweet clover. Coumarin derivatives are used both therapeutically and as rodenticides. Warfarin (Coumadin) is used widely as a therapeutic anticoagulant but is no longer popular as a rodenticide because rats and mice have become resistant. The most common anticoagulant rodenticides available today contain long-acting **"superwarfarins"** such as brodifacoum, diphacinone, bromadiolone, chlorophacinone, difenacoum, pindone, and valone, which have profound and prolonged anticoagulant effects.

I. **Mechanism of toxicity.** All these compounds inhibit hepatic synthesis of the vitamin K–dependent coagulation factors II, VII, IX, and X. Only the synthesis of new factors is affected, and the anticoagulant effect is delayed until currently circulating factors have been degraded. Peak effects usually are not observed for 2–3 days because of the long half-lives of factors IX and X (24–60 hours).

**A.** The duration of anticoagulant effect after a single dose of **warfarin** is usually 2–7 days. (See also Table II–59, p 382.)

**B. Superwarfarin** products may continue to produce significant anticoagulation for weeks to months after a single ingestion.

**II. Toxic dose.** The toxic dose is highly variable.

**A.** Generally, a single small ingestion of **warfarin** (eg, 10–20 mg) will not cause serious intoxication (most warfarin-based rodenticides contain 0.05% warfarin). In contrast, chronic or repeated ingestion of even small amounts (eg, 2 mg/day) can produce significant anticoagulation. Patients with hepatic dysfunction, malnutrition, or a bleeding diathesis are at greater risk.

**B. Superwarfarins** are extremely potent and can have prolonged effects even after a single small ingestion (ie, as little as 1 mg in an adult). However, in a large study of accidental superwarfarin ingestions in children, no serious cases of anticoagulation occurred.

**C.** Multiple **drug interactions** are known to alter the anticoagulant effect of warfarin. The following website was compiled by the British National Formulary and lists drug-drug interactions with warfarin: http://www.drugintel.com/physicians/coumadin_warfarin_drug_interactions.htm.

**III. Clinical presentation.** Excessive anticoagulation may cause ecchymoses, subconjunctival hemorrhage, bleeding gums, or evidence of internal hemorrhage (eg, hematemesis, melena, or hematuria). The most immediately life-threatening complications are massive GI bleeding and intracranial hemorrhage.

**A.** Anticoagulant effects may be apparent within 8–12 hours, but with superwarfarins peak effects commonly are delayed for up to 2 days after ingestion.

**B.** Evidence of continuing anticoagulant effects may persist for days, weeks, or even months with superwarfarin products.

**IV. Diagnosis** is based on the history and evidence of anticoagulant effects. It is important to identify the exact product ingested to ascertain whether a superwarfarin is involved.

**A. Specific levels. Brodifacoum** levels are available through commercial laboratories and may be useful in making the diagnosis and determining the endpoint for vitamin K therapy. Levels less than 4–10 ng/mL are not expected to interfere with coagulation.

1. An anticoagulant effect is best quantified by baseline and daily repeated measurement of the **prothrombin time** (PT) and calculation of the **International Normalized Ratio** (INR), which may not be elevated until 1–2 days after ingestion. A normal PT 48 hours after exposure rules out significant ingestion.
2. Blood levels of clotting factors II, VII, IX, and X will be decreased, but these specific measurements are not usually necessary.

**B. Other useful laboratory studies** include CBC and blood type and cross-match. The partial thromboplastin time and platelet count may be useful in ruling out other causes of bleeding.

**V. Treatment**

**A. Emergency and supportive measures.** If significant bleeding occurs, be prepared to treat shock with transfusions of blood and fresh frozen plasma and obtain immediate neurosurgical consultation if intracranial bleeding is suspected.

1. Take care not to precipitate hemorrhage in severely anticoagulated patients; prevent falls and other trauma. If possible, avoid the use of nasogastric or endotracheal tubes or central intravenous lines.
2. Avoid drugs that may enhance bleeding or decrease metabolism of the anticoagulant (see Table II–58 and http://www.drugintel.com/physicians/coumadin_warfarin_drug_interactions.htm).

**B. Specific drugs and antidotes. Vitamin $K_1$** (phytonadione, see p 518) but ***not vitamin $K_3$*** (menadione) effectively restores the production of clotting factors. It should be given if there is evidence of significant anticoagulation.

**TABLE II–58. WARFARIN INTERACTIONS (SELECTED EXAMPLES)**

| Increased anticoagulant effect | Decreased anticoagulant effect |
|---|---|
| Allopurinol | Barbiturates |
| Amiodarone | Carbamazepine |
| Anabolic/androgenic steroids | Cholestyramine |
| Anticoagulant/antiplatelet drugs | Glutethimide |
| Chloral hydrate | Nafcillin |
| Cimetidine | Oral contraceptives |
| Disulfiram | Phenytoin |
| Ginkgo biloba | Rifampin |
| Nonsteroidal anti-inflammatory agents | |
| Quinidine | |
| Salicylates | |
| Sulfonamides | |

**Note:** This list represents *only a small sample* of drugs that may interfere with warfarin's pharmacokinetics and anticoagulant action.

***Note,*** however, that if it is given prophylactically after an acute ingestion, the 48-hour prothrombin time cannot be used to determine the severity of the overdose, and it is suggested that the patient be monitored for a minimum of 5 days after the last vitamin $K_1$ dose.

1. Because vitamin K will not begin to restore clotting factors for 6 or more hours (peak effect 24 hours), patients with active hemorrhage may require **fresh frozen plasma** or **fresh whole blood.** Recombinant activated factor VII (Novoseven™) has been advocated as an alternative to fresh frozen plasma for rapid reversal of warfarin-induced anticoagulation. The optimal dose is unknown, but doses of 35–120 mcg/kg have been used in clinical trials, with the higher dose reported to be optimal in reversing patients with INR values up to 5.
2. Administer **oral vitamin $K_1$** every 6 hours (see p 518). Doses of up to 800 mg daily have been required to maintain a satisfactory INR. Vitamin K can also be administered subcutaneously or IV, but these routes are not recommended. ***Caution:*** Vitamin K–mediated reversal of anticoagulation may be dangerous for patients who require constant anticoagulation (eg, for prosthetic heart valves). Very minute doses should be given if a partial effect is desired.
3. **Prolonged dosing** of vitamin K may be required for several weeks in patients who have ingested a long-acting superwarfarin product.

**C. Decontamination** (see p 45). Administer activated charcoal orally if conditions are appropriate (see Table I–38, p 51). Gastric lavage is not necessary after small to moderate ingestions if activated charcoal can be given promptly and should be avoided in a person who is already anticoagulated.

**D. Enhanced elimination.** There is no role for enhanced elimination procedures.

TABLE II–59. PHARMACOKINETIC DATA[a]

| Drug | Onset (hr) | Peak (hr) | Half-Life (hr) | Active Metabolite | Half-Life of Active Metabolite (hr) | Vd (L/kg) | % Protein Binding | Enhanced Elimination | Comments |
|---|---|---|---|---|---|---|---|---|---|
| Abacavir | | Rapid | 1.54 +/– 0.63 | | | 0.86 +/– 0.15 | 50 | | Metabolism by alcohol dehydrogen-ase |
| Acebutolol | 1–3 | 2–3 | 3–6 | Yes | 8–13 | 3 | 10–26 | HD | |
| Acetaminophen | 0.5 | 0.5–2 | 1–3 | | | 0.8–1 | 10–30 | HD | S |
| Acetazolamide | 1 | 1–4 | 1.5–8 | | | | | | |
| Acetohexamide | 2 | 4 | 1.3 | Yes | | | 65–90 | | |
| Acrivastine | Rapid | 1–2 | 1.5–3.5 | Yes | | | 50 | | |
| Acyclovir | | 1.5–2 | 2.5–3.3 | | | 0.66–0.8 | 15 | HD | HD not usually needed |
| Alatrofloxacin | | | 9.4 – 12.7 | Yes | | 1.2–1.4 | 76 | | |
| Albuterol | 0.25–0.5 | 1–2 | 2–5 | | | 2 | 10 | | S |
| Alprazolam | Intermediate | 1–2 | 6.3–26.9 | | | 0.9–1.6 | 80 | | |
| Alprenolol | 0.5 | 2–4 | 2–3 | Yes | 1 | 3–6 | 80 | | |
| Amantadine | 1–4 | 1–4 | 7–37 | | | 4–8 | 60–70 | HD | HD in patients with no renal function |
| Amikacin | | 1 | 2–3 | | | 24 L | 0–11 | HD, PD | |
| Amiloride | 2 | 3–10 | 21–144 | | | 5 | 23 | | |
| Amiodarone | | | 26–107 days | Yes | 61 days | 1.3–66 | 95 | | |
| Amitriptyline | 1–2 | 4 | 9–25 | Yes | 18–35 | 8 | 95 | | |
| Amlodipine | | 6–9 | 30–50 | | | 21 | 95 | | |
| Amobarbital | < 1 | 2 | 10–40 | | | 0.9–1.4 | 59 | HD, HP, PD, MDAC | |

| | | | | | | | | | |
|---|---|---|---|---|---|---|---|---|---|
| Amoxapine | | 1–2 | 8–30 | Yes | 30 | 0.9–1.2 | 90 | | |
| Amoxicillin | | 1 | 1.3 | | | 0.41 | 18 | | |
| Amphetamine | | 1–3 | 7–14 | Yes | | 3.5–6 | 16 | | Route-dependent kinetics |
| Ampicillin | | 1 | 1.5 | | | 0.28 | 18 | | |
| Amprenavir | | 1–2 | 7.1–10.6 | | | 430 L | 90 | | |
| Anisotropine | | 5–6 | | | | | | | |
| Aprobarbital | < 1 | 12 | 14–34 | | | | 20–55 | HD, HP, PD, MDAC | |
| Aspirin | 0.4 | 1–2 | 2-4.5 | Yes | 2–3 | 0.1–0.3 | 50–80 | HD, HP | S; dose-dependent kinetics |
| Astemizole | | 1–4 | 20–24 | Yes | 10–12 days | 250 | 97 | | |
| Atazanavir | | 2.5 | 6.5–7.9 | | | | 86 | | Fecal elimination primarily |
| Atenolol | 2–3 | 2–4 | 4–10 | | | 50–75 L | 5 | HD | |
| Atropine | Rapid | Rapid | 2–4 | | | 2 | 5–23 | | |
| Azatidine | | 3–4 | 9 | | | | | | |
| Azelastine | | 2–3 | 22 | Yes | 54 | 14.5 | 88 | | |
| Azide | 1 min | | | | | | | | Duration 0.25 hours |
| Azithromycin | 2–3 | 2.4–4 | 68 | | | 23–31 | 7–50 | | |
| Bacitracin | | 1–2 IM | | | | | | | Renal elimination |
| Baclofen | 0.5–1 | 2–3 | 2.5–4 | | | 1–2.5 | 30–36 | | |
| Benazepril | 2–6 | 0.5–1 | 0.6 | Yes | 22 | 8.7 L | 97 | | |
| Bendroflumethiazide | 2 | 4 | 3–4 | | | | | | |
| Benzphetamine | | 3–4 | 6–12 | Yes | 4–14 | | | | Metabolized to amphetamine / meth-amphetamine |

(*continued*)

TABLE II–59. PHARMACOKINETIC DATA[a] (CONTINUED)

| Drug | Onset (hr) | Peak (hr) | Half-Life (hr) | Active Metabolite | Half-Life of Active Metabolite (hr) | Vd (L/kg) | % Protein Binding | Enhanced Elimination | Comments |
|---|---|---|---|---|---|---|---|---|---|
| Benzthiazide | 2 | 4–6 | | | | | | | |
| Benztropine | 1–2 | 4–6 | 4–6.5 | | | | | | |
| Bepridil | 2–3 | | 24 | Yes | | 8 | 99 | | |
| Betaxolol | 2–3 | 2–6 | 12–22 | | | 5–13 | 55 | HD | |
| Biperiden | | 1.5 | 18–24 | | | 24 | | | |
| Bisoprolol | | 3 | 8–12 | | | 3 | 30 | | |
| Bretylium | < 0.1 | 1–2 | 5–14 | | | 5.9 | 5 | | |
| Bromfenac | 0.5 | 1–3 | 1–2 | | | 0.15 | 99 | | |
| Bromocriptine | | 1.4 | 6–50 | | | | 90–96 | | |
| Brompheniramine | Rapid | 2–5 | 25 | | | 12 | | | S |
| Bumetanide | 0.5–1 | 1–2 | 2 | | | 13–25 | 95 | | |
| Bupivacaine | < 0.1 | 0.5–1 | 2–5 | | | 0.4–1 | 82–96 | | |
| Bupropion | | 2 | 16 | Yes | 20–24 | 20 | 80 | | S |
| Buspirone | | 0.67–1.5 | 2–4 | Yes | 2 | 5.3 | 95 | | |
| Butabarbital | < 1 | 0.5–1.5 | 35–50 | | | | 26 | HD, HP, PD, MDAC | |
| Butanediol (BD) | | | | Yes | | | | | Metabolized to GHB |
| Butorphanol | < 0.2 | 0.5–1.0 | 5–6 | | | 7–8 | 83 | | |
| Caffeine | 0.25–0.75 | 0.5–2 | 3–10 | Yes | 2–16 | 0.7–0.8 | 36 | MDAC, HP, HD | |
| Candesartan | 2–4 | 3–4 | 9 | | | 0.13 | > 99 | | |

| | | | | | | | | | |
|---|---|---|---|---|---|---|---|---|---|
| Captopril | 0.5 | 0.5–1.5 | 1.9 | | | 0.7 | 25–30 | HD | |
| Carbamazepine | | 6–24 | 5–55 | Yes | 5–10 | 1.4–3 | 75 | MDAC, HP, HD | S |
| Carbenicillin | | 1 | 1.0–1.5 | | | 0.18 | 50 | | |
| Carbinoxamine | | | 10–20 | | | 0.25 | 0 | | |
| Carisoprodol | 0.5 | 1–4 | 1.5–8 | Yes | 8–17 | | | | |
| Carprofen | | 1–3 | 4–10 | | | | 99 | | |
| Carteolol | 1 | 3–6 | 6 | Yes | 8–12 | | 25–30 | | |
| Carvedilol | 1 | 4–7 | 6–10 | Yes | | 120 L | 98 | | |
| Cefaclor | | 0.75–1 | 0.6–0.9 | | | 0.36 | 60–85 | HD | |
| Cefamandole | | 0.2 IV; 0.5–2 IM | 0.5 IV; 1 IM | | | 0.145 | 56–78 | | |
| Cefazolin | | | 1.5–2 | | | 0.14 | 60–80 | | |
| Cefditoren pivoxil | | 1.5–3 | 1.2–2 | | | | 90 | | |
| Cefmetazole | | | 1.2 | | | | 65 | | |
| Cefoperazone | | | 1.5–2.5 | | | 0.15 | 82–93 | | |
| Cefotetan | | < 0.5 IV; 1–3 hr IM | 3–4.6 | | | | 88–90 | | |
| Ceftriaxone | | 0.5 | 5.8–8.7 | | | 5.78–13.5 | 85–95 | | Extensive bile excretion |
| Celecoxib | | 2–3 | 11 | | | 400 L | 97 | | |
| Cephaloridine | | 0.5 | 0.8 | | | | | PD | |
| Cephalothin | | 0.5 | | Yes | | 0.24 | 65–79 | | 70% renal eliminated unchanged |
| Cetirizine | Rapid | 1 | 8 | | | 0.5 | 93 | | |

(*continued*)

TABLE II–59. PHARMACOKINETIC DATA[a] (CONTINUED)

| Drug | Onset (hr) | Peak (hr) | Half-Life (hr) | Active Metabolite | Half-Life of Active Metabolite (hr) | Vd (L/kg) | % Protein Binding | Enhanced Elimination | Comments |
|---|---|---|---|---|---|---|---|---|---|
| Chloral hydrate | 0.5–1 | 0.25–0.5 | 0.07 | Yes | 8–11 | 0.6 | 35–41 (trichloroethanol) | | |
| Chloramphenicol | | 1 | 4 | | | 0.57–1.55 | 60 | HP | |
| Chlordiazepoxide | Intermediate | 0.5–4 | 5–30 | Yes | 18–96 | 0.3 | 96 | | |
| Chloroquine | | 2 | 2 months | Yes | 35–67 days | 115–285 | 55 | | |
| Chlorothiazide | 2 | 4 | 1–2 | | | 0.2 | 95 | | |
| Chlorphenesin | | 2 | 3.5 | | | 1.27 | | | |
| Chlorpheniramine | 1 | 2–6 | 12–43 | | | 2.5–7.5 | 70 | | S |
| Chlorpromazine | 0.5–1 | 2–4 | 8–30 | Yes | 4–12 | 8–160 | 90–99 | | S |
| Chlorpropamide | 1 | 3–6 | 25–48 | | | 0.13–0.23 | 60–90 | HP | |
| Chlorprothixene | 1.5–2 | 2.5–3 | 8–12 | Yes | 20–40 | 10–25 | | | |
| Chlorthalidone | 2–3 | 2–6 | 40–65 | | | 3.9 | 75 | | |
| Chlorzoxazone | 1 | 1–2 | 1 | | | | | | |
| Cidofovir | | | | | | 0.41–0.54 | < 6 | | |
| Cinnarizine | | 2–4 | 3–6 | | | | | | |
| Ciprofloxacin | | 1–2 | 4 | | | | 20–40 | | |
| Clarithromycin | | 2–4 | 3–4 | Yes | 5–9 | 243–266 L | 42–50 | | |

| | | | | | | | | | |
|---|---|---|---|---|---|---|---|---|---|
| Clemastine | Rapid | 3–5 | 21 | | | 13 | | | |
| Clidinium | 1 | | 2–20 | | | | | | |
| Clindamycin | | 0.75 | 2.4–3 | Yes | | | > 90 | | |
| Clomipramine | | 3–4 | 20–40 | Yes | 54–77 | 10–20 | 97 | | |
| Clonazepam | Intermediate | 1–4 | 18–50 | | | 3.2 | 85 | | |
| Clonidine | 0.5–1 | 2–4 | 5–13 | | | 3–5.5 | 20–40 | | |
| Clorazepate | Fast | 1–2 | 2.3 | Yes | 40–120 | 0.2–1.3 | 97–98 | | |
| Clozapine | | 2 | 8–13 | | | 0.5–3 | 97 | | |
| Cocaine | | 0.5 | 1 | Yes | 4–5 | 2–2.7 | 10 | | Route dependent kinetics |
| Codeine | < 0.5 | 0.5–1.0 | 2–4 | Yes | 2–4 | 3.5 | 20 | | |
| Colchicine | | 0.5–1 | 4.4–31 | | | 2 | 30–50 | | Symptoms delayed 2–12 hrs in OD |
| Coumadin | 24–72 | 3–7 days | 36–72 | Yes | 20–90 | 0.15 | 99 | | |
| Cyclobenzaprine | 1 | 3–4 | 24–72 | | | | 93 | | |
| Cyproheptadine | 2–3 | 6–9 | 16 | | | | | | |
| Dapsone | 2–4 | 4–8 | 10–50 | Yes | | 1.5 | 70–90 | MDAC, HP | |
| Daptomycin | | | 8–9 | | | 0.092–0.12 | 90–95 | HD, PD | |
| Delavirdine | | 1 | 2–11 | | | | 98 | | |
| Darifenacin | | 7 | 12–20 | | | 163 L | 98 | | S |
| Demeclocycline | | | 10–17 | | | 1–2 | 40–80 | | |
| Desipramine | | 3–6 | 12–24 | Yes | 22 | 22–60 | 80 | | |
| Desloratadine | 1 | 3 | 27 | Yes | 25–30 | | 82 | | |

(*continued*)

TABLE II–59. PHARMACOKINETIC DATA[a] (CONTINUED)

| Drug | Onset (hr) | Peak (hr) | Half-Life (hr) | Active Metabolite | Half-Life of Active Metabolite (hr) | Vd (L/kg) | % Protein Binding | Enhanced Elimination | Comments |
|---|---|---|---|---|---|---|---|---|---|
| Dexbrompheniramine |  |  | 22 |  |  |  |  |  |  |
| Dexfenfluramine | 1.5–8 | 1.5–8.0 | 17–20 | Yes | 32 | 12 |  |  |  |
| Dextroamphetamine | 1–1.5 | 1–3 | 10–12 |  |  | 6 | 16 |  | S |
| Dextromethorphan | < 0.5 | 2.5 | 3 | Yes | 3–6 | 5–6 |  |  | S |
| Diazepam | Very fast | 0.5–2 | 20–80 | Yes | 40–120 | 1.1 | 98 |  |  |
| Diazoxide | 1 | 3–5 | 24 |  |  |  | 90 | HD, PD |  |
| Dichlorphenamide | 1 | 2–4 |  |  |  |  |  |  |  |
| Diclofenac | 0.2 | 1–3 | 2 |  |  | 0.1–0.5 | 99 |  | S |
| Dicyclomine | 1–2 | 1.5 | 2–10 |  |  | 3.7 |  |  | S |
| Didanosine |  | 0.25–1.5 | 1.5 +/– 0.4 |  |  | 1.08 +/– 0.22 | < 5 |  |  |
| Diethylpropion |  | 2 | 2.5–6 | Yes | 4–8 |  |  |  | S |
| Diflunisal | 1 | 2–3 | 8–12 |  |  | 0.1 | 99 |  |  |
| Digitoxin | 2–4 | 10 | 5–8 days | Yes | 30–50 | 0.5 | 95 | MDAC |  |
| Digoxin | 1–2 | 6–12 | 30–50 | Yes |  | 5–10 | 25 |  |  |
| Dihydroergotamine | 0.5 | 0.5–3 | 2–4 | Yes |  | 15 | 90 |  | In overdose, vasospasm may last for weeks |
| Diltiazem | 1 | 2–4 | 4–6 | Yes | 11 | 5.3 | 77–93 |  | S |
| Dimenhydrinate | < 0.5 |  |  |  |  |  |  |  |  |
| Diphenhydramine | < 0.5 | 1–4 | 2–8 |  |  | 5 | 85 |  |  |
| Diphenoxylate | 1 | 2 | 2.5 | Yes | 3–14 | 324 L |  |  |  |

| | | | | | | | | | |
|---|---|---|---|---|---|---|---|---|---|
| Disopyramide | | | 4–10 | | | 0.6–1.3 | 35–95 | HP, HD | |
| Disulfiram | 3–12 | 8–12 | 7–8 | Yes | 9–22 | | 96 | | |
| Doxazosin | 4–8 | 2–5 | 8–22 | | | 1–3.4 | 98–99 | | |
| Doxepin | | 2 | 8–15 | Yes | 28–52 | 9–33 | 80 | | |
| Doxylamine | | 2–3 | 10 | | | 2.7 | | | |
| Dronabinol | 0.5–1 | 1–4 | 20–30 | Yes | | 10 | 90–99 | | Half-life longer in chronic users |
| Efavirenz | | 3–5 | 40–76 | | | | 99 | | |
| Emtricitabine | Rapid | 1–2 | 10 | | | | < 4 | HD | Renal elimination primarily |
| Enalapril | 1 | 1 | 1.3 | Yes | 11 | | 50–60 | HD | |
| Encainide | | 1 | 2–11 | | | 2.7–4.3 | 70–85 | | |
| Enfuvirtide | | 4 | 3.8 ± 0.6 | | | 5.5 ± 1.1 | 92 | | |
| Ephedrine | 0.25–1 | | 3–4 | | | 2.6–3.1 | | | |
| Eprosartan | | 1–2 | 5–9 | | | 308 L | 98 | | |
| Ergonovine | < 1 | 2–3 | | | | | | | |
| Ergotamine | | 1–3 | 3–12 | | | 1.8 | | | In overdose, vasospasm may last for weeks |
| Erythromycin | | 1 | 1.4 | | | | 70 | | |
| Esmolol | < 1 min IV | 5 min IV | 9 min IV | | | 3.4 | 55 | | |
| Estazolam | Fast | 2 | 8–28 | | | | 93 | | |
| Eszopiclone | | 1 | 6 | | | | 52–59 | | |
| Ethacrynic acid | 0.5 | 2 | 2–4 | Yes | | | | | |
| Ethchlorvynol | 0.5 | 1–2 | 10–20 | | | 3–4 | 35–50 | | |

(*continued*)

TABLE II–59. PHARMACOKINETIC DATA[a] (CONTINUED)

| Drug | Onset (hr) | Peak (hr) | Half-Life (hr) | Active Metabolite | Half-Life of Active Metabolite (hr) | Vd (L/kg) | % Protein Binding | Enhanced Elimination | Comments |
|---|---|---|---|---|---|---|---|---|---|
| Etidocaine | < 0.1 | 0.25–0.5 | 1.5 | | | 1.9 | 96 | | |
| Etodolac | 0.5 | 1–2 | 7 | | | 0.36 | 99 | | S |
| Famciclovir | | | 2–2.3 | Yes | 2.5 | 0.91–1.25 | < 20 | | Metabolized to active penciclovir |
| Felbamate | | | 20–23 | | | 0.67–0.83 | 23 | | |
| Felodipine | 2–5 | 2–4 | 11–16 | | | 9.7 | 99 | | |
| Fenfluramine | 1–2 | 2–4 | 10–30 | Yes | | 12–16 | | | |
| Fenoldopam | 0.25 | 0.5–2 | 0.16 | | | 0.6 | | | |
| Fenoprofen | 0.5 | 2 | 3 | | | | 99 | | |
| Fentanyl | < 0.25 | < 0.5 | 1–5 | | | 4 | 80 | | |
| Fexofenadine | Rapid | 2–3 | 14 | | | 12 | 60–70 | | |
| Flavoxate | 1 | 1.5 | | Yes | | | | | |
| Flecainide | | 3 | 14–15 | | | 9 | 40–68 | HD | |
| Flunitrazepam | 0.33 | < 4 | 20 | | | 3.3–5.5 | 78 | | |
| Fluoride | < 1.0 | 0.5–1.0 | 2–9 | | | 0.5–0.7 | | | S |
| Fluoxetine | | 6–8 | 70 | Yes | 4–16 days | 1000–7200 L | 94 | | |
| Fluphenazine | < 1 | 1–3 | 12–19 | Yes | | | 99 | | |
| Flurazepam | < 0.75 | 0.5–1 | 2–3 | Yes | 47–100 | 3.4 | 97 | | |
| Fluvoxamine | | 5 | 15 | | | 25 | 77 | | |
| Fosamprenavir | | Rapid | | Yes (amprenavir) | 7.7 | | 90 | | Rapidly hydrolyzed to amprenavir in the gut |

| | | | | | | | | | |
|---|---|---|---|---|---|---|---|---|---|
| Foscarnet | | | 3.3–4 | | | 0.41–0.52 | 14–17 | | Active tubular secretion |
| Fosinopril | 1 | 3–4 | < 1 | Yes | 11.5–12 | 10 L | 89–99 | | |
| Fosphenytoin | | | | Yes | 7–60 | 4.3–10.8 | > 95 | MDAC, HP | Converted to phenytoin within 0.25 hrs |
| Furosemide | 0.5 | 1–2 | 1 | | | 0.11 | 99 | | |
| Gabapentin | | 1–3 | 5–7 | | | 0.8 | < 3 | HD | |
| Gamma butyrolactone (GBL) | 0.33 hr | | | Yes | < 1 | | | | Metabolized to GHB |
| Gamma hydroxybu-tyrate (GHB) | 0.25 | < 1 | < 1 | | | | | | Zero order kinetics |
| Ganciclovir | | 1.8 (3 with food) | 4.8 oral; 3.5 IV | | | 0.74 | 1–2 | HD | |
| Gatifloxacin | | 1–2 | 7–14 | | | | | | > 70% excreted unchanged |
| Gentamicin | | 0.5 | 2 | | | 0.25 | < 10 | | |
| Glimepiride | 2–3 | | 5–9 | Yes | 3 | | > 99 | | |
| Glipizide | 0.5 | 1–2 | < 24 | | | 0.11 | 97–99 | | S |
| Glipizide, extended-release form | 2–3 | 6–12 | 24 | | | 0.11 | 97–99 | | |
| Glutethimide | 0.5 | 1–6 | 10–12 | | | 2.7 | 35–59 | | |
| Glyburide [micronized form] | 0.5 | 4 [2–3] | 5–10 | Yes | | | 99 | | |
| Glycopyrrolate | | 0.5–5 | 0.5–2 | | | 0.6 | | | |
| Grepafloxacin | | 2–5 | 15.7 ± 4.2 | | | 5–8 | | | |

(*continued*)

TABLE II–59. PHARMACOKINETIC DATA[a] (CONTINUED)

| Drug | Onset (hr) | Peak (hr) | Half-Life (hr) | Active Metabolite | Half-Life of Active Metabolite (hr) | Vd (L/kg) | % Protein Binding | Enhanced Elimination | Comments |
|---|---|---|---|---|---|---|---|---|---|
| Guanabenz | 1 | 2–5 | 7–14 | | | 7.4–13.4 | 90 | | |
| Guanfacine | 2 | 1.5–4 | 12–24 | | | 6.3 | 72 | | |
| Haloperidol | 1 | 2–6 | 13–35 | Yes | | 18–30 | > 90 | | S |
| Heroin | | 0.2 | 1–2 | Yes | 2–4 | | 40 | | Rapidly hydrolyzed to morphine |
| Hydralazine | < 0.5 | 0.5–1 | 3–5 | Yes | 2 | 1.6 | 88–90 | | |
| Hydrazoic acid | Rapid | | | | | | | | Duration 0.25 h |
| Hydrochlorothiazide | 2 | 4 | 2.5 | | | 0.83 | 64 | | |
| Hydrocodone | | 1–2 | 3–4 | Yes | 1.5–4 | 3–5 | 6–8 | | |
| Hydroflumethiazide | 2 | 4 | 17 | | | | | | |
| Hydromorphone | 0.5 | 1 | 1–4 | | | 1.2 | 35 | | |
| Hydroxychloroquine | | | 40 days | Yes | | 580–815 | 45 | | |
| Hydroxyzine | < 0.5 | 2–4 | 20–25 | Yes | 8 | 19 | | | |
| Hyoscyamine | 0.5 | 0.5–1 | 3–5 | | | | 50 | | S |
| Ibuprofen | 0.5 | 1–2 | 1.5–2.5 | | | 0.12–0.2 | 90–99 | | |
| Imipramine | | 1–2 | 11–25 | Yes | 12–24 | 10–20 | 70–90 | | |
| Indapamide | 1–2 | 2–3 | 14–18 | | | | 75 | | |
| Indinavir | | 0.8 | 1.8 | | | | 60 | | |
| Indomethacin | 0.5 | 1–2 | 3–11 | | | 0.3–0.9 | 99 | | |
| Indoramin | | 1–2 | 1–2 | | | 7.4 | 72–92 | | |
| Insulin, aspart | 0.25 | 1–3 | | | | | | | Duration 3–5 h |

| | | | | | | | | | |
|---|---|---|---|---|---|---|---|---|---|
| Insulin, glargine | 1.5 | Sustained effect | | | | | | | Duration 22–24 h |
| Insulin, glulisine | 0.3 | 0.6–1 | | | | | | | Duration 5 h |
| Insulin, isophane (NPH) | 1–2 | 8–12 | | | | | | | Duration 18–24 h |
| Insulin, lispro | 0.25 | 0.5–1.5 | | | | | | | Duration 6–8 h |
| Insulin, protamine zinc (PZI) | 4–8 | 14–20 | | | | | | | Duration 36 h |
| Insulin, rapid zinc (semilente) | 0.5 | 4–7 | | | | | | | Duration 12–16 h |
| Insulin, zinc (lente) | 1–2 | 8–12 | | | | | | | Duration 18–24 h |
| Insulin, regular | 0.5–1 | 2–3 | | | | | | | Duration 8–12 h |
| Ipratropium | | 1.5–3 | 2–4 | | | | | | |
| Irbesartan | 2 | 1.5–2 | 11–15 | | | 53–93 L | 90 | | |
| Isoniazid | < 1 | 1–2 | 0.5–4 | | | 0.6–0.76 | 0–10 | HD, PD | |
| Isopropanol | < 1 | < 1 | 2.5–6 | Yes | | 0.6 | | | |
| Isosorbide dinitrate | < 0.2 | < 0.5–1 | 1–4 | Yes | 4–5 | 48–473 L | Minor | | |
| Isosorbide mononitrate | < 1 | 0.5–2 | 6–7 | | | 0.7 | < 4 | | S |
| Isradipine | 1–2 | 2–3 | 8 | | | 3 | 95 | | S |
| Kanamycin | | 1 | 2–3 | | | 0.19 | 0–3 | | |
| Ketamine | < 1 min (IV) | | 2–4 | Yes | | 3.1 | 27 | | Duration 0.6–1 h |
| Ketoprofen | | 1–2 | 2–4 | | | 0.1 | 99 | | S |
| Ketorolac | | 1 | 4–6 | | | 0.15–0.3 | 99 | | |

(*continued*)

TABLE II–59. PHARMACOKINETIC DATA[a] (CONTINUED)

| Drug | Onset (hr) | Peak (hr) | Half-Life (hr) | Active Metabolite | Half-Life of Active Metabolite (hr) | Vd (L/kg) | % Protein Binding | Enhanced Elimination | Comments |
|---|---|---|---|---|---|---|---|---|---|
| Labetalol | 1–2 | 2–4 | 6–8 | | | 5–9 | 50 | | |
| Lamivudine | | | 5–7 | | | 1.3 | | | Primarily renal |
| Lamotrigine | | 2.2–3 | 22–36 | | | 0.9–1.3 | 55 | | |
| Levetiracetam | 1 | 1 | 6–8 | | | 0.7 | < 10 | HD | |
| Levobunolol | | 3 | 5–6 | Yes | 7 | 5.5 | | | |
| Levothyroxine ($T_4$) | | 10–20 days | 6–7 days | Yes | 2 days | 8.7–9.7 L | | | |
| L–Hyoscyamine | 0.5 | 0.5–1 | 3–12 | | | | 50 | HD, PD | |
| Lidocaine | | | 1–2 | | | 12 | 40–80 | | |
| Lincomycin | | 1 | 4.4–6.4 | | | 38 L | 72 | | |
| Linezolid | | 1–2 | 4.2–5.4 | | | 40–50 L | 31 | HD | |
| Liothyronine ($T_3$) | 2–4 | 2–3 days | 2 days | | | 41–45 L | | | |
| Lisinopril | 1 | 6–8 | 12 | | | 1.6 | Minimal | HD | |
| Lithium carbonate | | 2–6 | 14–30 | | | 0.7–1.4 | 0 | HD, CVVHD, CAVHD | S |
| Loperamide | 0.5–1 | 3–5 | 9–14 | | | | 97 | | |
| Lopinavir | | 4 | 5–6 | | | | 98–99 | | |
| Loratadine | 1 | 2 | 12–15 | Yes | 28 | 120 | 97 | | |
| Lorazepam | Intermediate | 2–4 | 10–20 | | | 1–1.3 | 85 | | |
| Losartan | | 1 | 2 | Yes | 6–9 | 34 L | 98.7 | | |
| Loxapine | 0.5 | 1–2 | 5–14 | Yes | 8–30 | | | | |

| | | | | | | | | | |
|---|---|---|---|---|---|---|---|---|---|
| Lysergic acid (LSD) | 0.5–2 | 1–2 | 3 | | | 0.27 | 80 | | |
| Magnesium | 1–3 | 1–2 | 4–5 | | | 0.5 | 34 | HD | |
| Maprotiline | | 8–16 | 21–50 | Yes | | 18–22 | 90 | | |
| Mazindol | 0.5–1 | 2 | 30–50 | Yes | 5.2 days | | | | |
| Meclizine | 1–2 | | 6 | | | | | | |
| Meclofenamate | | 0.5–1 | 1–3 | | | 0.3 | 99 | | |
| Mefenamic acid | | 2–4 | 2 | | | | 99 | | |
| Mefloquine | | 6–24 | 20 days | | | 13–29 | 98 | | |
| Meloxicam | | 5–6; second peak at 12–14 h | 15–20 | | | 10 L | 99.4 | Cholestyramine, MDAC | Second peak level suggests gastrointestinal recirculation |
| Meperidine | < 1 | 1–2 | 2–5 | Yes | 15–30 | 3.7–4.2 | 55–75 | | |
| Mephobarbital | 0.5–2 | | 10–70 | Yes | 80–120 | 2.6 | 40–60 | HD, HP, PD, MDAC | Metabolized to phenobarbital |
| Meprobamate | < 1 | 1–3 | 10–11 | | | 0.7 | 20 | | |
| Mesoridazine | | 4–6 | 5–15 | Yes | | 3–6 | 75–91 | | |
| Metaldehyde | 1–3 | | 27 | | | | | | Depolymerizes to acetaldehyde |
| Metaproterenol | 1 | 2 | 3–7 | | | 6 | 10 | | S |
| Metaxalone | 1 | 2 | 2–3 | | | | | | |
| Metformin | | 2 | 2–6 | | | 26–1952 L | Negligible | HD | S. Reported Vd varies widely. |
| Methadone | 0.5–1.0 | 2–4 | 20–30 | | | 3.6 | 80 | | |
| Methamphetamine | | 1–3 | 6–15 | Yes | 7–24 | 3.5–5 | | | |

(*continued*)

TABLE II–59. PHARMACOKINETIC DATA[a] (CONTINUED)

| Drug | Onset (hr) | Peak (hr) | Half-Life (hr) | Active Metabolite | Half-Life of Active Metabolite (hr) | Vd (L/kg) | % Protein Binding | Enhanced Elimination | Comments |
|---|---|---|---|---|---|---|---|---|---|
| Methaqualone | | 1–2 | 20–60 | | | 2.4–6.4 | 80 | | |
| Methazolamide | 2–4 | 6–8 | 14 | | | | 55 | | |
| Methicillin | | 1 | 0.5 | | | 0.43 | 28–49 | | |
| Methocarbamol | 0.5 | 1–2 | 1–2 | | | | | | |
| Methohexital | < 0.2 IV | < 0.1 | 3–5 | | | 1–2.6 | 83 | HD, HP | |
| Methscopolamine | 1 | | | | | | | | |
| Methyclothiazide | 1–2 | 6 | | | | | | | |
| Methyldopa | 3–6 | 6–9 | 2–14 | | | 0.6 | 10 | | |
| Methylene-dioxymethamphet-amine (MDMA) | 0.3–1 | | 7.6 | Yes | | | | | 65% renally eliminated unchanged within 24 hours. |
| Methylphenidate | | 1–3 | 2–7 | Yes | 4 | 12–33 | 15 | | S |
| Methyprylon | 0.75 | 1–2 | 7–11 | Yes | | 0.6–1.5 | 60 | | |
| Methysergide | 24–48 | | 10 | | | | | | In overdose, vasospasm may last for weeks |
| Metolazone | 1 | 2 | 6–20 | | | | 95 | | |
| Metoprolol | 1 | 1.5–2 | 3–7 | | | 5.6 | 12 | | S |
| Metronidazole | | 1–2 | 8.5 | 6–14 | Yes | 10 | < 20 | HD | |
| Mexiletine | | 2–3 | 10–12 | | | 5–7 | 50–70 | | |
| Mezlocillin | | 0.5 | 0.8–1.1 | | | 0.14–0.26 | 16–42 | | |
| Mibefradil | 1–2 | 2–6 | 17–25 | | | 130–190 L | 99 | | |
| Midazolam | | 0.2–2.7 | 2.2–6.8 | Yes | 1–1.3 | 1.2–2 | 97 | | |

| | | | | | | | | | |
|---|---|---|---|---|---|---|---|---|---|
| Miglitol | | 2–3 | 2 | | | 0.18 | <4 | | |
| Minocycline | | 1–4 | 11–26 | | | 1–2 | 55–75 | | |
| Minoxidil | 1 | 2–8 | 3–4 | Yes | | 2.8–3.3 | Minimal | HD | |
| Mirtazapine | | 1.5–2 | 20–40 | Yes | 25 | 107 L | 85 | | |
| Moclobemide | | 1–2 | 2–4.6 | Yes | | 1.2 | 50 | | |
| Moexipril | 1 | 1.5 | 1 | Yes | 2–10 | 183 L | 50–70 | | |
| Moricizine | 2 | 0.5–2 | 1.5–3.5 | Yes | 3 | 8–11 | 95 | | |
| Morphine | < 1 | < 1 | 2–4 | | | 3–4 | 95 | | S |
| Moxalactam | | | 2–2.5 | | | | 80–86 | | |
| Nabumetone | | 4–12 | 24 | Yes | | | 99 | | |
| Nadolol | 3–4 | 4 | 10–24 | | | 2 | 30 | HD | |
| Nafcillin | | 1 | 1 | | | 1.1 | 84–90 | | |
| Nalbuphine | < 0.2 | 0.5–1.0 | 5 | | | 3–14 | | | |
| Nalidixic acid | | 2–4 | 1.1–2.5 | | | | 93 | | |
| Naloxone | 2 min IV | 0.25–0.5 IV | 0.5–1.5 | | | 3.6 | 54 | | Duration 1–4 hours |
| Naltrexone | | 1 | 4–10 | Yes | 4–13 | 3 | 20 | | Duration 24–72 |
| Naproxen | | 2–4 | 12–17 | | | 0.16 | 99 | | S |
| Nateglinide | 0.25 | 1–2 | 1.5–3 | Yes | | | 97–99 | | |
| Nefazodone | | 0.5–2 | 3 | Yes | 2–33 | 0.2–0.9 | 99 | | |
| Nelfinavir | | 2–4 | 3–5 | | | 2–7 | | | |
| Nevirapine | | 4 | 25–45 | | | 1.2 | 60 | | |

(*continued*)

TABLE II–59. PHARMACOKINETIC DATA[a] (CONTINUED)

| Drug | Onset (hr) | Peak (hr) | Half-Life (hr) | Active Metabolite | Half-Life of Active Metabolite (hr) | Vd (L/kg) | % Protein Binding | Enhanced Elimination | Comments |
|---|---|---|---|---|---|---|---|---|---|
| Niacin | < 1 | 3–4 | | Yes | | | | | S |
| Nicardipine | 0.5 | 0.5–2 | 8 | | | 0.7 | 95 | | S |
| Nicotine | | | 1–4 | Yes | 10–40 | 2–3 | 5–20 | | Kinetics varies with formulation. Half-life is urine pH dependent. |
| Nifedipine | 0.5 | 1 | 2–5 | | | 0.8–2.2 | 95 | | S |
| Nisoldipine | | 1–3 | 4 | Yes | | 4–5 | 99 | | S |
| Nitrendipine | 1–2 | 2 | 2–20 | | | 6 | 98 | | |
| Nitrofurantoin | | | 0.3 | | | | 25–60 | | |
| Nitroprusside | 1 min IV | 1 min IV | 3–11 min | | | | | | |
| Norfloxacin | | 1 | 3–4 | | | | 10–15 | | |
| Nortriptyline | | 7 | 18–35 | Yes | | 15–27 | 93 | | |
| Olanzapine | | 6 | 21–54 | Yes | 59 | 1000 L | 93 | | |
| Orphenadrine | | 2–4 | 14–16 | | | | 20 | | |
| Oxaprozin | | 2–4 | 42–50 | | | 0.16–0.24 | 99 | | |
| Oxazepam | Slow | 2–4 | 5–20 | | | 0.4–0.8 | 87 | | |
| Oxcarbazepine | | 4.5 | 2 | Yes | 9 | 0.7 | | | |
| Oxybutynin | 0.5–1 | 1–3 | 1–12 | Yes | 4–10 | 2.7 | | | S |
| Oxycodone | < 0.5 | 1 | 2–5 | Yes | | 1.8–3.7 | | | |
| Oxymetazoline | < 0.5 | | 5–8 | | | | | | |
| Oxyphenbutazone | | | 27–64 | | | | 90 | MDAC | |
| Oxyphencyclimine | | 4 | 13 | | | | | | |

| | | | | | | | | | |
|---|---|---|---|---|---|---|---|---|---|
| Oxprenolol | 2 | 3 | 1–3 | | | 1.2 | 70–80 | | S |
| Paraldehyde | < 0.3 | 0.5–1 | 6–7 | | | 0.9–1.7 | | | |
| Paroxetine | | 3–8 | 21 | | | 8.7 | 95 | | |
| Pemoline | | 2–4 | 9–14 | | | 0.2–0.6 | 40–50 | | |
| Penbutolol | 1–3 | 1.5–3 | 17–26 | Yes | 9–54 | 32–42 L | 80–98 | | |
| Penciclovir | | | | | | 1.5 | < 20 | | Parent drug is famciclovir |
| Penicillin | | 1 | 0.5 | | | | 60–80 | HD, CHP | |
| Pentazocine | < 0.5 | 1–2 | 2–3 | | | 4.4–8.0 | 65 | | |
| Pentobarbital | 0.25 | 0.5–2 | 15–50 | | | 0.5–1 | 45–70 | HD, HP | |
| Pergolide | | 1–2 | 27 | Yes | | | 90 | | |
| Perindopril | 1.5 | 1 | 0.8–1 | Yes | 3–120 | 0.22 | 60 | HD | |
| Perphenazine | | 3–6 | 8–12 | Yes | | 10–35 | | | |
| Phencyclidine | < 0.1 | 0.5 | 1 (30–100 in adipose) | Yes | | 6.0 | 65 | | Duration 1–2 days |
| Phendimetrazine | 1 | 1–3 | 5–12.5 | Yes | 8 | | 15 | | S |
| Pheniramine | | 1–2.5 | 16–19 | | | 2 | | | |
| Phenmetrazine | | 2–5 | 8 | | | | | | |
| Phenobarbital | < 0.1 | 0.5–2 | 80–120 | | | 0.5–0.9 | 20–50 | MDAC, HD, HP | |
| Phenoxybenzamine | 1 (IV) | | 24 | | | | | | |
| Phentermine | | 4 | 7–24 | | | 3–4 | | | S |
| Phentolamine | 1 min (IV) | | 19 min | | | | < 72 | | |
| Phenylbutazone | | 2–3 | 50–100 | Yes | 27–64 | 0.14 | 98 | MDAC | |

(*continued*)

TABLE II–59. PHARMACOKINETIC DATA[a] (CONTINUED)

| Drug | Onset (hr) | Peak (hr) | Half-Lfe (hr) | Active Metabolite | Half-Life of Active Metabolite (hr) | Vd (L/kg) | % Protein Binding | Enhanced Elimination | Comments |
|---|---|---|---|---|---|---|---|---|---|
| Phenylephrine | 0.25 IV | | 2–3 | | | 5 | | | |
| Phenylpropanolamine | 1 | 1–3 | 3–7 | | | 2.5–5 | | | S |
| Phenyltoloxamine | 1 | 2–3 | | | | | | | |
| Phenytoin | | 1.5–3 | 7–60 | | | 0.5–1 | > 90 | MDAC, CHP | S; zero–order kinetics at high levels; half-life is concentration dependent |
| Pindolol | 1–3 | 2 | 3–4 | | | 1.2–2 | 40–60 | | |
| Pioglitazone | | 2–4 | 3–7 | Yes | 16–24 | 0.63 | >99 | | |
| Piperacillin | | 0.5 | 0.6–1.2 | | | 0.29 | 22 | | |
| Piroxicam | | 0.5 | 45–50 | | | 0.13 | 99 | Cholestyramine, and MDAC | |
| Polymyxin B | | | 4.3–6 | | | | | | |
| Prazosin | 2–4 | 2–4 | 2–4 | Yes | | 0.6–1.7 | 95 | | |
| Primaquine | | 1–2 | 3–8 | Yes | 22–30 | 269 +/– 121 L | | | Accumulation with chronic use |
| Primidone | | | 3.3–12 | Yes | 29–120 | 0.4–1.0 | 20–30 | HD, HP, PD, MDAC | Metabolized to PEMA / phenobarbital |
| Procainamide | | 1–2 | 3–5 | Yes | 5–7 | 1.5–2.5 | 15 | HP, HD | S |
| Procarbazine | | 1 | 0.2 IV | | | | | | |
| Prochlorperazine | 0.5 | 2–4 | 7–23 | Yes | | 12–18 | | | S |
| Procyclidine | | 1–2 | 7–16 | | | 1.1 | | | |
| Promethazine | 0.5 | 2–3 | 7–16 | | | 171 | 93 | | |
| Propafenone | | 2–3 | 2–10 | | | 1.9–3 | 77–97 | | |

| | | | | | | | | | |
|---|---|---|---|---|---|---|---|---|---|
| Propantheline | < 1 | 6 | 1–9 | | | | | | |
| Propoxyphene | 0.5–1.0 | 2–3 | 6–12 | Yes | 30–36 | 12–26 | | | |
| Propranolol | 1–2 | 2–4 | 2–6 | Yes | 5–7.5 | 6 | 93 | | S |
| Protriptyline | | 25 | 54–92 | | | 22 | 92 | | |
| Pseudoephedrine | 0.5 | 3 | 5–8 | | | 2.5–3 | 20 | | S |
| Pyrazinamide | | 2 | 9–10 | | | | 10 | HD | |
| Pyridoxine | < 1 | 1–2 | 15–20 days | Yes | | | | | |
| Quazepam | | 2 | 39 | Yes | 70–75 | 5–8.6 | > 95 | | |
| Quetiapine | | 1.5 | 6 | | | 6–14 | 83 | | |
| Quinacrine | | 1–3 | 5 days | | | 620 | | | |
| Quinapril | 1 | 0.5–2 | 0.8 | Yes | 2 | | 97 | | |
| Quinidine | 0.5 | 1–3 | 6–8 | Yes | | 2–3 | 70–90 | | S |
| Quinine | | 1–3 | 8–14 | | | 1.2–1.7 | 80 | | |
| Ramipril | 2 | 0.7–2 | 1–5 | Yes | 13–17 | | 73 | HD | |
| Repaglinide | 0.5 | 1–1.5 | 1–1.5 | | | 0.44 | 98 | | |
| Rifampin | | 2–4 | 1.5–5 | Yes | | 1.6 | 89 | | |
| Risperidone | | 1–2 | 20–30 | Yes | 21–30 | | 90 | | |
| Risperidone | | 1.0 | 3–16 | Yes | 20–22 | | 90 | | |
| Ritodrine | | 1 | 1–2 | Yes | 15 | 0.7 | 32 | | |
| Ritonavir | | 2–4 | | | | | | | Excreted renally and in feces |
| Rofecoxib | | 2–3 | 17 | | | 86–91 L | 87 | | |
| Rosiglitazone | | 1–3.5 | 3–4 | | | 0.25 | 99.8 | | |

*(continued)*

TABLE II–59. PHARMACOKINETIC DATA[a] (CONTINUED)

| Drug | Onset (hr) | Peak (hr) | Half-Life (hr) | Active Metabolite | Half-Life of Active Metabolite (hr) | Vd (L/kg) | % Protein Binding | Enhanced Elimination | Comments |
|---|---|---|---|---|---|---|---|---|---|
| Saquinavir | | | | | | 700 L | 90 | | |
| Scopolamine | 0.5 | 1 | 3 | | | 1.5 | | | |
| Secobarbital | 0.25 | 1–6 | 15-40 | | | 1.5–1.9 | 45–70 | HD, HP, PD, MDAC | |
| Selegiline | 0.5–1 | 0.5–2 | 0.3–1.2 | Yes | 7–20 | | 94 | | |
| Sertraline | | 4–8 | 28 | Yes | 60–100 | 20 | 99 | | |
| Solifenacin succinate | | 3-8 | 45–68 | Yes | | 600 L | 98 | | |
| Sotalol | 1–2 | 2–3 | 5–15 | | | 1.6–2.4 | < 5 | HD | |
| Sparfloxacin | | 0.4–6 | 16–30 | | | 3.1–4.7 | 45 | | |
| Spectinomycin | | 1 | 1.2–2.8 | | | | | | |
| Spironolactone | 24 | 24–48 | 2 | Yes | 16.5 | | 95 | | |
| Stavudine | | 1 | 1.44 oral; 1.15 IV | | | 58 L | Negligible | | Active tubular secretion |
| Streptomycin | | 1 | 2.5 | | | | | | |
| Strychnine | 0.5 | | 10–16 | | | 13 | | | |
| Sulfamethoxazole | | | 9–12 | | | 0.21 | 70 | HD | |
| Sulindac | | 2 | 7–16 | Yes | 16 | | 98 | | |
| Tamsulosin | 4–8 | 4–8 | 9–13 | | | 0.2 | 99 | | S |
| Telmisartan | 3 | 0.5–1 | 24 | | | 500 L | 99.5 | | |
| Temazepam | Intermediate | 1.2–1.6 | 3.5–18.4 | | | 0.6–1.3 | 96 | | |
| Tenofovir | | 1 | 17 | | | 1.2–1.3 | 7.2 | | Active tubular secretion |
| Terazosin | 3 | 1 | 9–12 | | | 25–30 L | 90–94 | | |

| | | | | | | | | | |
|---|---|---|---|---|---|---|---|---|---|
| Terbutaline | 0.5–1 | 3 | 4–16 | | | 1.5 | 15 | | |
| Terfenadine | 1–2 | 2–4 | 6–8.5 | Yes | 8.5 | | 97 | | |
| Tetracycline | | | 6–12 | | | 1–2 | 65 | HD | |
| Tetrahydrozoline | 0.25–1 | | 1.2–4 | | | | | | |
| Theophylline | 0.5–1 | | 4–6 | | | 0.5 | 40 | HP, HD, MDAC | S |
| Thiopental | < 0.1 | < 0.1 | 8–10 | | | 1.4–6.7 | 72–86 | HD, HP | |
| Thioridazine | | 1–2 | 10–36 | Yes | 1–2 | 18 | 96 | | |
| Thiothixene | 1–2 | 1–3 | 34 | | | | | | |
| Thyroid, desiccated | 2 days | 8–10 days | 2–7 days | Yes | 2 days | | 99 | | |
| Tiagabine | Rapid | 1 | 7–9 | | | | 96 | | |
| Ticarcillin | | 0.5 | 1–1.2 | | | 0.22 | 45 | | |
| Tigecycline | | | 37–67 | | | | | | |
| Timolol | | 0.5–3 | 2–4 | | | 1.5 | < 10 | | |
| Tipranavir | | 2 | 5.5 | | | 7.7–10.2 | > 99.9 | | Fecal elimination primarily |
| Tizanidine | | 1.5 | 2.5 | | | 2.4 | 30 | | |
| Tobramycin | | 0.5 | 2–2.5 | | | | 0–3 | | |
| Tocainide | | 1–2 | 11–15 | | | 2–4 | 10–22 | HD | |
| Tolazamide | 1 | 4–6 | 7 | Yes | | | | | |
| Tolazoline | | | 3–10 | | | 1.61 | | | |
| Tolbutamide | 1 | 5–8 | 4.5–6.5 | | | | 80–99 | | |
| Tolmetin | | 1 | 1 | | | 0.13 | 99 | | |
| Tolterodine | Rapid | 1 | 2–3 | Yes | 3 | 0.9–1.6 | 96 | | S |

(continued)

TABLE II–59. PHARMACOKINETIC DATA[a] (CONTINUED)

| Drug | Onset (hr) | Peak (hr) | Half-Life (hr) | Active Metabolite | Half-Life of Active Metabolite (hr) | Vd (L/kg) | % Protein Binding | Enhanced Elimination | Comments |
|---|---|---|---|---|---|---|---|---|---|
| Topiramate | Rapid | 1.8–4.3 | 21 | | | 0.6–0.8 | 13–17 | HD | |
| Torsemide | 0.5–1 | 1–4 | 2–4 | | | 0.14 | 97 | | |
| Tramadol | 1 | 2–3 | 6 | Yes | 7.5 | 2.6–2.9 | 20 | | |
| Trandolapril | | 0.5–2 | 0.6–1.6 | Yes | 16–24 | 18 L | 80 | | |
| Tranylcypromine | | 0.7–3.5 | 1.5–3.5 | Yes | | 3 | | | |
| Trazodone | | 0.5–2 | 3–9 | Yes | | 0.6 | 90–95 | | |
| Triamterene | 2–4 | 2–8 | 1.5–2 | Yes | 3 | 2.5 | 65 | | |
| Triazolam | Fast | 1–2 | 1.5–5.5 | | | 0.7–1.5 | 78–89 | | |
| Trichlormethiazide | 2 | 4 | 2–7 | | | | | | |
| Trifluoperazine | | 2–5 | 5–18 | Yes | | | 90–99 | | |
| Trihexyphenidyl | 1 | 2–3 | 3–10 | | | | | | S |
| Trimazosin | 1 | 1 | 2.7 | Yes | | | 99 | | |
| Trimeprazine | | 3.5–4.5 | 4–8 | | | | | | |
| Trimethobenzamide | 0.5 | 1 | 1 | | | 0.5 | | | |
| Trimethoprim | | 1–4 | 8–11 | | | | 44 | HP | |
| Trimipramine | | 2 | 15–30 | Yes | | 31 | 95 | | |
| Tripelennamine | 0.5 | 2–3 | 3–5 | | | 9–12 | | | S |
| Triprolidine | | 1.5–2.5 | 3–5 | | | | | | |
| Trospium chloride | | 5–6 | 15–21 | | | 395 L | 50–85 | | |
| Trovafloxacin | | 1–2 | 9.1–12.7 | Yes | | 1.2–1.4 | 76 | | |
| Urapidil | < 0.4 | | 5 | Yes | 12.5 | 0.4–0.77 | 75–80 | | S |

| | | | | | | | | | |
|---|---|---|---|---|---|---|---|---|---|
| Valacyclovir | | 0.5 | | Yes | 2.5–3.3 | | | | Prodrug, converted to acyclovir |
| Valdecoxib | | 3 | 8–11 | Yes | | 86 L | 98 | | |
| Valproic acid | | | 5–20 | Yes | | 0.1–0.5 | 80–95 | HD, HP | S |
| Valsartan | 2 | 2–4 | 6 | | | 17 L | 95 | | |
| Vancomycin | | 1 | 4–6 | | | 0.3–0.7 | 55 | | |
| Venlafaxine | | 1–2 | 5 | Yes | 11 | 6–7 | 30 | | S |
| Verapamil | 0.5–2 | 6–8 | 2–8 | Yes | 10–19 | 4.7 | 83–92 | | S |
| Vidarabine | | | | Yes | 2.4–3.3 | | 20–30 | HD | |
| Vigabatrin | Rapid | 2 | 4–8 | | | 0.8 | Negligible | | |
| Zalcitabine | | | 1–3 | | | 0.534 | | | Renal excretion primarily |
| Zaleplon | 1.5 | 1 | 1 | | | 1.4 | 45–75 | | |
| Zidovudine (AZT) | | 0.5–1.5 | 1 | | | 1.6 | 34–38 | | |
| Ziprasidone | | 4.5 | 4–10 | | | 1.5–2.3 | > 99 | | |
| Zolpidem | 1 | 1.6 | 1.4–4.5 | | | 0.54 | 92.5 | | |
| Zonisamide | | 2–6 | 50–68 | | | 1.45 | 40 | | |

[a]Data provided are based on therapeutic dosing, not overdose. In general, after overdose, the peak effect is delayed and the half-life and duration of effect are prolonged. Changes may occur in the volume of distribution and the percent protein bound. Kinetics may vary depending on the formulation.

Key to abbreviations: S = sustained-release formulations are available and may lead to delayed absorption and prolonged effect; HD = hemodialysis; HP = hemoperfusion; PD = peritoneal dialysis; CHP = charcoal hemoperfusion; MDAC = multiple-dose activated charcoal; CVVHD = continuous venovenous hemodiafiltration; CAVHD = continuous arteriovenous hemodiafiltration.

The apparent volume of distribution (Vd) is reported in liters per kilogram (L/kg) unless the field specifically states liters only (L).

Table compiled by Ilene B. Anderson, PharmD.

# SECTION III. **Therapeutic Drugs and Antidotes**

*Thomas E. Kearney, PharmD*

## INTRODUCTION

This section provides detailed descriptions of antidotes and other therapeutic agents used in the management of a poisoned patient. For each agent, a summary is provided of its pharmacologic effects, clinical indications, adverse effects and contraindications, use in pregnancy, dosage, available formulations, and recommended minimum stocking levels for the hospital pharmacy. This section covers agents routinely utilized in the management of poisoning and has been augmented to include antidotal treatment for agents used in chemical and nuclear terrorism and for exotic snake venoms as well as some antidotes that are not commercially available in the United States.

**I. Use of antidotes in pregnancy.** It is always prudent to avoid or minimize drug exposure during pregnancy, and physicians are often reluctant to use an antidote for fear of fetal harm. This reluctance, however, must be tempered with a case-by-case risk-benefit analysis of use of the particular therapeutic agent. An acute drug overdose or poisoning in pregnancy may threaten the life of the mother as well as the fetus, and the antidote or therapeutic agent, despite unknown or questionable effects on the fetus, may have lifesaving benefit. The inherent toxicity and large body burden of the drug or toxic chemical involved in the poisoning may far exceed those of the therapeutic agent or antidote.

With most agents discussed in this section, there is little or no information about their use in pregnant patients. The **Food and Drug Administration (FDA)** has established five categories of required labeling to indicate the potential for teratogenicity (see Table III–1). The distinction between categories depends mainly on the amount and reliability of animal and human data and the risk-benefit assessment for use of a specific agent. Note that the categorization may be based on anticipated chronic or repeated use and may not be relevant to a single or brief antidotal treatment.

**II. Hospital stocking.** The hospital pharmacy should maintain the medical staff–approved stock of antidotes and other emergency drugs. Surveys of hospitals consistently have demonstrated inadequate stocks of antidotes. Many antidotes are used only infrequently, have a short shelf life, or are expensive. There have also been disruptions and delays in the supply of antidotes from manufacturers as well as discontinuation of some products (eg, multidose glucagon). The optimal and most cost-effective case management of poisonings, however, requires having adequate supplies of antidotes readily available. Fortunately, only a minimal acquisition and maintenance cost is required to stock many of these drugs adequately. Other cost reduction strategies may include employment of an institutional approval and utilization review process (eg, requiring local poison center approval for the use of selected costly antidotes), seeking arrangements with suppliers to replace expired and unused antidotes (note that some manufacturers have such a policy), and redistribution of soon-to-expire antidotes. In addition, some antidotes (eg, DMPS) may be available only through compounding pharmacies; therefore, they may not be listed by wholesalers and require additional diligence to ensure the purity of the product (since the drug may be supplied by multiple foreign sources and require extemporaneous preparation).

**A.** The basis for our **suggested minimum stocking level** is a combination of factors to anticipate the highest total dose of a drug generally given during a 24-hour period as quoted in the literature, the maximum manufacturer's recommended or tolerated daily dose, and estimation of these quantities for a 70-kg adult.

**B.** Larger quantities of a drug may be needed in unusual situations (eg, chemical terrorism), particularly if multiple patients are treated simultaneously or for extended

**TABLE III–1. FDA PREGNANCY CATEGORIES FOR TERATOGENIC EFFECTS**

| FDA Pregnancy Category | Definition |
| --- | --- |
| A | Adequate and well-controlled studies in pregnant women have failed to demonstrate a risk to the fetus in the first trimester, and there is no evidence of a risk later in pregnancy. The possibility of fetal harm appears remote. |
| B | Either (1) animal reproduction studies have failed to demonstrate any adverse effect (other than a decrease in fertility) but there are no adequate and well-controlled studies in pregnant women or (2) animal studies have shown an adverse effect that has not been confirmed by adequate and well-controlled studies in pregnant women. The possibility of fetal harm is probably remote. |
| C | Either (1) animal reproduction studies have shown an adverse effect on the fetus and there are no adequate and well-controlled human studies or (2) there are no animal or human studies. The drug should be given only if the potential benefit outweighs the potential risk to the fetus. |
| D | There is positive evidence of human fetal risk based on adverse reaction data from investigational or marketing experience or human studies, but the potential risks may be acceptable in light of potential benefits (eg, use in a life-threatening situation for which safer drugs are ineffective or unavailable). |
| X | Studies in animals or humans have demonstrated fetal abnormalities, there is positive evidence of fetal risk based on human experience, or both, and the risk of using the drug in a pregnant patient outweighs any possible benefit. The drug in contraindicated in women who are or may become pregnant. |

Reference: *Code of Federal Regulations,* title 21, section 201.57 (April 1, 1990).

periods. Hospitals in close proximity may wish to explore the practicality of sharing or pooling stocks but should carefully consider the logistics of such arrangements (eg, transferring stocks after hours or on weekends). Hospitals should be linked with regional emergency response plans for hazardous (and nuclear/biological/chemical terrorism) materials and mass-casualty incidents and the mobilization of local and national antidote stockpiles (ie, Strategic National Stockpile).

## ▶ ACETYLCYSTEINE (*N*-ACETYLCYSTEINE [NAC])

*Thomas E. Kearney, PharmD*

**I. Pharmacology.** Acetylcysteine (*N*-acetylcysteine [NAC]) is a mucolytic agent that acts as a sulfhydryl group donor, substituting for the liver's usual sulfhydryl donor, glutathione. It rapidly binds (detoxifies) the highly reactive electrophilic intermediates of metabolism or it may enhance the reduction of the toxic intermediate, NAPQI, to the parent, acetaminophen. It is most effective in preventing acetaminophen-induced liver injury when given early in the course of intoxication (within 8 to 10 hours), but may also be of benefit in reducing the severity of liver injury by several proposed mechanisms (improved blood flow and oxygen delivery, modified cytokine production, free radical or oxygen scavenging) even when given after 24 hours. This proposed role of NAC as a glutathione precursor, direct sulfhydryl binding agent, and antioxidant has also been the basis for its investigational use for poisonings from agents associated with a free radical or oxidative stress mechanism of toxicity or that bind to sulfhydryl groups. It may be used empirically when the severity of ingestion is unknown or serum concentrations of the ingested drug are not immediately available.

**II. Indications**

**A.** Acetaminophen overdose.

**B.** Case reports of or investigational use in carbon tetrachloride, chloroform, acrylonitrile, doxorubicin, arsenic, gold, amanitin mushroom, carbon monoxide, chromium, cyanide, paraquat, and methyl mercury poisoning.

**C.** Pennyroyal oil and clove oil poisoning (case reports). The mechanism of hepatic injury by pennyroyal oil and clove oil are similar to that of acetaminophen, and empiric use of NAC seems justified for any significant pennyroyal oil or clove oil ingestion.

**D.** Cisplatin nephrotoxicity and prevention of radiocontrast-induced nephropathy.

**III. Contraindications.** Known acute hypersensitivity or IgE-mediated anaphylaxis (rare). Anaphylactoid reactions, while similar in clinical effects, may be prevented or ameliorated as discussed below.

**IV. Adverse effects**

**A.** Acetylcysteine typically causes nausea and vomiting when given **orally.** If the dose is vomited, it should be repeated. The dose calculation and proper dilution (to 5%) should be verified (this effect may be dose and concentration dependent). Use of a gastric tube, slower rate of administration, and a strong antiemetic agent (eg, metoclopramide, p 475; ondansetron, p 489) may be necessary.

**B.** Rapid **intravenous** administration can cause flushing, rash, angioedema, hypotension, and bronchospasm (anaphylactoid reaction). Death (status epilepticus, intracranial hypertension) was reported in a 30-month-old child accidentally receiving a massive dose intravenously (2,450 mg/kg over 6 hours, 45 minutes), and fatal bronchospasm occurred in an adult with severe asthma. Reactions might be reduced by giving each dose slowly (over at least 60 minutes) in a dilute (3–4%) solution (this effect is dose and concentration dependent) and exercising extreme caution in asthmatics (avoid IV use or carefully titrate with more dilute solutions and slower infusion rates). If an anaphylactoid reaction occurs, stop the infusion immediately and treat with diphenhydramine (see p 442) if urticaria and or angioedema is present, and epinephrine (see p 448) for more serious reactions (shock, bronchoconstriction). Once symptoms have resolved, the infusion may be recommenced at a slower infusion rate (by further dilution and given over at least 1 hour). Note: dilutional hyponatremia and seizures developed in a 3-year-old after IV administration from excess free water (see pediatric dilution precautions below).

**C. Use in pregnancy.** FDA category B. (See Table III–1) There is no evidence for teratogenicity. Use of this drug to treat acetaminophen overdose is considered beneficial to both mother and developing fetus. However, maternal hypotension or hypoxia due to a serious anaphylactoid reaction from IV administration may harm the fetus.

**V. Drug or laboratory interactions**

**A.** Activated charcoal adsorbs acetylcysteine and may interfere with its systemic absorption. When both are given orally together, data suggest that peak acetylcysteine levels are decreased by about 30% and that the time to reach peak level may be delayed. However, these effects are not considered clinically important.

**B.** NAC can produce a false-positive test for ketones in the urine.

**VI. Dosage and method of administration**

**A. Oral loading dose.** Give 140 mg/kg of the 10% (1.4 ml/kg) or 20% (0.7 ml/kg) solution diluted to approximately 5% in juice or soda to enhance palatability: dilute the loading dose of 10% NAC with 1.4 mL/kg of juice or soda (for 20% NAC dilute with 2 mL/kg of juice/soda). (See Table III–2 for oral dilution guidelines)

**B. Maintenance oral dose.** Give 70 mg/kg (as a 5% solution) every 4 hours. To make an approximately 5% solution, dilute the maintenance dose of 10% NAC (0.7 mL/kg) with 0.7 mL/kg of juice or soda (for 20% NAC dilute 0.35 mL/kg with 1

**TABLE III–2. DILUTION GUIDELINES FOR ORAL ADMINISTRATION OF NAC**

| | Volume of NAC | Approximate volume of soda/juice needed to make 5% solution |
|---|---|---|
| **Loading Dose (140mg/kg)** | | |
| Using 20% NAC (200 mg/ml) solution | 0.7 mL/kg | 2 mL/kg |
| Using 10% NAC (100 mg/ml) solution | 1.4 mL/kg | 1.4 mL/kg |
| **Maintenance dose (70 mg/kg)** | | |
| Using 20% NAC (200 mg/ml) solution | 0.35 mL/kg | 1 mL/kg |
| Using 10% NAC (100 mg/ml) solution | 0.7 mL/kg | 0.7 mL/kg |

mL/kg of juice/soda). (See Table III–2 for oral dilution guidelines). The conventional protocol for treatment of acetaminophen poisoning in the United States calls for 17 doses of oral NAC given over approximately 72 hours. However, successful shorter protocols in Canada and Europe utilize intravenous NAC for only 20 hours for uncomplicated poisonings without evidence of liver injury treated within 8 hours of ingestion. We use a shorter oral NAC regimen consisting of the usual loading dose followed by 70 mg/kg every 4 hours for five doses (20 hours). If there is evidence of hepatic toxicity, NAC should be continued until resolution of toxic effects (ie, liver function tests are clearly improving).

**C.** An **intravenous** preparation (Acetadote, Cumberland Pharmaceuticals) was approved in 2004 by the U.S. FDA and is indicated if the patient is unable to tolerate the oral formulation because of vomiting, ileus, intestinal obstruction, or other GI problems.

1. The package insert recommends the following 20 hour regimen for uncomplicated poisonings treated within 8 hours (in adults): 150 mg/kg in 200 mL of 5% dextrose in water ($D_5W$) over 15 minutes, followed by 50 mg/kg in 500 mL of $D_5W$ over 4 hours and then 100 mg/kg in 1000 mL of $D_5W$ over 16 hours. However, anaphylactoid reactions have been reported (including death in an obese asthma patient, whose dose was based on total body weight rather than ideal body weight) and we usually recommend that the loading dose be given over at least 45–60 minutes. (see Table III–3 for IV Acetadote administration guidelines and precautions)
2. Pediatric patients should have an alternate dilution volume or use of a saline-containing solution to avoid over-hydration and hyponatremia (see Table III–3 for IV Acetadote administration guidelines and precautions).
3. Many patients can be switched to an oral regimen after the first 1–2 IV doses, if vomiting has ceased.
4. If Acetadote is not available, then the oral preparation may be administered by the IV route (using an inline micropore filter).

   Contact a medical toxicologist or regional poison center ([800] 222-1222) for advice and see the formulations section below for preparation and administration.

**D. Dosage during dialysis.** Although acetylcysteine is removed during dialysis, no change in dosage is necessary.

**E. Dosage for prevention of radiocontrast-induced nephropathy.** Give 600 mg of PO NAC twice on the day before and the day of the procedure (4 doses total). This is coupled with IV hydration using 1/2 NS at 1 mL/kg/h for 12 hours before and after the administration of the contrast agent.

**VII. Formulations**

**A. Oral** The usual formulation is as a 10% (100-mg/mL) or 20% (200-mg/mL) solution, supplied as an inhaled mucolytic agent (Mucomyst, or generic). This

**TABLE III–3. DILUTION GUIDELINES FOR INTRAVENOUS ADMINISTRATION OF ACETADOTE**

| | Dose of Acetadote (20% = 200 mg/mL solution) | Volume of diluent ($D_5W$)[b] needed. | Duration of infusion |
|---|---|---|---|
| Loading Dose (150 mg/kg) | 0.75 mL/kg[a] | 3 mL/kg (pediatrics) up to 200 mL (adults) | Recommend over at least 45–60 minutes to reduce risk of anaphylactoid reactions. |
| First Maintenance dose (50 mg/kg) | 0.25 mL/kg | 1 mL/kg (pediatrics) up to 500 ml (adults) | Over 4 hours. |
| Second Maintenance dose (100 mg/kg) | 0.5 mL/kg | 2 mL/kg (pediatrics) up to 1000 ml (adults) | Over 16 hours. |

[a]We suggest use of ideal body weight for loading dose calculation in patients with morbid obesity (BMI > 40).
[b]Manufacturer indicates that NAC is also stable in 0.45% NS @ room temperature for 24 hours.

form is available through most hospital pharmacies or respiratory therapy departments. This preparation is ***not*** FDA approved for parenteral use. In rare circumstances when intravenous administration of this preparation is required and Acetadote is not available, dilute the loading dose to a 3–4% solution (In $D_5W$), use a micropore (0.22-micron) filter, and administer over 45–60 minutes. To make a 4% solution, dilute the loading dose of 10% NAC (1.4 mL/kg = 140 mg/kg) with 2.1 mL/kg of $D_5W$ (for 20% NAC dilute 0.7 mL/kg with 2.8 mL/kg of $D_5W$).

**B.** The new intravenous formulation (Acetadote) is available as a 20% solution in 30 mL (200 mg/mL) vials in a carton of 4 vials. Note: special precautions are needed to avoid accidental overdose or over-dilution with $D_5W$ in pediatric patients (see Table III–3 for IV Acetadote administration guidelines and precautions).

**C. Suggested minimum stocking level** for treatment of a 70-kg adult for the first 24 hours: 20% (oral) solution, 7 vials (30 mL each) and or 20% (IV) solution, 1 carton of 4 vials (30 ml each). We suggest that both preparations be stocked and that the oral solution be used preferentially in most cases.

## ▶ ANTIVENOM, CROTALINAE (RATTLESNAKE)

*Richard F. Clark, MD*

**I. Pharmacology.** Although two antivenoms are still available for the treatment of crotaline envenomation in some parts of the United States, the older product, Crotalinae polyvalent antivenom (equine) (Antivenom Crotalinae Polyvalent, Wyeth-Ayerst), largely has been replaced by the newer Crotalinae polyvalent immune Fab (ovine) (CroFab®, Protherics). To produce the polyvalent Fab antivenom, sheep are hyperimmunized with pooled venom from four North American snakes: *Crotalus adamanteus, C atrox, C scutulatus,* and *A piscivorus.* Papain then is added to the pooled serum product collected from the donor animals to cleave the immunogenic Fc fragment from the IgG antibody. The result is an affinity-purified Fab fragment antivenom. After administration, the antivenom is distributed widely throughout the body, where it binds to venom.

**II. Indications.** Antivenom is used for treatment of significant envenomation by Crotalinae species (see Table III–4 and p 344).

**III. Contraindications.** Known hypersensitivity to the antivenom or to horse serum is a relative contraindication for the Wyeth product; antivenom may still be indicated for severe envenomation despite a patient history of allergic reaction. Known hypersensitivity to sheep or sheep serum, or to papain or papayas, is a contraindication for the Protherics product (CroFab).

**IV. Adverse effects**

**A.** Immediate hypersensitivity reactions (including life-threatening anaphylaxis) may occur from both products, even in patients with no history of animal serum sensitivity and negative skin test results. Skin testing is **not** indicated with CroFab, and immediate hypersensitivity reactions appear to be less common.

**B.** Mild flushing and wheezing can occur within the first 30 minutes of intravenous administration and often will improve after slowing of the rate of infusion.

**C.** Delayed hypersensitivity (serum sickness) occurs in over 75% of patients who receive more than four vials of Wyeth antivenom and virtually all patients who receive more than 12 vials. Onset occurs in 5–14 days. CroFab administration can also lead to delayed hypersensitivity reactions, but this may be much less common than with the Wyeth product.

**D. Use in pregnancy.** FDA category C (indeterminate). (See p Table III–1.) There are no data on teratogenicity. Anaphylactic reaction resulting in shock or hypoxemia in the mother could conceivably adversely affect the fetus. However, severe envenomation of the mother should be treated aggressively to limit venom effects that could affect the fetus or placenta.

**V. Drug or laboratory interactions.** There are no known interactions.

**VI. Dosage and method of administration.** The initial dose is based on the severity of symptoms, not on body weight (Table III–4). Children may require doses as large as or larger than those for adults. The endpoint of antivenom therapy is the reversal of systemic manifestations (eg, shock, coagulopathy, and paresthesias) and the halting of progressive edema and pain. Repeat 4–6 vial increments of Fab antivenom (or 5–10 vial increments of Wyeth antivenom) per hour until progression of symptoms is halted. In some severe cases, large quantities of antivenom may be required, and in some cases, laboratory blood-clotting parameters may be refractory to even large doses. However, most cases can at least be stabilized with aggressive antivenom therapy. Antivenom may be effective up to 3 days or more after envenomation. If you suspect envenomation by the Mojave rattlesnake (*Crotalus scutulatus*) and symptoms are present, especially increased serum creatine phosphokinase (CPK) level, administer 10 vials of Wyeth antivenom or 4 vials of CroFab even when there is minimal swelling or local pain.

**A.** Treat all patients in an intensive care or monitored setting.

**B.** Before skin tests or antivenom administration, insert at least one and preferably two secure intravenous lines.

**TABLE III–4. INITIAL DOSE OF CROTALINAE ANTIVENOM**

| Severity of Envenomation | Initial Dose (vials): Antivenom Crotalinae Polyvalent (Wyeth) | Initial Dose (vials): CroFab (Protherics) |
|---|---|---|
| None or minimal | None | None |
| Mild (local pain and swelling) | 5 | 4 |
| Moderate (proximal progression of swelling, ecchymosis, mild systemic symptoms) | 10 | 4–6 |
| Severe (hypotension, rapidly progressive swelling and ecchymosis, coagulopathy) | 15 | 8 |

C. Perform the skin test for horse serum sensitivity for the Wyeth product (**not** indicated with CroFab), using a 1:10 dilution of antivenom (some experts prefer this method) or the sample of horse serum provided in the antivenom kit (follow package instructions). Do ***not*** perform the skin test unless signs of envenomation are present and imminent antivenom therapy is anticipated. If the skin test is positive, reconsider the need for antivenom as opposed to supportive care but do not abandon antivenom therapy if it is needed. Even if the skin test is negative, anaphylaxis may still occur unpredictably.

D. If antivenom is used in a patient with a positive skin test, pretreat with intravenous diphenhydramine (see p 442) and cimetidine (or another $H_2$ blocker; see p 433) and have ready at the bedside a preloaded syringe containing epinephrine (1:10,000 for intravenous use) in case of anaphylaxis. Dilute the antivenom 1:10 to 1:1000 before administration and give each vial very slowly at first (ie, over 30–45 minutes), increasing the rate of infusion as tolerated.

E. Reconstitute the lyophilized vial of either product with the 10 mL of diluent provided or sterile saline and gently swirl for 10–30 minutes to solubilize the material. Avoid shaking, which may destroy the immunoglobulins (as indicated by foam formation). Further dilution with 50–200 mL of saline may facilitate solubilization.

F. Administer antivenom by the intravenous route only. Start slowly, increasing the rate as tolerated. In nonallergic individuals, 5–10 vials of Wyeth antivenom or 4–6 vials of CroFab can be diluted in 250–500 mL saline and given over 60–90 minutes.

G. If there is an inadequate response to the initial dose, give an additional 4 vials of CroFab (5–10 vials of Wyeth) over 60 minutes, or give an additional 6 vials of CroFab if signs of severe envenomation are still present. Repeat in 4- to 6-vial increments (5–10 vials of Wyeth) per hour until the progression of symptoms is halted.

H. Recurrence of symptoms of envenomation may occur with use of either antivenom but may be more common with CroFab owing to its shorter half-life within the body of the Fab molecule. Recurrence after CroFab usually is manifested 12–36 hours after stabilization is achieved with the initial dosing of CroFab. Repeating laboratory tests and observing for progression of swelling therefore are recommended for 24 hours or more when CroFab antivenom is used. The repeat administration of CroFab in 2-vial (or more if needed) increments is recommended if recurrence occurs. As an alternative, the package insert suggests consideration of repeat 2-vial dosing every 6 hours for 3 additional doses in severe envenomations.

VII. **Formulations**

A. **Antivenom Crotalinae (formerly Crotalidae) polyvalent or Crotalinae polyvalent immune Fab.** Supplies can be located by a regional poison center ([800] 222-1222).

B. The **suggested minimum stocking level** to treat a 70-kg adult for the first 24 hours is 20 vials of Wyeth antivenom or 12 vials of CroFab.

## ▶ ANTIVENOM, *LATRODECTUS MACTANS* (BLACK WIDOW SPIDER)

*Richard F. Clark, MD*

I. **Pharmacology.** To produce the antivenom, horses are hyperimmunized with *Latrodectus mactans* (black widow spider) venom. The lyophilized protein product from pooled equine sera contains antibodies specific to certain venom fractions as well as residual serum proteins such as albumin and globulins. After intravenous administration, the antivenom distributes widely throughout the body, where it binds to venom.

**II. Indications**

**A.** Black widow envenomation–induced severe hypertension or muscle cramping that is not alleviated by muscle relaxants, analgesics, or sedation; consider particularly in patients at the extremes of age (ie, younger than 1 year or older than 65 years).

**B.** Black widow envenomation in **pregnancy** may cause abdominal muscle spasms severe enough to threaten spontaneous abortion or early onset of labor.

**III. Contraindications.** Known hypersensitivity to horse serum.

**IV. Adverse effects**

**A.** Immediate hypersensitivity may occur rarely, including life-threatening anaphylaxis.

**B.** Delayed-onset serum sickness may occur after 10–14 days but is rare owing to the small volume of antivenom used in most cases.

**C. Use in pregnancy.** FDA category C (indeterminate). There are no data on teratogenicity. An anaphylactic reaction resulting in shock or hypoxemia in the mother could conceivably affect the fetus adversely (see Table III–1).

**V. Drug or laboratory interactions.** No known interactions.

**VI. Dosage and method of administration.** Generally, one vial of antivenom is sufficient to treat black widow envenomation in adults or children. The antivenom is dosed on the basis of symptoms, not on patient weight.

**A.** Treat all patients in an emergency department or intensive care setting.

**B.** Before a skin test or antivenom administration, insert at least one and preferably two secure intravenous lines.

**C.** Perform a skin test for horse serum sensitivity by using a 1:10 dilution of antivenom (some experts prefer this method) or the sample of horse serum provided in the antivenom kit (according to package instructions). Do ***not*** perform the skin test unless signs of envenomation are present and imminent antivenom therapy is anticipated. If the skin test is positive, reconsider the need for antivenom as opposed to supportive care but do not abandon antivenom therapy if it is needed. Even if the skin test is negative, anaphylaxis may occur unpredictably.

**D.** If antivenom is used in a patient with horse serum sensitivity, pretreat with intravenous diphenhydramine (see p 442) and cimetidine (or another $H_2$ blocker; see p 433), and have ready at the bedside a preloaded syringe containing epinephrine (1:10,000 for intravenous use) in case of anaphylaxis. Dilute the antivenom (1:10 to 1:1000) and administer it very slowly in these cases.

**E.** Reconstitute the lyophilized product to 2.5 mL with the supplied diluent, using gentle swirling for 15–30 minutes to avoid shaking and destroying the immunoglobulins (as indicated by the formation of foam).

**F.** Dilute this solution to a total volume of 10–50 mL with normal saline.

**G.** Administer the diluted antivenom slowly over 15–30 minutes. One or two vials are sufficient in most cases.

**VII. Formulations**

**A.** Lyophilized antivenom (*L mactans*), 6000 units, contains 1:10,000 thimerosal as a preservative. Note product also listed as antivenin (*Latrodectus mactans*).

**B.** The **suggested minimum stocking level** to treat a 70-kg adult for the first 24 hours is one vial.

## ► ANTIVENOM, *MICRURUS FULVIUS* (CORAL SNAKE), AND EXOTIC ANTIVENOMS

*Richard F. Clark, MD*

**I. Pharmacology.** To produce the antivenom for North American coral snake bites, horses are hyperimmunized with venom from *Micrurus fulvius,* the eastern coral snake. The lyophilized protein preparation from pooled equine sera contains IgG antibodies to venom fractions as well as residual serum proteins. Administered intravenously, the antibodies distribute widely throughout the body, where they bind the target venom.

**Exotic antivenoms.** Companies outside the United States produce a variety of antivenoms for exotic snakebites. Most of these products treat snakebites by elapids, since this family of snakes causes the most severe envenomations worldwide. The vast majority are still whole-antibody products derived from horses. A few are produced as Fab fragments, or the slightly larger $Fab_2$ molecule (cleaved with pepsin instead of papain). In both of these cases, the Fc is removed from the solution. Many foreign antivenom products are polyvalent, a mixture of antivenoms for several species.

**II. Indications**

**A.** Envenomation by the eastern coral snake (*M fulvius*) or the Texas coral snake (*M fulvius tenere*).

**B.** ***May not be effective*** for envenomation by the western, Arizona, or Sonora coral snake (*M euryxanthus*).

**III. Contraindications.** Known hypersensitivity to *Micrurus* antivenom or to horse serum is a relative contraindication; if a patient with significant envenomation needs the antivenom, it should be given with caution. Antivenoms produced outside of the United States may be made from horse or sheep serum.

**IV. Adverse effects**

**A.** Immediate hypersensitivity, including life-threatening anaphylaxis, may occur even after a negative skin test for horse serum sensitivity.

**B.** Delayed hypersensitivity (serum sickness) may occur 1–3 weeks after antivenom administration, with the incidence and severity depending on the total quantity of antivenom administered.

**C. Use in pregnancy.** FDA category C (indeterminate). There are no data on teratogenicity. Anaphylactic reactions resulting in shock or hypoxemia in expectant mothers could conceivably affect the fetus adversely. This should be weighed against the potential detrimental effect of the venom on both the placenta and the fetus (see Table III–1).

**D. Exotic antivenoms.** All the whole-antibody preparations carry the same risk of immediate and delayed allergy as US-produced whole-IgG antivenoms.

**V. Drug or laboratory interactions.** There are no known interactions.

**VI. Dosage and method of administration.** Generally, the recommended initial dose of *Micrurus* antivenom is three to five vials. The drug is most effective if given before the onset of signs or symptoms of envenomation. An additional three to five vials may be given, depending on the severity of neurologic manifestations but not on body weight (children may require doses as large as or even larger than those for adults).

The recommended dose of exotic snake antivenom will vary. With other elapids, such as cobras, the antivenom is also more effective if given early in the course of the envenomation.

**A.** Treat all patients in an intensive care unit setting.

**B.** Before a skin test or antivenom administration, insert at least one and preferably two secure intravenous lines.

**C.** Perform a skin test for horse serum sensitivity, using a 1:10 dilution of antivenom (some experts prefer this method) or the sample of horse serum provided in the antivenom kit (according to package instructions). If the skin test is positive, reconsider the need for antivenom as opposed to supportive care but do not abandon antivenom therapy if it is needed. Even if the skin test is negative, anaphylaxis may occur unpredictably.

Antivenoms to exotic species may not contain skin-testing solutions. A small amount (0.1 mL) of antivenom can be used as a skin test for these preparations, or this step may be omitted (especially in the case of Fab and $Fab_2$ antivenoms).

**D.** If antivenom is used in a patient with a positive skin test, pretreat with intravenous diphenhydramine (see p 442) and cimetidine (or another $H_2$ blocker; p

433) and have ready at the bedside a preloaded syringe containing epinephrine (1:10,000 for intravenous use) in case of anaphylaxis. Dilute the antivenom (1:10 to 1:1000) and administer very slowly in these cases.

**E.** Reconstitute the lyophilized *Micrurus* antivenom with 10 mL of the diluent supplied, gently swirling for 10–30 minutes. Avoid shaking the preparation because this may destroy the immunoglobulins (as indicated by the formation of foam). Dilution with 50–200 mL of saline may aid solubilization.

**F.** Administer the antivenom intravenously over 15–30 minutes per vial.

**G. Exotic elapids.** Envenomation by exotic elapids, such as cobras, mambas, and all the poisonous snakes of Australia, would be expected to produce the same or a worse degree of neurotoxicity as is seen in envenomation from coral snakes from the United States, and require antivenom administration as soon as possible. It is conceivable that bites from snakes within the same family could respond to antivenom made from venom of another snake in that family. Therefore, if type-specific antivenom is not available for a severe snakebite, same-family antivenom may be substituted with some possible efficacy. Regional poison centers (1-800-222-1222) may be able to assist in obtaining exotic antivenoms from collectors or zoos.

**VII. Formulations**

**A.** Antivenom (*M fulvius*) vial of lyophilized powder with 0.25% phenol and 0.005% thimerosal as preservatives. Note that this product is also listed as antivenin (*Micrurus fulvius*).

**B. Suggested minimum stocking level** to treat a 70-kg adult for the first 24 hours is 5–10 vials.

## ▶ APOMORPHINE

*Thomas E. Kearney, PharmD*

**I. Pharmacology.** Apomorphine is an alkaloid salt derived from morphine that is a dopaminergic agonist with minimal analgesic properties but marked emetic efficacy. Vomiting is produced by direct stimulation of the medullary chemoreceptor trigger zone. After subcutaneous administration, emesis occurs within an average of 5 minutes; oral administration is ***not*** recommended because of erratic absorption. In 2004, the FDA approved apomorphine for the treatment of hypomobility episodes associated with Parkinson's disease.

**II. Indications.** Apomorphine previously was used for induction of emesis in the acute management of oral poisoning, but it has been abandoned because of its potential for respiratory depression. The drug is not discussed further in this book, but it remains popular in veterinary practice.

## ▶ ATROPINE AND GLYCOPYRROLATE

*Richard J. Geller, MD, MPH*

**I. Pharmacology.** Atropine and glycopyrrolate are parasympatholytic agents that competitively block the action of acetylcholine at muscarinic receptors. Atropine is a naturally occurring tertiary amine that crosses the blood-brain barrier and shares significant structural and functional similarity with scopolamine, homatropine, and ipratropium. Glycopyrrolate is a synthetic quaternary amine that crosses the blood-brain barrier poorly and is less likely than atropine to cause altered mental status or tachycardia. Desired therapeutic effects for treating poisoning include decreased secretions from salivary and other glands, decreased bronchorrhea and wheezing, decreased intestinal secretion and peristalsis, increased heart rate, and enhanced atrioventricular conduction. The elimination half-life of atropine is 2–4 hours (longer in children), with approximately 50% excreted unchanged in urine. Glycopyrrolate is excreted unchanged primarily in the bile and urine.

**II. Indications**

**A.** Correction of bronchorrhea and excessive oral and GI tract secretions associated with organophosphate and carbamate insecticide intoxication. Glycopyrrolate may be especially useful in managing peripheral cholinergic symptoms in cholinesterase inhibitor poisoning. Although glycopyrrolate will not reverse CNS toxicity associated with cholinesterase inhibitor poisoning, it also will not cause the CNS side effects seen with large doses of atropine, which are difficult to distinguish from the toxic effects of cholinesterase inhibitors.

**B.** Acceleration of the rate of sinus node firing and AV nodal conduction velocity in the presence of drug-induced AV conduction impairment (eg, caused by digitalis, beta blockers, calcium antagonists, organophosphorus or carbamate insecticides, or physostigmine).

**C.** Reversal of central (by atropine) and peripheral (by atropine and glycopyrrolate) muscarinic symptoms in patients with intoxication by *Clitocybe* or *Inocybe* mushroom species.

**D.** When neostigmine or pyridostigmine is used to reverse nondepolarizing neuromuscular blockade, glycopyrrolate is the preferred agent to block unwanted muscarinic effects (neuromuscular blockers, see p 480).

**III. Contraindications**

All these contraindications are relative, and in some clinical situations benefit exceeds possible harm.

**A.** Patients with hypertension, tachyarrhythmias, thyrotoxicosis, congestive heart failure, coronary artery disease, valvular heart disease, and other illnesses who might not tolerate a rapid heart rate. Patients with severe cholinesterase inhibitor poisoning are often tachycardic. Atropine should not be withheld and may lower the heart rate (by improving oxygenation). Glycopyrrolate may also be helpful (due to its lessened propensity to cause a tachycardia).

**B.** Angle-closure glaucoma in which papillary dilation may increase intraocular pressure. (May be used safely if the patient is being treated with a miotic.)

**C.** Partial or complete obstructive uropathy.

**D.** Myasthenia gravis.

**E.** Obstructive diseases of the GI tract, severe ulcerative colitis, bacterial infections of the GI tract.

**IV. Adverse effects**

**A.** Adverse effects include dry mouth, blurred vision, cycloplegia, mydriasis, palpitations, tachycardia, aggravation of angina, congestive heart failure (CHF), and constipation. Urinary retention is common, and a Foley catheter may be needed. Duration of effects may be prolonged (several hours). Additionally, CNS anticholinergic toxicity (delirium) may occur with the large doses of atropine needed to treat cholinesterase inhibitor poisoning.

**B.** Atropine doses of less than 0.5 mg (in adults) and those administered by very slow intravenous push may result in paradoxic slowing of heart rate.

**C. Use in pregnancy.** Atropine is FDA category C (indeterminate). It readily crosses the placenta. However, this does not preclude its acute, short-term use for a seriously symptomatic patient (see p 407). Glycopyrrolate is FDA category B and crosses the placenta poorly.

**V. Drug or laboratory interactions**

**A.** Atropinization may occur more rapidly if atropine and pralidoxime are given concurrently to patients with organophosphate or carbamate insecticide poisoning.

**B.** Atropine and glycopyrrolate have an additive effect with other antimuscarinic and antihistaminic compounds.

**C.** Slowing of GI motility may delay absorption of orally ingested materials.

**VI. Dosage and method of administration**

**A. Cholinesterase inhibitor poisoning** (eg, organophosphate or carbamate insecticides, "nerve agents").

1. **Atropine.** For adults, begin with 0.5–2 mg IV; for children, give 0.02 mg/kg IV. (The drug may also be given via the intratracheal route; dilute the dose in normal saline to a total volume of 1–2 mL.) Double the dose every 5 minutes until satisfactory atropinization is achieved. (Decreased secretions and wheezing, increased heart rate.) Severely poisoned patients may require very large doses (eg, up to 100 mg over a few hours) of atropine determined by chemical titration and control of muscarinic symptoms. In mass-casualty situations, atropine can be given IM. It may also be administered by ophthalmic and inhalation routes for reversal of topical effects from gas or mist exposures.
2. **Glycopyrrolate.** Initial IV dose for adults is 1–2 mg (children: 0.025 mg/kg).
3. **Other agents.** If mass-casualty situation depletes the local supply of atropine and glycopyrrolate, other muscarinic receptor antagonist agents such as scopolamine (tertiary) and ipratropium (quaternary) may be considered.
4. **Therapeutic endpoints.** The goal of therapy is the drying of bronchial secretions (this endpoint may be reached prematurely if the patient is dehydrated) and reversal of wheezing and significant bradycardia. Recrudescence of symptoms may occur, and in severe poisonings several grams of atropine may be required and may be administered by constant IV infusion or with larger bolus doses and/or more frequent intervals (eg, 3–5 minutes).

**B. Drug-induced bradycardia.** Atropine is usually the drug of choice in this circumstance. For adults, give 0.5–1 mg IV; for children, give 0.02 mg/kg IV up to a maximum of 0.5 mg and 1 mg in adolescents. Repeat as needed. Note that 3 mg is a fully vagolytic dose in adults. If a response is not achieved by 3 mg, the patient is unlikely to benefit from further treatment unless bradycardia is caused by excessive cholinergic effects (eg, carbamate or organophosphate overdose).

**VII. Formulations**

**A. Parenteral.** Atropine sulfate injection, 0.05-, 0.1-, 0.3-, 0.4-, 0.5-, 0.6-, 0.8-, 1-, and 1.2-mg/mL solutions. (Atropine has been stockpiled by the Strategic National Stockpile (SNS) program as 20-mL vials of the 0.4 mg/mL solution and combined (2 mg per dose) with pralidoxime (600 mg per dose) in the Mark 1 auto-injector kits.) Use preservative-free formulations when massive doses are required. Glycopyrrolate injection (Robinul, others), 0.2 mg/mL in 1-, 2-, 5-, and 20-mL vials (some with 0.9% benzyl alcohol).

**B.** The **suggested minimum stocking level** to treat a 70-kg adult for the first 24 hours is 1 g atropine and 20 mg glycopyrrolate (higher amounts may be needed if this is the sole antimuscarinic agent).

## ► BAL (DIMERCAPROL)

*Michael J Kosnett, MD, MPH*

**I. Pharmacology.** BAL (British anti-Lewisite, dimercaprol, 2,3-dimercaptopropanol) is a dithiol chelating agent that is used in the treatment of poisoning by the heavy metals arsenic, mercury, lead, and gold. Because the vicinal thiol groups are unstable in aqueous solution, the drug is supplied as a 10% solution (100 mg/mL) in peanut oil that also contains 20% (200 mg/mL) benzyl benzoate. It is administered by deep IM injection. Most of the drug is absorbed within 1 hour and undergoes widespread distribution to most tissues. BAL, or its in vivo biotransformation product(s), is believed to form complexes with selected toxic metals, thereby minimizing the metal's reaction with endogenous ligands and increasing its excretion in urine.

In a study of humans treated with BAL after exposure to arsenicals, peak urinary arsenic excretion occurred in 2–4 hours and then declined rapidly.

**II. Indications**

**A.** Acute inorganic **arsenic** poisoning. Limited data suggest it may also be useful in the early stages of arsine poisoning (ie, during the first 24 hours).

**B. Mercury** poisoning (except monoalkyl mercury). BAL is most effective in preventing renal damage if it is administered within 4 hours after acute ingestion of inorganic mercury salts; its value in averting or treating the acute or chronic neurologic effects of elemental mercury vapor is unknown.

**C. Lead** poisoning (except alkyl lead compounds). BAL has been used concomitantly with calcium EDTA (p 446) in the treatment of pediatric lead encephalopathy, where the joint regimen has been associated with an accelerated decline in blood lead levels and increased urinary lead excretion. ***Note:*** BAL is not for use as a single-drug regimen in lead poisoning.

**D. Gold.** BAL has been associated with an increase in urinary gold excretion and clinical improvement in patients treated for adverse dermatologic, hematologic, or neurologic complications of pharmaceutical gold preparations.

**III. Contraindications**

**A.** Because BAL is dispensed in peanut oil, avoid use in patients with peanut allergy.

**B.** Use with caution in patients with hepatic and renal impairment. A few reports suggest that dimercaprol or its metabolites are dialyzable and that BAL increases the dialysis clearance of mercury in patients with renal failure.

**C.** BAL has caused hemolysis in patients with G-6-PD deficiency.

**D.** Because it is given by IM injection, use with caution in patients with thrombocytopenia or coagulopathies.

**IV. Adverse effects**

**A.** Local pain at injection site; sterile or pyogenic abscess formation.

**B.** Dose-related hypertension, with or without tachycardia. Onset, 15–30 minutes; duration, 2 hours. Use with caution in hypertensive patients.

**C. Other adverse symptoms.** Nausea and vomiting, headache; burning sensations in the eyes, lips, mouth, and throat sometimes accompanied by lacrimation, rhinorrhea, or salivation; myalgias; paresthesias; fever (particularly in children); a sensation of constriction in the chest; and generalized anxiety. Central nervous system depression and seizures have occurred in overdose.

**D. Use in pregnancy.** FDA category C (indeterminate) (see p 407). High doses of BAL are teratogenic and embryotoxic in mice. The safety of BAL in human pregnancy is not established, although it has been used in a pregnant patient with Wilson's disease without apparent harm. It should be used in pregnancy only for life-threatening acute intoxication.

**E. Redistribution of metals to the brain.** Despite its capacity to increase survival in acutely poisoned animals, BAL has been associated with redistribution of mercury and arsenic into the brain. Avoid use in chronic elemental mercury poisoning or alkyl (eg, methyl) mercury poisoning, where the brain is a key target organ.

**V. Drug or laboratory interactions**

**A.** Because a toxic complex with iron may be formed, avoid concurrent iron replacement therapy.

**B.** BAL may abruptly terminate gold therapy–induced remission of rheumatoid arthritis.

**VI. Dosage and method of administration (adults and children)**

**A. Arsenic, mercury, and gold poisoning.** Give BAL, 3 mg/kg deep intramuscular injection every 4–6 hours for 2 days, then every 12 hours for up to 7–10 days if the patient remains symptomatic and/or metal levels remain highly elevated. In patients with severe arsenic or mercury poisoning, an initial dose of up to 5 mg/kg may be used. Consider changing to oral succimer (p 510) or oral unithiol (p 515) once the patient is stable and able to absorb an oral formulation. ***Note:*** Intravenous unithiol (see p 515) has a more favorable therapeutic index than BAL and may be a preferable alternative in the treatment of acute arsenic or mercury intoxication.

**B. Lead encephalopathy** (only in conjunction with calcium EDTA therapy [see p 446]). For acute pediatric lead encephalopathy, some clinicians initiate treatment with BAL, 3–4 mg/kg IM (75 mg/$m^2$), followed in 4 hours by concomitant use of calcium EDTA and BAL, 3–4 mg/kg (75 mg/$m^2$) every 4–6 hours for up to 3 days.

**C. Arsine poisoning** (see p 119). Consider the use of BAL, 3 mg/kg IM every 4–6 hours for 1 day, if it can be begun within 24 hours of the onset of arsine poisoning.

**D. Lewisite burns to the eye**. Create a 5% solution of BAL by diluting the 10% ampule 1:1 in vegetable oil and *immediately* apply to the surface of the eye and conjunctivae. Parenteral treatment may also be necessary to treat systemic effects (see p 373).

**VII. Formulations**

**A. Parenteral** (for deep IM injection only; must ***not*** be given as IV). BAL in oil, 100 mg/mL, 3-mL ampules.

**B.** The **suggested minimum stocking level** to treat a 70-kg adult for the first 24 hours is 1800 mg (six ampules).

# ▶ BENZODIAZEPINES (DIAZEPAM, LORAZEPAM, AND MIDAZOLAM)

*Thomas E. Kearney, PharmD*

**I. Pharmacology**

**A.** Benzodiazepines potentiate inhibitory GABA neuronal activity in the CNS. Pharmacologic effects include reduction of anxiety, suppression of seizure activity, CNS depression (possible respiratory arrest when given rapidly intravenously), and inhibition of spinal afferent pathways to produce skeletal muscle relaxation.

**B.** In addition, diazepam has been reported to antagonize the cardiotoxic effect of chloroquine (the mechanism is unknown, but diazepam may compete with chloroquine for fixation sites on cardiac cells).

**C.** Benzodiazepines generally have little effect on the autonomic nervous system or cardiovascular system. However, enhancement of GABA neurotransmission may blunt sympathetic discharge (and lower blood pressure associated with sympathomimetic intoxications), and diazepam may have an effect on choline transport and acetylcholine turnover in the CNS this may be part of the basis for its beneficial effect for nerve agent poisoning (eg, Sarin, VX).

**D. Pharmacokinetics.** All these agents are well absorbed orally, but diazepam is not well absorbed intramuscularly. The drugs are eliminated by hepatic metabolism, with serum elimination half-lives of 1–50 hours. The duration of CNS effects is determined by the rate of drug redistribution from the brain to peripheral tissues. Active metabolites further extend the duration of effect of diazepam.

1. **Diazepam.** Onset of action is fast after intravenous injection but slow to intermediate after oral or rectal administration. The half-life is greater than 24 hours, although anticonvulsant effects and sedation are often shorter as a result of redistribution from the CNS.
2. **Lorazepam.** Onset is intermediate after intramuscular dosing. The elimination half-life is 10–20 hours, and anticonvulsant effects are generally longer than those for diazepam.

3. **Midazolam.** Onset is rapid after intramuscular or intravenous injection and intermediate after nasal application or ingestion. The half-life is 1.5–3 hours, and the duration of effects is very short owing to rapid redistribution from the brain. However, sedation may persist for 10 hours or longer after prolonged infusions as a result of saturation of peripheral sites and slowed redistribution.

**II. Indications**

A. **Anxiety and agitation.** Benzodiazepines often are used for the treatment of anxiety or agitation (eg, caused by sympathomimetic or hallucinogenic drug intoxication).

B. **Convulsions.** All three drugs can be used for the treatment of acute seizure activity or status epilepticus resulting from idiopathic epilepsy or convulsant drug overdose. Midazolam and lorazepam have the advantage of rapid absorption after intramuscular injection. Lorazepam also has a longer duration of anticonvulsant action than do the other two agents.

C. **Hypertension.** These drugs can be used for the initial treatment of sympathomimetic-induced hypertension.

D. **Muscle relaxant.** These drugs can be used for relaxation of excessive muscle rigidity and contractions (eg, caused by strychnine poisoning or black widow spider envenomation or rigidity syndromes with hyperthermia or dyskinesias or tetanus).

E. **Chloroquine poisoning.** Diazepam may antagonize cardiotoxicity.

F. **Alcohol or sedative-hypnotic withdrawal.** Diazepam and lorazepam are used to abate symptoms and signs of alcohol and hypnosedative withdrawal (eg, anxiety, tremor, and seizures).

G. **Conscious sedation.** Midazolam is used to induce sedation and amnesia during brief procedures and in conjunction with neuromuscular paralysis for endotracheal intubation.

H. **Nerve agents.** These drugs can be used for the treatment of agitation, muscle fasciculations, and seizures associated with nerve agent poisoning (see p 372). They may have an additive or synergistic effect with other nerve agent antidotes (2-PAM, atropine).

**III. Contraindications.** Do not use in patients with a known sensitivity to benzodiazepines.

**IV. Adverse effects**

A. Central nervous system–depressant effects may interfere with evaluation of neurologic function. They also may cause a paradoxic reaction (restlessness, agitation) in less than 1% of patients (adults and children). Flumazenil (see p 452) has been used successfully to manage this effect.

B. Excessive or rapid intravenous administration may cause respiratory arrest.

C. The drug may precipitate or worsen hepatic encephalopathy.

D. Rapid or large-volume IV administration may cause cardiotoxicity similar to that seen with phenytoin (see p 304) because of the diluent propylene glycol. Continuous infusions with this vehicle may also result in a hyperlactatemia, increased osmolar gap, and renal dysfunction. Several products also contain up to 2% benzyl alcohol as a preservative.

E. **Use in pregnancy.** FDA category D. All these drugs readily cross the placenta. However, this does not preclude their acute, short-term use for a seriously symptomatic patient (see p 407).

**V. Drug or laboratory interactions**

A. Benzodiazepines will potentiate the CNS–depressant effects of opioids, ethanol, and other sedative-hypnotic and depressant drugs.

B. **Flumazenil** (see p 452) will reverse the effects of benzodiazepines and may trigger an acute abstinence syndrome in patients who use the drugs chronically. Patients who have received flumazenil will have an unpredictable but reduced or absent response to benzodiazepines.

C. Diazepam may produce a false-positive glucose reaction with Clinistix and Diastix test strips.

**VI. Dosage and method of administration**

**A. Anxiety or agitation; muscle spasm or hyperactivity; hypertension**

1. **Diazepam.** Give 0.1–0.2 mg/kg (usual doses: children > 5 years and adults 2–10 mg; children > 30 days to 5 years 1–2 mg) IV initially (no faster than 5 mg/min in adults; administer over 3 minutes in children), depending on severity (tetanus requires higher doses); may repeat every 1–4 hours as needed. The oral dose is 0.1–0.3 mg/kg (adults 2–10 mg; lower doses for geriatric patients not to exceed 2.5 mg and less frequent intervals; children > 6 months 1–2.5 mg). Doses should be adjusted to tolerance and response. ***Caution:*** Do ***not*** give intramuscularly because of erratic absorption and pain on injection. Use lorazepam or midazolam if IM administration is necessary.
2. **Lorazepam.** Give 1–2 mg (children: 0.04 mg/kg IV) not to exceed 2 mg/min or 0.05 mg/kg IM (maximum 4 mg). The usual adult oral dose is 2–6 mg daily.
3. **Midazolam.** Give 0.05 mg/kg (up to 0.35 mg/kg for anesthesia induction) IV over 20–30 seconds (usual adult doses vary from 1 mg to a maximum of 5 mg given in increments of 2.5 mg every 2 minutes; lower dose in geriatric patients with maximum at 3.5 mg) or 0.07–0.1 mg/kg IM. Repeat after 10–20 minutes if needed. Continuous infusions have also been used to maintain effect with initial rates of 0.02–0.1 mg/kg/h (usual adult dose 1–7 mg/h; children 1–2 mcg/kg/min) and then titrated to effect. ***Caution:*** There have been several reports of respiratory arrest and hypotension after rapid intravenous injection, especially when midazolam is given in combination with opioids. Prolonged continuous infusion may lead to persistent sedation after the drug is discontinued because midazolam accumulates in tissues.

**B. Convulsions.** ***Note:*** If convulsions persist after initial doses of benzodiazepines, consider alternative anticonvulsant drugs such as phenobarbital (see p 494), phenytoin (p 496), pentobarbital (p 493),and propofol (p 502). Also, see treatment of seizures (p 22).

1. **Diazepam.** Give 0.1–0.2 mg/kg IV, not to exceed 5 mg/min, every 5–10 minutes (usual initial doses: adult, 5–10 mg; children ≥ 5 years, 1–2 mg; children ≤5 years, 0.2–0.5 mg), to a maximum total of 30 mg (adults) or 5 mg (young children) or 10 mg (older children).
2. **Lorazepam.** Give 1–2 mg (neonates, 0.05–0.1 mg/kg; older children, 0.04 mg/kg) IV, not to exceed 2 mg/min; repeat if needed after 5–10 minutes. Usual dose for status epilepticus is up to 4 mg slow IV push over 2 minutes (dilute with an equal volume of saline). The drug can also be given IM (0.05 mg/kg, maximum 4 mg), with onset of effects after 6–10 minutes.
3. **Midazolam.** Give 0.05 mg/kg (up to 0.2 mg/kg for refractory status epilepticus) IV over 20–30 seconds or 0.1–0.2 mg/kg IM; this may be repeated if needed after 5–10 minutes or maintained with a continuous infusion (see note above). The drug is absorbed rapidly after IM injection and can be used when IV access is not readily available.

**C. Chloroquine and hydroxychloroquine intoxication.** There is reported improvement of cardiotoxicity with **high-dose** administration of **diazepam** at 1–2 mg/kg IV (infuse over 30 minutes) followed by an infusion of 2 mg/kg/24 hours. ***Caution:*** This probably will cause apnea; the patient must be intubated, and ventilation must be controlled.

**D. Alcohol withdrawal syndrome**

1. **Diazepam.** Administer 5–10 mg IV initially, then 5 mg every 10 minutes until the patient is calm. Large doses may be required to sedate patients with severe withdrawal. The oral dose is 10–20 mg initially, repeated every 1–2 hours until calm.
2. **Lorazepam.** Administer 1–2 mg IV initially, then 1 mg every 10 minutes until the patient is calm. Large doses may be required to sedate patients in severe withdrawal. (***Note:*** Multidose vials may contain diluents and pre-

servatives such as propylene glycol and benzyl alcohol, which can be toxic in high doses.) The usual oral dose is 2–4 mg, repeated every 1–2 hours until calm.

**VII. Formulations**

**A. Parenteral**

1. **Diazepam** (Valium, others): 5-mg/mL solution, 2-mL prefilled syringes. 10 mg IM autoinjector (ComboPen) for nerve agent poisoning; note caution above.
2. **Lorazepam** (Ativan, others): 2- and 4-mg/mL solutions; 1 mL in 2-mL syringe for dilution and 10 mL multidose vials.
3. **Midazolam** (Versed): 1- and 5-mg/mL solutions; 1-, 2-, 5-, and 10-mL vials.

**B. Oral**

1. **Diazepam** (Valium, others): 2-, 5-, and 10-mg tablets.
2. **Lorazepam** (Ativan, others): 0.5-, 1-, and 2-mg tablets; 2 mg/mL oral solution.

**C. Suggested minimum stocking levels** to treat a 70-kg adult for the first 24 hours:

1. **Diazepam,** 200 mg.
2. **Lorazepam,** 24 mg.
3. **Midazolam,** 50 mg (two vials of 5 mg/mL, 5 mL each, or equivalent).

## ► BENZTROPINE

*Thomas E. Kearney, PharmD*

**I. Pharmacology.** Benztropine is an antimuscarinic agent with pharmacologic activity similar to that of atropine. The drug also exhibits antihistaminic properties. Benztropine is used for the treatment of parkinsonism and the control of extrapyramidal side effects associated with neuroleptic use.

**II. Indications.** Benztropine is an alternative in adults to diphenhydramine (the drug of choice for children) for the treatment of acute dystonic reactions associated with neuroleptics or metoclopramide. It has a longer duration of action than does diphenhydramine and is administered twice daily. ***Note:*** It is not effective for tardive dyskinesia or neuroleptic malignant syndrome (see p 22).

**III. Contraindications**

**A.** Angle-closure glaucoma.

**B.** Obstructive uropathy (prostatic hypertrophy).

**C.** Myasthenia gravis.

**D.** Not recommended for children under 3 years by the manufacturer; alternatively, use diphenhydramine (see p 442) or consider benztropine if the patient is unresponsive or hypersensitive to diphenhydramine and is experiencing a severe or life-threatening situation (eg, dystonic laryngeal or pharyngeal spasms).

**E.** Tardive dyskinesia

**F.** Known hypersensitivity

**IV. Adverse effects**

**A.** Adverse effects include sedation, blurred vision, tachycardia, urinary hesitancy or retention, and dry mouth. Adverse effects are minimal after single doses.

**B. Use in pregnancy.** FDA category C (indeterminate). However, this does not preclude its acute, short-term use for a seriously symptomatic patient (see p 407).

**V. Drug or laboratory interactions**

**A.** Benztropine has additive effects with other drugs that exhibit antimuscarinic properties (eg, antihistamines, phenothiazines, cyclic antidepressants, and disopyramide).

**B.** Slowing of GI motility may delay or inhibit absorption of certain drugs.

**VI. Dosage and method of administration**

**A. Parenteral.** Give 1–2 mg IV or IM (children 3 years old, 0.02 mg/kg and 1 mg maximum). May repeat dose in 15 minutes if unresponsive.

**B. Oral.** Give 1–2 mg PO every 12 hours (children 3 years old, 0.02 mg/kg and 1 mg maximum) for 2–3 days to prevent recurrence of symptoms. Maximum recommended dose for adults is 6 mg/day.

**VII. Formulations**

**A. Parenteral.** Benztropine mesylate (Cogentin), 1 mg/mL, 2-mL ampules.

**B. Oral.** Benztropine mesylate (Cogentin, generic), 0.5-, 1-, and 2-mg tablets.

**C.** The **suggested minimum stocking level** to treat a 70-kg adult for the first 24 hours is 6 mg (three ampules, 2 mL each).

# ▶ BICARBONATE, SODIUM

*Thomas E. Kearney, PharmD*

**I. Pharmacology**

**A.** Sodium bicarbonate is a buffering agent that reacts with hydrogen ions to correct acidemia and produce alkalemia. Urinary alkalinization from renally excreted bicarbonate ions enhances the renal elimination of certain acidic drugs (eg, salicylate, chlorpropamide, chlorophenoxy herbicides, fluoride, and phenobarbital) and helps prevent renal tubular damage from deposition of myoglobin in patients with rhabdomyolysis as well as from precipitation (by enhancing solubility) of methotrexate with high-dose therapy. In addition, maintenance of a normal or high serum pH may prevent intracellular distribution of salicylate and formate (a toxic metabolite of methanol).

**B.** The sodium ion load and alkalemia produced by hypertonic sodium bicarbonate reverse the sodium channel–dependent membrane-depressant ("quinidine-like") effects of several drugs (eg, tricyclic antidepressants, type Ia and type Ic antiarrhythmic agents, propranolol, propoxyphene, cocaine, and diphenhydramine).

**C.** Alkalinization causes an intracellular shift of potassium and is used for the acute treatment of hyperkalemia.

**D.** Sodium bicarbonate given orally or by gastric lavage forms an insoluble salt with iron and theoretically may help prevent absorption of ingested iron tablets (unproved).

**E.** Neutralization of acidic substances to prevent caustic injury usually is not recommended because of the potential for an exothermic reaction, generation of gas, and lack of evidence that tissue injury is minimized.

**F.** Case series of organophosphate (OP) poisonings in regions lacking sufficient access to traditional antidotes (oximes, atropine) have suggested beneficial outcomes from high-dose IV bicarbonate therapy (5 mEq/kg over 60 minutes, then 5–6 mEq/kg/day). The authors of those studies theorize that alkalinization may enhance degradation of OPs. It may also enhance the efficacy of 2-PAM (rat model).

**II. Indications**

**A.** Severe metabolic acidosis resulting from intoxication by methanol, ethylene glycol, or salicylates or from excessive lactic acid production (eg, resulting from status epilepticus or shock).

**B.** To produce urinary alkalinization, enhance elimination of certain acidic drugs (salicylate, phenobarbital, chlorpropamide, chlorophenoxy herbicides-2,4-D), and to prevent nephrotoxicity from the renal deposition of myoglobin after severe rhabdomyolysis or precipitation of methotrexate. (Although enhanced elimination may be achieved, it is uncertain if clinical outcomes are improved with this therapy.) Also recommended by REAC/TS for internal contamination of uranium from radiation emergencies to prevent acute tubular necrosis (see Radiation, p 327).

C. Cardiotoxicity with impaired ventricular depolarization (as evidenced by a prolonged QRS interval) caused by tricyclic antidepressants, type Ia or type Ic antiarrhythmics, and other membrane-depressant drugs (see Table II–7, p 90). ***Note:*** *Not effective* for dysrhythmias associated with abnormal repolarization (prolonged QT interval and torsade de pointes).

**III. Contraindications.** The following contraindications are relative:

**A.** Significant metabolic or respiratory alkalemia or hypernatremia.

**B.** Severe pulmonary edema associated with volume overload.

**C.** Intolerance to sodium load (renal failure, CHF).

**IV. Adverse effects**

**A.** Excessive alkalemia: impaired oxygen release from hemoglobin, hypocalcemic tetany, and paradoxic intracellular acidosis (from elevated $pCO_2$ concentrations) and hypokalemia.

**B.** Hypernatremia and hyperosmolality. Caution with rapid infusion of hypertonic solutions in neonates and young children.

**C.** Aggravation of CHF and pulmonary edema.

**D.** Extravasation leading to tissue inflammation and necrosis (product is hypertonic).

**E.** May exacerbate QT prolongation and associated dysrhythmias (eg, torsade de pointes) as a result of electrolyte shifts (hypokalemia).

**F. Use in pregnancy.** FDA category C (indeterminate). However, this does not preclude its acute, short-term use for a seriously symptomatic patient (see p 407).

**V. Drug or laboratory interactions.** Do not mix with other parenteral drugs because of the possibility of drug inactivation or precipitation.

**VI. Dosage and method of administration (adults and children)**

**A. Metabolic acidemia.** Give 0.5–1 mEq/kg IV bolus; repeat as needed to correct serum pH to at least 7.2. For salicylates, methanol, or ethylene glycol, raise the pH to at least 7.4–7.5.

**B. Urinary alkalinization.** Give 44–100 mEq in 1 L of 5% dextrose in 0.25% normal saline or 88–150 mEq in 1 L of 5% dextrose at 2–3 mL/kg/h (adults 150–200 mL/h). Check urine pH frequently and adjust flow rate to maintain urine pH level at 7–8.5. ***Note:*** Hypokalemia and fluid depletion prevent effective urinary alkalinization; add 20–40 mEq of potassium to each liter unless renal failure is present. Prevent excessive systemic alkalemia (keep blood pH < 7.55) and hypernatremia. Monitor urine pH and serum electrolytes hourly.

**C. Cardiotoxic ("membrane-stabilizing") drug intoxication.** Give 1–2 mEq/kg IV bolus over 1–2 minutes; repeat as needed to improve cardiotoxic manifestations (eg, prolonged QRS interval, wide-complex tachycardia, hypotension) and maintain serum pH at 7.45–7.55. There is no evidence that constant infusions are as effective as boluses given as needed.

**VII. Formulations**

**A.** Several products are available, ranging from 4.2% (0.5 mEq/mL preferred for neonates and young children) to 7.5% (0.89 mEq/mL) to 8.4% (1 mEq/mL) in volumes of 10–500 mL. The most commonly used formulation available in most emergency "crash carts" is 8.4% ("hypertonic") sodium bicarbonate, 1 mEq/mL, in 50-mL ampules or prefilled syringes.

**B.** The **suggested minimum stocking level** to treat a 70-kg adult for the first 24 hours is 10 ampules or syringes (approximately 500 mEq).

## ▶ BOTULINUM ANTITOXIN

*Raymond Y. Ho, PharmD*

**I. Pharmacology.** Botulinum antitoxin contains concentrated equine-derived antibodies directed against the toxins produced by the various strains of *Clostridium* *botulinum* (A, B, and E). The antitoxin is currently available in the bivalent (A, B) and monovalent (E) forms. The monovalent (E) form provides coverage for botulism from fish sources and is available only through an investigational new drug (IND) protocol. If type F is suspected, the CDC advises that there is variable cross-reactivity with type E antitoxin. An equine-derived heptavalent formulation has been developed for bioterrorism preparedness. It covers toxin types A, B, C, D, E, F, and G and is available only through an IND protocol. In October 2003, a human-derived botulism immune globulin (IgG antibodies), BabyBIG, was approved for the treatment of infant botulism caused by toxins A and B. The antibodies bind and inactivate freely circulating botulinum toxins but do ***not*** remove toxin that is already bound to nerve terminals. Because antitoxin will not reverse established paralysis once it occurs, it must be administered before paralysis sets in. Treatment within 24 hours of the onset of symptoms may shorten the course of intoxication and prevent progression to total paralysis.

**II. Indications.** The equine-derived botulinum antitoxin is used to treat clinical botulism (see p 136) from food-borne, wound, or intestinal colonization in children or adults to prevent the progression of neurologic manifestations. With the recent approval of the human-derived immune globulin, the equine-derived antitoxin is generally not recommended for treatment of infant botulism.

**III. Contraindications.**

**A. Equine-derived antibodies.** No absolute contraindications. Known hypersensitivity to botulinum antitoxin or horse serum requires extreme caution if this product is given.

**B. Human-derived immune globulin.** BabyBIG should not be given to patients with a prior history of severe reaction to human immunoglobulin products. BabyBIG contains trace amounts of immunoglobulin A. Individuals with selective immunoglobulin A deficiency may develop anaphylactic reactions to subsequent administration of blood products with immunoglobulin A.

**IV. Adverse effects**

**A. Equine-derived antibodies.** Immediate hypersensitivity reactions (anaphylaxis) resulting from the equine source of antibodies.

**B. Human-derived immune globulin.** Mild transient erythematous rashes of face and trunk are reported commonly. Minor reactions such as flu-like symptoms similar to those seen with the use of other IGIV products were observed. Infusion rate–related reactions ranging from mild flushing to severe anaphylaxis may occur.

**C. Use in pregnancy.** There are no data on teratogenicity. Anaphylactic reaction resulting in shock or hypoxemia in the mother could conceivably affect the fetus adversely.

**V. Drug or laboratory interactions.** No known interactions with equine-derived antibodies. Human-derived immune globulin preparations contain antibodies that may interfere with the immune response to live vaccines such as polio, measles, mumps, and rubella.

**VI. Dosage and method of administration**

**A.** For suspected or established clinical botulism, give one 10-mL vial diluted 1:10 in 0.9% saline (normal saline) and administer by slow IV infusion. A second vial may be administered in 2 to 4 hours if signs or symptoms worsen but is usually not necessary as the neutralizing antibodies (half-life of 5–8 days) far exceed the levels of circulating toxin. For heptavalent antitoxin, the IND protocol outlines the necessary steps for administration.

**B.** Perform a skin test prior to administration according to the package instructions. If the patient has known sensitivity to horse serum or demonstrates a positive skin test, provide desensitization as indicated in the package insert. Even if the skin test is negative, anaphylaxis may occur unpredictably. Pretreat the patient with diphenhydramine (see p 442), 1–2 mg/kg IV, and cimetidine, 300 mg IV (or other $H_2$ blocker, p 433), and have epinephrine (p 448) ready in case anaphylaxis occurs.

C. In cases of infant botulism, the recommended dosage for BabyBIG is 1 mL/kg (50mg/kg) as a single intravenous infusion as soon as a clinical diagnosis of infant botulism is made. BabyBIG should be administered intravenously at 0.5 mL/kg/hr (25 mg/kg/h). The rate may be increased to 1.0 mL/kg/h (50 mg/kg/h) if no untoward reaction occurs 15 minutes after the initial infusion rate. Do not exceed this rate of administration because of the risk for infusion-related anaphylaxis. The half-life of injected BabyBIG is approximately 28 days in infants, and a single intravenous infusion is expected to provide a protective level of neutralizing antibodies for 6 months.

**VII. Formulations**

A. **Parenteral.** Bivalent botulinum antitoxin or botulism antitoxin bivalent (equine) (7500 IU type A, 5500 IU type B) and monovalent botulinum antitoxin (8500 IU type E); available through the Centers for Disease Control (CDC), telephone (404) 639-3356 (weekdays) or (404) 639-2888 (after hours) or contact your local health department (for reporting and to facilitate access to antitoxin). BabyBIG is supplied in a single-dose, 6-mL vial containing 100 mg ± 20 mg lyophilized immunoglobulin for reconstitution. Reconstituted BabyBIG should be used within 2 hours. To obtain or determine the availability of BabyBIG for suspected infant botulism, contact the Infant Botulism Treatment and Prevention Program (IBTPP) at (510) 231-7600. More information is available at www.infantbotulism.org.

B. **Suggested minimum stocking level.** Not relevant; available only through federal (CDC) or state (California) government.

## ▶ BRETYLIUM

*Thomas E. Kearney, PharmD*

I. **Pharmacology.** Bretylium is a quaternary ammonium compound that is an effective type III antifibrillatory drug and also suppresses ventricular ectopic activity. It increases the threshold for ventricular fibrillation and reduces the disparity in action potential duration between normal and ischemic tissue, which is believed to abolish the boundary currents responsible for reentrant arrhythmias. Its pharmacologic actions are complex. Initially, norepinephrine is released from sympathetic neurons; this is followed by a block of further norepinephrine release. In addition, norepinephrine uptake is inhibited at adrenergic neurons. The result is a transient increase in heart rate, blood pressure, and cardiac output that may last from a few minutes to 1 hour. Subsequent adrenergic blockade produces vasodilation, which may result in hypotension.

**II. Indications**

A. **Prophylaxis and treatment of ventricular fibrillation.** Bretylium may be particularly effective in hypothermic patients.

B. **Ventricular tachycardia resistant to other antiarrhythmic agents.** However, it has not been proved beneficial for drug- or chemical-induced ventricular dysrhythmias.

**III. Contraindications**

A. Use with extreme caution in patients with intoxication by digitalis, chloral hydrate, or halogenated hydrocarbons, because the initial release of catecholamines may aggravate arrhythmias.

B. Use with extreme caution in patients with arrhythmias caused by intoxication with cyclic antidepressants or type Ia or type Ic antiarrhythmic agents because of additive cardiac depression.

C. Use with extreme caution in patients with severe pulmonary hypertension or aortic stenosis.

D. Not recommended for children under 12 years old.

**IV. Adverse effects**

A. Hypotension (both supine and orthostatic).

B. Nausea and vomiting from rapid intravenous administration.
C. Transient hypertension and worsening of arrhythmias may be caused by initial catecholamine release.
D. **Use in pregnancy.** FDA category C (indeterminate). However, this does not preclude its acute, short-term use for a seriously symptomatic patient (see p 407).

V. **Drug or laboratory interactions**

A. The pressor effect of sympathomimetic amines may be enhanced with initial catecholamine release.
B. Cardiac-depressant effects may be additive with other antiarrhythmic drugs, particularly type Ia and type Ic drugs.

VI. **Dosage and method of administration**

A. **For ventricular fibrillation,** give 5 mg/kg IV over 1 minute (in addition to cardiopulmonary resuscitation and defibrillation). If this is not effective, administration may be repeated with 10 mg/kg.
B. **For ventricular tachycardia,** give adults and children older than 12 years 5–10 mg/kg IV over 8–10 minutes or IM, repeated as necessary at 15-minute intervals to a maximum dose of 30 mg/kg; repeat every 6 hours as needed.
C. **The continuous infusion rate** after the loading dose is 1–2 mg/min (children ≥12 years old, 20–30 mcg/kg/min).

VII. **Formulations**

A. **Parenteral.** Bretylium tosylate (various), 50 mg/mL: 10-mL ampules, vials, and syringes; 500 (2 mg/mL) and 1000 (4 mg/mL) mg premixed in 250-mL 5% dextrose solutions.
B. The **suggested minimum stocking level** to treat a 70-kg adult for the first 24 hours is six 10-mL vials.

## ▶ BROMOCRIPTINE

*Thomas E. Kearney, PharmD*

I. **Pharmacology.** Bromocriptine mesylate is a semisynthetic derivative of the ergopeptide group of ergot alkaloids with dopaminergic agonist effects. It also has minor alpha-adrenergic antagonist properties. The dopaminergic effects account for its inhibition of prolactin secretion and its beneficial effects in the treatment of parkinsonism, neuroleptic malignant syndrome (NMS; see p 22), and cocaine craving as well as its adverse effect profile and drug interactions. A key limitation is the inability to administer bromocriptine by the parenteral route coupled with poor bioavailability (only about 6% of an oral dose is absorbed). In addition, the onset of therapeutic effects (eg, alleviation of muscle rigidity, hypertension, and hyperthermia) in the treatment of NMS may take several hours to days.

II. **Indications**

A. Treatment of NMS caused by neuroleptic drugs (eg, haloperidol and other antipsychotics) or levodopa withdrawal. ***Note:*** If the patient has significant hyperthermia (eg, rectal or core temperature ≥40°C [104°F]), bromocriptine should be considered secondary and adjunctive therapy to immediate measures such as neuromuscular paralysis and aggressive external cooling.
B. Bromocriptine has been used experimentally to alleviate craving for cocaine. However, a Cochrane database review (2003) concluded that current research does not support the use of dopamine agonists for treatment of cocaine dependence. ***Caution:*** There is one case report of a severe adverse reaction (hypertension, seizures, and blindness) when bromocriptine was used in a cocaine abuser during the postpartum period.
C. ***Note:*** Bromocriptine is ***not*** considered appropriate first-line therapy for acute drug-induced extrapyramidal or parkinsonian symptoms (see p 26).

III. **Contraindications**

A. Uncontrolled hypertension or toxemia of pregnancy.

B. Known hypersensitivity to the drug.

C. A relative contraindication is a history of angina, myocardial infarction, stroke, vasospastic disorders (eg, Raynaud's disease), or bipolar affective disorder. In addition, there is no published experience in children less than 7 years old. Children may achieve higher blood levels and require lower doses.

IV. **Adverse effects.** Most adverse effects are dose-related and of minor clinical consequence; some are unpredictable.

A. The most common side effect is nausea. Epigastric pain, dyspepsia, and diarrhea also have been reported.

B. Hypotension (usually transient) and syncope may occur at the initiation of treatment, and hypertension may occur later. Other cardiovascular effects include dysrhythmias (with high doses), exacerbation of angina and vasospastic disorders such as Raynaud's disease, and intravascular thrombosis resulting in acute myocardial infarction (one case report).

C. Nervous system side effects vary considerably and include headache, drowsiness, fatigue, hallucinations, mania, psychosis, agitation, seizures, and cerebrovascular accident. Multiple interrelated risk factors include dose, concurrent drug therapy, and preexisting medical and psychiatric disorders.

D. Rare effects include pulmonary toxicity (infiltrates, pleural effusion, and thickening) and myopia with long-term, high-dose treatment (months). There has been one case of retroperitoneal fibrosis.

E. **Use in pregnancy.** FDA category B (see p 407). This drug has been used therapeutically during the last trimester of pregnancy for treatment of a pituitary tumor. It has been shown to inhibit fetal prolactin secretion, and it may precipitate premature laband inhibit lactation in the mother.

V. **Drug or laboratory interactions**

A. Bromocriptine may accentuate hypotension in patients receiving antihypertensive drugs.

B. Theoretically, this drug may have additive effects with other ergot alkaloids, and its potential to cause peripheral vasospasm may be exacerbated by propranolol.

C. Bromocriptine may reduce ethanol tolerance.

D. There has been one case report of apparent serotonin syndrome (see p 22) in a patient with Parkinson's disease who received levodopa and carbidopa.

VI. **Dosage and method of administration for NMS.** In adults, administer 2.5–10 mg orally or by gastric tube 3–4 times daily (average adult dose 5 mg every 8 hours). May increase to a maximum of 20 mg every 6 hours. The pediatric dose is unknown (one case report of 0.08 mg/kg every 8 hours in a 7-year-old; the tablets were mixed in a 2.5-mg/10 mL slurry and given by feeding tube). Use small, frequent dosing to minimize nausea.

A. A therapeutic response usually is achieved with total daily doses of 5–30 mg.

B. Continue treatment for 7–10 days after control of rigidity and fever, then slowly taper the dose over 3 days (to prevent recurrence). Several days of therapy may be required for complete reversal of NMS.

VII. **Formulations**

A. **Oral.** Bromocriptine mesylate (Parlodel, others), 2.5-mg scored (SnapTabs) tablets and 5-mg capsules.

B. The **suggested minimum stocking level** to treat a 70-kg adult for the first 24 hours is 30 mg, or one 30-tablet (SnapTabs) package.

## ▶ CALCIUM

*Binh T. Ly, MD, and Jennifer Hannum, MD*

I. **Pharmacology**

A. Calcium is a cation that is necessary for the normal functioning of a variety of enzymes and organ systems, including muscle and nerve tissue. Hypocalcemia, or a blockade of calcium's effects, may cause muscle cramps, tetany, and ventricular fibrillation. Antagonism of calcium-dependent channels results in hypotension, bradycardia, and atrioventricular block.

**B.** Calcium ions rapidly bind to fluoride ions, abolishing their toxic effects.

**C.** Calcium can reverse the negative inotropic effects of calcium antagonists; however, depressed automaticity and AV nodal conduction velocity and vasodilation may not respond to calcium administration.

**D.** Calcium stabilizes cardiac cell membranes in hyperkalemic states.

**II. Indications**

**A.** Symptomatic hypocalcemia resulting from intoxication by fluoride, oxalate, or the intravenous anticoagulant citrate.

**B.** Hydrofluoric acid exposure (see p 222).

**C.** Hypotension in the setting of calcium channel antagonist (eg, verapamil) overdose (see p 143).

**D.** Severe hyperkalemia with cardiac manifestations (relatively contraindicated in the setting of digitalis toxicity; see III.B, below).

**E.** Symptomatic hypermagnesemia.

**III. Contraindications**

**A.** Hypercalcemia except in the setting of calcium channel antagonist poisoning, where hypercalcemia may be desirable.

**B.** Although controversial, calcium is relatively contraindicated in the setting of intoxication with cardiac glycosides (***may*** aggravate digitalis-induced ventricular tachydysrhythmias) and should be reserved for life-threatening situations.

**C.** ***Note:*** Calcium *chloride* salt should ***not*** be used for intradermal, subcutaneous, or intra-arterial injection because it is highly concentrated and may result in further tissue damage.

**IV. Adverse effects**

**A.** Tissue irritation, particularly with calcium chloride salt; extravasation may cause local irritation or necrosis.

**B.** Hypercalcemia, especially in patients with diminished renal function.

**C.** Hypotension, bradycardia, syncope, and cardiac dysrhythmias caused by rapid intravenous administration.

**D.** Neuromuscular weakness.

**E.** Constipation caused by orally administered calcium salts.

**F. Use in pregnancy.** FDA category C (indeterminate). This does not preclude its acute, short-term use for a seriously symptomatic patient (see p 407).

**V. Drug or laboratory interactions**

**A.** Inotropic and dysrhythmogenic effects of digitalis may be potentiated by calcium. The use of intravenous calcium in the setting of cardiac glycoside toxicity is not absolutely contraindicated, but indications remain controversial.

**B.** A precipitate will form with solutions containing soluble salts of carbonates, phosphates, or sulfates and with various antibiotics.

**VI. Dosage and method of administration.** ***Note:*** Calcium chloride contains nearly three times the amount of $Ca^{2+}$ per milliliter of 10% solution compared with the same concentration of calcium gluconate. A 10% solution of calcium chloride contains 27.2 mg/mL of elemental calcium. A 10% solution of calcium gluconate contains 9 mg/mL of elemental calcium.

**A. Oral fluoride ingestion.** Administer calcium-containing antacid (calcium carbonate) orally to complex fluoride ions.

**B. Symptomatic hypocalcemia, hyperkalemia.** Give 10% calcium gluconate, 10–20 mL (children, 0.2–0.3 mL/kg), or 10% calcium chloride, 5–10 mL (children, 0.1–0.2 mL/kg), slowly IV. Repeat as needed every 5–10 minutes.

**C. Calcium antagonist poisoning.** Start with doses as described above. *High-dose calcium* therapy has been reported to be effective in some cases of severe calcium channel blocker overdose. Corrected calcium concentrations of approximately 1.5 to 2 times normal have correlated with improved cardiac function. In the setting of calcium channel antagonist overdose, as much as 30 g of calcium gluconate has been given over 10 hours, resulting in a serum calcium concentration of 23.8 mg/dL, which was tolerated without adverse effect. However, not all patients will tolerate extreme elevations in serum calcium concentrations. Administer calcium as multiple boluses (eg, 1 g every 10–20 minutes) or as a continuous infusion (eg, 20–50 mg/kg/h). Serum calcium concentrations should be measured every 1–2 hours during therapy with high-dose calcium.

**D. Dermal hydrofluoric acid exposure.** For any exposure involving the hand or fingers, obtain immediate consultation from an experienced hand surgeon or medical toxicologist. Regardless of the specific therapy chosen, systemic narcotic analgesics should be strongly considered strongly as adjunctive therapy.

1. **Topical.** Calcium concentrations for topical therapy have ranged from 2.5 to 33%; the optimal concentration has not been determined. Most commonly, a 2.5% gel is prepared by combining 1 g of calcium gluconate per 40 g (approximately 40 mL) of water-soluble base material (Surgilube, K-Y Jelly). A 32.5% gel can be made by compounding a slurry of ten 650-mg calcium carbonate tablets in 20 mL of water-soluble lubricant. For exposures involving the hand or fingers, place the gel in a large surgical latex glove to serve as an occlusive dressing to maximize skin contact. Topical calcium gluconate treatment is much more effective if applied within 3 hours of the injury.
2. For **subcutaneous** injection (when topical treatment fails to relieve pain), inject 5–10% calcium gluconate (***not*** chloride) SC intralesionally and perifocally (0.5–1 mL/cm$^2$ of affected skin), using a 27-gauge or smaller needle. This can be repeated two to three times at 1- to 2-hour intervals if pain is not relieved. No more than 0.5 mL should be injected into each digit.
3. **Bier block technique:**
   a. Establish distal IV access in the affected extremity (eg, dorsum of the hand).
   b. Exsanguinate the extremity by elevation for 5 minutes. Alternatively, an Esmarch bandage may be utilized by wrapping from the distal to proximal extremity.
   c. Inflate a blood pressure cuff to just above systolic blood pressure. The arm can then be lowered or the bandage removed.
   d. With the cuff kept inflated, infuse 25–50 mL of a 2% calcium gluconate solution (10 mL of 10% calcium gluconate diluted with 40 mL of $D_5W$) into the empty veins.
   e. After 20–25 minutes, slowly release the cuff over 3–5 minutes.
   f. Repeat if pain persists or use the intra-arterial infusion.
4. For **intra-arterial** administration, dilute 10 mL of 10% calcium gluconate with 50 mL of $D_5W$ and infuse over 4 hours either through the brachial or the radial artery catheter. The patient should be monitored closely over the next 4–6 hours, and if pain recurs, a second infusion should be given. Some authors have reported 48–72 hours of continuous infusion.

**E. Other sites of hydrofluoric acid exposure**

1. **Nebulized** 2.5% calcium gluconate has been reported for cases of inhalational hydrofluoric acid exposure. Inhalational exposure should be considered with dermal exposures of > 5% total body surface area. Add 1.5 mL of 10% calcium gluconate to 4.5 mL of sterile water to make a 2.5% solution.
2. **Ocular** administration of 1% calcium gluconate solutions every 4–6 hours has been utilized for 24–48 hours but is of unproven efficacy compared with irrigation with saline or water. Higher concentrations of calcium gluconate may worsen corrosive injury to ocular structures. Ophthalmology consultation should be obtained.

**VII. Formulations**

**A. Oral.** Calcium carbonate; suspension, tablets, or chewable tablets; 300–800 mg.

B. **Parenteral.** Calcium gluconate (10%), 10 mL (1 g contains 4.5 mEq calcium); calcium chloride (10%), 10 mL (1 g contains 13.6 mEq).
C. **Topical.** Calcium gluconate gel (2.5%) in 25-g and 30-g tubes but none of these commercially available formulations has been approved by the FDA.
D. The **suggested minimum stocking level** to treat a 70-kg adult for the first 24 hours is 20–30 vials (1 g each) of 10% calcium gluconate and 10–15 vials (1 g each) of 10% calcium chloride.

## ▶ L-CARNITINE (LEVOCARNITINE)

*Christine A. Haller, MD*

I. **Pharmacology**
   A. Levocarnitine (L-carnitine) is an endogenous carboxylic acid that is involved in transport of long-chain fatty acids into cellular mitochondria for energy metabolism (Krebs cycle). L-carnitine is ubiquitous in diets rich in meats and dairy products and is also synthesized in the body from the amino acids lysine and methionine. Although dietary deficiencies are rare, hypocarnitinemia can result from certain medical conditions and inborn errors of metabolism and in patients receiving multiple anticonvulsant medications. It is hypothesized that valproic acid (VPA; see p 363) induces carnitine deficiency, thereby disrupting mitochondrial function and resulting in ammonia accumulation. Carnitine-deficient states may result in production of hepatotoxic VPA metabolites via microsomal oxidation. L-carnitine supplementation has been shown to be beneficial in both the prevention and the treatment of hyperammonemia associated with VPA therapy, and carnitine may improve the outcome in cases of VPA–induced hepatotoxicity and coma. However, there is no consensus on the optimal dose or route of administration (oral vs. parenteral) of L-carnitine.
   B. L-carnitine is also sold as a dietary supplement with a wide range of unproven claims ranging from improved sperm motility to prevention of Alzheimer's disease. It is postulated that carnitine supplementation enhances fat utilization during exercise, thereby improving endurance and promoting weight loss. However, published studies have failed to show that supraphysiologic doses of L-carnitine have any benefit in well-nourished individuals. Because the FDA does not regulate dietary supplements, the safety of L-carnitine supplements cannot be guaranteed (see Herbal Products, p 215).

II. **Indications**
   A. Hyperammonemia, encephalopathy, and hepatotoxicity related to VPA therapy.
   B. Low plasma free carnitine concentrations (reference range 19–60 mcmol/L) or total carnitine (reference range 30–73 mcmol/L) in patients taking valproic acid.
   C. Acute VPA overdose (see p 363) or supratherapeutic plasma VPA concentrations.
   D. Primary or secondary carnitine deficiency.
   E. Infants and children < 2 years of age receiving VPA as part of a multianticonvulsant drug regimen.

III. **Contraindications.** None known.

IV. **Adverse effects**
   A. Dose-related nausea, vomiting, diarrhea, and fishy body odor.
   B. Seizures have been reported in patients receiving oral and IV L-carnitine.
   C. **Use in pregnancy.** Category B (see p 407). No adequate studies have been conducted in pregnant women. It is not known if this drug is secreted in human breast milk.

V. **Drug or laboratory interactions.** None known.

**VI. Dosage and method of administration**

**A. Severe valproate-induced hepatotoxicity, hyperammonemia, coma, or acute valproic acid overdose.** Early intervention with IV (rather than oral) L-carnitine has been associated with better outcomes. Administer L-carnitine intravenously in a dose of 100 mg/kg by infusion or slow bolus injection over 2–3 minutes. An equivalent dose may be given every 8 hours to severely ill patients.

**B. Drug-induced carnitine deficiency and asymptomatic hyperammonemia.** Give orally 50–100 mg/kg/day in two to three divided doses, with a maximum of 3 g per day.

**VII. Formulations**

**A. Oral**. Levocarnitine (Carnitor, L-carnitine); 330- and 500-mg tablets; 250-mg capsules; and oral solution (1 g/10 mL) in 118-mL multiple-use containers.

**B. Parenteral**. Levocarnitine (Carnitor, others); injection of single-dose (5 mL) vials and amps containing 1 g L-carnitine per vial or amp.

**C. The suggested minimum stocking level** to treat a severely ill 70-kg adult for the first 24 hours is 7 g (seven vials).

## ▶ CHARCOAL, ACTIVATED

*Thomas E. Kearney, PharmD*

**I. Pharmacology.** Activated charcoal, by virtue of its large surface area, adsorbs many drugs and toxins. Highly ionic salts (eg, iron, lithium, and cyanide) and small polar molecules (eg, alcohols) are poorly adsorbed. Repeated oral doses of activated charcoal can increase the rate of elimination of some drugs that have a small volume of distribution and that undergo enterogastric or enterohepatic recirculation (eg, digitoxin) or diffuse into the GI lumen from the intestinal circulation (eg, phenobarbital and theophylline). See also discussion in Section I, p 50. Co-administration with cathartics is of unproven benefit and is associated with risks (see Section IV).

**II. Indications**

**A.** Activated charcoal is used orally after an ingestion to limit drug or toxin absorption. Although traditionally given after the stomach has been emptied by ipecac-induced emesis or gastric lavage, it is now more common practice and studies support that it may be used alone for most ingestions. However, evidence for benefit in the clinical setting does not exist, and some toxicologists advise against its routine use. Use in the home after a childhood exposure is controversial and of unproven benefit.

**B.** Repeated doses of activated charcoal may be indicated to enhance elimination of some drugs if (1) more rapid elimination will benefit the patient (and the benefits outweigh the risks of repeated doses; see IV.C and V.C, below) and (2) more aggressive means of removal (eg, hemodialysis and hemoperfusion) are not immediately indicated or available (see p 56). However, it has not been proved to improve patient outcome in clinical studies.

**C.** Repeated doses of activated charcoal may be useful when the quantity of drug or toxin ingested is greater than one-tenth of the usual charcoal dose (eg, an aspirin ingestion of more than 6–10 g) or when surface contact with the drug is hindered (eg, pharmacobezoars and wrapped or packaged drugs).

**III. Contraindications**

**A.** Gastrointestinal ileus or obstruction may prevent the administration of more than one or two doses.

**B.** Acid or alkali ingestions unless other drugs have also been ingested (charcoal makes endoscopic evaluation more difficult).

**C.** Use of charcoal-sorbitol mixtures should be avoided in children (risk of hypernatremia and dehydration).

**D.** Obtunded patients at risk for aspiration of charcoal (need intact or protected airway).

**IV. Adverse effects**

**A.** Constipation (may be prevented by coadministration of a cathartic).

**B.** Distension of the stomach, emesis (in particular if mixed with sorbitol) with potential risk of aspiration.

**C.** Diarrhea, dehydration, hypermagnesemia, and hypernatremia resulting from coadministered cathartics, especially with repeated doses of charcoal and cathartics or even after a single large dose of a premixed sorbitol-containing charcoal product.

**D.** Intestinal bezoar with obstruction (in particular with multidoses given to patients with impaired bowel motility).

**E.** Corneal abrasions have occurred when spilled in the eyes.

**F. Use in pregnancy.** Activated charcoal is not systemically absorbed. Diarrhea resulting in shock or hypernatremia in the mother could conceivably affect the fetus adversely.

**V. Drug or laboratory interactions**

**A.** Activated charcoal may reduce, prevent, or delay the absorption of orally administered antidotes or other drugs (eg, acetylcysteine).

**B.** The adsorptive capacity of activated charcoal may be diminished by the concurrent ingestion of ice cream, milk, or sugar syrup; the clinical significance is unknown but is probably minor.

**C.** Repeated doses of charcoal may enhance the elimination of some necessary therapeutic drugs (eg, anticonvulsants).

**VI. Dosage and method of administration**

**A. Initial dose.** Activated charcoal, 1 g/kg (adult dose 50–100 g; child < 5 years, 10–25 g) orally or via gastric tube, is administered, or if the quantity of toxin ingested is known, 10 times the amount of ingested toxin by weight is given. For massive overdoses (eg, 60–100 g of aspirin), this may need to be given in divided doses over 1–2 days.

**B. Repeat-dose charcoal.** Activated charcoal, 15–30 g (0.25–0.5 g/kg) every 2–4 hours or hourly (adults, average rate of 12.5 g/h; children, rate of 0.2 g/kg/h), is given orally or by gastric tube. (The optimal regimen and dose are unknown, but more frequent dosing to include continuous gastric infusion may be advantageous.) May administer a small dose of cathartic with every second or third charcoal dose (benefit is unproven). Do ***not*** use a cathartic with every activated charcoal dose. Endpoints for repeat-dose charcoal therapy include clinical improvement and declining serum drug level; the usual empiric duration is 24–48 hours.

**C.** For patients with nausea or vomiting, administer antiemetics (metoclopramide, p 475, or ondansetron, p 489) and consider giving the charcoal by gastric tube.

**VII. Formulations**

**A.** There are a variety of formulations and a large number of brands of activated charcoal. It is available as a powder, pellets, a liquid aqueous suspension (preferable), and a liquid suspension in sorbitol or propylene glycol.

**B.** The **suggested minimum stocking level** to treat a 70-kg adult for the first 24 hours is three bottles containing 50 g of activated charcoal each. Preferred stock is the plain aqueous suspension.

## ▶ CIMETIDINE AND OTHER $H_2$ BLOCKERS

*Thomas E. Kearney, PharmD*

**I. Pharmacology.** Cimetidine, ranitidine, famotidine, and nizatidine are selective competitive inhibitors of histamine on $H_2$ receptors. These receptors modulate smooth muscle, vascular tone, and gastric secretions and may be involved in clinical effects associated with anaphylactic and anaphylactoid reactions as well as ingestion of histamine or histamine-like substances (eg, scombroid fish poisoning). Cimetidine, as an inhibitor of cytochrome P-450 enzymes, has been proposed or studied in animals as an agent to block the production of toxic intermediate metabolites (eg, acetaminophen, carbon tetrachloride, halothane, *Amanita* mushroom poisoning), but this has not been shown to be beneficial for human poisonings or toxicity. It is also an inhibitor of alcohol dehydrogenase (see Drug or Laboratory Interactions below) and has been suggested for use in patients with an atypical aldehyde dehydrogenase enzyme to minimize a disulfiram ("Oriental flushing") reaction from acute alcohol ingestion.

**II. Indications**

**A.** Adjunctive with $H_1$ blockers such as diphenhydramine (see p 442) in the management and prophylactic treatment of anaphylactic and anaphylactoid reactions (see Antivenoms, pp 410–415).

**B.** Adjunctive with $H_1$ blockers such as diphenhydramine (see p 442) in the management of scombroid fish poisoning (p 204).

**C. Ranitidine** has been used to reduce vomiting associated with theophylline poisoning. Because cimetidine may interfere with hepatic elimination of theophylline, it should not be used.

**III. Contraindications.** Known hypersensitivity to $H_2$ blockers.

**IV. Adverse effects**

**A.** Headache, drowsiness, fatigue, and dizziness have been reported but are usually mild.

**B.** Confusion, agitation, hallucinations, and even seizures have been reported with cimetidine use in the elderly, the severely ill, and patients with renal failure. A case was reported of a dystonic reaction after IV cimetidine administration.

**C.** A reversible, dose-dependent rise in serum alanine aminotransferase (ALT) activity has been reported with nizatidine, a related agent. Hepatitis has also occurred with ranitidine.

**D.** Cardiac dysrhythmias (bradycardia, tachycardia) and hypotension have been associated with rapid IV bolus of cimetidine and ranitidine (rare).

**E.** Severe delayed hypersensitivity after high oral doses of cimetidine (case report).

**F.** Preparations containing the preservative benzyl alcohol have been associated with "gasping syndrome" in premature infants.

**V. Drug or laboratory interactions**

**A.** Cimetidine, and to a lesser extent ranitidine, reduces hepatic clearance and prolongs the elimination half-life of several drugs as a result of inhibition of cytochrome P-450 activity and reduction of hepatic blood flow. Examples of drugs affected include phenytoin, theophylline, phenobarbital, cyclosporine, morphine, lidocaine, calcium channel blockers, tricyclic antidepressants, and warfarin.

**B.** Cimetidine, ranitidine, and nizatidine inhibit gastric mucosal alcohol dehydrogenase and therefore increase the systemic absorption of ethyl alcohol.

**C.** Increased gastric pH may inhibit the absorption of some pH-dependent drugs, such as ketoconazole, ferrous salts, and tetracyclines.

**VI. Dosage and method of administration.** In general, there are no clinically proven advantages of any one of the $H_2$ blockers, although cimetidine is more likely to be associated with drug-drug interactions. The lowest-strength dosage forms are available over the counter, and several oral dosage form options (chewable tablets, oral solutions) may enhance palatability. See Table III–5 for oral and parenteral doses.

**VII. Formulations**

**A. Cimetidine (Tagamet, others)**

1. **Oral.** 200-, 300-, 400-, and 800-mg tablets; 300-mg/5 mL oral solution (contains parabens and propylene glycol).
2. **Parenteral.** 150 mg/mL in 2- and 8-mL vials (Tagamet preparation has 0.5% phenol); premixed 300 mg in 50 mL saline (6 mg/mL).

TABLE III–5. CIMETIDINE, FAMOTIDINE, NIZATIDINE, AND RANITIDINE

| Drug | Route | Dose[a] |
|---|---|---|
| Cimetidine | PO | 300 mg every 6–8 h or 400 mg every 12 h (maximum 2400 mg/day). Children: 10 mg/kg single dose; 20–40 mg/kg/day. |
| | IV, IM | 300 mg IV or IM every 6–8 h. For IV administration, dilute in normal saline to a total volume of 20 mL and give over 2 min or longer. Children: 10 mg/kg. |
| Famotidine | PO | 20–40 mg once or twice daily (as much as 160 mg every 6 h has been used). |
| | IV | 20 mg IV every 12 h (dilute in normal saline to a total volume of 5–10 mL). |
| Ranitidine | PO | 150 mg twice daily (up to 6 g/day has been used). |
| | IV, IM | 50 mg IV or IM every 6–8 h. For IV use, dilute in normal saline to a total volume of 20 mL and inject over 5 min or longer. |
| Nizatidine | PO | 150 mg once to twice daily (or 300 mg once daily). |

[a]Note: May need to reduce dose in patients with renal dysfunction.

B. **Famotidine (Pepcid, Pepcid AC, Pepcid RPD)**
   1. **Oral.** 10-, 20-, and 40-mg tablets; 10-mg chewable tablets and gelcaps; 20- and 40-mg disintegrating tablets; 40-mg/5 mL oral suspension (powder to be reconstituted).
   2. **Parenteral.** 10 mg/mL in 1- and 2-mL single-dose and 4-, 20-, and 50-mL multidose vials (may contain mannitol or benzyl alcohol); premixed 20 mg in 50 mL saline.

C. **Ranitidine (Zantac, others)**
   1. **Oral.** 75-, 150-, and 300-mg tablets and capsules; 15 mg/mL in 10 mL syrup (may contain alcohol and parabens); and 25- and 150-mg effervescent tablets.
   2. **Parenteral.** 1.0 mg/mL in 50-mL container; 25 mg/mL in 2- and 6-mL vials (with phenol).

D. **Nizatidine (Axid, others)**
   1. **Oral.** 75-mg tablets and 150- and 300-mg capsules.
   2. **Parenteral.** Not available in this dosage form.

E. The **suggested minimum stocking levels** to treat a 70-kg adult for the first 24 hours (all are parenteral dose form) are the following:
   1. **Cimetidine.** 1200 mg (8-mL vial).
   2. **Famotidine.** 40 mg (4-mL multidose vial).
   3. **Ranitidine.** 250 mg (10-mL vial).

# ► CYPROHEPTADINE

*F. Lee Cantrell, PharmD*

I. **Pharmacology.** Cyproheptadine is a first-generation, histamine-1 blocker with nonspecific serotonin (5-HT) antagonism. The administration of cyproheptadine to patients with serotonin syndrome appears to antagonize excessive stimulation of 5-HT1A and 5-HT2 receptors, resulting in improvements in clinical symptoms (based on anecdotal case reports).

II. **Indications. Cyproheptadine** may be beneficial in alleviating mild to moderate symptoms in cases of suspected serotonin syndrome (see p 21).

**III. Contraindications**

- **A.** Known hypersensitivity to cyproheptadine.
- **B.** Angle-closure glaucoma.
- **C.** Stenosing peptic ulcer.
- **D.** Symptomatic prostatic hypertrophy.
- **E.** Bladder neck obstruction.
- **F.** Pyloroduodenal obstruction.

**IV. Adverse effects**

- **A.** Transient mydriasis and urinary retention may result from anticholinergic properties.
- **B. Use in pregnancy.** FDA category B (see p 407). Unlikely to cause harm with short-term therapy.

**V. Drug or laboratory interactions.** Additive anticholinergic effects when given with other antimuscarinic drugs.

**VI. Dosage and method of administration (adults and children)**

- **A. Oral.** The initial dose is 4–8 mg orally and can be repeated every 1–4 hours as needed until symptoms resolve or a maximum daily dose of 32 mg is reached (children: 0.25 mg/kg/day divided every 6 hours with a maximum of 12 mg/day).

**VII. Formulations**

- **A. Oral.** Cyproheptadine hydrochloride (Periactin, others), 4-mg tablets, 2 mg/5 mL syrup.
- **B.** The **suggested minimum stocking level** to treat a 70-kg adult for the first 24 hours is one bottle (4 mg, 100 tablets).

## ▶ DANTROLENE

*Thomas E. Kearney, PharmD*

**I. Pharmacology.** Dantrolene relaxes skeletal muscle by inhibiting the release of calcium from the sarcoplasmic reticulum, thereby reducing actin-myosin contractile activity. Dantrolene can help control hyperthermia that results from excessive muscle hyperactivity, particularly when hyperthermia is caused by a defect within the muscle cell (eg, malignant hyperthermia). Dantrolene is not a substitute for other temperature-controlling measures (eg, sponging and fanning).

**II. Indications**

- **A.** The primary indication for dantrolene is malignant hyperthermia (see p 21).
- **B.** Dantrolene may be useful in treating hyperthermia and rhabdomyolysis caused by drug-induced muscular hyperactivity that is not controlled by usual cooling measures or neuromuscular paralysis.
- **C.** Theoretically, dantrolene is not expected to be effective for hyperthermia caused by conditions other than muscular hyperactivity, such as increased metabolic rate (eg, salicylate or dinitrophenol poisoning), neuroleptic malignant syndrome (NMS), impaired heat dissipation (eg, anticholinergic syndrome),and environmental exposure (heat stroke). However, there is anecdotal evidence (case reports or case-control studies) of benefit for the management of NMS, MAO inhibitor (phenelzine poisoning)–induced hyperthermia, dinitrophenol-induced hyperthermia, muscle rigidity from baclofen withdrawal, hypertonicity from carbon monoxide poisoning, tetanus, and black widow spider envenomation.

**III. Contraindications.** No absolute contraindications exist. Patients with muscular weakness or respiratory impairment must be observed closely for possible respiratory arrest.

**IV. Adverse effects**

- **A.** Muscle weakness, which may aggravate respiratory depression.
- **B.** Drowsiness, fatigue, dizziness, photosensitivity, and diarrhea.

C. **Black box warning.** Potential for fatal hepatotoxicity (hypersensitivity hepatitis) reported after chronic therapy. May also be dose-related (more common with 800 mg/day). Transaminases are elevated in about 10% of patients treated with dantrolene.

D. IV administration associated with pulmonary edema (mannitol may contribute), phlebitis, and urticaria (avoid extravasation).

E. **Use in pregnancy.** FDA category C (indeterminate). This does not preclude its acute, short-term use for a seriously symptomatic patient (see p 407).

V. **Drug or laboratory interactions**

A. Dantrolene may have additive CNS–depressant effects with sedative and hypnotic drugs.

B. Dantrolene and verapamil coadministration is associated with hyperkalemia (case report).

C. Each 20-mg vial of Dantrium contains 3 g of mannitol; this should be taken into consideration as it may have additive effects with any mannitol given to treat rhabdomyolysis. Use only sterile water (without bacteriostatic agent) to reconstitute. Incompatible with $D_5W$ and NS.

VI. **Dosage and method of administration (adults and children)**

A. **Parenteral.** Give 1 mg/kg rapidly IV; this may be repeated as needed every 5–10 minutes to a maximum total dose of 10 mg/kg. Satisfactory response usually is achieved with an average total dosage of 2.5 mg/kg.

B. **Oral.** To prevent recurrence of hyperthermia, administer 1–2 mg/kg intravenously or orally (up to 100 mg maximum) four times a day for 2–3 days. Daily dose not to exceed 400 mg (see black box warning). For prevention (patients at risk for malignant hyperthermia), give 1–2 days prior to surgery and give the last dose 3–4 hours before surgery or give IV at 2.5-mg/kg infused over 1 hour and 1 hour prior to anesthesia.

VII. **Formulations**

A. **Parenteral.** Dantrolene sodium (Dantrium), 20 mg of lyophilized powder for reconstitution (after reconstitution, protect from light and use within 6 hours to ensure maximal activity). Each 20-mg vial contains 3 g of mannitol (see adverse effects and interactions).

B. **Oral.** Dantrolene sodium (Dantrium) in 25-, 50-, and 100-mg capsules.

C. The **suggested minimum stocking level** to treat a 70-kg adult for the first 24 hours is thirty-five 20-mg vials.

## ▶ DEFEROXAMINE

*David L. Irons, PharmD*

I. **Pharmacology.** Deferoxamine is a specific chelating agent for iron. It binds free iron and, to some extent, loosely bound iron (eg, from ferritin or hemosiderin). Iron bound to hemoglobin, transferrin, cytochrome enzymes, and all other sites is not affected. The red iron-deferoxamine (ferrioxamine) complex is water soluble and is excreted renally, where it imparts an orange-pink, or "vin rosé," color to the urine. One hundred milligrams of deferoxamine is capable of binding 8.5 mg of elemental iron and 4.1 mg of aluminum in vitro. Deferoxamine and both the aluminoxamine and ferrioxamine complexes are dialyzable. The basic science literature supports the use of the drug, but clinical evidence of efficacy and safety is lacking.

II. **Indications**

A. Deferoxamine is used to treat iron intoxication (see p 230) when the serum iron is greater than 450–500 mcg/dL or when clinical signs of significant iron intoxication exist (eg, shock, acidosis, severe gastroenteritis, or numerous radiopaque tablets visible in the GI tract by x-ray).

B. Deferoxamine sometimes is used as a "test dose" to determine the presence of free iron by observing for the characteristic vin rosé color in the urine; however, a change in urine color is not a reliable indicator.

**C.** Deferoxamine has also been used for treatment of aluminum toxicity in patients with renal failure.

**III. Contraindications.** No absolute contraindications to deferoxamine use exist in patients with serious iron poisoning. The drug should be used with caution in patients with known sensitivity to deferoxamine and patients with renal failure/anuria who are not receiving hemodialysis.

**IV. Adverse effects**

**A.** Hypotension or an anaphylactoid-type reaction may occur from very rapid intravenous bolus administration; this can be avoided by limiting the rate of administration to 15 mg/kg/h.

**B.** Local pain, induration, and sterile abscess formation may occur at intramuscular injection sites. Large intramuscular injections may also cause hypotension.

**C.** The ferrioxamine complex may itself cause hypotension and may accumulate in patients with renal impairment; hemodialysis may be necessary to remove the ferrioxamine complex.

**D.** Deferoxamine, as a siderophore, promotes the growth of certain bacteria such as *Yersinia enterocolitica* and may predispose patients to *Yersinia* sepsis.

**E.** Infusions exceeding 24 hours have been associated with pulmonary complications (acute respiratory distress syndrome).

**F. Use in pregnancy.** FDA category C (indeterminate). Although deferoxamine is a teratogen in animals, it has relatively poor placental transfer, and there is no evidence that short-term treatment is harmful in human pregnancy (see p 407). More important, failure to treat a serious acute iron intoxication may result in maternal and fetal morbidity or death.

**V. Drug or laboratory interactions.** Deferoxamine may interfere with determinations of serum iron (falsely low) and total iron-binding capacity (falsely high). It may chelate and remove aluminum from the body.

**VI. Dosage and method of administration**

**A.** The intravenous route is preferred in all cases. In children or adults, give deferoxamine at an infusion rate generally not to exceed 15 mg/kg/h (although rates up to 40–50 mg/kg/h have been given in patients with massive iron intoxication). This correlates to a binding of 1.3 mg/kg/h when administered at 15 mg/kg/h. The maximum cumulative daily dose generally should not exceed 6 g (doses up to 16 g have been tolerated). The endpoints of therapy include loss of vin rosé–colored urine, a serum iron level less than 350 mcg/dL, and resolution of clinical signs of intoxication.

**B.** Oral complexation is ***not*** recommended.

**C.** Intramuscular injection is ***not*** recommended. If the patient is symptomatic, use the intravenous route. If the patient is not symptomatic but serious toxicity is expected to occur, intravenous access is essential (eg, for fluid boluses), and intravenous dosing provides more reliable administration.

**VII. Formulations**

**A. Parenteral.** Deferoxamine mesylate (Desferal), vials containing 500 mg and 2 g of lyophilized powder.

**B.** The **suggested minimum stocking level** to treat a 70-kg adult for the first 24 hours is 12 (500-mg) vials.

## ▶ DIAZOXIDE

*Thomas E. Kearney, PharmD*

**I. Pharmacology**

**A.** Diazoxide, a nondiuretic thiazide, is a direct arterial vasodilator that formerly was used to treat severe hypertension. Heart rate and cardiac output increase owing to a reflex response to decreased peripheral vascular resistance. The duration of the hypotensive effect ranges from 3 to 12 hours, although the elimination half-life is 20–40 hours.

**B.** Diazoxide has been used in the treatment of oral hypoglycemic overdose because it increases serum glucose by inhibiting insulin secretion, diminishing peripheral glucose utilization, and enhancing hepatic glucose release. However, octreotide (see p 488) has become the preferred agent because of its safety and efficacy.

**II. Indications**

**A.** Management of an acute hypertensive crisis, although other antihypertensive agents are preferred (see Phentolamine, p 495; Nitroprusside, p 485; and Labetalol, p 466).

**B.** Oral hypoglycemic overdose when serum glucose concentrations cannot be maintained adequately by intravenous 5% dextrose infusions and the preferred agent, octreotide, is unavailable or intolerable to the patient (known hypersensitivity).

**III. Contraindications**

**A.** Hypertension associated with aortic stenosis, aortic coarctation, hypertrophic cardiomyopathy, or arteriovenous shunt.

**B.** Known hypersensitivity to thiazides or other sulfonamide derivatives.

**IV. Adverse effects**

**A.** Hypotension or excessive blood pressure reduction must be avoided in patients with compromised cerebral or cardiac circulation.

**B.** Fluid retention from prolonged therapy may compromise patients with congestive heart failure.

**C.** Hyperglycemia may occur, particularly in patients with diabetes or hepatic dysfunction.

**D. Use in pregnancy.** FDA category C (indeterminate). This drug has caused skeletal, cardiac, and pancreatic abnormalities in animals, but no adequate human data exist. Use of this drug near term may cause hyperbilirubinemia and altered carbohydrate metabolism in a fetus or neonate, and intravenous administration during labor may cause cessation of uterine contractions. These cautions, however, do not necessarily preclude acute, short-term use of the drug for a seriously symptomatic patient (see p 407).

**V. Drug or laboratory interactions**

**A.** The hypotensive effect is potentiated by concomitant therapy with diuretics or beta-adrenergic blockers.

**B.** Diazoxide displaces warfarin from protein-binding sites and may transiently potentiate its anticoagulant effects.

**C.** Diazoxide can increase phenytoin metabolism.

**VI. Dosage and method of administration (adults and children)**

**A. For oral hypoglycemic-induced hypoglycemia:**

1. Give a 0.1–2 mg/kg/h infusion; initiate at a lower infusion rate and titrate up as needed. Hypotension is minimized by keeping the patient supine and increasing the infusion rate slowly. Duration of therapy has ranged from 22 to 60 hours.
2. An oral dosing regimen of 3–8 mg/kg/day divided into two to three doses is recommended for children and adults. If refractory, may require higher doses of up to 10 to 15 mg/kg/day (200 mg every 4 hours has been used).

**B. For hypertensive crisis,** give 1–3 mg/kg IV (150 mg maximum) or 50 to 100 mg total every 5–15 minutes as needed. ***Note:*** The use of a 300-mg rapid bolus is no longer recommended.

**VII. Formulations**

**A. Parenteral.** Diazoxide (Hyperstat), 15 mg/mL in 20-mL ampules.

**B. Oral.** Diazoxide (Proglycem), 50-mg/mL oral suspension (with alcohol and parabens).

**C.** The **suggested minimum stocking levels** to treat a 70-kg adult for the first 24 hours: parenteral, two vials (20 mL each); oral, 30 mL of suspension.

# ▶ DIGOXIN-SPECIFIC ANTIBODIES

*Thomas E. Kearney, PharmD*

I. **Pharmacology.** Digoxin-specific antibodies are produced in immunized sheep and have a high binding affinity for digoxin and, to a lesser extent, digitoxin and other cardiac glycosides. The Fab fragments used to treat poisoning are derived by cleaving the whole antibodies. The Fab fragment binds free digoxin. Once the digoxin-Fab complex is formed, the digoxin molecule is no longer pharmacologically active. The complex enters the circulation, is renally eliminated and cleared by the reticuloendothelial system, and has a half-life of 14–20 hours (may increase 10-fold with renal impairment). Reversal of signs of digitalis intoxication usually occurs within 30–60 minutes of administration (average initial response 19 minutes), with complete reversal varying up to 24 hours (average 88 minutes). There are two commercially available products, Digibind and DigiFab, that should be considered therapeutic equivalents. The decision to use either product may be based on availability and cost.

II. **Indications.** Digoxin-specific antibodies are used for life-threatening arrhythmias or hyperkalemia (≥5 mEq/L) caused by acute and chronic cardiac glycoside intoxication (see p 155). Treatment should be based on elevated levels as well as the presence of significant symptoms (eg, hyperkalemia, ventricular arrhythmias, bradyarrhythmias, and hypotension).

III. **Contraindications.** No contraindications are known. Caution is warranted in patients with known sensitivity to ovine (sheep) products; a skin test for hypersensitivity may be performed in such patients, using diluted reconstituted drug. There are no reports of hypersensitivity reactions in patients who have received the drug more than once (although this is a theoretical risk). Product may contain traces of papain; therefore, caution is advised in patients with allergies to papain, chymopapain, papaya extracts, and the pineapple enzyme bromelain.

IV. **Adverse effects**

A. Monitor the patient for potential hypersensitivity reactions and serum sickness. A dose- and rate-related (anaphylactoid) reaction may occur with rapid IV administration.

B. In patients with renal insufficiency and impaired clearance of the digitalis-Fab complex, a delayed rebound of free serum digoxin levels may occur for up to 130 hours.

C. Removal of the inotropic effect of digitalis may exacerbate preexisting heart failure.

D. With removal of the digitalis effect, patients with preexisting atrial fibrillation may develop an accelerated ventricular response.

E. Removal of the digitalis effect may reactivate sodium-potassium ATPase and shift potassium into cells, causing a drop in the serum potassium level.

F. **Use in pregnancy.** FDA category C (indeterminate). This does not preclude its acute, short-term use for a seriously symptomatic patient (see p 407).

V. **Drug or laboratory interactions**

A. Digoxin-specific Fab fragments will bind other cardiac glycosides, including digitoxin, ouabain, oleander glycosides, and possibly glycosides in lily-of-the-valley, strophanthus, squill, and toad venom (*Bufo* spp cardenolides).

B. The digoxin-Fab complex cross-reacts with the antibody commonly utilized in quantitative immunoassay techniques. This results in falsely high serum concentrations of digoxin owing to measurement of the inactive Fab complex (total serum digoxin levels may increase 10- to 21-fold). However, some assays and procedures may measure free digoxin levels, which may be useful for patients with renal impairment (to monitor a rebound in free serum digoxin levels after administration of Fab fragments).

VI. **Dosage and method of administration.** Each vial of either digoxin-immune Fab product binds 0.5 mg of digoxin.

A. **Complete neutralization/equimolar dosing; known level or amount in-**

**TABLE III–6. APPROXIMATE DIGOXIN-FAB DOSE IF AMOUNT INGESTED IS KNOWN**

| Tablets Ingested (0.125-mg size) | Tablets Ingested (0.25-mg size) | Approximate Dose Absorbed (mg) | Recommended Dose (no. vials) |
|---|---|---|---|
| 5 | 2.5 | 0.5 | 1 |
| 10 | 5 | 1 | 2 |
| 20 | 10 | 2 | 4 |
| 50 | 25 | 5 | 10 |
| 100 | 50 | 10 | 20 |

**gested.** Estimation of the dose of Fab is based on the body burden of digitalis. This may be calculated if the approximate amount ingested is known (Table III–6) or if the steady-state (postdistributional) serum drug concentration is known (Table III–7). (The steady-state serum drug concentration should be determined at least 12–16 hours after the last dose.) ***Note:*** The calculation of digoxin body burden is based on an estimated volume of distribution for digoxin of approximately 5–6 L/kg; however, other estimates for the Vd range as high as 8 L/kg. If the patient fails to respond to the initial treatment, the dose may have to increase by an additional 50%.

**B. Empiric dosing (unknown level and severe toxicity).** If the amount ingested or the postdistributional level is not known and the patient has life-threatening dysrhythmias, dosing may have to be empiric. The manufacturer recommends that 20 (10 for children) and 6 vials be given empirically for acute and chronic overdoses, respectively. However, average dose requirements are 10 and 5 vials for acute and chronic digoxin intoxication, respectively.

**C. Titration dosing.** Theoretically, Fab may be used to neutralize a *portion* of the digoxin body burden to reverse toxicity but maintain therapeutic benefits. The Fab dose can be estimated by subtracting the desired digoxin level from the measured postdistributional level before completing the calculation. Alternately, if the patient is hemodynamically stable, the drug can be given empirically, 1-3 vials at a time, titrating to clinical effect. A proposed strategy has been to infuse the initial or loading dose over 1 hour and then allow 1 hour after the end of the infusion period to assess the need for additional doses. However, partial dosing has been associated with recurrences of symptoms in some digoxin-poisoned patients.

**D.** Reconstitute the drug according to the package instructions and administer intravenously over 30 minutes, using a 0.22-micron membrane filter. Note that longer infusion periods (1–7 hours) have been suggested to optimize

**TABLE III–7. APPROXIMATE DIGOXIN-FAB DOSE BASED ON SERUM CONCENTRATION AT STEADY STATE (AFTER EQUILIBRATION)**

**Digoxin:**[a] number of digoxin-Fab vials = $\dfrac{\text{serum digoxin (ng/mL)} \times \text{body weight (kg)}}{100}$

**Digitoxin:** number of digoxin-Fab vials = $\dfrac{\text{serum digitoxin (ng/mL)} \times \text{body weight (kg)}}{1000}$

[a]This calculation provides a quick estimate of the number of vials needed but could underestimate the actual need because of variations in the volume of distribution (5–7 L/kg). Be prepared to increase dose by 50% if clinical response to initial dose is not satisfactory.

binding to Fab. It may also be given as a rapid bolus for immediately life-threatening arrhythmias.

**VII. Formulations**

**A. Parenteral.** Digibind, 38 mg of lyophilized digoxin-specific Fab fragments per vial. DigiFab, 40 mg of lyophilized digoxin-specific Fab fragments per vial.

**B.** The **suggested minimum stocking level** to treat a 70-kg adult for the first 24 hours is 20 vials of either product.

# ▶ DIPHENHYDRAMINE

*Thomas E. Kearney, PharmD*

**I. Pharmacology.** Diphenhydramine is an antihistamine with anticholinergic, antitussive, antiemetic, and local anesthetic properties. The antihistaminic property affords relief from itching and minor irritation caused by plant-induced dermatitis and insect bites and, when used as pretreatment, provides partial protection against anaphylaxis caused by animal serum–derived antivenoms or antitoxins. Drug-induced extrapyramidal symptoms respond to the anticholinergic effect of diphenhydramine. The effects of diphenhydramine are maximal at 1 hour after intravenous injection and last up to 7 hours. The drug is eliminated by hepatic metabolism, with a serum half-life of 3–7 hours.

**II. Indications**

**A.** Relief of symptoms caused by excessive histamine effect (eg, ingestion of scombroid-contaminated fish or niacin and rapid intravenous administration of acetylcysteine). Diphenhydramine may be combined with cimetidine or another $H_2$ histamine receptor blocker (see p 433).

**B.** Pretreatment before administration of animal serum–derived antivenoms or antitoxins, especially in patients with a history of hypersensitivity or with a positive skin test. Diphenhydramine can be combined with cimetidine or another $H_2$ histamine receptor blocker.

**C.** Neuroleptic drug–induced extrapyramidal symptoms and priapism (one case report).

**D.** Pruritus caused by poison oak, poison ivy, or minor insect bites.

**III. Contraindications**

**A.** Angle-closure glaucoma.

**B.** Prostatic hypertrophy with obstructive uropathy.

**C.** Concurrent therapy with monoamine oxidase inhibitors.

**IV. Adverse effects**

**A.** Sedation, drowsiness, and ataxia may occur. Paradoxic excitation is possible in small children.

**B.** Excessive doses may cause flushing, tachycardia, blurred vision, delirium, toxic psychosis, urinary retention, and respiratory depression.

**C.** Some preparations may contain sulfite preservatives, which can cause allergic-type reactions in susceptible persons.

**D.** Diphenhydramine may exacerbate dyskinetic movement disorders as a result of increased dopamine (eg, amphetamine or cocaine intoxication) or decreased cholinergic effects in the CNS.

**E.** Extravasation from an IV dose of 500 mg into arm soft tissue resulted in a chronic regional pain syndrome (case report). Local necrosis from subcutaneous route.

**F. Use in pregnancy.** FDA category B (see p 407). Fetal harm is extremely unlikely.

**V. Drug or laboratory interactions**

**A.** Additive sedative effect with opioids, ethanol, and other sedatives.

**B.** Additive anticholinergic effect with other antimuscarinic drugs.

**VI. Dosage and method of administration**

**A. Pruritus.** Give 25–50 mg PO every 4–6 hours (children, 5 mg/kg/day in divided doses; usual oral doses for ages 6–12 years are 12.5 to 25 mg every 4–6 hours and for ages 2 to 6 years they are 6.25 mg every 4–6 hours); maximum daily dose, 37.5 mg (children age 2–6 years), 150 mg (children age 6–12 years), and 300 mg (adult). The drug may also be applied topically, although systemic absorption and toxicity have been reported, especially when used on large areas with blistered or broken skin.

**B. Pretreatment before antivenom administration.** Give 50 mg (children, 0.5–1 mg/kg) IV; if possible, it should be given at least 15–20 minutes before antivenom use. Rate of IV administration should not exceed 25-mg/min.

**C. Drug-induced extrapyramidal symptoms.** Give 50 mg (children, 0.5–1 mg/kg) IV (at a rate not to exceed 25 mg/minute) or deep IM; if there is no response within 30–60 minutes, repeat dose to a maximum 100 mg (adults). Provide oral maintenance therapy, 25–50 mg (children, 0.5–1 mg/kg; usual oral dose if < 9 kg, 6.25 to 12.5 mg, and if > 9 kg, 12.5 to 25-mg) every 4–6 hours for 2–3 days to prevent recurrence; maximum daily dose, 300 mg (children) and 400 mg (adults).

**VII. Formulations**

**A. Oral.** Diphenhydramine hydrochloride (Benadryl, others), 25- and 50-mg tablets and capsules, 12.5-mg chewable tablets; elixir, syrup, and oral solution, 12.5 mg/5 mL.

**B. Parenteral.** Diphenhydramine hydrochloride (Benadryl, others), 50 mg/mL in 1-mL cartridges, amps, steri-vials, and syringes, and in 10-mL steri-vials (may contain benzethonium chloride) .

**C.** The **suggested minimum stocking level** to treat a 70-kg adult for the first 24 hours is one vial (50 mg/mL, 10 mL each) or eight vials (50 mg/mL, 1 mL each).

## ▶ DOPAMINE

*Neal L. Benowitz, MD*

**I. Pharmacology.** Dopamine is an endogenous catecholamine and the immediate metabolic precursor of norepinephrine. It stimulates alpha- and beta-adrenergic receptors directly and indirectly. In addition, it acts on specific dopaminergic receptors. Its relative activity at these various receptors is dose related. At low infusion rates (1–5 mcg/kg/min), dopamine stimulates beta-1 activity (increased heart rate and contractility) and increases renal and mesenteric blood flow through dopaminergic agonist activity. At high infusion rates (10–20 mcg/kg/min), alpha-adrenergic stimulation predominates, resulting in increased peripheral vascular resistance. Dopamine is not effective orally. After IV administration, its onset of action occurs within 5 minutes, and the duration of effect is less than 10 minutes. The plasma half-life is about 2 minutes.

**II. Indications**

**A.** Dopamine is used to increase blood pressure, cardiac output, and urine flow in patients with shock who have not responded to intravenous fluid challenge, correction of hypothermia, or reversal of acidosis.

**B.** Low-dose infusion is most effective for hypotension caused by venodilation or reduced cardiac contractility; high-dose dopamine is indicated for shock resulting from decreased peripheral arterial resistance.

**III. Contraindications**

**A.** Tachyarrhythmias or ventricular fibrillation and uncorrected hypovolemia.

**B.** High-dose infusion is relatively contraindicated in the presence of peripheral arterial occlusive disease with thrombosis and in patients with ergot poisoning (see p 187).

**IV. Adverse effects**

**A.** Severe hypertension, which may result in intracranial hemorrhage, pulmonary edema, or myocardial necrosis.

**B.** Aggravation of tissue ischemia, resulting in gangrene (with high-dose infusion).

**C.** Ventricular arrhythmias, especially in patients intoxicated by halogenated or aromatic hydrocarbon solvents or anesthetics.

**D.** Tissue necrosis after extravasation (see VI.A, below, for treatment of extravasation).

**E.** Anaphylactoid reaction induced by sulfite preservatives in sensitive patients.

**F. Use in pregnancy.** FDA category C (indeterminate). There may be a dose-related effect on uterine blood flow. This does not preclude its acute, short-term use for a seriously symptomatic patient (see p 407).

**V. Drug or laboratory interactions**

**A.** Enhanced pressor response may occur in the presence of cocaine and cyclic antidepressants owing to inhibition of neuronal reuptake.

**B.** Enhanced pressor response may occur in patients taking monoamine oxidase inhibitors owing to inhibition of neuronal metabolic degradation.

**C.** Chloral hydrate and halogenated hydrocarbon anesthetics may enhance the arrhythmogenic effect of dopamine, owing to sensitization of the myocardium to effects of catecholamines.

**D.** Alpha- and beta-blocking agents antagonize the adrenergic effects of dopamine; haloperidol and other dopamine antagonists may antagonize the dopaminergic effects.

**E.** There may be a reduced pressor response in patients with depleted neuronal stores of catecholamines (eg, chronic disulfiram or reserpine use).

**VI. Dosage and method of administration (adults and children)**

**A. Avoid extravasation.** ***Caution:*** The intravenous infusion must be free flowing, and the infused vein should be observed frequently for signs of subcutaneous infiltration (pallor, coldness, and induration). If extravasation occurs, immediately infiltrate the affected area with phentolamine (see p 495), 5–10 mg in 10–15 mL of normal saline (children, 0.1–0.2 mg/kg; maximum 10 mg total) via a fine (25- to 27-gauge) hypodermic needle; improvement is evidenced by hyperemia and return to normal temperature. Topical nitrates and infiltration of terbutaline have also been reported to be successful for treatment of extravasation involving other catecholamines.

**B.** For **predominantly inotropic effects,** begin with 1 mcg/kg/min and increase infusion rate as needed to 5–10 mcg/kg/min.

**C.** For **predominantly vasopressor effects,** infuse 10–20 mcg/kg/min and increase as needed. Doses above 50 mcg/kg/min may result in severe peripheral vasoconstriction and gangrene.

**VII. Formulations.**

**A.** Dopamine hydrochloride (Intropin and others): as a concentrate for admixture to intravenous solutions (40-, 80-, and 160-mg/mL in 5-mL amps, 5- and 10-mL vials or syringes, and 20-mL vials) or premixed parenteral product for injection (0.8, 1.6, and 3.2 mg/mL in 5% dextrose). All contain sodium bisulfite as a preservative.

**B.** The **suggested minimum stocking level** to treat a 70-kg adult for the first 24 hours is approximately 1800–2000 mg (two to three vials, 160 mg/mL, 5 mL each).

## ► DTPA

*Cindy Burkhardt, PharmD*

**I. Pharmacology.** Diethylenetriaminepentaacetate (Zn-DTPA and Ca-DTPA) is a chelating agent that is used in a calcium or zinc salt form and functions by forming a chelate with metal ions (plutonium, americium, curium) that then can be excreted in urine. DTPA has a plasma half-life of 20–60 minutes and is distributed in the extracellular space. It has a small amount of protein binding and does not undergo significant metabolism or tissue accumulation. The use of Ca-DTPA within one hour of contamination resulted in a 10-fold higher rate of elimination of plutonium compared with Zn-DTPA. Ca-DTPA is more effective than Zn-DTPA when given within 24 hours after internal contamination.

**II. Indications.** DTPA is FDA indicated for internal contamination with plutonium, americium, and curium. It has also been used for treatment of internal contamination with californium and berkelium.

**III. Contraindications**

- **A.** Known hypersensitivity to the agent.
- **B.** DTPA should not be used in uranium or neptunium exposures as it may increase bone deposition of these elements.
- **C.** Ca-DTPA should not be used in patients with renal failure, nephrotic syndrome, or bone marrow suppression.

**IV. Adverse effects**

- **A.** Nausea, vomiting, and diarrhea.
- **B.** Fever, chills and myalgias.
- **C.** Life-threatening side effects are distinctly uncommon, with no serious toxicity in human subjects after 4500 administrations of Ca-DTPA and 1000 administrations of Zn-DTPA.
- **D. Use in pregnancy.** FDA category C (Ca-DTPA) and category B (Zn-DTPA); Zn-DTPA may be used in pregnancy, though fetal risks are not completely known (see p 407).

**V. Drug or laboratory interactions**

- **A.** There are no major known drug interactions.
- **B.** There does not appear to be a decrement of body trace elements associated with the use of DTPA.

**VI. Dosage and method of administration**

- **A.** Upon known exposure, usual therapy would involve Ca- or Zn-DTPA given in a 1-g dosage as soon as possible. This may be given IV over 3–5 minutes in an undiluted form or may be diluted in 100–250 cc of NS, LR, or 5% dextrose in water. Administration time should not exceed 2 hours. Initial dose for pediatric patients is 14 mg/kg, not to exceed 1 g.
- **B.** It is preferable to give Ca-DTPA for the initial dose since it is more effective than Zn-DTPA during the first 24 hours. After 24 hours, Zn-DTPA and Ca-DTPA are equally effective. If Ca-DTPA is not available or is contraindicated in a patient, the same dose of Zn-DTPA may be substituted.
- **C.** After the initial dose of Ca-DTPA, treatment with 1 g of Zn-DTPA daily should be continued. If Zn-DTPA is not available, maintenance treatment can be continued with Ca-DTPA along with mineral supplements containing zinc if necessary. Treatment may be continued for days, months, or years depending on body burden and individual response to therapy. Generally given until the excretion enhancement factor (EEF) approaches 1.
- **D.** IM dosing generally is not recommended owing to significant pain with injection.
- **E.** Pregnant women should only be treated with Zn-DTPA.
- **F.** Nebulization in a 1:1 dilution is safe and effective for persons only contaminated only via inhalation. The intravenous route should be used if multiple routes of internal contamination occurred or the route is unknown.

**VII. Formulations**

- **A. Parenteral or nebulization.** Pentetate Calcium Trisodium Injection (Ca-DTPA); Pentetate Zinc Trisodium Injection (Zn-DTPA).One gram in 5 cc of diluent (200 mg/cc) packaged in single-use clear glass ampules. This is provided in boxes of 10 ampules for each salt (Ca-DTPA and Zn-DTPA) by Akorn Inc.
- **B.** The **suggested minimum stocking level** to treat a 70-kg adult for the first 24 hours is one ampule (1 gram) of DTPA. It is advisable to stock both Ca-DTPA and Zn-DTPA. DTPA is kept in the Strategic National Stockpile (SNS) at the

CDC. The Radiation Emergency Assistance Center (REAC/TS), can be contacted for information on obtaining DTPA and its recommended dosing ([865] 576-3131, on the Internet at www.orau.gov/reacts).

## ► EDTA, CALCIUM (CALCIUM DISODIUM EDTA, CALCIUM DISODIUM EDETATE, CALCIUM DISODIUM VERSENATE)

*Michael J. Kosnett, MD, MPH*

I. **Pharmacology.** Calcium EDTA has been used as a chelating agent to enhance elimination of certain toxic metals, principally lead. The elimination of endogenous metals, including zinc, manganese, iron, and copper, may also occur to a lesser extent. The plasma half-life of the drug is 20–60 minutes, and 50% of the injected dose is excreted in urine within 1 hour. Increased urinary excretion of lead begins within 1 hour of EDTA administration and is followed by a decrease in whole-blood lead concentration over the course of treatment. Calcium EDTA mobilizes lead from soft tissues and from a fraction of the larger lead stores present in bone. In persons with high body lead burdens, cessation of EDTA chelation often is followed by an upward rebound in blood lead levels as bone stores equilibrate with lower soft-tissue levels. ***Note:*** Calcium EDTA should ***not*** be confused with sodium EDTA (edetate disodium), which occasionally is used to treat life-threatening severe hypercalcemia.

II. **Indications**

A. Calcium EDTA has been used to decrease blood lead concentrations and increase urinary lead excretion in individuals with symptomatic lead intoxication and in asymptomatic persons with high blood lead levels. Although clinical experience associates calcium EDTA chelation with relief of symptoms (particularly lead colic) and decreased mortality, controlled clinical trials demonstrating therapeutic efficacy are lacking, and treatment recommendations have been largely empiric.

B. Calcium EDTA may have possible utility in poisoning by zinc, manganese, and certain heavy radioisotopes.

III. **Contraindications.** Since calcium EDTA increases renal excretion of lead, anuria is a relative contraindication. Accumulation of EDTA increases the risk of nephropathy, especially in volume-depleted patients. In patients with moderate renal insufficiency, reduce the dose in relative proportion to the deficit in creatinine clearance. The use of EDTA in conjunction with hemodialysis or hemofiltration has been reported in patients with renal failure.

IV. **Adverse effects**

A. Nephrotoxicity (eg, acute tubular necrosis, proteinuria, and hematuria) may be minimized by adequate hydration, establishment of adequate urine flow, avoidance of excessive doses, and limitation of continuous administration to 5 or fewer days. Laboratory assessment of renal function should be performed daily during treatment for severe intoxication and after the second and fifth days in other cases.

B. **Black box warning:** In individuals with lead encephalopathy, rapid or high-volume infusions may exacerbate increased intracranial pressure. In such cases, it is preferable to use lower-volume, more concentrated solutions for intravenous infusions. Alternatively, intramuscular injection may be considered.

C. Local pain may occur at intramuscular injection sites. Lidocaine (1 mL of 1% lidocaine per mL of EDTA concentrate) may be added to intramuscular injections to decrease discomfort.

D. **Inadvertent use of sodium EDTA** (edetate disodium) may cause serious **hypocalcemia**.

**E.** Calcium EDTA may result in short-term zinc depletion, which has uncertain clinical significance.

**F. Use in pregnancy.** The safety of calcium EDTA in human pregnancy has not been established, although uncomplicated use late in pregnancy has been reported. Fetal malformations with high doses have been noted in animal studies, possibly as a consequence of zinc depletion. If severe lead poisoning necessitates use during pregnancy, maternal zinc supplementation should be considered.

**V. Drug or laboratory interactions.** Intravenous infusions may be incompatible with 10% dextrose solutions, amphotericin, or hydralazine.

**VI. Dosage and method of administration for lead poisoning (adults and children).** ***Note:*** Administration of EDTA should never be a substitute for removal from lead exposure. In adults, the federal OSHA lead standard requires removal from occupational lead exposure of any worker with a single blood lead concentration in excess of 60 mcg/dL or an average of three successive values in excess of 50 mcg/dL. (However, recent declines in background lead levels and concern about adverse health effects of lower-level exposure support removal at even lower levels.) ***Prophylactic chelation,*** defined as the routine use of chelation to prevent elevated blood lead concentrations or to lower blood lead levels below the standard in asymptomatic workers, ***is not* permitted.** Consult the local or state health department or OSHA (see Table IV–3, p 535) for more detailed information.

**A. Lead poisoning with encephalopathy, acute lead colic, or blood lead levels greater than 150 mcg/dL:**

1. **Adults:** 2–4 g (or 30–50 mg/kg) IV per 24 hours as a continuous infusion (diluted to 2–4 mg/mL in normal saline or 5% dextrose). Courses of treatment should not exceed 5 days.
2. **Children:** 1000–1500 mg/m$^2$ per 24 hours as a continuous IV infusion (diluted to 2–4 mg/mL in normal saline or 5% dextrose). Some clinicians advocate that treatment of patients with lead encephalopathy, particularly children, be initiated along with a single dose of BAL (dimercaprol; see p 417), followed 4 hours later by the concomitant administration of BAL and calcium EDTA. BAL is discontinued after 3 days; EDTA may be continued for up to 5 consecutive days.

**B. Symptomatic lead poisoning without encephalopathy or colic.** Administer calcium EDTA at an adult dose of 2–4 g (or 30–50 mg/kg) IV per 24 hours or at a pediatric dose of 1000–1500 mg/m$^2$/day (approximately 20–30 mg/kg as a continuous IV infusion, diluted to 2–4 mg/mL) for 3–5 days.

**C.** Although intravenous administration is preferable, the daily dose (see above) may be administered by deep intramuscular injection in two or three divided doses (every 8–12 hours).

**D.** Because EDTA enhances urinary lead excretion, provide adequate fluids to maintain urine flow (optimally 1–2 mL/kg/h). However, avoid overhydration, which may aggravate cerebral edema.

**E.** Treatment courses should be separated by a minimum of 2 days, and an interval of 2 or more weeks may be indicated to assess the extent of post-treatment rebound in blood lead levels. An additional course of calcium EDTA treatment may be considered based on the basis of post-treatment blood lead concentrations and the persistence or recurrence of symptoms.

**F.** Consider changing to oral succimer (see p 510) or oral unithiol (p 515) after 3 to 5 days of calcium EDTA treatment provided that encephalopathy or colic has resolved, the blood lead level has fallen to less than 100 mcg/dL, and the patient is able to absorb an oral formulation.

**G.** Single-dose EDTA chelation lead mobilization tests have been advocated by some clinicians to evaluate body lead burden or assess the need for a full course of treatment in patients with moderately elevated blood lead levels, but the value and necessity of these tests are controversial.

**H.** Oral EDTA therapy is ***not*** recommended for prevention or treatment of lead poisoning, because it may *increase* the absorption of lead from the GI tract.

**VII. Formulations**

**A. Parenteral.** Calcium disodium edetate (Versenate), 200 mg/mL, 5-mL ampules. For intravenous infusion, dilute to 2–4 mg/mL in normal saline or 5% dextrose solution.

**B.** The **suggested minimum stocking level** to treat a 70-kg adult for the first 24 hours is three boxes (six ampules per box, 18 g).

# ▶ EPINEPHRINE

*Neal L. Benowitz, MD*

**I. Pharmacology.** Epinephrine is an endogenous catecholamine with alpha- and beta-adrenergic agonist properties that is used primarily in emergency situations to treat anaphylaxis or cardiac arrest. Beneficial effects include inhibition of histamine release from mast cells and basophils, bronchodilation, positive inotropic effects, and peripheral vasoconstriction. Epinephrine is not active after oral administration. Subcutaneous injection produces effects within 5–10 minutes, with peak effects at 20 minutes. Intravenous or inhalational administration produces much more rapid onset. Epinephrine is inactivated rapidly in the body, with an elimination half-life of 2 minutes.

**II. Indications**

**A.** Anaphylaxis and anaphylactoid reactions.

**B.** Epinephrine occasionally is used for hypotension resulting from overdose by beta blockers, calcium antagonists, and other cardiac-depressant drugs.

**III. Contraindications**

**A.** Tachyarrhythmias or ventricular fibrillation and uncorrected hypovolemia.

**B.** Epinephrine is relatively contraindicated in patients with organic heart disease, peripheral arterial occlusive vascular disease with thrombosis, or ergot poisoning (see p 187).

**C.** Narrow-angle glaucoma.

**IV. Adverse effects**

**A.** Anxiety, restlessness, tremor, and headache.

**B.** Severe hypertension, which may result in intracranial hemorrhage, pulmonary edema, or myocardial necrosis or infarction.

**C.** Use with caution in patients intoxicated by halogenated or aromatic hydrocarbon solvents and anesthetics, because these agents may sensitize the myocardium to the arrhythmogenic effects of epinephrine.

**D.** Tissue necrosis after extravasation or intra-arterial injection.

**E.** Aggravation of tissue ischemia, resulting in gangrene.

**F.** Anaphylactoid reaction, which may occur owing to the bisulfite preservative in patients with sulfite hypersensitivity.

**G.** Hypokalemia, hypophosphatemia, hyperglycemia, and leukocytosis may occur owing to the beta-adrenergic effects of epinephrine.

**H. Use in pregnancy.** FDA category C (indeterminate). Epinephrine is teratogenic in animals, crosses the placenta, can cause placental ischemia, and may suppress uterine contractions, but these effects do not preclude its acute, short-term use for a seriously symptomatic patient (see p 407).

**V. Drug or laboratory interactions**

**A.** An enhanced arrhythmogenic effect may occur when epinephrine is given to patients with chloral hydrate overdose or anesthetized with cyclopropane or halogenated general anesthetics.

**B.** Use in patients taking propranolol and other nonselective beta blockers may produce severe hypertension owing to blockade of beta-2–mediated vasodilation, resulting in unopposed alpha-mediated vasoconstriction.

- **C.** Cocaine and cyclic antidepressants may enhance stimulant effects owing to inhibition of neuronal epinephrine reuptake.
- **D.** Monoamine oxidase inhibitors may enhance pressor effects because of decreased neuronal epinephrine metabolism.
- **E.** Digitalis intoxication may enhance the arrhythmogenicity of epinephrine.

**VI. Dosage and method of administration**

- **A.** ***Caution:*** **Avoid extravasation.** The intravenous infusion must be free flowing, and the infused vein should be observed frequently for signs of subcutaneous infiltration (pallor, coldness, or induration).
  1. If extravasation occurs, immediately infiltrate the affected area with phentolamine (see p 495), 5–10 mg in 10–15 mL of normal saline (children, 0.1–0.2 mg/kg; maximum 10 mg total) via a fine (25- to 27-gauge) hypodermic needle; improvement is evidenced by hyperemia and return to normal temperature.
  2. Alternatively, topical application of nitroglycerin paste and infiltration of terbutaline have been reported to be successful.
- **B. Mild to moderate allergic reaction.** Give 0.3–0.5 mg SC or IM (children, 0.01 mg/kg of 1:1000 solution or 1:200 suspension; maximum 0.5 mg). May be repeated after 10–15 minutes if needed.
- **C. Severe anaphylaxis.** Give 0.05–0.1 mg IV (0.5–1 mL of a 1:10,000 solution) every 5–10 minutes (children, 0.01 mg/kg; maximum 0.1 mg) or an IV infusion at 1–4 mcg/min. If intravenous access is not available, the endotracheal route may be used; give 0.5 mg (5 mL of a 1:10,000 solution) down the endotracheal tube.
- **D. Hypotension.** Infuse at 1 mcg/min; titrate upward every 5 minutes as necessary. If the patient has refractory hypotension and is on a beta-adrenergic blocking drug, consider glucagon (see p 456).

**VII. Formulations**

- **A. Parenteral.** Epinephrine hydrochloride (Adrenalin, EpiPen, others), 0.01 mg/mL (1:100,000), 0.1 mg/mL (1:10,000), in 10-mL prefilled syringes and vials; 0.5 mg/mL (1:2000) in 0.3-mL single-dose autoinjectors, and 1 mg/mL (1:1000) in 1-mL ampules, 30-mL vials, and 0.3-mL single-dose autoinjectors. Most preparations contain sodium bisulfite or sodium metabisulfite as a preservative.
- **B.** The **suggested minimum stocking level** to treat a 70-kg adult for the first 24 hours is 10 mg (10 ampules, 1:1000, 1 mL, or equivalent).

## ▶ ESMOLOL

*Thomas E. Kearney, PharmD*

**I. Pharmacology.** Esmolol is a short-acting, IV, cardioselective beta-adrenergic blocker with no intrinsic sympathomimetic or membrane-depressant activity. In usual therapeutic doses, it causes little or no bronchospasm in patients with asthma. Esmolol produces peak effects within 6–10 minutes of administration of an intravenous bolus. It is hydrolyzed rapidly by red blood cell esterases, with an elimination half-life of 9 minutes; therapeutic and adverse effects disappear within 30 minutes after the infusion is discontinued.

**II. Indications**

- **A.** Rapid control of supraventricular and ventricular tachyarrhythmias and hypertension, especially if caused by excessive sympathomimetic activity (eg, stimulant drugs, hyperthyroid state).
- **B.** Reversal of hypotension and tachycardia caused by excessive beta-adrenergic activity resulting from theophylline or caffeine overdose.
- **C.** Control of ventricular tachyarrhythmias caused by excessive myocardial catecholamine sensitivity (eg, chloral hydrate and chlorinated hydrocarbon solvents).

**III. Contraindications**

A. Contraindications include hypotension, bradycardia, and congestive heart failure secondary to intrinsic cardiac disease or cardiac-depressant effects of drugs and toxins (eg, cyclic antidepressants and barbiturates).

B. Hypertension caused by alpha-adrenergic or generalized stimulant drugs (eg, cocaine, amphetamines), unless esmolol is coadministered with a vasodilator (eg, nitroprusside or phentolamine). Paradoxic hypertension may result from an unopposed alpha effect, although it is less likely than that associated with the use of a non-specific beta-adrenergic blocker (propranolol).

**IV. Adverse effects**

A. Hypotension and bradycardia may occur, especially in patients with intrinsic cardiac disease or cardiac-depressant drug overdose.

B. Bronchospasm may occur in patients with asthma or chronic bronchospasm, but it is less likely than with propranolol or other nonselective beta blockers and is rapidly reversible after the infusion is discontinued.

C. Esmolol may mask physiologic responses to hypoglycemia (tremor, tachycardia, and glycogenolysis) and therefore should be used with caution in patients with diabetes.

D. **Use in pregnancy.** FDA category C (indeterminate). This does not preclude its short-term use for a seriously symptomatic patient (see p 407). High-dose infusion may contribute to placental ischemia.

**V. Drug or laboratory interactions**

A. Esmolol may transiently increase the serum digoxin level by 10–20%, but the clinical significance of this is unknown.

B. Recovery from succinylcholine-induced neuromuscular blockade may be delayed slightly (5–10 minutes). Similarly, esmolol metabolism may be inhibited by anticholinesterase agents (eg, organophosphates).

C. Esmolol is not compatible with sodium bicarbonate solutions.

**VI. Dosage and method of administration**

A. Dilute before intravenous injection to a final concentration of 10 mg/mL with 5% dextrose, lactated Ringer's injection, or saline solutions.

B. Give as an intravenous infusion, starting at 0.025–0.05 mg/kg/min and increasing as needed up to 0.2 mg/kg/min (average dose 0.1 mg/kg/min). Steady-state concentrations are reached approximately 30 minutes after each infusion adjustment. A loading dose of 0.5 mg/kg should be given over 1 minute if more rapid onset of clinical effects (5–10 minutes) is desired.

C. Infusion rates greater than 0.2 mg/kg/min are likely to produce excessive hypotension. At rates greater than 0.3 mg/kg/min, the beta-blocking effects lose their beta-1 selectivity.

**VII. Formulations**

A. **Parenteral.** Esmolol hydrochloride (Brevibloc), 2.5 g in 10-mL ampules (250 mg/mL), 100 mg in 10-mL vials (10 mg/mL), and 20 mg/mL (double strength) in 5-mL vials and 100-mL bags.

B. The **suggested minimum stocking level** to treat a 70-kg adult for the first 24 hours is 2 ampules (250 mg/mL, 10 mL) or 25 vials (10 mg/mL, 10 mL).

## ► ETHANOL

*Thomas E. Kearney, PharmD*

I. **Pharmacology.** Ethanol (ethyl alcohol) acts as a competitive substrate for the enzyme alcohol dehydrogenase, preventing the metabolic formation of toxic metabolites from methanol or ethylene glycol. Blood ethanol concentrations of 100 mg/dL, or at least a 1:4 molar ratio of ethanol to toxic alcohol/glycol, effectively saturate alcohol dehydrogenase and prevent further methanol and ethylene glycol metabolism (see also Fomepizole, p 454). Ethanol is well absorbed from the

GI tract when given orally, but the onset is more rapid and predictable when it is given intravenously. The elimination of ethanol is zero order; the average rate of decline is 15 mg/dL/h. However, this is highly variable and will be influenced by prior chronic use of alcohol, recruitment of alternate metabolic pathways, and concomitant hemodialysis (eg, to remove methanol or ethylene glycol).

**II. Indications.** Suspected **methanol** (methyl alcohol, see p 260) or **ethylene glycol** (see p 193) poisoning with:

**A.** A suggestive history of ingestion of a toxic dose but no available blood concentration measurements;

**B.** Metabolic acidosis and an unexplained elevated osmolar gap (see p 32); or

**C.** A serum methanol or ethylene glycol concentration ≥20 mg/dL.

**D. Note:** Since the introduction of fomepizole (4-methylpyrazole, see p 454), a potent inhibitor of alcohol dehydrogenase, most patients with ethylene glycol or methanol poisoning probably will be treated with this drug instead of ethanol, particularly in cases involving small children, patients taking disulfiram, patients with pancreatitis, and hospitals lacking laboratory support to perform rapid ethanol levels (for monitoring treatment). Ethanol is more difficult to dose, requires more monitoring, and has a greater risk of adverse effects. Studies suggest that despite the higher acquisition costs for fomepizole, it may be more cost-effective than ethanol.

**E.** Other substances that are metabolized by alcohol dehydrogenase to toxic metabolites include propylene glycol, diethylene glycol, triethylene glycol, glycol ethers (eg, ethylene glycol ethyl ether, ethylene glycol butyl ether), and 1,4-butanediol. The criteria for ethanol therapy and evidence for improved outcomes are lacking for these substances.

**III. Contraindications.** Use of interacting drugs, which may cause disulfiram-type reaction (see V.B, below).

**IV. Adverse effects**

**A.** Nausea, vomiting, and gastritis may occur with oral administration. Ethanol may also exacerbate pancreatitis.

**B.** Inebriation, sedation, and hypoglycemia (particularly in children and malnourished adults) may occur.

**C.** Intravenous use sometimes is associated with local phlebitis (especially with ethanol solutions 10%). Hyponatremia may result from large doses of sodium-free intravenous solutions.

**D.** Acute flushing, palpitations, and postural hypotension may occur in patients with atypical aldehyde dehydrogenase enzyme (up to 50–80% of Japanese, Chinese, and Korean individuals).

**E. Use in pregnancy.** FDA category C (indeterminate). Ethanol crosses the placenta. Chronic overuse in pregnancy is associated with birth defects (fetal alcohol syndrome). The drug reduces uterine contractions and may slow or stop labor. However, these effects do not preclude its acute, short-term use for a seriously symptomatic patient (see p 407).

**V. Drug or laboratory interactions**

**A.** Ethanol potentiates the effect of CNS–depressant drugs and hypoglycemic agents.

**B. Disulfiram reaction** (see p 184), including flushing, palpitations, and postural hypotension, may occur in patients taking disulfiram as well as a variety of other medications (eg, metronidazole, furazolidone, procarbazine, chlorpropamide, some cephalosporins, and *Coprinus* mushrooms). In such cases, fomepizole is the recommended alternative to ethanol treatment.

**C.** Drugs or chemicals metabolized by alcohol dehydrogenase (eg, chloral hydrate, isopropyl alcohol) also have impaired elimination. Fomepizole and ethanol mutually inhibit each other's metabolism.

**VI. Dosage and method of administration.** Obtain serum ethanol levels after the loading dose and frequently during maintenance therapy to ensure a concentration of 100–150 mg/dL (eg, every 1–2 hours until goal achieved, eg, level = 100

**TABLE III–8. ETHANOL DOSING (ADULTS AND CHILDREN)**

| | Intravenous[c] | | Oral |
|---|---|---|---|
| **Dose** | **5%** | **10%** | **50%** |
| Loading[a] | 15 mL/kg | 7.5 mL/kg | 2 mL/kg |
| Maintenance[b] | 2–4 mL/kg/h | 1–2 mL/kg/h | 0.2–0.4 mL/kg/h |
| Maintenance during hemodialysis[b] | 4–7 mL/kg/h | 2–3.5 mL/kg/h | 0.4–0.7 mL/kg/h |

[a]If the patient's serum ethanol level is greater than 0, reduce the loading dose in a proportional manner. Multiply the calculated loading dose by the following factor:

$$\frac{100 - [\text{patient's serum ethanol in mg/dL}]}{100}$$

[b]Doses may vary on the individual. Chronic alcoholics have a higher rate of ethanol elimination, and maintenance doses should be adjusted to maintain an ethanol level of approximately 100 mg/dL.
[c]Infuse intravenous loading dose over 20–30 minutes or longer.

mg/dL, or after change in infusion rate and then every 2–4 hours during the maintenance dosing).

**A.** Ethanol may be given orally or intravenously. The desired serum concentration is 100 mg/dL (20 mmol/L); this can be achieved by giving approximately 750 mg/kg (Table III–8) as a loading dose, followed by a maintenance infusion of approximately 100–150 mg/kg/h (give a larger dose to chronic alcoholics). A 10% ethanol solution is preferred for IV (to minimize fluids, but it may require central venous access in children), and a solution of less than 30% (usually 20% given for palatability and absorption) is preferred for oral administration.

**B.** Increase the infusion rate to 175–250 mg/kg/h (larger dose for chronic alcoholics) during hemodialysis to offset the increased rate of ethanol elimination. Alternatively, ethanol may be added to the dialysate.

**VII. Formulations**

**A. Oral.** Pharmaceutical-grade ethanol (96% USP). ***Note:*** Commercial liquor may be used orally if pharmaceutical-grade ethanol is not available; administer 160 mL/kg divided by the "proof" of the liquor (eg, if using 80 proof liquor, give 2.0 mL/kg). Mix with juice and dilute to a concentration of 20%.

**B. Parenteral.** Ethanol 5% in 5% dextrose solution; 10% in 5% dextrose solution in 1000 mL.

**C.** The **suggested minimum stocking level** to treat a 70-kg adult for the first 24 hours is three bottles (10% ethanol, 1 L each).

## ► FLUMAZENIL

*Walter H. Mullen, PharmD*

**I. Pharmacology.** Flumazenil (Romazicon) is a highly selective competitive inhibitor of CNS benzodiazepine receptors. It has no demonstrable benzodiazepine agonist activity and no significant toxicity even in high doses. It has no effect on alcohol or opioid receptors, and it does not reverse alcohol intoxication. Flumazenil is most effective parenterally (high first-pass effect with oral administration). After intravenous administration, the onset of benzodiazepine reversal occurs within 1–2 minutes, peaks at 6–10 minutes, and lasts for 1–5 hours, depending on the dose of flumazenil and the degree of preexisting benzodiazepine effect. It is eliminated by hepatic metabolism, with a serum half-life of approximately 1 hour.

**II. Indications**

**A.** Rapid reversal of benzodiazepine overdose–induced coma and respiratory depression, both as a diagnostic aid and as a potential substitute for endotracheal intubation. Rule out high-risk patients (see below). Lowest-risk patients include patients with a known iatrogenic exposure, toddler ingestion, and patients with a paradoxic response (characterized by agitation or excitement and excessive movement or restlessness) to a benzodiazepine where reversal of effect is desired.

**B.** Postoperative or postprocedure reversal of benzodiazepine sedation.

**C.** Flumazenil may reverse CNS depression from certain non–benzodiazepine sedatives and hypnotics, eg, zolpidem (Ambien) and zaleplon (Sonata).

**III. Contraindications**

**A.** Known hypersensitivity to flumazenil or benzodiazepines.

**B.** Suspected serious tricyclic antidepressant or other proconvulsant overdose.

**C.** Benzodiazepine use for control of a potentially life-threatening condition (eg, status epilepticus or increased intracranial pressure).

**IV. Adverse effects**

**A.** Anxiety, agitation, headache, dizziness, nausea, vomiting, tremor, and transient facial flushing.

**B.** Rapid reversal of benzodiazepine effect in patients with benzodiazepine addiction or high tolerance may result in an acute withdrawal state, including hyperexcitability, tachycardia, and seizures (rarely reported).

**C.** Seizures or arrhythmias may be precipitated in patients with a serious cyclic antidepressant or other proconvulsant overdose.

**D.** Flumazenil has precipitated arrhythmias in a patient with a mixed benzodiazepine and chloral hydrate overdose.

**E.** Other risks include resedation and aspiration.

**F. Use in pregnancy.** FDA category C (indeterminate). This does not preclude its acute, short-term use for a seriously symptomatic patient (see p 407).

**V. Drug or laboratory interactions.** No known interactions. Flumazenil does not appear to alter the kinetics of benzodiazepines or other drugs.

**VI. Dosage and method of administration**

**A. Benzodiazepine overdose.** Titrate the dosage until the desired response is achieved.

1. Administer 0.2 mg IV over 30 seconds (pediatric dose not established; start with 0.01 mg/kg). If there is no response, give 0.3 mg. If there still is no response, give 0.5 mg and repeat every 30 seconds if needed to a total maximum dose of 3 mg (1 mg in children).
2. Because effects last only 1–5 hours, continue to monitor the patient closely for resedation. If multiple repeated doses are needed, consider a continuous infusion (0.2–1 mg/h).

**B. Reversal of conscious sedation or anesthetic doses of benzodiazepine.** A dose of 0.2 mg given intravenously is usually sufficient and may be repeated, titrating up to 1 mg.

**VII. Formulations**

**A. Parenteral.** Flumazenil (Romazicon), 0.1 mg/mL, 5- and 10-mL vials with parabens and EDTA.

**B.** The **suggested minimum stocking level** to treat a 70-kg adult for the first 24 hours is 10 vials (0.1 mg/mL, 10 mL).

## ► FOLIC ACID

*F. Lee Cantrell, PharmD*

**I. Pharmacology.** Folic acid is a B-complex vitamin that is essential for protein synthesis and erythropoiesis. In addition, the administration of folate to patients with methanol poisoning may enhance the conversion of the toxic metabolite formic acid to carbon dioxide and water, based on studies in folate-deficient primates. ***Note:*** Folic acid requires metabolic activation and is not effective for the treatment of poisoning by dihydrofolate reductase inhibitors (eg, methotrexate and trimethoprim). Leucovorin (see p 468) is the proper agent in these situations.

**II. Indications.** Adjunctive treatment for methanol poisoning.

**III. Contraindications.** No known contraindications.

**IV. Adverse effects.**

- **A.** Rare allergic reactions have been reported after intravenous administration.
- **B. Use in pregnancy.** FDA category A (see p 407). Folic acid is a recommended supplement.

**V. Drug or laboratory interactions.** This agent may decrease hydantoin levels by enhancing their metabolism.

**VI. Dosage and method of administration.** The dose required for methanol or ethylene glycol poisoning is not established, although 50 mg IV (children, 1 mg/kg) every 4 hours for six doses has been recommended.

**VII. Formulations.**

- **A. Parenteral.** Sodium folate (Folvite), 5 mg/mL, 10-mL vials.
- **B.** The **suggested minimum stocking level** to treat a 70-kg adult for the first 24 hours is six vials (5 mg/mL, 10 mL each).

## ▶ FOMEPIZOLE (4-METHYLPYRAZOLE, 4-MP)

*Thomas E. Kearney, PharmD*

**I. Pharmacology**

- **A.** Fomepizole (4-methylpyrazole) is a potent competitive inhibitor of alcohol dehydrogenase, the first enzyme in the metabolism of ethanol and other alcohols. Fomepizole can prevent the formation of toxic metabolites after methanol or ethylene glycol ingestion. Furthermore, early treatment with fomepizole for ethylene glycol or methanol poisoning (before the presence of a significant acidosis) may obviate the need for dialysis. Since the introduction of fomepizole, most patients with ethylene glycol or methanol poisoning probably will be treated with this drug instead of ethanol, particularly in cases involving small children, patients taking disulfiram, patients with altered consciousness and ingestion of multiple substances, patients with pancreatitis or active liver disease, and hospitals lacking laboratory support to perform rapid ethanol levels (for monitoring treatment). Economic models have suggested that fomepizole may be more cost-effective than ethanol despite the high acquisition cost of fomepizole.
- **B.** Fomepizole is eliminated mainly via zero-order kinetics, but P-450 metabolism can undergo autoinduction within 2–3 days. The drug is dialyzable. It is well absorbed and has been used successfully with PO administration but is not approved by this route in the United States.

**II. Indications** are similar to those for ethanol (see p 450): suspected or confirmed **methanol** (methyl alcohol; see p 260) or **ethylene glycol** (see p 193) poisoning with one or more of the following:

- **A.** A reliable history of ingestion of a toxic dose but no available blood concentration measurements (when used empirically, allows a 12-hour "window" after one dose to assess the patient);
- **B.** Metabolic acidosis and an unexplained elevated osmolar gap (see p 32); or
- **C.** Serum methanol or ethylene glycol concentration ≥20 mg/dL.
- **D.** Other substances that are metabolized by alcohol dehydrogenase to toxic metabolites include propylene glycol, diethylene glycol, triethylene glycol, glycol ethers (eg, ethylene glycol ethyl ether, ethylene glycol butyl ether), and 1,4-butanediol. The criteria for fomepizole therapy and evidence for improved

outcomes are lacking for all these substances. However, case reports of poisonings from some of these other glycols (eg, propylene glycol, diethylene glycol) have suggested benefit when fomepizole therapy is coupled with dialysis to remove the potentially toxic parent compound and concomitantly prevent the formation of toxic metabolites.

**E.** Disulfiram reaction (or risk of): to halt progression or production of acetaldehyde, assuming that ethanol is still present (based on case reports).

**III. Contraindications.** History of allergy to the drug or to other pyrazoles.

**IV. Adverse effects**

**A.** Venous irritation and phlebosclerosis after intravenous injection of the undiluted product.

**B.** Headache, nausea, and dizziness are the most commonly reported side effects. Less common effects are vomiting, tachycardia, hypotension, feeling of inebriation, rash, fever, and eosinophilia.

**C.** Transient non-dose-dependent elevation of hepatic transaminases has been reported after multiple doses.

**D.** Although safety and effectiveness in children have not been established by the manufacturer, fomepizole has been used successfully and reported for pediatric poisonings (as young as 8 months).

**E. Use in pregnancy.** FDA category C (indeterminate). Has been used in pregnant patients without immediate adverse effects on the mother or fetus (see p 407).

**V. Drug or laboratory interactions**

**A.** Drugs or chemicals metabolized by alcohol dehydrogenase (eg, chloral hydrate, ethanol, isopropyl alcohol) will also have impaired elimination. Fomepizole and ethanol mutually inhibit each other's metabolism.

**B.** Drugs or chemicals metabolized by cytochrome P-450 enzymes may compete with fomepizole for elimination. Also, induction of P-450 activity by these drugs or by fomepizole may alter metabolism.

**VI. Dosage and method of administration.** ***Note:*** The interval between the initial dose and subsequent maintenance doses, 12 hours, provides an opportunity to confirm the diagnosis with laboratory testing.

**A. Initial dose.** Give a loading dose of 15 mg/kg (up to 1 g). Dilute in at least 100 mL of normal saline or 5% dextrose and infuse intravenously slowly over 30 minutes. (Oral administration may be considered for patients lacking IV access.) Patients > 100 kg may receive a loading dose of 1500 mg (one vial) to avoid wastage from opening a second vial of fomepizole. However, it is unknown if sufficient enzyme blockade will be achieved in all patients, and additional doses are recommended if there is evidence of a worsening acidosis. ***Note:*** The drug may solidify at room temperature and should be inspected visually prior to administration. If there is any evidence of solidification, hold the vial under a stream of warm water or roll between the hands.

**B. Maintenance therapy.** Give 10 mg/kg every 12 hours for four doses, then increase to 15 mg/kg (to offset increased metabolism resulting from autoinduction) until methanol or ethylene glycol serum levels are below 20 mg/dL.

**C. Adjustment for hemodialysis.** To offset loss of fomepizole during dialysis, increase the frequency of dosing to every 4 hours. (***Note:*** With newer high-flux hemodialysis equipment, fomepizole half-life averages 1.7 hours compared with 3 hours with standard dialysis.)

**VII. Formulations**

**A. Parenteral.** Fomepizole (Antizol, Jazz Pharmaceuticals): 1 g/mL in 1.5-mL vials, prepackaged in tray packs containing four vials.

**B.** The **suggested minimum stocking level** to treat a 70-kg adult for the first 24 hours is four vials. ***Note:*** Jazz Pharmaceuticals has announced that it will replace free of charge any expired vials of fomepizole if returned within 6 months of the expiration date.

# ▶ GLUCAGON

*Thomas E. Kearney, PharmD*

I. **Pharmacology.** Glucagon is a polypeptide hormone that stimulates the formation of adenyl cyclase, which in turn increases the intracellular concentration of cyclic adenosine monophosphate (cAMP). This results in enhanced glycogenolysis and an elevated serum glucose concentration, vascular smooth-muscle relaxation, and positive inotropic, chronotropic, and dromotropic effects. These effects occur independently of beta-adrenergic stimulation (glucagon has a separate receptor on the myocardium). It may also increase arachidonic acid levels in cardiac tissue via an active metabolite, miniglucagon. Arachidonic acid improves cardiac contractility owing to its effects on calcium. Glucagon is destroyed in the GI tract and must be given parenterally. After intravenous administration, effects are seen within 1–2 minutes and persist for 10–20 minutes. The serum half-life is about 3–10 minutes. ***Note:*** Glucagon usually is not considered first-line therapy for hypoglycemia because of its slow onset of action and reliance on glycogen stores. Instead, use glucose (see p 457) if it is available.

II. **Indications**

A. Hypotension, bradycardia, or conduction impairment caused by beta-adrenergic blocker intoxication (see p 131). Also consider in patients with hypotension associated with anaphylactic or anaphylactoid reactions who may be on beta-adrenergic blocking agents.

B. Possibly effective for severe cardiac depression caused by intoxication with calcium antagonists, tricyclic antidepressants, quinidine, or other types Ia and Ic antiarrhythmic drugs. Because of the benign side-effect profile of glucagon, consider its early empiric use in any patient with myocardial depression (bradycardia, hypotension, or low cardiac output) who does not respond rapidly to usual measures.

C. To facilitate passage of obstructed gastric foreign bodies (eg, drug packets) through the pylorus into the intestine (based on a case report).

III. **Contraindications.** Known hypersensitivity to the drug (rare) or pheochromocytoma or insulinoma.

IV. **Adverse effects**

A. Hyperglycemia, hypokalemia.

B. Nausea and vomiting by delaying gastric emptying and hypotonicity. May affect GI decontamination (activated charcoal, whole-bowel irrigation).

C. **Use in pregnancy.** FDA category B. Fetal harm is extremely unlikely (see p 407).

V. **Drug or laboratory interactions.** Concurrent administration of epinephrine potentiates and prolongs the hyperglycemic and cardiovascular effects of glucagon. It is unknown if glucagon interferes with the effectiveness of insulin and glucose therapy for severe calcium antagonist poisoning. Note that glucagon stimulates endogenous insulin secretion.

VI. **Dosage and method of administration.** Give 3–10 mg IV (may also titrate with 0.05 mg/kg boluses or 3–5 mg given over 1–2 minutes and repeated every 3 minutes until response or a total of 10 mg), followed by 1–5 mg/h infusion (children, 0.15 mg/kg IV or titrate with 0.05 mg/kg every 3 minutes, followed by 0.05–0.1 mg/kg/h). Up to 10 mg/h infusions have been used for adults. For very large doses, consider using sterile water or $D_5W$ to reconstitute rather than the glycerine-containing diluent provided with the drug (eg, add 4 mg glucagon to 50 mL $D_5W$ for continuous infusion). Note that the optimal duration of therapy is not known and that tachyphylaxis may occur with prolonged infusions (case report with infusion duration > 24 hours).

VII. **Formulations.** ***Note:*** Glucagon is no longer available in 10-mg vials; instead, the 1-mg kits must be used at a considerably higher cost to attain adequate dosing for the management of poisonings.

A. **Parenteral.** Glucagon Emergency (or Diagnostic) Kit, 1 unit (approximately 1 mg, with 1-mL syringe diluent with glycerine), and GlucaGen (Glucagon Hydrochloride) Diagnostic Kit (1 mg with 1 mL sterile water for diluent).

B. The **suggested minimum stocking level** to treat a 70-kg adult for the first 24 hours is 100 mg (100 kits, 1 unit each).

## ► GLUCOSE

*Thomas E. Kearney, PharmD*

I. **Pharmacology.** Glucose is an essential carbohydrate that is used as a substrate for energy production within the body. Although many organs use fatty acids as an alternative energy source, the brain is totally dependent on glucose as its major energy source; thus, hypoglycemia may cause serious brain injury rapidly. Dextrose administered with insulin shifts potassium intracellularly and maintains euglycemia for treatment of calcium antagonist poisoning (hyperinsulinemia-euglycemia [HIE] therapy).

II. **Indications**

A. Hypoglycemia.

B. Empiric therapy for patients with stupor, coma, or seizures who may have unsuspected hypoglycemia.

C. Used with an insulin infusion for severe calcium antagonist poisoning (see p 143), beta-blocker poisoning (see p 131), and hyperkalemia (p 37).

III. **Contraindications.** No absolute contraindications for empiric treatment of comatose patients with possible hypoglycemia. However, hyperglycemia and (possibly) recent ischemic brain injury may be aggravated by excessive glucose administration.

IV. **Adverse effects**

A. Hyperglycemia and serum hyperosmolality.

B. Local phlebitis and cellulitis after extravasation (occurs with concentrations ≥10%) from the intravenous injection site.

C. Administration of a large glucose load may precipitate acute Wernicke-Korsakoff syndrome in thiamine-depleted patients. For this reason, thiamine (see p 513) is given routinely along with glucose to alcoholic or malnourished patients.

D. Administration of large volumes of sodium-free dextrose solutions may contribute to fluid overload, hyponatremia, hypokalemia, and mild hypophosphatemia.

E. **Use in pregnancy.** FDA category C (indeterminate). This does not preclude its acute, short-term use for a seriously symptomatic patient (see p 407).

V. **Drug or laboratory interactions.** No known interactions.

VI. **Dosage and method of administration**

A. As empiric therapy for coma, give 50–100 mL of 50% dextrose (equivalent to 25–50 g glucose) slowly (eg, about 3 mL/min) via a secure intravenous line (children, 2–4 mL/kg of 25% dextrose; do ***not*** use 50% dextrose in children).

B. Persistent hypoglycemia (eg, resulting from poisoning by sulfonylurea agent) may require repeated boluses of 25% (for children) or 50% dextrose and infusion of 5–10% dextrose, titrated as needed. Consider the use of octreotide (see p 488) in such situations. Note that glucose can stimulate endogenous insulin secretion, which may exacerbate a hyperinsulinemia (resulting in wide fluctuations of blood glucose levels while treating sulfonylurea poisonings).

C. **Hyperinsulinemia-euglycemia** therapy usually requires an initial dextrose bolus (unless the patient's initial blood glucose is > 250 mg/dL) followed by a dextrose infusion at a rate of 0.5 g/kg/h using a 5% to 50% dextrose solution (if > 25% dextrose solution, administer via a central line) as needed to maintain euglycemia while infusing insulin (see p 461).

**VII. Formulations**

A. **Parenteral.** Dextrose (d-Glucose) injection, 50%, 50-mL ampules, vials, and prefilled injector; 25% dextrose, 10-mL syringes; various solutions of 2.5–70% dextrose, some in combination with saline or other crystalloids.

B. The **suggested minimum stocking level** to treat a 70-kg adult for the first 24 hours is four prefilled injectors (50% and 25%) and four bottles or bags (5% and 10%, 1 L each).

## ▶ HALOPERIDOL AND DROPERIDOL

*Thomas E. Kearney, PharmD*

I. **Pharmacology.** Haloperidol and droperidol are butyrophenone neuroleptic drugs that are useful for the management of acutely agitated psychotic patients and as antiemetics. They have strong central antidopaminergic activity and weak anticholinergic and anti–alpha-adrenergic effects. Haloperidol is well absorbed from the GI tract and by the intramuscular route. Droperidol is available only for parenteral use and is also well absorbed by the intramuscular route. Droperidol has a more predictable and rapid onset of 3–10 minutes, and both have peak pharmacologic effects that occur within 30–40 minutes of an intramuscular injection. Both drugs are metabolized principally by the liver. The serum half-life for haloperidol is 12–24 hours.

II. **Indications**

A. **Haloperidol** is used for the management of acute agitated functional psychosis or extreme agitation induced by stimulants or hallucinogenic drugs, especially when drug-induced agitation has not responded to a benzodiazepine.

B. **Droperidol** had been recognized to a have more rapid onset and greater efficacy than haloperidol (for agitation and psychosis as well as an antiemetic for drug- or toxin-induced nausea and vomiting). However, its role in routine therapy is uncertain because of reports of deaths and a new "black box" warning about QT prolongation (see IV.D, below). Therefore, other antiemetic drugs (eg, metoclopramide, see p 475, and ondansetron, see p 489) should be considered as first-line drugs to control persistent nausea and vomiting.

III. **Contraindications**

A. Severe CNS depression in the absence of airway and ventilatory control.

B. Severe parkinsonism.

C. Known hypersensitivity to haloperidol or droperidol.

D. Prolonged QTc interval (prior to droperidol administration, a 12-lead ECG is recommended).

IV. **Adverse effects**

A. Haloperidol and droperidol produce less sedation and less hypotension than chlorpromazine but are associated with a higher incidence of extrapyramidal side effects.

B. Rigidity, diaphoresis, and hyperpyrexia may be a manifestation of neuroleptic malignant syndrome (see p 21) induced by haloperidol, droperidol, and other neuroleptic agents.

C. Haloperidol lowers the seizure threshold and should be used with caution in patients with known seizure disorder or those who have ingested a convulsant drug.

D. Large doses of haloperidol can prolong the QT interval and cause torsade de pointes (see p 14). The FDA recently added a **black box warning** for droperidol that QT prolongation and torsade de pointes have occurred at or below recommended doses.

E. Both drugs may cause orthostatic hypotension and tachycardia.

F. Some oral haloperidol tablets contain tartrazine dye, which may precipitate allergic reactions in susceptible patients.

**G. Use in pregnancy.** FDA category C (indeterminate). These drugs are teratogenic and fetotoxic in animals and cross the placenta. Their safety in human pregnancy has not been established (see p 407).

**V. Drug or laboratory interactions**

**A.** Haloperidol and droperidol potentiate CNS–depressant effects of opioids, antidepressants, phenothiazines, ethanol, barbiturates, and other sedatives.

**B.** Combined therapy with lithium may increase the risk of neuroleptic malignant syndrome (see p 21).

**VI. Dosage and method of administration**

**A. Oral.** Give 2–5 mg of haloperidol PO; repeat once if necessary; usual daily dose is 3–5 mg two to three times daily (children  3 years old, 0.05–0.15 mg/kg/day or 0.5 mg in two to three divided doses).

**B. Parenteral.** ***Caution:*** Monitor the QT interval continuously and treat torsade de pointes if it occurs (see p 14).

1. **Haloperidol.** Give 2–5 mg of haloperidol IM; may repeat once after 20–30 minutes and hourly if necessary (children  3 years old, same as orally). Haloperidol is not approved for intravenous use in the United States, but that route has been used widely and is apparently safe (except the decanoate salt formulation, which is a depo product for monthly deep IM injections only).
2. **Droperidol.** Usual adult dose for delirium is 5 mg IM, and sedative dose is 2.5–5.0 mg IM (initial maximum dose of 2.5 mg with additional 1.25-mg doses titrated to desired effect). For antiemetic effects, usually given 30–60 minutes as a premedication, 2.5–10 mg (children 0.088–0.165 mg/kg) slowly IV or IM. Note: See warnings above; use alternative antiemetics as first-line therapy.

**VII. Formulations**

**A. Haloperidol**

1. **Oral.** Haloperidol (Haldol), 0.5-, 1-, 2-, 5-, 10-, and 20-mg tablets, 2-mg (as lactate)/mL concentrate in 15 and 120 mL, and 5- and 10-mL unit dose.
2. **Parenteral.** Haloperidol (Haldol), 5 (as lactate) mg/mL, 1-mL ampules, syringes, and vials, and 2-, 2.5-, and 10-mL vials.

**B. Droperidol** (Inapsine, others), 2.5 mg/mL, 1- and 2-mL ampules or vials.

**C.** The **suggested minimum stocking level** to treat a 70-kg adult for the first 24 hours is two vials of haloperidol (5 mg/mL, 10 mL each) and three vials of droperidol (2.5 mg/mL, 2 mL each).

## ▶ HYDROXOCOBALAMIN

*Kathryn H. Meier, PharmD*

**I. Pharmacology.** Hydroxocobalamin and cyanocobalamin are synthetic forms of vitamin B12 that are used for the treatment of pernicious anemia. Hydroxocobalamin has been recognized as an antidote for cyanide poisoning for over 45 years. Hydroxocobalamin immediately exchanges its hydroxyl group with free cyanide in the plasma to produce the nontoxic cyanocobalamin. When administered to patients with cyanide poisoning, it rapidly improves heart rate, systolic blood pressure, and acidemia. Well-designed animal studies suggest enhanced antidotal efficacy when hydroxocobalamin is used with thiosulfate (see p 514). In normal individuals, hydroxocobalamin has a plasma half-life of 3–20 hours. In patients with cyanide poisoning, the half-life is 14–24 hours, and the complexed compound, cyanocobalamin, has a half-life of 6–12 hours. Oral absorption is extremely poor; intranasal absorption occurs with very small doses.

**II. Indications**

**A.** Treatment of acute cyanide poisoning or patients suspected to be at high risk for cyanide poisoning (eg, smoke inhalation victims). ***Note:*** See VII, p 460.

B. Prophylaxis against cyanide poisoning during nitroprusside infusion.

III. **Contraindications.** Do not use in patients with a known hypersensitivity to this drug.

IV. **Adverse effects**

A. After antidotal doses, body fluids become pink or red after hydroxocobalamin administration; this subsides within 2–7 days.

B. Nausea, vomiting, hypertension, and mild muscle twitching or spasms have been reported occasionally.

C. Allergic reactions have not been reported with acute intravenous therapy for cyanide poisoning. However, allergic reactions have been reported when it has been used for chronic IM therapy.

D. **Use in pregnancy.** No assigned FDA category; no reported experience with use during pregnancy is available. This does not preclude its acute, short-term use for a seriously symptomatic patient (see p 407), and it is probably preferable to nitrite administration for cyanide poisoning.

V. **Drug or laboratory interactions.** Coloration of the serum sample can interfere with the following laboratory tests: falsely decreased aspartate aminotransferase (AST) and creatinine and falsely increased magnesium and bilirubin. Consider sampling for these prior to hydroxocobalamin administration.

VI. **Dosage and method of administration.** ***Note:*** Not available in the United States in a form sufficiently concentrated to provide an adequate dose for cyanide poisoning.

A. **Acute cyanide poisoning.** Give 5 g (children 70 mg/kg) by IV infusion over 30 minutes; 5 g of hydroxocobalamin will neutralize approximately 40 mcmol/L (1.04 mg/L) of cyanide in blood. Doses up to 20 g have been used. Based on animal studies, administration of hydroxocobalamin with thiosulfate (see p 514) may improve outcome.

B. **Prophylaxis during nitroprusside infusion.** Administer 25 mg/h IV. ***Note:*** Low-strength (1 mg/mL) injection products in the United States may contain the preservative parabens. Unknown safety if a parabens-containing product is used.

VII. **Formulations**

A. **Parenteral (United States).** Hydroxocobalamin, 1 mg/mL IM; 10- and 30-mL vials (may contain parabens). The United States does not have a formulation practical for treating acute cyanide poisoning at this time. EMD Pharmaceuticals, Durham, NC, currently has licensing and is developing Cyanokit for the US market.

B. **Parenteral (non-United States).** Cyanokit contains two of the following: 2.5-g vial of freeze-dried hydroxocobalamin, 100-mL vials of sterile 0.9% sodium chloride, and a transfer device. Designed for potential field use. Available in Europe from Merck.

C. The **suggested minimum stocking level (outside the United States)** to treat a 70-kg adult for acute cyanide poisoning is three Cyanokits (equivalent to 15 g). Note that fires often involve several victims and would require multiple kits.

## ▶ INAMRINONE (FORMERLY AMRINONE)

*F. Lee Cantrell, PharmD*

I. **Pharmacology.** Inamrinone is a positive inotropic agent with vasodilator activity. It is not a beta-adrenergic receptor agonist, and its exact mechanism of action is unknown. It appears to work by inhibiting myocardial cell phosphodiesterase activity, thereby increasing cellular concentrations of cyclic AMP. Cardiac afterload and preload are reduced owing to a direct vasodilator effect.

II. **Indications.** Inamrinone may be useful as a third-line inotropic agent for patients with beta-blocker, mixed beta- and alpha-blocker (eg, labetalol), or calcium antagonist overdose when intravenous fluids, atropine, beta agonists, and glucagon have failed to restore cardiac output and blood pressure.

**III. Contraindications.** Known hypersensitivity to inamrinone or sulfites (used as a preservative).

**IV. Adverse effects**

**A.** Hypotension may result from direct vasodilator effects, especially in patients who are volume depleted. Give adequate intravenous fluids prior to and with inamrinone administration.

**B.** The formulation contains sodium metabisulfite as a preservative, which can cause acute allergic-like reactions in patients (especially asthmatics) who are sensitive to sulfites.

**C.** Inamrinone may aggravate outflow obstruction in patients with hypertrophic subaortic stenosis.

**D.** Inamrinone affects platelet survival time, resulting in a dose- and time-dependent thrombocytopenia.

**E. Use in pregnancy.** FDA category C (indeterminate). Animal studies are conflicting, and there are no good human data (see p 407). Use only if the benefit justifies the potential risk (eg, a severe beta-blocker or calcium antagonist overdose unresponsive to other measures).

**F.** Name changed from amrinone to inamrinone to prevent confusion with amiodarone.

**V. Drug or laboratory interactions.** The positive inotropic effects of inamrinone are additive with other inotropic agents, including digitalis glycosides. These drugs can be used together, but the patient should be monitored for cardiac dysrhythmias.

**VI. Dosage and method of administration**

**A.** The initial dose is 0.75 mg/kg as a bolus over 2–3 minutes. This is followed by an infusion at 5–10 mcg/kg/min.

**B.** The manufacturer recommends that the total daily dose not exceed 10 mg/kg. However, up to 18 mg/kg/day has been given to some patients.

**VII. Formulations**

**A.** Inamrinone lactate: 5 mg/mL in 20-mL ampules containing 0.25 mg/mL sodium metabisulfite as a preservative.

**B. Suggested minimum stocking level** to treat a 70-kg adult for the first 24 hours is 10 ampules.

## ▶ INSULIN

*Kathleen Birnbaum, PharmD*

**I. Pharmacology**

**A.** Insulin, a hormone secreted by the beta cells of the pancreas, promotes cellular uptake of glucose into skeletal and cardiac muscles and adipose tissue. Insulin shifts potassium intracellularly.

**B.** The mechanism by which insulin-dextrose (hyperinsulinemia-euglycemia) therapy improves inotropy and increases peripheral vascular resistance is not known. Calcium antagonists inhibit insulin secretion by blocking the L-type calcium channels of pancreatic islet cells and induce insulin resistance. Insulin may reverse the hyperglycemia, hypoinsulinemia, and acidosis commonly observed in calcium antagonist poisoning. In calcium antagonist and beta-adrenergic blocker overdose, myocardial metabolism shifts from free fatty acid to carbohydrate metabolism. Insulin stimulates myocardial metabolism and inhibits free fatty acid metabolism. Insulin may also improve glucose uptake by cardiac myocytes.

**C.** Human regular insulin is biosynthetically prepared using recombinant DNA technology. The onset of action to decrease blood glucose for regular insulin is 30 minutes to 1 hour, and the duration of action is 5–8 hours. The serum half-life of regular insulin is 4–5 minutes after IV administration.

**II. Indications**

**A.** Hyperglycemia and diabetic ketoacidosis.

**B.** Severe hyperkalemia (p 37).

**C.** Administered with dextrose for hypotension induced by calcium antagonists (p 143) and beta-adrenergic blockers (p 131). Improved hemodynamics has been reported in a small number of patients with calcium antagonist toxicity. Insulin-dextrose treatment can improve cardiovascular function after beta-adrenergic overdose in animals, but its use has not been reported in humans with beta-adrenergic toxicity.

**III. Contraindications.** Known hypersensitivity to the drug (less frequent with human insulin than with animal-derived insulin).

**IV. Adverse effects**

**A.** Hypoglycemia.

**B.** Hypokalemia.

**C.** Lipohypertrophy or lipoatrophy at injection site (more common with repeated use).

**D. Use in pregnancy.** FDA category B (see p 407). Human insulin does not cross the placental barrier.

**V. Drug or laboratory interactions.**

**A.** Hypoglycemia may be potentiated by ethanol, sulfonylureas, and salicylates.

**B.** Corticosteroids (by decreasing peripheral insulin resistance and promoting gluconeogenesis), glucagon (by enhanced glycogenolysis), and epinephrine (via beta-adrenergic effects) may antagonize the effects of insulin.

**VI. Dosage and method of administration**

**A. Hyperglycemia.** Administer regular insulin 5–10 U IV initially, followed by infusion of 5–10 U/h, while monitoring the effect on serum glucose levels (children: 0.1 U/kg initially and then 0.1 U/kg/h).

**B. Hyperkalemia.** Administer regular insulin 0.1 U/kg IV with 50 mL of 50% dextrose (children: 0.1 U/kg insulin with 2 mL/kg of 25% dextrose).

**C. Hypotension** from calcium antagonists and beta-adrenergic blockers unresponsive to conventional therapy (**hyperinsulinemia-euglycemia therapy**):

1. **Bolus** of regular human insulin 1 U/kg IV. If blood glucose < 200 mg/dL, give 50 mL (25 g) of 50% dextrose IV (children: 0.25 g/kg of 25% dextrose).
2. **Continuous infusion.** Dilute 500 U of regular human insulin in 500 mL 0.9% saline (1 U/mL insulin concentration). Follow bolus with 0.5–1 U/kg/h insulin infusion titrated to blood pressure ≥ 100 mm Hg systolic. Begin 10% dextrose infusion and administer dextrose boluses as needed to maintain glucose between 100–200 mg/dL.
3. **Monitoring.** Measure blood glucose at least every 15–30 minutes for the first 4 hours until blood glucose is maintained at 100–200 mg/dL for 4 hours, then every hour. Monitor blood glucose hourly for several hours after the insulin infusion is discontinued since reactive hypoglycemia may occur. Monitor potassium hourly initially and then at least every 4 to 6 hours. Replete potassium as needed to maintain potassium > 2.5 mEq/dL. Magnesium and phosphorus levels may also fluctuate.
4. **Onset of Effect**. Hemodynamic improvement may not occur for more than 30 minutes. Increase insulin infusion after 30–60 minutes if no improvement in blood pressure occurs.
5. **Duration of Therapy**. Duration of insulin-dextrose treatment has varied from a single insulin bolus to infusions lasting 6 hours to 4 days. Average insulin infusion duration is 24–31 hours.
6. ***Note:*** Optimal insulin dosage is not known. An inadvertent bolus of 10 U/kg was administered without adverse effects. Infusions have ranged from 0.1 U/kg/h to 2 U/kg/h.

VII. **Formulations**

A. **Parenteral.** Human regular insulin (Humulin R, Novulin R), 100 U/mL, 10-mL vials. Only human regular insulin can be administered intravenously.

B. The **suggested minimum stocking level** to treat a 70-kg adult for the first 24 hours is two 10-mL vials.

## ▶ IODIDE (POTASSIUM IODIDE, KI)

*Freda Rowley, PharmD*

I. **Pharmacology.** Iodine-131 is a product of fission reactions and is likely to be a major form of internal radioactive contamination after a major nuclear reactor accident or weapon detonation. Potassium iodide (KI) blocks thyroid gland uptake of the radioactive isotopes of iodine (to prevent thyroid cancer) by both diluting the radioactive iodine and "filling" the gland with nontoxic iodine. For optimal protection, KI should be administered before or at the time of exposure to inhaled radioactive iodines but will have protective effects if initiated up to 3 or 4 hours after exposure. If the exposure to radioactive iodines persists, daily administration is indicated.

II. **Indications.** Potassium iodide is indicated for prevention of uptake of radioactive isotopes of iodine by the thyroid gland; therefore, when a public health emergency has occurred in which sufficient exposure to radioactive iodine is likely, potassium iodide is indicated. ***Note:*** KI should be used only when and if directed by federal, state, or local public health officials.

III. **Contraindications**

A. Known iodine allergy. Persons with the rare disorder of dermatitis herpetiformis and hypocomplementemic vasculitis are at increased risk of sensitivity.

B. Iodine may be used in pregnancy and in infants and children, but safety has not been established clearly (see IV, below).

IV. **Adverse effects**

A. GI upset, diarrhea, burning of throat, metallic taste in mouth, and, rarely, sialoadenitis (inflammation of the salivary glands). These effects become more common as duration of therapy and dosing increase.

B. Allergic reactions ranging from skin rashes to respiratory distress may occur, though life-threatening reactions are very uncommon.

C. Iodine-induced thyrotoxicosis, hypothyroidism, and goiter may occur, but incidence is probably less than 2% even if therapy is used for a longer duration.

D. A bluish skin discoloration involving sweat glands may occur after large doses of iodine-containing products.

E. **Use in pregnancy.** FDA category D (see p 407). Crosses the placental barrier and may cause hypothyroidism and goiter in the fetus. Risk is minimal with short-term use (eg, 10 days) and when given long periods before term.

F. **Use in Neonates**. Because of the increased risk of hypothyroidism in neonates (< 1 month old), thyroid function tests should be monitored.

V. **Drug or laboratory interactions**

A. Synergistic hypothyroid activity with lithium.

B. TSH and free $T_4$ monitoring of thyroid function is reliable in the setting of standard dosing of potassium iodide. Recommended in all neonates treated with KI.

C. Risk of hyperkalemia with prolonged use along with other potassium supplements and potassium-sparing medications (eg, spironolactone). However, the daily dose of potassium from KI is only about 3–4 mEq.

VI. **Dosage and method of administration**

A. There are various dosing guidelines, including those recommended by the US Food and Drug Administration and the World Health Organization (WHO). Public health officials should decide on the regimen they will use in a specific situation. See http://www.fda.gov/cder/guidance/5386fnl.htm for a guidance document from the FDA's Center for Drug Evaluation and Research.

**B.** Generally for adults > 18 years, 130 mg orally every day is recommended. Oral daily doses for other ages: adolescents and children (from 3–18 years), 65 mg; 1 month–3 years, 32 mg; 0–1 month, 16 mg. Children who are adult size (approaching 150 pounds) should be given an adult dose of 130 mg.

**C.** Duration of therapy may be from 1 day to many weeks, depending on public health recommendations.

**VII. Formulations**

**A. Oral** (Thyro-Block, others). Scored tablets (130 mg and 65 mg) of potassium iodide. Formulations of potassium iodide syrups (325 mg KI/5 mL) and oral solutions such as Lugol's solution (5% iodine and 10% KI) may be found.

**B.** Potassium iodide solution can be made from crushed KI tablets for use in children and adults unable to swallow tablets. Prepare with a 130-mg tablet (or two 65-mg tablets) crushed and mixed with 4 teaspoons (20 mL) of water until dissolved, then 4 teaspoons (20 mL) of chocolate milk, orange juice, soda, or baby formula. This results in a 130 mg per 8 teaspoonfuls (40 mL) solution. Plain water or low-fat milk may not adequately mask the salty, unpleasant taste of KI tablets. The solution will keep up to 7 days in the refrigerator. The FDA recommends that the solution be prepared weekly and the unused portion discarded. (Reference: FDA's Center for Drug Evaluation and Research Home Preparation Procedure for Emergency Administration of Potassium Iodide Tablets to Infants and Small Children: http://ww.fda.gov/cder/drugprepare/kiprep.htm).

**C.** The **suggested minimum stocking level** to treat a 70-kg adult for the first 24 hours is one 130-mg tablet.

## ▶ IPECAC SYRUP

*Jon Lorett, PharmD*

**I. Pharmacology.** Ipecac syrup is a mixture of plant-derived alkaloids, principally emetine and cephaeline, that produce emesis by direct irritation of the stomach and stimulation of the central chemoreceptor trigger zone. Vomiting occurs in 90% of these patients, usually within 20–30 minutes. Depending on the time after ingestion of the toxin, ipecac-induced emesis removes 15–50% of the stomach contents. There is no evidence that the use of ipecac improves the clinical outcome in poisoned patients, and it should not be administered routinely in their management.

**II. Indications.** For a more complete discussion of gastric decontamination, see p 47.

**A.** The use of ipecac syrup may be beneficial in rare situations in which there is substantial risk of serious toxicity, no existing or likely risk of a contraindication to its use, no alternative therapy available for gastric decontamination, and an expected delay of more than 1 hour for medical care in a heath-care facility. It should not be administered if it will adversely affect a more definitive treatment that might be provided in a hospital setting.

**B.** In health-care facilities, the use of ipecac may delay the administration or reduce the effectiveness of activated charcoal, oral antidotes, and whole-bowel irrigation. Thus, its routine administration in the emergency department has been abandoned.

**III. Contraindications**

**A.** Comatose or obtunded mental state.

**B.** Ingestion of a caustic or corrosive substance or sharp object.

**C.** Ingestion of petroleum distillates or hydrocarbons (see p 219).

**D.** Ingestion of a drug or toxin likely to result in abrupt onset of seizures or coma (eg, tricyclic antidepressants, strychnine, camphor, nicotine, cocaine, amphetamines, isoniazid).

**E.** Severe hypertension.

**F.** Patients at high risk for hemorrhagic diathesis (eg, coagulopathy or esophageal varices).

**IV. Adverse effects**

- **A.** Persistent GI upset after emesis may significantly delay administration of activated charcoal or other oral antidotes.
- **B.** Severe and repeated vomiting may cause esophageal (Mallory-Weiss) tears, pneumomediastinum, hemorrhagic gastritis, or intracranial hemorrhage.
- **C.** Vomiting may stimulate the vagal reflex, resulting in bradycardia or atrioventricular block.
- **D.** Drowsiness occurs in about 20% and diarrhea in 25% of children.
- **E.** Single ingestions of therapeutic doses of ipecac syrup are not toxic (the formerly used fluid extract was more potent), and failure to induce vomiting does not require removal of the ipecac. However, **chronic repeated ingestion** of ipecac (eg, in patients with bulimia) may result in accumulation of cardiotoxic alkaloids and lead to fatal cardiomyopathy and arrhythmias.
- **F. Use in pregnancy.** FDA category C (indeterminate) (see p 407). There is minimal systemic absorption, but it may induce uterine contractions in late pregnancy.

**V. Drug or laboratory interactions**

- **A.** Ipecac syrup potentiates nausea and vomiting associated with the ingestion of other gastric irritants.
- **B.** Ipecac syrup is adsorbed in vitro by activated charcoal; however, ipecac still produces vomiting when given concurrently with charcoal.
- **C.** Ipecac syrup contains 1.5–2% ethanol, which may cause an adverse reaction in patients taking disulfiram (see p 184) or other agents that have disulfiram-like effects (eg, metronidazole and *Coprinus* mushrooms).

**VI. Dosage and method of administration**

- **A. Children 6–12 months old.** Give 5–10 mL. ***Note:*** Not recommended for non–health-care facility use in this age group.
- **B. Children 1–12 years old.** Give 15 mL.
- **C. Adults and children over 12 years old.** Give 30 mL.
- **D.** Follow ipecac administration with 4–8 oz of water or clear liquid. If emesis does not occur within 30 minutes, repeat the dose of ipecac and fluid.

**VII. Formulations**

- **A.** Ipecac syrup, 30 mL.
- **B.** With the availability of more effective means of gastric decontamination and a lack of evidence that ipecac improves clinical outcome, there is no need to stock ipecac in the hospital setting.

# ► ISOPROTERENOL

*Thomas E. Kearney, PharmD*

**I. Pharmacology.** Isoproterenol is a catecholamine-like drug that stimulates beta-adrenergic receptors (beta-1 and -2). Its pharmacologic properties include positive inotropic and chronotropic cardiac effects, peripheral vasodilation, and bronchodilation. Isoproterenol is not absorbed orally and shows variable and erratic absorption from sublingual and rectal sites. The effects of the drug are terminated rapidly by tissue uptake and metabolism; effects persist only a few minutes after intravenous injection.

**II. Indications**

- **A.** Severe bradycardia or conduction block resulting in hemodynamically significant hypotension (see p 15). ***Note:*** After beta-blocker overdose, even exceedingly high doses of isoproterenol may not overcome the pharmacologic blockade of beta receptors, and glucagon (see p 456) is the preferred agent.
- **B.** To increase heart rate and thereby abolish polymorphous ventricular tachycardia (torsade de pointes) associated with QT interval prolongation (see p 14).

**III. Contraindications**

- **A.** Do not use isoproterenol for ventricular fibrillation or ventricular tachycardia (other than torsade de pointes).
- **B.** Use with extreme caution in the presence of halogenated or aromatic hydrocarbon solvents or anesthetics or chloral hydrate.

**IV. Adverse effects**

- **A.** Increased myocardial oxygen demand may result in angina pectoris or acute myocardial infarction.
- **B.** Peripheral beta-2-adrenergic–mediated vasodilation may worsen hypotension.
- **C.** The drug may precipitate ventricular arrhythmias.
- **D.** Sulfite preservative in some parenteral preparations may cause hypersensitivity reactions.
- **E.** Hypokalemia may occur secondary to beta-2-adrenergic–mediated intracellular potassium shift.
- **F. Use in pregnancy.** FDA category C (indeterminate). This does not preclude its acute, short-term use for a seriously symptomatic patient (see p 407). However, it may cause fetal ischemia and also can reduce or stop uterine contractions.

**V. Drug or laboratory interactions**

- **A.** Additive beta-adrenergic stimulation occurs in the presence of other sympathomimetic drugs, theophylline, and glucagon.
- **B.** Administration in the presence of cyclopropane, halogenated anesthetics, or other halogenated or aromatic hydrocarbons may enhance the risk of ventricular arrhythmias because of sensitization of the myocardium to the arrhythmogenic effects of catecholamines.
- **C.** Digitalis-intoxicated patients are more prone to develop ventricular arrhythmias when isoproterenol is administered.
- **D.** Beta blockers may interfere with the action of isoproterenol by competitive blockade at beta-adrenergic receptors.

**VI. Dosage and method of administration**

- **A.** For intravenous infusion, use a solution containing 4 mcg/mL (dilute 5 mL of 1:5,000 solution in 250 mL $D_5W$), and begin with 0.5–1 mcg/min infusion (children, 0.1 mcg/kg/min) and increase as needed for desired effect or as tolerated (by monitoring for arrhythmias). For emergency treatment, the infusion rate may start at 5 mcg/min. The usual upper dosage is 20 mcg/min (1.5 mcg/kg/min in children), but as much as 200 mcg/min has been given in adults with propranolol overdose. Preparations will degrade (and turn dark) with exposure to light, air, or heat.
- **B.** For IV bolus, the usual adult dose is 20–60 mcg (1–3 mL of a 1:50,000 solution) and repeat bolus doses of 10–200 mcg. If a dilute solution is not available, make a solution of 1:50,000 (20 mcg/mL) by diluting 1 mL of the 1:5000 solution to a volume of 10 mL with normal saline or $D_5W$.

**VII. Formulations**

- **A. Parenteral.** Isoproterenol hydrochloride (Isuprel, others), 20 mcg/mL (1:50,000) in 10 mL with needle or 200 mcg/mL (1:5,000) in 1- and 5-mL amps and 5- and 10-mL vials, which all contain sodium bisulfite or sodium metabisulfite as a preservative.
- **B.** The **suggested minimum stocking level** to treat a 70-kg adult for the first 24 hours is 10 (10-mL) vials.

## ► LABETALOL

*Thomas E. Kearney, PharmD*

**I. Pharmacology.** Labetalol is a mixed alpha- and beta-adrenergic antagonist; after intravenous administration, the nonselective beta-antagonist properties are approximately sevenfold greater than the alpha-1 antagonist activity. Hemodynamic effects generally include decreases in heart rate, blood pressure, and systemic vascular resistance. Atrioventricular conduction velocity may be decreased. After intravenous injection, hypotensive effects are maximal within 10–15 minutes and persist for about 2–4 hours. The drug is eliminated by hepatic metabolism and has a half-life of 5–6 hours.

**II. Indications.** Labetalol may be used to treat hypertension accompanied by tachycardia associated with stimulant drug overdose (eg, cocaine or amphetamines). ***Note:*** Hypertension with bradycardia suggests excessive alpha-mediated vasoconstriction (see pp 17, 323); in this case, a pure alpha blocker such as phentolamine (p 495) is preferable, because the reversal of beta-2–mediated vasodilation may worsen hypertension. In addition, it may have an unpredictable effect on coronary vascular tone; other agents, such as nitroglycerin, may be preferable for stimulant-induced coronary vasoconstriction.

**III. Contraindications**

**A.** Asthma.

**B.** Congestive heart failure.

**C.** Atrioventricular block.

**IV. Adverse effects**

**A.** Paradoxic hypertension may result when labetalol is used in the presence of stimulant intoxicants that have strong mixed alpha- and beta-adrenergic agonist properties (eg, cocaine, amphetamines) owing to the relatively weak alpha-antagonist properties of labetalol compared with its beta-blocking ability. (This has been reported with propranolol but not with labetalol.)

**B.** Orthostatic hypotension and negative inotropic effects may occur.

**C.** Dyspnea and bronchospasm may result, particularly in asthmatics.

**D.** Nausea, abdominal pain, diarrhea, tremors, dizziness, and lethargy have been reported.

**E. Use in pregnancy.** FDA category C (indeterminate). This does not preclude its acute, short-term use for a seriously symptomatic patient (see p 407).

**V. Drug or laboratory interactions**

**A.** Additive blood pressure lowering with other antihypertensive agents, halothane, or nitroglycerin.

**B.** Cimetidine increases the oral bioavailability of labetalol.

**C.** Labetalol is incompatible with 5% sodium bicarbonate injection (forms a precipitate).

**D.** Labetalol may cause false-positive elevation of urinary catecholamine levels and can produce a false-positive test for amphetamines on urine drug screening.

**VI. Dosage and method of administration**

**A. Adult.** Give 20-mg slow (over 2 minutes) IV bolus initially; repeat with 40- to 80-mg doses at 10-minute intervals until blood pressure is controlled or a cumulative dose of 300 mg is achieved (most patients will respond to total doses of 50–200 mg). Alternatively, administer a constant infusion of 0.5–2 mg/min (adjust rate) until blood pressure is controlled or a 300-mg cumulative dose is reached. After this, give oral labetalol starting at 100 mg twice daily.

**B. Children older than 12 years.** Initial dose of 0.25 mg/kg is given intravenously over 2 minutes.

**VII. Formulations**

**A. Parenteral.** Labetalol hydrochloride (Normodyne, Trandate), 5 mg/mL, 20- and 40-mL multidose vials (with EDTA and parabens as preservative), and 4- and 8-mL prefilled syringes.

**B. Oral.** Labetalol hydrochloride (Normodyne, Trandate, others), 100-, 200-, and 300-mg tablets.

**C.** The **suggested minimum stocking level** to treat a 70-kg adult for the first 24 hours is two vials (5 mg/mL, 40 mL each).

# ▶ LEUCOVORIN CALCIUM

*Kathy Birnbaum, PharmD*

I. **Pharmacology.** Leucovorin (folinic acid or citrovorum factor) is a metabolically functional form of folic acid. Unlike folic acid, leucovorin does not require reduction by dihydrofolate reductase, and therefore it can participate directly in the one-carbon transfer reactions necessary for purine biosynthesis and cellular DNA and RNA production. In animal models of methanol intoxication, replacement of a deficiency of leucovorin and folic acid can reduce morbidity and mortality by catalyzing the oxidation of the highly toxic metabolite formic acid to nontoxic products. However, there is no evidence that administration of these agents in the absence of a deficiency is effective.

II. **Indications**

A. **Folic acid antagonists (eg, methotrexate, trimethoprim, and pyrimethamine).** ***Note:*** Leucovorin treatment is essential because cells are incapable of utilizing folic acid owing to inhibition of dihydrofolate reductase.

B. **Methanol poisoning.** Leucovorin is an alternative to folic acid.

III. **Contraindications.** No known contraindications.

IV. **Adverse effects**

A. Allergic reactions as a result of prior sensitization have been reported.

B. Hypercalcemia from the calcium salt may occur (limit infusion rate to 16 mL/min).

C. **Use in pregnancy.** FDA category C (indeterminate). This does not preclude its acute, short-term use in a seriously symptomatic patient (see p 407).

V. **Drug or laboratory interactions.** Leucovorin bypasses the antifolate effect of methotrexate.

VI. **Dosage and method of administration**

A. **Methotrexate poisoning. *Note:*** *Efficacy depends on early administration; the drug should be given within 1 hour of poisoning if possible.* Administer intravenously a dose equal to or greater than the dose of methotrexate. If the dose is large but unknown, administer 75 mg (children, 10 mg/m$^2$/dose) and then 12 mg every 6 hours for four doses. Serum methotrexate levels can be used to guide subsequent leucovorin therapy (Table III–9). Do not use oral therapy.

B. **Other folic acid antagonists.** Administer 5–15 mg/day IM, IV, or PO for 5–7 days.

C. **Methanol poisoning.** For adults and children, give 1 mg/kg (up to 50–70 mg) IV every 4 hours for one to two doses. Oral folic acid is given thereafter at the same dosage every 4–6 hours until resolution of symptoms and adequate elimination of methanol from the body (usually 2 days). Although leucovorin

**TABLE III–9. LEUCOVORIN DOSE DETERMINATION (AFTER THE FIRST 24 HOURS)**

| Methotrexate Concentration (mcmol/L) | Hours After Methotrexate Exposure | Leucovorin Dose[a] (Adults and Children) |
|---|---|---|
| 0.1–1 | 24 | 10–15 mg/m$^2$ every 6 hours for 12 doses |
| 1–5 | 24 | 50 mg/m$^2$ every 6 hours until the serum level is less than 0.1 mcmol/L |
| 5–10 | 24 | 100 mg/m$^2$ every 6 hours until the serum level is less than 0.1 mcmol/L |

Reference: Methotrexate Management, in Rumack BH et al (eds.); *Poisindex.* Denver, 1989.

[a]If serum creatinine increases by 50% in the first 24 hours after methotrexate, increase the dose frequency to every 3 hours until the methotrexate level is less than 5 mcmol/L

could be used safely for the entire course of treatment, it is no more effective than folic acid and its cost does not justify such prolonged use in place of folic acid.

**VII. Formulations**

A. **Parenteral.** Leucovorin calcium (Folinic Acid, Citrovorum Factor), 3- and 10-mg/mL vials; 50, 100, and 350 mg for reconstitution (use sterile water rather than the diluent provided, which contains benzyl alcohol).

B. **Oral.** Leucovorin calcium (various), 5-, 15-, and 25-mg tablets.

C. The **suggested minimum stocking level** to treat a 70-kg adult for the first 24 hours is two 100-mg vials or one 350-mg vial.

## ▶ LIDOCAINE

*Thomas E. Kearney, PharmD*

**I. Pharmacology**

A. Lidocaine is a local anesthetic and a type Ib antiarrhythmic agent. It inhibits fast sodium channels and depresses automaticity within the His-Purkinje system and the ventricles but has a variable effect and may shorten the effective refractory period and action potential duration. Conduction within ischemic myocardial areas is depressed, abolishing reentrant circuits. Unlike quinidine and related drugs, lidocaine exerts a minimal effect on the automaticity of the sinoatrial node and on conduction through the AV node and does not decrease myocardial contractility or blood pressure in usual doses. It also has rapid "on-off" binding to sodium channels (to allow reactivation of the channel) and competes with other sodium channel blockers (that are slow to release and block the channel throughout the cardiac cycle). This may account for its antiarrhythmic effect with poisonings from other sodium channel blockers (type 1a antiarrhythmics, tricyclic antidepressants).

B. The oral bioavailability of lidocaine is poor owing to extensive first-pass hepatic metabolism (although systemic poisoning is possible from ingestion). After intravenous administration of a single dose, the onset of action is within 60–90 seconds and the duration of effect is 10–20 minutes. The elimination half-life of lidocaine is approximately 1.5–2 hours; active metabolites have elimination half-lives of 2–10 hours. Lidocaine clearance declines with continuous infusions and may be attributable to its metabolite monoethylglycinexylidide (MEGX). Drug accumulation may occur in patients with congestive heart failure or liver or renal disease.

**II. Indications.** Lidocaine is used for the control of ventricular arrhythmias arising from poisoning by a variety of cardioactive drugs and toxins (eg, digoxin, cyclic antidepressants, stimulants, and theophylline). Patients with atrial arrhythmias usually do not respond to this drug.

**III. Contraindications**

A. The presence of nodal or ventricular rhythms in the setting of third-degree AV or intraventricular block. These are usually reflex escape rhythms that may provide lifesaving cardiac output, and abolishing them may result in asystole.

B. Hypersensitivity to lidocaine or other amide-type local anesthetics (rare).

**IV. Adverse effects**

A. Excessive doses produce dizziness, confusion, agitation, and seizures.

B. Conduction defects, bradycardia, and hypotension may occur with extremely high serum concentrations or in patients with underlying conduction disease.

C. **Use in pregnancy.** FDA category B. Fetal harm is extremely unlikely (see p 407).

**V. Drug or laboratory interactions**

A. Cimetidine and propranolol may decrease the hepatic clearance of lidocaine.

B. Lidocaine may produce additive effects with other local anesthetics. In severe cocaine intoxication, lidocaine theoretically may cause additive neuronal depression.

**VI. Dosage and method of administration (adults and children)**

**A.** Administer 1–1.5 mg/kg (usual adult dose 50–100 mg; children, 1 mg/kg) IV bolus at a rate of 25–50 mg/min, followed by infusion of 1–4 mg/min (20–50 mcg/kg/min) to maintain serum concentrations of 1.5–5 mg/L.

**B.** If significant ectopy persists after the initial bolus, repeat doses of 0.5 mg/kg IV can be given if needed at 10-minute intervals (to a maximum 300 mg or 3 mg/kg total dose; children may be given repeat 1 mg/kg doses every 5–10 minutes to a maximum of 5 mg/kg).

**C.** In patients with congestive heart failure or liver disease, use half the recommended maintenance infusion dose.

**VII. Formulations**

**A. Parenteral.** Lidocaine hydrochloride for cardiac arrhythmias (Xylocaine, others). Direct IV: 1% (10 mg/mL), 2% (20 mg/mL) in 5-mL ampules and prefilled syringes, and 5- to 50-mL vials; 4%, 10%, and 20% in 1- and 2-g single-dose vials or additive syringes for preparing intravenous infusions; 0.2% (in 500 and 1000 mL), 0.4% (in 250 and 500 mL), and 0.8% (in 250 and 500 mL) in $D_5W$ solutions prepared for infusions.

**B.** The **suggested minimum stocking level** to treat a 70-kg adult for the first 24 hours is 10 prefilled 100-mg syringes and six 1-g vials for infusions.

# ► MAGNESIUM

*R. David West, PharmD*

**I. Pharmacology**

**A.** Magnesium is the fourth most common cation in the body and is the second most abundant intracellular cation after potassium. Magnesium plays an essential role as an enzymatic cofactor in a number of biochemical pathways, including energy production from adenosine triphosphate (ATP).

**B.** Magnesium has a direct effect on the $Na^+,K^+$-ATPase pump in both cardiac and nerve tissues. Further, magnesium has some calcium-blocking activity and may indirectly antagonize digoxin at the myocardial $Na^+,K^+$-ATPase pump.

**C.** Magnesium modifies skeletal and smooth-muscle contractility. Infusions can cause vasodilation, hypotension, and bronchodilation. It can reduce or abolish seizures of toxemia.

**D.** Magnesium is primarily an intracellular ion, and only 1% is in the extracellular fluid. A low serum Mg level under 1.2 mg/dL may indicate a net body deficit of 5000 mg or more.

**E.** Hypomagnesemia can be associated with a number of acute or chronic disease processes (malabsorption, pancreatitis, diabetic ketoacidosis). It may result from chronic diuretic use or alcoholism. It is a potentially serious, life-threatening consequence of hydrofluoric acid poisoning.

**II. Indications**

**A.** Replacement therapy for patients with hypomagnesemia.

**B.** Torsade de pointes ventricular tachycardia (see p 14).

**C.** Other arrhythmias suspected to be related to hypomagnesemia. Magnesium may be helpful in selected patients with cardiac glycoside toxicity but is not a substitute for digoxin-specific Fab fragments.

**D.** Barium ingestions (see p 126). Magnesium sulfate can be used orally to convert soluble barium to insoluble, nonabsorbable barium sulfate if given early.

**III. Contraindications**

**A.** Magnesium should be administered cautiously in patients with renal impairment to avoid the potential for serious hypermagnesemia.

**B.** Heart block and bradycardia.

**IV. Adverse effects**

**A.** Flushing, sweating, hypothermia.

B. Depression of deep tendon reflexes, flaccid paralysis, respiratory paralysis.
C. Depression of cardiac function, hypotension, bradycardia, general circulatory collapse (in particular with rapid administration).
D. Gastrointestinal upset and diarrhea with oral administration.
E. **Use in pregnancy.** FDA category A. Magnesium sulfate is used commonly used as a agent for premature labor (see p 407).

V. **Drug or laboratory interactions**
A. General CNS depressants. Additive effects may occur when CNS depressants are combined with magnesium infusions.
B. Neuromuscular blocking agents. Concomitant administration of magnesium with neuromuscular blocking agents may enhance and prolong their effect. Dose adjustment may be needed to avoid prolonged respiratory depression.

VI. **Dosage and method of administration (adults and children)**
A. Magnesium can be given orally, IV, or by IM injection. When it is given parenterally, the IV route is preferred and the sulfate salt generally is used.
B. Magnesium dosing is highly empiric and is guided by both clinical response and the estimated total body deficit of Mg based on serum levels.
C. **Adults:** Give 1 g (8.12 mEq) every 6 hours IV for four doses. For severe hypomagnesemia, doses as high as 1 mEq/kg/24 h or 8–12 g/day in divided doses have been used. Magnesium sulfate can be diluted in $D_5W$ or NS 50–100 mL and infused over 5–60 minutes. **Children:** Give 25–50 mg/kg/dose IV for three to four doses. Maximum single dose should not exceed 2000 mg (16 mEq). Higher dosages of 100 mg/kg/dose IV have also been employed.
D. For treatment of life-threatening arrhythmias (ventricular tachycardia or fibrillation associated with hypomagnesemia) in adults, give 1–2 g (8–16 mEq) IV, which can be given over 1–2 minutes. It should be diluted to 20% or less and infused no faster than 1 g/min (see IV, above). It can also be administered as a loading dose of 1–2 g (8–16 mEq) IV diluted in 50–100 mL of $D_5W$ or NS and infused over 5 to 60 minutes. A common regimen for adults is 2 g IV over 20 minutes.
E. For soluble barium ingestions, magnesium sulfate can be given to form insoluble, poorly absorbed barium sulfate. Adults should receive 30 g orally or by lavage, and children 250 mg/kg. Magnesium sulfate should not be given IV in these cases.

VII. **Formulations.**
A. **Parenteral**. Magnesium sulfate vials, 50% (4.06 mEq/mL, 500 mg/mL) in volumes of 2 mL, 10 mL, 20 mL, and 50 mL where 2 mL is equivalent to 1 g or 8.12 mEq Also available in 10% (0.8 mEq/mL) and 12.5% (1 mEq/mL) in 20- and 50-mL ampules and vials as well as large-volume premix bags. Magnesium chloride injection is also available but is used less commonly.
B. **Oral.** A large number of oral dosage forms are available, formulated in both immediate and sustained-release formulations.
C. The **suggested minimum stocking level** to treat a 70-kg adult for the first 24 hours is at least 12 g of parenteral magnesium sulfate.

## ▶ MANNITOL

*Gary W. Everson, PharmD*

I. **Pharmacology**
A. Mannitol is an osmotically active solute diuretic. Mannitol inhibits water reabsorption at the loop of Henle and the proximal tubule. The increase in urine output usually is accompanied by an increase in solute excretion. In addition, mannitol transiently increases serum osmolality and decreases CSF pressure by creating an osmotic gradient between brain tissue and the vascular compartment. Water moves across this gradient into the blood vessels, lowering the CSF pressure and decreasing intracranial pressure.

   B. Mannitol may reverse the effects of ciguatoxin by inhibiting ciguatoxin-induced opening of sodium channels and reducing cellular excitability. Mannitol may also increase the dissociation of ciguatoxin from its binding sites on cell membranes.
   C. In the past, mannitol was used to induce "forced diuresis" for some poisonings (eg, phenobarbital, salicylate) to enhance their renal elimination, but it has been abandoned because of lack of efficacy and potential risks (cerebral and pulmonary edema).

II. **Indications**
   A. Proposed as a treatment for neurologic and neurosensory manifestations caused by ciguatera poisoning (see p 204).
   B. Possible adjunctive agent in treating severe vitamin A toxicity associated with increased intracranial pressure (pseudotumor cerebri).
   C. Sometimes used as an adjunct to fluid therapy for acute oliguria resulting from massive rhabdomyolysis (see p 26).

III. **Contraindications**
   A. Severe dehydration.
   B. Acute intracranial bleeding.
   C. Pulmonary edema.
   D. Anuria associated with severe renal disease.

IV. **Adverse effects**
   A. Mannitol may cause excessive expansion of intravascular space when administered in high concentrations at a rapid rate. This may result in congestive heart failure and pulmonary edema.
   B. Mannitol causes movement of intracellular water to the extracellular space and can produce both transient hyperosmolality and hyponatremia.
   C. Oligoanuric renal failure has occurred in patients receiving mannitol. Low-dose mannitol appears to result in renal vasodilating effects, whereas high doses (> 200 g/day) may produce renal vasoconstriction.
   D. **Use in pregnancy.** FDA category C (indeterminate). This does not preclude its acute, short-term use in a seriously symptomatic patient (see p 407).

V. **Drug or laboratory interactions.** No known interactions.

VI. **Dosage and method of administration**
   A. **Ciguatera poisoning.** Recommended dose is 1 g/kg administered IV over 30–45 minutes. Reportedly most effective when given within 1–2 days of exposure, but case reports describe alleged benefit up to 8 weeks after exposure. Ciguatera poisoning may be accompanied by dehydration that must be treated with intravenous fluids prior to the administration of mannitol.
   B. **Vitamin A–induced pseudotumor cerebri.** Give 0.25 g/kg up to 1 g/kg administered intravenously.

VII. **Formulations**
   A. **Parenteral.** Mannitol 10% (500 mL, 1000 mL); 15% (150 mL, 500 mL); 20% (250 mL, 500 mL); 25% (50-mL vials and syringes).
   B. The **suggested minimum stocking level** to treat a 70-kg adult for the first 24 hours is approximately 70 g (500 mL of 20% mannitol).

## ▶ METHOCARBAMOL

*Thomas E. Kearney, PharmD*

I. **Pharmacology.** Methocarbamol is a centrally acting muscle relaxant. It does not directly relax skeletal muscle and does not depress neuromuscular transmission or muscle excitability; muscle relaxation is probably related to its sedative effects. After intravenous administration, the onset of action is nearly immediate. Elimination occurs by hepatic metabolism, with a serum half-life of 0.9–2.2 hours.

**II. Indications**

A. Control of painful muscle spasm caused by black widow spider envenomation (see p 347). Methocarbamol should be used as an adjunct to other medications (eg, morphine, diazepam) that are considered more effective.

B. Management of muscle spasm caused by mild tetanus (see p 353) or strychnine (see p 350) poisoning.

**III. Contraindications**

A. Known hypersensitivity to the drug.

B. History of epilepsy (intravenous methocarbamol may precipitate seizures).

**IV. Adverse effects**

A. Dizziness, drowsiness, nausea, flushing, and metallic taste may occur.

B. Extravasation from an intravenous site may cause phlebitis and sloughing. Do not administer subcutaneously.

C. Hypotension, bradycardia, and syncope have occurred after intramuscular or intravenous administration. Keep the patient in a recumbent position for 10–15 minutes after injection.

D. Urticaria and anaphylactic reactions have been reported.

E. **Use in pregnancy.** There is no reported experience, and no FDA category has been assigned.

**V. Drug or laboratory interactions**

A. Methocarbamol produces additive sedation with alcohol and other CNS depressants.

B. Methocarbamol may cause false-positive urine 5-hydroxyindole acetic acid (5-HIAA) and vanillylmandelic acid (VMA) results.

C. The urine may turn brown, black, or blue after it stands.

**VI. Dosage and method of administration**

A. **Parenteral**

1. Administer 1 g (children, 15 mg/kg) IV over 5 minutes, followed by 0.5 g in 250 mL of 5% dextrose (children, 10 mg/kg in 5 mL of 5% dextrose) over 4 hours. Repeat every 6 hours to a maximum of 3 g daily.
2. For tetanus, higher doses are usually recommended. Give 1–2 g IV initially, no faster than 300 mg/min; if needed, use a continuous infusion up to a total of 3 g.
3. The usual intramuscular dose is 500 mg every 8 hours for adults and 10 mg/kg every 8 hours for children. Do not inject more than 5 mL into the gluteal region. Do not give subcutaneously.

B. **Oral.** Switch to oral administration as soon as tolerated. Give 0.5–1 g (children, 10–15 mg/kg) PO or by gastric tube every 6 hours. The maximum dose is 1.5 g every 6 hours; for tetanus, the maximum adult dose is 24 g/day.

**VII. Formulations**

A. **Parenteral.** Methocarbamol (Robaxin, others), 100 mg/mL in 10-mL vials.

B. **Oral.** Methocarbamol (Robaxin, others), 500- and 750-mg tablets.

C. The **suggested minimum stocking level** to treat a 70-kg adult for the first 24 hours is 24 vials (100 mg/mL, 10 mL each).

## ▶ METHYLENE BLUE

*Fabian Garza, PharmD*

**I. Pharmacology.**

A. Methylene blue is a thiazine dye that increases the conversion of methemoglobin to hemoglobin. Methylene blue is reduced via methemoglobin reductase and nicotinamide adenosine dinucleotide phosphate (NADPH) to leukomethylene blue, which in turn reduces methemoglobin. Glucose-6-phospate dehydrogenase is essential for generation of NADPH and is thus essential for the function of methylene blue as an antidote. Therapeutic effect is seen within 30 minutes. Methemoglobin is excreted in bile and urine, which may turn blue or green.

**B.** Methylene blue has been used to treat ifosfamide-induced encephalopathy, but the exact pathophysiologic mechanisms responsible are not known. Methylene blue may reverse the neurotoxic effects of the ifosfamide metabolites.

**II. Indications.**

**A.** Methylene blue is used to treat methemoglobinemia (see p 262), in which the patient has symptoms or signs of hypoxemia (eg, dyspnea, confusion, or chest pain) or has a methemoglobin level greater than 30%. ***Note:*** Methylene blue is not effective for sulfhemoglobinemia.

**B.** Methylene blue has been used to reverse and prevent ifosfamide-related encephalopathy.

**III. Contraindications**

**A.** G6PD deficiency. Treatment with methylene blue is ineffective and may cause hemolysis.

**B.** Severe renal failure.

**C.** Known hypersensitivity to methylene blue.

**D.** Methemoglobin reductase deficiency.

**E.** Reversal of nitrite-induced methemoglobinemia for treatment of cyanide poisoning.

**IV. Adverse effects**

**A.** Gastrointestinal upset, headache, and dizziness may occur.

**B.** Excessive doses of methylene blue (≥7 mg/kg) can actually cause methemoglobinemia by directly oxidizing hemoglobin. Doses greater than 15 mg/kg are associated with hemolysis, particularly in neonates. May also dye secretions and mucous membranes and interfere with clinical findings of cyanosis.

**C.** Long-term administration may result in marked anemia.

**D.** Extravasation may result in local tissue necrosis.

**E.** **Use in pregnancy.** FDA category C (indeterminate). This does not preclude its acute, short-term use for a seriously symptomatic patient (see p 407).

**V. Drug or laboratory interactions.**

**A.** No known drug interactions, but the intravenous preparation should not be mixed with other drugs.

**B.** Transient false-positive methemoglobin levels of about 15% are produced by dosages of 2 mg/kg of methylene blue. It may also alter pulse oximeter readings.

**VI. Dosage and method of administration (adults and children)**

**A. Methemoglobinemia**

1. Administer 1–2 mg/kg (0.1–0.2 mL/kg of 1% solution) IV slowly over 5 minutes. May be repeated in 30–60 minutes.
2. Simultaneous administration of dextrose may be warranted to provide adequate NAD and NADPH co-factors.
3. If no response after two doses, do not repeat dosing; consider G6PD deficiency or methemoglobin reductase deficiency.
4. Patients with continued production of methemoglobin from a long-acting oxidant stress (eg, dapsone) may require repeated dosing every 6–8 hours for 2–3 days.
5. Flush IV line with 15–30 mL of normal saline to reduce incidence of local pain.

**B. Ifosfamide encephalopathy**

1. *Prophylaxis:* Administer 50 mg PO or IV (slowly over 5 minutes) every 6 to 8 hours while receiving ifosfamide.
2. **Treatment:** Administer 50 mg IV (slowly over 5 minutes) every 4–6 hours until symptoms resolve.

**VII. Formulations**

**A.** **Parenteral.** Methylene blue injection 1% (10 mg/mL).

**B.** The **suggested minimum stocking level** to treat a 70-kg adult for the first 24 hours is five ampules (10 mg/mL, 10 mL each).

# ► METOCLOPRAMIDE

*Judith A. Alsop, PharmD*

I. **Pharmacology.** Metoclopramide is a dopamine antagonist with antiemetic activity at the chemoreceptor trigger zone. It also accelerates GI motility and facilitates gastric emptying. The onset of effect is 1–3 minutes after intravenous administration, and therapeutic effects persist for 1–2 hours after a single dose. The drug is excreted primarily by the kidney. The elimination half-life is about 5–6 hours but may be as long as 14.8 hours in patients with renal insufficiency and 15.4 hours in patients with cirrhosis.

II. **Indications**

A. Metoclopramide is used to prevent and control persistent nausea and vomiting, particularly when the ability to administer activated charcoal (eg, treatment of theophylline poisoning) or another oral antidotal therapy (eg, acetylcysteine for acetaminophen poisoning) is compromised.

B. Theoretical (unproved) use to stimulate bowel activity in patients with ileus who require repeat-dose activated charcoal or whole-bowel irrigation.

III. **Contraindications**

A. Known hypersensitivity to the drug; possible cross-sensitivity with procainamide.

B. Mechanical bowel obstruction or intestinal perforation.

C. Pheochromocytoma (metoclopramide may cause hypertensive crisis).

IV. **Adverse effects**

A. Sedation, restlessness, fatigue, and diarrhea may occur.

B. Extrapyramidal reactions may result, particularly with high-dose treatment. Pediatric patients appear to be more susceptible. These reactions may be prevented by pretreatment with diphenhydramine (see p 442).

C. May increase the frequency and severity of seizures in patients with seizure disorders.

D. Parenteral formulations that contain sulfite preservatives may precipitate bronchospasm in susceptible individuals.

E. **Use in pregnancy.** FDA category B. Not likely to cause harm when used as short-term therapy (see p 407).

V. **Drug or laboratory interactions**

A. Additive sedation in the presence of other CNS depressants.

B. Risk of extrapyramidal reactions may be increased in the presence of other dopamine antagonist agents (eg, haloperidol and phenothiazines).

C. In one study involving hypertensive patients, metoclopramide enhanced the release of catecholamines. As a result, the manufacturer advises cautious use in hypertensive patients and suggests that the drug should not be used in patients taking monoamine oxidase inhibitors.

D. Agitation, diaphoresis, and extrapyramidal movement disorder were reported in two patients taking selective serotonin reuptake inhibitors (sertraline, venlafaxine) who received IV metoclopramide.

E. The drug may enhance the absorption of ingested drugs by promoting gastric emptying.

F. Anticholinergic agents may inhibit bowel motility effects.

G. Numerous IV incompatibilities: calcium gluconate, sodium bicarbonate, cimetidine, furosemide, and many antibiotic agents (eg, ampicillin, chloramphenicol, erythromycin, penicillin G, potassium, tetracycline).

VI. **Dosage and method of administration**

A. **Low-dose therapy.** Effective for mild nausea and vomiting. Give 10–20 mg IM or slowly IV (children, 0.1 mg/kg/dose).

B. **High-dose therapy.** For control of severe or persistent vomiting. For adults and children, give 1–2 mg/kg IV infusion over 15 minutes in 50 mL dextrose or saline. May be repeated twice at 2- to 3-hour intervals.

1. Metoclopramide is most effective if given before emesis or 30 minutes before administration of a nausea-inducing drug (eg, acetylcysteine).

2. If no response to initial dose, may give additional 2 mg/kg and repeat every 2–3 hours up to maximum 12 mg/kg total dose.
3. Pretreatment with 50 mg (children, 1 mg/kg) of diphenhydramine (see p 442) helps prevent extrapyramidal reactions.
4. Reduce dose by one-half in patients with renal insufficiency.

**VII. Formulations**

A. **Parenteral.** Metoclopramide hydrochloride (Reglan, others), 5 mg/mL; 2-, 10-, 30-, 50-, and 100-mL vials. Also available in preservative-free 2-, 10-, and 30-mL vials and 2- and 10-mL ampules.

B. The **suggested minimum stocking level** to treat a 70-kg adult for the first 24 hours is 1000 mg (four vials, 50 mL each, or equivalent).

## ▶ MORPHINE

*Thomas E. Kearney, PharmD*

I. **Pharmacology.** Morphine is the principal alkaloid of opium and is a potent analgesic and sedative agent. In addition, it decreases venous tone and systemic vascular resistance, resulting in reduced preload and afterload. Morphine is absorbed variably from the GI tract and usually is used parenterally. After intravenous injection, peak analgesia is attained within 20 minutes and usually lasts 3–5 hours. Morphine is eliminated by hepatic metabolism, with a serum half-life of about 3 hours; however, the clearance of morphine is slowed and the duration of effect is prolonged in patients with renal failure resulting from accumulation of the active metabolite morphine-6-glucuronide.

**II. Indications**

A. Severe pain associated with black widow spider envenomation, rattlesnake envenomation, or other bites or stings.
B. Pain caused by corrosive injury to the eyes, skin, or GI tract.
C. Pulmonary edema resulting from congestive heart failure. Chemical-induced noncardiogenic pulmonary edema is ***not*** an indication for morphine therapy.

**III. Contraindications**

A. Known hypersensitivity to morphine.
B. Respiratory or CNS depression with impending respiratory failure unless the patient is already intubated or equipment and trained personnel are standing by for intervention if necessary with intubation or the reversal agent naloxone (see p 477).
C. Suspected head injury. Morphine may obscure or cause exaggerated CNS depression.

**IV. Adverse effects**

A. Respiratory and CNS depression may result in respiratory arrest. Depressant effects may be prolonged in patients with liver disease and chronic renal failure. Risk factors or co-morbidities for morphine-induced respiratory depression include naïve user lacking tolerance, hypothyroidism, morbid obesity, and sleep apnea syndrome. Note that tidal volume may be depressed without perceptible changes in respiratory rate and that these effects are influenced by external stimuli (eg, noise, manipulation).
B. Hypotension may occur owing to decreased systemic vascular resistance and venous tone.
C. Nausea, vomiting, and constipation may occur.
D. Bradycardia, wheezing, flushing, pruritus, urticaria, and other histamine-like effects may occur.
E. Sulfite preservative in some parenteral preparations may cause hypersensitivity reactions.
F. **Use in pregnancy.** FDA category C (indeterminate). This does not preclude its acute, short-term use in a seriously symptomatic patient (see p 407).

**V. Drug or laboratory interactions**

**A.** Additive depressant effects with other opioid agonists, ethanol and other sedative-hypnotic agents, tranquilizers, and antidepressants.

**B.** Morphine is physically incompatible with solutions containing a variety of drugs, including aminophylline, phenytoin, phenobarbital, and sodium bicarbonate.

**VI. Dosage and method of administration**

**A.** Morphine may be injected subcutaneously, intramuscularly, or intravenously. The oral and rectal routes produce erratic absorption and are not recommended for use in acutely ill patients.

**B.** The usual initial dose is 2–10 mg IV (may dilute with 4-5 mL sterile water and give slowly over 4–5 minutes as well as titrate in small increments, 1–4 mg, every 5 minutes) or 10–15 mg SC or IM, with maintenance analgesic doses of 5–20 mg every 4 hours. The pediatric dose is 0.1–0.2 mg/kg every 4 hours. Note that the dosage range may vary and risk factors for respiratory depression should be carefully considered. In particular, exercise caution in morbidly obese patients. Remember that peak analgesic (and toxic) effects may be delayed (by an average of 20 minutes for IV), and naloxone should be immediately accessible if respiratory depression occurs.

**VII. Formulations**

**A. Parenteral.** Morphine sulfate for injection; variety of available concentrations from 0.5 to 50 mg/mL. Note that some preparations contain sulfites as a preservative.

**B.** The **suggested minimum stocking level** to treat a 70-kg adult for the first 24 hours is 150 mg.

## ▶ NALOXONE AND NALMEFENE

*Terry Carlson, PharmD*

**I. Pharmacology.** Naloxone and nalmefene are pure opioid antagonists that competitively block mu, kappa, and delta opiate receptors within the CNS. They have no opioid agonist properties and can be given safely in large doses without producing respiratory or CNS depression. ***Naltrexone*** is another potent competitive opioid antagonist that is active orally and is used to prevent recidivism in patients detoxified from opioid abuse. It has also been used to reduce craving for alcohol. It is ***not*** used for the acute reversal of opioid intoxication and will not be discussed further in this handbook.

**A. Naloxone,** a synthetic *N*-allyl derivative of oxymorphone, undergoes extensive first-pass metabolism and is not effective orally but may be given subcutaneously, intramuscularly, intravenously, or even endotracheally. After intravenous administration, opioid antagonism occurs within 1–2 minutes and persists for approximately 1–4 hours. The plasma half-life ranges from 31–80 minutes.

**B. Nalmefene,** an injectable methylene analog of naltrexone, was approved in 1995. It is 4 times more potent than naloxone at mu receptors and slightly more potent at kappa receptors. It has a longer elimination half-life (ranging from approximately 8–11 hours after IV dosing) and a duration of action of 1–4 hours (see Table III–10). The prolonged effects of nalmefene are related to the slow dissociation from the opioid receptor, which is not reflected in the area under the curve (AUC) plasma curve.

**II. Indications**

**A.** Reversal of acute opioid intoxication manifested by coma, respiratory depression, or hypotension.

**B.** Empiric therapy for stupor or coma suspected to be caused by opioid overdose.

**TABLE III–10. CHARACTERISTICS OF NALOXONE AND NALMEFENE**

| | Naloxone | Nalmefene |
|---|---|---|
| **Elimination half-life** | 60–90 min | 10–13 h |
| **Duration of action** | 1 h | 1–4 h[a] |
| **Metabolism** | Liver (glucuronidation) | Liver (glucuronidation) |
| **Advantages** | Lower cost; shorter action; more human experience | Longer duration lowers risk of recurrent respiratory depression for most (but not all) opioids |
| **Disadvantages** | More frequent dosing or constant infusion | Cost; may cause prolonged opioid withdrawal |

[a]High doses (eg, > 6 mg) may increase the duration of action but are not recommended at this time.

**C.** Anecdotal reports suggest that high-dose naloxone may partially reverse the CNS and respiratory depression associated with clonidine (see p 168), ethanol (see p 189), benzodiazepine (see p 129), or valproic acid (see p 363) overdoses, although these effects are inconsistent.

**III. Contraindications.** Do not use in patients with a known hypersensitivity to either agent (may have cross-sensitivity).

**IV. Adverse effects.** Human studies have documented an excellent safety record for both drugs. Volunteers have received up to 24 mg of nalmefene intravenously and 50 mg orally.

**A.** Use in opiate-dependent patients may precipitate acute withdrawal syndrome. This may be more protracted with nalmefene. Neonates of addicted mothers may have more severe withdrawal symptoms, including seizures. Aggressive use of opiate antagonists in so-called rapid opioid detoxification (ROD) and ultra-rapid opioid detoxification (UROD) has been associated with marked increases in plasma corticotropin, cortisol, sympathetic activity, and catecholamine levels; pulmonary edema; acute renal failure; ventricular bigeminy; psychosis; delirium; and deaths.

**B.** Pulmonary edema or ventricular fibrillation occasionally has occurred shortly after naloxone administration in opioid-intoxicated patients. Pulmonary edema has also been associated with postanesthetic use of naloxone, especially when catecholamines and large fluid volumes have been administered. Pulmonary edema has been reported after IV nalmefene.

**C.** Reversing the sedative effects of an opioid may amplify the toxic effects of other drugs. For example, agitation, hypertension, and ventricular irritability have occurred after naloxone administration to persons high on a “speedball” (heroin plus cocaine or methamphetamine).

**D.** Seizures have been associated with nalmefene use in animal studies but have not been reported in humans.

**E.** There has been one case report of hypertension after naloxone administration in a patient with clonidine overdose.

**F. Use in pregnancy.** FDA category B (see p 407). Naloxone- or nalmefene-induced drug withdrawal syndrome may precipitate labor in an opioid-dependent mother.

**V. Drug or laboratory interactions.** Naloxone and nalmefene antagonize the analgesic effect of opioids. Naloxone is not associated with a positive enzymatic urine screen for opiates. A 2-mg IV dose of nalmefene was not associated with a false-positive urine test (Emit II assay) in one study.

**VI. Dosage and method of administration for suspected opioid-induced coma**

**A. Naloxone.** Administer 0.4–2 mg IV; repeat at 2- to 3-minute intervals until desired response is achieved. Titrate carefully in opioid-dependent patients (start at 0.05 mg). The dose for children is the same as that for adults.

1. The total dose required to reverse the effects of the opioid is highly variable and is dependent on the concentration and receptor affinity of the opioid. Some drugs (eg, propoxyphene, diphenoxylate/atropine [Lomotil], buprenorphine, pentazocine, and the fentanyl derivatives) do not respond to usual doses of naloxone. However, if no response is achieved by a total dose of 10–15 mg, the diagnosis of opioid overdose should be questioned.
2. ***Caution:*** Resedation can occur when the naloxone wears off in 1–2 hours. Repeated doses of naloxone may be required to maintain reversal of the effects of opioids with prolonged elimination half-lives (eg, methadone) or sustained-release formulations or when packets or vials have been ingested.
3. **Infusion.** Give 0.4–0.8 mg/h in normal saline or 5% dextrose, titrated to clinical effect (in infants, start with 0.04–0.16 mg/kg/h). Another method is to estimate two-thirds of the initial dose needed to awaken the patient and give that amount each hour.

**B. Nalmefene.** In a non-opioid-dependent adult, give an initial dose of 0.5 mg/70 kg, followed by 1.0 mg/70 kg 2–5 minutes later. No added benefit of dosage higher than 1.5 mg/70 kg has been established. If opioid dependency is suspected, give a challenge dose of 0.1 mg/70 kg, followed by a 2-minute wait for signs or symptoms of opioid withdrawal (nausea, chills, myalgia, dysphoria, abdominal cramps, joint pain). If there is no indication of withdrawal, give standard doses. The effect of the drug may be prolonged in patients with end-stage renal failure or hepatic disease.

1. Dosage, safety, and efficacy in children have not been established. However, it has been shown to be safe and effective in reversing procedural sedation in children when given in postoperative incremental doses of 0.25 mcg/kg every 2–5 minutes to a maximum total dose of 1 mcg/kg. Nalmefene pharmacokinetics in children is similar to that in adults.
2. As with naloxone, the total dose required to reverse the effects of the opioid is highly variable.
3. ***Caution:*** The duration of action of nalmefene will vary with the half-life and concentration of the opioid being reversed, the presence of other sedating drugs, and the dose of nalmefene. Smaller doses of nalmefene may have a shorter duration because of rapid redistribution of the drug out of the brain. Fully reversing doses (1–1.5 mg in a 70-kg person) have been shown to last several hours. However, this may not be long enough for patients who have overdosed on a long-acting opioid such as methadone or have ingested a drug-containing condom or packet with unpredictable breakage and absorption.

**C.** ***Note:*** Although both drugs can be given by the intramuscular or subcutaneous route, absorption is erratic and incomplete. Naloxone is not effective orally. Huge doses of nalmefene have been used orally in experimental studies, but this route is not recommended at this time.

**VII. Formulations**

**A. Naloxone** hydrochloride (Narcan): 0.02, 0.4, or 1 mg/mL; 1-, 2-, or 10-mL syringes, ampules, or vials. The **suggested minimum stocking level** to treat a 70-kg adult for the first 24 hours is 30 mg (three vials, 1 mg/mL, 10 mL each, or equivalent).

**B. Nalmefene** hydrochloride (Revex): 100 mcg in 1-mL ampules (blue label); 1 mg/mL in 2-mL vials (green label); syringes containing 2 mL of 1 mg/mL nalmefene. The **suggested minimum stocking level** to treat a 70-kg adult for the first 24 hours is 16 mg (eight vials, 1 mg/mL, 2 mL each, or equivalent).

# ▶ NEUROMUSCULAR BLOCKERS

*Thomas E. Kearney, PharmD*

**I. Pharmacology**

**A.** Neuromuscular blocking agents produce skeletal muscle paralysis by inhibiting the action of acetylcholine at the neuromuscular junction. **Depolarizing agents** (eg, succinylcholine; Table III–11) depolarize the motor end plate and block recovery; transient muscle fasciculations occur with the initial depolarization. **Nondepolarizing agents** (atracurium, pancuronium, and others; Table III–11) are classified as either a benzylisoquinolinium diester (eg, mivacurium, atracurium) or an aminosteroid (eg, vecuronium, rocuronium) and competitively block the action of acetylcholine at the motor end plate; therefore, no initial muscle fasciculations occur. They also block acetylcholine at sympathetic ganglia, and this may result in hypotension.

**B.** The neuromuscular blockers produce complete muscle paralysis with no depression of CNS function (they are positively charged and water-soluble compounds that do not cross the brain-blood barrier rapidly). Thus, patients who are conscious will remain awake but unable to move and patients with status epilepticus may continue to have CNS seizure activity despite flaccid paralysis. Furthermore, the neuromuscular blockers do not relieve pain or anxiety.

**C.** Succinylcholine produces the most rapid onset of effects, with total paralysis within 30–60 seconds after intravenous administration. It is hydrolyzed rapidly by plasma cholinesterases, and its effects dissipate in 10–20 minutes. Rocuronium, a nondepolarizing agent, also offers a rapid onset for rapid-sequence intubations. Onset and duration of several other neuromuscular blockers are described in Table III–11.

**II. Indications**

**A.** Neuromuscular blockers are used to abolish excessive muscular activity, rigidity, or peripheral seizure activity when continued hyperactivity may produce or aggravate rhabdomyolysis and hyperthermia. Examples of such situations include the following. ***Note:*** The preferred agent for these conditions is a nondepolarizing agent.

1. Drug overdoses involving stimulants (eg, amphetamines, cocaine, phencyclidine, monoamine oxidase inhibitors) or strychnine.
2. Tetanus.
3. Hyperthermia associated with muscle rigidity or hyperactivity (eg, status epilepticus, neuroleptic malignant syndrome, or serotonin syndrome; see p 20). ***Note:*** Neuromuscular blockers are not effective for malignant hyperthermia (see p 21); in fact, inability to induce paralysis with these agents should suggest the diagnosis of malignant hyperthermia.

**B.** Neuromuscular blockers provide prompt flaccid paralysis to facilitate orotracheal intubation. The preferred agents for this purpose are rapid-onset agents such as succinylcholine, rapacurium, mivacurium, rocuronium, and vecuronium. They also are used to treat laryngospasm.

**III. Contraindications**

**A.** Lack of preparedness or inability to intubate the trachea and ventilate the patient after total paralysis ensues. Proper equipment and trained personnel must be assembled before the drug is given.

**B.** Known history of malignant hyperthermia. Succinylcholine use is associated with malignant hyperthermia in susceptible patients (incidence, approximately 1 in 50,000 in adults and 1 in 10,000 in children).

**C.** Known hypersensitivity or anaphylactic reaction (non-dose-related) to agent or preservative (eg, benzyl alcohol). Succinylcholine is implicated most commonly, but anaphylaxis has been reported with rocuronium, atracurium, mivacurium, and cisatracurium.

**D.** Known history of or at high risk for succinylcholine-induced hyperkalemia. (See IV.D. below.)

**TABLE III–11. SELECTED NEUROMUSCULAR BLOCKERS**

| Drug | Onset | Duration[a] | Dose (all are intravenous) |
|---|---|---|---|
| **Depolarizing** | | | |
| Succinylcholine | 0.5–1 min | 2–3 min | 0.6 mg/kg[b] (children: 1 mg/kg[c]) over 10–20 seconds; repeat as needed. |
| **Nondepolarizing** | | | |
| Atracurium | 3–5 min | 20–45 min | 0.4–0.5 mg/kg (children < 2 years: 0.3–0.4 mg/kg). |
| Cisatracurium | 1.5–2 min | 55–61 min | 0.15–0.2 mg/kg (children 2–12 years: 0.1 mg/kg), then 1–3 mcg/kg/min to maintain blockade. |
| Pancuronium | 2–3 min | 35–45 min | 0.06–0.1 mg/kg; then 0.01–0.02 mg/kg every 20–40 min as needed to maintain blockade. |
| Rocuronium | 0.5–3 min | 22–94 min | 0.6–1 mg/kg; then 0.01 mg/kg/min to maintain blockade. |
| Vecuronium | 1–2 min | 25–40 min | For children > 1 year and adults: 0.08–0.1 mg/kg bolus, then 0.01–0.02 mg/kg every 10–20 min to maintain blockade. |
| Doxacurium | 5–7 min | 56–160 min | 0.05–0.08 mg/kg (children 0.03–0.05 mg/kg), then 0.005–0.01 mg/kg every 30–45 min to maintain blockade (children may require more frequent dosing). |
| Pipecuronium | 3–5 min | 17–175 min | 0.05–0.1 mg/kg (adjust for renal function); then 0.01–0.015 mg/kg every 17–175 min (children may be less sensitive and require more frequent dosing). |
| Mivacurium | 2–4 min | 13–23 min | 0.15–0.25 mg/kg (children 0.2 mg/kg), then 0.1 mg/kg every 15 min, or by continuous infusion and start with 0.01 mg/kg/min and maintain with average adult dose of 0.006–0.007 mg/kg/min (children 0.014 mg/kg/min). |

[a]For most agents, onset and duration are dose- and age-dependent. With succinylcholine or mivacurium, effects may be prolonged in patients who have genetic plasma cholinesterase deficiency or organophosphate intoxication.
[b]To prevent fasciculations, administer a small dose of a nondepolarizing agent (eg, pancuronium, 0.01 mg/kg) 2–3 min before the succinylcholine.
[c]Pretreat children with atropine at 0.005–0.01 mg/kg to prevent bradycardia or atrioventricular block.

**IV. Adverse effects**

**A.** Complete paralysis results in respiratory depression and apnea.

**B.** Succinylcholine can stimulate vagal nerves, resulting in sinus bradycardia and AV block. Children are particularly sensitive to vagotonic effects (can prevent with atropine).

**C.** Muscle fasciculations may cause increased intraocular and intragastric pressure (the latter may result in emesis and aspiration of gastric contents). Rhabdomyolysis and myoglobinuria may be observed, especially in children.

**D.** Succinylcholine may produce hyperkalemia in patients with neuropathy, myopathy, recent severe burns, or head and spinal cord injury (this risk is maximal a few months after the injury). There is one case report of a patient with wound botulism. The mechanism is increased extrajunctional muscle acetylcholine receptors and may also occur with prolonged use of nondepolarizing agents.

**E.** Clinically significant histamine release with bronchospasm may occur, especially with succinylcholine, mivacurium, and rapacuronium (which was withdrawn from the market). It is more common with smokers and patients with reversible airway disease.

**F.** Neuromuscular blockade is potentiated by hypokalemia and hypocalcemia (nondepolarizing agents) and by hypermagnesemia (depolarizing and nondepolarizing agents).

**G.** Prolonged effects may occur after succinylcholine use in patients with genetic deficiency of plasma cholinesterase.

**H.** Prolonged effects may occur in patients with neuromuscular disease (eg, myasthenia gravis, Eaton-Lambert syndrome) or resistance (eg, myasthenia gravis and succinylcholine).

**I.** Tachycardia caused by vagal block and sympathomimetic effects from pancuronium and high-dose rocuronium.

**J.** Neuropathies, myopathies, and persistent muscular weakness associated with prolonged use owing to chemical denervation.

**K. Use in pregnancy.** FDA category C (indeterminate). This does not preclude their acute, short-term use in a seriously ill patient (see p 407).

**V. Drug or laboratory interactions**

**A.** Actions of the nondepolarizing agents are potentiated by ether, methoxyflurane, and enflurane and are inhibited or reversed by anticholinesterase agents (eg, neostigmine, physostigmine, and carbamate and organophosphate insecticides).

**B.** Organophosphate or carbamate (see p 292) insecticide intoxication may potentiate or prolong the effect of succinylcholine.

**C.** Numerous drugs may potentiate neuromuscular blockade. These drugs include calcium antagonists, dantrolene, aminoglycoside antibiotics, propranolol, membrane-stabilizing drugs (eg, quinidine), magnesium, lithium, and thiazide diuretics.

**D.** Anticonvulsants (carbamazepine and phenytoin) and theophylline may delay the onset and shorten the duration of action of some nondepolarizing agents. Carbamazepine has additive effects, and reduction of the neuromuscular blocker dose may be required.

**E.** Dysrhythmias are possible with myocardial sensitizers (eg, halothane) and sympathetic stimulating agents (eg, pancuronium).

**VI. Dosage and method of administration** (see Table III–11)

**VII. Formulations**

**A. Succinylcholine chloride** (Anectine® and others), 20 and 50 mg/mL; 10-mL vials (with parabens and benzyl alcohol) and ampules; 100 mg in 5-mL syringe; 500 mg and 1 g (powder for infusion). The **suggested minimum stocking level** to treat a 70-kg adult for the first 24 hours is two vials of each concentration.

B. **Atracurium besylate** (Tracrium), 10 mg/mL in 5-mL single-dose and 10-mL multidose vials (with benzyl alcohol). The **suggested minimum stocking level** to treat a 70-kg adult for the first 24 hours is four 10-mL vials.

C. **Cisatracurium besylate** (Nimbex), 2 mg/mL in 5- and 10-mL vials; 10 mg/mL in 20-mL vials (with benzyl alcohol). The **suggested minimum stocking level** to treat a 70-kg adult for the first 24 hours is one 20-mL vial or the equivalent.

D. **Pancuronium bromide** (Pavulon, others), 1 and 2 mg/mL in 2-, 5-, and 10-mL vials, ampules (some with benzyl alcohol), and syringes. The **suggested minimum stocking level** to treat a 70-kg adult for the first 24 hours is eight vials (2 mg/mL, 5 mL each).

E. **Rocuronium bromide** (Zemuron), 10 mg/mL in 5- and 10-mL vials. The **suggested minimum stocking level** to treat a 70-kg adult for the first 24 hours is seven vials.

F. **Vecuronium bromide** (Norcuron, others), 10-mg and 20-mg vials of lyophilized powder for reconstitution (Norcuron contains mannitol, and diluent may contain benzyl alcohol). The **suggested minimum stocking level** to treat a 70-kg adult for the first 24 hours is three vials.

G. **Doxacurium chloride** (Nuromax), 1 mg/mL in 5-mL vials (with benzyl alcohol). The **suggested minimum stocking level** to treat a 70-kg adult for the first 24 hours is three vials.

H. **Pipecuronium bromide** (Arduan) 10 mg in 10-mL vials (powder for injection). The **suggested minimum stocking level** to treat a 70-kg adult for the first 24 hours is two vials.

I. **Mivacurium chloride** (Mivacron) 0.5 mg/mL and 2 mg/mL in 5- and 10-mL single-use vials. The **suggested minimum stocking level** to treat a 70-kg adult for the first 24 hours is four 10-mL vials or the equivalent.

## ► NICOTINAMIDE (NIACINAMIDE)

*Thomas E. Kearney, PharmD*

I. **Pharmacology.** Nicotinamide (niacinamide, vitamin $B_3$), one of the B vitamins, is required for the functioning of the coenzymes nicotinamide adenine dinucleotide (NAD) and nicotinamide adenine dinucleotide phosphate (NADP). NAD and NADP are responsible for energy transfer reactions. Niacin deficiency, which results in pellagra, can be corrected with nicotinamide.

II. **Indications.** Nicotinamide is used to prevent the neurologic and endocrinologic toxicity associated with the ingestion of Vacor (PNU), a rodenticide that is believed to act by antagonizing nicotinamide (see p 362). The best results are achieved when nicotinamide therapy is instituted within 3 hours of ingestion. It may also be effective for treatment of Vacor analogs such as alloxan and streptozocin.

III. **Contraindications.** No known contraindications.

IV. **Adverse effects**

A. Headache and dizziness.

B. Hyperglycemia.

C. Hepatotoxicity (reported after chronic use with daily dose ≥3 g).

D. **Use in pregnancy.** No assigned FDA category. This does not preclude its acute, short-term use in a seriously symptomatic patient (see p 407).

V. **Drug or laboratory interactions.** No known interactions.

VI. **Dosage and method of administration (adults and children).** ***Note:*** The parenteral preparation is no longer available in the United States. The oral form may be substituted but is of unknown efficacy.

A. Give 500 mg IV initially, followed by 100–200 mg IV every 4 hours for 48 hours. Then give 100 mg orally 3–5 times daily for 2 weeks. If clinical deterioration from the Vacor progresses during initial therapy with nicotinamide, change the dosing interval to every 2 hours. The maximum suggested daily dose is 3 g.

B. ***Note:*** Nicotinic acid (niacin) is ***not*** a substitute for nicotinamide in the treatment of Vacor ingestions.

**VII. Formulations**

A. **Parenteral.** Niacinamide, 100 mg/mL (not available in the United States).

B. **Oral.** Niacinamide, 100- and 500-mg tablets, is available without a prescription. The **suggested minimum stocking level** to treat a 70-kg adult for the first 24 hours is 3 g.

# ▶ NITRITE, SODIUM AND AMYL

*Walter H. Mullen, PharmD*

I. **Pharmacology.** Sodium nitrite injectable solution and amyl nitrite crushable ampules for inhalation are components of the cyanide antidote package. The value of nitrites as an antidote to cyanide poisoning is twofold: They oxidize hemoglobin to methemoglobin, which binds free cyanide, and they may enhance endothelial cyanide detoxification by producing vasodilation. Inhalation of an ampule of amyl nitrite produces a methemoglobin level of about 5%. Intravenous administration of a single dose of sodium nitrite is anticipated to produce a methemoglobin level of about 20–30%.

**II. Indications**

A. Symptomatic cyanide poisoning (see p 176). Nitrites are not usually used for empiric treatment unless cyanide is suspected very strongly, and they are not recommended for smoke inhalation victims.

B. Nitrites are possibly effective for hydrogen sulfide poisoning if given within 30 minutes of exposure (see p 224).

**III. Contraindications**

A. Significant preexisting methemoglobinemia (> 40%).

B. Severe hypotension is a relative contraindication as it may be worsened by nitrites.

C. Administration to patients with concurrent carbon monoxide poisoning is a relative contraindication; generation of methemoglobin may further compromise oxygen transport to the tissues. Hydroxocobalamin (see p 459) has supplanted the use of nitrites for smoke inhalation victims (patients often have mixed carbon monoxide and cyanide poisoning) in countries where it is available.

**IV. Adverse effects**

A. Headache, facial flushing, dizziness, nausea, vomiting, tachycardia, and sweating may occur. These side effects may be masked by the symptoms of cyanide poisoning.

B. Rapid intravenous administration may result in hypotension.

C. Excessive and potentially fatal methemoglobinemia may result.

D. **Use in pregnancy.** No assigned FDA category. These agents may compromise blood flow and oxygen delivery to the fetus and may induce fetal methemoglobinemia. Fetal hemoglobin is more sensitive to the oxidant effects of nitrites. However, this does not preclude their acute, short-term use for a seriously symptomatic patient (see p 407).

**V. Drug or laboratory interactions**

A. Hypotension may be exacerbated by the concurrent presence of alcohol or other vasodilators or any antihypertensive agent.

B. Methylene blue should not be administered to a cyanide-poisoned patient because it may reverse nitrite-induced methemoglobinemia and theoretically result in release of free cyanide ions. However, it may be considered when severe and life-threatening excessive methemoglobinemia is present.

C. Binding of methemoglobin to cyanide (cyanomethemoglobin) may lower the measured free methemoglobin level.

**TABLE III–12. PEDIATRIC DOSING OF SODIUM NITRITE BASED ON HEMOGLOBIN CONCENTRATION**

| Hemoglobin (g/dL) | Initial Dose (mg/kg) | Initial Dose of 3% Sodium Nitrite (mL/kg) |
|---|---|---|
| 7 | 5.8 | 0.19 |
| 8 | 6.6 | 0.22 |
| 9 | 7.5 | 0.25 |
| 10 | 8.3 | 0.27 |
| 11 | 9.1 | 0.3 |
| 12 | 10 | 0.33 |
| 13 | 10.8 | 0.36 |
| 14 | 11.6 | 0.39 |

**VI. Dosage and method of administration**

**A. Amyl nitrite crushable ampules.** Crush one to two ampules in gauze, cloth, or a sponge and place under the nose of the victim, who should inhale deeply for 30 seconds. Rest for 30 seconds, then repeat. Each ampule lasts about 2–3 minutes. If the victim is receiving respiratory support, place the ampules in the facemask or port access to the endotracheal tube. Stop ampule use when administering intravenous sodium nitrite.

**B. Sodium nitrite parenteral**

1. **Adults.** Administer 300 mg of sodium nitrite (10 mL of 3% solution) IV over 3–5 minutes.
2. **Children.** Give 0.15–0.33 mL/kg to a maximum of 10 mL. Pediatric dosing should be based on the hemoglobin concentration if it is known (see Table III–12). If anemia is suspected or hypotension is present, start with the lower dose, dilute in 50–100 mL of saline, and give over at least 5 minutes.
3. Oxidation of hemoglobin to methemoglobin occurs within 30 minutes. If no response to treatment occurs within 30 minutes, an additional half-size dose of intravenous sodium nitrite may be given.

**VII. Formulations**

**A. Amyl nitrite.** A component of the cyanide antidote package, 0.3 mL in crushable ampules, 12 per kit. The drug may also be acquired separately in Aspirols. ***Note:*** The ampules have a shelf life of only 1 year and may disappear because of the potential for abuse (as "poppers").

**B. Sodium nitrite parenteral.** A component of the cyanide antidote package, 300 mg in 10 mL of sterile water (3%), two ampules per kit.

**C.** The **suggested minimum stocking level** to treat a 70-kg adult for the first 24 hours is two cyanide antidote packages or the equivalent (one package should be kept in the emergency department). Available from Taylor Pharmaceuticals.

## ▶ NITROPRUSSIDE

*Thomas E. Kearney, PharmD*

**I. Pharmacology.** Nitroprusside is an ultra-short-acting titratable parenteral hypotensive agent that acts by directly relaxing vascular smooth muscle as a nitric oxide donor. Both arterial dilation and venous dilation occur; the effect is more marked in patients with hypertension. A small increase in heart rate may be observed in hypertensive patients. Intravenous administration produces nearly immediate onset of action, with a duration of effect of 1–10 minutes. Resistance may occur with high renin activity. Nitroprusside is metabolized rapidly, with a serum half-life of about 1–2 minutes. Cyanide is produced during metabolism and is converted to the less toxic thiocyanate. Thiocyanate has a half-life of 2–3 days and accumulates in patients with renal insufficiency.

**II. Indications**

**A.** Rapid control of severe hypertension (eg, in patients with stimulant intoxication or monoamine oxidase inhibitor toxicity).

**B.** Arterial vasodilation in patients with ergot-induced peripheral arterial spasm.

**III. Contraindications**

**A.** Compensatory hypertension, for example, in patients with increased intracranial pressure (eg, hemorrhage or mass lesion) or patients with coarctation of the aorta. If nitroprusside is required in such patients, use with extreme caution.

**B.** Use with caution in patients with hepatic insufficiency, because cyanide metabolism may be impaired.

**IV. Adverse effects**

**A.** Nausea, vomiting, headache, and sweating may be caused by excessively rapid lowering of blood pressure.

**B. Cyanide toxicity,** manifested by altered mental status and metabolic (lactic) acidosis, may occur with rapid high-dose infusion (10–15 mcg/kg/min) for periods of 1 hour or longer. Patients with depleted thiosulfate stores (eg, malnourished) may have elevated cyanide levels at lower infusion rates. Continuous intravenous infusion of hydroxocobalamin, 25 mg/h (see p 459), or thiosulfate (p 514) has been used to limit cyanide toxicity. If severe cyanide toxicity occurs, discontinue the nitroprusside infusion and consider antidotal doses of thiosulfate and sodium nitrite (p 484) or high-dose hydroxocobalamin (p 459).

**C. Thiocyanate intoxication,** manifested by disorientation, delirium, muscle twitching, and psychosis, may occur with prolonged high-dose nitroprusside infusions (usually ≥3 mcg/kg/min for 48 hours or longer), particularly in patients with renal insufficiency (may occur at rates as low as 1 mcg/kg/min). Thiocyanate production is also enhanced by co-administration of sodium thiosulfate. Monitor thiocyanate levels if the nitroprusside infusion lasts more than 1–2 days; toxicity is associated with thiocyanate levels of 50 mg/L or greater. Usually treat by lowering the infusion rate or discontinuing the use of nitroprusside. Thiocyanate is removed effectively by hemodialysis.

**D.** Rebound hypertension may be observed after sudden discontinuance.

**E.** Methemoglobinemia may be observed in patients receiving more than 10 mg/kg but is typically not severe.

**F. Use in pregnancy.** FDA category C (indeterminate; see p 407). It may cross the placenta and may affect uterine blood flow; however, it has been used successfully in pregnant women.

**V. Drug or laboratory interactions.** A hypotensive effect is potentiated by other antihypertensive agents and inhalational anesthetics.

**VI. Dosage and method of administration**

**A.** Use only in an emergency or intensive care setting with the capability of frequent or continuous blood pressure monitoring.

**B.** Dissolve 50 mg of sodium nitroprusside in 3 mL of 5% dextrose; then dilute this solution in 250, 500, or 1000 mL of 5% dextrose to achieve a concentration of 200, 100, or 50 mcg/mL, respectively. Protect the solution from light to avoid photodegradation (as evidenced by a color change) by covering the bottle and tubing with paper or aluminum foil.

**C.** Start with an intravenous infusion rate of 0.3 mcg/kg/min with a controlled infusion device and titrate to desired effect. The average dose is 3 mcg/kg/min in children and adults (range 0.5–10 mcg/kg/min).

**1.** The maximum rate should not exceed 10 mcg/kg/min to avoid the risk of acute cyanide toxicity. If there is no response after 10 minutes at the maximum rate, discontinue the infusion and use an alternative vasodilator (eg, phentolamine; see p 495).

2. Sodium thiosulfate (see p 514) has been added in a ratio of 10 mg thiosulfate to 1 mg nitroprusside to reduce or prevent cyanide toxicity.

**VII. Formulations**

- **A. Parenteral.** Nitroprusside sodium (Nitropress and others), 50 mg of lyophilized powder for reconstitution in 2- and 5-mL vials.
- **B.** The **suggested minimum stocking level** to treat a 70-kg adult for the first 24 hours is 24 vials.

## ▶ NOREPINEPHRINE

*Neal L. Benowitz, MD*

**I. Pharmacology.** Norepinephrine is an endogenous catecholamine that stimulates mainly alpha-adrenergic receptors. It is used primarily as a vasopressor to increase systemic vascular resistance and venous return to the heart. Norepinephrine is also a weak beta-1-adrenergic receptor agonist, and it may increase heart rate and cardiac contractility in patients with shock. Norepinephrine is not effective orally and is absorbed erratically after subcutaneous injection. After intravenous administration, the onset of action is nearly immediate, and the duration of effect is 1–2 minutes after the infusion is discontinued.

**II. Indications.** Norepinephrine is used to increase blood pressure and cardiac output in patients with shock caused by venodilation, low systemic vascular resistance, or both. Hypovolemia, depressed myocardial contractility, hypothermia, and electrolyte imbalance should be corrected first or concurrently.

**III. Contraindications**

- **A.** Uncorrected hypovolemia.
- **B.** Norepinephrine is relatively contraindicated in patients with peripheral arterial occlusive vascular disease with thrombosis or ergot poisoning (see p 187).

**IV. Adverse effects**

- **A.** Severe hypertension, which may result in intracranial hemorrhage, pulmonary edema, or myocardial necrosis.
- **B.** Aggravation of tissue ischemia, resulting in gangrene.
- **C.** Tissue necrosis after extravasation.
- **D.** Anxiety, restlessness, tremor, and headache.
- **E.** Anaphylaxis induced by sulfite preservatives in sensitive patients. Use with extreme caution in patients with known hypersensitivity to sulfite preservatives.
- **F.** Use with caution in patients intoxicated by chloral hydrate or halogenated or aromatic hydrocarbon solvents or anesthetics.
- **G. Use in pregnancy.** This drug crosses the placenta and can cause placental ischemia and reduce uterine contractions.

**V. Drug or laboratory interactions**

- **A.** Enhanced pressor response may occur in the presence of cocaine and cyclic antidepressants owing to inhibition of neuronal reuptake.
- **B.** Enhanced pressor response may occur in patients taking monoamine oxidase inhibitors owing to inhibition of neuronal metabolic degradation.
- **C.** Alpha- and beta-blocking agents may antagonize the adrenergic effects of norepinephrine.
- **D.** Anticholinergic drugs may block reflex bradycardia, which normally occurs in response to norepinephrine-induced hypertension, enhancing the hypertensive response.
- **E.** Chloral hydrate overdose and cyclopropane and halogenated or aromatic hydrocarbon solvents and anesthetics may enhance myocardial sensitivity to the arrhythmogenic effects of norepinephrine.

**VI. Dosage and method of administration**

**A. *Caution:* Avoid extravasation.** The intravenous infusion must be free flowing, and the infused vein should be observed frequently for signs of infiltration (pallor, coldness, or induration).

1. If extravasation occurs, immediately infiltrate the affected area with phentolamine (see p 495), 5–10 mg in 10–15 mL of normal saline (children, 0.1–0.2 mg/kg; maximum 10 mg) via a fine (25- to 27-gauge) hypodermic needle; improvement is evidenced by hyperemia and return to normal temperature.
2. Alternatively, topical application of nitroglycerin paste and infiltration of terbutaline have been reported successful.

**B. Intravenous infusion.** Begin at 4–8 mcg/min (children, 1–2 mcg/min or 0.1 mcg/kg/min) and increase as needed every 5–10 minutes.

**VII. Formulations.** Norepinephrine bitartrate is oxidized rapidly on exposure to air; it must be kept in its airtight ampule until immediately before use. If the solution appears brown or contains a precipitate, do not use it. The stock solution must be diluted in 5% dextrose or 5% dextrose-saline for infusion; usually, a 4-mg ampule is added to 1 L of fluid to provide 4 mcg/mL of solution.

**A. Parenteral.** Norepinephrine bitartrate (Levophed), 1 mg/mL, 4-mL ampule. Contains sodium bisulfite as a preservative.

**B.** The **suggested minimum stocking level** to treat a 70-kg adult for the first 24 hours is five ampules.

## ► OCTREOTIDE

*Thomas E. Kearney, PharmD*

**I. Pharmacology**

**A.** Octreotide is a synthetic polypeptide and a long-acting analog of somatostatin. It significantly antagonizes pancreatic insulin release and is useful for the management of poisonings from drug-induced endogenous secretion of insulin-, oral sulfonylurea–, and quinine-induced hyperinsulinemic and hypoglycemic poisonings.

**B.** Octreotide also suppresses pancreatic function, gastric acid secretion, and biliary and GI tract motility.

**C.** As a polypeptide, it is bioavailable only by parenteral administration (intravenously or subcutaneously). Approximately 30% of octreotide is excreted unchanged in the urine, and it has an elimination half-life of 1.7 hours. Its half-life may be increased in patients with renal dysfunction and in the elderly.

**II. Indications.** Oral sulfonylurea hypoglycemic overdose (see p 93) and quinine-induced hypoglycemia (p 327) when serum glucose concentrations cannot be maintained by an intravenous 5% dextrose infusion. It may also be considered a first-line agent along with dextrose since it can reduce glucose requirements and prevent rebound hypoglycemia in patients with sulfonylurea poisoning. This agent is preferred over diazoxide (p 438). It is uncertain whether octreotide has a role with exogenous insulin poisoning, and it has a theoretical disadvantage of blocking counterregulatory reactions (prevents glucagon and growth hormone secretion) to hypoglycemia.

**III. Contraindications.** Hypersensitivity to the drug (anaphylactic shock has occurred).

**IV. Adverse effects.** In general, the drug is well tolerated. Patients may experience pain or burning at the injection site. For the most part, the adverse effect profile is based on long-term therapy for other disease states.

**A.** The suppressive effects on the biliary tract may lead to significant gallbladder disease (cholelithiasis) and pancreatitis.

**B.** Gastrointestinal effects (diarrhea, nausea, discomfort) may occur in 5–10% of users. Headache, dizziness, and fatigue have also been observed.

C. Cardiac effects may include bradycardia, conduction abnormalities (QT prolongation), hypertension, and exacerbation of congestive heart failure. These effects have been observed primarily in patients treated for acromegaly.

D. **Use in pregnancy.** FDA category B. Not likely to cause harm with short-term therapy (see p 407).

V. **Drug or laboratory interactions**

A. Octreotide may inhibit the absorption of dietary fats and cyclosporine.

B. The drug depresses vitamin $B_{12}$ levels and can lead to abnormal Schilling's test results.

VI. **Dosage and method of administration**

A. **Oral sulfonylurea overdose.** Give 50–100 mcg (children: 4–5 mcg/kg/day divided every 6 hours) by subcutaneous or intravenous injection once or every 6–12 hours as needed (some sulfonylurea poisonings may require days of therapy). Infusions up to 125 mcg/h have been used (see note below). Most patients require approximately 24 hours of therapy and do not experience recurrent hypoglycemia upon discontinuation of octreotide. Monitor for recurrent hypoglycemia for 24 hours after termination of octreotide therapy.

B. **Quinine-induced hypoglycemia.** A dose of 50 mcg/h has been used in adult patients with malaria.

C. Subcutaneous injection sites should be rotated.

D. For IV administration, dilute in 50 mL normal saline or 5% dextrose and infuse over 15–30 min. Alternatively, the dose may be given IV push over 3 min.

E. ***Note:*** Optimal dosage regimen is not known. For other indications, daily doses up to 1500 mcg are utilized (120 mg has been infused over 8 hours without severe adverse effects).

VII. **Formulations**

A. **Parenteral.** Octreotide acetate (Sandostatin, generic): 0.05, 0.1, and 0.5 mg/mL in 1-mL ampules and vials; 0.2 and 1 mg/mL in 5-mL multidose vials. ***Note:*** Avoid use of the long-acting agent Sandostatin LAR Depot. This product is for once-a-month dosing in patients with acromegaly.

B. The **suggested minimum stocking level** to treat a 70-kg adult for the first 24 hours is two (1-mL) ampules or vials (0.1 mg/mL) or one (5-mL) multidose vial (0.2 mg/mL).

## ▶ ONDANSETRON

*Judith A. Alsop, PharmD*

I. **Pharmacology.** Ondansetron is a selective serotonin 5-$HT_3$ receptor antagonist with powerful antiemetic activity both centrally at the chemoreceptor trigger zone and peripherally at vagal nerve terminals. The onset is about 30 minutes after an intravenous dose and 60–90 minutes after an oral dose. The drug is metabolized extensively in the liver. The elimination half-life is 3–5.5 hours, increasing to as long as 20 hours in patients with severe liver disease.

II. **Indications.** Ondansetron is used to treat intractable nausea and vomiting, particularly when the ability to administer activated charcoal or antidotal therapy (eg, *N*-acetylcysteine) is compromised.

III. **Contraindications.** Known hypersensitivity to the drug.

IV. **Adverse effects**

A. Bronchospasm, hypersensitivity, and anaphylactoid reactions (rare).

B. Cardiac arrhythmias, tachycardia, angina, and chest pain (rare).

C. Anxiety, headache, drowsiness, fatigue, fever, and dizziness.

D. Extrapyramidal reactions may occur.

E. Diarrhea and constipation are both reported.

F. Seizures, hypoxia (rare).

G. Transient blindness (rare).

**H. Use in pregnancy.** FDA category B. Not likely to cause harm when used as short-term therapy (see p 407).

**V. Drug or laboratory interactions**

**A.** Extrapyramidal reactions are more likely in patients who are also taking haloperidol or other central dopamine-blocking drugs.

**B.** Anticholinergic agents may inhibit bowel motility.

**C.** Increased liver transaminases have been reported.

**D.** The risk of QT prolongation and cardiotoxicity is increased when ondansetron is used with patients also receiving droperidol.

**E.** Numerous IV incompatibilities: aminophylline, potassium chloride, sodium bicarbonate, furosemide, lorazepam, dexamethasone, methylprednisolone, sodium succinate, thiopental.

**VI. Dosage and method of administration. Adults:** Give 8 mg or 0.15 mg/kg IV in 50 mL normal saline or 5% dextrose. This may be repeated twice at 4-hour intervals. *Alternative high-dose therapy:* 32 mg in 50 mL saline or dextrose administered over 15 minutes. (Do not repeat this dose.) **Pediatrics**: Give 0.15 mg/kg IV. This may be repeated twice at 4-hour intervals.

**A.** Ondansetron is most effective when given at least 30 minutes before its antiemetic properties are needed.

**B.** Do not exceed a total daily dose of 8 mg in patients with severe liver disease.

**C.** Ondansetron does not require dilution and can be given by direct intravenous injection over a period of at least 30 seconds, preferably 2–3 minutes.

**D.** Intramuscular use is not recommended.

**VII. Formulations**

**A. Parenteral.** Ondansetron hydrochloride (Zofran): 2 mg/mL in 2-mL single-dose vials and 20-mL multidose vials. Also available as 32 mg in a 50-mL premixed container.

**B.** The **suggested minimum stocking level** to treat a 70-kg adult for the first 24 hours is 32 mg.

## ▶ OXYGEN AND HYPERBARIC OXYGEN

*Kent R. Olson, MD*

**I. Pharmacology.** Oxygen is a necessary oxidant to drive biochemical reactions. Room air contains 21% oxygen. Hyperbaric oxygen (HBO) (100% oxygen delivered to the patient in a pressurized chamber at 2–3 atm of pressure) may be beneficial for patients with severe carbon monoxide (CO) poisoning. It can hasten the reversal of CO binding to hemoglobin and intracellular myoglobin, can provide oxygen independent of hemoglobin, and may have protective actions in reducing postischemic brain damage. Randomized controlled studies have reported conflicting outcomes with HBO treatment, but there appears to be at least a marginal benefit in preventing subtle neuropsychiatric sequelae.

**II. Indications**

**A.** Supplemental oxygen is indicated when normal oxygenation is impaired because of pulmonary injury, which may result from aspiration (chemical pneumonitis) or inhalation of toxic gases. The $PO_2$ should be maintained at 70–80 mm Hg or higher if possible.

**B.** Supplemental oxygen usually is given empirically to patients with altered mental status or suspected hypoxemia.

**C.** Oxygen (100%) is indicated for patients with carbon monoxide poisoning, to increase the conversion of carboxyhemoglobin and carboxymyoglobin to hemoglobin and myoglobin, and to increase oxygen saturation of the plasma and subsequent delivery to tissues.

**D.** Hyperbaric oxygen may be beneficial for patients with severe carbon monoxide poisoning, although the clinical evidence is mixed. Potential indications include history of loss of consciousness; metabolic acidosis, age over 50 years, pregnancy, carboxyhemoglobin level greater than 25%, and cerebellar dysfunction (eg, ataxia).

E. HBO has also been advocated for treatment of poisoning by carbon tetrachloride, cyanide, and hydrogen sulfide and for severe methemoglobinemia, but the experimental and clinical evidence is scanty.

**III. Contraindications**

A. In **paraquat** poisoning, oxygen may contribute to lung injury. In fact, slightly *hypoxic* environments (10–12% oxygen) have been advocated to reduce the risk of pulmonary fibrosis from paraquat.

B. Relative contraindications to hyperbaric oxygen therapy include a history of recent middle ear or thoracic surgery, untreated pneumothorax, seizure disorder, and severe sinusitis.

**IV. Adverse effects.** ***Caution:*** Oxygen is extremely flammable.

A. Prolonged high concentrations of oxygen are associated with pulmonary alveolar tissue damage. In general, the fraction of inspired oxygen ($FIO_2$) should not be maintained at greater than 80% for more than 24 hours.

B. Oxygen therapy may increase the risk of retrolental fibroplasia in neonates.

C. Administration of high oxygen concentrations to patients with severe chronic obstructive pulmonary disease and chronic carbon dioxide retention who are dependent on hypoxemia to provide a drive to breathe may result in respiratory arrest.

D. Hyperbaric oxygen treatment can cause hyperoxic seizures, aural trauma (ruptured tympanic membrane), and acute anxiety resulting from claustrophobia. Seizures are more likely at higher atmospheric pressures (eg, 3 atm or greater).

E. Oxygen may potentiate toxicity via enhanced generation of free radicals with some chemotherapeutic agents (eg, bleomycin, Adriamycin, and daunorubicin).

F. **Use in pregnancy.** No known adverse effects.

**V. Drug or laboratory interactions.** None known.

**VI. Dosage and method of administration**

A. **Supplemental oxygen.** Provide supplemental oxygen to maintain a $PO_2$ of at least 70–80 mm Hg. If a $PO_2$ greater than 50 mm Hg cannot be maintained with an $FIO_2$ of at least 60%, consider positive end-expiratory pressure or continuous positive airway pressure.

B. **Carbon monoxide poisoning**. Provide 100% oxygen by tight-fitting mask or via endotracheal tube. Consider **hyperbaric oxygen therapy** if the patient has serious poisoning (see Indications, above) and the patient can be treated within 6 hours of the exposure. Consult with a poison center ([800] 222-1222) or a hyperbaric specialist to determine the location of the nearest HBO facility. Usually, three HBO treatments at 2.5–3 atm are recommended over a 24-hour period.

**VII. Formulations**

A. **Nasal cannula.** Provides 24–40% oxygen, depending on the flow rate and patient's breathing pattern.

B. **Ventimask.** Provides variable inspired oxygen concentrations from 24 to 40%.

C. **Nonrebreathing reservoir mask.** Provides 60–90% inspired oxygen concentrations.

D. **Hyperbaric oxygen.** One hundred percent oxygen can be delivered at a pressure of 2–3 atm.

## ▶ PENICILLAMINE

*Thomas E. Kearney, PharmD*

**I. Pharmacology.** Penicillamine is a derivative of penicillin that has no antimicrobial activity but effectively chelates some heavy metals, such as lead, mercury, and copper. It has been used as adjunctive therapy after initial treatment with calcium EDTA (see p 446) or BAL (dimercaprol; p 417), although its use largely has been replaced by the oral chelator succimer (DMSA, p 510) because of its poor safety profile. Penicillamine is well absorbed orally, and the penicillamine-metal complex is eliminated in the urine. No parenteral form is available.

**II. Indications**

**A.** Penicillamine may be used to treat heavy metal poisoning caused by lead (if the patient is intolerant to succimer, penicillamine may be used alone for minor intoxication or as adjunctive therapy after calcium EDTA or BAL in moderate to severe intoxication), mercury (after initial BAL therapy and if intolerant of succimer), and copper (succimer may be an alternative for mild to moderate poisoning).

**B.** For lead or mercury poisoning, oral succimer (see p 510) is preferable, as it may result in greater metal excretion with fewer adverse effects.

**C.** For copper poisoning (see p 174) and treatment of Wilson's disease to remove copper deposits in tissues.

**III. Contraindications**

**A.** Penicillin allergy is a contraindication (penicillamine products may be contaminated with penicillin).

**B.** Renal insufficiency is a relative contraindication because the complex is eliminated only through the urine.

**C.** Concomitant administration with other hematopoietic-depressant drugs (eg, gold salts, immunosuppressants, antimalarial agents, and phenylbutazone) is not recommended.

**D.** Cadmium poisoning. It may increase renal levels of cadmium and the potential for nephrotoxicity.

**IV. Adverse effects**

**A.** Hypersensitivity reactions: rash, pruritus, drug fever, hematuria, antinuclear antibodies, and proteinuria.

**B.** Leukopenia, thrombocytopenia, hemolytic anemia, aplastic anemia, and agranulocytosis.

**C.** Hepatitis and pancreatitis.

**D.** Anorexia, nausea, vomiting, epigastric pain, and impairment of taste.

**E.** The requirement for pyridoxine is increased, and the patient may require daily supplementation (see p 508).

**F. Use in pregnancy.** Birth defects have been associated with its use during pregnancy. No assigned FDA category (see p 407).

**V. Drug or laboratory interactions**

**A.** Penicillamine may potentiate the hematopoietic-depressant effects of drugs such as gold salts, immunosuppressants, antimalarial agents, and phenylbutazone.

**B.** Several drugs (eg, antacids and ferrous sulfate) and food can reduce GI absorption of penicillamine substantially.

**C.** Penicillamine may produce a false-positive test for ketones in the urine.

**VI. Dosage and method of administration**

**A.** Penicillamine should be taken on an empty stomach at least 1 hour before or 3 hours after meals and at bedtime.

**B.** The usual dose is 20–30 mg/kg/day, administered in three or four divided doses. The usual starting dose in adults is 250 mg four times daily. Initiating treatment at 25% of this dose and gradually increasing to the full dose over 2–3 weeks may minimize adverse reactions. The maximum adult daily dose is 2 g. In children with mild to moderate lead poisoning, a lower dose, 15 mg/kg/day, has been shown to maintain efficacy at lowering blood levels and minimizing adverse effects.

**C.** Weekly measurement of urinary and blood concentrations of the intoxicating metal is indicated to assess the need for continued therapy. Treatment for as long as 3 months has been tolerated.

**VII. Formulations.** ***Note:*** Although the chemical derivative *N*-acetylpenicillamine may demonstrate better CNS and peripheral nerve penetration, it is not currently available in the United States.

- **A. Oral.** Penicillamine (Cuprimine, Depen), 125- and 250-mg capsules; 250-mg titratable tablets.
- **B.** The **suggested minimum stocking level** to treat a 70-kg adult for the first 24 hours is 1500 mg.

# ▶ PENTOBARBITAL

*Thomas E. Kearney, PharmD*

**I. Pharmacology.** Pentobarbital is a short-acting barbiturate with anticonvulsant as well as sedative-hypnotic properties. It is used as a third-line drug in the treatment of status epilepticus. It also may reduce intracranial pressure in patients with cerebral edema by inducing vasoconstriction. After intravenous administration of a single dose, the onset of effect occurs within about 1 minute and lasts about 15 minutes. Pentobarbital demonstrates a biphasic elimination pattern; the half-life of the initial phase is 4 hours, and the terminal phase half-life is 35–50 hours. Effects are prolonged after termination of a continuous infusion.

**II. Indications**

- **A.** Pentobarbital is used for the management of status epilepticus that is unresponsive to conventional anticonvulsant therapy (eg, diazepam, phenytoin, or phenobarbital). If the use of pentobarbital for seizure control is considered, consultation with a neurologist is recommended.
- **B.** It is used to manage elevated intracranial pressure in conjunction with other agents.
- **C.** It may be used therapeutically or diagnostically for patients with suspected alcohol or sedative-hypnotic drug withdrawal syndrome.

**III. Contraindications**

- **A.** Known sensitivity to the drug.
- **B.** Manifest or latent porphyria.

**IV. Adverse effects**

- **A.** Central nervous system depression, coma, and respiratory arrest may occur, especially with rapid bolus or excessive doses.
- **B.** Hypotension may result, especially with rapid intravenous infusion.
- **C.** Laryngospasm and bronchospasm have been reported after rapid intravenous injection, although the mechanism is unknown.
- **D. Use in pregnancy.** FDA category D (possible fetal risk). Pentobarbital readily crosses the placenta, and chronic use may cause hemorrhagic disease of the newborn (owing to vitamin K deficiency) or neonatal dependency and withdrawal syndrome. However, these potential effects do not preclude its acute, short-term use in a seriously symptomatic patient (see p 407).

**V. Drug or laboratory interactions**

- **A.** Pentobarbital has additive CNS and respiratory depression effects with other barbiturates as well as sedative and opioid drugs.
- **B.** Hepatic enzyme induction generally is not encountered with acute pentobarbital overdose, although it may occur within 24–48 hours.
- **C.** Clearance may be enhanced by hemoperfusion, requiring supplemental doses during the procedure.

**VI. Dosage and method of administration**

- **A. Intermittent intravenous bolus.** Give 100 mg IV slowly over at least 2 minutes; repeat as needed at 2-minute intervals to a maximum dose of 300–500 mg (children, 1–3 mg/kg IV, repeated as needed to a maximum total of 5–6 mg/kg or 150–200 mg).

**B. Continuous intravenous infusion.** Administer a loading dose of 5–6 mg/kg IV over 1 hour (not to exceed 50 mg/min; children, 1 mg/kg/min), followed by maintenance infusion of 0.5–3 mg/kg/h titrated to the desired effect. For treatment of status epilepticus, use loading dose of 5–15 mg/kg given by IV infusion over 1 to 2 hours, monitor blood pressure (vasopressor support may be required, eg, dopamine) and provide respiratory support, and follow with maintenance infusion. Electroencephalographic achievement of burst suppression usually occurs with a serum pentobarbital concentration of 25–40 mcg/mL.

**C. Oral.** The oral regimen for treatment of barbiturate or other sedative-drug withdrawal syndrome is administration of 200 mg orally, repeated every hour until signs of mild intoxication appear (eg, slurred speech, drowsiness, and nystagmus). Most patients respond to 600 mg or less. Repeat the total initial dose every 6 hours as needed. Phenobarbital is an alternative (see p 494).

**VII. Formulations**

**A. Parenteral.** Pentobarbital sodium (Nembutal and others), 50 mg/mL in 1- and 2-mL tubes and vials and 20- and 50-mL vials.

**B. Oral.** Capsules (50 and 100 mg) and suppositories (30, 60, 120, and 200 mg). Also available as an elixir equivalent to 20 mg/5 mL.

**C.** The **suggested minimum stocking level** to treat a 70-kg adult for the first 24 hours is two vials, 50 mL each, or the equivalent.

## ▶ PHENOBARBITAL

*Thomas E. Kearney, PharmD*

**I. Pharmacology.** Phenobarbital is a barbiturate commonly used as an anticonvulsant. Because of the delay in onset of the therapeutic effect of phenobarbital, diazepam (see p 419) is usually the initial agent for parenteral anticonvulsant therapy. After an oral dose of phenobarbital, peak brain concentrations are achieved within 10–15 hours. Onset of effect after intravenous administration usually occurs within 5 minutes, although peak effects may take up to 30 minutes. Therapeutic plasma levels are 15–35 mg/L. The drug is eliminated by metabolism and renal excretion, and the elimination half-life is 48–100 hours.

**II. Indications**

**A.** Control of tonic-clonic seizures and status epilepticus, generally as a second- or third-line agent after diazepam or phenytoin has been tried. ***Note:*** For treatment of drug-induced seizures, especially seizures caused by theophylline, phenobarbital often is tried before phenytoin.

**B.** Management of withdrawal from ethanol and other sedative-hypnotic drugs.

**III. Contraindications**

**A.** Known sensitivity to barbiturates.

**B.** Manifest or latent porphyria.

**IV. Adverse effects**

**A.** Central nervous system depression, coma, and respiratory arrest may result, especially with rapid bolus or excessive doses.

**B.** Hypotension may result from rapid intravenous administration. This can be prevented by limiting the rate of administration to less than 50 mg/min (children, 1 mg/kg/min).

**C. Use in pregnancy.** FDA category D (possible fetal risk). Phenobarbital readily crosses the placenta, and chronic use may cause hemorrhagic disease of the newborn (owing to vitamin K deficiency) or neonatal dependency and withdrawal syndrome. However, these potential effects do not preclude its acute, short-term use in a seriously symptomatic patient (see p 407).

**V. Drug or laboratory interactions**

**A.** Phenobarbital has additive CNS and respiratory depression effects with other sedative drugs.

**B.** Hepatic enzyme induction with chronic use, although this is ***not*** encountered with acute phenobarbital dosing.

**C.** Extracorporeal removal techniques (eg, hemodialysis, hemoperfusion, and repeat-dose activated charcoal; see p 50) may enhance the clearance of phenobarbital, possibly requiring supplemental dosing to maintain therapeutic levels.

**VI. Dosage and method of administration**

**A. Parenteral.** Administer slowly intravenously (rate ≤50 mg/min; children, ≤1 mg/kg/min) until seizures are controlled or the loading dose of 10–15 mg/kg is achieved. For status epilepticus, give 15–20 mg/kg IV over 10–15 minutes, not to exceed 100 mg/minute (children have required as much as 30 mg/kg in the first 24 hours to treat status epilepticus). Slow the infusion rate if hypotension develops. Intermittent infusions of 2 mg/kg every 5–15 minutes may diminish the risk of respiratory depression or hypotension. For alcohol withdrawal seizures, initial dose of 260 mg, then 130 mg every 30 minutes until signs of mild intoxication (see below).

1. If intravenous access is not immediately available, phenobarbital may be given intramuscularly; the initial dose in adults and children is 3–5 mg/kg IM.
2. It may also be given by the intraosseous route.

**B. Oral.** For treatment of barbiturate or sedative drug withdrawal, give 60–120 mg orally and repeat every hour until signs of mild intoxication appear (eg, slurred speech, drowsiness, and nystagmus).

**VII. Formulations**

**A. Parenteral.** Phenobarbital sodium (Luminal and others), 30, 60, 65, and 130 mg/mL in 1-mL Tubex syringes, vials, and ampules.

**B. Oral.** 15-, 16-, 30-, 60-, 90-, and 100-mg tablets; 16-mg capsule; also elixir (15 and 20 mg/5 mL).

**C.** The **suggested minimum stocking level** to treat a 70-kg adult for the first 24 hours is 16 ampules (130 mg each) or the equivalent.

## ► PHENTOLAMINE

*Thomas E. Kearney, PharmD*

**I. Pharmacology.** Phentolamine is a competitive presynaptic and postsynaptic alpha-adrenergic receptor blocker that produces peripheral vasodilation. By acting on both venous and arterial vessels, it decreases total peripheral resistance and venous return. It also may stimulate beta-adrenergic receptors, causing cardiac stimulation. Phentolamine has a rapid onset of action (usually 2 minutes) and a short duration of effect (approximately 15–20 minutes).

**II. Indications**

**A.** Hypertensive crisis associated with stimulant drug overdose (eg, amphetamines, cocaine, or ephedrine). Also an adjunct for cocaine-induced acute coronary syndrome to reverse coronary artery vasoconstriction.

**B.** Hypertensive crisis resulting from interaction between monoamine oxidase inhibitors and tyramine or other sympathomimetic amines.

**C.** Hypertensive crisis associated with sudden withdrawal of sympatholytic antihypertensive drugs (eg, clonidine).

**D.** Extravasation of vasoconstrictive agents (eg, epinephrine, norepinephrine, and dopamine).

**III. Contraindications.** Use with extreme caution in patients with intracranial hemorrhage or ischemic stroke; excessive lowering of blood pressure may aggravate brain injury.

**IV. Adverse effects**

**A.** Hypotension and tachycardia may occur from excessive doses.

**B.** Anginal chest pain and cardiac arrhythmias may occur.

C. Slow intravenous infusion (≤0.3 mg/min) may result in transient increased blood pressure caused by stimulation of beta-adrenergic receptors.

D. **Use in pregnancy.** No assigned FDA category. However, this does not preclude its acute, short-term use in a seriously symptomatic patient (see p 407).

V. **Drug or laboratory interactions.** Additive or synergistic effects may occur with other antihypertensive agents, especially other alpha-adrenergic antagonists (eg, prazosin, terazosin).

VI. **Dosage and method of administration**

A. **Parenteral.** Give 1–5 mg IV (children, 0.02–0.1 mg/kg) as a bolus; repeat at 5- to 10-minute intervals as needed to lower blood pressure to a desired level (usually 100 mm Hg diastolic in adults and 80 mm Hg diastolic in children, but this may vary with the clinical situation).

B. **Catecholamine extravasation.** Infiltrate 5–10 mg in 10–15 mL of normal saline (children, 0.1–0.2 mg/kg; maximum 10 mg) into an affected area with a fine (25- to 27-gauge) hypodermic needle; improvement is evidenced by hyperemia and return to normal temperature.

VII. **Formulations**

A. **Parenteral.** Phentolamine mesylate, 5 mg in 2-mL vials (with mannitol).

B. The **suggested minimum stocking level** to treat a 70-kg adult for the first 24 hours is 20 vials.

## ▶ PHENYTOIN AND FOSPHENYTOIN

*Grant D. Lackey, PharmD*

I. **Pharmacology.** The neuronal membrane-stabilizing actions of phenytoin make this a popular drug for sustained control of acute and chronic seizure disorders and a useful drug for certain cardiac arrhythmias. Because of the relatively slow onset of anticonvulsant action, phenytoin usually is administered after diazepam. At serum concentrations considered therapeutic for seizure control, phenytoin acts similarly to lidocaine to reduce ventricular premature depolarization and suppress ventricular tachycardia. After intravenous administration, peak therapeutic effects are attained within 1 hour. The therapeutic serum concentration for seizure control is 10–20 mg/L. Elimination is nonlinear, with an apparent half-life averaging 22 hours. **Fosphenytoin,** a prodrug of phenytoin for intravenous use, is converted to phenytoin after injection, with a conversion half-life of 8–32 minutes.

II. **Indications**

A. Control of generalized tonic-clonic seizures or status epilepticus. However, benzodiazepines (p 419) and phenobarbital (p 494) are generally more effective for treating drug-induced seizures.

B. Control of cardiac arrhythmias, particularly those associated with digitalis intoxication.

III. **Contraindications.** Known hypersensitivity to phenytoin or other hydantoins.

IV. **Adverse effects.**

A. Rapid intravenous phenytoin administration (greater than 50 mg/min in adults or 1 mg/kg/min in children) may produce hypotension, AV block, and cardiovascular collapse, probably owing to the propylene glycol diluent. Fosphenytoin is readily soluble and does not contain propylene glycol, and a hypotensive response is not common.

B. Extravasation of phenytoin may result in local tissue necrosis and sloughing. Phenytoin may induce the "purple glove syndrome" (edema, discoloration, and pain) after peripheral IV administration. This can occur hours after infusion, in the absence of clinical signs of extravasation, and can lead to limb ischemia and necrosis from a compartment syndrome. Risk factors include elderly patients receiving large multiple doses, use of small IV catheters, high infusion rates, and use of the same catheter site for two or more IV push doses. Extravasation problems have not been observed with fosphenytoin.

C. Drowsiness, ataxia, nystagmus, and nausea may occur.

D. **Use in pregnancy.** No assigned FDA category. Congenital malformations (fetal hydantoin syndrome) and hemorrhagic disease of the newborn have occurred with chronic use. However, this does not preclude its acute, short-term use in a seriously symptomatic patient (see p 407).

V. Drug or laboratory interactions.

A. The various drug interactions associated with chronic phenytoin dosing (ie, accelerated metabolism of other drugs) are not applicable to its acute emergency use.

B. Extracorporeal removal methods (eg, hemoperfusion and repeat-dose activated charcoal) will enhance phenytoin clearance. Supplemental dosing may be required during such procedures to maintain therapeutic levels.

VI. **Dosage and method of administration.**

A. **Parenteral.**

1. **Phenytoin.** Administer a loading dose of 15–20 mg/kg IV slowly at a rate not to exceed 50 mg/min (1 mg/kg/min in children). It may be diluted in 50–150 mL of normal saline with the use of an in-line filter. Phenytoin has been administered via the intraosseous route in children. Do ***not*** administer by the intramuscular route.
2. **Fosphenytoin.** Dosage is based on the phenytoin equivalent: 750 mg of fosphenytoin is equivalent to 500 mg of phenytoin. (For example, a loading dose of 1 g phenytoin would require a dose of 1.5 g fosphenytoin.) Dilute twofold to 10-fold in 5% dextrose or normal saline and administer no faster than 225 mg/min.

B. **Maintenance oral phenytoin dose.** Give 5 mg/kg/d as a single oral dose of capsules or twice daily for other dosage forms and in children. Monitor serum phenytoin levels.

VII. **Formulations.**

A. **Parenteral.** Phenytoin sodium, 50 mg/mL, 2- and 5-mL ampules and vials. Fosphenytoin sodium (Cerebyx), 150 mg (equivalent to 100 mg phenytoin) in 2-mL vials or 750 mg (equivalent to 500 mg phenytoin) in 10-mL vials.

B. **Oral.** Phenytoin sodium (Dilantin and others), 30-mg and 50-mg chewable tablets and 100-mg capsule.

C. The **suggested minimum stocking level** to treat a 70-kg adult for the first 24 hours is six vials (50 mg/mL, 5 mL each) or the equivalent.

## ▶ PHYSOSTIGMINE AND NEOSTIGMINE

*Thomas E. Kearney, PharmD*

I. **Pharmacology.** Physostigmine and neostigmine are carbamates and reversible inhibitors of acetylcholinesterase, the enzyme that degrades acetylcholine. They increase concentrations of acetylcholine, causing stimulation of both muscarinic and nicotinic receptors. The tertiary amine structure of physostigmine allows it to penetrate the blood-brain barrier and exert central cholinergic effects as well. Neostigmine, a quaternary ammonium compound, is unable to penetrate the CNS. Owing to cholinergic stimulation of the brainstem's reticular activating system, physostigmine has nonspecific analeptic (arousal) effects. After parenteral administration of physostigmine, the onset of action is within 3–8 minutes and the duration of effect is usually 30–90 minutes. The elimination half-life is 15–40 minutes. Neostigmine has a slower onset of 7–11 minutes and longer duration of effect of 60–120 minutes.

II. **Indications**

A. Physostigmine is used for the management of severe anticholinergic syndrome (agitated delirium, urinary retention, severe sinus tachycardia, or hyperthermia with absent sweating) from antimuscarinic agents (eg, benztropine, atropine, jimson weed or [*Datura*], diphenhydramine). See p 85 for discussion of anticholinergic toxicity. Although there are anecdotal case reports of its use to treat delirium and coma associated with GHB, baclofen, and several atypical antipsychotic (olanzapine, clozapine, quetiapine) agents, its safety and efficacy are uncertain with these intoxications.

B. Physostigmine is sometimes used diagnostically to differentiate functional psychosis from anticholinergic delirium.

C. Neostigmine is used primarily to reverse the effect of nondepolarizing neuromuscular blocking agents.

**III. Contraindications**

A. Physostigmine should ***not*** be used as an antidote for cyclic antidepressant overdose because it may worsen cardiac conduction disturbances, cause bradyarrhythmias or asystole, and aggravate or precipitate seizures.

B. Do ***not*** use physostigmine with concurrent use of depolarizing neuromuscular blockers (eg, succinylcholine).

C. Known hypersensitivity to agent or preservative (eg, benzyl alcohol, bisulfite).

D. Relative contraindications may include: bronchospastic disease or asthma, peripheral vascular disease, intestinal and bladder blockade, parkinsonian syndrome, and cardiac conduction defects (AV Block).

**IV. Adverse effects**

A. Bradycardia, heart block, and asystole.

B. Seizures (particularly with rapid administration or excessive dose of physostigmine).

C. Nausea, vomiting, hypersalivation, and diarrhea.

D. Bronchorrhea and bronchospasm (caution in asthmatics).

E. Fasciculations and muscle weakness.

F. **Use in pregnancy.** FDA category C (see p 407). Transient weakness has been noted in neonates whose mothers were treated with physostigmine for myasthenia gravis.

**V. Drug or laboratory interactions**

A. May potentiate agents metabolized by the cholinesterase enzyme (eg, depolarizing neuromuscular blocking agents—succinylcholine, cocaine, esmolol), cholinesterase inhibitors (eg, organophosphate and carbamate insecticides), and other cholinergic agents (eg, pilocarpine).

B. They may inhibit or reverse the actions of nondepolarizing neuromuscular blocking agents (eg, pancuronium, vecuronium, etc). Neostigmine is used therapeutically for this purpose.

C. They may have additive depressant effects on cardiac conduction in patients with cyclic antidepressant, beta-adrenergic antagonist, and calcium antagonist overdoses.

D. Physostigmine, through its nonspecific analeptic effects, may induce arousal in patients with GHB, opioid, benzodiazepine, sedative-hypnotic intoxication, or ketamine and propofol-induced anesthesia.

**VI. Dosage and method of administration**

A. **Physostigmine.** Parenteral: 0.5–2 mg slow (≤1 mg/min as adverse effects may be related to rapid administration) IV push (children, 0.02 mg/kg and given ≤0.5 mg/min) while a cardiac monitor is used to monitor the patient; repeat as needed every 10–30 minutes (symptoms may recrudesce due to the short half-life of physostigmine). Usual adult total dose is 4 mg. Atropine (see p 415) should be kept nearby to reverse excessive muscarinic stimulation and given at 1/2 the physostigmine dose (adults: 1–4 mg; children: 1 mg). Do ***not*** administer physostigmine intramuscularly or as a continuous intravenous infusion.

B. **Neostigmine.** Parenteral: 0.5–2 mg slow IV push (children: 0.025–0.08 mg/kg/dose) and repeat as required (total dose rarely exceeds 5 mg). Premedicate with glycopyrrolate (0.2 mg per mg of neostigmine; usual adult dose 0.2–0.6 mg; child 0.004–0.02 mg/kg) or atropine (0.4 mg per mg of neostigmine; usual adult dose 0.6–1.2 mg; child 0.01–0.04 mg/kg) several minutes before or simultaneously with neostigmine to prevent muscarinic effects (bradycardia, secretions).

**VII. Formulations**

**A. Parenteral.** Physostigmine salicylate (Antilirium), 1 mg/mL in 2-mL ampules (contains benzyl alcohol and bisulfite). Neostigmine methylsulfate (Prostigmine, others), 1:1000, 1:2000, 1:4000 in 1- and 10-mL ampules and vials (contains phenol or parabens).

**B.** The **suggested minimum stocking level** to treat a 70-kg adult for the first 24 hours is 10 ampules (2 mL each) for physostigmine and one 10-mL vial of 1:2000 or equivalent for neostigmine.

## ▶ POTASSIUM

*Judith A. Alsop, PharmD*

**I. Pharmacology.** Potassium is the primary intracellular cation, which is essential for maintenance of acid-base balance, intracellular tonicity, transmission of nerve impulses, contraction of cardiac, skeletal, and smooth muscle, and maintenance of normal renal function (and ability to alkalinize urine). Potassium also acts as an activator in many enzyme reactions and participates in many physiological processes such as carbohydrate metabolism, protein synthesis, and gastric secretion. Potassium is critical in regulating nerve conduction and muscle contraction, especially in the heart. A variety of toxins cause alterations in serum potassium levels (see Table I–27, p 37).

**II. Indications**

**A.** For treatment or prevention of hypokalemia (see p 37).

**B.** Supplement to bicarbonate therapy (see p 423) for alkalinization of urine.

**III. Contraindications**

**A.** Potassium should be administered cautiously in patients with renal impairment or impairment of renal excretion of potassium (ACE inhibitor toxicity and hypoaldosteronism, potassium-sparing diuretics) to avoid the potential for serious hyperkalemia.

**B.** Potassium should be administered cautiously in patients with impairment of intracellular transport of potassium (due to inhibition of Na-K ATPase pump with cardiac glycosides or inhibition of beta-adrenergic transport with beta blockers). Administration of potassium may lead to large incremental rises in serum levels.

**C.** Potassium should be administered cautiously in patients with intracellular spillage of potassium (rhabdomyolysis, hemolysis).

**D.** Potassium should be administered cautiously in patients with severe acute dehydration.

**IV. Adverse effects**

**A.** Nausea, vomiting, abdominal pain, and diarrhea with oral administration.

**B. Parenteral administration**. ***Note:*** DO NOT use undiluted injectable potassium preparations: direct injection can be lethal if given too rapidly; pain at the injection site and phlebitis may occur, especially during infusion of solutions containing greater than 30 mEq/L.

**C.** Hyperkalemia is the most serious adverse reaction (see p 37).

**D. Use in pregnancy.** FDA category C (indeterminate) (see p 407).

**V. Drug or laboratory interactions**

**A.** Drug interactions, see Contraindications, above.

**B.** Numerous IV incompatibilities: mannitol, diazepam, dobutamine, ergotamine, fat emulsion, nitroprusside, ondansetron, phenytoin, penicillin G sodium, promethazine, streptomycin.

**C.** Serum potassium levels may be fictitiously elevated if the blood sample is hemolyzed.

**VI. Dosage and method of administration (adults and children)**

**A.** The dose is variable and depends on the serum potassium level and severity of symptoms. The normal serum potassium level is 3.5–5 mEq/L. For parenteral administration, potassium must be diluted (see Adverse Effects, above).

**B.** The usual daily adult maintenance dose is 40–80 mEq. The usual daily pediatric maintenance dose is 2–3 mEq/kg or 40 mEq/$m^2$.

**C.** Potassium depletion resulting in a 1-mEq/L decrease in serum potassium may require 100–200 mEq for replacement to restore body stores. This replacement requirement will be offset with changes or corrections in intracellular transport (reversal of methylxanthine or beta-adrenergic agonist toxicity).

**D.** For a serum potassium of 2.5 mEq/L or greater, the maximum infusion rate of potassium in adults is 10 mEq/h, maximum concentration is 40 mEq/L, and maximum dose is 200 mEq per 24 hours. Do not exceed 1 mEq/kg/hr or 30 mEq per dose for IV use in pediatric patients. Adjust volume of fluid to body size of patient

**E.** For a serum potassium of less than 2.0 mEq/L, the maximum infusion rate of potassium in adults is 40 mEq/h, although infusions of 50 mEq/h have been used for short periods of time with constant EKG monitoring and frequent determination of laboratory values. The maximum concentration is 80 mEq/L, and maximum dose is 400 mEq per 24 hours.

**F.** Continuous cardiac monitoring with frequent laboratory monitoring is essential during administration of IV potassium.

**VII. Formulations**

**A.** Potassium acetate injection: 2 mEq/mL in 20-, 50-, and 100-mL vials; 4 mEq/mL in 50-mL vials.

**B.** Potassium chloride for injection concentrate: 2 mEq/mL in 250 and 500 mL; 10 mEq in 5-, 10-, 50-, and 100-mL vials and 5-mL additive syringes; 20 mEq in 10- and 20-mL vials, 10-mL additive syringes, and 10-mL ampules; 30 mEq in 15-, 20-, 30-, and 100-mL vials and 20-mL additive syringes; 40 mEq in 20-, 30-, 50-, and 100-mL vials, 20-mL ampules, and 20-mL additive syringes; 60 mEq in 30-mL vials; and 90 mEq in 30-mL vials.

**C.** The **suggested minimum stocking level** to treat a 70-kg adult for the first 24 hours is 500 mEq.

## ▶ PRALIDOXIME (2-PAM) AND OTHER OXIMES

*Richard J. Geller, MD, MPH*

**I. Pharmacology.** Oximes reverse acetylcholinesterase (AChE) inhibition by reactivating the phosphorylated cholinesterase enzyme and protecting the enzyme from further inhibition. Although this effect is most pronounced with organophosphate pesticides, positive clinical results have been seen with carbamate insecticides that have nicotinic toxicity and variably with cholinesterase inhibitors formulated as "nerve gas" chemical weapons. The clinical effects of oximes are most apparent at nicotinic receptors, with reversal of skeletal muscle weakness and muscle fasciculations. Their impact on muscarinic symptoms (salivation, sweating, bradycardia, and bronchorrhea) is significantly less pronounced than that of the antimuscarinic agents atropine and glycopyrrolate, along with which oximes invariably are administered (see p 415).

**A.** Pralidoxime chloride (2-PAM) is the only oxime currently approved for use in the United States. Oximes differ in their effectiveness against specific agents, doses, and side-effect profiles. In the United Kingdom, the methanesulfonate salt of pralidoxime, P2S, is used. In other European countries and South Africa, TMB4 and obidoxime (Toxogonin) are employed. 2-PAM methiodide is used in Japan. HI-6 is a promising oxime long under development.

**B.** Oximes are effective when given before the enzyme has been bound irreversibly ("aged") by the organophosphate, although they may have additional modes of action. The rate of aging varies considerably with each organophosphorus compound. For dimethylphosporylated AChE (eg, from dichlorvos, Malathion poisoning), the aging half-life is approximately 3.7 hours, whereas for diethylphosphorylated AChE (eg, from diazinon or parathion poisoning), the aging half-life is approximately 33 hours. For some chemical warfare agents, aging may occur in several minutes (soman-phosphorylated AChE aging half-life is about 2–6 minutes). However, late therapy with 2-PAM is appropriate (even several days after exposure), especially in patients poisoned with diethylating compounds and by fat-soluble compounds (eg, fenthion, demeton) that can be released from tissue stores over days, causing continuous or recurrent intoxication.

**C.** "Nerve" agents prepared as chemical warfare weapons, such as sarin, soman, tabun, and VX, are mechanistically similar to AChE-inhibiting insecticides. However, they are far more potent and are responsive only to certain oximes. Pralidoxime is not effective against tabun, for example, but trimedoxime (TMB4) may be. Current oxime research seeking agents with broader activity against nerve agents is evaluating the H oximes HLO-7 and HI-6.

**D.** Inadequate dosing of 2-PAM may be linked to the "intermediate syndrome," which is characterized by prolonged muscle weakness.

**E.** Peak plasma concentrations are reached within 5–15 minutes after intravenous 2-PAM administration. Pralidoxime is eliminated by renal excretion and hepatic metabolism, with a half-life of 0.8–2.7 hours.

**II. Indications**

**A.** Oximes are used to treat poisoning caused by cholinesterase inhibitor insecticides and nerve agents, ie, organophosphates, mixtures of organophosphorus and carbamate insecticides, and pure carbamate insecticide intoxication with nicotinic-associated symptoms. Pralidoxime has low toxicity, is possibly ineffective if treatment is delayed until after the cholinesterase enzyme has aged, is able to reverse nicotinic as well as muscarinic effects, and can reduce atropine requirements. For these reasons, pralidoxime should be used early and empirically for suspected cholinesterase inhibitor poisoning.

**B.** With carbamate poisoning, cholinesterase inhibition spontaneously resolves without "aging" of the enzyme. As a result, many references state that pralidoxime is not needed for carbamate poisoning. However, spontaneous reversal of enzyme inhibition may take up to 30 hours, and case reports suggest that pralidoxime is effective in human carbamate poisoning. Data suggesting increased toxicity of pralidoxime in carbaryl (Sevin) poisoning are based on limited animal studies, and the results are not generalizable to humans.

**III. Contraindications**

**A.** Use in patients with myasthenia gravis may precipitate a myasthenic crisis; however, in severe suspected cholinesterase inhibitor poisoning, benefit may exceed anticipated risk.

**B.** Use with caution and in reduced doses in patients with renal impairment.

**IV. Adverse effects**

**A.** Nausea, headache, dizziness, drowsiness, diplopia, and hyperventilation may occur.

**B.** Rapid intravenous administration may result in tachycardia, laryngospasm, muscle rigidity, and transient neuromuscular blockade. Hypertension, which is reversible with drug cessation or by administration of phentolamine, 5 mg IV, is also ascribed to rapid infusion.

**C. Use in pregnancy.** FDA category C (indeterminate). This does not preclude its acute, short-term use in a seriously symptomatic patient (see p 407).

**V. Drug or laboratory interactions**

**A. Muscarinic blockade** may occur more quickly when atropine (or glycopyrrolate) and pralidoxime are administered concurrently.

**B.** Red blood cell cholinesterase (ChE) activity is reactivated more readily reactivated by pralidoxime than by plasma ChE.

**VI. Dosage and method of administration.** For pralidoxime, the intravenous route is preferred. Intramuscular or subcutaneous injection is possible when the intravenous route is not immediately available. The Mark 1 autoinjector kit contains

600 mg pralidoxime (and 2 mg atropine) for IM use in the event of nerve gas attack.

**A. Initial dose.** Give 1–2 g (children, 25–50 mg/kg up to 1 g) as a continuous intravenous infusion in 100 mL of saline (1–2 mL/kg) over 15–30 minutes. Repeat the initial dose after 1 hour if muscle weakness or fasciculations are not relieved. Several grams may be required in some cases.

**B. Immediate field treatment of nerve agent poisoning** is accomplished with intramuscular 2-PAM. The dose is 600 mg IM for mild to moderate symptoms and up to 1800 mg for severe poisonings. The Mark I autoinjector kit contains 600 mg 2-PAM and 2 mg atropine and is designed for self-administration

**C. Maintenance infusion.** Because of the short half-life of 2-PAM and the longer duration of many organophosphorus compounds, toxicity frequently recurs, requiring repeated doses.

1. Discrete intermittent boluses may result in wide fluctuation in serum levels and erratic clinical effects. Therefore, after the initial dose it is preferable to give 2-PAM as a continuous intravenous infusion in a 1% solution (1 g in 100 mL saline) at a rate of 200–500 mg/h (children, 5–10 mg/kg/h) and titrate to the desired clinical response.
2. Despite earlier recommendations that 2-PAM should be given for only 24 hours, therapy may have to be continued for several days, particularly when long-acting, lipid-soluble organophosphates are involved. Gradually reduce the dose and carefully observe the patient for signs of recurrent muscle weakness or other signs of toxicity.
3. ***Note:*** 2-PAM may accumulate in patients with renal insufficiency.

**VII. Formulations**

**A. Parenteral.** Pralidoxime chloride (2-PAM, Protopam), 1 g with 20 mL sterile water.

**B.** The **suggested minimum stocking level** to treat a 70-kg adult for the first 24 hours is 12 vials. ***Note:*** In agricultural areas or urbanized regions preparing for possible accidental or terrorist release of a large amount of cholinesterase inhibitor agent, much larger stockpiling may be appropriate. Pralidoxime has been stockpiled by the Strategic National Stockpile (SNS) program as Mark I autoinjector kits and 1-g vials of pralidoxime chloride.

## ▶ PROPOFOL

*Richard Lynton, MD*

**I. Pharmacology**

**A.** Propofol (2,6-diisopropylphenol) is a sedative-hypnotic agent in a class of alkyl phenol compounds. It is an oil at room temperature, is highly lipid soluble, and is administered as an emulsion. It is also an antioxidant, anticonvulsant, and anti-inflammatory agent; reduces intracranial pressure; and has bronchodilator properties. Propofol's site of action is at the $GABA_A$ receptor, where it activates the chloride channel. There may also be some action at the glutamate and glycine receptor sites. Propofol is an antagonist at the *N*-methyl-D-aspartate (NMDA) receptor. It is also an inhibitor of cytochrome P-450 enzymes.

**B.** On infusion, its effects are seen within less than 3 minutes and peak concentrations are reached in less than 20 minutes.

**C.** It is highly protein bound, with a volume of distribution of 2–5 L/kg after a single infusion and 25–60 L/kg after a continuous infusion of longer than 7 days. Propofol has a high clearance rate estimated at 1.5–2.2 L/min. This clearance rate exceeds hepatic blood flow and suggests extrahepatic metabolism.

**D.** Propofol is metabolized rapidly in the liver by conjugation to glucuronide and sulfate intermediates that are water soluble and inactive. This occurs predominantly via oxidation by cytochrome P-450 2B6. P-450 isoforms 2A6, 2C8, 2C18, 2C19, and 1A2 are also involved in its metabolism to a lesser extent. There is minimal enterohepatic circulation, and less than 1% is excreted unchanged.

**II. Indications**

**A.** Propofol is most useful when the goal of anesthesia or sedation is rapid induction and recovery. It can be used for the induction and maintenance of anesthesia.

**B.** Propofol is useful in the intensive care unit for sedation of mechanically ventilated patients, especially patients with severe head injuries. It may also be beneficial for conscious sedation in certain settings.

**C.** Propofol may be effective as an adjunct anesthetic agent for refractory alcohol or other sedative-hypnotic withdrawal syndromes (such as GHB and barbiturates) and can also be used to treat status epilepticus.

**D.** Propofol has been used in rapid opiate detoxification protocols.

**III. Contraindications**

**A.** Not approved for pediatric patients less than 3 years of age who require sedation for mechanical ventilation. Several deaths have been reported when propofol was used in this setting.

**B.** It may be contraindicated for patients with seizure disorders (risk of seizures while weaning from therapy) and those with underlying hyperlipidemic states.

**C.** Hypersensitivity to propofol or additives such as sulfites and allergy to soybean or eggs.

**IV. Adverse effects**

**A.** Pain at the injection site can occur (use larger veins or premedicate with lidocaine).

**B.** Hypotension, bradycardia, supraventricular tachydysrhythmias, conduction disturbances, cough, and bronchospasm may occur.

**C.** Rapid infusion rates and anesthetic doses require respiratory support. Avoid rapid bolus doses in the elderly because of the higher risk of hypotension, bradycardia, apnea, and airway obstruction.

**D.** Anesthetic doses may be associated with myoclonus, posturing, and seizure-like movement phenomena (jerking, thrashing). Seizures have been noted when patients were weaned from propofol. Allergic reactions to metabisulfite are possible. Bacterial infections have also been noted.

**E. Propofol infusion syndrome,** a condition of lactic acidosis, renal failure, rhabdomyolysis, and cardiovascular collapse, has been reported after prolonged high-dose infusion in both pediatric and adult populations. Prolonged use (> 48 hours), infusion rates greater than 5mg/kg/h, and concomitant catecholamine administration (with or without steroids) have been implicated as risk factors.

**F.** Acute pancreatitis with single or prolonged use can occur. Hyperlipidemia can also occur after prolonged use.

**G.** Though it is not thought of as a drug of abuse, propofol abuse has been reported.

**H.** Urine may be discolored green or dark green.

**I. Use in pregnancy.** FDA category B. Propofol crosses the placenta and may be associated with neonatal CNS depression (see p 407).

**V. Drug or laboratory interactions**

**A.** An additive effect with other CNS depressants may result in lower propofol dosage requirements if given concomitantly. Through its inhibition of cytochrome P-450 2C9, 2D6, and 3A4, propofol may increase levels of midazolam, diazepam, and other opiates such as sufentanyl and alfentanyl, causing respiratory depression, bradycardia, and hypotension.

**B.** Propofol levels may be increased by lidocaine, bupivacaine, and halothane, producing an increased hypnotic effect.

**C.** Concurrent use with succinylcholine may result in bradycardia.

**VI. Dosage and method of administration.** Propofol currently is administered as an intravenous medication only, and the dosage must be individualized and titrated.

A. For **induction anesthesia,** give 1–2.5 mg/kg (slow infusion rate of about 40 mg every 10 seconds). If titrating with intermittent bolus doses (usually 40-mg increments), allow approximately 2 minutes for peak effect. In pediatric patients (3 to 16 years of age), give 2.5–3.5mg/kg over 20–30 seconds. For maintenance anesthesia, the dose should be titrated between 50 and 150 mcg/kg/min (or 3–9 mg/kg/h) and may be supplemented with intermittent bolus doses of 25–50 mg. Healthy pediatric patients (2 months–16 years) have been administered continuous infusion doses ranging between 7.5–18 mg/kg/h. After initial induction dose, may require a higher continuous infusion dose of up to 200 mcg/kg/min (or 12 mg/kg/h) for the first 10–15 minutes.

B. For **sedation,** use a lower dosage range of 25–75 mcg/kg/min (or 1.5–4.5 mg/kg/h) or titrate with intermittent bolus doses of 10–20 mg, then maintain with 25–50 mcg/kg/min (or 1.5–3 mg/kg/h).

C. Pediatric patients may require a higher dose: 2.5–3.5 mg/kg induction dose, followed immediately by 200–300 mcg/kg/min (or 12–18 mg/kg/h) for about 30 minutes, then 125–150 mcg/kg/min (or 7.5–9 mg/kg/h).

D. For patients older than 60 years of age, a lower induction dose of 1–1.5 mg/kg (infuse about 20 mg every 10 seconds) is recommended.

E. For rapid opiate detoxification, patients are given 2–4 mg/kg (or 6 mg/kg/h with intermittent bolus doses of 0.3–0.5 mg/kg) followed by maintenance of 3.5–6 mg/kg/h (usually for 5–8 hours). This is coupled with a neuromuscular blocker, and an opiate antagonist (naloxone or naltrexone) is administered after anesthesia is achieved.

**VII. Formulations**

A. **Parenteral.** Propofol (Diprivan) 1% (10 mg/mL) emulsion in 10% soybean oil with 2.25% glycerol and 1.25% purified egg phospholipid in 20-, 50-, or 100-mL vials and a 50-mL prefilled syringe. Contains disodium EDTA or sodium metabisulfite as a preservative. A 2% (20 mg/mL) emulsion has been formulated to provide the same amount of drug with less lipid concentration but has not been approved in the United States. ***Note:*** Propofol is provided as a ready- to-use preparation, but if dilution is necessary, use only $D_5W$ and do not dilute to concentrations less than 2 mg/mL.

B. The **suggested minimum stocking level** to treat a 70-kg adult for the first 24 hours is 2.5 g (provides anesthesia for a 6-hour interval).

## ▶ PROPRANOLOL

*Thomas E. Kearney, PharmD*

I. **Pharmacology.** Propranolol is a nonselective beta-adrenergic blocker that acts on beta-1 receptors in the myocardium and beta-2 receptors in the lung, vascular smooth muscle, and kidney. Within the myocardium, propranolol depresses heart rate, conduction velocity, myocardial contractility, and automaticity. Although propranolol is effective orally, for toxicologic emergencies it usually is administered by the intravenous route. After intravenous injection, the onset of action is nearly immediate and the duration of effect is 10 minutes to 2 hours, depending on the cumulative dose. The drug is eliminated by hepatic metabolism, with a half-life of about 2–3 hours. Propranolol also has antagonistic properties at the 5-$HT1_A$ receptor and has been used to treat serotonin syndrome with mixed success (anecdotal case reports).

**II. Indications**

A. To control excessive sinus tachycardia or ventricular arrhythmias caused by catecholamine excess (eg, theophylline or caffeine), sympathomimetic drug intoxication (eg, amphetamines, pseudoephedrine, or cocaine), or excessive myocardial sensitivity (eg, chloral hydrate, freons, or chlorinated and other hydrocarbons).

**B.** To control hypertension in patients with excessive beta-1–mediated increases in heart rate and contractility; used in conjunction with a vasodilator (eg, phentolamine) in patients with mixed alpha- and beta-adrenergic hyperstimulation.

**C.** To raise diastolic blood pressure in patients with hypotension caused by excessive beta-2–mediated vasodilation (eg, theophylline or metaproterenol).

**D.** May ameliorate or reduce beta-adrenergic–mediated electrolyte and other metabolic abnormalities (eg, hypokalemia, hyperglycemia, and lactic acidosis).

**E.** Serotonin syndrome (see p 21).

**III. Contraindications**

**A.** Use with extreme caution in patients with asthma, congestive heart failure, sinus node dysfunction, or another cardiac conduction disease and in those receiving calcium antagonists and other cardiac-depressant drugs.

**B.** Do not use as a single therapy for hypertension resulting from sympathomimetic overdose. Propranolol produces peripheral vascular beta blockade, which may abolish beta-2–mediated vasodilation and allow unopposed alpha-mediated vasoconstriction, resulting in paradoxic worsening of hypertension; coronary artery constriction may cause or exacerbate acute coronary syndrome.

**IV. Adverse effects**

**A.** Bradycardia and sinus and atrioventricular block.

**B.** Hypotension and congestive heart failure.

**C.** Bronchospasm in patients with asthma or bronchospastic chronic obstructive pulmonary disease. ***Note:*** Propranolol (in *small* intravenous doses) has been used successfully in asthmatic patients overdosed on theophylline or beta-2 agonists without precipitating bronchospasm.

**D. Use in pregnancy.** FDA category C (indeterminate). Propranolol may cross the placenta, and neonates delivered within 3 days of administration of this drug may have persistent beta-adrenergic blockade. However, this does not preclude its acute, short-term use in a seriously symptomatic patient (see p 407).

**V. Drug or laboratory interactions**

**A.** Propranolol may allow unopposed alpha-adrenergic stimulation in patients with mixed adrenergic stimulation (eg, epinephrine surge in patients with acute hypoglycemia, pheochromocytoma, or cocaine or amphetamine intoxication), resulting in severe hypertension or end-organ ischemia.

**B.** Propranolol has an additive hypotensive effect with other antihypertensive agents.

**C.** This drug may potentiate competitive neuromuscular blockers (see p 480).

**D.** Propranolol has additive depressant effects on cardiac conduction and contractility when given with calcium antagonists.

**E.** Cimetidine reduces hepatic clearance of propranolol.

**F.** Propranolol may worsen vasoconstriction caused by ergot alkaloids.

**VI. Dosage and method of administration**

**A. Parenteral.** Give 0.5–3 mg slow IV not to exceed 1 mg/min (children 0.01–0.1 mg/kg slow IV over 5 minutes; maximum 1 mg/dose) while monitoring heart rate and blood pressure; dose may be repeated as needed after 5–10 minutes. The dose required for complete beta receptor blockade is about 0.2 mg/kg. For serotonin syndrome, give 1 mg IV not to exceed 1 mg/min (children 0.1 mg/kg/dose over 10 min; maximum 1 mg/dose) every 2–5 minutes until a maximum of 5 mg. May repeat at 6- to 8-hour intervals.

**B. Oral.** Oral dosing may be initiated after the patient is stabilized; the dosage range is about 1–5 mg/kg/day in three or four divided doses for both children and adults. For serotonin syndrome, an adult dose of 20 mg every 8 hours has been used.

**VII. Formulations**

**A. Parenteral.** Propranolol hydrochloride (Inderal and others), 1 mg/mL in 1-mL ampules, vials, and prefilled syringes.

B. **Oral.** Propranolol hydrochloride (Inderal and others), 60-, 80-, 120-, and 160-mg sustained-release capsules; 10-, 20-, 40-, 60-, 80-, and 90-mg tablets; 4-, 8-, and 80-mg/mL oral solution and concentrate.

C. The **suggested minimum stocking level** to treat a 70-kg adult for the first 24 hours is 10 ampules or syringes.

## ▶ PROTAMINE

*Thomas E. Kearney, PharmD*

I. **Pharmacology.** Protamine is a cationic protein obtained from fish sperm that rapidly binds to and inactivates heparin. The onset of action after intravenous administration is nearly immediate (30–60 seconds) and lasts up to 2 hours. It also partially neutralizes low-molecular-weight heparins (LMWHs) and can act as an anticoagulant by inhibiting thromboplastin.

II. **Indications**

A. Protamine is used for the reversal of the anticoagulant effect of heparin when an excessively large dose has been administered inadvertently. Protamine generally is not needed for treatment of bleeding during standard heparin therapy because discontinuance of the heparin infusion is generally sufficient.

B. Protamine may be used for reversal of regional anticoagulation in the hemodialysis circuit in cases in which anticoagulation of the patient would be contraindicated (ie, active GI or CNS bleeding).

III. **Contraindications**

A. Do not give protamine to patients with known sensitivity to the drug. Diabetic patients who have used protamine insulin may be at the greatest risk for hypersensitivity reactions.

B. Protamine reconstituted with benzyl alcohol should not be used in neonates because of suspected toxicity from the alcohol.

IV. **Adverse effects**

A. Rapid intravenous administration is associated with hypotension, bradycardia, and anaphylactoid reactions. Have epinephrine (see p 448), diphenhydramine (p 442), and cimetidine or another $H_2$ blocker (p 433) ready. Reaction may be prevented by avoiding high infusion rates of > 5 mg/min.

B. A rebound effect caused by heparin may occur within 8 hours of protamine administration.

C. Excess doses may lead to anticoagulation and the risk of bleeding.

D. **Use in pregnancy.** FDA category C (indeterminate). Maternal hypersensitivity reaction or hypotension could result in placental ischemia. However, this does not preclude its acute, short-term use for a seriously symptomatic patient (see p 407).

V. **Drug or laboratory interactions.** No known drug interactions other than the reversal of the effect of heparin.

VI. **Dosage and method of administration**

A. Administer protamine by slow intravenous injection over at least 1–3 minutes, not to exceed 50 mg in a 10-minute period.

B. The dose of protamine depends on the total dose and the time since administration of heparin.

1. If immediately after heparin administration, give 1–1.5 mg of protamine for each 100 units of heparin.
2. If 30–60 minutes after heparin administration, give only 0.5–0.75 mg of protamine for each 100 units of heparin.
3. If 2 hours or more after heparin administration, give only 0.25–0.375 mg of protamine for each 100 units of heparin.
4. If heparin was being administered by constant infusion, give 25–50 mg of protamine.

**C.** If the patient is overdosed with an unknown quantity of heparin, give an empiric dose of 25–50 mg over 15 minutes (to minimize hypotension) and determine the activated partial thromboplastin time (aPTT) after 5–15 minutes and for up to 2–8 hours to determine the need for additional doses.

**D. For an overdose of a low-molecular-weight heparin:**

1. **Dalteparin or tinazaparin.** Give 1 mg of protamine for every 100 anti-factor Xa international units of dalteparin and tinzaparin.
2. **Enoxaparin.** Give 1 mg of protamine for each 1 mg of enoxaparin.
3. If the overdose amount is unknown, consider an empiric dose of 25–50 mg given over 15 minutes. The anti-Xa:IIa factor ratios vary for LMWH products, and if they are high, as with a LMW heparinoid (eg, danaparoid), protamine may be ineffective. Anti-factor Xa activity levels and aPTT values are usually not completely reversed, but the hemorrhagic effect may be neutralized. LMWHs have longer half-lives (4–6 hours) and accumulate with renal insufficiency; therefore, coagulopathies may persist and protamine should be considered even several hours after the overdose.

**VII. Formulations**

**A. Parenteral.** Protamine sulfate, 50 mg in 5-mL vials or 250 mg in 25-mL vials.

**B.** The **suggested minimum stocking level** to treat a 70-kg adult for the first 24 hours is one 25 mL vial.

# ▶ PRUSSIAN BLUE

*Sandra A. Hayashi, PharmD*

**I. Pharmacology.** Insoluble Prussian blue (ferric hexacyanoferrate) has been used to treat radioactive and nonradioactive cesium and thallium poisonings. Owing to the long half-lives of these isotopes, ingestion can pose significant long-term health risks. Insoluble Prussian blue binds thallium and cesium in the gut as they undergo enterohepatic recirculation, enhancing fecal excretion. Proposed mechanisms of binding include chemical cation exchange, physical adsorption, and mechanical trapping within the crystal lattice structure. Insoluble Prussian blue is not absorbed across the intact GI wall.

**II. Indications.** Known or suspected internal contamination by:

**A.** Radioactive cesium (eg, $^{137}Cs$) and nonradioactive cesium.

**B.** Radioactive thallium (eg, $^{201}Tl$) and nonradioactive thallium.

**III. Contraindications.** There are no absolute contraindications. The efficacy of the agent relies on a functioning GI tract; thus, ileus may preclude its use and effectiveness.

**IV. Adverse effects**

**A.** Upset stomach and constipation.

**B.** May bind other elements, causing electrolyte or nutritional deficits, such as asymptomatic hypokalemia.

**C.** Does not treat the complications of radiation exposure.

**D.** Blue discoloration of feces (and teeth if capsules are opened).

**E. Use in pregnancy.** FDA category C (indeterminate) (see p 407). Since Prussian blue is not absorbed from the GI tract, effects on the fetus are not expected.

**V. Drug or laboratory interactions**

**A.** No major interactions.

**B.** May decrease absorption of tetracycline.

**VI. Dosage and method of administration.**

**A.** Adults and adolescents: Usual dose is 3 g orally TID (9 g daily), although higher doses (> 10 g daily) are often used for acute thallium poisoning (particularly if thallium is present in the GI tract). Doses may be decreased to 1 to 2 g TID when internal radioactivity is reduced and to improve patient tolerance.

B. Pediatrics (2–12 years): 1 g orally TID.
C. Capsules may be opened and mixed with food or water for those who have difficulty swallowing. However, this may cause blue discoloration of the mouth and teeth.
D. Co-ingestion with food may increase effectiveness by stimulating bile secretion.
E. Treatment should continue for a minimum of 30 days. The duration of treatment should be guided by the level of contamination as measured by the amount of residual whole-body radioactivity.

**VII. Formulations**

A. Oral: Insoluble Prussian blue powder (Radiogardase™), 0.5 g in gelatin capsules, packaged in an amber bottle of 30 capsules each.
B. The **suggested minimum stocking level** to treat a 70-kg adult for the first month is 540 capsules (18 bottles, 30 capsules each) based on a daily dose of 9 G. At this time, the minimum order is 25 bottles. Prussian blue is kept in the Strategic National Stockpile (SNS) at the CDC. The Radiation Emergency Assistance Center (REAC/TS), can be contacted for information on obtaining Prussian blue and its recommended dosing ([865] 576-3131, on the Internet at www.orau.gov/reacts).

## ▶ PYRIDOXINE (VITAMIN $B_6$)

*Thomas E. Kearney, PharmD*

I. **Pharmacology.** Pyridoxine (vitamin $B_6$) is a water-soluble B-complex vitamin that acts as a cofactor in many enzymatic reactions. Overdose involving isoniazid or other monomethylhydrazines (eg, *Gyromitra* mushrooms) may cause seizures by interfering with pyridoxine utilization in the brain, and pyridoxine given in high doses can control these seizures rapidly and may hasten consciousness. It can also correct the lactic acidosis secondary to isoniazid-induced impaired lactate metabolism. In ethylene glycol intoxication, pyridoxine may enhance metabolic conversion of the toxic metabolite glyoxylic acid to the nontoxic product glycine. Pyridoxine is well absorbed orally but usually is given intravenously for urgent uses. The biologic half-life is about 15–20 days.

II. **Indications**

A. Acute management of seizures caused by intoxication with isoniazid (see p 233), hydrazine, *Gyromitra* mushrooms (p 272), or possibly cycloserine. Pyridoxine may act synergistically with diazepam (p 419).
B. Adjunct to therapy for ethylene glycol intoxication.
C. May improve dyskinesias induced by levodopa.

III. **Contraindications.** Use caution in patients with known sensitivity to pyridoxine or parabens preservative.

IV. **Adverse effects**

A. Usually no adverse effects are noted from acute dosing of pyridoxine.
B. Chronic excessive doses may result in peripheral neuropathy (see p 30).
C. Use of the 1-mL vials may cause mild CNS depression owing to the preservative if 50 or more vials (to deliver 5 g or more of pyridoxine) are administered (equivalent to 250 mg or more of chlorobutanol).
D. **Use in pregnancy.** FDA category A (see p 407). However, chronic excessive use in pregnancy has resulted in pyridoxine withdrawal seizures in neonates.

V. **Drug or laboratory interactions.** No adverse interactions are associated with acute dosing.

VI. **Dosage and method of administration**

A. **Isoniazid poisoning.** Give 1 g of pyridoxine intravenously for each gram of isoniazid known to have been ingested (as much as 52 g has been administered and tolerated). Dilute in 50 mL dextrose or saline and give over 5 minutes (rate of 1 g/min). If the ingested amount is unknown, administer 4–5 g IV empirically and repeat every 5–20 minutes as needed.

B. **Monomethylhydrazine poisoning.** Give 25 mg/kg IV; repeat as necessary.

C. **Ethylene glycol poisoning.** Give 50 mg IV or IM every 6 hours until intoxication is resolved.

D. **Cycloserine poisoning.** A dosage of 300 mg/day has been recommended.

VII. **Formulations**

A. **Parenteral.** Pyridoxine hydrochloride (various), 100 mg/mL (10% solution) in 1- and 30-mL vials (1-mL vial contains the preservative chlorobutanol, and 30-mL vial contains parabens). ***Note:*** Only one US company, Legere Pharmaceuticals (Scottsdale, AZ; phone: 800-528-3144), manufactures and distributes the 3-g (30-mL) vials. See adverse effects above regarding use of the 1-mL vials.

B. The **suggested minimum stocking level** to treat a 70-kg adult for the first 24 hours is 20 g (7 vials, 30 mL each, or the equivalent).

## ▶ SILYMARIN OR MILK THISTLE (*SILYBUM MARIANUM*)

*Christine A. Haller, MD*

I. **Pharmacology.** Extracts of the milk thistle plant have been used since ancient times to treat a variety of liver and gallbladder diseases, including cholestasis, jaundice, cirrhosis, acute and chronic hepatitis, and primary malignancies, and to protect the liver against toxin-induced injury. The extract of the ripe seeds and leaves contains 70–80% of the active flavonoid silymarin, which is composed chiefly of silybin A and B. The hypothesized mechanism of action of silymarin, supported by in vitro and animal studies, is twofold: alteration of hepatocyte cell membrane permeability, preventing toxin penetration, and increased ribosomal protein synthesis, promoting hepatocyte regeneration. Although the efficacy of milk thistle for toxin-induced liver injury in humans has not been established clearly, it has been associated with reduced liver damage when administered within 48 hours of *Amanita phalloides* ingestion. Competitive inhibition of *A. phalloides* toxin receptor binding has been demonstrated. One study also showed preservation of hepatic glutathione stores in rats exposed to high levels of acetaminophen.

Silymarin also is reported to have antifibrotic, anti-inflammatory, and antioxidant activity and may have therapeutic efficacy in the treatment of prostate and skin cancer. There is preliminary evidence that milk thistle constituents may also protect against the nephrotoxic effects of drugs such as acetaminophen, cisplatin, and vincristine.

II. **Indications.** Unproven but possibly effective as adjuvant therapy in cases of acute hepatic injury caused by *Amanita phalloides* mushroom ingestion, acetaminophen toxicity, and potentially other chemical and drug-induced liver diseases. Silymarin is available in the United States and Europe as a parenteral drug, and milk thistle extracts can also be purchased as over-the-counter dietary supplements for oral use.

III. **Contraindications.** None reported.

IV. **Adverse effects** are few and generally mild.

A. Nausea, diarrhea, abdominal fullness or pain, flatulence, and anorexia may occur.

B. Milk thistle is a member of the *Asteraceae* (daisy) family and can cause an allergic reaction in ragweed-sensitive individuals, including rash, urticaria, pruritus, and anaphylaxis.

C. **Use in pregnancy.** FDA category B. Insufficient reliable information is available (see p 407).

V. **Drug or laboratory interactions.** Although milk thistle has been shown to induce slight cytochrome P-450 enzyme inhibition in vitro, significant drug interactions with milk thistle extract have not been demonstrated in humans.

**VI. Dosage and method of administration**

**A.** Oral doses used in published studies have ranged from 280 to 800 mg/day of standardized silymarin. A typical dose used for toxic hepatitis is 420 mg/day in two or three oral doses.

**B.** Intravenous dosing for *Amanita phalloides* mushroom poisoning is 20–50 mg/kg over 24 hours divided into four infusions. Each intravenous dose is administered over 2 hours.

**VII. Formulations**

**A. Oral.** In the United States, milk thistle extract is available as a nonprescription dietary supplement (eg, Thisilyn). Oral pharmaceutical formulations available in Europe include Legalon (standardized to contain 70% silymarin) and Silibide (isolated silibinin complexed with phosphatidylcholine). Because silymarin is poorly water soluble, milk thistle tea is not considered an effective preparation.

**B. Parenteral.** An injectable preparation of 50 mg/mL silymarin is now available in the United States (Apothecare 1-800-969-6601).

# ▶ SUCCIMER (DMSA)

*Michael J Kosnett, MD, MPH*

**I. Pharmacology**

**A.** Succimer (meso-2,3-dimercaptosuccinic acid [DMSA]) is a chelating agent that is used in the treatment of intoxication from several heavy metals. A water-soluble analog of BAL (dimercaprol; see p 413), succimer enhances the urinary excretion of lead and mercury. Its effect on elimination of the endogenous minerals calcium, iron, and magnesium is insignificant. Minor increases in zinc and copper excretion may occur. In an animal model, oral succimer was not associated with a significant increase in GI absorption of lead; the effect of oral succimer on GI absorption of mercury and arsenic is not known.

**B.** After oral administration, peak blood concentrations occur in approximately 3 hours. Distribution is predominantly extracellular, and in the blood it is extensively bound (> 90%) to plasma proteins. Succimer is eliminated primarily in the urine, where 80–90% appears as mixed disulfides, mainly 2:1 or 1:1 cysteine-succimer adducts. Studies suggest that these adducts, rather than the parent drug, may be responsible for metal chelating activity in vivo. The elimination half-life of transformed succimer is approximately 2–4 hours. Renal clearance may be diminished in the setting of pediatric lead intoxication.

**II. Indications**

**A.** Succimer is approved for treatment of **lead** intoxication, where it is associated with increased urinary excretion of the metal and concurrent reversal of metal-induced enzyme inhibition. Oral succimer is comparable to parenteral calcium EDTA (see p 446) in decreasing blood lead concentrations. Although succimer treatment has been associated with subjective clinical improvement, controlled clinical trials demonstrating therapeutic efficacy have not been reported. A recent large, randomized, double-blind placebo-controlled trial of succimer in children with blood lead concentrations between 25 and 44 mcg/dL found no evidence of benefit on clinical outcome or long-term blood lead reduction.

**B.** Succimer is protective against the acute lethal and nephrotoxic effects of **mercuric salts** in animal models and increases urinary mercury excretion in animals and humans. It therefore may have clinical utility in the treatment of human poisoning by inorganic mercury.

**C.** Succimer is protective against acute lethal effects of **arsenic** in animal models and may have potential utility in acute human arsenic poisoning.

**III. Contraindications.** History of allergy to the drug. Because succimer and its transformation products undergo renal elimination, safety and efficacy in patients with severe renal insufficiency are uncertain. There is no available evidence that succimer increases hemodialysis clearance of toxic metals in anuric patients.

**IV. Adverse effects**

**A.** Gastrointestinal disturbances including anorexia, nausea, vomiting, and diarrhea are the most common side effects and occur in less than 10% of patients. There may be a mercaptan-like odor to the urine; this has no clinical significance.

**B.** Mild, reversible increases in liver transaminases have been observed in 6–10% of patients.

**C.** Rashes, some requiring discontinuation of treatment, have been reported in less than 5% of patients.

**D.** Isolated cases of mild to moderate neutropenia have been reported.

**E.** Minimal increases (less than twofold) in urinary excretion of zinc and copper have been observed and have minor or no clinical significance.

**F. Use in pregnancy.** FDA category C (indeterminate). Succimer has produced adverse fetal effects when administered to pregnant animals in amounts one to two orders of magnitude greater than recommended human doses. However, succimer has also diminished the adverse effects of several heavy metals in animal studies. Its effect on human pregnancy has not been determined (see p 407).

**V. Drug or laboratory interactions.** No known interactions. Concurrent administration with other chelating agents has not been studied adequately.

**VI. Dosage and method of administration (adults and children)**

**A. Lead poisoning.** Availability in the United States is limited to an oral formulation (100-mg capsules) officially approved by the FDA for use in children with blood lead levels ≥45 mcg/dL. However, DMSA can also lower lead concentrations in adults. ***Note:*** Administration of DMSA should never be a substitute for removal from lead exposure. In adults, the federal OSHA lead standard requires removal from occupational lead exposure of any worker with a single blood lead concentration in excess of 60 mcg/dL or an average of three successive values in excess of 50 mcg/dL; however, recent data suggest that removal at lower blood lead levels may be warranted. ***Prophylactic chelation,*** defined as the routine use of chelation to prevent elevated blood lead concentrations or lower blood lead levels below the standard in asymptomatic workers, ***is not permitted.*** Consult the local or state health department or OSHA (see Table IV–3, p 535) for more detailed information.

1. Give 10 mg/kg (or 350 mg/m$^2$ in children) orally every 8 hours for 5 days and then give the same dose every 12 hours for 2 weeks.
2. An additional course of treatment may be considered. based on posttreatment blood lead levels and the persistence or recurrence of symptoms. Although blood lead levels may decline by more than 50% during treatment, patients with high body lead burdens may experience rebound to within 20% of pretreatment levels as bone stores equilibrate with tissue levels. Check blood lead levels 1 and 7–21 days after chelation to assess the extent of rebound and/or the possibility of reexposure.
3. Experience with oral succimer for severe lead intoxications (ie, lead encephalopathy) is very limited. In such cases, consideration should be given to parenteral therapy with calcium EDTA (see p 446).

**B. Mercury and arsenic poisoning**

1. Intoxication by inorganic mercury compounds and arsenic compounds may result in severe gastroenteritis and shock. In such circumstances, the capacity of the gut to absorb orally administered succimer may be impaired severely, and use of an available parenteral agent such as unithiol (see p 506) or BAL (p 413) may be preferable.
2. Give 10 mg/kg (or 350 mg/m$^2$) orally every 8 hours for 5 days and then give the same dose every 12 hours for 2 weeks. Extending the duration of treatment in the presence of continuing symptoms or high levels of urinary metal excretion should be considered but is of undetermined value.

VII. **Formulations**

A. **Oral.** Succimer, *meso*-2,3-dimercaptosuccinic acid, DMSA (Chemet), 100-mg capsules in bottles of 100.

B. **Parenteral.** A parenteral form of DMSA (sodium 2,3-dimercaptosuccinate), infused at a dose of 1–2 g per day, has been in use in the People's Republic of China but is not available in the United States.

C. The **suggested minimum stocking level** to treat a 70-kg adult for the first 24 hours is 21 capsules.

# ▶ TETANUS TOXOID AND IMMUNE GLOBULIN

*John H. Tegzes, VMD*

I. **Pharmacology.** Tetanus is caused by tetanospasmin, a protein toxin produced by *Clostridium tetani* (see Tetanus, p 353).

A. **Tetanus toxoid** uses modified tetanospasmin, which has been made nontoxic but still retains the ability to stimulate the formation of antitoxin. Tetanus toxoid provides active immunization to those with known, complete tetanus immunization histories as well as those with unknown or incomplete histories.

B. Human **tetanus immune globulin** (antitoxin) provides passive immunity by neutralizing circulating tetanospasmin and unbound toxin in a wound. It does not have an effect on toxin that already is bound to neural tissue, and tetanus antibody does not penetrate the blood-brain barrier.

II. **Indications.** All wound injuries require consideration of tetanus prevention and treatment. This includes animal and insect bites and stings, injections from contaminated hypodermic needles, deep puncture wounds (including high-pressure, injection-type chemical exposures such as those from paint guns), burns, and crush wounds.

A. **Tetanus toxoid prophylaxis** (active immunization) is given as a primary series of three doses in childhood. The first and second doses are given 4 to 8 weeks apart, and the third dose is given 6 to 12 months after the second. A booster dose is required every 10 years.

1. **Unknown or incomplete history** of a previous primary series of three doses: tetanus toxoid is indicated for all wounds, including clean minor wounds.
2. **Known complete histories** of a primary series of three doses: tetanus toxoid is indicated for clean, minor wounds if it has been longer than 10 years since the last dose and for all other wounds if it has been longer than 5 years since the last dose.

B. **Tetanus immune globulin** (passive immunization) is indicated for persons with tetanus. Antitoxin also is indicated as prophylaxis for wounds that are neither clean nor minor in persons who have unknown or incomplete histories of the primary three-dose series of tetanus toxoid.

III. **Contraindications**

A. **Toxoid**

1. History of a severe allergic reaction (acute respiratory distress and collapse) after a previous dose of tetanus toxoid.
2. History of encephalopathy within 72 hours of a previous dose of tetanus toxoid.
3. Precautions should be taken in individuals with histories of fever greater than 40.5°C (104.9°F) within 48 hours of a previous dose, collapse or shock-like state within 48 hours of a previous dose, or seizures within 3 days of a previous dose.

B. **Antitoxin.** The *equine* tetanus antitoxin is contraindicated in persons who have had previous hypersensitivity or serum sickness reactions to other equine-derived products. Preferably, use the *human* tetanus immune globulin product in all cases if it is available.

**IV. Adverse effects of the toxoid**

**A.** Local effects, including pain, erythema, and induration at the injection site. These effects are usually self-limiting and do not require therapy.

**B.** Exaggerated local (Arthus-like) reactions. These unusual reactions may present as extensive painful swelling from the shoulder to the elbow. They generally occur in individuals with preexisting very high serum tetanus antitoxin levels.

**C.** Severe systemic reactions such as generalized urticaria, anaphylaxis, and neurologic complications have been reported. A few cases of peripheral neuropathy and Guillain-Barré syndrome have also been reported.

**D. Use in pregnancy.** FDA category C (indeterminate). Tetanus toxoid may be used during pregnancy. Pregnant patients not previously vaccinated should receive the three-dose primary series (see p 407).

**V. Drug or laboratory interactions.** None.

**VI. Dosage and method of administration**

**A. Tetanus toxoid**

**1.** Adult Td consists of tetanus toxoid, 5 LF U/0.5 mL, and diphtheria toxoid, adsorbed 2 LF U/0.5 mL up to 12.5 LF U/0.5 mL. A 0.5-mL dose is given intramuscularly. Adult Td is used for routine boosters and primary vaccination in persons 7 years old and older. Three doses constitute a primary series of Td. The first two doses are separated by a minimum of 4 weeks, with the third dose given 6–12 months after the second. Boosters are given every 10 years thereafter.

**2.** In children less than 7 years old, primary tetanus immunization is with tetanus toxoid in combination with diphtheria toxoid and acellular pertussis (DTaP). Pediatric DT (without pertussis) also may be used when there is a contraindication to pertussis vaccine. At least 4 weeks should separate the first and second and the second and third doses. A fourth dose should be given no less than 6 months after the third dose. All doses are 0.5 mL given intramuscularly and usually contain tetanus toxoid 5 LF U/0.5 mL.

**B. Antitoxin.** Human tetanus immune globulin is given at 3000–5000 units intramuscularly, in divided doses, for the treatment of tetanus in children and adults, with part of the dose infiltrated around the wound. Doses of 250–500 units intramuscularly are given for postexposure prophylaxis.

**VII. Formulations**

**A. Adult.** Tetanus toxoid 5 LF U/0.5 mL in combination with diphtheria toxoid, adsorbed 2 LF U/0.5 mL, supplied in 0.5-mL single-dose vials; tetanus toxoid 5 LF U/0.5 mL in combination with diphtheria toxoid, adsorbed 6.6 LF U/0.5 mL to 12.5 LF U/0.5 mL, supplied in 5-mL multidose vials.

**B. Pediatric.** Pediatric DT, 0.5-mL single-dose vials, and 5-mL multidose vials; DTaP, containing diphtheria toxoid 6.7 LF U/0.5 mL, tetanus toxoid 5 LF U/0.5 mL, and pertussis vaccine 4 protective units/0.5 mL.

**C. Human tetanus immune globulin.** Supplied in single-dose vials containing 250 units.

**D.** The **suggested minimum stocking level** to treat a 70-kg adult for the first 24 hours is a single-dose vial of Td and immune globulin.

## ▶ THIAMINE (THIAMIN, VITAMIN $B_1$)

*Thomas E. Kearney, PharmD*

**I. Pharmacology.** Thiamine (vitamin $B_1$) is a water-soluble vitamin that acts as an essential cofactor for various pathways of carbohydrate metabolism. Thiamine also acts as a cofactor in the metabolism of glyoxylic acid (produced in ethylene glycol intoxication). Thiamine deficiency may result in beriberi and Wernicke-

Korsakoff syndrome. Thiamine is absorbed rapidly after oral, intramuscular, or intravenous administration. However, parenteral administration is recommended for initial management of thiamine deficiency syndromes.

**II. Indications**

**A.** Empiric therapy to prevent and treat Wernicke-Korsakoff syndrome in alcoholic or malnourished patients. This also includes any patient presenting with an altered mental status of unknown etiology. Thiamine should be given concurrently with glucose in such patients.

**B.** Adjunctive treatment in patients poisoned with ethylene glycol to possibly enhance the detoxification of glyoxylic acid.

**III. Contraindications.** Use caution in patients with known sensitivity to thiamine or preservatives.

**IV. Adverse effects**

**A.** Anaphylactoid reactions, vasodilation, hypotension, weakness, and angioedema after rapid intravenous injection. This may be attributable to the vehicle or contaminates of thiamine preparations in the past; rare reaction with new preparations.

**B.** Acute pulmonary edema in patients with beriberi owing to a sudden increase in vascular resistance.

**C. Use in pregnancy.** FDA category A for doses up to the recommended daily allowance (RDA) and category C for pharmacologic doses (see p 407).

**V. Drug or laboratory interactions.** Theoretically, thiamine may enhance the effect of neuromuscular blockers, although the clinical significance is unclear.

**VI. Dosage and method of administration.** Parenteral, 100 mg (children, 50 mg) slow IV (over 5 minutes) or IM; may repeat every 8 hours at doses of 5–100 mg. For Wernicke's encephalopathy, follow with daily parenteral doses of 50–100 mg until the patient is taking a regular diet. Doses as high as 1 g over the first 12 hours have been given to patients with acute Wernicke-Korsakoff syndrome.

**VII. Formulations**

**A. Parenteral.** Thiamine hydrochloride (various), 100 mg/mL, in 1- and 2-mL Tubex and multiple-dose vials (vials may contain benzyl alcohol).

**B.** The **suggested minimum stocking level** to treat a 70-kg adult for the first 24 hours is 1 g (five 2-mL multiple-dose vials or the equivalent).

# ▶ THIOSULFATE, SODIUM

*Cindy Burkhardt, PharmD*

**I. Pharmacology.** Sodium thiosulfate is a sulfur donor that promotes the conversion of cyanide to the less toxic thiocyanate by the sulfur transferase enzyme rhodanese. Unlike nitrites, thiosulfate is essentially nontoxic and may be given empirically in suspected cyanide poisoning. Well-designed animal studies suggest enhanced antidotal efficacy when hydroxocobalamin is used with thiosulfate.

**II. Indications**

**A.** May be given alone or in combination with nitrites (see p 279) or hydroxocobalamin (see p 459) in patients with acute cyanide poisoning.

**B.** Empiric treatment of possible cyanide poisoning associated with smoke inhalation.

**C.** Prophylaxis during nitroprusside infusions (see p 485).

**D.** Extravasation of mechlorethamine (infiltrate locally; see pp 101 and 102).

**E.** Bromate salt ingestion (unproved).

**III. Contraindications.** No known contraindications.

**IV. Adverse effects**

**A.** Intravenous infusion may produce burning sensation, muscle cramping and twitching, and nausea and vomiting.

**B. Use in pregnancy.** FDA category C (indeterminate). This does not preclude its acute, short-term use in a seriously symptomatic patient (see p 407).

**V. Drug or laboratory interactions.** Thiosulfate falsely lowers measured cyanide concentrations in several methods.

**VI. Dosage and method of administration**

**A. For cyanide poisoning.** Administer 12.5 g (50 mL of 25% solution) IV at 2.5–5 mL/min. The pediatric dose is 400 mg/kg (1.6 mL/kg of 25% solution) up to 50 mL. Half the initial dose may be given after 30–60 minutes if needed.

**B. For prophylaxis during nitroprusside infusions.** The addition of 10 mg thiosulfate for each milligram of nitroprusside in the intravenous solution has been reported to be effective, although physical compatibility data are not available.

**VII. Formulations**

**A. Parenteral.** As a component of the cyanide antidote package, thiosulfate sodium, 25% solution, 50 mL. Also available separately in vials and ampules containing 2.5 g/10 mL or 1 g/10 mL.

**B.** The **suggested minimum stocking level** to treat a 70-kg adult for the first 24 hours is two cyanide antidote packages (one should be kept in the emergency department). Available from Taylor Pharmaceuticals.

## ▶ UNITHIOL (DMPS)

*Michael J. Kosnett, MD, MPH*

**I. Pharmacology.** Unithiol (DMPS; 2,3-dimercaptopropanol-sulfonic acid), a dimercapto chelating agent that is a water-soluble analog of BAL (see p 417), is used in the treatment of poisoning by several heavy metals, principally mercury, arsenic, and lead. Available on the official formularies of Russia and former Soviet countries since 1958 and in Germany since 1976, unithiol has been legally available from compounding pharmacists in the United States since 1999. The drug can be administered orally and parenterally. Oral bioavailability is approximately 50%, with peak blood concentrations occurring in approximately 3.7 hours. It is bound extensively to plasma proteins, mainly albumin. More than 80% of an intravenous dose is excreted in the urine, 10% as unaltered unithiol and 90% as transformed products, predominantly cyclic DMPS sulfides. The elimination half-life for total unithiol is approximately 20 hours. Unithiol and/or its in vivo biotransformation products form complexes with a variety of inorganic and organic metal compounds, increasing excretion of the metal in the urine and decreasing its concentration in various organs, particularly the kidney. Unlike BAL, unithiol does not redistribute mercury to the brain.

**II. Indications**

**A.** Unithiol has been used primarily in the treatment of intoxication by **mercury**, **arsenic**, and **lead**. In animal models, unithiol has averted or reduced the acute toxic effects of inorganic mercury salts and inorganic arsenic when administered promptly (minutes to hours) after exposure. Unithiol is associated with a reduction in tissue levels of mercury, arsenic, and lead in experimental animals, and it increases the excretion of those metals in humans. However, randomized, double-blind, placebo-controlled clinical trials demonstrating therapeutic efficacy in acute or chronic heavy metal poisoning have not been reported.

**B.** Animal studies and a few case reports suggest that unithiol may have utility in the treatment of poisoning by **bismuth** compounds.

**III. Contraindications**

**A.** History of allergy to the drug.

**B.** Because renal excretion is the predominant route of elimination of unithiol and its metal complexes, caution is warranted in administering unithiol to patients with severe renal insufficiency. Use of unithiol as an adjunct to hemodialysis or hemofiltration in patients with anuric renal failure caused by mercury salts and bismuth has been reported.

**IV. Adverse effects**

- **A.** The German manufacturer (Heyl) notes a low overall incidence (< 4%) of adverse side effects.
- **B.** Self-limited, reversible allergic dermatologic reactions such as exanthems and urticaria have been the most commonly reported adverse effect. Isolated cases of major allergic reactions, including erythema multiforme and Stevens-Johnson syndrome, have been reported.
- **C.** Because rapid intravenous administration may be associated with vasodilation and transient hypotension, intravenous injections of unithiol should be administered slowly, over a 15- to 20-minute interval.
- **D.** Unithiol increases the urinary excretion of copper and zinc, an effect that is not anticipated to be clinically significant in patients without preexisting deficiency of these trace elements.
- **E. Use in pregnancy**. Unithiol did not exhibit teratogenicity or other developmental toxicity in animal studies. Although protection against the adverse reproductive effects of selected toxic metals has been demonstrated in pregnant animals, there is insufficient clinical experience with the use of unithiol in human pregnancy.

**V. Drug or laboratory interactions.**

- **A.** Aqueous solutions of unithiol for intravenous injection should not be mixed with other drugs or minerals. Oral preparations should not be consumed simultaneously with mineral supplements.
- **B.** Unithiol has been shown to form a complex with an arsenic metabolite ($MMA^{III}$), which then is excreted in the urine. Laboratory techniques that use hydride reduction to measure urinary arsenic and its metabolites ("speciation") may not detect this complex. However, the complex will contribute to measurement of "total urinary arsenic."

**VI. Dosage and method of administration.** Unithiol may be administered by the oral, intramuscular, and intravenous routes. The intravenous route should be reserved for treatment of severe acute intoxication by inorganic mercury salts or arsenic when compromised GI or cardiovascular status may interfere with rapid or efficient absorption from the GI tract. In animal models, oral unithiol did not increase the GI absorption of mercuric chloride.

- **A. Severe acute poisoning by inorganic mercury or arsenic**. Administer 3–5 mg/kg every 4 hours by slow intravenous infusion over 20 minutes. If, after several days, the patient's GI and cardiovascular status have stabilized, consider changing to oral unithiol, 4–8 mg/kg every 6–8 hours.
- **B. Symptomatic poisoning by lead (without encephalopathy).** Oral unithiol, 4–8 mg/kg orally every 6–8 hours, may be considered an alternative to succimer (see p 510). ***Note:*** Parenteral therapy with EDTA (see p 440) is preferable for the treatment of severe lead intoxication (lead encephalopathy or lead colic) and for patients with extremely high blood lead concentrations (eg, blood lead >150 mcg/dL).
- **C.** Mobilization or "chelation challenge" tests measuring an increase in urinary excretion of mercury and arsenic after a single dose of unithiol have been described, but their diagnostic or prognostic value has not been established.

**VII. Formulations**

- **A.** In the United States, compounding pharmacists (including hospital inpatient pharmacies) may obtain bulk quantities of pharmaceutical-grade unithiol and dispense it as injection solutions for infusion (usually 50 mg/mL in sterile water). Capsules (typically in 100- or 300-mg sizes) may also be prepared in an oral dose form. Note that bulk unithiol must be obtained outside the United States, and such supplies should have a certificate of analysis to assure product purity.
- **B.** The **suggested minimum stocking level** to treat a 70-kg adult for the first 24 hours is 2100 mg.

## ▶ VASOPRESSIN

*Ben Tsutaoka, PharmD*

**I. Pharmacology**

**A.** Vasopressin is a peptide hormone that is synthesized in the hypothalamus. The primary stimuli for endogenous physiologic release are hyperosmolality, hypotension, and hypovolemia. It is used in the critical care setting for severe catecholamine-resistant vasodilatory shock, in which case it acts as a potent vasoconstrictor. Conditions in which vasopressin has shown to be beneficial include septic shock, postcardiotomy shock, milrinone-induced hypotension, and the late phase of hemorrhagic shock. There is insufficient and conflicting human and animal data to recommend its use routinely to manage shock from poisoning. Further data are needed to define its risks, benefits, and optimum dose. Increases in arterial pressure should be evident within the first hour. Its serum half-life is less than 15 minutes.

**II. Indications**

**A.** ***Note:*** Vasopressin should not be used as a first-line agent to treat hypotension. It is used as add-on therapy to treat severe vasodilatory hypotension that is unresponsive or refractory to one or more adrenergic agents (eg, high-dose dopamine, epinephrine, norepinephrine, phenylephrine). There are only four case reports in the medical literature in which vasopressin was used for overdose. The drug poisonings treated in those patients were amlodipine, caffeine, milrinone, and amitriptyline. Animal models of verapamil toxicity have not demonstrated any hemodynamic or survival benefit.

**B.** As a means to reduce adrenergic agent requirements while treating vasodilatory hypotension.

**III. Contraindications**

**A.** Vasopressin infusion should be discontinued if there is a decrease in the cardiac index and/or stroke volume. ***Note:*** Serious consideration should be given to monitoring cardiac indexes invasively via a pulmonary artery catheter to titrate hemodynamic effects and dosing.

**B.** Use with extreme caution if there is evidence of decreased cardiac output despite adequate intravascular volume or evidence of cardiogenic shock.

**C.** Vasopressin should be used cautiously in treating an overdose of an agent that has myocardial depressant effects (eg, calcium channel blockers, beta blockers).

**IV. Adverse effects**

**A. Negative inotropic effect.**

1. Vasopressin has been shown to result in a decrease in the cardiac index. This may be attributed to an increase in systemic vascular resistance and afterload on a depressed myocardium or may be related in part to a compensatory decrease in heart rate. Dobutamine and milrinone have been used in conjunction with vasopressin in attempts to attenuate this negative inotropic effect.

**B. Ischemia** (especially at doses > 0.05 U/minute)

1. Cardiac arrest has been reported at doses > 0.05 U/min.
2. Ischemic skin lesions of the distal extremities and trunk and lingual regions.
3. Mesenteric ischemia and hepatitis may occur.

**C. Thrombocytopenia**

**D. Use in pregnancy.** FDA category B (see p 407). There are no reports linking the use of vasopressin with congenital defects. Vasopressin and the related synthetic agents desmopressin and lypressin have been used during pregnancy to treat diabetes insipidus.

**V. Dosage and method of administration**

**A.** Intravenous infusion at 0.01–0.04 U/min. Vasopressin should be diluted with normal saline or 5% dextrose in water to a final concentration of 0.1–1 U/mL.

Doses higher than 0.04 U/min are not recommended and may be associated with a greater incidence of adverse effects (see above). Administration through central venous access is recommended to minimize the risk of extravasation. Local skin necrosis has occurred when vasopressin was infused through a peripheral venous catheter.

**B.** Once an adequate blood pressure is achieved and stabilized, steps should be taken to reduce the doses of adrenergic agents and vasopressin gradually.

**VI. Formulations**

**A.** Vasopressin (Pitressin™ and others): 20 U/mL, 0.5-, 1-, and 10-mL vials.

**B.** The **suggested minimum stocking level** to treat a 70-kg adult for the first 24 hours is 60 U (six vials of 0.5 mL, three vials of 1 mL, or one vial of 10 mL).

## ► VITAMIN $K_1$ (PHYTONADIONE)

*Thomas E. Kearney, PharmD*

**I. Pharmacology.** Vitamin $K_1$ is an essential cofactor in the hepatic synthesis of coagulation factors II, VII, IX, and X. In adequate doses, vitamin $K_1$ reverses the inhibitory effects of coumarin and indanedione derivatives on the synthesis of these factors. ***Note:*** **Vitamin $K_3$ (menadione) is *not* effective** in reversing excessive anticoagulation caused by these agents. After parenteral vitamin $K_1$ administration, there is a 6- to 8-hour delay before vitamin K–dependent coagulation factors begin to achieve significant levels, and peak effects are not seen until 1–2 days after the initiation of therapy. The duration of effect is 5–10 days. The response to vitamin $K_1$ is variable, and the optimal dosage regimen is unknown; it is influenced by the potency and amount of the ingested anticoagulant, vitamin K pharmacokinetics, and the patient's hepatic biosynthetic capability. Fresh frozen plasma or whole blood is indicated for immediate control of serious hemorrhage.

**II. Indications**

**A.** Excessive anticoagulation caused by coumarin and indanedione derivatives, as evidenced by elevated prothrombin time. Vitamin $K_1$ is ***not*** indicated for empiric treatment of anticoagulant ingestion, as most cases do not require treatment, and its use will delay the onset of an elevated prothrombin time as a marker of a toxic ingestion.

**B.** Vitamin K deficiency (eg, malnutrition, malabsorption, or hemorrhagic disease of the newborn) with coagulopathy.

**C.** Hypoprothrombinemia resulting from salicylate intoxication.

**III. Contraindications.** Do not use in patients with known hypersensitivity to vitamin K or preservatives.

**IV. Adverse effects**

**A. Black box warning**: Anaphylactoid reactions have been reported after intravenous administration and have been associated with fatalities. Intravenous use should be restricted to true emergencies; the patient must be monitored closely in an intensive care setting.

**B.** Intramuscular administration in anticoagulated patients may cause large, painful hematomas. This can be avoided by using the oral or subcutaneous route.

**C.** Patients receiving anticoagulants for medical reasons (eg, deep vein thrombosis or prosthetic heart valves) may experience untoward effects from complete reversal of their anticoagulation status. Preferably, such patients should receive small quantities of fresh frozen plasma or extremely small titrated doses (0.5–1 mg) of vitamin K until the prothrombin time is in the desired therapeutic range (eg, 1.5–2 times normal). Adjunctive anticoagulation with heparin may be required until the desired prothrombin time is achieved.

**D. Use in pregnancy.** FDA category C (indeterminate). Vitamin $K_1$ crosses the placenta readily. However, this does not preclude its acute, short-term use in a seriously symptomatic patient (see p 407).

**V. Drug or laboratory interactions.** Empiric use after an acute anticoagulant overdose will delay (for up to several days) the onset of elevation of prothrombin time, and this may give a false impression of insignificant ingestion in a case of serious "superwarfarin" overdose (see p 379).

**VI. Dosage and method of administration**

**A. Oral.** The usual dose of vitamin $K_1$ (***not*** menadione or vitamin $K_3$) is 10–50 mg two to four times a day in adults and 5–10 mg (or 0.4 mg/kg/dose) two to four times a day in children. Recheck the prothrombin time after 48 hours and increase the dose as needed. ***Note:*** Very high daily doses (7 mg/kg per day or more) have been required in adults with brodifacoum poisoning; in addition, treatment for several weeks or months may be needed because of the long duration of effect of the "superwarfarin." Because the only available oral vitamin $K_1$ formulation is 5 mg, high-dose treatment may require patients to ingest up to 100 pills per day, and long-term compliance with the regimen is often problematic.

**B. Parenteral injection** is an alternative route of administration but is not likely to result in more rapid reversal of anticoagulant effects and is associated with potentially serious side effects. If hemorrhage is present, use fresh frozen plasma for rapid replacement of coagulation factors. Subcutaneous administration is preferred over IM injection, although both can cause hematomas. The maximum volume is 5 mL or 50 mg per dose per injection site. The adult dose is 10–25 mg, and that for children is 1–5 mg; this may be repeated in 6–8 hours. Switch to oral therapy as soon as possible. Intravenous administration is used only rarely because of the risk of an anaphylactoid reaction. The usual dose is 10–25 mg (0.6 mg/kg in children under 12 years), depending on the severity of anticoagulation, diluted in preservative-free dextrose or sodium chloride solution. Give slowly at a rate not to exceed 1 mg/min or 5% of the total dose per minute, whichever is slower.

**VII. Formulations.** ***Note:*** Do ***not*** use menadione (vitamin $K_3$).

**A. Parenteral.** Phytonadione (AquaMEPHYTON and others), 2 mg/mL in 0.5-mL ampules and prefilled syringes, and 10 mg/mL in 1-mL ampules (ampules contain fatty acid derivative and benzyl alcohol).

**B. Oral.** Phytonadione (Mephyton), 5-mg tablets.

**C.** The **suggested minimum stocking level** to treat a 70-kg adult for the first 24 hours is 100 mg (20 tablets and ten 1-mL (10 mg) ampules or the equivalent).

# SECTION IV. ENVIRONMENTAL AND OCCUPATIONAL TOXICOLOGY

## ▶ EMERGENCY MEDICAL RESPONSE TO HAZARDOUS MATERIALS INCIDENTS

*Kent R. Olson, MD, and R. Steven Tharratt, MD*

With the constant threat of accidental releases of hazardous materials and the potential use of chemical weapons by terrorists, local emergency response providers must be prepared to handle victims who may be contaminated with chemical substances. Many local jurisdictions have developed hazardous-materials (HazMat) teams that usually are composed of fire and paramedical personnel who are trained to identify hazardous situations quickly and take the lead in organizing a response. Health-care providers such as ambulance personnel, nurses, physicians, and local hospital officials should participate in emergency response planning and drills with their local HazMat team before a chemical disaster occurs.

I. **General considerations.** The most important elements of successful medical management of a hazardous-materials incident are as follows:
   - A. Use extreme caution when dealing with unknown or unstable conditions.
   - B. Rapidly assess the potential hazard severity of the substances involved.
   - C. Determine the potential for secondary contamination of downstream personnel and facilities.
   - D. Perform any needed decontamination at the scene ***before*** victim transport, if possible.

II. **Organization.** Chemical accidents are managed under the **Incident Command System.** The Incident Commander or Scene Manager is usually the senior representative of the agency that has primary traffic investigative authority, but authority may be delegated to a senior fire or health official. The first priorities of the Incident Commander are to secure the area, establish a command post, create hazard zones, and provide for the decontamination and immediate prehospital care of any victims. However, hospitals must be prepared to manage victims who leave the scene before teams arrive and may arrive at the emergency department unannounced, possibly contaminated, and needing medical attention.
   - A. **Hazard Zones** (Figure IV–1) are determined by the nature of the spilled substance and wind and geographic conditions. In general, the command post and support area are located upwind and uphill from the spill, with sufficient distance to allow rapid escape if conditions change.
     1. The **Exclusion Zone** (also known as the "hot" or "red" zone) is the area immediately adjacent to the chemical incident. This area may be extremely hazardous to persons without appropriate protective equipment. Only properly trained and equipped personnel should enter this zone, and they may require vigorous decontamination when leaving the area.
     2. The **Contamination Reduction Zone** (also known as the "warm" or "yellow" zone) is where victims and rescuers are decontaminated before undergoing further medical assessment and prehospital care. Patients in the Exclusion and Contamination Reduction Zones generally receive only rudimentary first aid such as cervical spine stabilization and placement on a backboard.
     3. The **Support Zone** (also known as the "cold" or "green" zone) is where the Incident Commander, support teams, press, medical treatment areas, and ambulances are situated. It is usually upwind, uphill, and a safe distance from the incident.
   - B. **Medical officer.** A member of the HazMat team should already have been designated to be in charge of health and safety. This person is responsible, with

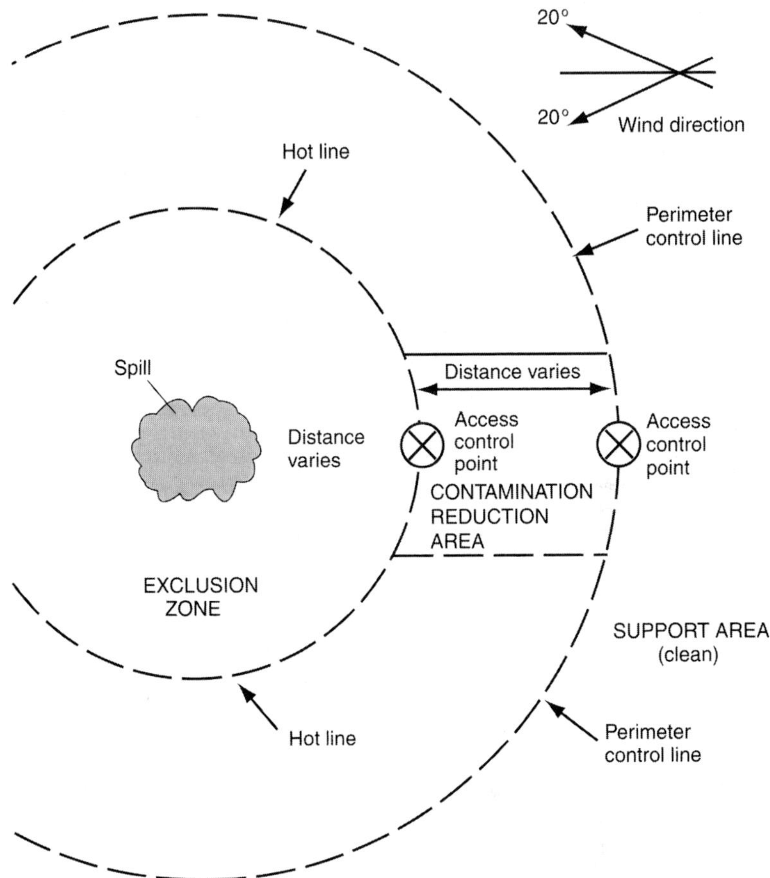


**FIGURE IV–1.** Control zones at a hazardous-materials incident site.

help from the technical reference specialist, for determining the nature of the chemicals, the likely severity of their health effects, the need for specialized personal protective gear, the type and degree of decontamination required, and the supervision of triage and prehospital care. In addition, the medical officer, with the site safety officer, supervises the safety of response workers at the emergency site and monitors entry to and exit from the spill site.

**III. Assessment of hazard potential.** Be prepared to recognize dangerous situations and respond appropriately. The potential for toxic or other types of injury depends on the chemicals involved, their toxicity, their chemical and physical properties, the conditions of exposure, and the circumstances surrounding their release. Be aware that a substance's reactivity, flammability, explosiveness, or corrosiveness may be a source of greater hazard than its systemic toxicity. Do not depend on your senses for safety even though sensory input (eg, smell) may give clues to the nature of the hazard.

**A. Identify the substances involved.** Make inquiries and look for labels, warning placards, and shipping papers.

1. The **National Fire Protection Association (NFPA)** has developed a labeling system for describing chemical hazards that is widely used (Figure IV–2).

2. The **US Department of Transportation** (**DOT**) has developed a system of warning placards for vehicles carrying hazardous materials. The DOT placards usually bear a four-digit substance identification code and a single-digit hazard classification code (Figure IV–3). Identification of the substance from the four-digit code can be provided by the regional poison control center, CHEMTREC, or the DOT manual (see B, below).
3. **Shipping papers,** which may include Material Safety Data Sheets (MSDS), usually are carried by a driver or pilot or may be found in the truck cab or pilot's compartment.

B. **Obtain toxicity information.** Determine the acute health effects and obtain advice on general hazards, decontamination procedures, and medical management of victims. Resources include the following:

1. **Regional poison control centers** ([800] 222-1222). The regional poison control center can provide information on immediate health effects, the need for decontamination or specialized protective gear, and specific treatment, including the use of antidotes. The regional center can also provide consultation with a medical toxicologist.
2. **CHEMTREC** ([800] 424-9300). Operated by the Chemical Manufacturers' Association, this 24-hour hotline can provide information on the identity and hazardous properties of chemicals and, when appropriate, can put the caller in touch with industry representatives and medical toxicologists.
3. See Table IV–4 (p 542) and specific chemicals covered in Section II of this manual.

**NATIONAL FIRE PROTECTION ASSOCIATION**
**IDENTIFICATION OF THE FIRE HAZARDS OF MATERIALS**

NFPA 704

Hazard Signal System

Flammability (Red)

4 – Highly flammable and volatile
3 – Highly flammable
2 – Flammable
1 – Low flammability
0 – Does not burn

Health hazard (Blue)

4 – Extremely hazardous
3 – Moderately hazardous
2 – Hazardous
1 – Slightly hazardous
0 – No health hazard

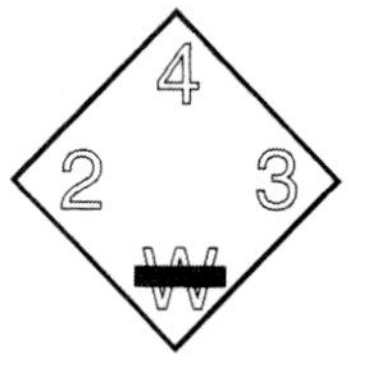


Reactivity (Yellow)

4 – Highly explosive, detonates easily
3 – Explosive, less readily detonated
2 – Violently reactive but does not detonate
1 – Not violently reactive
0 – Normally stable

Other hazards

☢ – Radioactive

OX – Oxidizer

W – Water-reactive

**FIGURE IV–2.** National fire Protection Association (NFPA) identification of the hazards of materials. (Modified and reproduced, with permission, from *Fire Protection Guide on Hazardous Materials*, 9th ed. National Fire Protection Association, 1986.) (*continued on p 523*)

| Signal | Identification of Health Hazard Color Code: BLUE — Type of Possible Injury | Signal | Identification of Flammability Color Code: RED — Susceptibility of Materials to Burning | Signal | Identification of Reactivity (Stability) Color Code: YELLOW — Susceptibility to Release of Energy |
|---|---|---|---|---|---|
| 4 | Materials which on very short exposure could cause death or major residual injury even though prompt medical treatment were given. | 4 | Materials which will rapidly or completely vaporize at atmospheric pressure and normal ambient temperature, or which are readily dispersed in air and which will burn readily. | 4 | Materials which in themselves are readily capable of detonation or of explosive decomposition or reaction at normal temperatures and pressures. |
| 3 | Materials which on short exposure could cause serious temporary or residual injury even though prompt medical treatment were given. | 3 | Liquids and solids that can be ignited under almost all ambient temperature conditions. | 3 | Materials which in themselves are capable of detonation or explosive reaction but require a strong initiating source or which must be heated under confinement before initiation or which react explosively with water. |
| 2 | Materials which on intense or continued exposure could cause temporary incapacitation or possible residual injury unless prompt medical treatment is given. | 2 | Materials must be moderately heated or exposed to relatively high ambient temperatures before ignition can occur. | 2 | Materials that readily undergo violent chemical change at elevated temperatures and pressures; includes materials that react violently with water. |
| 1 | Materials which on exposure would cause irritation but only minor residual injury even if no treatment is given. | 1 | Materials that must be preheated before ignition can occur. | 1 | Materials which in themselves are normally stable, but which can become unstable at elevated temperatures and pressures. |
| 0 | Materials which on exposure under fire conditions would offer no hazard beyond that of ordinary combustible material. | 0 | Materials that will not burn. | 0 | Materials which in themselves are normally stable, even under fire exposure conditions, and which are not reactive with water. |

**FIGURE IV–2.** (Continued) National Fire Protection Association (NFPA) identification of the hazards of materials.

**EXAMPLE OF PLACARD AND PANEL WITH ID NUMBER**

The Identification Number (ID No.) may be displayed on placards or on orange panels on tanks. Check the sides of the transport vehicle if the ID number is not displayed on the ends of the vehicle.

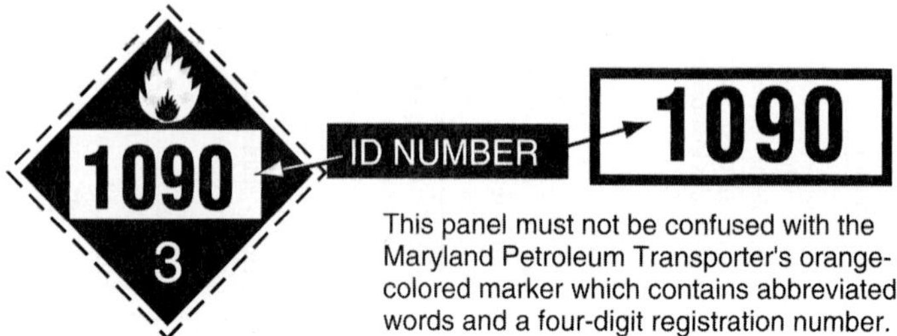
1090
3
ID NUMBER
1090
This panel must not be confused with the Maryland Petroleum Transporter's orange-colored marker which contains abbreviated words and a four-digit registration number.

**FIGURE IV–3.** Example of US Department of Transportation (DOT) vehicle warning placard and panel with DOT identification number.

4. A variety of texts, journals, and computerized information systems are available but are of uneven scope or depth. See the reference list at the end of this section.

C. **Recognize dangerous environments.** In general, environments likely to expose the rescuer to the same conditions that caused grave injury to the victim are not safe for unprotected entry. **These situations require trained and properly equipped rescue personnel.** Examples include the following:
   1. Any indoor environment where the victim was rendered unconscious or otherwise disabled.
   2. Environments causing acute onset of symptoms in rescuers, such as chest tightness, shortness of breath, eye or throat irritation, coughing, dizziness, headache, nausea, and loss of coordination.
   3. Confined spaces such as large tanks or crawl spaces. (Their poor ventilation and small size can result in extremely high levels of airborne contaminants. In addition, such spaces permit only a slow or strenuous exit, which may become physically impossible for an intoxicated individual.)
   4. Spills involving substances with poor warning properties or high vapor pressures, especially when they occur in an indoor or enclosed environment. Substances with poor warning properties can cause serious injury without any warning signs of exposure such as smell and eye irritation. High vapor pressures increase the likelihood that dangerous air concentrations may be present. Also note that gases or vapors with a density greater than that of air may become concentrated in low-lying areas.

D. **Determine the potential for secondary contamination.** Although the threat of secondary contamination of emergency response personnel, equipment, and downstream facilities *may* be significant, it varies widely, depending on the chemical, its concentration, and whether basic decontamination has been performed already. Not all toxic substances carry a risk of downstream contamination even though they may be extremely hazardous to rescuers in the hot zone. Exposures involving inhalation only and no external contamination do not pose a risk of secondary contamination.
   1. Examples of substances with **no significant risk** for secondary contamination of personnel outside the hot zone are **gases,** such as carbon monoxide, arsine, and chlorine, and **vapors,** such as those from xylene, toluene, and perchloroethylene.

2. Examples of substances that have **significant potential** for secondary contamination and require aggressive decontamination and protection of downstream personnel include potent organophosphorus insecticides, oily nitro compounds, and highly radioactive compounds such as cesium and plutonium.
3. In many cases involving substances with a high potential for secondary contamination, this risk can be minimized by removing grossly contaminated clothing and thoroughly cleansing the body in the contamination reduction corridor, including soap or shampoo wash. After these measures are followed, only rarely will the members of the downstream medical team face significant persistent personal threat to their health from an exposed victim.

IV. **Personal protective equipment.** Personal protective equipment includes chemical-resistant clothing and gloves and protective respiratory gear. The use of such equipment should be supervised by experts in industrial hygiene or others with appropriate training and experience. Equipment that is incorrectly selected, improperly fitted, poorly maintained, or inappropriately used may provide a false sense of security and may fail, resulting in serious injury.

A. **Protective clothing** may be as simple as a disposable apron or as sophisticated as a fully encapsulated chemical-resistant suit. However, no chemical-resistant clothing is completely impervious to all chemicals over the full range of exposure conditions. Each suit is rated for its resistance to specific chemicals, and many are also rated for chemical breakthrough time.

B. **Protective respiratory gear** may be a simple paper mask, a cartridge filter respirator, or a positive-pressure air-supplied respirator. Respirators must be properly fitted for each user.

1. **A paper mask** may provide partial protection against gross quantities of airborne dust particles but does not prevent exposure to gases, vapors, and fumes.
2. **Cartridge filter respirators** filter certain chemical gases and vapors out of the ambient air. They are used only when the toxic substance is known to be adsorbed by the filter, the airborne concentration is low, and there is adequate oxygen in the ambient air.
3. **Air-supplied respirators** provide an independent source of clean air. They may be fully self-contained units or masks supplied with air by a long hose. A **self-contained breathing apparatus** (SCBA) has a limited duration of air supply, from 5 to 30 minutes. Users must be fitted for their specific gear.

V. **Victim management.** Victim management includes rapid stabilization and removal from the Exclusion Zone, initial decontamination, delivery to emergency medical services personnel at the Support Zone perimeter, and medical assessment and treatment in the support area. Usually only the HazMat team or other fire department personnel with appropriate training and protective gear will be responsible for rescue from the hot zone, where skin and respiratory protection may be critical. Emergency medical personnel without specific training and appropriate equipment must not enter the hot zone unless it is determined to be safe by the Incident Commander and the medical officer.

A. **Stabilization in the Exclusion Zone.** If there is suspicion of trauma, the patient should be placed on a backboard, with a cervical collar applied if appropriate. Position the patient so that the airway remains open. Gross contamination may be brushed off the patient. No further medical intervention can be expected from rescuers who are wearing bulky suits, masks, and heavy gloves. Therefore, every effort should be made to get a seriously ill patient out of this area as quickly as possible. Victims who are ambulatory should be directed to walk to the contamination reduction area.

B. **Initial decontamination.** Gross decontamination may take place in the Exclusion Zone (eg, brushing off chemical powder and removing soaked clothing), but most decontamination occurs in the contamination reduction corridor before the victim is transferred to waiting emergency medical personnel in the support area. Do not delay critical treatment while decontaminating the victim unless the nature of the contaminant makes such treatment too dangerous. Consult a regional poison control center ([800] 222-1222) for specific advice on decontamination. See also Section I, p 45.

1. Remove contaminated clothing and flush exposed skin, hair, or eyes with copious plain water from a high-volume, low-pressure fire hose. For oily substances, additional washing with soap or shampoo may be required. Ambulatory, cooperative victims may be able to perform their own decontamination.
2. For eye exposures, remove contact lenses if present and irrigate eyes with plain water or, if available, normal saline dribbled from an intravenous bag. Continue irrigation until symptoms resolve or, if the contaminant is an acid or base, until the pH of the conjunctival sac is nearly normal (pH 6–8).
3. Double bag and save all removed clothing and jewelry.
4. Collect runoff water if possible, but generally rapid flushing of exposed skin or eyes should not be delayed because of environmental concerns. Remember that protection of health takes precedence over environmental concerns in a hazardous-materials incident.
5. For ingestions, if the material ingested is a suspected corrosive substance or the patient is experiencing painful swallowing or has oral burns, give the patient a glass of water to drink.
6. In the majority of incidents, basic victim decontamination as outlined above will substantially reduce or eliminate the potential for secondary contamination of downstream personnel or equipment. Procedures for cleaning equipment are contaminant-specific and depend on the risk of chemical persistence as well as toxicity.

C. **Treatment in the support area.** Once the patient is decontaminated (if required) and released into the support area, triage, basic medical assessment, and treatment by emergency medical providers may begin. In the majority of incidents, once the victim has been removed from the hot zone and is stripped and flushed, there is little or no risk of secondary contamination of these providers, and sophisticated protective gear is not necessary. Simple surgical latex gloves, a plain apron, or disposable outer clothing is generally sufficient.

1. Maintain a patent airway and assist breathing if necessary (see pp 1–7). Administer supplemental oxygen.
2. Provide supportive care for shock (see p 31), arrhythmias (pp 13–15), coma (p 18), or seizures (p 22).
3. Treat with specific antidotes if appropriate and available.
4. Further skin, hair, or eye washing may be necessary. If the victim ingested a toxic substance, consider oral administration of **activated charcoal** (see p 51).
5. Take notes on the probable or suspected level of exposure for each victim, the initial symptoms and signs, and the treatment provided. For chemicals with delayed toxic effects, this could be lifesaving.

VI. **Ambulance transport and hospital treatment.** For skin or inhalation exposures, no special precautions should be required if adequate decontamination has been carried out in the field prior to transport.

A. **Patients who have ingested toxic substances** may vomit en route; carry a large plastic bag–lined basin and extra towels to soak up and immediately isolate spillage. Vomitus may contain the original toxic material or even toxic gases created by the action of stomach acid on the substance (eg, hydrogen cyanide from ingested cyanide salts). When performing gastric lavage in the emergency department, isolate gastric washings (eg, with a closed-wall suction container system).

**B.** For unpredictable situations in which **a contaminated victim arrives at the hospital before decontamination,** it is important to have a strategy ready that will minimize exposure of hospital personnel:

1. Ask the local HazMat team to set up a contamination reduction area outside the hospital emergency department entrance. However, keep in mind that all teams may already be committed and not available to assist.
2. Prepare in advance a hose with 29.4°C (85°F) water, soap, and an old gurney for rapid decontamination ***outside*** the emergency department entrance. Have a child's inflatable pool or another container ready to collect water runoff, if possible. However, do not delay patient decontamination if water runoff cannot be contained easily.
3. Do not bring patients soaked with liquids into the emergency department until they have been stripped and flushed outside, as the liquids may emit gas vapors and cause illness among hospital staff.
4. For incidents involving radioactive materials or other highly contaminating substances that are not volatile, utilize the hospital's radiation accident protocol, which generally will include the following:
   a. Restricted access zones.
   b. Isolation of ventilation ducts leading out of the treatment room to prevent spreading of the contamination throughout the hospital.
   c. Paper covering for floors and use of absorbent materials if liquids are involved.
   d. Protective clothing for hospital staff (gloves, paper masks, shoe covers, caps, and gowns).
   e. Double bagging and saving all contaminated clothing and equipment.
   f. Monitoring to detect the extent and persistence of contamination (ie, using a Geiger counter for radiation incidents).
   g. Notifying appropriate local, state, and federal offices of the incident and obtaining advice on laboratory testing and decontamination of equipment.

**VII. Summary.** The emergency medical response to a hazardous-materials incident requires prior training and planning to protect the health of response personnel and victims.

**A.** Response plans and training should be flexible. The level of hazard and the required actions vary greatly with the circumstances at the scene and the chemicals involved.

**B.** First responders should be able to do the following:

1. Recognize potentially hazardous situations.
2. Take steps to protect themselves from injury.
3. Obtain accurate information about the identity and toxicity of each chemical substance involved.
4. Use appropriate protective gear.
5. Perform victim decontamination before transport to a hospital.
6. Provide appropriate first aid and advanced supportive measures as needed.
7. Coordinate their actions with other responding agencies such as the HazMat team, police and fire departments, and regional poison control centers.

**Useful Resources:**

ATSDR Medical Management Guidelines for Chemical Exposures: http://www.atsdr.cdc.gov/mmg.html. (An excellent resource for planning as well as emergency care, including prehospital and hospital management and guidelines for triage and decontamination.)

*Emergency Response Guidebook.* US Department of Transportation, Washington, DC, 2004. Available online at http://hazmat.dot.gov/pubs/erg/gydebook.htm.

*Fire Protection Guide to Hazardous Materials.* National Fire Protection Association, Batterymarch Park, MA, 2001.

NIOSH Pocket Guide to Occupational Hazards: http://www.cdc.gov/niosh/npg/npgd0000.html. (An excellent summary of workplace exposure limits and other useful information about the most common industrial chemicals.)

# ▶ EVALUATION OF THE PATIENT WITH OCCUPATIONAL CHEMICAL EXPOSURE

*Paul D. Blanc, MD, MSPH*

This chapter highlights common toxicologic problems in the workplace. Occupationally related disease is seen commonly in the outpatient setting. Estimates of the proportion of occupationally related medical problems in primary care practices range up to 15–20%, although this includes many patients with musculoskeletal complaints. However, approximately 5% of all symptomatic poison control center consultations are occupational in nature, suggesting a large number of chemical exposures. The largest single referring group for these calls is emergency medicine specialists.

I. **General considerations**
   A. **Occupational illness is rarely pathognomonic.** The connection between illness and workplace factors is typically obscure unless a specific effort is made to link exposure to disease.
      1. Massive or catastrophic events leading to acute onset of symptoms, such as an irritant gas release, are relatively uncommon.
      2. For most workplace exposures, symptom onset is more often insidious, following a subacute or chronic pattern, as in heavy metal poisoning.
      3. Long latency, often years, between exposure and disease makes linking cause and effect even more difficult, for example, in chronic lung disease or occupationally related cancer.
   B. **Occupational evaluation frequently includes legal and administrative components**
      1. Occupational illness, even if suspected but not established, may be a reportable illness in certain states (eg, in California through the Doctor's First Report system).
      2. Establishing quantifiable documentation of adverse effects at the time of exposure may be critical to future attribution of impairment (for example, spirometric evaluation soon after an irritant inhalant exposure).
      3. Although workers' compensation is in theory a straightforward "no-fault" insurance system, in practice it is often arcane and adversarial. It is important to remember that the person being treated is the patient, not the employer or a referring attorney.

II. **Components of the occupational exposure history**
   A. **Job and job process**
      1. Ask specifics about the job. Do not rely on descriptions limited to a general occupation or trade such as "machinist," "painter," "electronics worker," or "farmer."
      2. Describe the industrial process and equipment used on the job. If power equipment is used, ascertain how it is powered to assess carbon monoxide exposure risk.
      3. Determine whether the work process utilizes a closed (eg, a sealed reaction vat) system or an open system and what other processes or work stations are nearby. Work under a lab hood may be an effectively "closed" system, but not if the window is raised too far or if the airflow is not calibrated.
      4. Find out who does maintenance and how often it is done.
   B. **Level of exposure**
      1. Ask whether dust or mist can be seen in the air at the worksite. If so, question whether coworkers or nearby objects can be seen clearly (very high levels actually obscure sight). A history of dust-laden sputum or nasal discharge at the end of the work shift is also a marker of heavy exposure.
      2. Ask whether work surfaces are dusty or damp and whether the paint at the worksite is peeling or discolored (eg, from a corrosive atmosphere).
      3. Determine whether strong smells or tastes are present and, if so, whether they diminish over time, suggesting olfactory fatigue.

4. Find out whether there is any special ventilation system and where the fresh air intake is located (toxins actually can be recirculated by a poorly placed air intake system).
5. Establish whether the person has direct skin contact with the materials worked with, especially solvents or other liquid chemicals.
6. Confined-space work can be especially hazardous. Examples of such spaces include ship holds, storage tanks, and underground vaults.

C. **Personal protective gear** (see p 525). Respiratory system and skin protection may be essential for certain workplace exposures. Just as important as the availability of equipment are its proper selection and use.
   1. **Respiratory protection.** A disposable paper-type mask is inadequate for most exposures. A screw-in cartridge-type mask for which the cartridges are rarely changed is also unlikely to be effective. For an air-supplied respirator with an air supply hose, ascertain the location of the air intake.
   2. **Skin protection.** Gloves and other skin protection should be impervious to the chemical(s) used.

D. **Temporal aspects of exposure**
   1. The most important question is whether there have been any changes in work processes, products used, or job duties that could be temporally associated with the onset of symptoms.
   2. Patterns of recurring symptoms linked to the work schedule can be important, for example, if symptoms are different on the first day of the work week, at the end of the first shift of the week, at the end of the work week, or on days off or vacation days.

E. **Other aspects of exposure**
   1. It is critical to assess whether anyone else from the workplace is also symptomatic and, if so, to identify that person's precise job duties.
   2. Eating in work areas can result in exposure through ingestion; smoking on the job can lead to inhalation of native materials or toxic pyrolysis products.
   3. Determine whether a uniform is provided and who launders it. For example, family lead poisoning can occur through work clothes brought home for laundering. After certain types of contamination (eg, with pesticides), a uniform should be destroyed, not laundered and reused.
   4. Find out how large the worksite is, since small operations are often the most poorly maintained. An active work safety and health committee suggests that better general protection is in place.

F. **Common toxic materials of frequent concern that are commonly addressed in the occupational exposure history**
   1. **Two-part glues, paints, or coatings** that must be mixed just prior to use, such as urethanes and epoxides. These reactive polymers are often irritants or sensitizers.
   2. **Solvents or degreasers,** especially if exposure is high enough to cause dizziness, nausea, headache, or a sense of intoxication.
   3. **Respirable dusts,** including friable insulation or heat-resistant materials, and sand or quartz dust, especially from grinding or blasting.
   4. **Combustion products or fumes** from fires, flame cutting, welding, and other high-temperature processes.

G. Identifying the specific chemical exposures involved may be difficult because the worker may not know or may not have been told their precise identification. Even the manufacturer may be uncertain because components of the chemical mixture were obtained elsewhere or because exposure is due to undetermined process by-products. Finally, the exposure may have occurred long before. Aids to exposure identification include the following:
   1. **Product labels.** Obtain product labels as a first step. However, the label alone is unlikely to provide detailed information.
   2. **Material safety data sheets.** Contact the manufacturer directly for a material safety data sheet (MSDS). These must be provided upon a physi-

cian's request in cases of suspected illness. Do not take no for an answer. You may need to supplement the MSDS information through direct discussion with a technical person working for the supplier.

3. **Computerized databases.** Consult computerized databases (Poisindex, TOMES, NIOSHTIC, others) for further information. Regional poison control centers ([800] 222-1222) can be extremely useful.
4. **DOT identification placards.** In cases of transportation release, Department of Transportation (DOT) identification placards may be available (see p 524).
5. **Industrial exposure data.** Rarely, detailed industrial hygiene data may be available to delineate specific exposures and exposure levels in cases of ongoing, chronic exposure.
6. **Existing process exposure data.** Often, exposure is assumed on the basis of known specific exposures linked to certain work processes. Selected types of exposure are listed in Table IV–1.

III. **Organ-specific occupational toxidromes.** A list of *Ten Leading Causes of Occupational Injuries and Illnesses* has been published by the National Institute for Occupational Safety and Health (NIOSH). This list, organized generally by organ system, is included in Table IV–2, along with additional disorders not on the original NIOSH list.

A. **Occupational lung diseases**

1. In acute pulmonary injury from **inhaled irritants,** exposure is typically brief and intense; initial symptom onset occurs within minutes to 24–48 hours after exposure. The responses to irritant exposure, in increasing severity, are mucous membrane irritation, burning eyes and runny nose, tracheobronchitis, hoarseness, cough, laryngospasm, bronchospasm, and pulmonary edema progressing to adult respiratory distress syndrome (ARDS). Lower-water-solubility gases (nitrogen dioxide, ozone, and phosgene) may produce little upper airway mucous membrane irritation. Any irritant (high or low solubility) can cause pulmonary edema after sufficient exposure.
2. **Heavy metal** pneumonitis is clinically similar to irritant inhalation injury. As with low-solubility gases, upper-airway mucous membrane irritation is minimal; thus, the exposure may have poor warning properties. Offending agents include cadmium, mercury, and, in limited industrial settings, nickel carbonyl.
3. **Febrile inhalational syndromes** are acute, self-limited flu-like syndromes that include **metal fume fever** (caused by galvanized-metal fumes), **polymer fume fever** (after thermal breakdown of certain fluoropolymers), and "**organic dust toxic syndrome**" (ODTS) (after heavy exposure to high levels of organic dust such as occurs in shoveling wood chip mulch). In none of these syndromes is lung injury marked. The presence of hypoxemia or lung infiltrates suggests an alternative diagnosis.
4. **Work-related asthma** is a common occupational problem. Classic occupational asthma typically occurs after sensitization to either high-molecular-weight chemicals (eg, inhaled foreign proteins) or small chemicals that appear to act as haptens (the most common of which are urethane isocyanates such as **toluene diisocyanate** [TDI]). After acute, high-level irritant inhalations, for example, of **chlorine,** a chronic irritant-induced asthma may persist (sometimes called reactive airways dysfunction syndrome [RADS]).
5. **Chronic fibrotic occupational lung diseases** include **asbestosis** (see p 121), **silicosis, coal workers' pneumoconiosis,** and a few other less common fibrotic lung diseases associated with occupational exposures to substances such as **beryllium** and hard metal (**cobalt-tungsten carbide**). These conditions occur after years of exposure and have a long latency, although patients may present for evaluation after an acute exposure. Referral for follow-up surveillance is appropriate if exposure is anticipated to be long term.

**TABLE IV–1. SELECTED JOB PROCESSES AT HIGH RISK OF SPECIFIC TOXIC EXPOSURES**

| Job Process | Exposure |
|---|---|
| Aerospace and other specialty metal work | Beryllium |
| Artificial nail application | Methacrylate |
| Artificial nail removal | Acetonitrile, nitroethane |
| Artificial leather making, fabric coating | Dimethylformamide |
| Auto body painting | Isocyanates |
| Battery recycling | Lead fumes and dust |
| Carburetor cleaning (car repair) | Methylene chloride |
| Cement manufacture | Sulfur dioxide |
| Commercial refrigeration | Ammonia, sulfur dioxide |
| Concrete application | Chromic acid |
| Custodial work | Chlorine (hypochlorite + acid mixes) |
| Dry cleaning | Chlorinated hydrocarbon solvents |
| Epoxy glue and coatings use | Trimellitic anhydride |
| Explosives work | Nitrate oxidants |
| Fermentation operation | Carbon dioxide |
| Fire fighting | Carbon monoxide, cyanide, acrolein |
| Fumigation | Methyl bromide, Vikane (sulfuryl fluoride), phosphine |
| Furniture refinishing | Methylene chloride |
| Gas-shielded welding | Nitrogen dioxide |
| Gold refining | Mercury vapor |
| Hospital sterilizer work | Ethylene oxide, glutaraldehyde |
| Indoor fork lift or compressor operation | Carbon monoxide |
| Manure pit operation | Hydrogen sulfide |
| Metal degreasing | Chlorinated hydrocarbon solvents |
| Metal plating | Cyanide, acid mists |
| Microelectronics chip etching | Hydrofluoric acid |
| Microelectronic chip doping | Arsine gas, diborane gas |
| Paper pulp work | Chlorine, chlorine dioxide, ozone |
| Pool and hot tub disinfection | Chlorine, bromine |
| Pottery glazing and glassmaking | Lead dust |
| Radiator repair | Lead fumes |
| Rayon manufacturing | Carbon disulfide |
| Rubber cement glue use | *n*-Hexane, other solvents |
| Rocket and jet fuel work | Hydrazine, monomethylhydrazine |
| Sandblasting, concrete finishing | Silica dust |
| Sewage work | Hydrogen sulfide |
| Silo work with fresh silage | Nitrogen dioxide |
| Sheet-metal flame cutting or brazing | Cadmium fumes |
| Structural paint refurbishing | Lead fumes and dust |
| Tobacco harvesters | Nicotine |
| Water treatment or purification | Chlorine, ozone |
| Welding galvanized steel | Zinc oxide fumes |
| Welding solvent-contaminated metal | Phosgene |

**TABLE IV–2. LEADING WORK-RELATED DISEASES AND INJURIES AND THEIR RELEVANCE TO CLINICAL TOXICOLOGY**

| Work-Related Conditions | NIOSH* | Relevance | Examples of Relevant Conditions |
|---|---|---|---|
| Occupational lung disease | Yes | High | Irritant inhalation |
| Musculoskeletal | Yes | Low | Chemical-related Raynaud's syndrome |
| Cancer | Yes | Moderate | Acute leukemia |
| Trauma | Yes | Low | High-pressure injury |
| Cardiovascular disease | Yes | Moderate | Carbon monoxide ischemia |
| Disorders of reproduction | Yes | Low | Spontaneous abortion |
| Neurotoxic disorders | Yes | High | Acetylcholinesterase inhibition |
| Noise-induced hearing loss | Yes | Low | Potential drug interactions |
| Dermatologic conditions | Yes | Moderate | Hydrofluoric acid burn |
| Psychologic disorders | Yes | Moderate | Postexposure stress disorder |
| Hepatic injury | No | High | Chemical hepatitis |
| Renal disease | No | Moderate | Acute tubular necrosis |
| Hematologic conditions | No | High | Methemoglobinemia |
| Physical exposures | No | Low | Radiation sickness |
| Systemic illness | No | High | Cyanide toxicity |

*NIOSH = National Institute for Occupational Safety and Health list of 10 leading conditions.

6. **Hypersensitivity pneumonitis** (also called **allergic alveolitis**) includes a group of diseases caused by chronic exposure to organic materials, especially thermophilic bacteria. The most common of these is **"farmer's lung."** Although the process is chronic, acute illness can occur in a sensitized host after heavy exposure to the offending agent. In such cases the illness may need to be differentiated from exposure to an irritant inhalant leading to acute lung injury.

B. **Musculoskeletal** conditions, including acute mechanical trauma, are the most common occupational medicine problem but rarely have direct toxicologic implications.
   1. **Raynaud's syndrome** may be associated rarely with chemical exposure (eg, vinyl chloride monomer).
   2. **High-pressure injection injuries** (eg, from paint spray guns) are important not because of systemic toxicity resulting from absorption of an injected substance (eg, paint thinner) but because of extensive irritant-related tissue necrosis. Emergency surgical evaluation of such cases is mandatory.

C. **Occupational cancer** is a major public concern and often leads to referral for toxicologic evaluation. A variety of different cancers have been associated with workplace exposure, some more strongly than others. Identifying the chemical causes of cancer has proved a great challenge for occupational toxicologists and epidemiologists. Often, the practitioner is faced with an individual patient who seeks an assessment of the relative attribution of disease caused by chemical exposures in that particular case for purposes of gaining compensation or establishing liability. This process, however, tends to be far removed from the acute care setting, and clinical oncology management is not affected directly by such etiologic considerations.

D. **Cardiovascular disease**

1. **Atherosclerotic** cardiovascular disease is associated with **carbon disulfide.** This chemical solvent is used in rayon manufacturing and in specialty applications and research laboratories. It is also a principal metabolite of **disulfiram.**
2. **Carbon monoxide** at high levels can cause myocardial infarction in otherwise healthy individuals and, at lower levels, can aggravate ischemia in the face of established atherosclerotic heart disease (ASHD). Chronic exposure to carbon monoxide may also be associated with ASHD. Many jurisdictions automatically grant workers' compensation to fire fighters or police officers with ASHD, regarding it as a "stress-related" occupational disease. This is related to social policy rather than established epidemiologic risk.
3. **Nitrate withdrawal–induced** coronary artery spasm has been reported among workers heavily exposed to nitrates during munitions manufacturing.
4. **Hydrocarbon solvents,** especially chlorinated hydrocarbons, and chlorofluorocarbon propellants all enhance the sensitivity of the myocardium to catecholamine-induced dysrhythmias.

E. **Adverse reproductive outcomes** have been associated with or implicated in occupational exposures to **heavy metals** (lead and organic mercury), hospital chemical exposures (including **anesthetic and sterilizing gases**), and **dibromochloropropane** (a soil fumigant now banned in the United States).

F. **Occupational neurotoxins**

1. **Acute** central nervous system (CNS) toxicity can occur with many pesticides (including both cholinesterase-inhibiting and chlorinated hydrocarbons). The CNS is also the target of **methyl bromide** (a structural fumigant; see p 139). Cytotoxic and anoxic asphyxiant gases (eg, carbon monoxide, cyanide, and hydrogen sulfide) all cause acute CNS injury. **Hydrocarbon solvents** (see p 219) are typically CNS depressants at high exposure levels.
2. **Chronic** CNS toxicity is the hallmark of heavy metals. This includes inorganic forms (**arsenic, lead,** and **mercury**) and organic forms (tetraethyl lead and methyl mercury). Chronic **manganese** (see p 251) exposure can cause psychosis and parkinsonism. Postanoxic injury, especially from **carbon monoxide** (p 157), can also lead to parkinsonism.
3. Established causes of **peripheral neuropathy** include lead, arsenic, mercury, carbon disulfide (mentioned earlier in connection with ASHD), *n*-hexane, and certain organophosphates.

G. **Occupational ototoxicity** is common but is usually noise-induced rather than chemical-related. Preexisting noise-induced hearing loss may magnify the impact of common ototoxic drugs.

H. **Occupational skin disorders**

1. Allergic and irritant contact dermatitis and acute caustic chemical or acid injuries are the most common toxin-related skin problems. Systemic toxicity may occur but is not a common complicating factor.
2. **Hydrofluoric acid** burns present a specific set of management problems (see p 222). Relevant occupations include not only the microelectronics industry but also maintenance or repair jobs in which hydrofluoric acid–containing rust removers are used.

I. **Work-related psychological disorders** include a heterogeneous mix of diagnoses. Among these diagnoses, "posttraumatic stress disorder" and "mass psychogenic illness" can be extremely relevant to medical toxicology because these patients may believe that their symptoms have a chemical etiology. After reasonable toxicologic causes have been excluded, psychological diagnoses should be considered when nonspecific symptoms or multiple somatic complaints cannot be linked to abnormal signs or physiologic effects.

J. **Occupational chemical hepatotoxins** (see also p 39)
   1. Causes of acute chemical hepatitis include exposure to industrial solvents such as **halogenated hydrocarbons** (methylene chloride, trichloroethylene, and trichloroethane), carbon tetrachloride (only rarely encountered in modern industry), and **dimethylformamide, dinitropropane,** and **dimethylacetamide.** The jet and rocket fuel components **hydrazine** and **monomethylhydrazine** are also potent hepatotoxins.
   2. Other hepatic responses that can be occupationally related include steatosis, cholestatic injury, hepatoportal sclerosis, and hepatic porphyria. The acute care provider should always consider a toxic chemical etiology in the differential diagnosis of liver disease.

K. **Renal diseases**
   1. **Acute tubular necrosis** can follow high-level exposure to a number of toxins, although the more common exposure scenario is a suicide attempt rather than workplace inhalation.
   2. **Interstitial nephritis** is associated with chronic exposure to heavy metals, whereas hydrocarbon exposure has been associated epidemiologicly with **glomerular nephritis,** particularly Goodpasture's disease.

L. **Hematologic toxicity**
   1. Industrial oxidants are an important potential cause of chemically induced **methemoglobinemia** (see p 262), especially in the dyestuff and munitions industries.
   2. **Bone marrow** is an important target organ for certain chemicals, such as **benzene** and **methyl cellosolve.** Both can cause pancytopenia. Benzene exposure also causes leukemia in humans. **Lead** causes anemia through interference with hemoglobin synthesis.
   3. **Arsine gas** is a potent cause of massive hemolysis. It is of industrial importance in microelectronics manufacturing.

M. **Nonchemical physical exposures** in the workplace are important because they can cause systemic effects that mimic chemical toxidromes. The most important example is **heat stress,** which is a major occupational health issue. Other relevant nonchemical, work-related physical exposure types include **ionizing radiation, nonionizing radiation** (such as ultraviolet, infrared, and microwave exposure), and **increased barometric pressure** (eg, among caisson workers). Except for extremes of exposure, the adverse effects of these physical factors generally are associated with chronic conditions.

N. **Systemic poisons** fit poorly into organ system categories but are clearly of major importance in occupational toxicology. Prime examples are the cytotoxic asphyxiants **hydrogen cyanide** (especially in metal plating and metal refining) (see p 176), **hydrogen sulfide** (important as a natural by-product of organic material breakdown) (p 224), and **carbon monoxide** (principally encountered as a combustion by-product but also a metabolite of the solvent methylene chloride) (p 151). **Arsenic** (p 115) is a multiorgan toxin with a myriad of effects. It has been used widely in agriculture and is an important metal smelting by-product. A systemic **disulfiram reaction** (p 184) can occur as a drug interaction with coexposure to certain industrial chemicals. Toxicity from **dinitrophenol,** an industrial chemical that uncouples oxidative phosphorylation, is also best categorized as a systemic effect.

IV. **Laboratory testing**

A. Testing for specific occupational toxins has a limited but important role. Selected tests are listed in the descriptions of specific substances in Section II of this book.

B. For significant irritant inhalation exposures, in addition to assessing oxygenation and chest radiographic status, early spirometric assessment is often important.

C. General laboratory testing for chronic exposure assessment should be driven by the potential organ toxicity delineated previously. Standard recommendations

**TABLE IV–3. REGIONAL OFFICES OF THE OCCUPATIONAL SAFETY AND HEALTH ADMINISTRATION (OSHA)**

| Region | Regional Office | Phone Number | States Served |
|---|---|---|---|
| I | Boston | (617) 565-9860 | Connecticut, Maine, Massachusetts, New Hampshire, Rhode Island, Vermont |
| II | New York City | (212) 337-2378 | New York, New Jersey, Puerto Rico, Virgin Islands |
| III | Philadelphia | (215) 596-1201 | Delaware, District of Columbia, Maryland, Pennsylvania, Virginia, West Virginia |
| IV | Atlanta | (404) 562-2300 | Alabama, Florida, Georgia, Kentucky, Mississippi, North Carolina, South Carolina, Tennessee |
| V | Chicago | (312) 353-2220 | Illinois, Indiana, Michigan, Minnesota, Ohio, Wisconsin |
| VI | Dallas | (214) 767-4731 | Arkansas, Louisiana, New Mexico, Oklahoma, Texas |
| VII | Kansas City | (816) 426-5861 | Iowa, Kansas, Missouri, Nebraska |
| VIII | Denver | (303) 844-1600 | Colorado, Montana, North Dakota, South Dakota, Utah, Wyoming |
| IX | San Francisco | (415) 975-4310 | Arizona, California, Hawaii, Nevada, Guam |
| X | Seattle | (206) 553-5930 | Alaska, Idaho, Oregon, Washington |

(eg, in NIOSH criteria documents) often include a complete blood count, electrolytes, tests of renal and liver function, and periodic chest radiographic and pulmonary function studies.

**V. Treatment**

**A.** Elimination or reduction of further exposure is a key treatment intervention in occupational toxicology. This includes prevention of exposure of coworkers. The **Occupational Safety and Health Administration (OSHA)** may be of assistance and should be notified immediately about an ongoing, potentially life-threatening workplace exposure situation. Contact information for regional OSHA offices is listed in Table IV–3. Workplace modification and control, especially the substitution of less hazardous materials, should always be the first line of defense. Worker-required personal protective equipment is, in general, less preferred.

**B.** The medical treatment of occupational toxic illness should follow the general principles outlined earlier in this section and in Sections I and II of this book. In particular, the use of specific antidotes should be undertaken in consultation with a regional poison control center ([800] 222-1222) or other specialists. This is particularly true before chelation therapy is initiated for heavy metal poisoning.

Blanc PD, Balmes JR: History and physical examination. In: Harber P, Schenker M, Balmes JR, eds. *Occupational and Environmental Respiratory Diseases.* St. Louis: CV Mosby, 1995:28–38.

## ▶ THE TOXIC HAZARDS OF INDUSTRIAL AND OCCUPATIONAL CHEMICALS

*Paul D. Blanc, MD, MSPH, Patricia Hess Hiatt, BS, and Kent R. Olson, MD**

Basic information on the toxicity of many of the most commonly encountered and toxicologically significant industrial chemicals is provided in Table IV–4. The table is intended to expedite the recognition of potentially hazardous exposure situations and

*This chapter and Table IV–4 were originally conceived and created by Frank J. Mycroft, PhD.

therefore provides information such as vapor pressures, warning properties, physical appearance, occupational exposure standards and guidelines, and hazard classification codes, which may also be useful in the assessment of an exposure situation. Table IV–4 is divided into three sections: **health hazards, exposure guidelines,** and **comments.** To use the table correctly, it is important to understand the scope and limitations of the information it provides.

The chemicals included in Table IV–4 were selected on the basis of the following criteria: (1) toxic potential, (2) prevalence of use, (3) public health concern, and (4) availability of adequate toxicologic, regulatory, and physical- and chemical-property information. Several governmental and industrial lists of "hazardous chemicals" were used. A number of chemicals were omitted because no toxicologic information could be found, there are no regulatory standards, or they have very limited use. Chemicals that were of specific interest, those with existing exposure recommendations, and those of high use (even if of low toxicity) were included.

I. **Health hazard information.** The health hazards section of Table IV–4 focuses primarily on the basic hazards associated with possible inhalation of or skin exposure to chemicals in a workplace. It is based almost entirely on the occupational health literature. Most of our understanding of the potential effects of chemicals on human health is derived from occupational exposures, the levels of which are typically many times greater than those of environmental exposures. Moreover, the information in Table IV–4 unavoidably emphasizes *acute* health effects. Much more is known about the acute effects of chemicals on human health than about their chronic effects. The rapid onset of symptoms after exposure makes the causal association more readily apparent for acute health effects.

A. The table is *not* a comprehensive source of the toxicology and medical information needed to manage a severely symptomatic or poisoned patient. Medical management information and advice for specific poisonings are found in Section I (see emergency evaluation, p 1, and pulmonary and skin decontamination, p 45) and Section II (see caustics and corrosives, p 157; gases, p 212; and hydrocarbons, p 219).

B. **Hydrocarbons,** which are defined broadly as chemicals containing carbon and hydrogen, make up the majority of substances in Table IV–4. Hydrocarbons have a wide range of chemical structures and, not surprisingly, a variety of toxic effects. There are a few common features of hydrocarbon exposure, and the reader is directed to Section II, p 219, for information on general diagnosis and treatment. Some common features include the following:

1. **Skin.** Dermatitis caused by defatting or removal of oils in the skin is common, especially with prolonged contact. Some agents can cause frank burns.
2. **Arrhythmias.** Many hydrocarbons, most notably fluorinated, chlorinated, and aromatic compounds, can sensitize the heart to the arrhythmogenic effects of epinephrine, resulting in premature ventricular contractions (PVCs), ventricular tachycardia, or fibrillation. Even simple aliphatic compounds such as butane occasionally can cause this effect.
   a. Because arrhythmias may not occur immediately, cardiac monitoring for 24 hours is recommended for all victims who have had significant hydrocarbon exposure (eg, syncope, coma, and arrhythmias).
   b. Ventricular arrhythmias preferably are treated with a beta-adrenergic blocker (eg, esmolol [p 449] or propranolol [p 504]) rather than lidocaine, procainamide, or amiodarone.
3. **Pulmonary aspiration** of most hydrocarbons, especially those with relatively high volatility and low viscosity (eg, gasoline, kerosene, and naphtha), can cause severe chemical pneumonitis.

C. **Carcinogens.** To broaden the scope of the table, findings from human and animal studies relating to the carcinogenic or reproductive toxicity of a chemical are included when available. The **International Agency for Research on**

**Cancer** (**IARC**) is the foremost authority in evaluating the carcinogenic potential of chemical agents for humans. The overall IARC evaluations are provided, when available, in the health hazards section of the table. The following IARC ratings are based primarily on human and animal data:

1. **IARC 1** substances are considered human carcinogens; generally there is sufficient epidemiologic information to support a causal association between exposure and human cancer.
2. **IARC 2** compounds are suspected of being carcinogenic to humans, based on a combination of data from animal and human studies. Group IARC 2 is subdivided into two parts:
   a. An **IARC 2A** rating indicates that a chemical is *probably* carcinogenic to humans. Most often there is limited evidence of carcinogenicity in humans combined with sufficient evidence of carcinogenicity in animals.
   b. **IARC 2B** indicates that a chemical is *possibly* carcinogenic to humans. This category may be used when there is limited evidence from epidemiologic studies and less than sufficient evidence for carcinogenicity in animals. It also may be used when there is inadequate evidence of carcinogenicity in humans and sufficient evidence in animals.
3. **IARC 3** substances cannot be classified in regard to their carcinogenic potential for humans because of inadequate data.
4. If a chemical is described in the table as carcinogenic but an IARC category is not given, IARC has not classified the chemical but other sources (eg, US Environmental Protection Agency and California Department of Health Services Hazard Evaluation Service and Information System) consider it carcinogenic.

D. **Problems in assessing health hazards.** The nature and magnitude of the health hazards associated with occupational or environmental exposures to any chemical depend on its intrinsic toxicity and the conditions of exposure.

1. Characterization of these hazards is often difficult. Important considerations include the potency of the agent, the route of exposure, the level and temporal pattern of exposure, genetic susceptibility, overall health status, and life-style factors that may alter individual sensitivities (eg, alcohol consumption may cause "degreaser's flush" in workers exposed to trichloroethylene). Despite their value in estimating the likelihood and potential severity of an effect, quantitative measurements of the level of exposure are not often available.
2. Hazard characterizations cannot address undiscovered or unappreciated health effects. The limited information available on the health effects of most chemicals makes this a major concern. For example, among the more than 5 million compounds known to science, only about 100,000 are listed in the *Registry of the Toxic Effects of Chemical Substances* (RTECS) published by the National Institute for Occupational Safety and Health (NIOSH). Among these 100,000 substances, fewer than 5000 have any toxicity studies relating to their potential tumorigenic or reproductive effects in animals or humans. Because of these gaps, the absence of information does not imply the absence of hazard.
3. The predictive value of animal findings for humans is sometimes uncertain. For many effects, however, there is considerable concordance between test animals and humans.
4. The developmental toxicity information presented here is not a sufficient basis on which to make clinical judgments as to whether a given exposure might affect a pregnancy adversely. For most chemicals known to have adverse effects on fetal development in test animals, there are insufficient epidemiologic data in humans. The predictive value of these animal findings for humans, who typically are exposed to levels much lower than those used in animal tests, is thought to be poor. In general, so little is known about the effects of substances on fetal development that it is pru-

dent to manage all chemical exposures conservatively. The information here is presented solely to identify those compounds for which available data further indicate the need to control exposures.

**II. Exposure guidelines and National Fire Protection Association rankings**

A. **Threshold limit values (TLVs)** are workplace exposure guidelines established by the American Conference of Governmental Industrial Hygienists (ACGIH), a professional society. Although the ACGIH has no regulatory authority, its recommendations are highly regarded and widely followed by the occupational health community. The toxicologic basis for each TLV varies. A TLV may be based on such diverse effects as respiratory sensitization, sensory irritation, narcosis, and asphyxia. Therefore, the TLV is not a relative index of toxicity. Because the degree of health hazard is a continuous function of exposure, TLVs are not fine lines separating safe from dangerous levels of exposure. The *Documentation of the Threshold Limit Values*, which is published by the ACGIH and describes in detail the rationale for each value, should be consulted for specific information on the toxicologic significance of a particular TLV. Common units for a TLV are parts of a chemical per million parts of air (**ppm**) and milligrams of a chemical per cubic meter of air (**mg/m$^3$**). **At standard temperature and pressure, TLV values in ppm can be converted to their equivalent concentrations in mg/m$^3$** by multiplying the TLV in ppm by the molecular weight (MW) in milligrams of the chemical and dividing the result by 22.4 (one mole of gas displaces 22.4 L of air at standard temperature and pressure):

$$\text{mg}/\text{m}^3 = \frac{\text{ppm} \times \text{MW}}{22.4}$$

1. The **threshold limit value time-weighted average (TLV-TWA)** refers to airborne contaminants and is the time-weighted average concentration to which nearly all workers may be exposed repeatedly during a normal 8-hour workday and 40-hour work week without an adverse effect. Unless otherwise indicated, the values listed under the ACGIH TLV heading are the TLV-TWA values. Because TLV-TWA values often are set to protect against worker discomfort, nonspecific minor health complaints such as eye or throat irritation, cough, headache, and nausea may indicate overexposure.
2. The **threshold limit value ceiling (TLV-C)** is the airborne concentration that should not be exceeded during any part of a working exposure. Ceiling guidelines often are set for rapidly acting agents for which an 8-hour time-weighted average exposure limit would be inappropriate. TLV-Cs are listed under the ACGIH TLV heading and are noted by a "(**C**)."
3. Compounds for which **skin contact** is a significant route of exposure are designated with an "**S**." This could refer to potential corrosive effects or systemic toxicity owing to skin absorption.
4. The ACGIH classifies some substances as being ***confirmed*** **(A1) or *suspected*** **(A2) human carcinogens or animal carcinogens (A3)**. These designations are also provided in the table. The ACGIH does not consider A3 carcinogens likely to cause human cancer.
5. The TLVs are heavily based on workplace exposures and conditions occurring within the United States. Their application, which requires training in industrial hygiene, therefore is limited to similar exposures and conditions.

B. **OSHA regulations** are standards for exposure to airborne contaminants that are set and enforced by OSHA, an agency of the federal government.

1. The **permissible exposure limit (PEL)** set by OSHA is closely analogous to the ACGIH TLV-TWA. In fact, when OSHA was established in 1971, it formally adopted the 1969 ACGIH TLVs for nearly all of its PELs. In 1988, OSHA updated the majority of its PELs by adopting the 1986 TLVs. These revised PELs were printed in the 1990 edition of this manual. However, in early 1993, the 1988 PEL revisions were voided as a result of legal chal-

lenges, and the earlier values were restored. Because these restored values cannot be assumed reliably to protect worker health and because the values may change again as a result of further administrative or legislative action, the PELs are not printed in this edition.

2. Substances that are specifically **regulated as carcinogens** by OSHA are indicated by "**OSHA CA**" under the ACGIH TLV heading. For these carcinogens, additional regulations apply. The notation "**NIOSH CA**" in the TLV column identifies the chemicals that NIOSH recommends be treated as potential human carcinogens.
3. Some states operate their own occupational health and safety programs in cooperation with OSHA. In these states, stricter standards may apply.

C. **Immediately dangerous to life or health** (**IDLH**) represents "a maximum concentration from which one could escape within 30 minutes without any escape-impairing symptoms or any irreversible health effects." The IDLH values originally were set jointly by OSHA and NIOSH for the purpose of respirator selection. They have been updated by NIOSH.

D. **Emergency Response Planning Guidelines** (**ERPGs**) have been developed by the American Industrial Hygiene Association (AIHA) for 70 specific substances. The values generally are based on limited human experience as well as available animal data and should be considered estimates. Although these values are printed in the IDLH column, they have different meanings:

1. **ERPG-1** is "the maximum air concentration below which it is believed nearly all individuals could be exposed for up to 1 hour without experiencing other than mild transient adverse health effects or perceiving a clearly defined objectionable odor."
2. **ERPG-2** is "the maximum air concentration below which it is believed that nearly all individuals could be exposed for up to 1 hour without experiencing or developing irreversible or other serious health effects or symptoms which could impair their abilities to take protective action."
3. **ERPG-3** is "the maximum air concentration below which it is believed that nearly all individuals could be exposed for up to 1 hour without experiencing or developing life-threatening health effects."
4. The ERPGs were developed for purposes of emergency planning and response. They are not exposure guidelines and do not incorporate the safety factors normally used in establishing acceptable exposure limits. Reliance on the ERPGs for exposures lasting longer than 1 hour is not safe.

E. **National Fire Protection Association** (**NFPA**) **codes** are part of the system created by the NFPA for identifying and ranking the potential fire hazards of materials. The system has three principal categories of hazard: **health** (**H**), **flammability** (**F**), and **reactivity** (**R**). Within each category, hazards are ranked from four (4), indicating a severe hazard, to zero (0), indicating no special hazard. The NFPA rankings for each substance are listed under their appropriate headings. The criteria for rankings within each category are found in Figure IV–2, p 522.

1. The NFPA health hazard rating is based on both the intrinsic toxicity of a chemical and the toxicities of its combustion or breakdown products. The overall ranking is determined by the greater source of health hazard under fire or other emergency conditions. Common hazards from the ordinary combustion of materials are not considered in these rankings.
2. This system is intended to provide basic information to fire-fighting and emergency-response personnel. Its application to specific situations requires skill. Conditions at the scene, such as the amount of material involved and its rate of release, wind conditions, and the proximity to various populations and their health status, are as important as the intrinsic properties of a chemical in determining the magnitude of a hazard.

III. **Comments section.** The comment column of Table IV–4 provides supplementary information on the physical and chemical properties of substances that would be helpful in assessing their health hazards. Information such as physical state and appearance, vapor pressures, warning properties, and potential breakdown products is included.

A. Information on the **physical state and appearance** of a compound may help in its identification and indicate whether dusts, mists, vapors, or gases are likely means of airborne exposure. ***Note:*** For many products, especially pesticides, appearance, and some hazardous properties may vary with the formulation.

B. The **vapor pressure** of a substance determines its potential maximum air concentration and influences the degree of inhalation exposure or airborne contamination. Vapor pressures fluctuate greatly with temperature.
   1. Substances with high vapor pressures tend to volatilize more quickly and can reach higher maximum air concentrations than substances with low vapor pressures. Some substances have such low vapor pressures that airborne contamination is a threat only if they are finely dispersed in a dust or mist.
   2. Substances with a **saturated-air concentration** below their TLVs do not pose a significant vapor inhalation hazard. Vapor pressures can be converted roughly to saturated-air concentrations expressed in parts per million by multiplying by a factor of 1300. This is equivalent to dividing by 760 mm Hg and then multiplying the result by 1 million to adjust for the original units of parts per million (a pressure of 1 equals 760 mm Hg):

$$\text{ppm} = \frac{\text{Vapor pressure (mm Hg)}}{760} \times 10^6$$

C. **Warning properties** such as odor and sensory irritation can be valuable indicators of exposure. However, because of olfactory fatigue and individual differences in odor thresholds, the sense of smell is often unreliable in detecting many compounds. There is no correlation between the quality of an odor and its toxicity. Pleasant-smelling compounds are not necessarily less toxic than foul-smelling ones.
   1. The warning property assessments found in the table are based on OSHA evaluations. For the purpose of this manual, chemicals described as having *good* warning properties can be detected by smell or irritation at levels below the TLV by most individuals. Chemicals described as having *adequate* warning properties can be detected at air levels near the TLV. Chemicals described as having *poor* warning properties can be detected only at levels significantly above the TLV or not at all.
   2. Reported values for odor threshold in the literature vary greatly for many chemicals and are therefore uncertain. These differences make assessments of warning qualities difficult.

D. **Thermal-breakdown products.** Under fire conditions, many organic substances will break down to other toxic substances. The amounts, kinds, and distribution of breakdown products vary with the fire conditions and are not easily modeled. Information on the likely thermal-decomposition products is included because of their importance in the assessment of health hazards under fire conditions.
   1. In general, incomplete combustion of *any* organic material will produce some carbon monoxide (see p 151).
   2. The partial combustion of compounds containing sulfur, nitrogen, or phosphorus atoms will also release their oxides (see pp 352, 281, and 308).
   3. Compounds with chlorine atoms will release some hydrogen chloride or chlorine (see p 162) when exposed to high heat or fire; some chlorinated compounds may also generate phosgene (p 306).
   4. Compounds containing the fluorine atom are similarly likely to break down to yield some hydrogen fluoride (see p 222) and fluorine.
   5. Some compounds (eg, polyurethane) that contain an unsaturated carbon-nitrogen bond will release cyanide (see p 176) during their decomposition.

6. Polychlorinated aromatic compounds may yield polychlorinated dibenzodioxins and polychlorinated dibenzofurans (see p 183) when heated.
7. In addition, smoke from a chemical fire is likely to contain large amounts of the volatilized original chemical and still other poorly characterized partial-breakdown products.
8. The thermal-breakdown product information in Table IV–4 is derived primarily from data found in the literature and the general considerations described immediately above. Aside from the NFPA codes, Table IV–4 does not cover the chemical reactivity or compatibility of substances.

IV. **Summary.** Table IV–4 provides basic information that describes the potential health hazards associated with exposure to several hundred chemicals. The table is not a comprehensive listing of all the possible health hazards for each chemical. The information compiled here comes from a wide variety of respected sources (see the references that follow the table) and focuses on the more likely or commonly reported health effects. Publications from NIOSH, OSHA, ACGIH, the Hazard Evaluation System and Information Service of the State of California, and NFPA; major textbooks in the fields of toxicology and occupational health; and major review articles were the primary sources of the information here. Refer to the original sources for more complete information. Table IV–4 is intended primarily to guide users in the quick qualitative assessment of common toxic hazards. Its application to specific situations requires skill. Because of the many data gaps in the toxicology literature, exposures generally should be managed conservatively. Contact a regional poison control center ([800] 222-1222) or medical toxicologist for expert assistance in managing specific emergency exposures.

# TABLE IV–4. HEALTH HAZARD SUMMARIES FOR INDUSTRIAL AND OCCUPATIONAL CHEMICALS

Abbreviations and designations used in this table are defined as follows:

| | | |
|---|---|---|
| IARC | = | International Agency for Research on Cancer overall classification (see p 537): 1 = known human carcinogen; 2A = probable human carcinogen; 2B = possible human carcinogen; 3 = inadequate data available. |
| TLV | = | American Conference of Governmental Industrial Hygienists (ACGIH) threshold limit value 8-hour time- weighted average (TLV-TWA) air concentration (see p 538): A1 = ACGIH-confirmed human carcinogen; A2 = ACGIH-suspected human carcinogen; A3 = ACGIH animal carcinogen. |
| ppm | = | parts of chemical per million parts of air. |
| mg/m$^3$ | = | milligrams of chemical per cubic meter of air. |
| mppcf | = | million particles of dust per cubic foot of air. |
| (C) | = | ceiling air concentration (TLV-C) that should not be exceeded at any time. |
| S | = | skin absorption can be significant route of exposure. |
| SEN | = | potential for worker sensitization as a result of dermal contact or inhalation exposure. |
| NIOSH CA | = | Judged by National Institute for Occupational Safety and Health to be a known or suspected human carcinogen (see p 539). |
| OSHA CA | = | Regulated by the Occupational Safety and Health Administration as an occupational carcinogen (see p 539). |
| IDLH | = | Immediately Dangerous to Life or Health air concentration (see p 539). |
| LEL | = | For this substance, the IDLH value is set at 10% of the Lower Explosive Limit. |
| ERPG | = | Emergency Response Planning Guidelines air concentration values for a 1-hour period of exposure (see p 539). |
| NFPA Codes | = | National Fire Protection Association hazard classification codes (see p 522 and p 523): 0 (no hazard) <—> 4 (severe hazard) |

| | | |
|---|---|---|
| H | = | health hazard |
| F | = | fire hazard |
| R | = | reactivity hazard |
| Ox | = | oxidizing agent |
| W | = | water-reactive substance |

| Health Hazard Summaries | ACGIH TLV | IDLH | NFPA Codes H F R | Comments |
|---|---|---|---|---|
| **Acetaldehyde (CAS: 75-07-0):** Corrosive; severe burns to eyes and skin may occur. Vapors strongly irritating to eyes and respiratory tract; evidence for adverse effects on fetal development in animals. A carcinogen in test animals (IARC 2B). | 25 ppm (C), A3<br>NIOSH CA | 2000 ppm<br>ERPG-1: 10 ppm<br>ERPG-2: 200 ppm<br>ERPG-3: 1000 ppm | 3 4 2 | Colorless liquid. Fruity odor and irritation are both adequate warning properties. Vapor pressure is 750 mm Hg at 20°C (68°F). Highly flammable. |
| **Acetic acid (vinegar acid [CAS: 64-19-7]):** Concentrated solutions are corrosive; severe burns to eyes and skin may occur. Vapors strongly irritating to eyes and respiratory tract. | 10 ppm | 50 ppm<br>ERPG-1: 5 ppm<br>ERPG-2: 35 ppm<br>ERPG-3: 250 ppm | 3 2 0 | Colorless liquid. Pungent, vinegar-like odor and irritation both occur near the TLV and are adequate warning properties. Vapor pressure is 11 mm Hg at 20°C (68°F). Flammable. |

| | | | | |
|---|---|---|---|---|
| **Acetic anhydride (CAS: 108-24-7):** Corrosive; severe burns to eyes and skin may result. Dermal sensitization has been reported. Vapors highly irritating to eyes and respiratory tract. | 5 ppm | 200 ppm | 3 2 1 | Colorless liquid. Odor and irritation both occur below the TLV and are good warning properties. Vapor pressure is 4 mm Hg at 20°C (68°F). Flammable. Evolves heat upon contact with water. |
| **Acetone (dimethyl ketone, 2-propanone [CAS: 67-64-1]):** Vapors mildly irritating to eyes and respiratory tract. A CNS depressant at high levels. Eye irritation and headache are common symptoms of moderate overexposure. | 500 ppm | 2500 ppm [LEL] | 1 3 0 | Colorless liquid with a sharp, aromatic odor. Eye irritation is an adequate warning property. Vapor pressure is 266 mm Hg at 25°C (77°F). Highly flammable. |
| **Acetonitrile (methyl cyanide, cyanomethane, ethanenitrile [CAS: 75-05-8]):** Vapors mildly irritating to eyes and respiratory tract. Inhibits several metabolic enzyme systems. Dermal absorption occurs. Metabolized to cyanide (see p 176); fatalities have resulted. Symptoms include headache, nausea, vomiting, weakness, and stupor. Limited evidence for adverse effects on fetal development in test animals given large doses. | 20 ppm, S | 500 ppm | 2 3 0 | Colorless liquid. Ether-like odor, detectable at the TLV, is an adequate warning property. Vapor pressure is 73 mm Hg at 20°C (68°F). Flammable. Thermal breakdown products include oxides of nitrogen and cyanide. May be found in products for removing sculptured nails. |
| **Acetophenone (phenyl methyl ketone [CAS: 98-86-2]):** Direct contact mildly irritating to eyes and skin. A CNS depressant at high levels. | 10 ppm | | 1 2 0 | Widely used in industry (eg, textile coatings). |
| **Acetylene tetrabromide (tetrabromoethane [CAS: 79-27-6]):** Direct contact is irritating to eyes and skin. Vapors irritating to eyes and respiratory tract. Dermal absorption occurs. Highly hepatotoxic; liver injury can result from low-level exposures. | 1 ppm [proposed: 0.1 ppm] | 8 ppm | 3 0 1 | Viscous, pale yellow liquid. Pungent, chloroform-like odor. Vapor pressure is less than 0.1 mm Hg at 20°C (68°F). Not combustible. Thermal breakdown products include hydrogen bromide and carbonyl bromide. |

(*continued*)

TABLE IV–4. HEALTH HAZARD SUMMARIES FOR INDUSTRIAL AND OCCUPATIONAL CHEMICALS (CONTINUED)

| Health Hazard Summaries | ACGIH TLV | IDLH | NFPA Codes H F R | Comments |
|---|---|---|---|---|
| **Acrolein (acryaldehyde, 2-propenal [CAS: 107-02-8]):** Highly corrosive; severe burns to eyes or skin may result. Vapors extremely irritating to eyes, skin, and respiratory tract; pulmonary edema has been reported. Permanent pulmonary function changes may result. See p 212. (IARC 3). | 0.1 ppm (C), S | 2 ppm<br>ERPG-1: 0.1 ppm<br>ERPG-2: 0.5 ppm<br>ERPG-3: 3 ppm | 4 3 3 | Colorless to yellow liquid. An unpleasant odor. Eye irritation occurs at low levels and provides a good warning property. Formed in the pyrolysis of many substances. Vapor pressure is 214 mm Hg at 20°C (68°F). Highly flammable. |
| **Acrylamide (propenamide, acrylic amide [CAS: 79-06-1]):** Concentrated solutions are slightly irritating. Well absorbed by all routes. A potent neurotoxin causing peripheral neuropathy. Contact dermatitis also reported. Testicular toxicity in test animals. A carcinogen in test animals (IARC 2A). | 0.03 mg/m$^3$ (respirable fraction), S, A3<br>NIOSH CA | 60 mg/m$^3$ | 2 2 2 | Colorless solid. Vapor pressure is 0.007 mm Hg at 20°C (68°F). Not flammable. Decomposes around 80°C (176°F). Breakdown products include oxides of nitrogen. Monomer used in the synthesis of polyacrylamide plastics. |
| **Acrylic acid (propenoic acid [CAS: 79-10-7]):** Corrosive; severe burns may result. Vapors highly irritating to eyes, skin, and respiratory tract. Limited evidence of adverse effects on fetal development at high doses in test animals. Based on structural analogies, compounds containing the acrylate moiety may be carcinogens. (IARC 3). | 2 ppm, S | ERPG-1: 2 ppm<br>ERPG-2: 50 ppm<br>ERPG-3: 750 ppm | 3 2 2 | Colorless liquid with characteristic acrid odor. Vapor pressure is 31 mm Hg at 25°C (77°F). Flammable. Inhibitor added to prevent explosive self-polymerization. |
| **Acrylonitrile (cyanoethylene, vinyl cyanide, propenenitrile [CAS: 107-13-1]):** Direct contact can be strongly irritating to eyes and skin. Well absorbed by all routes. A CNS depressant at high levels. Metabolized to cyanide (see p 176). Moderate acute overexposure will produce headache, weakness, nausea, and vomiting. Evidence of adverse effects on fetal development at high doses in animals. A carcinogen in test animals with limited epidemiologic evidence for carcinogenicity in humans (IARC 2A2B). | 2 ppm, S, A3<br>OSHA CA<br>NIOSH CA | 85 ppm<br>ERPG-1: 10 ppm<br>ERPG-2: 35 ppm<br>ERPG-3: 75 ppm | 4 3 2 | Colorless liquid with a mild odor. Vapor pressure is 83 mm Hg at 20°C (68°F). Flammable. Polymerizes rapidly. Thermal decomposition products include hydrogen cyanide and oxides of nitrogen. Used in the manufacture of ABS and SAN resins. |
| **Alachlor (CAS: 15972-60-8):** Not an eye irritant. Slightly irritating to the skin. A skin sensitizer. | | | | Wide use as an herbicide. Colorless crystals. Vapor pressure is .000022 mm Hg at 25°C (77°F). |
| **Aldicarb (CAS: 116-06-3):** A potent carbamate-type cholinesterase inhibitor (see p 292). Well absorbed dermally (IARC 3). | | | | Absorption by fruits has caused human poisonings. |

| | | | | |
|---|---|---|---|---|
| **Aldrin (CAS: 309-00-2):** Chlorinated insecticide (see p 160). Minor skin irritant. Convulsant. Hepatotoxin. Well absorbed dermally. Limited evidence for carcinogenicity in test animals. (IARC 3). | 0.25 mg/m$^3$, S, A3 NIOSH CA | 25 mg/m$^3$ | | Tan to dark brown solid. A mild chemical odor. Vapor pressure is 0.000006 mm Hg at 20°C (68°F). Not flammable but breaks down, yielding hydrogen chloride gas. Most uses have been banned in US. |
| **Allyl alcohol (2-propen-1-ol [CAS: 107-18-6]):** Strongly irritating to eyes and skin; severe burns may result. Vapors highly irritating to eyes and respiratory tract. Systemic poisoning can result from dermal exposures. May cause liver and kidney injury. | 0.5 ppm, S | 20 ppm | 4 3 1 | Colorless liquid. Mustard-like odor and irritation occur near the TLV and serve as good warning properties. Vapor pressure is 17 mm Hg at 20°C (68°F). Flammable. Used in chemical synthesis and as a pesticide. |
| **Allyl chloride (3-chloro-1-propene [CAS: 107-05-1]):** Highly irritating to eyes and skin. Vapors highly irritating to eyes and respiratory tract. Well absorbed by the skin, producing both superficial and penetrating irritation and pain. Causes liver and kidney injury in test animals. Chronic exposures have been associated with reports of mild neuropathy. (IARC 3). | 1 ppm, A3 | 250 ppm ERPG-1: 3 ppm ERPG-2: 40 ppm ERPG-3: 300 ppm | 3 3 1 | Colorless, yellow, or purple liquid. Pungent, disagreeable odor and irritation occur only at levels far above the TLV. Vapor pressure is 295 mm Hg at 20°C (68°F). Highly flammable. Breakdown products include hydrogen chloride and phosgene. |
| **Allyl glycidyl ether (AGE [CAS: 106-92-3]):** Highly irritating to eyes and skin; severe burns may result. Vapors irritating to eyes and respiratory tract. Sensitization dermatitis has been reported. Hematopoietic and testicular toxicity occurs in test animals at modest doses. Well absorbed through the skin. | 1 ppm | 50 ppm | | Colorless liquid. Unpleasant odor. Vapor pressure is 2 mm Hg at 20°C (68°F). Flammable. |
| **Allyl propyl disulfide (onion oil [CAS: 2179-59-1]):** Mucous membrane irritant and lacrimator. | 0.5 ppm, SEN | | | Liquid with a pungent, irritating odor. A synthetic flavorant and food additive. Thermal breakdown products include sulfur oxide fumes. |
| **alpha-Alumina (aluminum oxide [CAS: 1344-28-1]):** Nuisance dust and physical irritant. | 10 mg/m$^3$ | | | |

(C) = ceiling air concentration (TLV-C); S = skin absorption can be significant; SEN = potential sensitizer; A1 = ACGIH-confirmed human carcinogen; A2 = ACGIH-suspected human carcinogen; NFPA Hazard Codes: H = health, F = fire, R = reactivity, Ox = oxidizer, W = water-reactive, 0 (none) <—> 4 (severe). ERPG = Emergency Response Planning Guideline. See p 539 for an explanation of definitions.

(*continued*)

TABLE IV–4. HEALTH HAZARD SUMMARIES FOR INDUSTRIAL AND OCCUPATIONAL CHEMICALS (CONTINUED)

| Health Hazard Summaries | ACGIH TLV | IDLH | NFPA Codes H F R | Comments |
|---|---|---|---|---|
| **Aluminum metal (CAS: 7429-90-5):** Dusts can cause mild eye and respiratory tract irritation. Long-term inhalation of large amounts of fine aluminum powders or fumes from aluminum ore (bauxite) has been associated with reports of pulmonary fibrosis (Shaver's disease). Acute exposures in aluminum refining ("pot room") have been associated with asthma-like responses. Industrial processes used to produce aluminum have been associated with an increased incidence of cancer in workers. | 10 mg/m³ (metal and oxide)<br><br>5 mg/m³ (pyrophoric powders, welding fumes)<br><br>2 mg/m³ (soluble salts, alkyls NOS) | | 0 3 1 (powder) | Oxidizes readily. Fine powders and flakes are flammable and explosive when mixed with air. Reacts with acids and caustic solutions to produce flammable hydrogen gas. |
| **Aluminum phosphide (CAS: 20859-73-8):** Effects caused by phosphine gas that is produced on contact with moisture. Severe respiratory tract irritant. See phosphides, p 307. | | | 4 4 2 W | Used as a structural fumigant as dry powder or pellet, similar to zinc phosphide. |
| **4-Aminodiphenyl (*p*-aminobiphenyl, *p*-phenylaniline [CAS: 92-67-1]):** Potent bladder carcinogen in humans (IARC 1). Causes methemoglobinemia (p 262). | S, A1<br>OSHA CA<br>NIOSH CA | | | Colorless crystals. |
| **2-Aminopyridine (CAS: 504-29-0):** Mild irritant. Potent CNS convulsant. Very well absorbed by inhalation and skin contact. Signs and symptoms include headache, dizziness, nausea, elevated blood pressure, and convulsions. | 0.5 ppm | 5 ppm | | Colorless solid with a distinctive odor and a very low vapor pressure at 20°C (68°F). Combustible. |
| **Amitrole (3-amino-1,2,4-triazole [CAS: 61-82-5]):** Mild irritant. Well absorbed by inhalation and skin contact. Shows antithyroid activity in test animals. Evidence of adverse effects on fetal development in test animals at high doses. A carcinogen in test animals (IARC 3). Overexposure can cause acute lung injury. | 0.2 mg/m³, A3<br>NIOSH CA | | | Used as an herbicide. Crystalline solid. Appearance and some hazardous properties vary with the formulation. |

| | | | | |
|---|---|---|---|---|
| **Ammonia (CAS: 7664-41-7):** Corrosive; severe burns to eyes and skin result. Vapors highly irritating to eyes and respiratory tract; pulmonary edema has been reported. Severe responses are associated with anhydrous ammonia or with concentrated ammonia solutions (see p 71). | 25 ppm | 300 ppm<br>ERPG-1: 25 ppm<br>ERPG-2: 150 ppm<br>ERPG-3: 750 ppm | 3 1 0 | Colorless gas or aqueous solution. Pungent odor and irritation are good warning properties. Anhydrous ammonia is flammable. Breakdown products include oxides of nitrogen. Although widely used in industry, concentrated forms are most frequently encountered in agriculture and from its use as a refrigerant. |
| ***n*-Amyl acetate (CAS: 628-63-7):** Defats the skin, producing a dermatitis. Vapors mildly irritating to eyes and respiratory tract. A CNS depressant at very high levels. Reversible liver and kidney injury may occur at very high exposures. | 50 ppm | 1000 ppm | 1 3 0 | Colorless liquid. Its banana-like odor detectable below the TLV is a good warning property. Vapor pressure is 4 mm Hg at 20°C (68°F). Flammable |
| ***sec*-Amyl acetate ($\alpha$-methylbutyl acetate [CAS: 628-38-0]):** Defats the skin, producing a dermatitis. Vapors irritating to eyes and respiratory tract. A CNS depressant at very high levels. Reversible liver and kidney injury may occur at high-level exposures. | 50 ppm | 1000 ppm | 1 3 0 | Colorless liquid. A fruity odor occurs below the TLV and is a good warning property. Vapor pressure is 7 mm Hg at 20°C (68°F). Flammable. |
| **Aniline (aminobenzene, phenylamine [CAS: 62-53-3]):** Mildly irritating to eyes upon direct contact, with corneal injury possible. Potent inducer of methemoglobinemia (see p 262). Well absorbed via inhalation and dermal routes. Limited evidence of carcinogenicity in test animals (IARC 3). | 2 ppm, S, A3<br>NIOSH CA | 100 ppm | 3 2 0 | Colorless to brown viscous liquid. Distinctive amine odor and mild eye irritation occur well below the TLV and are good warning properties. Vapor pressure is 0.6 mm Hg at 20°C (68°F). Combustible. Breakdown products include oxides of nitrogen. |
| ***o*-Anisidine (*o*-methoxyaniline [CAS: 29191-52-4]):** Mild skin sensitizer causing dermatitis. Causes methemoglobinemia (see p 262). Well absorbed through skin. Headaches and vertigo are signs of exposure. Possible liver and kidney injury. A carcinogen in test animals (IARC 2B). | 0.5 mg/m$^3$, S, A3<br>NIOSH CA | 50 mg/m$^3$ | 2 1 0 | Colorless, red, or yellow liquid with the fishy odor of amines. Vapor pressure is less than 0.1 mm Hg at 20°C (68°F). Combustible. Primarily used in the dyestuffs industry. |

(C) = ceiling air concentration (TLV-C); S = skin absorption can be significant; SEN = potential sensitizer; A1 = ACGIH-confirmed human carcinogen; A2 = ACGIH-suspected human carcinogen; NFPA Hazard Codes: H = health, F = fire, R = reactivity, Ox = oxidizer, W = water-reactive, 0 (none) <—> 4 (severe). ERPG = Emergency Response Planning Guideline. See p 539 for an explanation of definitions.

(*continued*)

TABLE IV–4. HEALTH HAZARD SUMMARIES FOR INDUSTRIAL AND OCCUPATIONAL CHEMICALS (CONTINUED)

| Health Hazard Summaries | ACGIH TLV | IDLH | NFPA Codes H F R | Comments |
|---|---|---|---|---|
| **Antimony and salts (antimony trichloride, antimony trioxide, antimony pentachloride [CAS: 7440-36-0]):** Dusts and fumes irritating to eyes, skin, and respiratory tract. Toxicity through contamination with silica or arsenic may occur. Antimony trioxide is carcinogenic in test animals with limited evidence for carcinogenicity among antimony trioxide production workers (IARC 2B). See also p 99. | 0.5 mg/m$^3$ (as Sb) | 50 mg/m$^3$ (as Sb) | 3 0 1 ($SbCl_5$)<br>4 0 1 ($SbF_5$) | The metal is silver-white and has a very low vapor pressure. Some chloride salts release HCl upon contact with air. |
| **ANTU (α-naphthylthiourea [CAS: 86-88-4]):** Well absorbed by skin contact and inhalation. Pulmonary edema and liver injury may result from ingestion. Repeated exposures can injure the thyroid and adrenals, producing hypothyroidism. Possible slight contamination with a2-naphthylamine, a human bladder carcinogen. | 0.3 mg/m$^3$ | 100 mg/m$^3$ | | Colorless to gray solid powder. Odorless. A rodenticide. Breakdown products include oxides of nitrogen and sulfur dioxide. |
| **Arsenic (CAS: 7440-38-2):** Irritating to eyes and skin; hyperpigmentation, hyperkeratoses, and skin cancers have been described. A general cellular poison. May cause bone marrow suppression, peripheral neuropathy, and gastrointestinal, liver, and cardiac injury. Some arsenic compounds have adverse effects on fetal development in test animals. Exposure linked to skin, respiratory tract, and liver cancer in workers (IARC 1). See also p 115. | 0.01 mg/m$^3$ (as As)<br>A1<br>OSHA CA, NIOSH CA | 5 mg/m$^3$ (as As) | | Elemental forms vary in appearance. Crystals are gray. Amorphous forms may be yellow or black. Vapor pressure is very low: about 1 mm Hg at 372°C (701°F). |
| **Arsine (CAS: 7784-42-1):** Extremely toxic hemolytic agent. Symptoms include abdominal pain, jaundice, hemoglobinuria, and renal failure. Low-level chronic exposures reported to cause anemia. See also p 119. | [proposed: 0.005 ppm]<br>NIOSH CA | 3 ppm<br>ERPG-2: 0.5 ppm<br>ERPG-3: 1.5 ppm | 4 4 2 | Colorless gas with an unpleasant garlic-like odor. Flammable. Breakdown products include arsenic trioxide and arsenic fumes. Used in the semiconductor industry. |
| **Asbestos (chrysotile, amosite, crocidolite, tremolite, anthophyllite):** Effects of exposure include asbestosis (fibrosis of the lung), lung cancer, mesothelioma, and possible digestive tract cancer (IARC 1). Signs of toxicity are usually delayed at least 15–30 years. See also p 121. | 0.1 fibers/cm$^3$ (respirable fibers), A1<br>OSHA CA, NIOSH CA | | | Fibrous materials. Not combustible. TLVs vary with type: amosite, 0.5 fibers/cm$^3$, A1; chrysotile, 2 fibers/cm$^3$, A1; crocidolite, 0.2 fibers/cm$^3$, A1; other forms, 2 fibers/cm$^3$, A1. |

| | | | | |
|---|---|---|---|---|
| **Asphalt fumes (CAS: 8052-42-4):** Vapors and fumes irritating to eyes, skin, and respiratory tract. Skin contact can produce hyperpigmentation, dermatitis, or photosensitization. Some constituents are carcinogenic in test animals. | 0.5 $mg/m^3$ (inhalable fraction) NIOSH CA | | | Smoke with an acrid odor. Asphalt is a complex mixture of parrafinic, aromatic, and heterocyclic hydrocarbons formed by the evaporation of lighter hydrocarbons from petroleum and the partial oxidation of the residue. |
| **Atrazine [2-chloro-4-ethylamino-6-isoprylamino-s-triazine] (CAS: 1912-24-9):** The most heavily used triazine herbicide. Skin and eye irritant. IARC 3. | 5 $mg/m^3$ | | | Colorless crystals with a neglibile vapor pressure. Slightly sensitive to light. |
| **Azinphos-methyl (Guthion [CAS: 86-50-0]):** Low-potency organophosphate anticholinesterase insecticide (see p 292). Requires metabolic activation. | 0.2 $mg/m^3$ (inhalable fraction & vapor), S, SEN | 10 $mg/m^3$ | | Brown waxy solid with a negligible vapor pressure. Not combustible. Breakdown products include sulfur dioxide, oxides of nitrogen, and phosphoric acid. |
| **Barium and soluble compounds (CAS: 7440-39-3):** Powders irritating to eyes, skin, and respiratory tract. Although not typical of workplace exposures, ingestion of soluble barium salts (as opposed to the insoluble medical compounds used in radiography) are associated with muscle paralysis. See also p 126. | 0.5 $mg/m^3$ (as Ba) | 50 $mg/m^3$ (as Ba) | | Most soluble barium compounds (eg, barium chloride, barium carbonate) are odorless white solids. Elemental barium spontaneously ignites on contact with air and reacts with water to form flammable hydrogen gas. |
| **Benomyl (methyl1-[butylcarbamoyl]-2-benzimidazolecarbamate, Benlate [CAS: 17804-35-2]):** A carbamate cholinesterase inhibitor (see p 292). Mildly irritating to eyes and skin. Of low systemic toxicity in test animals by all routes. Evidence of adverse effects on fetal development in test animals. | 10 $mg/m^3$ | | | White crystalline solid with a negligible vapor pressure at 20°C (68°F). Fungicide and miticide. Appearance and some hazardous properties vary with the formulation. |
| **Benzene (CAS: 71-43-2):** Vapors mildly irritating to eyes and respiratory tract. Well absorbed by all routes. A CNS depressant at high levels. Symptoms include headache, nausea, tremors, cardiac arrhythmias, and coma. Chronic exposure may result in hematopoietic system depression, aplastic anemia, and leukemia (IARC 1). See also p 127. | 0.5 ppm, S, A1 OSHA CA, NIOSH CA | 500 ppm<br>ERPG-1: 50 ppm<br>ERPG-2: 150 ppm<br>ERPG-3: 1000 ppm | 2 3 0 | Colorless liquid. Aromatic hydrocarbon odor. Vapor pressure is 75 mm Hg at 20°C (68°F). Flammable. The generic term "benzine" is often used for gasoline or gasoline-like solvents and may not equate with benzene-containing materials. |

(C) = ceiling air concentration (TLV-C); S = skin absorption can be significant; SEN = potential sensitizer; A1 = ACGIH-confirmed human carcinogen; A2 = ACGIH-suspected human carcinogen; NFPA Hazard Codes: H = health, F = fire, R = reactivity, Ox = oxidizer, W = water-reactive, 0 (none) <—> 4 (severe). ERPG = Emergency Response Planning Guideline. See p 539 for an explanation of definitions.

(*continued*)

TABLE IV–4. HEALTH HAZARD SUMMARIES FOR INDUSTRIAL AND OCCUPATIONAL CHEMICALS (CONTINUED)

| Health Hazard Summaries | ACGIH TLV | IDLH | NFPA Codes H F R | Comments |
|---|---|---|---|---|
| **Benzidine (*p*-diaminodiphenyl [CAS: 92-87-5]):** Extremely well absorbed by inhalation and through skin. Causes bladder cancer in exposed workers (IARC 1). | S, A1<br>OSHA CA, NIOSH CA | | | White or reddish solid crystals. Breakdown products include oxides of nitrogen. Found in dyestuffs, rubber industry, and analytic laboratories. |
| **Benzoyl peroxide (CAS: 94-36-0):** Dusts cause skin, eye, and respiratory tract irritation. A skin sensitizer. IARC 3. | 5 mg/m$^3$ | 1500 mg/m$^3$ | | White granules or crystalline solids with a very faint odor. Vapor pressure is negligible at 20°C (68°F). Strong oxidizer, reacting with combustible materials. Decomposes at 75°C (167°F). Unstable and explosive at high temperatures. |
| **Benzyl chloride ($\alpha$ chlorotoluene, [chloro-methyl]benzene [CAS: 100-44-7]):** Highly irritating to skin and eyes. A potent lacrimator. Vapors highly irritating to respiratory tract. Symptoms include weakness, headache, and irritability. May injure liver. Limited evidence for carcinogenicity and adverse effects on fetal development in test animals (IARC 2A). | 1 ppm, A3 | 10 ppm<br>ERPG-1: 1 ppm<br>ERPG-2: 10 ppm<br>ERPG-3: 25 ppm | 3 2 1 | Colorless liquid with a pungent odor. Vapor pressure is 0.9 mm Hg at 20°C (68°F). Combustible. Breakdown products include phosgene and hydrogen chloride. |
| **Beryllium (CAS: 7440-41-7):** Very high acute exposure to dusts and fumes causes eye, skin, and respiratory tract irritation. However, more important, chronic low-level exposures to beryllium oxide dusts can produce interstitial lung disease called berylliosis, which is a sarcoid-like condition that can have extrapulmonary manifestations. A carcinogen in test animals. There is limited evidence of carcinogenicity in humans (IARC1). | 0.002 mg/m$^3$, A1 [proposed: 0.00005 ppm, S, SEN, A1]<br>NIOSH CA | 4 mg/m$^3$ (as Be)<br>ERPG-2: 25 mcg/m$^3$<br>ERPG-3: 100 mcg/m$^3$ | 3 1 0 | Silver-white metal or dusts. Reacts with some acids to produce flammable hydrogen gas. Exposures have occurred in nuclear and aerospace workers; may be present in any specialty metal alloy manufacturing process. |
| **Biphenyl (diphenyl [CAS: 92-52-4]):** Fumes mildly irritating to eyes. Chronic overexposures can cause bronchitis and liver injury. Peripheral neuropathy and CNS injury have also been reported. | 0.2 ppm | 100 mg/m$^3$ | 2 1 0 | White crystals. Unusual but pleasant odor. Combustible. Previously used as antimold treatment for paper (for example, in wrapping citrus). An outbreak of parkinsonism has been reported in this context. |

| | | | | |
|---|---|---|---|---|
| **Borates (anhydrous sodium tetraborate, borax [CAS: 1303-96-4]):** Contact with dusts is highly irritating to eyes, skin, and respiratory tract. Contact with tissue moisture may cause thermal burns because hydration of borates generates heat. See also p 135. | 2 mg/m$^3$ (inhalable fraction) | | | White or light gray solid crystals. Odorless. |
| **Boron oxide (boric anhydride, boric oxide [CAS: 1303-86-2]):** Contact with moisture generates boric acid (see p 135). Direct eye or skin contact with dusts is irritating. Occupational inhalation exposure has caused sore throat and cough. Evidence for adverse effects on the testes in test animals. | 10 mg/m$^3$ | 2000 mg/m$^3$ | | Colorless glassy granules, flakes, or powder. Odorless. Not combustible. |
| **Boron tribromide (CAS: 10294-33-4):** Corrosive; decomposed by tissue moisture to hydrogen bromide (see p 135) and boric acid (see p 135). Severe skin and eye burns may result from direct contact. Vapors highly irritating to eyes and respiratory tract. | 1 ppm (C) | | 3 0 2<br>W | Colorless fuming liquid. Reacts with water, forming hydrogen bromide and boric acid. Vapor pressure is 40 mm Hg at 14°C (57°F). |
| **Boron trifluoride (CAS: 7637-07-2):** Corrosive; decomposed by tissue moisture to hydrogen fluoride (see p 135) and boric acid (see p 135). Severe skin and eye burns may result. Vapors highly irritating to eyes, skin, and respiratory tract. | 1 ppm (C) | 25 ppm<br>ERPG-1: 2 mg/ m$^3$<br>ERPG-2: 30 mg/ m$^3$<br>ERPG-3: 100 mg/ m$^3$ | 4 0 1 | Colorless gas. Dense white irritating fumes produced on contact with moist air. These fumes contain boric acid and hydrogen fluoride. |
| **Bromine (CAS: 7726-95-6):** Corrosive; severe skin and eye burns may result. Vapors highly irritating to eyes and respiratory tract; pulmonary edema may result. Measles-like eruptions may appear on the skin several hours after a severe exposure. | 0.1 ppm | 3 ppm<br>ERPG-1: 0.1 ppm<br>ERPG-2: 0.5 ppm<br>ERPG 3: 5 ppm | 3 0 0<br>Ox | Heavy red-brown fuming liquid. Odor and irritation thresholds are below the TLV and are adequate warning properties. Vapor pressure is 175 mm Hg at 20°C (68°F). Not combustible. Used as an alternative to chlorine in water purification (eg, hot tubs). |

(C) = ceiling air concentration (TLV-C); S = skin absorption can be significant; SEN = potential sensitizer; A1 = ACGIH-confirmed human carcinogen; A2 = ACGIH-suspected human carcinogen; NFPA Hazard Codes: H = health, F = fire, R = reactivity, Ox = oxidizer, W = water-reactive, 0 (none) <—> 4 (severe). ERPG = Emergency Response Planning Guideline. See p 539 for an explanation of definitions.

(*continued*)

TABLE IV–4. HEALTH HAZARD SUMMARIES FOR INDUSTRIAL AND OCCUPATIONAL CHEMICALS (CONTINUED)

| Health Hazard Summaries | ACGIH TLV | IDLH | NFPA Codes H F R | Comments |
|---|---|---|---|---|
| **Bromine pentafluoride (CAS: 7789-30-2):** Corrosive; severe skin and eye burns may result. Vapors extremely irritating to eyes and respiratory tract. Chronic overexposures caused severe liver and kidney injury in test animals. | 0.1 ppm | | 4 0 3<br>W, Ox | Pale yellow liquid. Pungent odor. Not combustible. Highly reactive, igniting most organic materials and corroding many metals. Highly reactive with acids. Breakdown products include bromine and fluorine. |
| **Bromoform (tribromomethane [CAS: 75-25-2]):** Vapors highly irritating to eyes and respiratory tract. Well absorbed by inhalation and skin contact. CNS depressant. Liver and kidney injury may occur. Two preliminary tests indicate that it may be an animal carcinogen (IARC 3). | 0.5 ppm, S, A3 | 850 ppm | | Colorless to yellow liquid. Chloroform-like odor and irritation are adequate warning properties. Vapor pressure is 5 mm Hg at 20°C (68°F). Not combustible. Thermal breakdown products include hydrogen bromide and bromine. |
| **1,3-Butadiene (CAS: 106-99-0):** Vapors mildly irritating. A CNS depressant at very high levels. Evidence of adverse effects on reproductive organs and fetal development in test animals. A very potent carcinogen in test animals; evidence of carcinogenicity in exposed workers (IARC 2A). | 2 ppm, A2<br>NIOSH CA | 2000 ppm [LEL]<br>ERPG-1: 10 ppm<br>ERPG-2: 200 ppm<br>ERPG-3: 5000 ppm | 2 4 2 | Colorless gas. Mild aromatic odor is a good warning property. Readily polymerizes. Inhibitor added to prevent peroxide formation. Used in the formation of styrene-butadiene and ABS plastics. |
| **2-Butoxyethanol (ethylene glycol monobutyl ether, butyl Cellosolve [CAS: 111-76-2]):** Liquid very irritating to eyes and slightly irritating to skin. Vapors irritating to eyes and respiratory tract. Mild CNS depressant. A hemolytic agent in test animals. Well absorbed dermally. Liver and kidney toxicity in test animals. Reproductive toxicity much less than that of certain other glycol ethers such as ethylene glycol monomethyl ether. See also p 193. (IARC 3). | 20 ppm, A3 | 700 ppm | | Colorless liquid with a mild ether-like odor. Irritation occurs below the TLV and is a good warning property. Vapor pressure is 0.6 mm Hg at 20°C (68°F). Flammable. |
| ***n*-Butyl acetate (CAS: 123-86-4):** Vapors irritating to eyes and respiratory tract. A CNS depressant at high levels. Limited evidence for adverse effects on fetal development in test animals. | 150 ppm | 1700 ppm [LEL]<br>ERPG-1: 5 ppm<br>ERPG-2: 200 ppm<br>ERPG-3: 3000 ppm | 1 3 0 | Colorless liquid. Fruity odor is a good warning property. Vapor pressure is 10 mm Hg at 20°C (68°F). Flammable. |

| | | | | |
|---|---|---|---|---|
| ***sec*-Butyl acetate (2-butanol acetate [CAS: 105-46-4]):** Vapors irritating to eyes and respiratory tract. A CNS depressant at high levels. | 200 ppm | 1700 ppm [LEL] | 1 3 0 | |
| ***tert*-Butyl acetate (*tert*-butyl ester of acetic acid [CAS: 540-88-5]):** Vapors irritating to eyes and respiratory tract. A CNS depressant at high levels. | 200 ppm | 1500 ppm [LEL] | | |
| ***n*-Butyl acrylate (CAS: 141-32-2):** Highly irritating to skin and eyes; corneal necrosis may result. Vapors highly irritating to eyes and respiratory tract. Based on structural analogies, compounds containing the acrylate moiety may be carcinogens (IARC 3). | 2 ppm, SEN | ERPG-1: 0.05 ppm<br>ERPG-2: 25 ppm<br>ERPG-3: 250 ppm | 2 2 2 | Colorless liquid. Vapor pressure is 3.2 mm Hg at 20°C (68°F). Flammable. Contains inhibitor to prevent polymerization. |
| ***n*-Butyl alcohol (CAS: 71-36-3):** Irritating upon direct contact. Vapors mildly irritating to eyes and respiratory tract. A CNS depressant at very high levels. Chronic occupational overexposures associated with hearing loss and vestibular impairment. | 20 ppm | 1400 ppm [LEL] | 1 3 0 | Colorless liquid. Strong odor and irritation occur below the TLV and are both good warning properties. Flammable. |
| ***sec*-Butyl alcohol (CAS: 78-92-2):** Vapors mildly irritating to eyes and respiratory tract. A CNS depressant at high levels. | 100 ppm | 2000 ppm | 1 3 0 | Colorless liquid. Pleasant odor occurs well below the TLV and is an adequate warning property. Vapor pressure is 13 mm Hg at 20°C (68°F). Flammable. |
| ***tert*-Butyl alcohol (CAS: 75-65-0):** Vapors mildly irritating to eyes and respiratory tract. A CNS depressant at high levels. | 100 ppm | 1600 ppm | 1 3 0 | Colorless liquid. Camphor-like odor and irritation occur slightly below the TLV and are good warning properties. Vapor pressure is 31 mm Hg at 20°C (68°F). Flammable. |
| **Butylamine (CAS: 109-73-9):** Caustic alkali. Liquid highly irritating to eyes and skin upon direct contact; severe burns may result. Vapors highly irritating to eyes and respiratory tract. May cause histamine release. | 5 ppm (C), S | 300 ppm | 3 3 0 | Colorless liquid. Ammonia or fish-like odor occurs below the TLV and is an adequate warning property. Vapor pressure is about 82 mm Hg at 20°C (68°F). Flammable. |

(C) = ceiling air concentration (TLV-C); S = skin absorption can be significant; SEN = potential sensitizer; A1 = ACGIH-confirmed human carcinogen; A2 = ACGIH-suspected human carcinogen; NFPA Hazard Codes: H = health, F = fire, R = reactivity, Ox = oxidizer, W = water-reactive, 0 (none) <—> 4 (severe). ERPG = Emergency Response Planning Guideline. See p 539 for an explanation of definitions.

(*continued*)

TABLE IV–4. HEALTH HAZARD SUMMARIES FOR INDUSTRIAL AND OCCUPATIONAL CHEMICALS (CONTINUED)

| Health Hazard Summaries | ACGIH TLV | IDLH | NFPA Codes H F R | Comments |
|---|---|---|---|---|
| ***tert*-Butyl chromate (CAS: 1189-85-1):** Liquid highly irritating to eyes and skin; severe burns may result. Vapors or mists irritating to eyes and respiratory tract. A liver and kidney toxin. By analogy to other Cr(VI) compounds, a possible carcinogen. | 0.1 mg/m$^3$ (C) (as $CrO_3$), S NIOSH CA | 15 mg/m$^3$ (as Cr VI) | | Liquid. Reacts with moisture. |
| ***n*-Butyl glycidyl ether (BGE, glycidylbutylether, 1,2-epoxy-3-butoxy propane [CAS: 2426-08-6]):** Liquid irritating to eyes and skin. Vapors irritating to the respiratory tract. A CNS depressant. Causes sensitization dermatitis upon repeated exposures. Testicular atrophy and hematopoietic injury at modest doses in test animals. | 3 ppm, S, SEN | 250 ppm | | Colorless liquid. Vapor pressure is 3 mm Hg at 20°C (68°F). |
| ***n*-Butyl lactate (CAS: 138-22-7):** Vapors irritating to eyes and respiratory tract. Workers have complained of sleepiness, headache, coughing, nausea, and vomiting. | 5 ppm | | 1 2 0 | Colorless liquid. Vapor pressure is 0.4 mm Hg at 20°C (68°F). Combustible. |
| ***n*-Butyl mercaptan (butanethiol [CAS: 109-79-5]):** Vapors mildly irritating to eyes and respiratory tract. Pulmonary edema occurred at high exposure levels in test animals. A CNS depressant at very high levels. Limited evidence for adverse effects on fetal development in test animals at high doses. | 0.5 ppm | 500 ppm | 2 3 0 | Colorless liquid. Strong, offensive garlic-like odor. Vapor pressure is 35 mm Hg at 20°C (68°F). Flammable. |
| ***o*-sec-Butylphenol (CAS: 89-72-5):** Irritating to skin upon direct, prolonged contact; burns have resulted. Vapors mildly irritating to eyes and respiratory tract. | 5 ppm, S | | | A liquid. |
| ***p*-tert-Butyltoluene (CAS: 98-51-1):** Mild skin irritant upon direct contact. Defatting agent causing dermatitis. Vapors irritating to eyes and respiratory tract. A CNS depressant. Limited evidence of adverse effects on fetal development in test animals at high doses. | 1 ppm | 100 ppm | | Colorless liquid. Gasoline-like odor and irritation occur below the TLV and are both good warning properties. Vapor pressure is less than 1 mm Hg at 20°C (68°F). Combustible. |
| **gamma-Butyrolactone (CAS: 96-48-0):** Little animal or human toxicity information. Some reports indicate human exposure similar to gamma-hydroxybutric acid (GHB), producing CNS and respiratory depression. IARC 3. | | | | Industrial solvent. Contained in some "acetone-free" nail polish removers (now restricted in US). Metabolized to GHB. Vapor pressure 1.5 mm Hg at 20°C (68°F). |

| | | | | |
|---|---|---|---|---|
| **Cadmium and compounds:** Acute fumes and dust exposures can injure the respiratory tract; pulmonary edema can occur. Chronic exposures associated primarily with kidney injury and lung injury. Adverse effects on the testes and on fetal development in test animals. Cadmium and some of its compounds are carcinogenic in test animals. Limited direct evidence for carcinogenicity in humans (IARC 12A). See also p 140. | 0.01 mg/m$^3$ (total dust, as Cd), 0.002 mg/m$^3$ (respirable fraction, as Cd) A2 NIOSH CA | 9 mg/m$^3$ (dust and fumes, as Cd) | | Compounds vary in color. Give off fumes when heated or burned. Generally poor warning properties. Metal has a vapor pressure of about 1 mm Hg at 394°C (741°F) and reacts with acids to produce flammable hydrogen gas. "Silver solder" typically contains cadmium. |
| **Calcium cyanamide (calcium carbimide, lime nitrogen [CAS: 156-62-7]):** Dusts highly irritating to eyes, skin, and respiratory tract. Causes sensitization dermatitis. Systemic symptoms include nausea, fatigue, headache, chest pain, and shivering. A disulfiram-like interaction with alcohol (see p 184), "cyanamide flush," may occur in exposed workers. See also cadmium, p 140. | 0.5 mg/m$^3$ | | | Gray crystalline material. Reacts with water, generating ammonia and flammable acetylene. |
| **Calcium hydroxide (hydrated lime, caustic lime [CAS: 1305-62-0]):** Corrosive (see p 157); severe eye and skin burns may result. Dusts moderately irritating to eyes and respiratory tract. | 5 mg/m$^3$ | | | White, deliquescent crystalline powder. Odorless. |
| **Calcium oxide (lime, quicklime, burnt lime [CAS: 1305-78-8]):** Corrosive (see p 157). Exothermic reactions with moisture. Highly irritating to eyes and skin upon direct contact. Dusts highly irritating to skin, eyes, and respiratory tract. | 2 mg/m$^3$ | 25 mg/m$^3$ | 3 0 1 | White or gray solid powder. Odorless. Hydration generates heat. |
| **Camphor, synthetic (CAS: 76-22-2):** Irritating to eyes and skin upon direct contact. Vapors irritating to eyes and nose; may cause loss of sense of smell. A convulsant at doses typical of overdose ingestion rather than industrial exposure. See also p 146. | 2 ppm | 200 mg/m$^3$ | 0 2 0 | Colorless glassy solid. Sharp, obnoxious, aromatic odor near the TLV is an adequate warning property. Vapor pressure is 0.18 mm Hg at 20°C (68°F). Combustible. |
| **Caprolactam (CAS: 105-60-2):** Highly irritating to eyes and skin upon direct contact. Vapors, dusts, and fumes highly irritating to eyes and respiratory tract. Convulsant activity in test animals. | 5 mg/m$^3$ (inhalable fraction and vapor) | | | White solid crystals. Unpleasant odor. Vapor pressure is 6 mm Hg at 120°C (248°F). Thermal breakdown products include oxides of nitrogen. |

(C) = ceiling air concentration (TLV-C); S = skin absorption can be significant; SEN = potential sensitizer; A1 = ACGIH-confirmed human carcinogen; A2 = ACGIH-suspected human carcinogen; NFPA Hazard Codes: H = health, F = fire, R = reactivity, Ox = oxidizer, W = water-reactive, 0 (none) <—> 4 (severe). ERPG = Emergency Response Planning Guideline. See p 539 for an explanation of definitions.

*(continued)*

TABLE IV–1. HEALTH HAZARD SUMMARIES FOR INDUSTRIAL AND OCCUPATIONAL CHEMICALS (CONTINUED)

| Health Hazard Summaries | ACGIH TLV | IDLH | NFPA Codes H F R | Comments |
|---|---|---|---|---|
| **Captafol (Difolatan [CAS: 2425-06-1]):** Dusts irritating to eyes, skin, and respiratory tract. A skin and respiratory tract sensitizer. May cause photoallergic dermatitis. Evidence for carcinogenicity in animal tests (IARC 2A). | 0.1 mg/m$^3$, S<br>NIOSH CA | | | White solid crystals. Distinctive, pungent odor. Fungicide. Thermal breakdown products include hydrogen chloride and oxides of nitrogen or sulfur. |
| **Carbaryl (1-naphthyl *N*-methylcarbamate, Sevin [CAS: 63-25-2]):** A carbamate-type cholinesterase inhibitor (see p 292). Evidence of adverse effects on fetal development in test animals at high doses (IARC 3). | 5 mg/m$^3$ | 100 mg/m$^3$ | | Colorless, white or gray solid. Odorless. Vapor pressure is 0.005 mm Hg at 20°C (68°F). Breakdown products include oxides of nitrogen and methylamine. |
| **Carbofuran (2,3-dihydro-2,2'-dimethyl-7-benzofuranylmethyl-carbamate, Furadan [CAS: 1563-66-2]):** A carbamate-type cholinesterase inhibitor (see p 292). Not well absorbed by skin contact. | 0.1 mg/m$^3$ (inhalable fraction and vapor) | | | White solid crystals. Odorless. Vapor pressure is 0.00005 mm Hg at 33°C (91°F). Thermal breakdown products include oxides of nitrogen. |
| **Carbon black (CAS: 1333-86-4):** Causes eye and respiratory irritation. A lung carcinogen in test animals (IARC 2B). | 3.5 mg/m$^3$<br>NIOSH CA | | | Extremely fine powdery forms of elemental carbon; may have adsorbed polycyclic organic hydrocarbons. |
| **Carbon disulfide (CAS: 75-15-0):** Vapors mildly irritating to eyes and respiratory tract. A CNS depressant causing coma at high concentrations. Well absorbed by all routes. Acute symptoms include headache, dizziness, nervousness, and fatigue. Neuropathies, parkinsonian syndromes, and psychosis may occur. A liver and kidney toxin. An atherogenic agent causing stroke and heart disease. Adversely affects male and female reproductive systems in test animals and humans. Evidence for adverse effects on fetal development in test animals. See also p 150. | [proposed: 1 ppm, S] | 500 ppm<br>ERPG-1: 1 ppm<br>ERPG-2: 50 ppm<br>ERPG-3: 500 ppm | 3 3 0 | Colorless to pale yellow liquid. Disagreeable odor occurs below the TLV and is a good warning property. Vapor pressure is 300 mm Hg at 20°C (68°F). Highly flammable. Major use in viscose rayon manufacture but is also used in chemical synthesis and as an industrial solvent. It was used in the past as an agricultural fumigant. |

| | | | | |
|---|---|---|---|---|
| **Carbon monoxide (CAS: 630-08-0):** Binds to hemoglobin, forming carboxyhemoglobin and causing cellular hypoxia. Persons with heart disease are more susceptible. Signs and symptoms include headache, dizziness, coma, and convulsions. Permanent CNS impairment and adverse effects on fetal development may occur after severe poisoning. See also p 151. | 25 ppm | 1200 ppm<br>ERPG-1: 200 ppm<br>ERPG-2: 350 ppm<br>ERPG-3: 500 ppm | 3 4 0 | Colorless, odorless gas. No warning properties. Important sources of exposure include indoor use of internal combustion engines, structural fires, and faulty space heaters. |
| **Carbon tetrabromide (tetrabromomethane [CAS: 558-13-4]):** Highly irritating to eyes upon direct contact. Vapors highly irritating to eyes and respiratory tract. The liver and kidneys are also likely target organs. | 0.1 ppm | | | White to yellow-brown solid. Vapor pressure is 40 mm Hg at 96°C (204°F). Nonflammable; thermal breakdown products may include hydrogen bromide and bromine. |
| **Carbon tetrachloride (tetrachloromethane [CAS 56-23-5]):** Mildly irritating upon direct contact. A CNS depressant. May cause cardiac arrhythmias. Highly toxic to kidney and liver. Alcohol abuse increases risk of liver toxicity. A carcinogen in test animals (IARC 2B). See also p 222. | 5 ppm, S, A2<br>NIOSH CA | 200 ppm<br>ERPG-1: 20 ppm<br>ERPG-2: 100 ppm<br>ERPG-3: 750 ppm | 3 0 0 | Colorless. Ether-like odor is a poor warning property. Vapor pressure is 91 mm Hg at 20°C (68°F). Not combustible. Breakdown products include hydrogen chloride, chlorine gas, and phosgene. |
| **Carbonyl fluoride ($COF_2$ [CAS: 353-50-41]):** Extremely irritating to eyes and respiratory tract; pulmonary edema may result. Toxicity results from its hydrolysis to hydrofluoric acid (see p 222). | 2 ppm | | | Colorless, odorless gas. Decomposes upon contact with water to produce hydrofluoric acid. |
| **Catechol (1,2-benzenediol [CAS: 120-80-9]):** Highly irritating upon direct contact; severe eye and deep skin burns result. Well absorbed by skin. Systemic toxicity similar to that of phenol (see p 303); however, catechol may be more likely to cause convulsions and hypertension. At high doses, renal and liver injury may occur. IARC 2B. | 5 ppm, S, A3 | | | Colorless solid crystals. |
| **Cesium hydroxide (cesium hydrate [CAS: 21351-79-1]):** Corrosive (see p 157). Highly irritating upon direct contact; severe burns may result. Dusts are irritating to eyes and respiratory tract. | 2 $mg/m^3$ | | | Colorless or yellow crystals that absorb moisture. Negligible vapor pressure. |

(C) = ceiling air concentration (TLV-C); S = skin absorption can be significant; SEN = potential sensitizer; A1 = ACGIH-confirmed human carcinogen; A2 = ACGIH-suspected human carcinogen; NFPA Hazard Codes: H = health, F = fire, R = reactivity, Ox = oxidizer, W = water-reactive, 0 (none) <—> 4 (severe). ERPG = Emergency Response Planning Guideline. See p 539 for an explanation of definitions.

(*continued*)

TABLE IV–4. HEALTH HAZARD SUMMARIES FOR INDUSTRIAL AND OCCUPATIONAL CHEMICALS (CONTINUED)

| Health Hazard Summaries | ACGIH TLV | IDLH | NFPA Codes H F R | Comments |
|---|---|---|---|---|
| **Chlordane (CAS: 57-74-9):** Irritating to skin. A CNS convulsant. Skin absorption is rapid and has caused convulsions and death. Hepatotoxic. Evidence of carcinogenicity in test animals (IARC 2B). See also p 160. | 0.5 mg/m$^3$, S, A3<br>NIOSH CA | 100 mg/m$^3$ | | Viscous amber liquid. Formulations vary in appearance. A chlorine-like odor. Vapor pressure is 0.00001 mm Hg at 20°C (68°F). Not combustible. Thermal breakdown products include hydrogen chloride, phosgene, and chlorine gas. EPA banned this insecticide in 1976. |
| **Chlorinated camphene (toxaphene [CAS: 8001-35-2]):** Moderately irritating upon direct contact. A CNS convulsant. Acute symptoms include nausea, confusion, tremors, and convulsions. Well absorbed by skin. Potential liver and kidney injury. See also p 160. | 0.5 mg/m$^3$, S, A3<br>NIOSH CA | 200 mg/m$^3$ | | Waxy amber-colored solid. Formulations vary in appearance. Turpentine-like odor. Vapor pressure is about 0.3 mm Hg at 20°C (68°F). Pesticide use banned in the US since 1990. |
| **Chlorinated diphenyl oxide (CAS: 55720-99-5):** Chloracne may result from even small exposures. A hepatotoxin in chronically exposed test animals. Signs and symptoms include gastrointestinal upset, jaundice, and fatigue. See also Dioxins (p 183). | 0.5 mg/m$^3$ | 5 mg/m$^3$ | | Waxy solid or liquid. Vapor pressure is 0.00006 mm Hg at 20°C (68°F). |
| **Chlorine (CAS: 7782-50-5):** Extremely irritating to eyes, skin, and respiratory tract; severe burns and pulmonary edema may occur. Symptoms include lacrimation, sore throat, headache, coughing, and wheezing. High concentrations may cause rapid tissue swelling and airway obstruction through laryngeal edema. See also p 162. | 0.5 ppm | 10 ppm<br>ERPG-1: 1 ppm<br>ERPG-2: 3 ppm<br>ERPG-3: 20 ppm | 4 0 0<br>Ox | Amber liquid or greenish-yellow gas. Irritating odor and irritation occur near the TLV and are both good warning properties. Can be formed when acid cleaners are mixed with hypochlorite bleach cleaners. |
| **Chlorine dioxide (chlorine peroxide [CAS: 10049-04-4]):** Extremely Irritating to eyes and respiratory tract. Symptoms and signs are those of chlorine gas above (see p 162). | 0.1 ppm | 5 ppm<br>ERPG-2: 0.5 ppm<br>ERPG-3: 3 ppm | | Yellow-green or orange gas or liquid. Sharp odor at the TLV is a good warning property. Reacts with water to produce perchloric acid. Decomposes explosively in sunlight, with heat, or with shock to produce chlorine gas. Bleaching agent widely used in paper industry. |

| | | | | |
|---|---|---|---|---|
| **Chlorine trifluoride (chlorine fluoride [CAS: 7790-91-2]):** Upon contact with moist tissues, hydrolyzes to chlorine (see p 162), hydrogen fluoride (see p 222), and chlorine dioxide. Extremely irritating to eyes, skin, and respiratory tract; severe burns or delayed pulmonary edema could result. | 0.1 ppm (C) | 20 ppm<br>ERPG-1: 0.1 ppm<br>ERPG-2: 1 ppm<br>ERPG-3: 10 ppm | 4 0 3<br>W, Ox | Greenish-yellow or colorless liquid or gas or white solid. Possesses a suffocating, sweet odor. Not combustible. Water-reactive, yielding hydrogen fluoride and chlorine gas. Used as incendiary and rocket fuel additive. |
| **Chloroacetaldehyde (CAS: 107-20-0):** Extremely corrosive upon direct contact; severe burns will result. Vapors extremely irritating to eyes, skin, and respiratory tract. | 1 ppm (C) | 45 ppm | | Colorless liquid with a pungent, irritating odor. Vapor pressure is 100 mm Hg at 20°C (68°F). Combustible. Readily polymerizes. Thermal breakdown products include phosgene and hydrogen chloride. |
| **alpha-Chloroacetophenone (tear gas, chemical Mace [CAS: 532-27-4]):** Extremely irritating to mucous membranes and respiratory tract. With extremely high inhalational exposures, lower respiratory injury is possible. A potent skin sensitizer. See also p 373. | 0.05 ppm | 15 mg/m$^3$ | 2 1 0 | Sharp, irritating odor and irritation occur near the TLV and are adequate warning properties. Vapor pressure is 0.012 mm Hg at 20°C (68°F). Mace is a common crowd control agent. |
| **Chlorobenzene (monochlorobenzene [CAS: 108-90-7]):** Irritating; skin burns may result from prolonged contact. Vapors irritating to eyes and respiratory tract. A CNS depressant. May cause methemoglobinemia (see p 262). Prolonged exposure to high levels has caused lung, liver, and kidney injury in test animals. | 10 ppm, A3 | 1000 ppm | 2 3 0 | Colorless liquid. Aromatic odor occurs below the TLV and is a good warning property. Vapor pressure is 8.8 mm Hg at 20°C (68°F). Flammable. Thermal breakdown products include hydrogen chloride and phosgene. |
| ***o*-Chlorobenzylidene malononitrile (tear gas, OCBM, CS [CAS: 2698-41-1]):** Highly irritating on direct contact; severe burns may result. Aerosols and vapors very irritating to mucous membranes and upper respiratory tract. With extremely high inhalational exposures, lower respiratory injury is possible. Potent skin sensitizer. Symptoms include headache, nausea and vomiting, severe eye and nose irritation, excess salivation, and coughing. See also p 373. | 0.05 ppm (C), S | 2 mg/m$^3$ | | White solid crystals. Pepper-like odor. Vapor pressure is much less than 1 mm Hg at 20°C (68°F). CS is a common crowd control agent. |

(C) = ceiling air concentration (TLV-C); S = skin absorption can be significant; SEN = potential sensitizer; A1 = ACGIH-confirmed human carcinogen; A2 = ACGIH-suspected human carcinogen; NFPA Hazard Codes: H = health, F = fire, R = reactivity, Ox = oxidizer, W = water-reactive, 0 (none) <—> 4 (severe). ERPG = Emergency Response Planning Guideline. See p 539 for an explanation of definitions.

*(continued)*

TABLE IV–4. HEALTH HAZARD SUMMARIES FOR INDUSTRIAL AND OCCUPATIONAL CHEMICALS (CONTINUED)

| Health Hazard Summaries | ACGIH TLV | IDLH | NFPA Codes H F R | Comments |
|---|---|---|---|---|
| **Chlorobromomethane (bromochloromethane, Halon 1011 [CAS: 74-97-5]):** Irritating upon direct contact. Vapors mildly irritating to eyes and respiratory tract. A CNS depressant. Disorientation, nausea, headache, seizures, and coma have been reported at high exposure. Chronic high doses caused liver and kidney injury in test animals. | 200 ppm | 2000 ppm | | Colorless to pale yellow liquid. Sweet, pleasant odor detectable far below the TLV. Vapor pressure is 117 mm Hg at 20°C (68°F). Thermal breakdown products include hydrogen chloride, hydrogen bromide, and phosgene. |
| **Chlorodifluoromethane (Freon 22 [CAS: 75-45-6]):** Irritating upon direct contact. Vapors mildly irritating to eyes and respiratory tract. A CNS depressant. High-level exposure may cause arrhythmias. There is evidence at high doses for adverse effects on fetal development in test animals (IARC 3). See also p 208. | 1000 ppm | | | Colorless, almost odorless gas. Nonflammable. Thermal breakdown products may include hydrogen fluoride. Widely used commercial refrigerant (eg, in seafood industry). |
| **Chloroform (trichloromethane [CAS: 67-66-3]):** Mildly irritating upon direct contact; dermatitis may result from prolonged exposure. Vapors slightly irritating to eyes and respiratory tract. A CNS depressant. High levels (15,000–20,000 ppm) can cause coma and cardiac arrhythmias. Can produce liver and kidney damage. Limited evidence of adverse effects on fetal development in test animals. A carcinogen in test animals (IARC 2B). See also p 153. | 10 ppm, A3<br>NIOSH CA | 500 ppm<br>ERPG-2: 50 ppm<br>ERPG-3: 5000 ppm | 2 0 0 | Colorless liquid. Pleasant, sweet odor. Not combustible. Vapor pressure is 160 mm Hg at 20°C (68°F). Breakdown products include hydrogen chloride, phosgene, and chlorine gas. |
| ***bis*(Chloromethyl) ether (BCME [CAS: 542-88-1]):** A human and animal carcinogen (IARC 1). | 0.001 ppm, A1<br>OSHA CA<br>NIOSH CA | ERPG-2: 0.1 ppm<br>ERPG-3: 0.5 ppm | | Colorless liquid with a suffocating odor. Vapor pressure is 100 mm Hg at 20°C (68°F). Used in the manufacture of ion-exchange resins. |
| **Chloromethyl methyl ether (CMME, methyl chloromethyl ether [CAS: 107-30-2]):** Vapors irritating to eyes and respiratory tract. Workers show increased risk of lung cancer, possibly owing to contamination of CMME with 1–7% BCME (IARC 1). (See above.) | A2<br>OSHA CA<br>NIOSH CA | ERPG-2: 1 ppm<br>ERPG-3: 10 ppm | | Combustible. Breakdown products include oxides of nitrogen and hydrogen chloride. Used in the manufacture of ion-exchange resins. |
| **4-Chloro-2-Methylphenoxyacetic acid [MCPA]. [CAS 94-75-7]** GI irritant with less toxicity than related phenoxherbicides 2,4-D and mecoprop (see p 163). | | | | White crystalline solid. |
| **1-Chloro-1-nitropropane (CAS: 600-25-9):** Based on animal studies, vapors highly irritating to eyes and respiratory tract and may cause pulmonary edema. High levels may cause injury to cardiac muscle, liver, and kidney. | 2 ppm | 100 ppm | — 2 3 | Colorless liquid. Unpleasant odor and tearing occur near the TLV and are good warning properties. Vapor pressure is 5.8 mm Hg at 20°C (68°F). |

| | | | | |
|---|---|---|---|---|
| **Chloropentafluoroethane (fluorocarbon 115 [CAS: 76-15-3]):** Irritating upon direct contact. Vapors mildly irritating to eyes and respiratory tract. Produces coma and cardiac arrhythmias, but only at very high levels in test animals. See also p 208. | 1000 ppm | | | Colorless, odorless gas. Thermal breakdown products include hydrogen fluoride and hydrogen chloride. |
| **Chloropicrin (trichloronitromethane [CAS: 76-06-2]):** Extremely irritating upon direct contact; severe burns may result. Vapors extremely irritating to eyes, skin, and respiratory tract; delayed pulmonary edema has been reported. Kidney and liver injuries have been observed in test animals. | 0.1 ppm | 2 ppm<br>ERPG-1: 0.1 ppm<br>ERPG-2: 0.3 ppm<br>ERPG-3: 1.5 ppm | 4 0 3 | Colorless, oily liquid. Sharp, penetrating odor and tearing occur near the TLV and are good warning properties. Vapor pressure is 20 mm Hg at 20°C (68°F). Breakdown products include oxides of nitrogen, phosgene, nitrosyl chloride, and chlorine gas. Used as a fumigant and also as an additive for its warning properties. |
| **beta-Chloroprene (2-chloro-1,3-butadiene [CAS: 126-99-8]):** Irritating upon direct contact. Vapors irritating to eyes and respiratory tract. A CNS depressant at high levels. Liver and kidneys are major target organs. Limited evidence for adverse effects on fetal development and male reproduction in test animals. Equivocal evidence of carcinogenicity in test animals (IARC 2B). | 10 ppm, S<br>NIOSH CA | 300 ppm | 2 3 0 | Colorless liquid with an ether-like odor. Vapor pressure is 179 mm Hg at 20°C (68°F). Highly flammable. Breakdown products include hydrogen chloride. Used in making neoprene. |
| ***o*-Chlorotoluene (2-chloro-1-methylbenzene [CAS: 95-49-8]):** In test animals, direct contact produced skin and eye irritation; high vapor exposures resulted in tremors, convulsions, and coma. By analogy to toluene and chlorinated compounds, may cause cardiac arrhythmias. | 50 ppm | | 2 2 0 | Colorless liquid. Vapor pressure is 10 mm Hg at 43°C (109°F). Flammable. |
| **Chlorpyrifos (Dursban, 0,0-diethyl-0-(3,5,6-trichloro-2-pyridinyl [CAS: 2921-88-2]):** An organophosphate-type cholinesterase inhibitor (see p 292). | 0.1 mg/m$^3$, S (inhalable fraction and vapor) | | | White solid crystals. Vapor pressure is 0.00002 mm Hg at 25°C (77°F). |

(C) = ceiling air concentration (TLV-C); S = skin absorption can be significant; SEN = potential sensitizer; A1 = ACGIH-confirmed human carcinogen; A2 = ACGIH-suspected human carcinogen; NFPA Hazard Codes: H = health, F = fire, R = reactivity, Ox = oxidizer, W = water-reactive, 0 (none) <—> 4 (severe). ERPG = Emergency Response Planning Guideline. See p 539 for an explanation of definitions.

(*continued*)

TABLE IV–4. HEALTH HAZARD SUMMARIES FOR INDUSTRIAL AND OCCUPATIONAL CHEMICALS (CONTINUED)

| Health Hazard Summaries | ACGIH TLV | IDLH | NFPA Codes H F R | Comments |
|---|---|---|---|---|
| **Chromic acid and chromates (chromium trioxide, sodium dichromate, potassium chromate):** Highly irritating upon direct contact; severe eye and skin ulceration (chrome ulcers) may result. Dusts and mists highly irritating to eyes and respiratory tract. Skin and respiratory sensitization (asthma) may occur. Chromium trioxide is a teratogen in test animals. Certain hexavalent chromium compounds are carcinogenic in test animals and humans (IARC 1). IARC 3 (chromium III compounds and chromium metal). See also p 166. | 0.5 mg/m$^3$ (Cr III compounds), 0.05 mg/m$^3$, A1 (water-soluble Cr VI, compounds), 0.01 mg/m$^3$, A1 (insoluble Cr IV compounds) NIOSH CA | 15 mg/m$^3$ (Cr VI) | | Soluble chromate compounds are water-reactive. Chromates are common components of cement in concrete fabrication. |
| **Chromium metal and insoluble chromium salts:** Irritating upon direct contact with skin and eyes; dermatitis may result. Ferrochrome alloys possibly associated with pneumonoconiotic changes. See also p 166. | 0.5 mg/m$^3$ (metal, as Cr), 0.01 mg/m$^3$, A1 (Cr VI compounds, as Cr) | 250 mg/m$^3$ (Cr II compounds)<br>25 mg/m$^3$ (Cr III compounds)<br>250 mg/m$^3$ (Cr metal) | | Chromium metal, silver luster; copper chromite, greenish-blue solid. Odorless. |
| **Chromyl chloride (CAS: 14977-61-8):** Hydrolyzes upon contact with moisture to produce chromic trioxide, HCl, chromic trichloride, and chlorine. Highly irritating upon direct contact; severe burns may result. Mists and vapors highly irritating to eyes and respiratory tract. Certain hexavalent chromium VI compounds are carcinogenic in test animals and humans. See also p 166. | 0.025 ppm NIOSH CA | | | Dark red fuming liquid. Water-reactive, yielding hydrogen chloride, chlorine gas, chromic acid, and chromic chloride. |
| **Coal tar pitch volatiles (particulate polycyclic aromatic hydrocarbons [CAS: 65996-93-2]):** Irritating upon direct contact. Contact dermatitis, acne, hypermelanosis, and photosensitization may occur. Fumes irritating to eyes and respiratory tract. A carcinogen in test animals and humans (IARC 1). | 0.2 mg/m$^3$, A1 NIOSH CA | 80 mg/m$^3$ | | A complex mixture composed of a high percentage of polycyclic aromatic hydrocarbons. A smoky odor. Combustible. Creosote is an important source of exposure. |

| | | | |
|---|---|---|---|
| **Cobalt and compounds:** Irritating upon direct contact; dermatitis and skin sensitization may occur. Fumes and dusts irritate the respiratory tract; chronic interstitial pneumonitis and respiratory tract sensitization reported. Cardiotoxicity associated with ingestion, but has not been well documented with occupational exposures. Evidence of carcinogenicity in test animals (IARC 2B). | 0.02 mg/m$^3$ (elemental and inorganic compounds, as Co) A3 | 20 mg/m$^3$ (as Co) | Elemental cobalt is a black or gray, odorless solid with a negligible vapor pressure. "Hard metal" used in specialty grinding and cutting is a tungsten carbide–cobalt amalgam and causes a specific (giant cell) pneumonitis pattern. |
| **Cobalt hydrocarbonyl (CAS: 16842-03-8):** In animal testing, overexposure produces symptoms similar to those of nickel carbonyl and iron pentacarbonyl. Effects include headache, nausea, vomiting, dizziness, fever, and pulmonary edema. | 0.1 mg/m$^3$ (as Co) | ERPG-2: 0.13 ppm<br>ERPG-3: 0.42 ppm | Flammable gas. |
| **Copper fumes, dusts, and salts:** Irritation upon direct contact varies with the compound. The salts are more irritating and can cause corneal ulceration. Allergic contact dermatitis is rare. Dusts and mists irritating to the respiratory tract; nasal ulceration has been described. Ingestion can cause severe gastroenteritis and hepatic injury. See also p 174. | [proposed: 0.1 mg/m$^3$ (elemental and copper oxides, as Cu, inhalable fraction) 0.05 mg/m$^3$ (soluble compounds, as Cu, respirable fraction)] | 100 mg/m$^3$ (as Cu) | Salts vary in color. Generally odorless. |
| **Cotton dust:** Chronic exposure causes a respiratory syndrome called byssinosis. Symptoms include cough and wheezing, typically appearing on the first day of the work week and continuing for a few days or all week, although they may subside within an hour after leaving work. Can lead to irreversible obstructive airway disease. A flu-like illness similar to metal fume fever (see p 259) also occurs among cotton workers ("Monday morning fever"). | 0.2 mg/m$^3$ | 100 mg/m$^3$ | Cotton textile manufacture is the principal source of exposure. "Card room" work (an early stage in cotton thread production) is the most significant source of exposure. |

(C) = ceiling air concentration (TLV-C); S = skin absorption can be significant; SEN = potential sensitizer; A1 = ACGIH-confirmed human carcinogen; A2 = ACGIH-suspected human carcinogen; NFPA Hazard Codes: H = health, F = fire, R = reactivity, Ox = oxidizer, W = water-reactive, 0 (none) <—> 4 (severe). ERPG = Emergency Response Planning Guideline. See p 539 for an explanation of definitions.

(*continued*)

TABLE IV–4. HEALTH HAZARD SUMMARIES FOR INDUSTRIAL AND OCCUPATIONAL CHEMICALS (CONTINUED)

| Health Hazard Summaries | ACGIH TLV | IDLH | NFPA Codes H F R | Comments |
|---|---|---|---|---|
| **Creosote (coal tar creosote [CAS: 8001-58-9]):** A primary irritant, photosensitizer, and corrosive. Direct eye contact can cause severe keratitis and corneal scarring. Prolonged skin contact can cause chemical acne, pigmentation changes, and severe penetrating burns. Exposure to the fumes or vapors causes irritation of mucous membranes and the respiratory tract. Systemic toxicity results from phenolic and cresolic constituents. Liver and kidney injury may occur with heavy exposure. A carcinogen in test animals. Some evidence for carcinogenicity in humans (IARC 2A). See also phenol, p 303. | NIOSH CA | | 2 2 0 | Oily, dark liquid. Appearance and some hazardous properties vary with the formulation. Sharp, penetrating smoky odor. Combustible. Creosote is produced by the fractional distillation of coal tar. See entry on coal tar pitch volatiles. Plant-derived "creosote" is a different material that was used as a medicinal agent in the past and does not have the same carcinogenic potential. |
| **Cresol (methylphenol, cresylic acid, hydroxymethylbenzene [CAS: 1319-77-3]):** Corrosive. Skin and eye contact can cause severe burns. Exposure may be prolonged owing to local anesthetic action on skin. Well absorbed by all routes. Dermal absorption is a major route of systemic poisoning. Induces methemoglobinemia (see p 262). CNS depressant. Symptoms include headache, nausea and vomiting, tinnitus, dizziness, weakness, and confusion. Severe lung, liver and kidney injury may occur. See also phenol, p 303. | 5 ppm, S | 250 ppm | 3 2 0 (*ortho*)<br>3 2 0 (*meta, para*) | Colorless, yellow, or pink liquid with a phenolic odor. Vapor pressure is 0.2 mm Hg at 20°C (68°F). Combustible. |
| **Crotonaldehyde (2-butenal [CAS: 4170-30-3]):** Highly irritating upon direct contact; severe burns may result. Vapors highly irritating to eyes and respiratory tract; delayed pulmonary edema may occur. Evidence for carcinogenicity in test animals (IARC 3). | 0.3 ppm (C), S, A3 | 50 ppm<br>ERPG-1: 2 ppm<br>ERPG-2: 10 ppm<br>ERPG-3: 50 ppm | 4 3 2 | Colorless to straw-colored liquid. Pungent, irritating odor occurs below the TLV and is an adequate warning property. A warning agent added to fuel gases. Vapor pressure is 30 mm Hg at 20°C (68°F). Flammable. Polymerizes when heated. |
| **Crufomate (4-*tert*-butyl-2-chlorophenyl *N*-methyl *O*-methylphosphoramidate [CAS: 299-86-5]):** An organophosphate cholinesterase inhibitor (see p 292). | 5 mg/m$^3$ | | | Crystals or yellow oil. Pungent odor. Flammable. |

| | | | | |
|---|---|---|---|---|
| **Cumene (isopropylbenzene [CAS: 98-82-8]):** Mildly irritating upon direct contact. A CNS depressant at moderate levels. Well absorbed through skin. Adverse effects in fetal development in rats at high doses. | 50 ppm | 900 ppm [LEL] | 2 3 1 | Colorless liquid. Sharp, aromatic odor below the TLV is a good warning property. Vapor pressure is 8 mm Hg at 20°C (68°F). Flammable. |
| **Cyanamide (carbodiimide [CAS: 420-04-2]):** Causes transient vasomotor flushing. Highly irritating and caustic to eyes and skin. Has a disulfiram-like interaction with alcohol, producing flushing, headache, and dyspnea (see p 184). | 2 mg/m$^3$ | | 4 1 3 | Combustible. Thermal breakdown products include oxides of nitrogen. Used as an agricultural chemical for plant growth regulation. |
| **Cyanide salts (sodium cyanide, potassium cyanide):** Potent and rapidly fatal metabolic asphyxiants that inhibit cytochrome oxidase and stop cellular respiration. Well absorbed through skin; caustic action can promote dermal absorption. See also p 176. | 5 mg/m$^3$ (C) (as cyanide), S | 25 mg/m$^3$ (as cyanide) | | Solids. Mild, almond-like odor. In presence of moisture or acids, hydrogen cyanide may be released. Odor is a poor indicator of exposure to hydrogen cyanide. May be generated in fires from the pyrolysis of such products such as polyurethane and polyacrylonitrile. |
| **Cyanogen (dicyan, oxalonitrile [CAS: 460-19-5]):** Hydrolyzes to release hydrogen cyanide and cyanic acid. Toxicity similar to that of hydrogen cyanide (see p 176). Vapors irritating to eyes and respiratory tract. | 10 ppm | | 4 4 2 | Colorless gas. Pungent, almond-like odor. Breaks down on contact with water to yield hydrogen cyanide and cyanate. Flammable. |
| **Cyanogen chloride (CAS: 506-77-4):** Vapors extremely irritating to eyes and respiratory tract; pulmonary edema may result. Cyanide interferes with cellular respiration (see p 176). | 0.3 ppm (C) | ERPG-2: 0.4 ppm<br>ERPG-3: 4 ppm | | Colorless liquid or gas with a pungent odor. Thermal breakdown products include hydrogen cyanide and hydrogen chloride. Formed by a reaction with hypochlorite in the treatment of cyanide-containing wastewater. |
| **Cyclohexane (CAS: 110-82-7):** Mildly irritating upon direct contact. Vapors irritating to eyes and respiratory tract. A CNS depressant at high levels. Chronically exposed test animals developed liver and kidney injury. | 100 ppm | 1300 ppm [LEL] | 1 3 0 | Colorless liquid with a sweet, chloroform-like odor. Vapor pressure is 95 mm Hg at 20°C (68°F). Highly flammable. |

(C) = ceiling air concentration (TLV-C); S = skin absorption can be significant; SEN = potential sensitizer; A1 = ACGIH-confirmed human carcinogen; A2 = ACGIH-suspected human carcinogen; NFPA Hazard Codes: H = health, F = fire, R = reactivity, Ox = oxidizer, W = water-reactive, 0 (none) <—> 4 (severe). ERPG = Emergency Response Planning Guideline. See p 539 for an explanation of definitions.

(*continued*)

TABLE IV–4. HEALTH HAZARD SUMMARIES FOR INDUSTRIAL AND OCCUPATIONAL CHEMICALS (CONTINUED)

| Health Hazard Summaries | ACGIH TLV | IDLH | NFPA Codes H F R | Comments |
|---|---|---|---|---|
| **Cyclohexanol (CAS: 108-93-0):** Irritating upon direct contact. Vapors irritating to eyes and respiratory tract. Well absorbed by skin. A CNS depressant at high levels. Based on animal tests, it may injure the liver and kidneys at high doses. | 50 ppm, S | 400 ppm | 1 2 0 | Colorless viscous liquid. Mild camphor-like odor. Irritation occurs near the TLV and is a good warning property. Vapor pressure is 1 mm Hg at 20°C (68°F). Combustible. |
| **Cyclohexanone (CAS: 108-94-1):** Irritating upon direct contact. Vapors irritate the eyes and respiratory tract. A CNS depressant at very high levels. Chronic, moderate doses caused slight liver injury in test animals. | 20 ppm, S, A3 | 700 ppm | 1 2 0 | Clear to pale yellow liquid with peppermint-like odor. Vapor pressure is 2 mm Hg at 20°C (68°F). Flammable. |
| **Cyclohexene (1,2,3,4-tetrahydrobenzene [CAS: 110-83-8]):** By structural analogy to cyclohexane, may cause respiratory tract irritation. A CNS depressant. | 300 ppm | 2000 ppm | 1 3 0 | Colorless liquid with a sweet odor. Vapor pressure is 67 mm Hg at 20°C (68°F). Flammable. Readily forms peroxides and polymerizes. |
| **Cyclohexylamine (aminocyclohexane [CAS: 108-91-8]):** Corrosive and highly irritating upon direct contact. Vapors highly irritating to eyes and respiratory tract. Pharmacologically active, possessing sympathomimetic activity. Weak methemoglobin-forming activity (see p 262). Very limited evidence for adverse effects on reproduction in test animals. Animal studies suggest brain, liver, and kidneys are target organs. | 10 ppm | | 3 3 0 | Liquid with an obnoxious, fishy odor. Flammable. |
| **Cyclonite (RDX, trinitrotrimethylenetriamine [CAS: 121-82-4]):** Dermal and inhalation exposures affect the CNS with symptoms of confusion, headache, nausea, vomiting, convulsions, and coma. Does not have nitrate-like toxicity. | 0.5 mg/m$^3$, S | | | Crystalline solid. Vapor pressure is negligible at 20°C (68°F). Thermal breakdown products include oxides of nitrogen. Explosive. |
| **Cyclopentadiene [CAS: 542-92-7]):** Mildly irritating upon direct contact. Vapors irritating to eyes and respiratory tract. A CNS depressant at high levels. Animal studies suggest some potential for kidney and liver injury at high doses. | 75 ppm | 750 ppm | | Colorless liquid. Sweet, turpentine-like odor. Irritation occurs near the TLV and is a good warning property. Vapor pressure is high at 20°C (68°F). Flammable. |

| | | | | |
|---|---|---|---|---|
| **Cyclopentane (CAS: 287-92-3]):** Mildly irritating upon direct contact. Vapors irritating to eyes and respiratory tract. A CNS depressant at very high levels. Solvent mixtures containing cyclopentane have caused peripheral neuropathy, although this may have been related to *n*-hexane in combination. | 600 ppm | | 1 3 0 | Colorless liquid with a faint hydrocarbon odor. Vapor pressure is about 400 mm Hg at 31°C (88°F). Flammable. |
| **DDT (dichlorodiphenyltrichloroethane [CAS: 50-29-3]):** Dusts irritating to eyes. Ingestion may cause tremor and convulsions. Chronic low-level exposure results in bioaccumulation. A carcinogen in test animals (IARC 2B). See also p 160. | 1 mg/m$^3$, A3 NIOSH CA | 500 mg/m$^3$ | | Colorless, white, or yellow solid crystals with a faint aromatic odor. Vapor pressure is 0.0000002 mm Hg at 20°C (68°F). Combustible. Banned for use in US in 1973. |
| **Decaborane (CAS: 17702-41-9):** A potent CNS toxin. Symptoms include headache, dizziness, nausea, loss of coordination, and fatigue. Symptoms may be delayed in onset for 1–2 days; convulsions occur in more severe poisonings. Systemic poisonings can result from dermal absorption. Animal studies suggest a potential for liver and kidney injury. | 0.05 ppm, S | 15 mg/m$^3$ | 3 2 1 | Colorless solid crystals with a pungent odor. Vapor pressure is 0.05 mm Hg at 25°C (77°F). Combustible. Reacts with water to produce flammable hydrogen gas. Used as a rocket fuel additive and as a rubber vulcanization agent. |
| **Demeton (Systox, mercaptophos [CAS: 8065-48-3]):** An organophosphate-type cholinesterase inhibitor (see p 292). | 0.05 mg/m$^3$ (inhalable fraction and vapor), S | 10 mg/m$^3$ | | A sulfur-like odor. A very low vapor pressure at 20°C (68°F). Thermal breakdown products include oxides of sulfur. |
| **Diacetone alcohol (4-hydroxy-4-methyl-2 pentanone [CAS: 123-42-2]):** Irritating upon direct contact. Vapors very irritating to eyes and respiratory tract. A CNS depressant at high levels. Possibly some hemolytic activity. | 50 ppm | 1800 ppm [LEL] | 1 2 0 | Colorless liquid with an agreeable odor. Vapor pressure is 0.8 mm Hg at 20°C (68°F). Flammable. |
| **Diazinon (0,*O*-diethyl *O*-2-isopropyl-4-methyl-6-pyrimidinylthiophosphate [CAS: 333-41-5]):** An organophosphate-type cholinesterase inhibitor (see p 292). Well absorbed dermally. Limited evidence for adverse effects on male reproduction and fetal development in test animals at high doses. | 0.01 mg/m$^3$ (inhalable fraction and vapor), S | | | Commercial grades are yellow to brown liquids with a faint odor. Vapor pressure is 0.00014 mm Hg at 20°C (68°F). Thermal breakdown products include oxides of nitrogen and sulfur. |

(C) = ceiling air concentration (TLV-C); S = skin absorption can be significant; SEN = potential sensitizer; A1 = ACGIH-confirmed human carcinogen; A2 = ACGIH-suspected human carcinogen; NFPA Hazard Codes: H = health, F = fire, R = reactivity, Ox = oxidizer, W = water-reactive, 0 (none) <—> 4 (severe). ERPG = Emergency Response Planning Guideline. See p 539 for an explanation of definitions.

(*continued*)

TABLE IV–4. HEALTH HAZARD SUMMARIES FOR INDUSTRIAL AND OCCUPATIONAL CHEMICALS (CONTINUED)

| Health Hazard Summaries | ACGIH TLV | IDLH | NFPA Codes H F R | Comments |
|---|---|---|---|---|
| **Diazomethane (azimethylene, diazirine [CAS: 334-88-3]):** Extremely irritating to eyes and respiratory tract; pulmonary edema has been reported. Immediate symptoms include cough, chest pain, and respiratory distress. A potent methylating agent and respiratory sensitizer. | 0.2 ppm, A2 | 2 ppm | | Yellow gas with a musty odor. Air mixtures and compressed liquids can be explosive when heated or shocked. |
| **Diborane (boron hydride [CAS: 19287-45-7]):** Extremely irritating to the respiratory tract; pulmonary edema may result. Repeated exposures have been associated with headache, fatigue, and dizziness; muscle weakness or tremors; and chills or fever. Animal studies suggest the liver and kidney are also target organs. | 0.1 ppm | 15 ppm<br>ERPG-2: 1 ppm<br>ERPG-3: 3 ppm | 4 4 3<br>W | Colorless gas. Obnoxious, nauseatingly sweet odor. Highly flammable. Water-reactive; ignites spontaneously with moist air at room temperatures. A strong reducing agent. Breakdown products include boron oxide fumes. Used in microelectronic industry. Reacts violently with halogenated extinguishing agents. |
| **1,2-Dibromo-3-chloropropane (DBCP [CAS: 96-12-8]):** Irritant of eyes and respiratory tract. Has caused sterility (aspermia, oligospermia) in overexposed men. Well absorbed by skin contact and inhalation. A carcinogen in test animals (IARC 2B). | OSHA CA<br>NIOSH CA | | | Brown liquid with a pungent odor. Combustible. Thermal breakdown products include hydrogen bromide and hydrogen chloride. No longer used as a pesticide in the US. |
| **1, 2-Dibromo-2,2-dichloroethyl dimethyl phosphate (Naled, Dibrom [CAS: 300-76-5]):** An organophosphate anticholinesterase agent (see p 292). Highly irritating upon contact; eye injury is likely. Dermal sensitization can occur. Well absorbed dermally; localized muscular twitching results within minutes of contact. | 0.1 mg/m$^3$ (inhalable fraction and vapor), S, SEN | 200 mg/m$^3$ | | Has a pungent odor. Vapor pressure is 0.002 mm Hg at 20°C (68°F). Not combustible. Thermal breakdown products include hydrogen bromide, hydrogen chloride, and phosphoric acid. |
| **Dibutyl phosphate (di-*n*-butyl phosphate [CAS: 107-66-4]):** A moderately strong acid likely to be irritating upon direct contact. Vapors and mists are irritating to the respiratory tract and have been associated with headache at low levels. | 1 ppm | 30 ppm | | Colorless to brown liquid. Odorless. Vapor pressure is much less than 1 mm Hg at 20°C (68°F). Decomposes at 100°C (212°F) to produce phosphoric acid fumes. |

| | | | | |
|---|---|---|---|---|
| **Dibutyl phthalate (CAS: 84-74-2):** Mildly irritating upon direct contact. Ingestion has produced nausea, dizziness, photophobia, and lacrimation but no permanent effects. Adverse effects on fetal development and male reproduction in test animals at very high doses. | 5 mg/$m^3$ | 4000 mg/$m^3$ | 0 1 0 | Colorless, oily liquid with a faint aromatic odor. Vapor pressure is less than 0.01 mm Hg at 20°C (68°F). Combustible. |
| **1, 2-Dichloroacetylene (CAS: 7572-29-4):** Vapors extremely irritating to eyes and respiratory tract; pulmonary edema may result. CNS toxicity includes nausea and vomiting, headache, involvement of trigeminal nerve and facial muscles, and outbreaks of facial herpes. Limited evidence for carcinogenicity in test animals (IARC 3). | 0.1 ppm (C), A3<br>NIOSH CA | | | Colorless liquid. |
| ***o*-Dichlorobenzene (1,2-dichlorobenzene [CAS: 95-50-1]):** Irritating upon direct contact; skin blisters and hyperpigmentation may result from prolonged contact. Vapor also irritating to eyes and respiratory tract. Highly hepatotoxic in test animals. Evidence for adverse effects on male reproduction in test animals (IARC 3). | 25 ppm | 200 ppm | 2 2 0 | Colorless to pale yellow liquid. Aromatic odor and eye irritation occur well below the TLV and are adequate warning properties. Thermal breakdown products include hydrogen chloride and chlorine gas. |
| ***p*-Dichlorobenzene (1,4-dichlorobenzene [CAS: 106-46-7]):** Irritating upon direct contact with the solid. Vapors irritating to eyes and respiratory tract. Systemic effects include headache, nausea, vomiting, and liver injury. The *ortho* isomer is more toxic to the liver. A carcinogen in test animals (IARC 2B). | 10 ppm, A3<br>NIOSH CA | 150 ppm | 2 2 0 | Colorless or white solid. Mothball odor and irritation occur near the TLV and are adequate warning properties. Vapor pressure is 0.4 mm Hg at 20°C (68°F). Combustible. Thermal breakdown products include hydrogen chloride. Used as a moth repellant. |
| **3,3'-Dichlorobenzidine (CAS: 91-94-1):** Well absorbed by the dermal route. Animal studies suggest that severe eye injury and respiratory tract irritation may occur. A potent carcinogen in test animals (IARC 2B). | S, A3<br>OSHA CA<br>NIOSH CA | | | Crystalline needles with a faint odor. |
| **Dichlorodifluoromethane (Freon 12, Fluorocarbon 12 [CAS: 75-71-8]):** Mild eye and respiratory tract irritant. Extremely high exposures (eg, 100,000 ppm) can cause coma and cardiac arrhythmias. See also p 208. | 1000 ppm | 15,000 ppm | | Colorless gas. Ether-like odor is a poor warning property. Vapor pressure is 5.7 mm Hg at 20°C (68°F). Not combustible. Decomposes slowly on contact with water or heat to produce hydrogen chloride, hydrogen fluoride, and phosgene. |

(C) = ceiling air concentration (TLV-C); S = skin absorption can be significant; SEN = potential sensitizer; A1 = ACGIH-confirmed human carcinogen; A2 = ACGIH-suspected human carcinogen; NFPA Hazard Codes: H = health, F = fire, R = reactivity, Ox = oxidizer, W = water-reactive, 0 (none) <—> 4 (severe). ERPG = Emergency Response Planning Guideline. See p 539 for an explanation of definitions.

(*continued*)

TABLE IV–4. HEALTH HAZARD SUMMARIES FOR INDUSTRIAL AND OCCUPATIONAL CHEMICALS (CONTINUED)

| Health Hazard Summaries | ACGIH TLV | IDLH | NFPA Codes H F R | Comments |
|---|---|---|---|---|
| **1,3-Dichloro-5,5-dimethylhydantoin (Halane, Dactin [CAS: 118-52-5]):** Releases hypochlorous acid and chlorine gas (see p 162) on contact with moisture. Direct contact with the dust or concentrated solutions irritating to eyes, skin, and respiratory tract. | 0.2 mg/m$^3$ | 5 mg/m$^3$ | | White solid with a chlorine-like odor. Odor and eye irritation occur below the TLV and are adequate warning properties. Not combustible. Thermal breakdown products include hydrogen chloride, phosgene, oxides of nitrogen, and chlorine gas. |
| **1,1-Dichloroethane (ethylidene chloride [CAS: 75-34-3]):** Mild eye and skin irritant. Vapors irritating to the respiratory tract. A CNS depressant at high levels. By analogy with its 1,2-isomer, may cause arrhythmias. Animal studies suggest some potential for kidney and liver injury. | 100 ppm | 3000 ppm | 2 3 0 | Colorless, oily liquid. Chloroform-like odor occurs at the TLV. Vapor pressure is 182 mm Hg at 20°C (68°F). Flammable. Thermal breakdown products include vinyl chloride, hydrogen chloride, and phosgene. |
| **1,2-Dichloroethane (ethylene dichloride [CAS: 107-06-2]):** Irritating upon prolonged contact; burns may occur. Well absorbed dermally. Vapors irritating to eyes and respiratory tract. A CNS depressant at high levels. May cause cardiac arrhythmias. Severe liver and kidney injury has been reported. A carcinogen in test animals (IARC 2B). | 10 ppm<br>NIOSH CA | 50 ppm<br>ERPG-1: 50 ppm<br>ERPG-2: 200 ppm<br>ERPG-3: 200 ppm | 2 3 0 | Flammable. Thermal breakdown products include hydrogen chloride and phosgene. |
| **1,1-Dichloroethylene (vinylidine chloride [CAS: 75-35-4]):** Irritating upon direct contact. Vapors very irritating to eyes and respiratory tract. A CNS depressant. May cause cardiac arrhythmias. In test animals, damages the liver and kidneys. Limited evidence of carcinogenicity in test animals (IARC 3). | 5 ppm<br>NIOSH CA | | 4 4 2 | Colorless liquid. Sweet, ether-like or chloroform-like odor occurs below the TLV and is a good warning property. Polymerizes readily. Also used as a copolymer with vinyl chloride. |
| **1,2-Dichloroethylene (1,2-dichloroethene, acetylene dichloride [CAS: 540-59-0]):** Vapors mildly irritating to respiratory tract. A CNS depressant at high levels; once used as an anesthetic agent. May cause cardiac arrhythmias. Low hepatotoxicity. | 200 ppm | 1000 ppm | 2 3 2 | Colorless liquid with a slightly acrid, ether-like or chloroform-like odor. Vapor pressure is about 220 mm Hg at 20°C (68°F). Thermal breakdown products include hydrogen chloride and phosgene. |
| **Dichloroethyl ether (bis[2-chloroethyl] ether, dichloroethyl oxide [CAS: 111-44-4]):** Irritating upon direct contact; corneal injury may result. Vapors highly irritating to respiratory tract. A CNS depressant at high levels. Dermal absorption occurs. Animal studies suggest the liver and kidneys are also target organs at high exposures. Limited evidence for carcinogenicity in test animals. | 5 ppm, S<br>NIOSH CA | 100 ppm | 3 2 1 | Colorless liquid. Obnoxious, chlorinated solvent odor occurs at the TLV and is a good warning property. Flammable. Breaks down on contact with water. Thermal breakdown products include hydrogen chloride. |

| | | | | |
|---|---|---|---|---|
| **Dichlorofluoromethane (fluorocarbon 21, Freon 21, Halon 112 [CAS: 75-43-4]):** Animal studies suggest much greater hepatotoxicity than most common chlorofluorocarbons. Causes CNS depression, respiratory irritation, and cardiac arrhythmias at very high air levels (eg, 100,000 ppm). Evidence for adverse effects on fetal development (preimplantation losses) in test animals at high levels. See also p 208. | 10 ppm | 5000 ppm | | Colorless liquid or gas with a faint ether-like odor. Thermal breakdown products include hydrogen chloride, hydrogen fluoride, and phosgene. |
| **1,1-Dichloro-1-nitroethane [CAS: 594-72-9]):** Based on animal studies, highly irritating upon direct contact. Vapors highly irritating to eyes, skin, and respiratory tract; pulmonary edema may result. In test animals, lethal doses also injured the liver, heart, and kidneys. | 2 ppm | 25 ppm | 2 2 3 | Colorless liquid. Obnoxious odor and tearing occur only at dangerous levels and are poor warning properties. Vapor pressure is 15 mm Hg at 20°C (68°F). |
| **2,4-Dichlorophenol [CAS: 120-83-2]:** Extremely toxic, but the mechanism of action in human fatalities has not been determined. | | | | Used as a chemical precursor in the manufacture of 2,4-dichlorophenoxyacetic acid (2,4-D). Exposure occurs through unintended releases in industrial settings. |
| **2,4-Dichlorophenoxyacetic acid (2,4-D [CAS: 94-75-9]):** Direct skin contact can produce a rash. Overexposed workers have rarely experienced peripheral neuropathy. Severe rhabdomyolysis and minor liver and kidney injury may occur. Adverse effects on fetal development at high doses in test animals. There are weak epidemiologic associations of phenoxy herbicides with soft tissue sarcomas. IARC 2B (chlorophenoxy herbicides). See also p 163. | 10 mg/m$^3$ | 100 mg/m$^3$ | | White to yellow crystals. Appearance and some hazardous properties vary with the formulation. Odorless. Vapor pressure is negligible at 20°C (68°F). Thermal breakdown products include hydrogen chloride and phosgene. |
| **1,3-Dichloropropene (1,3-dichloropropylene, Telone [CAS: 542-75-6]):** Based on animal studies, irritating upon direct contact. Well absorbed dermally. Vapors irritating to eyes and respiratory tract. In test animals, moderate doses caused severe injuries to the liver, pancreas, and kidneys. A carcinogen in test animals (IARC 2B). | 1 ppm, S, A3<br>NIOSH CA | | 2 3 0 | Colorless or straw-colored liquid. Sharp, chloroform-like odor. Polymerizes readily. Vapor pressure is 28 mm Hg at 25°C (77°F). Thermal breakdown products include hydrogen chloride and phosgene. |

(C) = ceiling air concentration (TLV-C); S = skin absorption can be significant; SEN = potential sensitizer; A1 = ACGIH-confirmed human carcinogen; A2 = ACGIH-suspected human carcinogen; NFPA Hazard Codes: H = health, F = fire, R = reactivity, Ox = oxidizer, W = water-reactive, 0 (none) <—> 4 (severe). ERPG = Emergency Response Planning Guideline. See p 539 for an explanation of definitions.

(*continued*)

TABLE IV–4. HEALTH HAZARD SUMMARIES FOR INDUSTRIAL AND OCCUPATIONAL CHEMICALS (CONTINUED)

| Health Hazard Summaries | ACGIH TLV | IDLH | NFPA Codes H F R | Comments |
|---|---|---|---|---|
| **2,2-Dichloropropionic acid (CAS: 75-99-0):** Corrosive upon direct contact with concentrate; severe burns may result. Vapors mildly irritating to eyes and respiratory tract. | 5 mg/m$^3$ (inhalable fraction) | | | Colorless liquid. The sodium salt is a solid. |
| **Dichlorotetrafluoroethane (fluorocarbon 114, Freon 114 [CAS: 76-14-2]):** Vapors may sensitize the myocardium to arrhythmogenic effects of epinephrine at modestly high air levels (25,000 ppm). Other effects at higher levels (100,000–200,000 ppm) include respiratory irritation and CNS depression. See also p 208. | 1000 ppm | 15,000 ppm | | Colorless gas with a mild ether-like odor. Thermal breakdown products include hydrogen chloride, hydrogen fluoride, and phosgene. |
| **Dichlorvos (DDVP, 2,2-dichlorovinyl dimethyl phosphate [CAS: 62-73-7]):** An organophosphate-type cholinesterase inhibitor (see p 292). Extremely well absorbed through skin. Evidence of carcinogenicity in test animals (IARC 2B). | 0.1 mg/m$^3$ (inhalable fraction and vapor), S, SEN | 100 mg/m$^3$ | | Colorless to amber liquid with a slight chemical odor. Vapor pressure is 0.032 mm Hg at 32°C (90°F). |
| **Dicrotophos (dimethyl *cis*-2-dimethylcarbamoyl-1-methylvinyl phosphate, Bidrin [CAS: 141-66-2]):** An organophosphate cholinesterase inhibitor (see p 292). Dermal absorption occurs. | 0.05 mg/m$^3$ (inhalable fraction and vapor), S | | | Brown liquid with a mild ester odor. |
| **Dieldrin (CAS: 60-57-1):** Minor skin irritant. Potent convulsant and hepatotoxin. Dermal absorption is a major route of systemic poisoning. Overexposures produce headache, dizziness, twitching, and convulsions. Limited evidence for adverse effects on fetal development and carcinogenicity in test animals (IARC 3). See also p 160. | 0.25 mg/m$^3$, S NIOSH CA | 50 mg/m$^3$ | | Light brown solid flakes with a mild chemical odor. Appearance and some hazardous properties vary with the formulation. Vapor pressure is 0.0000002 mm Hg at 32°C (90°F). Not combustible. |
| **Diesel exhaust:** A respiratory irritant. May act as an adjuvant to immunologic sensitization. Animal and epidemiologic studies provide evidence of pulmonary carcinogenicity (IARC 2A). | 100 mg/m$^3$, S, A3 (uncombusted liquid fuel) NIOSH CA | | | Diesel engines emit a complex mixture of gases, vapors, and respirable particles, including many polycyclic aromatic and nitroaromatic hydrocarbons and oxides of nitrogen, sulfur, and carbon, including carbon monoxide. |

| | | | | |
|---|---|---|---|---|
| **Diethylamine (CAS: 109-89-7):** Corrosive. Highly irritating upon direct contact; severe burns may result. Vapors highly irritating to eyes and respiratory tract; pulmonary edema may occur. Subacute animal studies suggest liver and heart may be target organs. | 5 ppm, S | 200 ppm | 3 3 0 | Colorless liquid. Fishy, ammonia-like odor occurs below the TLV and is a good warning property. Vapor pressure is 195 mm Hg at 20°C (68°F). Highly flammable. Thermal breakdown products include oxides of nitrogen. |
| **2-Diethylaminoethanol (*N,N*-diethylthanolamine, DEAE [CAS: 100-37-8]):** Based on animal studies, highly irritating upon direct contact and a skin sensitizer. Vapors likely irritating to eyes, skin, and respiratory tract. Reports of nausea and vomiting after a momentary exposure to 100 ppm. | 2 ppm, S | 100 ppm | 3 2 0 | Colorless liquid. Weak to nauseating ammonia odor. Flammable. Thermal breakdown products include oxides of nitrogen. |
| **Diethylenetriamine (DETA [CAS: 111-40-0]):** Corrosive; highly irritating upon direct contact; severe burns may result. Vapors highly irritating to eyes and respiratory tract. Dermal and respiratory sensitization can occur. | 1 ppm, S | | 3 1 0 | Viscous yellow liquid with an ammonia-like odor. Vapor pressure is 0.37 mm Hg at 20°C (68°F). Combustible. Thermal breakdown products include oxides of nitrogen. |
| **Diethyl ketone (3-pentanone [CAS: 96-22-0]):** Mildly irritating upon direct contact. Vapors mildly irritating to eyes and respiratory tract. | 200 ppm | | 1 3 0 | Colorless liquid with an acetone-like odor. Flammable. |
| **Diethyl sulfate (CAS: 64-67-5):** Strong eye and respiratory tract irritant. Sufficient evidence of carcinogenicity in test animals. Limited evidence (laryngeal cancers) in humans (IARC 2A). | | | 3 1 1 | An alkylating agent. Colorless oily liquid with a peppermint odor. |
| **Difluorodibromomethane (dibromodifluoromethane, Freon 12B2 [CAS: 75-61-6]):** Based on animal tests, vapors irritate the respiratory tract. A CNS depressant. By analogy to other freons, may cause cardiac arrhythmias. In test animals, high-level chronic exposures caused lung, liver, and CNS injury. See also p 208. | 100 ppm | 2000 ppm | | Heavy, volatile, colorless liquid with an obnoxious, distinctive odor. Vapor pressure is 620 mm Hg at 20°C (68°F). Not combustible. Thermal breakdown products include hydrogen bromide and hydrogen fluoride. |
| **Diglycidyl ether (di[2,3-epoxypropyl]-ether, DGE [CAS: 2238-07-5]):** Extremely irritating upon direct contact; severe burns result. Vapors highly irritating to eyes and respiratory tract; pulmonary edema may result. Testicular atrophy and adverse effects on the hematopoietic system at low doses in test animals. CNS depression also noted. An alkylating agent and a carcinogen in test animals. | 0.1 ppm NIOSH CA | 10 ppm | | Colorless liquid with a very irritating odor. Vapor pressure is 0.09 mm Hg at 25°C (77°F). |

(C) = ceiling air concentration (TLV-C); S = skin absorption can be significant; SEN = potential sensitizer; A1 = ACGIH-confirmed human carcinogen; A2 = ACGIH-suspected human carcinogen; NFPA Hazard Codes: H = health, F = fire, R = reactivity, Ox = oxidizer, W = water-reactive, 0 (none) <—> 4 (severe). ERPG = Emergency Response Planning Guideline. See p 539 for an explanation of definitions.

(*continued*)

TABLE IV–4. HEALTH HAZARD SUMMARIES FOR INDUSTRIAL AND OCCUPATIONAL CHEMICALS (CONTINUED)

| Health Hazard Summaries | ACGIH TLV | IDLH | NFPA Codes H F R | Comments |
|---|---|---|---|---|
| **Diisobutyl ketone (2,6-dimethyl-4-heptanone [CAS: 108-83-8]):** Mildly irritating upon direct contact. Vapors mildly irritate eyes and respiratory tract. A CNS depressant at high levels. | 25 ppm | 500 ppm | 1 2 0 | Colorless liquid with a weak, ether-like odor. Vapor pressure is 1.7 mm Hg at 20°C (68°F). |
| **Diisopropylamine (CAS: 108-18-9):** Corrosive. Highly irritating upon direct contact; severe burns may result. Vapors very irritating to eyes and respiratory tract. Workers exposed to levels of 25–50 ppm have complained of hazy vision, nausea, and headache. | 5 ppm, S | 200 ppm | 3 3 0 | Colorless liquid with an ammonia-like odor. Vapor pressure is 60 mm Hg at 20°C (68°F). Flammable. Thermal breakdown products include oxides of nitrogen. |
| **Dimethyl acetamide (DMAC [CAS: 127-19-5]):** Potent hepatotoxin. Inhalation and skin contact are major routes of absorption. Limited evidence for adverse effects on fetal development in test animals at high doses. | 10 ppm, S | 300 ppm | 2 2 0 | Colorless liquid with a weak ammonia-like odor. Vapor pressure is 1.5 mm Hg at 20°C (68°F). Combustible. Thermal breakdown products include oxides of nitrogen. |
| **Dimethylamine (DMA [CAS: 124-40-3]):** Corrosive upon direct contact; severe burns may result. Vapors extremely irritating to eyes and respiratory tract. Animal studies suggest liver is a target organ. | 5 ppm | 500 ppm<br>ERPG-1: 10.6 ppm<br>ERPG-2: 100 ppm<br>ERPG-3: 500 350 ppm | 3 4 0 | Colorless liquid or gas. Fishy or ammonia-like odor far below TLV is a good warning property. Flammable. Thermal breakdown products include oxides of nitrogen. |
| **4-Dimethylaminophenol (CAS: 619-60-3):** Potent oxidizer used to induce methemoglobinemia in some countries outside the US (especially Germany). | | | | |
| ***N,N*-Dimethylaniline (CAS: 121-69-7):** Causes methemoglobinemia (see p 262). A CNS depressant. Well absorbed dermally. Limited evidence for carcinogenicity in test animals (IARC 3). | 5 ppm, S | 100 ppm | 3 2 0 | Straw- to brown-colored liquid with an amine-like odor. Vapor pressure is less than 1 mm Hg at 20°C (68°F). Combustible. Thermal breakdown products include oxides of nitrogen. |
| **Dimethylcarbamoyl chloride (CAS: 79-44-7):** Rapidly hydrolyzed by moisture to dimethylamine, carbon dioxide, and hydrochloric acid. Expected to be extremely irritating upon direct contact or by inhalation. A carcinogen in test animals (IARC 2A). | A2<br>NIOSH CA | | | Liquid. Rapidly reacts with moisture to yield dimethylamine and hydrogen chloride. |

| | | | | |
|---|---|---|---|---|
| ***N,N*-Dimethylformamide (DMF [CAS: 68-12-2]):** Dermally well absorbed. Symptoms of overexposure include abdominal pain, nausea, and vomiting. This chemical is a potent hepatotoxin in humans. Interferes with ethanol to cause disulfiram-like reactions (see p 184). Limited epidemiologic association with an increased risk of testicular cancer (IARC 3). Limited evidence for adverse effects on fetal development in animals. | 10 ppm, S | 500 ppm<br>ERPG-1: 2 ppm<br>ERPG-2: 100 ppm<br>ERPG-3: 200 ppm | 1 2 0 | Colorless to pale yellow liquid. Faint ammonia-like odor is a poor warning property. Vapor pressure is 2.7 mm Hg at 20°C (68°F). Flammable. Thermal breakdown products include oxides of nitrogen. |
| ***1,1*-Dimethylhydrazine (DMH, UDMH [CAS: 57-14-7]):** Corrosive upon direct contact; severe burns may result. Vapors extremely irritating to eyes and respiratory tract; pulmonary edema may occur. Well absorbed through the skin. May cause methemoglobinemia (see p 262); may cause hemolysis. A potent hepatotoxin; a carcinogen in test animals (IARC 2B). | 0.01 ppm, S<br>NIOSH CA | 15 ppm | 4 3 1 | Colorless liquid with yellow fumes. Amine odor. Vapor pressure is 1.3 mm Hg at 20°C (68°F). Thermal breakdown products include oxides of nitrogen. |
| **Dimethylmercury (mercury dimethyl, [CAS 593-74-8]):** Extremely toxic liquid readily absorbed by inhalation or across intact skin; as little as 1–2 drops on a latex glove caused death in a research chemist. Neurotoxic effects include progressive ataxia, dysarthria, visual and auditory dysfunction, and coma. See also Mercury (p 253). | OSHA PEL for alkyl mercury compounds in general: 0.01 $mg/m^3$ | | | Colorless liquid with a weak, sweet odor. Density 3.2 g/mL. Vapor pressure 50–82 mm Hg at 20°C (68°F). Permeable through latex, neoprene, and butyl rubber gloves. (OSHA recommends Silver Shield laminate gloves under outer gloves.) |
| **Dimethyl sulfate (CAS: 77-78-1):** Powerful vesicant action; hydrolyzes to sulfuric acid and methanol. Extremely irritating upon direct contact; severe burns have resulted. Vapors irritating to eyes and respiratory tract; delayed pulmonary edema may result. Skin absorption is rapid. A carcinogen in test animals (IARC 2A). | 0.1 ppm, S, A3<br>NIOSH CA | 7 ppm | 4 2 0 | Colorless, oily liquid. Very mild onion odor is barely perceptible and is a poor warning property. Vapor pressure is 0.5 mm Hg at 20°C (68°F). Combustible. Thermal breakdown products include sulfur oxides. |
| ***N,N*-Dimethyl-p-toluidine (CAS: 99-97-8):** Oxidizing agent causing methemoglobinemia, presumably through its metabolite p-methylphenylhydroxylamine. See Methemoglobinemia p 262. | | | | Used as a polymerization accelerator for ethyl methacrylate monomer. Exposure has occurred through artificial (sculpted) nail application. |

(C) = ceiling air concentration (TLV-C); S = skin absorption can be significant; SEN = potential sensitizer; A1 = ACGIH-confirmed human carcinogen; A2 = ACGIH-suspected human carcinogen; NFPA Hazard Codes: H = health, F = fire, R = reactivity, Ox = oxidizer, W = water-reactive, 0 (none) <—> 4 (severe). ERPG = Emergency Response Planning Guideline. See p 539 for an explanation of definitions.

(*continued*)

TABLE IV–4. HEALTH HAZARD SUMMARIES FOR INDUSTRIAL AND OCCUPATIONAL CHEMICALS (CONTINUED)

| Health Hazard Summaries | ACGIH TLV | IDLH | NFPA Codes H F R | Comments |
|---|---|---|---|---|
| **Dinitrobenzene [CAS: 528-29-0 (ortho); 100-25-4 (para)]:** May stain tissues yellow upon direct contact. Vapors are irritating to respiratory tract. Potent inducer of methemoglobinemia (see p 262). Chronic exposures may result in anemia and liver damage. Injures testes in test animals. Very well absorbed through the skin. | 0.15 ppm, S | 50 mg/m$^3$ | 3 1 4 | Pale yellow crystals. Explosive; detonated by heat or shock. Vapor pressure is much less than 1 mm Hg at 20°C (68°F). Thermal breakdown products include oxides of nitrogen. |
| **Dinitro-o-cresol (2-methyl-4,6-dinitrophenol [CAS: 534-52-1]):** Highly toxic; uncouples oxidative phosphorylation in mitochondria, increasing metabolic rate and leading to fatigue, sweating, rapid breathing, tachycardia, and fever. Liver and kidney injury may occur. Symptoms may last for days, as it is excreted very slowly. May induce methemoglobinemia (see p 262). Poisonings may result from dermal exposure. Yellow-stained skin may mark exposure. | 0.2 mg/m$^3$, S | 5 mg/m$^3$ | | Yellow solid crystals. Odorless. Dust is explosive. Vapor pressure is 0.00005 mm Hg at 20°C (68°F). Thermal breakdown products include oxides of nitrogen. |
| **2,4-Dinitrophenol (CAS: 25550-58-7):** Potent uncoupler of oxidative phosphorylation. Initial findings include hypertension, fever, dyspnea, and tachypnea. May cause methemoglobinemia and harm liver and kidneys. May stain skin at point of contact. Limited evidence for adverse effects on fetal development. See also p 299. | | | | Industrial chemical and pesticide. Abused as a chemical dietary supplement for weight loss and in body building. Fatal hyperthermia has been reported. |
| **2,4-Dinitrotoluene (DNT [CAS: 25321-14-6]):** May cause methemoglobinemia (see p 262). Uncouples oxidative phosphorylation, leading to increased metabolic rate and hyperthermia, tachycardia, and fatigue. A hepatotoxin. May cause vasodilation; headache and drop in blood pressure are common. Cessation of exposure may precipitate angina pectoris in pharmacologically dependent workers. Well absorbed by all routes. May stain skin yellow. Injures testes in test animals and, possibly, exposed workers. A carcinogen in test animals. | 0.2 mg/m$^3$, A3, S NIOSH CA | 50 mg/m$^3$ | 3 1 3 | Orange-yellow solid (pure) or oily liquid with a characteristic odor. Explosive. Thermal breakdown products include oxides of nitrogen. Vapor pressure is 1 mm Hg at 20°C (68°F). |
| **1,4-Dioxane (1,4-diethylene dioxide [CAS: 123-91-1]):** Vapors irritating to eyes and respiratory tract. Inhalation or dermal exposures may cause gastrointestinal upset and liver and kidney injury. A carcinogen in test animals (IARC 2B). | 20 ppm, S, A3 NIOSH CA | 500 ppm | 2 3 1 | Colorless liquid. Mild ether-like odor occurs only at dangerous levels and is a poor warning property. Vapor pressure is 29 mm Hg at 20°C (68°F). Flammable. |

| | | | | |
|---|---|---|---|---|
| **Dioxathion (2,3-*p*-dioxanedithiol *S,S*-bis [*O,O*-diethyl phosphorodithioate] [CAS: 78-34-2]):** An organophosphate-type cholinesterase inhibitor (see p 298). Well absorbed dermally. | 0.1 mg/m$^3$ (inhalable fraction and vapor), S | | | Amber liquid. Vapor pressure is negligible at 20°C (68°F). Thermal breakdown products include oxides of sulfur. |
| **Dipropylene glycol methyl ether (DPGME [CAS: 34590-94-8]):** Mildly irritating to eyes upon direct contact. A CNS depressant at very high levels. | 100 ppm, S | 600 ppm | 0 2 0 | Colorless liquid with a mild ether-like odor. Nasal irritation is a good warning property. Vapor pressure is 0.3 mm Hg at 20°C (68°F). Combustible. |
| **Diquat (1,1-ethylene-2,2'-dipyridinium dibromide, Reglone, Dextrone [CAS: 85-00-7]):** Corrosive in high concentrations. Acute renal failure and reversible liver injury may occur. Chronic feeding studies caused cataracts in test animals. Although pulmonary edema might occur, unlike paraquat, pulmonary fibrosis has not been shown with human diquat exposures. See also p 297. | 0.5 mg/m$^3$ (total dust, inhalable fraction)<br>0.1 mg/m$^3$ (respirable dust), S | | | Yellow solid crystals. Appearance and some hazardous properties vary with the formulation. |
| **Disulfiram (tetraethylthiuram disulfide, Antabuse [CAS: 97-77-8]):** Inhibits aldehyde dehydrogenase, an enzyme involved in ethanol metabolism. Exposure to disulfiram and alcohol will produce flushing, headache, and hypotension. Disulfiram may also interact with other industrial solvents that share metabolic pathways with ethanol. Limited evidence for adverse effects on fetal development in test animals (IARC 3). See also p 184. | 2 mg/m$^3$ | | | Crystalline solid. Thermal breakdown products include oxides of sulfur. |
| **Disulfoton (*O,O*-diethyl-*S*-ethylmercapto-ethyl dithiophosphate [CAS: 298-04-4]):** An organophosphate-type cholinesterase inhibitor (see p 298). Dermally well absorbed. | 0.05 mg/m$^3$, S | | | Vapor pressure is 0.00018 mm Hg at 20°C (68°F). Thermal breakdown products include oxides of sulfur. |
| **Divinylbenzene (DVB, vinylstyrene [CAS: 1321-74-0]):** Mildly irritating upon direct contact. Vapors mildly irritating to eyes and respiratory tract. | 10 ppm | | 1 2 2 | Pale yellow liquid. Combustible. Must contain inhibitor to prevent explosive polymerization. |
| **Emery (corundum, impure aluminum oxide [CAS: 112-62-9]):** An abrasive, nuisance dust causing physical irritation to eyes, skin, and respiratory tract. | 10 mg/m$^3$ | | | Solid crystals of aluminum oxide. Often used for its abrasive properties (eg, emery cloth, emery wheel). |

(C) = ceiling air concentration (TLV-C); S = skin absorption can be significant; SEN = potential sensitizer; A1 = ACGIH-confirmed human carcinogen; A2 = ACGIH-suspected human carcinogen; NFPA Hazard Codes: H = health, F = fire, R = reactivity, Ox = oxidizer, W = water-reactive, 0 (none) <—> 4 (severe). ERPG = Emergency Response Planning Guideline. See p 539 for an explanation of definitions.

(*continued*)

TABLE IV–4. HEALTH HAZARD SUMMARIES FOR INDUSTRIAL AND OCCUPATIONAL CHEMICALS (CONTINUED)

| Health Hazard Summaries | ACGIH TLV | IDLH | NFPA Codes H F R | Comments |
|---|---|---|---|---|
| **Endosulfan (CAS: 115-29-7):** Inhalation and skin absorption are major routes of exposure. Symptoms include nausea, confusion, excitement, twitching, and convulsions. Animal studies suggest liver and kidney injury from very high exposures. Limited evidence for adverse effects on male reproduction and fetal development in animal studies. See also p 160. | 0.1 mg/m$^3$, S | | | Chlorinated hydrocarbon insecticide. Tan, waxy solid with a mild sulfur dioxide odor. Thermal breakdown products include oxides of sulfur and hydrogen chloride. |
| **Endrin (CAS: 72-20-8):** Endrin is the stereoisomer of dieldrin, and its toxicity is very similar. Well absorbed through skin. Overexposure may produce headache, dizziness, nausea, confusion, twitching, and convulsions. Adverse effects on fetal development in test animals (IARC 3). See also p 160. | 0.1 mg/m$^3$, S | 2 mg/m$^3$ | | Colorless, white, or tan solid. A stereoisomer of dieldrin. A mild chemical odor and negligible vapor pressure of 0.0000002 mm Hg at 20°C (68°F). Not combustible. Thermal breakdown products include hydrogen chloride. |
| **Environmental tobacco smoke:** Passive smoking causes respiratory irritation and small reductions in lung function. It increases severity and frequency of asthmatic attacks in children. May cause coughing, phlegm production, chest discomfort, and reduced lung function in adults. Causes developmental toxicity in infants and children and reproductive toxicity in adult females. Epidemiologic studies show passive smoking causes lung cancer (IARC 1). | | | | |
| **Epichlorohydrin (chloropropylene oxide [CAS: 106-89-8]):** Extremely irritating upon direct contact; severe burns may result. Vapors highly irritating to eyes and respiratory tract; pulmonary edema has been reported. Other effects include nausea, vomiting, and abdominal pain. Sensitization has been reported occasionally reported. Animal studies suggest a potential for liver and kidney injury. High doses reduce fertility in test animals. A carcinogen in test animals (IARC 2A). | 0.5 ppm, S, A3<br>NIOSH CA | 75 ppm<br>ERPG-1: 2 ppm<br>ERPG-2: 20 ppm<br>ERPG-3: 100 ppm | 3 3 2 | Colorless liquid. The irritating, chloroform-like odor is detectable only at extremely high exposures and is a poor warning property. Vapor pressure is 13 mm Hg at 20°C (68°F). Flammable. Thermal breakdown products include hydrogen chloride and and phosgene. |
| **EPN (*O-ethyl O-p*-nitrophenyl phenylphosphonothioate [CAS: 2104-64-5]):** An organophosphate-type cholinesterase inhibitor (see p 298). | 0.1 mg/m$^3$ (inhalable fraction), S | 5 mg/m$^3$ | | Yellow solid or brown liquid. Vapor pressure is 0.0003 mm Hg at 100°C (212°F). |

| | | | | |
|---|---|---|---|---|
| **Ethanolamine (2-aminoethanol [CAS: 141-43-5]):** Highly irritating upon direct contact; severe burns may result. Prolonged contact with skin is irritating. Animal studies suggest that at high levels, vapors are irritating to eyes and respiratory tract and liver and kidney injury may occur. Limited evidence for adverse effects on fetal development in animal studies. | 3 ppm | 30 ppm | 3 2 0 | Colorless liquid. A mild ammonia-like odor occurs at the TLV and is an adequate warning property. Vapor pressure is less than 1 mm Hg at 20°C (68°F). Combustible. Thermal breakdown products include oxides of nitrogen. |
| **Ethion (phosphorodithioic acid [CAS: 563-12-2]):** An organophosphate-type cholinesterase inhibitor (see p 193). Well absorbed dermally. | 0.05 mg/m$^3$ (inhalable fraction and vapor), S | | | Colorless, odorless liquid when pure. Technical products have an objectionable odor. Vapor pressure is 0.000002 mm Hg at 20°C (68°F). Thermal breakdown products include oxides of sulfur. |
| **2-Ethoxyethanol (ethylene glycol monoethyl ether, EGEE, Cellosolve [CAS: 110-80-5]):** Mildly irritating on direct contact. Skin contact is a major route of absorption. Overexposures may reduce sperm counts in men. A potent teratogen in both rats and rabbits. Large doses cause lung, liver, testes, kidney, and spleen injury in test animals. See also p 193. | 5 ppm, S | 500 ppm | 2 2 0 | Colorless liquid. Very mild, sweet odor occurs only at very high levels and is a poor warning property. Vapor pressure is 4 mm Hg at 20°C (68°F). |
| **2-Ethoxyethyl acetate (ethylene glycol monoethyl ether acetate, Cellosolve acetate):** Mildly irritating upon direct contact. May produce CNS depression and kidney injury. Skin contact is a major route of absorption. Metabolized to 2-ethoxyethanol. Adverse effects on fertility and fetal development in animals. See also p 193. | 5 ppm, S | 500 ppm | 2 2 0 | Colorless liquid. Mild ether-like odor occurs at the TLV and is a good warning property. Flammable. |
| **Ethyl acetate (CAS: 141-78-6):** Slightly irritating to eyes and skin. Vapors irritating to eyes and respiratory tract. A CNS depressant at very high levels. Metabolized to ethanol and acetic acid, so may have some of the fetotoxic potential of ethanol. | 400 ppm | 2000 ppm [LEL] | 1 3 0 | Colorless liquid. Fruity odor occurs at the TLV and is a good warning property. Vapor pressure is 76 mm Hg at 20°C (68°F). Flammable. |
| **Ethyl acrylate (CAS: 140-88-5):** Extremely irritating upon direct contact; severe burns may result. A skin sensitizer. Vapors highly irritating to eyes and respiratory tract. In animal tests, heart, liver, and kidney damage was observed at high doses. A carcinogen in test animals (IARC 2B). | 5 ppm<br>NIOSH CA | 300 ppm<br>ERPG-1: 0.01 ppm<br>ERPG-2: 30 ppm<br>ERPG-3: 300 ppm | 2 3 2 | Colorless liquid. Acrid odor occurs below the TLV and is a good warning property. Vapor pressure is 29.5 mm Hg at 20°C (68°F). Flammable. Contains an inhibitor to prevent dangerous self-polymerization. |

(C) = ceiling air concentration (TLV-C); S = skin absorption can be significant; SEN = potential sensitizer; A1 = ACGIH-confirmed human carcinogen; A2 = ACGIH-suspected human carcinogen; NFPA Hazard Codes: H = health, F = fire, R = reactivity, Ox = oxidizer, W = water-reactive, 0 (none) <—> 4 (severe). ERPG = Emergency Response Planning Guideline. See p 539 for an explanation of definitions.

(*continued*)

TABLE IV–4. HEALTH HAZARD SUMMARIES FOR INDUSTRIAL AND OCCUPATIONAL CHEMICALS (CONTINUED)

| Health Hazard Summaries | ACGIH TLV | IDLH | NFPA Codes H F R | Comments |
|---|---|---|---|---|
| **Ethyl alcohol (alcohol, grain alcohol, ethanol, EtOH [CAS: 64-17-5]):** At high levels, vapors irritating to eyes and respiratory tract. A CNS depressant at high levels of exposure. Strong evidence for adverse effects on fetal development in test animals and humans with chronic ingestion (fetal alcohol syndrome). See also p 189. | 1000 ppm | 3300 ppm [LEL] | 0 3 0 | Colorless liquid with a mild, sweet odor. Vapor pressure is 43 mm Hg at 20°C (68°F). Flammable. |
| **Ethylamine (CAS: 75-04-7):** Corrosive upon direct contact; severe burns may result. Vapors highly irritating to eyes, skin, and respiratory tract; delayed pulmonary edema may result. Animal studies suggest potential for liver and kidney injury at moderate doses. | 5 ppm, S | 600 ppm | 3 4 0 | Colorless liquid or gas with an ammonia-like odor. Highly flammable. Thermal breakdown products include oxides of nitrogen. |
| **Ethyl amyl ketone (5-methyl-3-heptanone [CAS: 541-85-5]):** Irritating to eyes upon direct contact. Vapors irritating to eyes and respiratory tract. A CNS depressant at high levels. | 25 ppm | 100 ppm | | Colorless liquid with a strong, distinctive odor. Flammable. |
| **Ethylbenzene (CAS: 100-41-4):** Mildly irritating to eyes upon direct contact. May cause skin burns upon prolonged contact. Dermally well absorbed. Vapors irritating to eyes and respiratory tract. A CNS depressant at high levels of exposure. IARC 2B. | 100 ppm, A3 | 800 ppm [LEL] | 2 3 0 | Colorless liquid. Aromatic odor and irritation occur at levels close to the TLV and are adequate warning properties. Vapor pressure is 7.1 mm Hg at 20°C (68°F). Flammable. |
| **Ethyl bromide (CAS: 74-96-4):** Irritating to skin upon direct contact. Irritating to respiratory tract. A CNS depressant at high levels and may cause cardiac arrhythmias. Former use as an anesthetic agent was discontinued because of fatal liver, kidney, and myocardial injury. Evidence for carcinogenicity in test animals. | 5 ppm, S, A3 | 2000 ppm | 2 1 0 | Colorless to yellow liquid. Ether-like odor detectable only at high, dangerous levels. Vapor pressure is 375 mm Hg at 20°C (68°F). Highly flammable. Thermal breakdown products include hydrogen bromide and bromine gas. |
| **Ethyl butyl ketone (3-heptanone [CAS: 106-35-4]):** Mildly irritating to eyes upon direct contact. Vapors irritating to eyes and respiratory tract. A CNS depressant at high levels. | 50 ppm | 1000 ppm | 1 2 0 | Colorless liquid. Fruity odor is a good warning property. Vapor pressure is 4 mm Hg at 20°C (68°F). Flammable. |

| | | | | |
|---|---|---|---|---|
| **Ethyl chloride (CAS: 75-00-3):** Mildly irritating to eyes and respiratory tract. A CNS depressant at high levels; has caused cardiac arrhythmias at anesthetic doses. Animal studies suggest the kidneys and liver are target organs at high doses. Structurally similar to the carcinogenic chloroethanes. | 100 ppm, A3, S | 3800 ppm [LEL] | 1 4 0 | Colorless liquid or gas with a pungent, ether-like odor. Highly flammable. Thermal breakdown products include hydrogen chloride and phosgene. |
| **Ethylene chlorohydrin (2-chloroethanol [CAS: 107-07-3]):** Irritating to eyes upon direct contact. Skin contact is extremely hazardous because it is not irritating and absorption is rapid. Vapors irritating to eyes and respiratory tract; pulmonary edema has been reported. Systemic effects include CNS depression, myocardiopathy, shock, and liver and kidney damage. | 1 ppm (C), S | 7 ppm | 4 2 0 | Colorless liquid with a weak ether-like odor. Vapor pressure is 5 mm Hg at 20°C (68°F). Combustible. Thermal breakdown products include hydrogen chloride and phosgene. |
| **Ethylenediamine (CAS: 107-15-3):** Highly irritating upon direct contact; burns may result. Respiratory and dermal sensitization may occur. Vapors irritating to eyes and respiratory tract. Animal studies suggest potential for kidney injury at high doses. | 10 ppm, S | 1000 ppm | 3 2 0 | Colorless viscous liquid or solid. Ammonia-like odor occurs at the PEL and is an adequate warning property. Vapor pressure is 10 mm Hg at 20°C (68°F). Flammable. Thermal breakdown products include oxides of nitrogen. |
| **Ethylene dibromide (1,2-dibromoethane, EDB [CAS: 106-93-4]):** Highly irritating upon direct contact; severe burns result. Highly toxic by all routes. Vapors highly irritating to eyes and respiratory tract. Severe liver and kidney injury may occur. A CNS depressant. Adverse effects on the testes in test animals and, possibly, humans. A carcinogen in test animals (IARC 2A). See p 193. | S, A3<br>NIOSH CA | 100 ppm | 3 0 0 | Colorless liquid or solid. Mild, sweet odor is a poor warning property. Vapor pressure is 11 mm Hg at 20°C (68°F). Not combustible. Thermal breakdown products include hydrogen bromide and bromine gas. Fumigant and chemical intermediate used in organic synthesis. |
| **Ethylene glycol (antifreeze [CAS: 107-21-1]):** A CNS depressant. Metabolized to oxalic and other acids; severe acidosis may result. Precipitation of calcium oxalate crystals in tissues can cause extensive injury. Adversely affects fetal development in animal studies at very high doses. Not well absorbed dermally. See also p 193. | 100 mg/m$^3$ (C) | | 1 1 0 | Colorless viscous liquid. Odorless with a very low vapor pressure. |

(C) = ceiling air concentration (TLV-C); S = skin absorption can be significant; SEN = potential sensitizer; A1 = ACGIH-confirmed human carcinogen; A2 = ACGIH-suspected human carcinogen; NFPA Hazard Codes: H = health, F = fire, R = reactivity, Ox = oxidizer, W = water-reactive, 0 (none) <—> 4 (severe). ERPG = Emergency Response Planning Guideline. See p 539 for an explanation of definitions.

(*continued*)

TABLE IV–4. HEALTH HAZARD SUMMARIES FOR INDUSTRIAL AND OCCUPATIONAL CHEMICALS (CONTINUED)

| Health Hazard Summaries | ACGIH TLV | IDLH | NFPA Codes H F R | Comments |
|---|---|---|---|---|
| **Ethylene glycol dinitrate (EGDN [CAS: 628-96-6]):** Causes vasodilation similar to other nitrite compounds. Headache, hypotension, flushing, palpitation, delirium, and CNS depression may occur. Well absorbed by all routes. Tolerance and dependence may develop to vasodilatory effects; cessation after repeated exposures may cause angina pectoris. Weak inducer of methemoglobinemia (see p 262). | 0.05 ppm, S | 75 mg/m$^3$ | | Yellow oily liquid. Vapor pressure is 0.05 mm Hg at 20°C (68°F). Explosive. |
| **Ethyleneimine (CAS: 151-56-4):** Strong caustic. Highly irritating upon direct contact; severe burns may result. Vapors irritating to eyes and respiratory tract; delayed-onset pulmonary edema may occur. Overexposures have resulted in nausea, vomiting, headache, and dizziness. Well absorbed dermally. A carcinogen in animals. | 0.5 ppm, S, A3<br>OSHA CA<br>NIOSH CA | 100 ppm | 4 3 3 | Colorless liquid with an amine-like odor. Vapor pressure is 160 mm Hg at 20°C (68°F). Flammable. Contains inhibitor to prevent explosive self-polymerization. |
| **Ethylene oxide (CAS: 75-21-8):** Highly irritating upon direct contact. Vapors irritating to eyes and respiratory tract; delayed pulmonary edema has been reported. A CNS depressant at very high levels. Chronic overexposures can cause peripheral neuropathy and possible permanent CNS impairment. Adverse effects on fetal development and fertility in test animals and limited evidence in humans. A carcinogen in animal studies. Limited evidence of carcinogenicity in humans (IARC 1). See also p 193. | 1 ppm, A2<br>OSHA CA<br>NIOSH CA | 800 ppm<br>ERPG-2: 50 ppm<br>ERPG-3: 500 ppm | 3 4 3 | Colorless. Highly flammable. Ether-like odor is a poor warning property. Important source of exposures is sterilization operations in health-care industry. |
| **Ethyl ether (diethyl ether, ether [CAS: 60-29-7]):** Vapors irritating to eyes and respiratory tract. A CNS depressant and anesthetic agent; tolerance may develop to this effect. Overexposure produces nausea, headache, dizziness, anesthesia, and respiratory arrest. Evidence for adverse effects on fetal development in test animals. | 400 ppm | 1900 ppm [LEL] | 1 4 1 | Colorless liquid. Ether-like odor occurs at low levels and is a good warning property. Vapor pressure is 439 mm Hg at 20°C (68°F). Highly flammable. |

| | | | | |
|---|---|---|---|---|
| **Ethyl formate (CAS: 109-94-4):** Slightly irritating to the skin upon direct contact. Vapors mildly irritating to eyes and upper respiratory tract. In test animals, very high levels caused rapid narcosis and pulmonary edema. | 100 ppm | 1500 ppm | 2 3 0 | Colorless liquid. Fruity odor and irritation occur near the TLV and are good warning properties. Vapor pressure is 194 mm Hg at 20°C (68°F). Highly flammable. |
| **Ethyl methylacrylate monomer (CAS: 97-63-2):** Irritant and sensitizing agent. | | | | Precusor of ethyl methacrylate polymers. Flammable. |
| **Ethyl mercaptan (ethanethiol [CAS: 75-08-1]):** Vapors mildly irritating to eyes and respiratory tract. Respiratory paralysis and CNS depression at very high levels. Headache, nausea, and vomiting likely owing to strong odor. | 0.5 ppm | 500 ppm | 2 4 0 | Colorless liquid. Penetrating, offensive, mercaptan-like odor. Vapor pressure is 442 mm Hg at 20°C (68°F). |
| ***N*-Ethylmorpholine (CAS: 100-74-3):** Irritating to eyes upon direct contact. Vapors irritating to eyes and respiratory tract. Workers exposed to levels near the TLV reported drowsiness and temporary visual distrubances, including corneal edema. Animal testing suggests potential for skin absorption. | 5 ppm, S | 100 ppm | 2 3 0 | Colorless liquid with ammonia-like odor. Vapor pressure is 5 mm Hg at 20°C (68°F). Flammable. Thermal breakdown products include oxides of nitrogen. |
| **Ethyl silicate (tetraethyl orthosilicate, tetraethoxysilane [CAS: 78-10-4]):** Irritating upon direct contact. Vapors irritating to eyes and respiratory tract. All human effects noted at vapor exposures above the odor threshold. In subchronic animal testing, high vapor levels produced liver, lung, and kidney damage and delayed-onset pulmonary edema. | 10 ppm | 700 ppm<br>ERPG-1: 25 ppm<br>ERPG-2: 100 ppm<br>ERPG-3: 300 ppm | 2 2 0 | Colorless liquid. Faint alcohol-like odor and irritation are good warning properties. Vapor pressure is 2 mm Hg at 20°C (68°F). Flammable. |
| **Fenamiphos (ethyl 3-methyl-4-[methylthio]-phenyl[1-methylethyl]phosphoramide [CAS: 22224-92-6]):** An organophosphate-type cholinesterase inhibitor (see p 193). Well absorbed dermally. | [proposed 0.05 mg/$m^3$, S] | | | Tan, waxy solid. Vapor pressure is 0.000001 mm Hg at 30°C (86°F). |
| **Fensulfothion (*O,O*-diethyl *O*-[4-(methyl-sulfinyl)phenyl]phosphorothioate [CAS: 115-90-2]):** An organophosphate-type cholinesterase inhibitor (see p 193). | 0.01 mg/$m^3$ (inhalable fraction and vapor), S | | | Brown liquid. |

(C) = ceiling air concentration (TLV-C); S = skin absorption can be significant; SEN = potential sensitizer; A1 = ACGIH-confirmed human carcinogen; A2 = ACGIH-suspected human carcinogen; NFPA Hazard Codes: H = health, F = fire, R = reactivity, Ox = oxidizer, W = water-reactive, 0 (none) <—> 4 (severe). ERPG = Emergency Response Planning Guideline. See p 539 for an explanation of definitions.

(*continued*)

TABLE IV–4. HEALTH HAZARD SUMMARIES FOR INDUSTRIAL AND OCCUPATIONAL CHEMICALS (CONTINUED)

| Health Hazard Summaries | ACGIH TLV | IDLH | NFPA Codes H F R | Comments |
|---|---|---|---|---|
| **Fenthion (*O,O*-dimethyl *O*-[3-methyl-4-(methylthio)phenyl]phosphorothioate [CAS: 55-38-9]):** An organophosphate-type cholinesterase inhibitor (see p 193). Highly lipid soluble; toxicity may be prolonged. Dermal absorption is rapid. | [proposed 0.05 mg/m3, S] | | | Yellow to tan viscous liquid with a mild garlic-like odor. Vapor pressure is 0.00003 mm Hg at 20°C (68°F). |
| **Ferbam (ferric dimethyldithiocarbamate [CAS: 14484-64-1]):** Thiocarbamates do not act through cholinesterase inhibition. Dusts irritating upon direct contact; causes dermatitis in persons sensitized to sulfur. Dusts are mild respiratory tract irritants. Limited evidence for adverse effects on fetal development in test animals (IARC 3). | 10 mg/m$^3$ | 800 mg/m$^3$ | | Odorless, black solid. Vapor pressure is negligible at 20°C (68°F). Thermal breakdown products include oxides of nitrogen and sulfur. Used as a fungicide. |
| **Ferrovanadium dust (CAS: 12604-58-9):** Mild irritant of eyes and respiratory tract. | 1 mg/m$^3$ | 500 mg/m$^3$ | | Odorless, dark-colored powders. |
| **Fipronil (CAS: 120068-37-3):** Phenylpyrazole insecticide, blocks GABA-gated chloride channels and can cause seizures. Mild irritant of eyes and respiratory tract. | | | | |
| **Fluoride dust (as fluoride):** Irritating to eyes and respiratory tract. Workers exposed to levels 10 mg/m$^3$ suffered nasal irritation and bleeding. Lower-level exposures have produced nausea and eye and respiratory tract irritation. Chronic overexposures may result in skin rashes. Fluorosis, a bone disease with chronic high-level fluoride ingestion, is not associated with occupational dust inhalation. See also p 199. | 2.5 mg/m$^3$ (as F) | 250 mg/m$^3$ (as F) | | Appearance varies with the compound. Sodium fluoride is a colorless to blue solid. |
| **Fluorine (CAS: 7782-41-4):** Rapidly reacts with moisture to form ozone and hydrofluoric acid. The gas is a severe eye, skin, and respiratory tract irritant; severe penetrating burns and pulmonary edema have resulted. Systemic hypocalcemia can occur with fluorine or hydrogen fluoride exposure. See also p 222. | 1 ppm | 25 ppm<br>ERPG-1: 0.5 ppm<br>ERPG-2: 5.0 ppm<br>ERPG-3: 20 ppm | 4 0 4<br>W | Pale yellow gas. Sharp odor is a poor warning property. Highly reactive; will ignite many oxidizable materials. Uses include rocket fuel oxidizer. |

| | | | | |
|---|---|---|---|---|
| **Fonofos (*O*-ethyl *S*-phenyl ethylphosphono-thiolothionate, Dyfonate [CAS: 944-22-9]):** An organophosphate-type cholinesterase inhibitor (see p 292). Highly toxic; oral toxicity in test animals ranged from 3 to 13 mg/kg for rats, and rabbits died after eye instillation. | [proposed: 0.1 mg/$m^3$ (inhalable fraction and vapor), S] | | | Vapor pressure is 0.00021 mm Hg at 20°C (68°F). Thermal breakdown products include oxides of sulfur. |
| **Formaldehyde (formic aldehyde, methanal, HCHO, formalin [CAS: 50-00-0]):** Highly irritating to eyes upon direct contact; severe burns result. Irritating to skin; may cause sensitization dermatitis. Vapors highly irritating to eyes and respiratory tract. Sensitization may occur. A carcinogen in test animals (IARC 1). See also p 206. | 0.3 ppm (C), SEN, A2<br>OSHA CA<br>NIOSH CA | 20 ppm<br>ERPG-1: 1 ppm<br>ERPG-2: 10 ppm<br>ERPG-3: 25 ppm | 3 4 0 (gas)<br>3 2 0 (formalin) | Colorless gas with a suffocating odor. Combustible. Formalin (15% methanol) solutions are flammable. |
| **Formamide (methanamide [CAS: 75-12-7]):** In animal tests, mildly irritating upon direct contact. Adverse effects on fetal development in test animals at very high doses. | 10 ppm, S | | 2 1 – | Clear, viscous liquid. Odorless. Vapor pressure is 2 mm Hg at 70°C (158°F). Combustible. Thermal breakdown products include oxides of nitrogen. |
| **Formic acid (CAS: 64-18-6):** Acid is corrosive; severe burns may result from contact of eyes and skin with concentrated acid. Vapors highly irritating to eyes and respiratory tract. Ingestion may produce severe metabolic acidosis (see methanol, p 260). | 5 ppm | 30 ppm | 3 2 0 | Colorless liquid. Pungent odor and irritation occur near the TLV and are adequate warning properties. Vapor pressure is 30 mm Hg at 20°C (68°F). Combustible. |
| **Furfural (bran oil [CAS: 98-01-1]):** Highly irritating upon direct contact; burns may result. Vapors highly irritating to eyes and respiratory tract; pulmonary edema may result. Animal studies indicate the liver is a target organ. Hyperreflexia and convulsions occur at large doses in test animals. IARC 3. | 2 ppm, S, A3 | 100 ppm<br>ERPG-1: 2 ppm<br>ERPG-2: 10 ppm<br>ERPG-3: 100 ppm | 3 2 0 | Colorless to light brown liquid. Almond-like odor occurs below the TLV and is a good warning property. Vapor pressure is 2 mm Hg at 20°C (68°F). Combustible. Thermal breakdown products include oxides of nitrogen. |
| **Furfuryl alcohol (CAS: 98-00-0):** Dermal absorption occurs. Vapors irritating to eyes and respiratory tract. A CNS depressant at high air levels. | 10 ppm, S | 75 ppm | 1 2 1 | Clear, colorless liquid. Upon exposure to light and air, changes color to red or brown. Vapor pressure is 0.53 mm Hg at 20°C (68°F). Combustible. |

(C) = ceiling air concentration (TLV-C); S = skin absorption can be significant; SEN = potential sensitizer; A1 = ACGIH-confirmed human carcinogen; A2 = ACGIH-suspected human carcinogen; NFPA Hazard Codes: H = health, F = fire, R = reactivity, Ox = oxidizer, W = water-reactive, 0 (none) <—> 4 (severe). ERPG = Emergency Response Planning Guideline. See p 539 for an explanation of definitions.

(*continued*)

TABLE IV–4. HEALTH HAZARD SUMMARIES FOR INDUSTRIAL AND OCCUPATIONAL CHEMICALS (CONTINUED)

| Health Hazard Summaries | ACGIH TLV | IDLH | NFPA Codes H F R | Comments |
|---|---|---|---|---|
| **Gasoline (CAS: 8006-61-9):** Although exact composition varies, the acute toxicity of all gasolines is similar. Vapors irritating to eyes and respiratory tract at high levels. A CNS depressant; symptoms include incoordination, dizziness, headaches, and nausea. Benzene (generally < 1%) is one significant chronic health hazard. Other additives such as ethylene dibromide and tetraethyl and tetramethyl lead are present in low amounts and may be absorbed through the skin. Very limited evidence for carcinogenicity in test animals. See also p 219. | 300 ppm, A3 NIOSH CA | | 1 3 0 | Clear to amber liquid with a characteristic odor. Highly flammable. Gasoline is sometimes used inappropriately used as a solvent. Substance abuse via inhalation has been reported. |
| **Germanium tetrahydride (CAS: 7782-65-2):** A hemolytic agent with effects similar to but less potent than those of arsine in animals. Symptoms include abdominal pain, hematuria, anemia, and jaundice. | 0.2 ppm | | | Colorless gas. Highly flammable. |
| **Glutaraldehyde (1,5-pentandial [CAS: 111-30-8]):** The purity and therefore the toxicity of glutaraldehyde vary widely. Allergic dermatitis may occur. Highly irritating on contact; severe burns may result. Vapors highly irritating to eyes and respiratory tract; respiratory sensitization may occur. In animal studies, the liver is a target organ at high doses. See p 110. | 0.05 ppm (C), SEN | | | Colorless solid crystals. Vapor pressure is 0.0152 mm Hg at 20°C (68°F). Can undergo hazardous self-polymerization. Commonly used as a sterilizing agent in medical settings. |
| **Glycidol (2,3-epoxy-1-propanol [CAS: 556-52-5]):** Highly irritating to eyes on contact; burns may result. Moderately irritating to skin and respiratory tract. Evidence for carcinogenicity and testicular toxicity in test animals (IARC 2A). | 2 ppm, A3 | 150 ppm | | Colorless liquid. Vapor pressure is 0.9 mm Hg at 25°C (77°F). Combustible. |
| **Glyphosate (CAS: 1071-83-6):** Herbicide. Intentional self-poisoning has caused acute noncardiogenic pulmonary edema, renal failure; toxic effects may result from the surfactant rather than from glyphosate itself. | | | | White or colorless solid. Odorless or slight amine odor; negligible vapor pressure. Stable to light and heat. |
| **Hafnium (CAS: 7440-58-6):** Based on animal studies, dusts are mildly irritating to eyes and skin. Liver injury may occur at very high doses. | 0.5 mg/m$^3$ | 50 mg/m$^3$ | | The metal is a gray solid. Other compounds vary in appearance. |

| Health Hazard Summaries | ACGIH TLV | IDLH | NFPA Codes H F R | Comments |
|---|---|---|---|---|
| **Heptachlor (CAS: 76-44-8):** CNS convulsant. Skin absorption is rapid and has caused convulsions and death. Hepatotoxic. Stored in fatty tissues. Limited evidence for adverse effects on fetal development in test animals at high doses. A carcinogen in test animals (IARC 2B). See also p 163. | 0.05 mg/m$^3$, S, A3 NIOSH CA | 35 mg/m$^3$ | | White or light tan, waxy solid with a camphor-like odor. Vapor pressure is 0.0003 mm Hg at 20°C (68°F). Thermal breakdown products include hydrogen chloride. Not combustible. Pesticide use banned by EPA in 1988. |
| ***n*-Heptane (CAS: 142-82-5):** Vapors only slightly irritating to eyes and respiratory tract. May cause euphoria, vertigo, CNS depression, and cardiac arrhythmias at high levels. | 400 ppm | 750 ppm | 1 3 0 | Colorless clear liquid. Mild gasoline-like odor occurs below the TLV and is a good warning property. Vapor pressure is 40 mm Hg at 20°C (68°F). Flammable. |
| **Hexachlorobutadiene (CAS: 87-68-3):** Based on animal studies, rapid dermal absorption is expected. The kidney is the major target organ. A carcinogen in test animals (IARC 3). | 0.02 ppm, S, A3 NIOSH CA | ERPG-1: 1 ppm ERPG-2: 3 ppm ERPG-3: 10 ppm | 2 1 1 | Heavy, colorless liquid. Thermal breakdown products include hydrogen chloride and phosgene. |
| **Hexachlorocyclopentadiene (CAS: 77-47-4):** Vapors extremely irritating to eyes and respiratory tract; lacrimation, salivation. In animal studies, a potent kidney and liver toxin. At higher levels the brain, heart, and adrenal glands were affected. Tremors occurred at high doses. | 0.01 ppm | | | Yellow to amber liquid with a pungent odor. Vapor pressure is 0.08 mm Hg at 20°C (68°F). Not combustible. |
| **Hexachloroethane (perchloroethane [CAS: 67-72-1]):** Hot fumes irritating to eyes, skin, and mucous membranes. Based on animal studies, causes CNS depression and kidney and liver injury at high doses. Limited evidence of carcinogenicity in test animals (IARC 2B). | 1 ppm, S, A3 NIOSH CA | 300 ppm | | White solid with a camphor-like odor. Vapor pressure is 0.22 mm Hg at 20°C (68°F). Not combustible. Thermal breakdown products include phosgene, chlorine gas, and hydrogen chloride. |
| **Hexachloronaphthalene (Halowax 1014 [CAS: 1335-87-1]):** Based on workplace experience, a potent toxin causing severe chloracne and severe, occasionally fatal, liver injury. Skin absorption can occur. | 0.2 mg/m$^3$, S | 2 mg/m$^3$ | | Light yellow solid with an aromatic odor. Vapor pressure is less than 1 mm Hg at 20°C (68°F). Not combustible. |
| **Hexamethylphosphoramide (CAS: 680-31-9):** Low-level exposures produced nasal cavity cancer in rats (IARC 2B). Adverse effects on the testes in test animals. | S, A3 NIOSH CA | | | Colorless liquid with an aromatic odor. Vapor pressure is 0.07 mm Hg at 20°C (68°F). Thermal breakdown products include oxides of nitrogen. |

(C) = ceiling air concentration (TLV-C); S = skin absorption can be significant; SEN = potential sensitizer; A1 = ACGIH-confirmed human carcinogen; A2 = ACGIH-suspected human carcinogen; NFPA Hazard Codes: H = health, F = fire, R = reactivity, Ox = oxidizer, W = water-reactive, 0 (none) <—> 4 (severe). ERPG = Emergency Response Planning Guideline. See p 539 for an explanation of definitions.

(*continued*)

TABLE IV–4. HEALTH HAZARD SUMMARIES FOR INDUSTRIAL AND OCCUPATIONAL CHEMICALS (CONTINUED)

| Health Hazard Summaries | ACGIH TLV | IDLH | NFPA Codes H F R | Comments |
|---|---|---|---|---|
| ***n*-Hexane (normal hexane [CAS: 110-54-3]):** Vapors mildly irritating to eyes and respiratory tract. A CNS depressant at high levels, producing headache, dizziness, and gastrointestinal upset. Occupational overexposures have resulted in peripheral neuropathies. Methyl ethyl ketone potentiates this toxicity. Testicular toxicity in animal studies. | 50 ppm, S | 1100 ppm [LEL] | 1 3 0 | Colorless, clear liquid with a mild gasoline odor. Vapor pressure is 124 mm Hg at 20°C (68°F). Highly flammable. |
| **Hexane isomers (other than *n*-hexane, isohexane, 2,3-demethylbutane):** Vapors mildly irritating to eyes and respiratory tract. A CNS depressant at high levels, producing headache, dizziness, and gastro intestinal upset. | 500 ppm | | | Colorless liquids with a mild petroleum odor. Vapor pressures are high at 20°C (68°F). Highly flammable. |
| ***sec*-Hexyl acetate (1,3-dimethylbutyl acetate [CAS: 108-84-9]):** At low levels, vapors irritating to eyes and respiratory tract. Based on animal studies, a CNS depressant at high levels. | 50 ppm | 500 ppm | 1 2 0 | Colorless liquid. Unpleasant fruity odor and irritation are both good warning properties. Vapor pressure is 4 mm Hg at 20°C (68°F). Flammable. |
| **Hexylene glycol (2-methyl-2,4-pentanediol [CAS: 107-41-5]):** Irritating upon direct contact; vapors irritating to eyes and respiratory tract. A CNS depressant at very high doses in animal studies. | 25 ppm (C) | | 1 1 0 | Liquid with a faint sweet odor. Vapor pressure is 0.05 mm Hg at 20°C (68°F). Combustible. |
| **Hydrazine (diamine [CAS: 302-01-2]):** Corrosive upon direct contact; severe burns result. Vapors extremely irritating to eyes and respiratory tract; pulmonary edema may occur. Highly hepatotoxic. A convulsant and hemolytic agent. Kidneys are also target organs. Well absorbed by all routes. A carcinogen in test animals (IARC 2B). | 0.01 ppm, S, A3<br>NIOSH CA | 50 ppm<br>ERPG-1: 0.5 ppm<br>ERPG-2: 5 ppm<br>ERPG-3: 30 ppm | 3 3 3<br>(vapors explosive) | Colorless, fuming, viscous liquid with an amine odor. Vapor pressure is 10 mm Hg at 20°C (68°F). Flammable. Thermal breakdown products include oxides of nitrogen. Used as a rocket fuel and in some military jet systems. |
| **Hydrogen bromide (HBr [CAS: 10035-10-6]):** Direct contact with concentrated solutions may cause corrosive acid burns. Vapors highly irritating to eyes and respiratory tract; pulmonary edema may result. | 2 ppm (C) | 30 ppm | 3 0 0 | Colorless gas or pressurized liquid. Acrid odor and irritation occur near the TLV and are adequate warning properties. Not combustible. |

| | | | | |
|---|---|---|---|---|
| **Hydrogen chloride (hydrochloric acid, muriatic acid, HCl [CAS: 7647-01-0]):** Direct contact with concentrated solutions may cause corrosive acid burns. Vapors highly irritating to eyes and respiratory tract; pulmonary edema has resulted. See p 212. | 2 ppm (C) | 50 ppm<br>ERPG-1: 3 ppm<br>ERPG-2: 20 ppm<br>ERPG-3: 150 ppm | 3 0 1 | Colorless gas with a pungent, choking odor. Irritation occurs near the TLV and is a good warning property. Not combustible. Contact with water, including atmospheric humidity, leads to formation of hydrochloric acid. |
| **Hydrogen cyanide (hydrocyanic acid, prussic acid, HCN [CAS: 74 90-8]):** A rapidly acting potent metabolic asphyxiant that inhibits cytochrome oxidase and stops cellular respiration. See also p 176. | 4.7 ppm (C), S | 50 ppm<br>ERPG-2: 10 ppm<br>ERPG-3: 25 ppm | 4 4 2<br>(vapors extremely toxic) | Colorless to pale blue liquid or colorless gas with a sweet, bitter almond smell that is an inadequate warning property even for those sensitive to it. Vapor pressure is 620 mm Hg at 20°C (68°F). Cyanide salts will release HCN gas with exposure to acids or heat. |
| **Hydrogen fluoride (hydrofluoric acid, HF [CAS: 7664-39-3]):** Produces severe, penetrating burns to eyes, skin, and deeper tissues upon direct contact with solutions. Onset of pain and erythema may be delayed as much as 12–16 hours. As a gas, highly irritating to the eyes and respiratory tract; pulmonary edema has resulted. Severe hypocalcemia may occur with overexposure. See p 222. | 3 ppm (C) (as F) | 30 ppm<br>ERPG-1: 2 ppm<br>ERPG-2: 20 ppm<br>ERPG-3: 50 ppm | 4 0 1 | Colorless fuming liquid or gas. Irritation occurs at levels below the TLV and is an adequate warning property. Vapor pressure is 760 mm Hg at 20°C (68°F). Not combustible. Commercial rust-removing products may contain HF, but generally at lower concentrations (< 10%). |
| **Hydrogen peroxide (CAS: 7722-84-1):** A strong oxidizing agent. Direct contact with concentrated solutions can produce severe eye damage and skin irritation, including erythema and vesicle formation. Vapors irritating to eyes, skin, mucous membranes, and respiratory tract. See also p 287. IARC 3. | 1 ppm, A3 | 75 ppm<br>ERPG-1: 10 ppm<br>ERPG-2: 50 ppm<br>ERPG-3: 100 ppm | 2 0 3<br>Ox (60% or greater)<br>2 0 1<br>Ox (40–60%) | Colorless liquid with a slightly sharp, distinctive odor. Vapor pressure is 5 mm Hg at 30°C (86°F). Because of instability, usually found in aqueous solutions (3% for home use, higher in some "health food" products and in industry). Not combustible but a very powerful oxidizing agent. |
| **Hydrogen selenide (CAS: 7783-07-5):** Vapors extremely irritating to eyes and respiratory tract. Systemic symptoms from low-level exposure include nausea and vomiting, fatigue, metallic taste in mouth, and a garlicky breath odor. Animal studies indicate hepatotoxicity. | 0.05 ppm | 1 ppm<br>ERPG-2: 0.2 ppm<br>ERPG-3: 2 ppm | | Colorless gas. The strongly offensive odor and irritation occur only at levels far above the TLV and are poor warning properties. Flammable. Water-reactive. |

(C) = ceiling air concentration (TLV-C); S = skin absorption can be significant; SEN = potential sensitizer; A1 = ACGIH-confirmed human carcinogen; A2 = ACGIH-suspected human carcinogen; NFPA Hazard Codes: H = health, F = fire, R = reactivity, Ox = oxidizer, W = water-reactive, 0 (none) <—> 4 (severe). ERPG = Emergency Response Planning Guideline. See p 539 for an explanation of definitions.

*(continued)*

TABLE IV–4. HEALTH HAZARD SUMMARIES FOR INDUSTRIAL AND OCCUPATIONAL CHEMICALS (CONTINUED)

| Health Hazard Summaries | ACGIH TLV | IDLH | NFPA Codes H F R | Comments |
|---|---|---|---|---|
| **Hydrogen sulfide (sewer gas [CAS: 7783-06-4]):** Vapors irritating to eyes and respiratory tract. At higher levels, a potent, rapid systemic toxin causing cellular asphyxia and death. Systemic effects of low-level exposure include headache, cough, nausea, and vomiting. See also p 224. | 10 ppm [proposed 1 ppm] | 100 ppm<br>ERPG-1: 0.1 ppm<br>ERPG-2: 30 ppm<br>ERPG-3: 100 ppm | 4 4 0 | Colorless gas. Although the strong rotten egg odor can be detected at very low levels, olfactory fatigue occurs. Odor is therefore a poor warning property. Flammable. Produced by the decay of organic material as may occur in sewers, manure pits, and fish processing. Fossil fuel production also may generate the gas. |
| **Hydroquinone (1,4-dihydroxybenzene [CAS: 123-31-9]):** Highly irritating to eyes upon direct contact. Chronic occupational exposures may cause partial discoloration and opacification of the cornea. Systemic effects reported result from ingestion and include tinnitus, headache, dizziness, gastrointestinal upset, CNS excitation, and skin depigmentation. May cause methemoglobinemia (see p 262). Limited evidence of carcinogenicity in test animals (IARC 3). | 2 mg/m$^3$, A3 | 50 mg/m$^3$ | 2 1 0 | White solid crystals. Vapor pressure is less than 0.001 mm Hg at 20°C (68°F). Combustible. |
| **2-Hydroxypropyl acrylate (HPA [CAS: 999-61-1]):** Highly irritating upon direct contact; severe burns may result. Vapors highly irritating to eyes and respiratory tract. Based on structural analogies, compounds containing the acrylate moiety may be carcinogens. | 0.5 ppm, S, SEN | | 3 1 2 | Combustible liquid. |
| **Indene (CAS: 95-13-6):** Repeated direct contact with the skin produced a dry dermatitis but no systemic effects. Vapors probably irritating to eyes and respiratory tract. Based on animal studies, high air levels may cause liver and kidney damage. | 10 ppm | | | Colorless liquid. |
| **Indium (CAS: 7440-74-6):** Based on animal studies, the soluble salts are extremely irritating to eyes upon direct contact. Dusts irritating to eyes and respiratory tract. In animal studies, indium compounds are highly toxic parenterally but much less toxic orally. | 0.1 mg/m$^3$ | | | Appearance varies with the compound. The elemental metal is a silver-white lustrous solid. |

| | | | | |
|---|---|---|---|---|
| **Iodine (CAS: 7553-56-2):** Extremely irritating upon direct contact; severe burns result. Vapors extremely irritating and corrosive to eyes and respiratory tract. Rarely, a skin sensitizer. Medicinal use of iodine-containing drugs has been associated with fetal goiter, a potentially life-threatening condition for a fetus or infant. Iodine causes adverse effects on fetal development in test animals. See also p 227. | 0.1 ppm (C) | 2 ppm<br>ERPG-1: 0.1 ppm<br>ERPG-2: 0.5 ppm<br>ERPG-3: 5 ppm | | Violet-colored solid crystals. Sharp, characteristic odor is a poor warning property. Vapor pressure is 0.3 mm Hg at 20°C (68°F). Not combustible. |
| **Iron oxide fume (CAS: 1309-37-1):** Fumes and dusts can produce a benign pneumoconiosis (siderosis) with shadows on chest radiographs. | 5 mg/m$^3$ (as Fe) [proposed 5 mg/m$^3$ (respirable fraction)] | 2500 mg/m$^3$ (as Fe) | | Red-brown fume with a metallic taste. Vapor pressure is negligible at 20°C (68°F). |
| **Iron pentacarbonyl (iron carbonyl [CAS: 13463-40-6]):** Acute toxicity resembles that of nickel carbonyl. Inhalation of vapors can cause lung and systemic injury without warning signs. Symptoms of overexposure include headache, nausea and vomiting, and dizziness. Symptoms of severe poisoning are fever, extreme weakness, and pulmonary edema; effects may be delayed for up to 36 hours. | 0.1 ppm | | | Colorless to yellow viscous liquid. Vapor pressure is 40 mm Hg at 30.3°C (86.5°F). Highly flammable. |
| **Isoamyl acetate (banana oil, 3-methyl butyl acetate [CAS: 123-92-2]):** May be irritating to skin upon prolonged contact. Vapors mildly irritating to eyes and respiratory tract. Symptoms in men exposed to 950 ppm for 0.5 hour included headache, weakness, dyspnea, and irritation of the nose and throat. A CNS depressant at high doses in test animals. | 50 ppm | 1000 ppm | 1 3 0 | Colorless liquid. Banana-like odor and irritation occur at low levels and are good warning properties. Vapor pressure is 4 mm Hg at 20°C (68°F). Flammable. |
| **Isoamyl alcohol (3-methyl-1-butanol [CAS: 123-51-3]):** Vapors irritating to eyes and respiratory tract. A CNS depressant at high levels. | 100 ppm | 500 ppm | 1 2 0 | Colorless liquid. Irritating alcohol-like odor and irritation are good warning properties. Vapor pressure is 2 mm Hg at 20°C (68°F). Flammable. |
| **Isobutyl acetate (2-methylpropyl acetate [CAS: 110-19-0]):** Vapors mildly irritating to eyes and respiratory tract. A CNS depressant at high levels. | 150 ppm | 1300 ppm [LEL] | 1 3 0 | Colorless liquid. Pleasant fruity odor is a good warning property. Vapor pressure is 13 mm Hg at 20°C (68°F). Flammable. |

(C) = ceiling air concentration (TLV-C); S = skin absorption can be significant; SEN = potential sensitizer; A1 = ACGIH-confirmed human carcinogen; A2 = ACGIH-suspected human carcinogen; NFPA Hazard Codes: H = health, F = fire, R = reactivity, Ox = oxidizer, W = water-reactive, 0 (none) <—> 4 (severe). ERPG = Emergency Response Planning Guideline. See p 539 for an explanation of definitions.

(*continued*)

TABLE IV–4. HEALTH HAZARD SUMMARIES FOR INDUSTRIAL AND OCCUPATIONAL CHEMICALS (CONTINUED)

| Health Hazard Summaries | ACGIH TLV | IDLH | NFPA Codes H F R | Comments |
|---|---|---|---|---|
| **Isobutyl alcohol (2-methyl-1 propanol [CAS: 78-83-1]):** A CNS depressant at high levels. | 50 ppm | 1600 ppm | 1 3 0 | Colorless liquid. Mild characteristic odor is a good warning property. Vapor pressure is 9 mm Hg at 20°C (68°F). Flammable. |
| **Isophorone (trimethylcyclohexenone [CAS: 78-59-1]):** Vapors irritating to eyes and respiratory tract. Workers exposed to 5–8 ppm complained of fatigue and malaise after 1 month. Higher exposures result in nausea, headache, dizziness, and a feeling of suffocation at 200–400 ppm. Limited evidence for adverse effects on fetal development in test animals. | 5 ppm (C), A3 | 200 ppm | 2 2 0 W | Colorless liquid with a camphor-like odor. Vapor pressure is 0.2 mm Hg at 20°C (68°F). Flammable. |
| **Isophorone diisocyanate (CAS: 4098-71-9):** Based on animal studies, extremely irritating upon direct contact; severe burns may result. By analogy with other isocyanates, vapors or mists likely to be potent respiratory sensitizers, causing asthma. See also p 232. | 0.005 ppm | | 2 2 1 W | Colorless to pale yellow liquid. Vapor pressure is 0.0003 mm Hg at 20°C (68°F). Possible thermal breakdown products include oxides of nitrogen and hydrogen cyanide. |
| **2-Isopropoxyethanol (isopropyl Cellosolve, ethylene glycol monoisopropyl ether [CAS: 109-59-1]):** Defatting agent causing dermatitis. May cause hemolysis. | 25 ppm, S | | | Clear colorless liquid with a characteristic odor. |
| **Isopropyl acetate (CAS: 108-21-4):** Vapors irritating to the eyes and respiratory tract. A weak CNS depressant. | 100 ppm | 1800 ppm | 1 3 0 | Colorless liquid. Fruity odor and irritation are good warning properties. Vapor pressure is 43 mm Hg at 20°C (68°F). Flammable. |
| **Isopropyl alcohol (isopropanol, 2-propanol [CAS: 67-63-0]):** Vapors produce mild eye and respiratory tract irritation. High exposures can produce CNS depression. See also p 234. | 200 ppm | 2000 ppm [LEL] | 1 3 0 | Rubbing alcohol. Sharp odor and irritation are adequate warning properties. Vapor pressure is 33 mm Hg at 20°C (68°F). Flammable. |

| | | | | |
|---|---|---|---|---|
| **Isopropylamine (2-aminopropane [CAS: 75-31-0]):** Corrosive upon direct contact; severe burns may result. Vapors highly irritating to the eyes and respiratory tract. Exposure to vapors can cause transient corneal edema. | 5 ppm | 750 ppm | 3 4 0 | Colorless liquid. Strong ammonia odor and irritation are good warning properties. Vapor pressure is 478 mm Hg at 20°C (68°F). Highly flammable. Thermal breakdown products include oxides of nitrogen. |
| **Isopropyl ether (diisopropyl ether [CAS: 108-20-3]):** A skin irritant upon prolonged contact with liquid. Vapors mildly irritating to the eyes and respiratory tract. A CNS depressant. | 250 ppm | 1400 ppm [LEL] | 1 3 1 | Colorless liquid. Offensive and sharp ether-like odor and irritation are good warning properties. Vapor pressure is 119 mm Hg at 20°C (68°F). Highly flammable. Contact with air causes formation of explosive peroxides. |
| **Isopropyl glycidyl ether (CAS: 4016-14-2):** Irritating upon direct contact. Allergic dermatitis may occur. Vapors irritating to eyes and respiratory tract. In animals, A CNS depressant at high oral doses; chronic exposures produced liver injury. Some glycidyl ethers possess hematopoietic and testicular toxicity. | 50 ppm | 400 ppm | | Flammable. Vapor pressure is 9.4 mm Hg at 25°C (77°F). |
| **Kepone (chlordecone [CAS: 143-50-0]):** Neurotoxin; overexposure causes slurred speech, memory impairment, incoordination, weakness, tremor, and convulsions. Causes infertility in males. Hepatotoxic. Well absorbed by all routes. A carcinogen in test animals. See also p 160. | NIOSH CA | | | A solid. Not manufactured in the US since 1978. |
| **Ketene (ethenone [CAS: 463-51-4]):** Vapors extremely irritating to the eyes and respiratory tract; pulmonary edema may result and can be delayed for up to 72 hours. Toxicity similar to that of phosgene (see p 306), of which it is the nonchlorinated analog, in both magnitude and time course. | 0.5 ppm | 5 ppm | | Colorless gas with a sharp odor. Polymerizes readily. Acetylating agent. Water-reactive. |

(C) = ceiling air concentration (TLV-C); S = skin absorption can be significant; SEN = potential sensitizer; A1 = ACGIH-confirmed human carcinogen; A2 = ACGIH-suspected human carcinogen; NFPA Hazard Codes: H = health, F = fire, R = reactivity, Ox = oxidizer, W = water-reactive, 0 (none) <—> 4 (severe). ERPG = Emergency Response Planning Guideline. See p 539 for an explanation of definitions.

(*continued*)

TABLE IV–4. HEALTH HAZARD SUMMARIES FOR INDUSTRIAL AND OCCUPATIONAL CHEMICALS (CONTINUED)

| Health Hazard Summaries | ACGIH TLV | IDLH | NFPA Codes H F R | Comments |
|---|---|---|---|---|
| **Lead (inorganic compounds, dusts, and fumes):** Toxic to CNS and peripheral nerves, kidneys, and hematopoietic system. Toxicity may result from acute or chronic exposures. Inhalation and ingestion are the major routes of absorption. Symptoms and signs include abdominal pain, anemia, mood or personality changes, and peripheral neuropathy. Encephalopathy may develop with high blood levels. Adversely affects reproductive functions in men and women. Adverse effects on fetal development in test animals. Such inorganic lead compounds are carcinogenic in animal studies (IARC 2A). See also p 237. | 0.05 mg/m$^3$, A3 | 100 mg/m$^3$ (as Pb) | | The elemental metal is dark gray. Vapor pressure is low, about 2 mm Hg at 1000°C (1832°F). Major industrial sources include smelting, battery manufacture, radiator repair, and glass and ceramic processing. |
| **Lead arsenate (CAS: 10102-48-4):** Most common acute poisoning symptoms are caused by arsenic, with lead being responsible for chronic toxicity. Symptoms include abdominal pain, headache, vomiting, diarrhea, nausea, itching, and lethargy. Liver and kidney damage may also occur. See both lead and arsenic, pp 237 and 115. | 0.15 mg/m$^3$ | | | White powder often dyed pink. Not combustible. |
| **Lead chromate (chrome yellow [CAS: 7758-97-6]):** Toxicity may result from both the chromium and the lead components. Lead chromate is a suspect human carcinogen owing to the carcinogenicity of hexavalent chromium and inorganic lead compounds. See both lead and hexavalent chromium, pp 237 and 166. | 0.05 mg/m$^3$ (as Pb)<br>0.012 mg/m$^3$ (as Cr), A2 | | | Yellow pigment in powder or crystal form. |
| **Lindane (gamma-hexachlorocyclohexane [CAS: 58-89-9]):** A CNS stimulant and convulsant. Vapors irritating to the eyes and mucous membranes and produce severe headaches and nausea. Well absorbed by all routes. Animal feeding studies have resulted in lung, liver, and kidney damage. May injure bone marrow. Equivocal evidence of carcinogenicity in test animals. See also p 160. | 0.5 mg/m$^3$, S, A3 | 50 mg/m$^3$ | | White crystalline substance with a musty odor if impure. Not combustible. Vapor is 0.0000094 mm Hg at 20°C (68°F). Use as a pesticide restricted by EPA to certified applicators. No longer used as a topical scabicide. |
| **Lithium hydride (CAS: 7580-67-8):** Strong vesicant and alkaline corrosive. Extremely irritating upon direct contact; severe burns result. Dusts extremely irritating to eyes and respiratory tract; pulmonary edema may develop. Symptoms of systemic toxicity include nausea, tremors, confusion, blurring of vision, and coma. | 0.025 mg/m$^3$ | 0.5 mg/m$^3$<br>ERPG-1: 0.025 mg/m$^3$<br>ERPG-2: 0.1 mg/m$^3$<br>ERPG-3: 0.5 mg/m$^3$ | 3 2 2<br>W | Off-white, translucent solid powder that darkens on exposure. Odorless. Very water-reactive, yielding highly flammable hydrogen gas and caustic lithium hydroxide. Finely dispersed powder may ignite spontaneously. |

| | | | | |
|---|---|---|---|---|
| **LPG (liquified petroleum gas [CAS: 68476-85-7]):** A simple asphyxiant and possible CNS depressant. Flammability dangers greatly outweigh toxicity concerns. See also hydrocarbons, p 219. | 1000 ppm | 2000 ppm [LEL] | | Colorless gas. An odorant usually is added as the pure product is odorless. Highly flammable. |
| **Magnesium oxide fume (CAS: 1309-48-4):** Slightly irritating to eyes and upper respiratory tract. There is little evidence to support magnesium oxide as a cause of metal fume fever (see p 259). | 10 mg/$m^3$ (inhalable fraction and vapor) | 750 mg/$m^3$ | | White fume. |
| **Malathion (*O,O*-dimethyl dithiophosphate of diethyl mercaptosuccinate [CAS: 121-75-5]):** An organophosphate-type cholinesterase inhibitor (see p 292). May cause skin sensitization. Absorbed dermally. IARC 3. | 1 mg/$m^3$ (inhalable fraction and vapor), S | 250 mg/$m^3$ | | Colorless to brown liquid with mild skunk-like odor. Vapor pressure is 0.00004 mm Hg at 20°C (68°F). Thermal breakdown products include oxides of sulfur and phosphorus. |
| **Maleic anhydride (2,5-furandione [CAS: 108-31-6]):** Extremely irritating upon direct contact; severe burns may result. Vapors and mists extremely irritating to eyes, skin, and respiratory tract. A skin and respiratory tract sensitizer (asthma) (IARC 3). | 0.1 ppm, SEN | 10 mg/$m^3$<br>ERPG-1: 0.02 mg/$m^3$<br>ERPG-2: 2 mg/$m^3$<br>ERPG-3: 20 mg/$m^3$ | 3 1 1 | Colorless to white solid. Strong, penetrating odor. Eye irritation occurs at the TLV and is an adequate warning property. Vapor pressure is 0.16 mm Hg at 20°C (68°F). Combustible. |
| **Mancozeb (CAS: 1018-01-7):** Fungicide. Based on animal testing and human experience, low toxicity. Produces dermatitis in some individuals. | | | | Yellow powder. Odorless. Negligible vapor pressure. Decomposes at high temperature. |
| **Manganese (CAS: 7439-96-5):** Chronic overexposure results in a CNS toxicity manifested as psychosis, which may be followed by a progressive toxicity similar to parkinsonism (Manganism). See also p 251. | 0.2 mg/$m^3$ (elemental and inorganic compounds, as Mn), S | 500 mg/$m^3$ (Mn compounds, as Mn) | | Elemental metal is a gray, hard, brittle solid. Other compounds vary in appearance. Exposure occurs in mining and milling of the metal, in ferromanganese steel production, and through electric arc welding. |
| **Manganese cyclopentadienyl tricarbonyl [CAS: 12079-65-1]:** MCT is an organic manganese compound used as a gasoline antiknock additive. See Manganese, p 251. | mg/$m^3$, S (as elemental Mn) | | | MCT is used in Canada but still under EPA review in the USA. |
| **Mecoprop (MCPP [CAS: 93-65-2]):** See chlorophenoxy herbicides, p 164. IARC 2B (chlorophenoxy herbicides). | | | | Colorless or white crystals and flakes. |

(C) = ceiling air concentration (TLV-C); S = skin absorption can be significant; SEN = potential sensitizer; A1 = ACGIH-confirmed human carcinogen; A2 = ACGIH-suspected human carcinogen; NFPA Hazard Codes: H = health, F = fire, R = reactivity, Ox = oxidizer, W = water-reactive, 0 (none) <—> 4 (severe). ERPG = Emergency Response Planning Guideline. See p 539 for an explanation of definitions.

(*continued*)

TABLE IV–4. HEALTH HAZARD SUMMARIES FOR INDUSTRIAL AND OCCUPATIONAL CHEMICALS (CONTINUED)

| Health Hazard Summaries | ACGIH TLV | IDLH | NFPA Codes H F R | Comments |
|---|---|---|---|---|
| **Mercury (quicksilver [CAS: 7439-97-6]):** Acute exposures to high vapor levels reported to cause toxic pneumonitis and pulmonary edema. Well absorbed by inhalation. Skin contact can produce irritation and sensitization dermatitis. Mercury salts but not metallic mercury are toxic primarily toxic to the kidneys by acute ingestion. High acute or chronic overexposures can result in CNS toxicity (erythrism, chronic renal disease, brain injury, and peripheral neuropathies. Some inorganic mercury compounds have adverse effects on fetal development in test animals. See also p 253. IARC 3. | 0.025 mg/$m^3$ (inorganic and elemental), S | 10 mg/$m^3$ ERPG-2: 0.25 ppm ERPG-3: 2 0.5 ppm | | Elemental metal is a dense, silvery liquid. Odorless. Vapor pressure is 0.0012 mm Hg at 20°C (68°F). Sources of exposure include small-scale gold refining operations by hobbyists and mercury-containing instruments. |
| **Mercury, alkyl compounds (dimethylmercury, diethyl mercury, ethylmercuric chloride, phenylmercuric acetate):** Well absorbed by all routes. Slow excretion may allow accumulation to occur. Readily crosses blood-brain barrier and placenta. Can cause kidney damage, organic brain disease, and peripheral neuropathy. Some compounds are extremely toxic. Methylmercury is teratogenic in humans. See also p 253. | 0.01 mg/$m^3$ (alkyl compounds, as Hg), S | 2 mg/$m^3$ (as Hg) | | Colorless liquids or solids. Many alkyl compounds have a disagreeable odor. Inorganic mercury can be converted to alkyl mercury compounds in the environment. Can accumulate in food chain. Phenylmercuric acetate use as a fungicide was banned from indoor paints in 1990. |
| **Mesityl oxide (4-methyl-3-penten-2-one [CAS: 141-79-7]):** Causes dermatitis upon prolonged contact. Vapors very irritating to eyes and respiratory tract. Based on animal tests, a CNS depressant and injures kidney and liver at high levels. | 15 ppm | 1400 ppm [LEL] | 2 3 1 | Colorless viscous liquid with a peppermint-like odor. Irritation is an adequate warning property. Vapor pressure is 8 mm Hg at 20°C (68°F). Flammable. Readily forms peroxides. |
| **Metam sodium (sodium methydithiocarbamate [CAS: 137-42-8]):** Soil pesticide. Skin, eye, mucous membrane, and respiratory tract irritant. | | | 2 1 0 | Olive green to light yellow liquid with fairly string sulfur-like odor. Miscible in water. Boiling point 110°C. Vapor pressure 21 mm Hg at 25°C (77°F). Reacts with water to yield methyl isothiocyanate, an irritant gas related to methyl isocyanate. Combustion may release oxides of sulfur and nitrogen. |
| **Methacrylic acid (2-methylpropenoic acid [CAS: 79-41-4]):** Corrosive upon direct contact; severe burns result. Vapors highly irritating to eyes and, possibly, respiratory tract. Based on structural analogies, compounds containing the acrylate moiety may be carcinogens. | 20 ppm | | 3 2 2 | Liquid with an acrid, disagreeable odor. Vapor pressure is less than 0.1 mm Hg at 20°C (68°F). Combustible. Polymerizes above 15°C (59°F), emitting toxic gases. |

| | | | | |
|---|---|---|---|---|
| **Methomyl (*S*-methyl *N* [(methylcarbamoyl)oxy] thioacetimidate, Lannate, Nudrin [CAS: 16752-77-5]):** A carbamate-type cholinesterase inhibitor (see p 244). | 2.5 mg/m$^3$ | | | A slight sulfur odor. Vapor pressure is 0.00005 mm Hg at 20°C (68°F). Thermal breakdown products include oxides of nitrogen and sulfur. |
| **Methoxychlor (dimethoxy-DDT, 2,2-bis(*p*-methoxyphenol)-1,1,1-trichloroethane [CAS: 72-43-5]):** A convulsant at very high doses in test animals. Limited evidence for adverse effects on male reproduction and fetal development in test animals at high doses (IARC 3). See also p 160. | 10 mg/m$^3$<br>NIOSH CA | 5000 mg/m$^3$ | | Colorless to tan solid with a mild fruity odor. Appearance and some hazardous properties vary with the formulation. Vapor pressure is very low at 20°C (68°F). |
| **2-Methoxyethanol (ethylene glycol monomethyl ether, methyl cellosolve [CAS: 109-86-4]):** Workplace overexposures have resulted in depression of the hematopoietic system and encephalopathy. Symptoms include disorientation, lethargy, and anorexia. Well absorbed dermally. Animal testing revealed testicular atrophy and teratogenicity at low doses. Overexposure associated with reduced sperm counts in workers. See also p 194. | 0.1 ppm, S | 200 ppm | 2 2 0 | Clear, colorless liquid with a faint odor. Vapor pressure is 6 mm Hg at 20°C (68°F). Flammable. |
| **2-Methoxyethyl acetate (ethylene glycol monomethyl ether acetate, methyl cellosolve acetate [CAS: 110-49-6]):** Mildly irritating to eyes upon direct contact. Dermally well absorbed. Vapors slightly irritating to the respiratory tract. A CNS depressant at high levels. Based on animal studies, may cause kidney damage, leukopenia, testicular atrophy, and birth defects. See also p 193. | 0.1 ppm, S | 200 ppm | 1 2 — | Colorless liquid with a mild, pleasant odor. Flammable. |
| **Methyl acetate (CAS: 79-20-9):** Vapors moderately irritating to the eyes and respiratory tract. A CNS depressant at high levels. Hydrolyzed to methanol in the body with possible consequent toxicity similar to that of methanol (see p 260). | 200 ppm | 3100 ppm [LEL] | 1 3 0 | Colorless liquid with a pleasant, fruity odor that is a good warning property. Vapor pressure is 173 mm Hg at 20°C (68°F). Flammable. |
| **Methyl acetylene (propyne [CAS: 74-99-7]):** A CNS depressant and respiratory irritant at very high air concentrations in test animals. | 1000 ppm | 1700 ppm [LEL] | 2 4 2 | Colorless gas with sweet odor. Flammable. |

(C) = ceiling air concentration (TLV-C); S = skin absorption can be significant; SEN = potential sensitizer; A1 = ACGIH-confirmed human carcinogen; A2 = ACGIH-suspected human carcinogen; NFPA Hazard Codes: H = health, F = fire, R = reactivity, Ox = oxidizer, W = water-reactive, 0 (none) <—> 4 (severe). ERPG = Emergency Response Planning Guideline. See p 539 for an explanation of definitions.

(*continued*)

TABLE IV–4. HEALTH HAZARD SUMMARIES FOR INDUSTRIAL AND OCCUPATIONAL CHEMICALS (CONTINUED)

| Health Hazard Summaries | ACGIH TLV | IDLH | NFPA Codes H F R | Comments |
|---|---|---|---|---|
| **Methyl acrylate (2-propenoic acid methyl ester [CAS: 96-33-3]):** Methacrylic acid. Highly irritating upon direct contact; severe burns may result. A skin sensitizer. Vapors highly irritating to the eyes and respiratory tract. Based on structural analogies, compounds containing the acrylate moiety may be carcinogens (IARC 3). | 2 ppm, S, SEN | 250 ppm | 3 3 2 | Colorless liquid with a sharp, fruity odor. Vapor pressure is 68.2 mm Hg at 20°C (68°F). Inhibitor included to prevent violent polymerization. Exposure can occur through artcifical (sculpted) nail application. |
| **Methylacrylonitrile (2-methyl-2-propenenitrile [CAS: 126-98-7]):** Mildly irritating upon direct contact. Well absorbed dermally. Metabolized to cyanide (see p 176). In animal tests, acute inhalation at high levels caused death without signs of irritation, probably by a mechanism similar to that of acrylonitrile. Lower levels produced convulsions and loss of motor control. | 1 ppm, S | | | Liquid. Vapor pressure is 40 mm Hg at 13°C (55°F). |
| **Methylal (dimethoxymethane [CAS: 109-87-5]):** Mildly irritating to eyes and respiratory tract. A CNS depressant at very high levels. Animal studies suggest a potential to injure heart, liver, kidneys, and lungs at very high air levels. | 1000 ppm | 2200 ppm [LEL] | 2 3 2 | Colorless liquid with pungent, chloroform-like odor. Highly flammable. |
| **Methyl alcohol (methanol, wood alcohol [CAS: 67-56-1]):** Mildly irritating to eyes and skin. Systemic toxicity may result from absorption by all routes. Toxic metabolites are formate and formaldehyde. A CNS depressant. Signs and symptoms include headache, nausea, abdominal pain, dizziness, shortness of breath, metabolic acidosis, and coma. Visual disturbances (optic neuropathy) range from blurred vision to blindness. See also p 260. | 200 ppm, S | 6000 ppm<br>ERPG-1: 200 ppm<br>ERPG-2: 1000 ppm<br>ERPG-3: 5000 ppm | 1 3 0 | Colorless liquid with a distinctive, sharp odor that is a poor warning property. Flammable. Found in windshield fluids and antifreezes. |
| **Methylamine (CAS: 74-89-5):** Corrosive. Vapors highly irritating to eyes, skin, and respiratory tract; severe burns and pulmonary edema may result. | 5 ppm | 100 ppm<br>ERPG-1: 10 ppm<br>ERPG-2: 100 ppm<br>ERPG-3: 500 ppm | 3 4 0 | Colorless gas with a fishy or ammonia-like odor. Odor is a poor warning property owing to olfactory fatigue. Flammable. |
| **Methyl-*n*-amyl ketone (2-heptanone [CAS: 110-43-0]):** Vapors are irritating to eyes and respiratory tract. A CNS depressant. Flammable. | 50 ppm | 800 ppm | 1 2 0 | Colorless or white liquid with a fruity odor. Vapor pressure is 2.6 mm Hg at 20°C (68°F). |

| | | | | |
|---|---|---|---|---|
| ***N*-methylaniline (CAS: 100-61-8):** A potent inducer of methemoglobinemia (see p 262). Well absorbed by all routes. Animal studies suggest potential for liver and kidney injury. | 0.5 ppm, S | | | Yellow to light brown liquid with a weak ammonia-like odor. Vapor pressure is less than 1 mm Hg at 20°C (68°F). Thermal breakdown products include oxides of nitrogen. |
| **Methyl bromide (bromomethane [CAS: 74-83-9]):** Causes severe irritation and burns upon direct contact. Vapors irritating to the lung; pulmonary edema may result. The CNS, liver, and kidneys are major target organs; acute poisoning causes nausea, vomiting, delirium, and convulsions. Both inhalation and skin exposure may cause systemic toxicity. Chronic exposures associated with peripheral neuropathy in humans. Evidence for adverse effects on fetal development in test animals. Limited evidence of carcinogenicity in test animals (IARC 3). See also p 264, and chloropicrin in this table. | 1 ppm, S<br>NIOSH CA | 250 ppm<br>ERPG-2: 50 ppm<br>ERPG-3: 200 ppm | 3 1 0 | Colorless liquid or gas with a mild chloroform-like odor that is a poor warning property. Chloropicrin, a lacrimator, often is added as a warning agent. Methyl bromide is a widely used fumigant in agriculture and in structural pesticide control. |
| **Methyl *n*-butyl ketone (MBK, 2-hexanone [CAS: 591-78-6]):** Vapors irritating to eyes and respiratory tract at high levels. A CNS depressant at high doses. Causes peripheral neuorpathy by a mechanism thought to be the same as that of *n*-hexane. Well absorbed by all routes. Causes testicular toxicity in animal studies. | 5 ppm, S | 1600 ppm | 2 3 0 | Colorless liquid with an acetone-like odor. Vapor pressure is 3.8 mm Hg at 20°C (68°F). Flammable. NIOSH recommended exposure limit is 1.0 ppm. |
| **Methyl chloride (CAS: 74-87-3):** Once used as an anesthetic. Symptoms include headache, confusion, ataxia, convulsions, and coma. Liver, kidney, and bone marrow are other target organs. Evidence for adverse effects on both the testes and fetal development in test animals at high doses. | 50 ppm, S<br>NIOSH CA | 2000 ppm<br>ERPG-2: 400 ppm<br>ERPG-3: 1000 ppm | 1 4 0 | Colorless gas with a mild, sweet odor that is a poor warning property. Highly flammable. |
| **Methyl-2-cyanoacrylate (CAS: 137-05-3):** Vapors irritating to the eyes and upper respiratory tract. May act as a sensitizer. A strong and fast-acting glue that can fasten body parts to each other or surfaces. Direct contact with the eye may result in mechanical injury if the immediate bonding of the eyelids is followed by forced separation. | 0.2 ppm | | | Colorless viscous liquid. Commonly, this compound and related ones are known as "super glues." |

(C) = ceiling air concentration (TLV-C); S = skin absorption can be significant; SEN = potential sensitizer; A1 = ACGIH-confirmed human carcinogen; A2 = ACGIH-suspected human carcinogen; NFPA Hazard Codes: H = health, F = fire, R = reactivity, Ox = oxidizer, W = water-reactive, 0 (none) <—> 4 (severe). ERPG = Emergency Response Planning Guideline. See p 539 for an explanation of definitions.

(*continued*)

TABLE IV–4. HEALTH HAZARD SUMMARIES FOR INDUSTRIAL AND OCCUPATIONAL CHEMICALS (CONTINUED)

| Health Hazard Summaries | ACGIH TLV | IDLH | NFPA Codes H F R | Comments |
|---|---|---|---|---|
| **Methylcyclohexane (CAS: 108-87-2):** Irritating upon direct contact. Vapors irritating to eyes and respiratory tract. A CNS depressant at high levels. Based on animal studies, some liver and kidney injury may occur at chronic high doses. | 400 ppm | 1200 ppm [LEL] | 2 3 0 | Colorless liquid with a faint benzene-like odor. Vapor pressure is 37 mm Hg at 20°C (68°F). Highly flammable. |
| ***o*-Methylcyclohexanone (CAS: 583-60-8):** Based on animal studies, irritating upon direct contact. Dermal absorption occurs. Vapors irritating to eyes and respiratory tract. A CNS depressant at high levels. | 50 ppm, S | 600 ppm | — 2 0 | Colorless liquid with mild peppermint odor. Irritation is a good warning property. Vapor pressure is about 1 mm Hg at 20°C (68°F). Flammable. |
| **Methyl demeton (*O,O*-dimethyl 2-ethylmercaptoethyl thiophosphate [CAS: 8022-00-2]):** An organophosphate-type cholinesterase inhibitor (see p 292). | 0.5 mg/m$^3$, S | | | Colorless to pale yellow liquid with an unpleasant odor. Vapor pressure is 0.00036 mm Hg at 20°C (68°F). Thermal breakdown products include oxides of sulfur and phosphorus. |
| **4,4'-Methylene-bis(2-chloroaniline) (MOCA [CAS: 101-14-4]):** A carcinogen in test animals (IARC 2A). Dermal absorption occurs. | 0.01 ppm, S, A2<br>NIOSH CA | | | Tan solid. Thermal breakdown products include oxides of nitrogen and hydrogen chloride. |
| **Methylene bis(4-cyclohexylisocyanate [CAS: 5124-30-1]):** A strong irritant and skin sensitizer. Based on analogy to other isocyanates, vapors are likely to be potent respiratory tract irritants and sensitizers. | 0.005 ppm | | | White to pale yellow solid flakes. Odorless. Possible thermal breakdown products include oxides of nitrogen and hydrogen cyanide. |
| **Methylene bisphenyl isocyanate (4,4-di-phenylmethane diisocyanate, MDI [CAS: 101-68-8]):** Irritating upon direct contact. Vapors and dusts highly irritating to eyes and respiratory tract. Potent respiratory tract sensitizer (asthma). IARC 3. | 0.005 ppm | 75 mg/m$^3$<br>ERPG-1: 0.2 mg/m$^3$<br>ERPG-2: 2 mg/m$^3$<br>ERPG-3: 25 mg/m$^3$ | 1 2 1<br>W | White to pale yellow flakes. Odorless. Vapor pressure is 0.05 mm Hg at 20°C (68°F). Possible thermal breakdown products include oxides of nitrogen and hydrogen cyanide. Component of urethanes. |

| | | | | |
|---|---|---|---|---|
| **Methylene chloride (methylene dichloride, dichloromethane [CAS: 75-09-2]):** Irritating upon prolonged direct contact. Dermal absorption occurs. Vapors irritating to eyes and respiratory tract. A CNS depressant. May cause cardiac arrhythmias. Liver and kidney injury at high concentrations. Converted to carbon monoxide in the body with resultant carboxyhemoglobin formation. A carcinogen in test animals (IARC 2B). See also p 266. | 50 ppm, A3<br>OSHA CA<br>NIOSH CA | 2300 ppm<br>ERPG-1: 200 ppm<br>ERPG-2: 750 ppm<br>ERPG-3: 4000 ppm | 2 1 0 | Heavy colorless liquid with a chloroform-like odor that is a poor warning property. Vapor pressure is 350 mm Hg at 20°C (68°F). Possible thermal breakdown products include phosgene and hydrogen chloride. Methylene chloride is a solvent with many industrial and commercial uses (eg, furniture strippers, carburetor cleaners). |
| **4,4'-Methylene dianiline (4,4'-diaminodiphenylmethane [CAS: 101-77-9]):** Vapors highly irritating to eyes and respiratory tract. Hepatotoxicity (cholestatic jaundice) observed in overexposed workers. Systemic toxicity may result from inhalation, ingestion, or skin contact. Methemoglobinemia (see p 262), kidney injury, retinal injury, and evidence of carcinogenicity in animals (IARC 2B). | 0.1 ppm, S, A3<br>NIOSH CA | | 3 1 0 | Light brown solid crystals with a faint amine odor. Combustible. Thermal breakdown products include oxides of nitrogen. |
| **Methyl ethyl ketone (2-butanone, MEK [CAS: 78-93-3]):** Vapors irritating to eyes and respiratory tract. A CNS depressant at high levels. Limited evidence for adverse effects on fetal development in test animals. Potentiates neurotoxicity of methyl butyl ketone and *n*-hexane. | 200 ppm | 3000 ppm | 1 3 0 | Colorless liquid with a mild acetone odor. Vapor pressure is 77 mm Hg at 20°C (68°F). Flammable. |
| **Methyl ethyl ketone peroxide (CAS: 1338-23-4):** Based on chemical reactivity, highly irritating upon direct contact; severe burns may result. Vapors or mists likely to be highly irritating to the eyes and respiratory tract. In animal tests, overexposure resulted in liver, kidney, and lung damage. | 0.2 ppm (C) | | | Colorless liquid with a characteristic odor. Shock sensitive. Breaks down above 50°C (122°F). Explodes upon rapid heating. May contain additives such as dimethyl phthalate, cyclohexanone peroxide, and diallylphthalate to add stability. |
| **Methyl formate (CAS: 107-31-3):** Vapors highly irritating to eyes and respiratory tract. A CNS depressant at high levels. Exposure has been associated with visual disturbances, including temporary blindness. | 100 ppm | 4500 ppm | 2 4 0 | Colorless liquid with a pleasant odor at high levels. Odor is a poor warning property. Vapor pressure is 476 mm Hg at 20°C (68°F). Highly flammable. |

(C) = ceiling air concentration (TLV-C); S = skin absorption can be significant; SEN = potential sensitizer; A1 = ACGIH-confirmed human carcinogen; A2 = ACGIH-suspected human carcinogen; NFPA Hazard Codes: H = health, F = fire, R = reactivity, Ox = oxidizer, W = water-reactive, 0 (none) <—> 4 (severe). ERPG = Emergency Response Planning Guideline. See p 539 for an explanation of definitions.

(*continued*)

TABLE IV–4. HEALTH HAZARD SUMMARIES FOR INDUSTRIAL AND OCCUPATIONAL CHEMICALS (CONTINUED)

| Health Hazard Summaries | ACGIH TLV | IDLH | NFPA Codes H F R | Comments |
|---|---|---|---|---|
| **Methylhydrazine (monomethylhydrazine [CAS: 60-34-4]):** Similar to hydrazine in toxic actions. Vapors likely to be highly irritating to the eyes and respiratory tract. Causes methemoglobinemia (see p 262). Potent hemolysin. Highly hepatotoxic. Causes kidney injury. A convulsant. A carcinogen in test animals. See also Mushrooms p 275. | 0.01 ppm, S, A3<br>NIOSH CA | 20 ppm | 4 3 2 | Colorless clear liquid. Vapor pressure is 36 mm Hg at 20°C (68°F). Flammable. In addition to potential industrial uses, exposure to methylhydrazine can occur from ingestion of false morel mushrooms. |
| **Methyl iodide: (iodomethane [CAS: 74-88-4]):** An alkylating agent. Based on chemical properties, likely to be highly irritating upon direct contact; severe burns may result. Dermal absorption is likely. Vapors highly irritating to respiratory tract; pulmonary edema has resulted. Neurotoxic; signs and symptoms include nausea, vomiting, dizziness, slurred speech, visual disturbances, ataxia, tremor, irritability, convulsions, and coma. Delusions and hallucinations may last for weeks during recovery. Severe hepatic injury may also occur. Limited evidence of carcinogenicity in test animals (IARC 3). | 2 ppm, S,<br>NIOSH CA | 100 ppm<br>ERPG-1: 25 ppm<br>ERPG-2: 50 ppm<br>ERPG-3: 125 ppm | | Colorless, yellow, red, or brown liquid. Not combustible. Vapor pressure is 375 mm Hg at 20°C (68°F). Thermal breakdown products include iodine and hydrogen iodide. |
| **Methyl isoamyl ketone (5-methyl-2-hexanone [CAS: 110-12-3]):** By analogy to other aliphatic-ketones, vapors are likely to be irritating to eyes and respiratory tract. Likely to be a CNS depressant. | 50 ppm | | 1 2 0 | Colorless liquid with a pleasant odor. Vapor pressure is 4.5 mm Hg at 20°C (68°F). Flammable. |
| **Methyl isobutyl ketone (4-methyl-2-pentanone, hexone [CAS: 108-10-1]):** Irritating to eyes upon direct contact. Vapors irritating to eyes and respiratory tract. Reported systemic symptoms in humans are weakness, dizziness, ataxia, nausea, vomiting, and headache. High-dose studies in animals suggest a potential for liver and kidney injury. | 50 ppm | 500 ppm | 2 3 1 | Colorless liquid with a mild odor. Vapor pressure is 7.5 mm Hg at 25°C (77°F). Flammable. |

| | | | | |
|---|---|---|---|---|
| **Methyl isocyanate (MIC [CAS: 624-83-9]):** Highly reactive; highly corrosive upon direct contact. Vapors extremely irritating to eyes, skin, and respiratory tract; severe burns and pulmonary edema have resulted. A sensitizing agent. Toxicity is not related to cyanide. Evidence that severe poisonings have adverse effects on fetal development. | 0.02 ppm, S | 3 ppm<br>ERPG-1: 0.025 ppm<br>ERPG-2: 0.25 ppm<br>ERPG-3: 1.5 ppm | 4 3 2<br>W | Colorless liquid with a sharp, disagreeable odor that is a poor warning property. Vapor pressure is 348 mm Hg at 20°C (68°F). Flammable. Reacts with water to release methylamine. Polymerizes upon heating. Thermal breakdown products include hydrogen cyanide and oxides of nitrogen. Used as a chemical intermediate in pesticide synthesis. MIC is not in urethanes. |
| **Methyl mercaptan (CAS: 74-93-1):** Causes delayed-onset pulmonary edema. CNS effects include narcosis and convulsions. Reported to have caused methemoglobinemia and hemolysis in a patient with G6PD deficiency. | 0.5 ppm | 150 ppm<br>ERPG-1: 0.005 ppm<br>ERPG-2: 25 ppm<br>ERPG-3: 100 ppm | 4 4 0 | Colorless liquid with an offensive rotten egg odor. Odor and irritation are good warning properties. |
| **Methyl methacrylate (CAS: 80-62-6):** Irritating upon direct contact. Vapors irritating to the eyes, skin, and respiratory tract. A sensitizer (asthma). At very high levels may produce headache, nausea, vomiting, dizziness. Limited evidence for adverse effects on fetal development in animal tests at very high doses (IARC 3). | 50 ppm, SEN | 1000 ppm | 2 3 2 | Colorless liquid with a pungent, acrid, fruity odor. Vapor pressure is 35 mm Hg at 20°C (68°F). Flammable. Contains inhibitors to prevent self-polymerization. Used in resin polymers, including medical applications. |
| **Methyl parathion (*O,O*-dimethyl *O-p*-nitro-phenylphosphorothioate [CAS: 298-00-0]):** A highly potent organophosphate cholinesterase inhibitor (see p 292). IARC 3. | 0.2 $mg/m^3$, S | | | Tan liquid with a strong garlic-like odor. Vapor pressure is 0.5 mm Hg at 20°C (68°F). Appearance may vary with formulation. |
| **Methyl propyl ketone (2-pentanone [CAS: 107-87-9]):** Vapors irritating to eyes and respiratory tract. Based on animal studies, a CNS depressant at high levels. | 200 ppm | 1500 ppm | 2 3 0 | Colorless liquid with a characteristic odor. Vapor pressure is 27 mm Hg at 20°C (68°F). Flammable. |
| **Methyl silicate (tetramethoxy silane [CAS: 681-84-5]):** Highly reactive; corrosive upon direct contact; severe burns and loss of vision may result. Vapors extremely irritating to eyes and respiratory tract; severe eye burns and pulmonary edema may result. | 1 ppm | ERPG-2: 10 ppm<br>ERPG-3: 20 ppm | | Colorless crystals. Reacts with water, forming silicic acid and methanol. |

(C) = ceiling air concentration (TLV-C); S = skin absorption can be significant; SEN = potential sensitizer; A1 = ACGIH-confirmed human carcinogen; A2 = ACGIH-suspected human carcinogen; NFPA Hazard Codes: H = health, F = fire, R = reactivity, Ox = oxidizer, W = water-reactive, 0 (none) <—> 4 (severe). ERPG = Emergency Response Planning Guideline. See p 539 for an explanation of definitions.

(*continued*)

TABLE IV–4. HEALTH HAZARD SUMMARIES FOR INDUSTRIAL AND OCCUPATIONAL CHEMICALS (CONTINUED)

| Health Hazard Summaries | ACGIH TLV | IDLH | NFPA Codes H F R | Comments |
|---|---|---|---|---|
| **alpha-Methylstyrene (CAS: 98-83-9):** Slightly irritating upon direct contact. Vapors irritating to eyes and respiratory tract. A CNS depressant at high levels. | 50 ppm | 700 ppm | 1 2 1 | Colorless liquid with a characteristic odor. Irritation is an adequate warning property. Vapor pressure is 1.9 mm Hg at 20°C (68°F). Flammable. |
| **Methyl tert butyl ether (MTBE [CAS: 1634-04-4]):** Vapors mildly irritating to eyes and respiratory tract. A CNS depressant; acute exposure at high levels can cause nausea, vomiting, dizziness, and sleepiness. Adverse effects on liver and kidney in test animals at high levels. Evidence for adverse effects on reproduction and carcinogenicity in test animals exposed to very high concentrations (IARC 3). | 50 ppm, A3 | | | A volatile colorless liquid at room temperature. Gasoline additive. Vapor pressure is 248 mm Hg at 25°C (77°F). |
| **Metribuzin (4-amino-6-[1,1-dimethylethyl]-3-[methylthio]-1,2,4-triazin-5 [4H]-one [CAS: 21087-64-9]):** Human data available reveal no irritation or sensitization after dermal exposure. In animal testing, was poorly absorbed through the skin and produced no direct skin or eye irritation. Repeated high doses caused CNS depression and liver and thryoid effects. | 5 mg/m$^3$ | | | Vapor pressure is 0.00001 mm Hg at 20°C (68°F). Thermal breakdown products include oxides of sulfur and nitrogen. |
| **Mevinphos (2-carbomethoxy-1-methylvinyl dimethyl phosphate, phosdrin [CAS: 7786-34-7]):** An organophosphate cholinesterase inhibitor (see p 292). Well absorbed by all routes. Repeated exposures to low levels can accumulate to produce symptoms. | 0.01 mg/m$^3$ (inhalable fraction and vapor), S | 4 ppm | | Colorless or yellow liquid with a faint odor. Vapor pressure is 0.0022 mm Hg at 20°C (68°F). Combustible. Thermal breakdown products include phosphoric acid mist. |
| **Mica (CAS: 12001-25-2):** Dusts may cause pneumoconiosis upon chronic inhalation. | 3 mg/m$^3$ (respirable fraction) | 1500 mg/m$^3$ | | Colorless solid flakes or sheets. Odorless. Vapor pressure is negligible at 20°C (68°F). Noncombustible. |

| | | | | |
|---|---|---|---|---|
| **Monocrotophos (dimethyl 2-methylcarbamoyl-1-methylvinyl phosphate [CAS: 6923-22-4]):** An organophosphate-type cholinesterase inhibitor (see p 292). Limited human data indicate it is well absorbed through the skin but is rapidly metabolized rapidly and excreted. | 0.05 mg/m$^3$ (inhalable fraction and vapor), S | | | Reddish-brown solid with a mild odor. |
| **Morpholine (tetrahydro-1,4-oxazine [CAS: 110-91-8]):** Corrosive; extremely irritating upon direct contact; severe burns may result. Well absorbed dermally. Vapors irritating to eyes and respiratory tract. Exposure to vapors has caused transient corneal edema. May cause severe liver and kidney injury. (IARC 3). | 20 ppm, S | 1400 ppm [LEL] | 3 3 0 | Colorless liquid with mild ammonia-like odor. Vapor pressure is 7 mm Hg at 20°C (68°F). Flammable. Thermal breakdown products include oxides of nitrogen. Found in some consumer polish and wax products. |
| **Monosodium methanearsonate (MSMA [CAS: 2163-80-6)].** Arsenical herbicide. Hepatoxin and auditory neurotoxin. | | | | Light yellow liquid. Odorless. |
| **Naphthalene (CAS: 91-20-3):** Highly irritating to eyes upon direct contact. Vapors are irritating to eyes and may cause cataracts upon chronic exposure. Dermally well absorbed. May induce methemoglobinemia (see p 262). Symptoms of overexposure include headache and nausea. IARC 2B. | 10 ppm, S | 250 ppm | 2 2 0 | White to brown solid. The mothball odor and respiratory tract irritation are good warning properties. Current mothball formulations in the US do not contain naphthalene. Vapor pressure is 0.05 mm Hg at 20°C (68°F). Combustible. |
| **beta-Naphthylamine (2-aminonaphthalene [CAS: 91-59-8]):** Acute overexposures can cause methemoglobinemia (see p 262) or acute hemorrhagic cystitis. Well absorbed through skin. Known human bladder carcinogen (IARC 1). | A1<br>OSHA CA<br>NIOSH CA | | | White to reddish crystals. Vapor pressure is 1 mm Hg at 108°C (226°F). Combustible. |
| **Nickel carbonyl (nickel tetracarbonyl [CAS: 13463-39-3]):** Inhalation of vapors can cause severe lung and systemic injury without irritant warning signs. Symptoms include headache, nausea, vomiting, fever, and extreme weakness. Based on animal studies, liver and brain damage may occur. Adverse effects on fetal development in test animals. A carcinogen in test animals. | 0.05 ppm (as Ni)<br>NIOSH CA | 2 ppm (as Ni) | 4 3 3 | Colorless liquid or gas. The musty odor is a poor warning property. Vapor pressure is 321 mm Hg at 20°C (68°F). Highly flammable. Exposures largely limited to nickel refining. |

(C) = ceiling air concentration (TLV-C); S = skin absorption can be significant; SEN = potential sensitizer; A1 = ACGIH-confirmed human carcinogen; A2 = ACGIH-suspected human carcinogen; NFPA Hazard Codes: H = health, F = fire, R = reactivity, Ox = oxidizer, W = water-reactive, 0 (none) <—> 4 (severe). ERPG = Emergency Response Planning Guideline. See p 539 for an explanation of definitions.

(*continued*)

TABLE IV–4. HEALTH HAZARD SUMMARIES FOR INDUSTRIAL AND OCCUPATIONAL CHEMICALS (CONTINUED)

| Health Hazard Summaries | ACGIH TLV | IDLH | NFPA Codes H F R | Comments |
|---|---|---|---|---|
| **Nickel metal and soluble inorganic salts (nickel chloride, nickel sulfate, nickel nitrate, nickel oxide):** May cause a severe sensitization dermatitis, "nickel itch," upon repeated contact. Fumes highly irritating to the respiratory tract. Some compounds have adverse effects on fetal development in test animals. Some compounds are human nasal and lung carcinogens (nickel compounds, IARC 1; nickel metal, IARC 2B). | 1.5 mg/m$^3$ (elemental)<br>0.1 mg/m$^3$ (soluble compounds), as Ni<br>0.2 mg/m$^3$, A1 (insoluble compounds), as Ni (inhalable fraction)<br>NIOSH CA | 10 mg/m$^3$ (as Ni) | | Gray metallic powder or green solids. All forms are odorless. |
| **Nicotine (CAS: 54-11-5):** A potent nicotinic cholinergic receptor agonist. Well absorbed by all routes of exposure. Symptoms include dizziness, confusion, weakness, nausea and vomiting, tachycardia and hypertension, tremors, convulsions, and muscle paralysis. Death from respiratory paralysis can be very rapid. Adverse effects on fetal development in animal studies. See also p 278. | 0.5 mg/m$^3$, S | 5 mg/m$^3$ | 4 1 0 | Pale yellow to dark brown viscous liquid with a fishy or amine-like odor. Vapor pressure is 0.0425 mm Hg at 20°C (68°F). Combustible. Thermal breakdown products include oxides of nitrogen. Although generally thought of in context of tobacco use and abstinence products, nicotine is a widely used pesticide. |
| **Nitric acid (aqua fortis, engraver's acid [CAS: 7697-37-2]):** Concentrated solutions corrosive to eyes and skin; very severe penetrating burns result. Vapors highly irritating to eyes and respiratory tract; pulmonary edema has resulted. Chronic inhalation exposure can produce bronchitis and erosion of the teeth. See also irritant gases, p 212. | 2 ppm | 25 ppm<br>ERPG-1: 1 ppm<br>ERPG-2: 6 ppm<br>ERPG-3: 78 ppm | 3 0 0<br>Ox (≤ 40%)<br>4 0 1<br>Ox (fuming) | Colorless, yellow, or red fuming liquid with an acrid, suffocating odor. Vapor pressure is approximately 62 mm Hg at 25°C (77°F). Not combustible. Interaction with organic materials can release nitrogen dioxide. |
| **Nitric oxide (NO, nitrogen monoxide [CAS: 10102-43-9]):** Nitric oxide slowly converts to nitrogen dioxide in air; eye and mucous membrane irritation and pulmonary edema are likely from nitrogen dioxide. Overexposures have been reported to result in acute and chronic obstructive airway disease. Based on animal studies, may cause methemoglobinemia (see p 262). Binds to hemoglobin at the same site as oxygen, and this may contribute to the toxicity. | 25 ppm | 100 ppm | | Colorless or brown gas. The sharp, sweet odor occurs below the TLV and is a good warning property. |

| | | | | |
|---|---|---|---|---|
| ***p*-Nitroaniline (CAS: 100-01-6):** Irritating to eyes upon direct contact; may injure cornea. Well absorbed by all routes. Overexposure results in headache, weakness, respiratory distress, and methemoglobinemia (see p 262). Liver damage may also occur. | 3 mg/m³, S | 300 mg/m³ | 3 1 2 | Yellow solid with an ammonia-like odor that is a poor warning property. Vapor pressure is much less than 1 mm Hg at 20°C (68°F). Combustible. Thermal breakdown products include oxides of nitrogen. |
| **Nitrobenzene (CAS: 98-95-3):** Irritating upon direct contact; sensitization dermatitis may occur. Well absorbed by all routes. Causes methemoglobinemia (see p 262). Symptoms include headache, cyanosis, weakness, and gastrointestinal upset. May injure liver. Injures testes in animals. Limited evidence for adverse effects on fetal development in animals. (IARC 2B). | 1 ppm, S, A3 | 200 ppm | 3 2 1 | Pale yellow to dark brown viscous liquid. Shoe polish–like odor is a good warning property. Vapor pressure is much less than 1 mm Hg at 20°C (68°F). Combustible. Thermal breakdown products include oxides of nitrogen. |
| ***p*-Nitrochlorobenzene (CAS: 100-00-5):** Irritating upon direct contact; sensitization dermatitis may occur upon repeated exposures. Well absorbed by all routes. Causes methemoglobinemia (see p 262). Symptoms include headache, cyanosis, weakness, and gastrointestinal upset. May cause liver and kidney injury. | 0.1 ppm, S, A3<br>NIOSH CA | 100 mg/m³ | 3 1 1 | Yellow solid with a sweet odor. Vapor pressure is 0.009 mm Hg at 25°C (77°F). Combustible. Thermal breakdown products include oxides of nitrogen and hydrogen chloride. |
| **4-Nitrodiphenyl (4-nitrobiphenyl [CAS: 92-93-3]):** Extremely well absorbed through skin. Produces bladder cancer in dogs and rabbits. Metabolized to 4-aminodiphenyl, which is a potent carcinogen in humans (IARC 3). | S, A2<br>OSHA CA<br>NIOSH CA | | | White solid with a sweet odor. Thermal breakdown products include oxides of nitrogen. |
| **Nitroethane (CAS: 79-24-3):** Based on high-exposure studies in animals, vapors are irritating to the respiratory tract. A CNS depressant. Can cause methemoglobinemia (see p 262). Causes liver injury at high levels of exposure in test animals. A structurally similar compound, 2-nitropropane, is a carcinogen. | 100 ppm | 1000 ppm | 1 3 3<br>(explodes on heating) | Colorless viscous liquid with a fruity odor that is a poor warning property. Vapor pressure is 15.6 mm Hg at 20°C (68°F). Flammable. Thermal breakdown products include oxides of nitrogen. |
| **Nitrogen dioxide (CAS: 10102-44-0):** Gases and vapors irritating to eyes and respiratory tract; fatal pulmonary edema has resulted. Initial symptoms include cough and dyspnea. Pulmonary edema may appear after a delay of several hours. The acute phase may be followed by a fatal secondary stage, with fever and chills, dyspnea, cyanosis, and delayed-onset pulmonary edema. See pp 212, 279. | 3 ppm | 20 ppm<br>ERPG-1: 1 ppm<br>ERPG-2: 15 ppm<br>ERPG-3: 30 ppm | 3 0 0<br>Ox | Dark brown fuming liquid or gas. Pungent odor and irritation occur only slightly above the TLV and are adequate warning properties. Vapor pressure is 720 mm Hg at 20°C (68°F). Important exposures include structural fires, silage (silo-filling), and gas-shielded (MIG or TIG) welding. |

(C) = ceiling air concentration (TLV-C); S = skin absorption can be significant; SEN = potential sensitizer; A1 = ACGIH-confirmed human carcinogen; A2 = ACGIH-suspected human carcinogen; NFPA Hazard Codes: H = health, F = fire, R = reactivity, Ox = oxidizer, W = water-reactive, 0 (none) <—> 4 (severe). ERPG = Emergency Response Planning Guideline. See p 539 for an explanation of definitions.

(*continued*)

TABLE IV–4. HEALTH HAZARD SUMMARIES FOR INDUSTRIAL AND OCCUPATIONAL CHEMICALS (CONTINUED)

| Health Hazard Summaries | ACGIH TLV | IDLH | NFPA Codes H F R | Comments |
|---|---|---|---|---|
| **Nitrogen trifluoride (nitrogen fluoride [CAS: 7783-54-2]):** Vapors may cause eye irritation. Based on animal studies, may cause methemoglobinemia (see p 262) and liver and kidney damage. | 10 ppm | 1000 ppm<br>ERPG-2: 400 ppm<br>ERPG-3: 800 ppm | | Colorless gas with a moldy odor that is a poor warning property. Not combustible. Highly reactive and explosive under a number of conditions. |
| **Nitroglycerin (glycerol trinitrate [CAS: 55-63-0]):** Causes vasodilation, including coronary arteries. Headache and drop in blood pressure are common. Well absorbed by all routes. Tolerance to vasodilation can occur; cessation of exposure may precipitate angina pectoris in pharmacologically dependent workers. See also p 279. | 0.05 ppm, S | 75 mg/m$^3$ | 2 2 4 | Pale yellow viscous liquid. Vapor pressure is 0.00026 mm Hg at 20°C (68°F). Highly explosive. |
| **Nitromethane (CAS: 75-52-5):** Based on high-dose animal studies, causes respiratory tract irritation, liver and kidney injury, and CNS depression with ataxia, weakness, convulsions, and, possibly, methemoglobinemia (see p 262). IARC 2B. | 20 ppm, A3 | 750 ppm | 1 3 4 | Colorless liquid with a faint fruity odor that is a poor warning property. Vapor pressure is 27.8 mm Hg at 20°C (68°F). Thermal breakdown products include oxides of nitrogen. |
| **1-Nitropropane (CAS: 108-03-2):** Vapors mildly irritating to eyes and respiratory tract. Liver and kidney injury may occur. | 25 ppm | 1000 ppm | 1 3 2<br>(may explode on heating) | Colorless liquid with a faint fruity odor that is a poor warning property. Vapor pressure is 7.5 mm Hg at 20°C (68°F). Flammable. Thermal breakdown products include oxides of nitrogen. |
| **2-Nitropropane (CAS: 79-46-9):** Mildly irritating, CNS depressant at high exposures. Highly hepatotoxic; fatalities have resulted. Renal toxicity also occurs. Well absorbed by all routes. Limited evidence for adverse effects on fetal development in test animals. A carcinogen in test animals (IARC 2B). | 10 ppm, A3<br>NIOSH CA | 100 ppm | 1 3 2<br>(may explode on heating) | Colorless liquid. Vapor pressure is 12.9 mm Hg at 20°C (68°F). Flammable. Thermal breakdown products include oxides of nitrogen. |
| ***N*-Nitrosodimethylamine (dimethylnitrosamine [CAS: 62-75-9]):** Overexposed workers suffered severe liver damage. Based on animal studies, well absorbed by all routes. A potent animal carcinogen producing liver, kidney, and lung cancers (IARC 2A). | S, A3<br>OSHA CA<br>NIOSH CA | | | Yellow viscous liquid. Combustible. |

| | | | | |
|---|---|---|---|---|
| **Nitrotoluene (*o*-, *m*-, *p*-nitrotoluene [CAS: 99-08-1]):** Weak inducer of methemoglobinemia (see p 262). By analogy to structurally similar compounds, dermal absorption is likely. IARC 3. | 2 ppm, S | 200 ppm | 3 1 1 | *Ortho* and *meta*, yellow liquid or solid. *Para,* yellow solid. All isomers have a weak, aromatic odor. Vapor pressure is approximately 0.15 mm Hg at 20°C (68°F). Thermal breakdown products include oxides of nitrogen. Intermediate in synthesis of dyestuffs and explosives. |
| **Nitrous oxide (CAS: 10024-97-2):** A CNS depressant. Hematopoietic effects from chronic exposure include megaloblastic anemia. Substance abuse has resulted in neuropathies. May have an adverse effect on human fertility and fetal development. See also p 283. | 50 ppm | | | Colorless gas. Sweet odor. Not combustible. Widely used as an anesthetic gas in dentistry, and a popular drug of abuse. |
| **Octachloronaphthalene (Halowax 1051 [CAS: 2234-13-1]):** By analogy to other chlorinated naphthalenes, workers overexposed by inhalation or skin contact may experience chloracne and liver damage. For chloracne, see also dioxins, p 183. | 0.1 mg/m$^3$, S | 0.1 mg/m$^3$ (effective IDLH) | | Pale yellow solid with an aromatic odor. Vapor pressure is less than 1 mm Hg at 20°C (68°F). Not combustible. Thermal breakdown products include hydrogen chloride. |
| **Octane (CAS: 111-65-9):** Vapors mildly irritating to eyes and respiratory tract. A CNS depressant at very high concentrations. | 300 ppm | 1000 ppm [LEL] | 0 3 0 | Colorless liquid. Gasoline-like odor and irritation are good warning properties. Vapor pressure is 11 mm Hg at 20°C (68°F). Flammable. |
| **Osmium tetroxide (osmic acid [CAS: 20816-12-0]):** Corrosive upon direct contact; severe burns may result. Fumes are highly irritating to eyes and respiratory tract. Based on high-dose animal studies, bone marrow injury and kidney damage may occur. | 0.0002 ppm (as Os) | 1 mg/m$^3$ (as Os) | | Colorless to pale yellow solid with a sharp and irritating odor like chlorine. Vapor pressure is 7 mm Hg at 20°C (68°F). Not combustible. Catalyst and laboratory reagent. |
| **Oxalic acid (ethanedioic acid [CAS: 144-62-7]):** A strong acid; corrosive to eyes and to skin upon direct contact (see p 157). Fumes irritating to respiratory tract. Highly toxic upon ingestion; precipitation of calcium oxalate crystals can cause hypocalcemia and renal damage. See also p 296. | 1 mg/m$^3$ | 500 mg/m$^3$ | 3 1 0 | Colorless or white solid. Odorless. Vapor pressure is less than 0.001 mm Hg at 20°C (68°F). |

(C) = ceiling air concentration (TLV-C); S = skin absorption can be significant; SEN = potential sensitizer; A1 = ACGIH-confirmed human carcinogen; A2 = ACGIH-suspected human carcinogen; NFPA Hazard Codes: H = health, F = fire, R = reactivity, Ox = oxidizer, W = water-reactive, 0 (none) <—> 4 (severe). ERPG = Emergency Response Planning Guideline. See p 539 for an explanation of definitions.

(*continued*)

TABLE IV–4. HEALTH HAZARD SUMMARIES FOR INDUSTRIAL AND OCCUPATIONAL CHEMICALS (CONTINUED)

| Health Hazard Summaries | ACGIH TLV | IDLH | NFPA Codes H F R | Comments |
|---|---|---|---|---|
| **Oxygen difluoride (oxygen fluoride, fluorine monoxide [CAS: 7783-41-7]):** Extremely irritating to the eyes, skin, and respiratory tract. Effects similar to those of hydrofluoric acid (see p 222) Based on animal studies, may also injure kidney, internal genitalia, and other organs. Workers have complained of severe headaches after low-level exposures. | 0.05 ppm (C) | 0.5 ppm | | Colorless gas with a strong and foul odor. Olfactory fatigue is common, so odor is a poor warning property. A strong oxidizing agent. |
| **Ozone (triatomic oxygen [CAS: 10028-15-6]):** Irritating to eyes and respiratory tract. Pulmonary edema has been reported. See also p 212. | 0.05 ppm (heavy work); 0.08 ppm (moderate work); 0.1 ppm (light work); 0.2 ppm (≤ 2 h) | 5 ppm | | Colorless or bluish gas. Sharp, distinctive odor is an adequate warning property. A strong oxidizing agent. Gas-shielded and specialty welding are potential sources of exposure, in addition to water purification and industrial bleaching operations. |
| **Paraquat (1,1'-dimethyl-4,4'-bipyridinium dichloride [CAS: 4687-14-7]):** Extremely irritating upon direct contact; severe corrosive burns may result. Well absorbed through skin. A potent toxin causing acute multiorgan failure as well as progressive fatal pulmonary fibrosis after ingestion. See also p 297. | 0.5 $mg/m^3$ 0.1 $mg/m^3$ (respirable fraction) | 1 $mg/m^3$ (total dust) 0.1 $mg/m^3$ (respirable fraction) | | Odorless white to yellow solid. Vapor pressure is negligible at 20°C (68°F). Not combustible. Thermal breakdown products include oxides of nitrogen and sulfur and hydrogen chloride. Although widely used as a herbicide, most deaths occur as a result of ingestion. |
| **Parathion (*O,O*-diethyl *O-p*-nitrophenyl phosphorothioate [CAS: 56-38-2]):** Highly potent organophosphate cholinesterase inhibitor (see p 292). Systemic toxicity has resulted from inhalation, ingestion, and dermal exposures. Evidence for adverse effects on fetal development in test animals at high doses (IARC 3). | 0.1 $mg/m^3$ (inhalable fraction and vapor), S | 10 $mg/m^3$ | | Yellow to dark brown liquid with garlic-like odor. Odor threshold of 0.04 ppm suggests it has good warning properties. Vapor pressure is 0.0004 mm Hg at 20°C (68°F). Thermal breakdown products include oxides of sulfur, nitrogen, and phosphorus. In the field, weathering/oxidation can convert parathion to the even more toxic organophosphate, paraoxon. |

| | | | | |
|---|---|---|---|---|
| **Pentaborane (CAS: 19624-22-7):** Highly irritating upon direct contact; severe burns may result. Vapors irritating to the respiratory tract. A potent CNS toxin; symptoms include headache, nausea, weakness, confusion, hyperexcitability, tremors, seizures, and coma. CNS effects may persist. Liver and kidney injury may also occur. | 0.005 ppm | 1 ppm | 4 4 2 | Colorless liquid. Vapor pressure is 171 mm Hg at 20°C (68°F). The pungent sour-milk odor occurring only at air levels well above the TLV is a poor warning property. May ignite spontaneously. Reacts violently with halogenated extinguishing media. Thermal breakdown products include boron acids. |
| **Pentachloronaphthalene (Halowax 1013 [CAS: 1321-64-8]):** Chloracne results from prolonged skin contact or inhalation. May cause severe, potentially fatal liver injury or necrosis by all routes of exposure. For chloracne, see also dioxins, p 183. | 0.5 mg/m$^3$, S | 0.5 mg/m$^3$ (effective IDLH) | | Pale yellow waxy solid with a pleasant aromatic odor. Odor threshold not known. Vapor pressure is less than 1 mm Hg at 20°C (68°F). Not combustible. Thermal breakdown products include hydrogen chloride fumes. |
| **Pentachlorophenol (Penta, PCP [CAS: 87-86-5]):** Irritating upon direct contact; burns may result. Vapors irritating to eyes and respiratory tract. A potent metabolic poison; uncouples oxidative phosphorylation. Well absorbed by all routes. Evidence for adverse effects on fetal development and carcinogenicity in test animals (IARC 2B). See also p 297. Case reports have associated PCP with bone marrow toxicity. | 0.5 mg/m$^3$, S, A3 | 2.5 mg/m$^3$ | 3 0 0 | Eye and nose irritation occur slightly above the TLV and are good warning properties. Vapor pressure is 0.0002 mm Hg at 20°C (68°F). Not combustible. Thermal breakdown products include hydrogen chloride, chlorinated phenols, and octachlorodibenzodioxin. Widely used as a wood preservative. Trace dioxin contamination can lead to chloracne. See page 183. |
| **Pentane (*n*-pentane [CAS: 109-66-0]):** Vapors mildly irritating to eyes and respiratory tract. A CNS depressant at high levels. | 600 ppm | 1500 ppm [LEL] | 1 4 0 | Colorless liquid with a gasoline-like odor that is an adequate warning property. Vapor pressure is 426 mm Hg at 20°C (68°F). Flammable. |
| **Petroleum distillates (petroleum naphtha, petroleum ether):** Vapors irritating to eyes and respiratory tract. A CNS depressant. If *n*-hexane, benzene, or other toxic contaminants are present, those hazards should be addressed. See also p 219. | | 1100 ppm [LEL] | 1 4 0 (petroleum ether) | Colorless liquid. Kerosene-like odor at levels below the TLV serves as a warning property. Highly flammable. Vapor pressure is about 40 mm Hg at 20°C (68°F). |

(C) = ceiling air concentration (TLV-C); S = skin absorption can be significant; SEN = potential sensitizer; A1 = ACGIH-confirmed human carcinogen; A2 = ACGIH-suspected human carcinogen; NFPA Hazard Codes: H = health, F = fire, R = reactivity, Ox = oxidizer, W = water-reactive, 0 (none) <—> 4 (severe). ERPG = Emergency Response Planning Guideline. See p 539 for an explanation of definitions.

(*continued*)

TABLE IV–4. HEALTH HAZARD SUMMARIES FOR INDUSTRIAL AND OCCUPATIONAL CHEMICALS (CONTINUED)

| Health Hazard Summaries | ACGIH TLV | IDLH | NFPA Codes H F R | Comments |
|---|---|---|---|---|
| **Phenol (carbolic acid, hydroxybenzene [CAS: 108-95-2]):** Corrosive acid and protein denaturant. Direct eye or skin contact causes severe tissue damage or blindness. Deep skin burns can occur without warning pain. Systemic toxicity by all routes; percutaneous absorption of vapor occurs. Vapors highly irritating to eyes and respiratory tract. Symptoms include nausea, vomiting, cardiac arrhythmias, circulatory collapse, convulsions, and coma. Toxic to liver and kidney. A tumor promoter. See also p 303 IARC 3. | 5 ppm, S | 250 ppm<br>ERPG-1: 10 ppm<br>ERPG-2: 50 ppm<br>ERPG-3: 200 ppm | 4 2 0 | Colorless to pink crystalline solid, or viscous liquid. Its odor has been described as being distinct, acrid, and aromatic or as being sweet and tarry. As the odor is detected at or below the TLV, it is a good warning property. Vapor pressure is 0.36 mm Hg at 20°C (68°F). Combustible. |
| **Phenylenediamine (*p*-diaminobenzene, *p*-aminoaniline [CAS: 106-50-3]):** Irritating upon direct contact. May cause skin and respiratory tract sensitization (asthma). Inflammatory reactions of larynx and pharynx have been noted often in exposed workers. IARC 3. | 0.1 mg/m$^3$, A3 | 25 mg/m$^3$ | — 1 0 | White to light purple or brown solid, depending on degree of oxidation. Combustible. Thermal breakdown products include oxides of nitrogen. |
| **Phenyl ether (diphenyl ether [CAS: 101-84-8]):** Mildly irritating upon prolonged direct contact. Vapors irritating to eyes and respiratory tract. Based on high-dose experiments in animals, liver and kidney damage may occur after ingestion. | 1 ppm | 100 ppm | | Colorless liquid or solid. Mildly disagreeable odor detected below the TLV serves as a good warning property. Vapor pressure is 0.02 mm Hg at 25°C (77°F). Combustible. |
| **Phenyl glycidyl ether (PGE, 1,2-epoxy-3-phenoxypropane [CAS: 122-60-1]):** Irritating upon direct contact. A skin sensitizer. Based on animal studies, vapors are very irritating to eyes and respiratory tract. In high-dose animal studies, a CNS depressant producing liver, kidney, spleen, testes, thymus, and hematopoietic system injury. A carcinogen in test animals (IARC 2B). | 0.1 ppm, S, SEN, A3<br>NIOSH CA | 100 ppm | | Colorless liquid with an unpleasant, sweet odor. Vapor pressure is 0.01 mm Hg at 20°C (68°F). Combustible. Readily forms peroxides. |
| **Phenylhydrazine (CAS: 100-63-0):** A strong base and corrosive upon direct contact. A potent skin sensitizer. Dermal absorption occurs. Vapors very irritating to eyes and respiratory tract. May cause hemolytic anemia with secondary kidney damage. Limited evidence of carcinogenicity in test animals. | 0.1 ppm, S, A3<br>NIOSH CA | 15 ppm | 3 2 0 | Pale yellow crystals or oily liquid with a weakly aromatic odor. Darkens upon exposure to air and light. Vapor pressure is less than 0.1 mm Hg at 20°C (68°F). Combustible. Thermal breakdown products include oxides of nitrogen. |

| | | | | |
|---|---|---|---|---|
| **Phenylphosphine (CAS: 638-21-1):** In animals, subchronic inhalation at 2 ppm caused loss of appetite, diarrhea, tremor, hemolytic anemia, dermatitis, and irreversible testicular degeneration. | 0.05 ppm (C) | | | Crystalline solid. Spontaneously combustible at high air concentrations. |
| **Phorate (*O,O*-diethyl S-(ethylthio)methyl phosphorodithioate, Thimet, Timet [CAS: 298-02-2]):** An organophosphate-type cholinesterase inhibitor (see p 292). Well absorbed by all routes. | 0.05 mg/m$^3$, (inhalable fraction and vapor), S | | | Clear liquid. Vapor pressure is 0.002 mm Hg at 20°C (68°F). |
| **Phosgene (carbonyl chloride, $COCl_2$ [CAS: 75-44-5]):** Extremely irritating to the lower respiratory tract. Exposure can be insidious because irritation and smell are inadequate as warning properties for pulmonary injury. Higher levels cause irritation of the eyes, skin, and mucous membranes. See also p 212. | 0.1 ppm | 2 ppm<br>ERPG-2: 0.2 ppm<br>ERPG-3: 1 ppm | 4 0 1 | Colorless gas. Sweet hay-like odor at low concentrations; sharp and pungent odor at high concentrations. Dangerous concentrations may not be detected by odor. |
| **Phosphine (hydrogen phosphide [CAS: 7803-51-2):** Extremely irritating to the respiratory tract; fatal pulmonary edema has resulted. A multisystem poison. Symptoms in moderately overexposed workers included diarrhea, nausea, vomiting, cough, headache, and dizziness. See also p 249. | 0.3 ppm | 50 ppm<br>ERPG-2: 0.5 ppm<br>ERPG-3: 5 ppm | 4 4 2 | Colorless gas. A fishy or garlic-like odor detected well below the TLV is considered to be a good warning property. May ignite spontaneously on contact with air. A common fumigant, generated on-site by aluminum or zinc phosphide and moisture. |
| **Phosphoric acid (CAS: 7664-38-2]):** A strong corrosive acid; severe burns may result from direct contact. Mist or vapors irritating to eyes and respiratory tract. | 1 mg/m$^3$ | 1000 mg/m$^3$ | 3 0 0 | Colorless, syrupy, odorless liquid. Solidifies at temperatures below 20°C (68°F). Vapor pressure is 0.03 mm Hg at 20°C (68°F). Not combustible. |
| **Phosphorus (yellow phosphorus, white phosphorus, P [CAS: 7723-14-0]):** Severe, penetrating burns may result upon direct contact. Material may ignite upon contact with skin. Fumes irritating to eyes and respiratory tract; pulmonary edema may occur. Potent hepatotoxin. Systemic symptoms include abdominal pain, jaundice, and garlic odor on the breath. Historically, chronic poisoning caused jaw bone necrosis (phossy jaw). See also p 308. | 0.1 mg/m$^3$ (yellow phosphorus) | 5 mg/m$^3$ | 4 4 2 | White to yellow, waxy or crystalline solid with acrid fumes. Flammable. Vapor pressure is 0.026 mm Hg at 20°C (68°F). Ignites spontaneously on contact with air. Thermal breakdown products include phosphoric acid fume. Historical exposures involved the match industry, which has long since substituted other forms of phosphorus. Current uses include munitions and pesticides. |

(C) = ceiling air concentration (TLV-C); S = skin absorption can be significant; SEN = potential sensitizer; A1 = ACGIH-confirmed human carcinogen; A2 = ACGIH-suspected human carcinogen; NFPA Hazard Codes: H = health, F = fire, R = reactivity, Ox = oxidizer, W = water-reactive, 0 (none) <—> 4 (severe). ERPG = Emergency Response Planning Guideline. See p 539 for an explanation of definitions.

(*continued*)

TABLE IV–4. HEALTH HAZARD SUMMARIES FOR INDUSTRIAL AND OCCUPATIONAL CHEMICALS (CONTINUED)

| Health Hazard Summaries | ACGIH TLV | IDLH | NFPA Codes H F R | Comments |
|---|---|---|---|---|
| **Phosphorus oxychloride (CAS: 10025-87-3):** Reacts with moisture to release phosphoric and hydrochloric acids; highly corrosive upon direct contact. Fumes extremely irritating to eyes and respiratory tract. Systemic effects include headache, dizziness, and dyspnea. Kidney toxicity may occur. | 0.1 ppm | | 4 0 2 W | Clear colorless to pale yellow, fuming liquid possessing a pungent odor. Vapor pressure is 40 mm Hg at 27.3°C (81°F). Not combustible. |
| **Phosphorus pentachloride (CAS: 10026-13-8):** Reacts with moisture to release phosphoric and hydrochloric acids; highly corrosive upon direct contact. Fumes extremely irritating to eyes and respiratory tract. | 0.1 ppm | 70 mg/m$^3$ | 3 0 2 W | Pale yellow solid with a hydrochloric acid-like odor. Not combustible. |
| **Phosphorus pentasulfide (CAS: 1314-80-3):** Rapidly reacts with moisture and moist tissues to form hydrogen sulfide (see p 224) and phosphoric acid. Severe burns may result from prolonged contact with tissues. Dusts or fumes extremely irritating to eyes and respiratory tract. Systemic toxicology is caused predominantly by hydrogen sulfide. | 1 mg/m$^3$ | 250 mg/m$^3$ | 2 1 2 W | Greenish-yellow solid with odor of rotten eggs. Olfactory fatigue reduces value of smell as a warning property. Thermal breakdown products include sulfur dioxide, hydrogen sulfide, phosphorus pentoxide, and phosphoric acid fumes. Ignites spontaneously in the presence of moisture. |
| **Phosphorus trichloride (CAS: 7719-12-2):** Reacts with moisture to release phosphoric and hydrochloric acids; highly corrosive upon direct contact. Fumes extremely irritating to eyes and respiratory tract. | 0.2 ppm | 25 ppm<br>ERPG-1: 0.5 ppm<br>ERPG-2: 3 ppm<br>ERPG-3: 15 ppm | 4 0 2 W | Fuming colorless to yellow liquid. Irritation provides a good warning property. Vapor pressure is 100 mm Hg at 20°C (68°F). Not combustible. |
| **Phthalic anhydride (phthalic acid anhydride [CAS: 85-44-9]):** Extremely irritating upon direct contact; chemical burns occur after prolonged contact. Dusts and vapors extremely irritating to respiratory tract. A potent skin and respiratory tract sensitizer (asthma). | 1 ppm, SEN | 60 mg/m$^3$ | 3 1 0 | White crystalline solid with choking odor at very high air concentrations. Vapor pressure is 0.05 mm Hg at 20°C (68°F). Combustible. Thermal breakdown products include phthalic acid fumes. |

| | | | | |
|---|---|---|---|---|
| **Picloram (4-amino-3,5,6-trichloropicolinic acid [CAS: 1918-02-1]):** Dusts mildly irritating to skin, eyes, and respiratory tract. Has low oral toxicity in test animals. Limited evidence of carcinogenicity in animals. | 10 mg/$m^3$ | | | White powder possessing a bleach-like odor. Vapor pressure is 0.0000006 mm Hg at 35°C (95°F). Thermal breakdown products include oxides of nitrogen and hydrogen chloride. |
| **Picric acid (2,4,6-trinitrophenol [CAS: 88-89-1]):** Irritating upon direct contact. Dust stains skin yellow and can cause sensitization dermatitis. Symptoms of low-level exposure are headache, dizziness, and gastrointestinal upset. May induce methemoglobinemia (see p 262). Ingestion can cause hemolysis, nephritis, and hepatitis. Staining of the conjunctiva and aqueous humor can give vision a yellow hue. A weak uncoupler of oxidative phosphorylation. | 0.1 mg/$m^3$ | 75 mg/$m^3$ | 3 4 4 | Pale yellow crystalline solid or paste. Odorless. Vapor pressure is much less than 1 mm Hg at 20°C (68°F). Decomposes explosively above 120°C (248°F). May detonate when shocked. Contact with metals, ammonia, or calcium compounds can form salts that are much more sensitive to shock detonation. |
| **Pindone (Pival, 2-pivaloyl-1,3-indanedione [CAS: 83-26-1]):** A vitamin K antagonist anticoagulant (see p 379). | 0.1 mg/$m^3$ | 100 mg/$m^3$ | | Bright yellow crystalline substance. |
| **Piperazine dihydrochloride (CAS: 142-64-3):** Irritating upon direct contact; burns may result. A moderate skin and respiratory sensitizer. Nausea, vomiting, and diarrhea are side effects of medicinal use. Overdosage has caused confusion, lethargy, coma, and seizures. | 5 mg/$m^3$ | | | White crystalline solid with a mild fishy odor. |
| **Piperidine (CAS: 110-89-4):** Highly irritating upon direct contact; severe burns may result. Vapors irritating to eyes and respiratory tract. Small doses initially stimulate autonomic ganglia; larger doses depress them. A 30–60 mg/kg dose may produce symptoms in humans. | | | 3 3 0 | Flammable. |
| **Platinum—soluble salts (sodium chloroplatinate, ammonium chloroplatinate, platinum tetrachloride):** Sensitizers causing asthma and dermatitis. Metallic platinum does not share these effects. Soluble platinum compounds are also highly irritating to eyes, mucous membranes, and respiratory tract. | 0.002 mg/$m^3$ (as Pt) | 4 mg/$m^3$ (as Pt) | | Appearance varies with the compound. Thermal breakdown products of some chloride salts include chlorine gas. Used as industrial catalysts and in specialized photographic applications. |

(C) = ceiling air concentration (TLV-C); S = skin absorption can be significant; SEN = potential sensitizer; A1 = ACGIH-confirmed human carcinogen; A2 = ACGIH-suspected human carcinogen; NFPA Hazard Codes: H = health, F = fire, R = reactivity, Ox = oxidizer, W = water-reactive, 0 (none) <—> 4 (severe). ERPG = Emergency Response Planning Guideline. See p 539 for an explanation of definitions.

(*continued*)

TABLE IV–4. HEALTH HAZARD SUMMARIES FOR INDUSTRIAL AND OCCUPATIONAL CHEMICALS (CONTINUED)

| Health Hazard Summaries | ACGIH TLV | IDLH | NFPA Codes H F R | Comments |
|---|---|---|---|---|
| **Polychlorinated biphenyls (chlorodiphenyls, Aroclor 1242, PCBs):** Exposure to high concentrations is irritating to eyes, nose, and throat. Chronically overexposed workers suffer from chloracne and liver injury. Reported symptoms are anorexia, gastrointestinal upset, and peripheral neuropathies. Some health effects may be caused by contaminants or thermal decomposition products. Adverse effects on fetal development and fertility in test animals. A carcinogen in test animals (IARC 2A). See also p 321. | 1 mg/m$^3$ (42% chlorine), S, NIOSH CA<br>0.5 mg/m$^3$ (54% chlorine), S, A3 NIOSH CA | 5 mg/m$^3$ (42% or 54% chlorine) | 2 1 0 | 42% chlorinated: a colorless to dark brown liquid with a slight hydrocarbon odor and a vapor pressure of 0.001 mm Hg at 20°C (68°F). 54% chlorinated: light yellow oily liquid with a slight hydrocarbon odor and a vapor pressure of 0.00006 mm Hg at 20°C (68°F). Thermal breakdown products include chlorinated dibenzofurans and chlorodibenzodioxins. Although no longer used, old transformers may still contain PCBs. |
| **Polytetrafluoroethylene decomposition products:** Overexposures result in polymer fume fever, a disease with flu-like symptoms including that include chills, fever, and cough. See also p 530. | | | | Produced by pyrolysis of Teflon and related materials. Perisofluorobutylene and carbonyl fluoride are among the pyrolysis products. |
| **Polyvinyl chloride decomposition products:** Fumes are irritating to the respiratory tract and may cause "meat wrapper's" asthma. | | | | Produced by the high-temperature partial breakdown of polyvinyl chloride plastics. Decomposition products include hydrochloric acid (see p 212). |
| **Portland cement (a mixture of mostly tricalcium silicate and dicalcium silicate with some alumina, calcium aluminate, and iron oxide):** Irritant of the eyes, nose, and skin; corrosive burns may occur. Long-term heavy exposure has been associated with dermatitis and bronchitis. | [proposed 1 mg/m$^3$ (inhalable fraction), A2] | 5000 mg/m$^3$ | | Gray powder. Odorless. Portland cement manufacture is typically is associated with sulfur dioxide exposure. |
| **Potassium hydroxide (KOH [CAS: 1310-58-3]):** A caustic alkali causing severe burns to tissues upon direct contact. Exposure to dust or mist causes eye, nose, and respiratory tract irritation. | 2 mg/m$^3$ (C) | | 3 0 1 | White solid that absorbs moisture. Vapor pressure is negligible at 20°C (68°F). Gives off heat and a corrosive mist when in contact with water. |
| **Propane (CAS: 74-98-6):** Simple asphyxiant. See also hydrocarbons, p 219. | 1000 ppm | 2100 ppm [LEL] | 1 4 0 | |

| | | | | |
|---|---|---|---|---|
| **Propargyl alcohol (2-propyn-1-ol [CAS: 107-19-7]):** Irritating to skin upon direct contact. Dermally well absorbed. A CNS depressant. Causes liver and kidney injury in test animals. | 1 ppm, S | | 4 3 3 | Light to straw-colored liquid with a geranium-like odor. Vapor pressure is 11.6 mm Hg at 20°C (68°F). Flammable. |
| **Propionic acid (CAS: 79-09-4):** Irritating to eyes and skin upon direct contact with concentrated solutions; burns may result. Vapors irritating to eyes, skin, and respiratory tract. A food additive of low systemic toxicity. | 10 ppm | | 3 2 0 | Colorless oily liquid with a pungent, somewhat rancid odor. Vapor pressure is 10 mm Hg at 39.7°C (103.5°F). Flammable. |
| **Propoxur (*o*-isopropoxyphenyl *N*-methylcarbamate, DDVP, Baygon [CAS: 114-26-1]):** A carbamate anticholinesterase insecticide (see p 292). Limited evidence for adverse effects on fetal development in test animals. | 0.5 mg/m$^3$, A3 | | | White crystalline solid with a faint characteristic odor. Vapor pressure is 0.01 mm Hg at 120°C (248°F). Common insecticide found in many OTC formulations. |
| ***n*-Propyl acetate (CAS: 109-60-4):** Vapors irritating to eyes and respiratory tract. Excessive inhalation may cause weakness, nausea, and chest tightness. Based on high-exposure studies in test animals, a CNS depressant. | 200 ppm | 1700 ppm | 1 3 0 | Colorless liquid. Mild fruity odor and irritant properties provide good warning properties. Vapor pressure is 25 mm Hg at 20°C (68°F). Flammable. |
| **Propyl alcohol (1-propanol [CAS: 71-23-8]):** Vapors mildly irritating to eyes and respiratory tract. A CNS depressant. See also isopropyl alcohol, p 234. | 200 ppm, A3 | 800 ppm | 1 3 0 | Colorless volatile liquid. Vapor pressure is 15 mm Hg at 20°C (68°F). Mild alcohol-like odor is an adequate warning property. |
| **Propylene dichloride (1,2-dichloropropane [CAS: 78-87-5]):** Vapors very irritating to eyes and respiratory tract. Causes CNS depression and severe liver and kidney damage at modest doses in animal studies. Testicular toxicity at high doses in test animals. | [proposed: 10 ppm, SEN] NIOSH CA | 400 ppm | 2 3 0 | Colorless liquid. Chloroform-like odor is considered an adequate warning property. Vapor pressure is 40 mm Hg at 20°C (68°F). Flammable. Thermal breakdown products include hydrogen chloride. An agricultural nematocide. |

(C) = ceiling air concentration (TLV-C); S = skin absorption can be significant; SEN = potential sensitizer; A1 = ACGIH-confirmed human carcinogen; A2 = ACGIH-suspected human carcinogen; NFPA Hazard Codes: H = health, F = fire, R = reactivity, Ox = oxidizer, W = water-reactive, 0 (none) <—> 4 (severe). ERPG = Emergency Response Planning Guideline. See p 539 for an explanation of definitions.

(*continued*)

TABLE IV–4. HEALTH HAZARD SUMMARIES FOR INDUSTRIAL AND OCCUPATIONAL CHEMICALS (CONTINUED)

| Health Hazard Summaries | ACGIH TLV | IDLH | NFPA Codes H F R | Comments |
|---|---|---|---|---|
| **Propylene glycol dinitrate (1,2-propylene glycol dinitrate, PGDN [CAS: 6423-43-4]):** Mildly irritating upon direct contact. Dermal absorption occurs. May cause methemoglobinemia (see p 262). Causes vasodilation, including coronary arteries. Headache and drop in blood pressure are common. Well absorbed by all routes. Tolerance to vasodilation can occur; cessation of exposure may precipitate angina pectoris in pharmacologically dependent workers. See also nitrates, p 279. | 0.05 ppm, S | | | Colorless liquid with an unpleasant odor. Thermal breakdown products include oxides of nitrogen. |
| **Propylene glycol monomethyl ether (1-methoxy-2-propanol [CAS: 107-98-2]):** Vapors very irritating to the eyes and possibly the respiratory tract. A mild CNS depressant. | 100 ppm | | 0 3 0 | Colorless, flammable liquid. |
| **Propylene imine (2-methylaziridine [CAS: 75-55-8]):** Very irritating upon direct contact; severe burns may result. Vapors highly irritating to eyes and respiratory tract. May also injure liver and kidneys. Well absorbed dermally. A carcinogen in test animals. | 2 ppm, S, A3<br>NIOSH CA | 100 ppm | | A fuming colorless liquid with a strong ammonia-like odor. Flammable. Thermal breakdown products include oxides of nitrogen. |
| **Propylene oxide (2-epoxypropane [CAS: 75-56-9]):** Highly irritating upon direct contact; severe burns result. Vapors highly irritating to eyes and respiratory tract. Based on high-dose animal studies, may cause CNS depression and peripheral neuropathy. A carcinogen in test animals (IARC 2B). | 2 ppm, SEN, A3<br>NIOSH CA | 400 ppm<br>ERPG-1: 50 ppm<br>ERPG-2: 250 ppm<br>ERPG-3: 750 ppm | 3 4 2 | Colorless liquid. Its sweet, ether-like odor is considered to be an adequate warning property. Vapor pressure is 442 mm Hg at 20°C (68°F). Highly flammable. Polymerizes violently. |
| ***n*-Propyl nitrate(nitric acid n-propyl ester [CAS: 627-13-4]):** Vasodilator causing headaches and hypotension. Causes methemoglobinemia (see p 262). See also nitrates, p 279. | 25 ppm | 500 ppm | 2 3 3<br>Ox (may explode on heating) | Pale yellow liquid with an unpleasant sweet odor. Vapor pressure is 18 mm Hg at 20°C (68°F). Flammable. Thermal breakdown products include oxides of nitrogen. |

| | | | | |
|---|---|---|---|---|
| **Pyrethrum (pyrethrin I or II; cinerin I or II; jasmolin I or II):** Dusts cause primary contact dermatitis and skin and respiratory tract sensitization (asthma). Of very low systemic toxicity. See also p 324. | 5 mg/m$^3$ | 5000 mg/m$^3$ | | Vapor pressure is negligible at 20°C (68°F). Combustible. Widely used insecticide. |
| **Pyridine (CAS: 110-86-1):** Irritating upon prolonged direct contact; occasional reports of skin sensitization. Vapors irritating to eyes and respiratory tract. A CNS depressant. Induces methemoglobinemia. Chronic ingestion of small amounts has caused fatal liver and kidney injury. Workers exposed to 6–12 ppm have complained of headache, dizziness, and gastrointestinal upset. Dermally well absorbed. IARC 3. | 1 ppm, A3 | 1000 ppm | 3 3 0 | Colorless or yellow liquid with a nauseating odor and a definite "taste" that serves as a good warning property. Vapor pressure is 18 mm Hg at 20°C (68°F). Flammable. Thermal breakdown products include oxides of nitrogen and cyanide. |
| **Pyrogallol (1,2,3-trihydroxybenzene; pyrogallic acid [CAS: 87-66-1]):** Highly irritating upon direct contact; severe burns may result. Potent reducing agent and general cellular poison. Causes methemoglobinemia (see p 262). Attacks heart, lungs, liver, kidneys, red blood cells, bone marrow, and muscle. Causes sensitization dermatitis. Deaths have resulted from the topical application of salves containing pyrogallol. | | | | White to gray odorless solid. |
| **Quinone (1,4-cyclohexadienedione, *p*-benzoquinone [CAS: 106-51-4]):** A severe irritant of the eyes and respiratory tract. May induce methemoglobinemia (see p 262). Acute overexposure to dust or vapors can cause conjunctival irritation and discoloration, corneal edema, ulceration, and scarring. Chronic exposures can permanently reduce visual acuity. Skin contact can cause irritation, ulceration, and pigmentation changes. IARC 3. | 0.1 ppm | 100 mg/m$^3$ | | Pale yellow crystalline solid. The acrid odor is not a reliable warning property. Vapor pressure is 0.1 mm Hg at 20°C (68°F). Sublimes when heated. |
| **Resorcinol (1,3-dihydroxybenzene [CAS: 108-46-3]):** Corrosive acid and protein denaturant; extremely irritating upon direct contact; severe burns result. May cause methemoglobinemia (see p 262). A sensitizer. Dermally well absorbed. See also phenol, p 303 IARC 3. | 10 ppm | | 1 0 | White crystalline solid with a faint odor. May turn pink on contact with air. Vapor pressure is 1 mm Hg at 108°C (226°F). Combustible. |

(C) = ceiling air concentration (TLV-C); S = skin absorption can be significant; SEN = potential sensitizer; A1 = ACGIH-confirmed human carcinogen; A2 = ACGIH-suspected human carcinogen; NFPA Hazard Codes: H = health, F = fire, R = reactivity, Ox = oxidizer, W = water-reactive, 0 (none) <—> 4 (severe). ERPG = Emergency Response Planning Guideline. See p 539 for an explanation of definitions.

(*continued*)

TABLE IV–4. HEALTH HAZARD SUMMARIES FOR INDUSTRIAL AND OCCUPATIONAL CHEMICALS (CONTINUED)

| Health Hazard Summaries | ACGIH TLV | IDLH | NFPA Codes H F R | Comments |
|---|---|---|---|---|
| **Ronnel (*O*,*O*-dimethyl-*O*-(2,4,5-trichlorophenyl) phosphorothioate, Fenchlorphos [CAS: 299-84-3]):** One of the least toxic organophosphate anticholinesterase insecticides (see p 292). | [proposed: 5 mg/m$^3$ (inhalable fraction and vapor)] | 300 mg/m$^3$ | | Vapor pressure is 0.0008 mm Hg at 20°C (68°F). Not combustible. Unstable above 149°C (300°F); harmful gases such as sulfur dioxide, dimethyl sulfide, and trichlorophenol may be released. |
| **Rotenone (tubatoxin, cube root, derris root, derrin [CAS: 83-79-4]):** Irritating upon direct contact. Dusts irritate the respiratory tract. A metabolic poison; depresses cellular respiration and inhibits mitotic spindle formation. Ingestion of large doses numbs oral mucosa and causes nausea and vomiting, muscle tremors, and convulsions. Chronic exposure caused liver and kidney damage in animal studies. Limited evidence for adverse effects on fetal development in animals at high doses. | 5 mg/m$^3$ | 2500 mg/m$^3$ | | White to red crystalline solid. Vapor pressure is negligible at 20°C (68°F). A natural pesticide extracted from plants such as cube, derris, and timbo. Odorless. Decomposes upon contact with air or light. Unstable to alkali. |
| **Sarin (GB [CAS: 107-44-8]):** Extremely toxic chemical warfare nerve agent (see p 373) by all routes of contact. Readily absorbed via respiratory tract and skin and eyes. A potent cholinesterase inhibitor with rapid onset of symptoms. Vapors highly irritating. | | | 4 1 1 | Clear, colorless liquid. Odorless. Most volatile of nerve agents. Vapor pressure is 2.1 mm Hg at 20°C (68°F). Not flammable. |
| **Selenium and inorganic compounds (as selenium):** Fumes, dusts, and vapors irritating to eyes, skin, and respiratory tract; pulmonary ecema may occur. Many compounds are well absorbed dermally. A general cellular poison. Chronic intoxication causes depression, nervousness, dermatitis, gastrointestinal upset, metallic taste in mouth and garlicky odor of breath, excess caries, and loss of fingernails or hair. The liver and kidneys are also target organs. Some selenium compounds have been found to cause birth defects and cancers in test animals. See also p 338. IARC 3. | 0. 2 mg/m$^3$ (as Se) | 1 mg/m$^3$ (as Se) | | Elemental selenium is a black, gray, or red crystalline or amorphous solid and is odorless. |
| **Selenium dioxide (selenium oxide [CAS: 7446-08-4]):** Strong vesicant; severe burns result from direct contact. Converted to selenious acid in the presence of moisture. Well absorbed dermally. Fumes and dusts very irritating to eyes and respiratory tract. See also p 338. | | | | White solid. Reacts with water to form selenious acid. |

| | | | | |
|---|---|---|---|---|
| **Selenium hexafluoride (CAS: 7783-79-1):** Vesicant. Reacts with moisture to form selenium acids and hydrofluoric acid; severe HF burns may result from direct contact (see p 339). Fumes highly irritating to eyes and respiratory tract; pulmonary edema may result. | 0.05 ppm | 2 ppm | | Colorless gas. Not combustible. |
| **Selenium oxychloride (CAS: 7791-23-3):** Strong vesicant. Direct contact can cause severe burns. Dermally well absorbed. Fumes extremely irritating to eyes and respiratory tract; delayed pulmonary edema may result. | | | | Colorless to yellow liquid. Hydrogen chloride and selenious acid fumes produced on contact with moisture. |
| **Silica, amorphous (diatomaceous earth, precipitated and gel silica):** Possesses little or no potential to cause silicosis. Most sources of amorphous silica contain quartz (see crystalline silica, below). If greater than 1% quartz is present, the quartz hazard must be addressed. When strongly heated (calcined) with limestone, diatomaceous earth becomes crystalline and can cause silicosis. Amorphous silica has been associated with lung fibrosis, but the role of crystalline silica contamination remains controversial. | [proposed: withdrawal of TLV due to insufficient data] | 3000 mg/m$^3$ | | White to gray powders. Odorless with a negligible vapor pressure. The TLV for dusts is 10 mg/m$^3$ if no asbestos and less than 1% quartz are present. |
| **Silica, crystalline (quartz; fused amorphous silica; cristobolite; tridymite; tripoli [CAS: 14464-46-1]):** Inhalation of dusts causes silicosis, a progressive, fibrotic scarring of the lung. Individuals with silicosis are much more susceptible to tuberculosis. Some forms of crystalline silica are carcinogenic (IARC 1). See p 287. | [proposed: 0.025 mg/m$^3$ (respirable fraction), A2] NIOSH CA | 25 mg/m$^3$ (cristobolite, tridymite)<br>50 mg/m$^3$ (quartz, tripoli) | | Colorless, odorless solid with a negligible vapor pressure. A component of many mineral dusts. |
| **Silicon (CAS: 7440-21-3):** A nuisance dust that does not cause pulmonary fibrosis. Parenteral exposure has been associated with systemic toxicity. | [proposed: withdrawal of TLV due to insufficient data] | | | Gray to black, lustrous needle-like crystals. Vapor pressure is negligible at 20°C (68°F). |

(C) = ceiling air concentration (TLV-C); S = skin absorption can be significant; SEN = potential sensitizer; A1 = ACGIH-confirmed human carcinogen; A2 = ACGIH-suspected human carcinogen; NFPA Hazard Codes: H = health, F = fire, R = reactivity, Ox = oxidizer, W = water-reactive, 0 (none) <—> 4 (severe). ERPG = Emergency Response Planning Guideline. See p 539 for an explanation of definitions.

(*continued*)

TABLE IV–4. HEALTH HAZARD SUMMARIES FOR INDUSTRIAL AND OCCUPATIONAL CHEMICALS (CONTINUED)

| Health Hazard Summaries | ACGIH TLV | IDLH | NFPA Codes H F R | Comments |
|---|---|---|---|---|
| **Silicon tetrachloride (tetrachlorosilane [CAS: 10026-04-7]):** Generates hydrochloric acid vapor upon contact with moisture; severe burns may result. Extremely irritating to eyes and respiratory tract; pulmonary edema may result. | | ERPG-1: 0.75 ppm<br>ERPG-2: 5 ppm<br>ERPG-3: 37 ppm | 3 0 2<br>W | Not combustible. |
| **Silver (CAS: 7440-22-4):** Silver compounds cause argyria, a blue-gray discoloration of tissues, which may be generalized throughout the viscera or localized to the conjunctiva, nasal septum, and gums. Some silver salts are corrosive upon direct contact with tissues. | 0.01 $mg/m^3$ (soluble compounds, as Ag)<br>0.1 $mg/m^3$ (metal) | 10 $mg/m^3$ (Ag compounds, as Ag) | | Compounds vary in appearance. Silver nitrate is a strong oxidizer. |
| **Sodium azide (hydrazoic acid, sodium salt; $NaN_3$ [CAS: 26628-22-8]):** Potent cellular toxin; inhibits cytochrome oxidase. Eye irritation, bronchitis, headache, hypotension, and collapse have been reported in overexposed workers. See also p 122. | 0.29 $mg/m^3$ (C) (as sodium azide)<br>0.11 ppm (C) (as hydrazoic acid vapor) | | | White, odorless, crystalline solid. |
| **Sodium bisulfide (NaSH [CAS: 16721-80-5]):** Decomposes in the presence of water to form hydrogen sulfide (see p 224) and sodium hydroxide (see p 157). Highly corrosive and irritating to eyes, skin, and respiratory tract. | | | | White crystalline substance with a slight odor of sulfur dioxide. |
| **Sodium bisulfite (sodium hydrogen sulfite, $NaHSO_3$ [CAS: 7631-90-5]):** Irritating to eyes, skin, and respiratory tract. Hypersensitivity reactions (angioedema, bronchospasm, or anaphylaxis) may occur. | 5 $mg/m^3$ | | | White crystalline solid with a slight sulfur dioxide odor and disagreeable taste. Widely used as a food and chemical preservative. |
| **Sodium fluoroacetate (compound 1080 [CAS: 62-74-8]):** A highly toxic metabolic poison. Metabolized to fluorocitrate, which prevents the oxidation of acetate in the Krebs cycle. Human lethal oral dose ranges from 2 to 10 mg/kg. See also p 200. | 0.05 $mg/m^3$, S | 2.5 $mg/m^3$ | | Fluffy white solid or a fine white powder. Sometimes dyed black. Hygroscopic. Odorless. Vapor pressure is negligible at 20°C (68°F). Not combustible. Thermal breakdown products include hydrogen fluoride. Has been used as a rodenticide. |
| **Sodium hydroxide (NaOH [CAS: 1310-73-2]):** A caustic alkali; may cause severe burns. Fumes or mists are highly irritating to eyes, skin, and respiratory tract. See also p 122. | 2 $mg/m^3$ (C) | 10 $mg/m^3$<br>ERPG-1: 0.5 $mg/m^3$<br>ERPG-2: 5 $mg/m^3$<br>ERPG-3: 50 $mg/m^3$ | 3 0 1<br>W | White solid that absorbs moisture. Odorless. Evolves great heat upon solution in water. Soda lye is an aqueous solution. |

| | | | | |
|---|---|---|---|---|
| **Sodium metabisulfite (sodium pyrosulfite [CAS: 7681-57-4]):** Very irritating to eyes and skin upon direct contact. Dusts irritating to eyes and respiratory tract; pulmonary edema may result. Hypersensitivity reactions may occur. | 5 mg/m$^3$ | | | White powder or crystalline material with a slight odor of sulfur dioxide. Reacts to form sulfur dioxide in the presence of moisture. |
| **Soman (GD [96-64-0]):** Extremely toxic chemical warfare nerve agent (see p 373) by all routes of contact. Readily absorbed via respiratory tract and skin and eyes. A potent cholinesterase inhibitor with rapid onset of symptoms. Vapors highly irritating. | | | 4 1 1 | Clear, colorless liquid. Slight camphor-like odor that is not an adequate indication of exposure. Vapor pressure is 0.4 mm Hg at 25°C (77°F). |
| **Stibine (antimony hydride [CAS: 7803-52-3]):** A potent hemolytic agent similar to arsine. Gases irritating to the lung; pulmonary edema may occur. Liver and kidney are secondary target organs. See also p 99. | 0.1 ppm | 5 ppm<br>ERPG-2: 0.5 ppm<br>ERPG-3: 1.5 ppm | 4 4 2 | Colorless gas. Odor similar to that of hydrogen sulfide but may not be a reliable warning property. Formed when acid solutions of antimony are treated with zinc or strong reducing agents. |
| **Stoddard solvent (mineral spirits, a mixture of aliphatic and aromatic hydrocarbons [CAS: 8052-41-3]):** Dermal absorption can occur. Vapors irritating to eyes and respiratory tract. A CNS depressant. Chronic overexposures associated with headache, fatigue, bone marrow hypoplasia, and jaundice. May contain a small amount of benzene. See also hydrocarbons, p 219. | 100 ppm | 20,000 mg/m$^3$ | 0 2 0 | Colorless liquid. Kerosene-like odor and irritation are good warning properties. Vapor pressure is approximately 2 mm Hg at 20°C (68°F). Flammable. |
| **Strychnine (CAS: 57-24-9):** Neurotoxin binds to inhibitory, postsynaptic glycine receptors, which results in excessive motor neuron activity associated with convulsions and muscular hyperrigidity leading to respiratory impairment or paralysis. See also p 350. | 0.15 mg/m$^3$ | 3 mg/m$^3$ | | White solid. Odorless. Vapor pressure is negligible at 20°C (68°F). Thermal breakdown products include oxides of nitrogen. Commonly used as a rodenticide (gopher bait). |
| **Styrene monomer (vinylbenzene [CAS: 100-42-5]):** Irritating upon direct contact. Dermal absorption occurs. Vapors irritating to respiratory tract. A CNS depressant. Symptoms include headache, nausea, dizziness, and fatigue. Cases of peripheral neuropathy have been reported. Limited evidence for adverse effects on fetal development and cancer in test animals (IARC 2B). | 20 ppm | 700 ppm<br>ERPG-1: 50 ppm<br>ERPG-2: 250 ppm<br>ERPG-3: 1000 ppm | 2 3 2 | Colorless viscous liquid. Sweet aromatic odor at low concentrations is an adequate warning property. Odor at high levels is acrid. Vapor pressure is 4.5 mm Hg at 20°C (68°F). Flammable. Inhibitor must be included to avoid explosive polymerization. Used in SBR, ABS, and SAN polymers. |

(C) = ceiling air concentration (TLV-C); S = skin absorption can be significant; SEN = potential sensitizer; A1 = ACGIH-confirmed human carcinogen; A2 = ACGIH-suspected human carcinogen; NFPA Hazard Codes: H = health, F = fire, R = reactivity, Ox = oxidizer, W = water-reactive, 0 (none) <—> 4 (severe). ERPG = Emergency Response Planning Guideline. See p 539 for an explanation of definitions.

(*continued*)

TABLE IV–4. HEALTH HAZARD SUMMARIES FOR INDUSTRIAL AND OCCUPATIONAL CHEMICALS (CONTINUED)

| Health Hazard Summaries | ACGIH TLV | IDLH | NFPA Codes H F R | Comments |
|---|---|---|---|---|
| **Subtilisins (proteolytic enzymes of *Bacillus subtilis* [CAS: 1395-21-7]):** Primary skin and respiratory tract irritants. Potent sensitizers causing primary bronchoconstriction and asthma. | 0.06 mcg/m³ (C) | | | Light-colored powder. Occupational asthma associated with introduction into detergent in a powder formulation. |
| **Sulfur dioxide (CAS: 7446-09-5):** Forms sulfurous acid upon contact with moisture. Strongly irritating to eyes and skin; burns may result. Extremely irritating to the respiratory tract; irritation of the upper airways has caused obstruction of the upper airways and pulmonary edema. Asthmatics are of documented increased sensitivity to the bronchoconstrictive effects of sulfur dioxide air pollution. See also p 352. IARC 3. | 2 ppm | 100 ppm<br>ERPG-1: 0.3 ppm<br>ERPG-2: 3 ppm<br>ERPG-3: 15 ppm | 3 0 0<br>(liquefied) | Colorless gas. Pungent, suffocating odor with a "taste" and irritative effects that are good warning properties. |
| **Sulfur hexafluoride (CAS: 2551-62-4):** Considered to be essentially a nontoxic gas. Asphyxiation by the displacement of air is suggested as the greatest hazard. | 1000 ppm | | | Odorless, colorless dense gas. May be contaminated with other fluorides of sulfur, including the highly toxic sulfur pentafluoride, which release HF or oxyfluorides on contact with moisture. |
| **Sulfuric acid (oil of vitriol, $H_2SO_4$ [CAS: 7664-93-9]):** Highly corrosive upon direct contact; severe burns may result. Breakdown may release sulfur dioxide (see p 146). Exposure to the mist can irritate the eyes, skin, and respiratory tract. | 0.2 mg/m³ (thoracic fraction), A2 (strong acid mists) | 15 mg/m³<br>ERPG-1: 2 mg/m³<br>ERPG-2: 10 mg/m³<br>ERPG-3: 30 mg/m³ | 3 0 2<br>W | Colorless to dark brown heavy, oily liquid. Odorless. Eye irritation may be an adequate warning property. A strong oxidizer. Addition of water creates strong exothermic reaction. Vapor pressure is less than 0.001 mm Hg at 20°C (68°F). |
| **Sulfur monochloride (CAS: 10025-67-9):** Forms hydrochloric acid and sulfur dioxide (see p 352) upon contact with water; direct contact can cause burns. Vapors highly irritating to the eyes, skin, and the respiratory tract. | 1 ppm (C) | 5 ppm | 3 1 1 | Fuming, amber to red oily liquid with a pungent, irritating, sickening odor. Eye irritation is a good warning property. Vapor pressure is 6.8 mm Hg at 20°C (68°F). Combustible. Breakdown products include hydrogen sulfide, hydrogen chloride, and sulfur dioxide. |

| | | | | |
|---|---|---|---|---|
| **Sulfur pentafluoride (disulfur decafluoride [CAS: 5714-22-7]):** Vapors are extremely irritating to the lungs; causes pulmonary edema at low levels (0.5 ppm) in test animals. | 0.01 ppm (C) | 1 ppm | | Colorless liquid or vapor with a sulfur dioxide-like odor. Vapor pressure is 561 mm Hg at 20°C (68°F). Not combustible. Thermal breakdown products include sulfur dioxide and hydrogen fluoride. |
| **Sulfur tetrafluoride ($SF_4$ [CAS: 7783-60-0]):** Readily hydrolyzed by moisture to form sulfur dioxide (see p 352) and hydrogen fluoride (see p 222). Extremely irritating to the respiratory tract; pulmonary edema may occur. Vapors also highly irritating to eyes and skin. | 0.1 ppm (C) | | | Colorless gas. Reacts with moisture to form sulfur dioxide and hydrogen fluoride. |
| **Sulfuryl fluoride (Vikane, $SO_2F_2$ [CAS: 2699-79-8]):** Irritating to eyes and respiratory tract; fatal pulmonary edema has resulted. Acute high exposure causes tremors and convulsions in test animals. Chronic exposures may cause kidney and liver injury and elevated fluoride. See also p 199. | 5 ppm | 200 ppm | | Colorless, odorless gas with no warning properties. Chloropicrin, a lacrimator, often is added to provide a warning property. Thermal breakdown products include sulfur dioxide and hydrogen fluoride. A widely used fumigant. |
| **Sulprofos (*O*-ethyl *O*-[4-(methylthio)phenyl] *S*-propylphosphorodithioate [CAS: 35400-43-2]):** An organophosphate anticholinesterase insecticide (see p 292). | 1 mg/m$^3$ | | | Tan-colored liquid with a characteristic sulfide odor. |
| **Tabun (GA [CAS: 77-81-6]):** Extremely toxic chemical warfare nerve agent (see p 373) by all routes of contact. Readily absorbed via respiratory tract and skin and eyes. A potent cholinesterase inhibitor with rapid onset of symptoms. Vapors are highly irritating. | | | 4 1 1 | Clear, colorless liquid. Slight fruity odor that is not an adequate indication of exposure. Vapor pressure is 0.037 mm Hg at 20°C (68°F). |
| **Talc, containing no asbestos fibers or crystalline silica (CAS: 14807-96-6):** A tissue irritant. Pulmonary aspiration may cause serious pneumonitis. IARC 3. | 2 mg/m$^3$ (respirable fraction; if talc contains asbestos fibers, see asbestos TLV) | 1000 mg/m$^3$ | | |
| **Tantalum compounds (as Ta):** Of low acute toxicity. Dusts mildly irritating to the lungs. | 5 mg/m$^3$ (metal and oxide dusts, as Ta) | 2500 mg/m$^3$ (metal and oxide dusts, as Ta) | | Metal is a gray-black solid, platinum-white if polished. Odorless. Tantalum pentoxide is a colorless solid. Used in aerospace and other specialty alloys. |

(C) = ceiling air concentration (TLV-C); S = skin absorption can be significant; SEN = potential sensitizer; A1 = ACGIH-confirmed human carcinogen; A2 = ACGIH-suspected human carcinogen; NFPA Hazard Codes: H = health, F = fire, R = reactivity, Ox = oxidizer, W = water-reactive, 0 (none) <—> 4 (severe). ERPG = Emergency Response Planning Guideline. See p 539 for an explanation of definitions.

(*continued*)

TABLE IV–4. HEALTH HAZARD SUMMARIES FOR INDUSTRIAL AND OCCUPATIONAL CHEMICALS (CONTINUED)

| Health Hazard Summaries | ACGIH TLV | IDLH | NFPA Codes H F R | Comments |
|---|---|---|---|---|
| **Tellurium and compounds (as Te):** Complaints of sleepiness, nausea, metallic taste, and garlicky odor on breath and perspiration associated with workplace exposures. Neuropathies have been noted in high-dose studies. Hydrogen telluride causes pulmonary irritation and hemolysis; however, its ready decomposition reduces likelihood of a toxic exposure. Some tellurium compounds are fetotoxic or teratogenic in test animals. | 0.1 mg/m$^3$ (as Te) | 25 mg/m$^3$ (as Te) | | Metallic tellurium is a solid with a silvery-white or grayish luster. |
| **Tellurium hexafluoride (CAS: 7783-80-4):** Slowly hydrolyzes to release hydrofluoric acid (see p 222) and telluric acid. Extremely irritating to the eyes and respiratory tract; pulmonary edema may occur. Has caused headaches, dyspnea, and garlicky odor on the breath of overexposed workers. | 0.02 ppm | 1 ppm | | Colorless gas. Offensive odor. Not combustible. Thermal breakdown products include hydrogen fluoride. |
| **Temephos (Abate, *O,O,O',O'*-tetramethyl *O,O*-thiodi-*p*-phenylene phosphorothioate [CAS: 3383-96-8]):** Primary irritant of eyes, skin, and respiratory tract; a moderately toxic organophosphate-type cholinesterase inhibitor (see p 292). Well absorbed by all routes. | 1 mg/m$^3$ (inhalable fraction and vapor), S | | | |
| **Terphenyls (diphenyl benzenes, triphenyls [CAS: 26140-60-3]):** Irritating upon direct contact. Vapors and mists irritating to respiratory tract; pulmonary edema has occurred at very high levels in test animals. Animal studies also suggest a slight potential for liver and kidney injury. | 5 mg/m$^3$ (C) | 500 mg/m$^3$ | 0 1 0 | White to light yellow crystalline solids. Irritation is a possible warning property. Vapor pressure is very low at 20°C (68°F). Combustible. Commercial grades are mixtures of *o-*, *m-*, *p-*isomers. |
| **2,3,7,8-Tetrachlorodibenzo-*p*-dioxin (TCDD [CAS 1746-01-6]):** See Dioxins (p 183). A potent form of acne (chloracne) is a specific marker of exposure. | NIOSH CA | | | White crystalline solid. A toxic contaminant of numerous chlorinated herbicides, including 2,4,5-T and 2,4-D. |
| **1,1,1,2-Tetrachloro-2,2-difluoroethane (halocarbon 112a; refrigerant 112a [CAS: 76-11-9]):** Of low acute toxicity. Very high air levels irritating to the eyes and respiratory tract. A CNS depressant at high levels. By anology to other freons, may cause cardiac arrhythmias. High-dose studies in animals suggest possible kidney and liver in jury. See also p 208. | 500 ppm | 2000 ppm | | Colorless liquid or solid with a slight ether-like odor. Vapor pressure is 40 mm Hg at 20°C (68°F). Not combustible. Thermal breakdown products include hydrogen chloride and hydrogen fluoride. |

| | | | | |
|---|---|---|---|---|
| **1,1,2,2-Tetrachloro-1,2-difluoroethane (halocarbon 112; refrigerant 112 [CAS: 76-12-0]):** Of low acute toxicity. Once used as an antihelminthic. Very high air levels cause CNS depression. Vapors mildly irritating. By analogy to other freons, may cause cardiac arrhythmias. See also p 208. | 500 ppm | 2000 ppm | | Colorless liquid or solid with a slight ether-like odor. Odor is of unknown value as a warning property. Vapor pressure is 40 mm Hg at 20°C (68°F). Not combustible. Thermal breakdown products include hydrogen chloride and hydrogen fluoride. |
| **1,1,2,2-Tetrachloroethane (acetylene tetrachloride [CAS: 79-34-5]):** Dermal absorption may cause systemic toxicity. Vapors irritating to the eyes and respiratory tract. A CNS depressant. By analogy to other chlorinated ethane derivatives, may cause cardiac arrhythmias. May cause hepatic or renal injury. Limited evidence of carcinogenicity in test animals (IARC 3). | 1 ppm, S, A3<br>NIOSH CA | 100 ppm | | Colorless to light yellow liquid. Sweet, suffocating, chloroform-like odor is a good warning property. Vapor pressure is 8 mm Hg at 20°C (68°F). Not combustible. Thermal breakdown products include hydrogen chloride and phosgene. |
| **Tetrachloroethylene (perchloroethylene [CAS: 127-18-4]):** Irritating upon prolonged contact; mild burns may result. Vapors irritating to eyes and respiratory tract. A CNS depressant. By analogy to other trichloroethylene and other chlorinated solvents, may cause arrhythmias. May cause liver and kidney injury. Chronic overexposure may cause short-term memory loss and personality changes. Limited evidence of adverse effects on reproductive function in males and fetal development in test animals. Evidence for carcinogenicity in test animals (IARC 2A). See also p 360. | 25 ppm, A3<br>NIOSH CA | 150 ppm<br>ERPG-1: 100 ppm<br>ERPG-2: 200 ppm<br>ERPG-3: 1000 ppm | 2 0 0 | Colorless liquid. Chloroform-like or ether-like odor and eye irritation are adequate warning properties. Vapor pressure is 14 mm Hg at 20°C (68°F). Not combustible. Thermal breakdown products include phosgene and hydrochloric acid. Used in the dry cleaning industry. |
| **Tetrachloronaphthalene (Halowax [CAS: 1335-88-2]):** Causes chloracne and jaundice. Stored in body fat. Dermal absorption occurs. For chloracne, see also dioxins, p 183. | 2 mg/m³ | 50 mg/m³ (effective IDLH) | | White to light yellow solid. Aromatic odor of unknown value as a warning property. Vapor pressure is less than 1 mm Hg at 20°C (68°F). Thermal breakdown products include hydrogen chloride and phosgene. |
| **Tetraethyl-di-thionopyrophosphate (TEDP, sulfotepp [CAS: 3689-24-5]):** An organophosphate anticholinesterase insecticide (see p 292). Well absorbed dermally. | 0.1 mg/m³ (inhalable fraction and vapor), S | 10 mg/m³ | | Yellow liquid with garlic odor. Not combustible. Thermal breakdown products include sulfur dioxide and phosphoric acid mist. |

(C) = ceiling air concentration (TLV-C); S = skin absorption can be significant; SEN = potential sensitizer; A1 = ACGIH-confirmed human carcinogen; A2 = ACGIH-suspected human carcinogen; NFPA Hazard Codes: H = health, F = fire, R = reactivity, Ox = oxidizer, W = water-reactive, 0 (none) <—> 4 (severe). ERPG = Emergency Response Planning Guideline. See p 539 for an explanation of definitions.

(*continued*)

TABLE IV–4. HEALTH HAZARD SUMMARIES FOR INDUSTRIAL AND OCCUPATIONAL CHEMICALS (CONTINUED)

| Health Hazard Summaries | ACGIH TLV | IDLH | NFPA Codes H F R | Comments |
|---|---|---|---|---|
| **Tetraethyl lead (CAS: 78-00-2):** A potent CNS toxin. Dermally well absorbed. Can cause psychosis, mania, convulsions, and coma. Reports of reduced sperm counts and impotence in overexposed workers. See also p 533. | 0.1 $mg/m^3$ (as Pb), S | 40 $mg/m^3$ (as Pb) | 3 2 3 | Colorless liquid. May be dyed blue, red, or orange. Slight musty odor of unknown value as a warning property. Vapor pressure is 0.2 mm Hg at 20°C (68°F). Combustible. Decomposes in light. As a gasoline additive, heavy exposure can occur through inappropriate use of gasoline as a solvent and in substance abuse. |
| **Tetraethylpyrophosphate (TEPP [CAS: 107-49-3]):** A potent organophosphate cholinesterase inhibitor (see p 292). Rapidly absorbed through skin. | 0.05 $mg/m^3$, S | 5 $mg/m^3$ | | Colorless to amber liquid with a faint fruity odor. Slowly hydrolyzed in water. Vapor pressure is 1 mm Hg at 140°C (284°F). Not combustible. Thermal breakdown products include phosphoric acid mist. |
| **Tetrahydrofuran (THF, diethylene oxide [CAS: 109-99-9]):** Mildly irritating upon direct contact. Vapors mildly irritating to eyes and respiratory tract. A CNS depressant at high levels. A liver and kidney toxin at high doses in test animals. | 50 ppm, S, A3 | 2000 ppm [LEL]<br>ERPG-1: 100 ppm<br>ERPG-2: 500 ppm<br>ERPG-3: 5000 ppm | 2 3 1 | Colorless liquid. The ether-like odor is detectable well below the TLV and provides a good warning property. Flammable. Vapor pressure is 145 mm Hg at 20°C (68°F). |
| **Tetramethyl lead (CAS: 75-74-1):** A potent CNS toxin thought to be similar to tetraethyl lead. See also p 533. | 0.15 $mg/m^3$ (as Pb), S | 40 $mg/m^3$ (as Pb) | 3 3 3 | Colorless liquid. May be dyed red, orange, or blue. Slight musty odor is of unknown value as a warning property. Vapor pressure is 22 mm Hg at 20°C (68°F). |
| **Tetramethyl succinonitrile (TMSN [CAS: 3333-52-6]):** A potent neurotoxin. Headaches, nausea, dizziness, convulsions, and coma have occurred in overexposed workers. | 0.5 ppm, S | 5 ppm | | Colorless, odorless solid. Thermal breakdown products include oxides of nitrogen. |
| **Tetranitromethane (CAS: 509-14-8):** Highly irritating upon direct contact; mild burns may result. Vapors extremely irritating to eyes and respiratory tract; pulmonary edema has been reported. May cause methemoglobinemia (see p 262). Liver, kidney, and CNS injury in test animals at high doses. Overexposure associated with headaches, fatigue, dyspnea. See also nitrates, p 279. IARC 2B. | 0.005 ppm, A3 | 4 ppm | | Colorless to light yellow liquid or solid with a pungent, acrid odor. Irritative effects are a good warning property. Vapor pressure is 8.4 mm Hg at 20°C (68°F). Not combustible. A weak explosive and oxidizer. Highly explosive in the presence of impurities. |

| | | | |
|---|---|---|---|
| **Tetrasodium pyrophosphate (CAS: 7722-88-5):** Alkaline; dusts are mild irritants of eyes, skin, and respiratory tract. | 5 mg/m$^3$ [proposed: withdrawal of TLV due to insufficient data] | | White powder. Alkaline in aqueous solution. |
| **Tetryl (nitramine, 2,4,6-trinitrophenylmethylnitramine [CAS: 479-45-8]):** Causes severe sensitization dermatitis. Dusts extremely irritating to the eyes and respiratory tract. Stains tissues bright yellow. May injure the liver and kidneys. Overexposures also associated with malaise, headache, nausea, and vomiting. | 1.5 mg/m$^3$ | 750 mg/m$^3$ | White to yellow solid. Odorless. A strong oxidizer. Vapor pressure is much less than 1 mm Hg at 20°C (68°F). Explosive used in detonators and primers. |
| **Thallium (CAS: 7440-28-0) and soluble compounds (thallium sulfate, thallium acetate, thallium nitrate):** A potent toxin causing diverse chronic effects, including psychosis, peripheral neuropathy, optic neuritis, alopecia, abdominal pain, irritability, and weight loss. Liver and kidney injury may occur. Ingestion causes severe hemorrhagic gastroenteritis. Absorption possible by all routes. See also p 354. | 0.1 mg/m$^3$ (as Tl), S | 15 mg/m$^3$ (as Tl) | Appearance varies with the compound. The elemental form is a bluish-white ductile heavy metal with a negligible vapor pressure. Thallium has been used as a rodenticide. |
| **Thioglycolic acid (mercaptoacetic acid [CAS: 68-11-1]):** Skin or eye contact with concentrated acid causes severe burns. Vapors irritating to eyes and respiratory tract. | 1 ppm, S | | Colorless liquid. Unpleasant mercaptan-like odor. Vapor pressure is 10 mm Hg at 18°C (64°F). Found in some cold-wave and depilatory formulations. |
| **Thiram (tetramethylthiuram disulfide [CAS: 137-26-8]):** Dusts mildly irritating to eyes, skin, and respiratory tract. A moderate allergen and a potent skin sensitizer. Has disulfiram-like effects in exposed persons who consume alcohol (see p 189). Experimentally a goitrogen. Adverse effects on fetal development in test animals at very high doses. IARC 3. | 1 mg/m$^3$ | 100 mg/m$^3$ | White to yellow powder with a characteristic odor. May be dyed blue. Vapor pressure is negligible at 20°C (68°F). Thermal breakdown products include sulfur dioxide and carbon disulfide. Used in rubber manufacture and as a fungicide. |

(C) = ceiling air concentration (TLV-C); S = skin absorption can be significant; SEN = potential sensitizer; A1 = ACGIH-confirmed human carcinogen; A2 = ACGIH-suspected human carcinogen; NFPA Hazard Codes: H = health, F = fire, R = reactivity, Ox = oxidizer, W = water-reactive, 0 (none) <—> 4 (severe). ERPG = Emergency Response Planning Guideline. See p 539 for an explanation of definitions.

(*continued*)

TABLE IV–4. HEALTH HAZARD SUMMARIES FOR INDUSTRIAL AND OCCUPATIONAL CHEMICALS (CONTINUED)

| Health Hazard Summaries | ACGIH TLV | IDLH | NFPA Codes H F R | Comments |
|---|---|---|---|---|
| **Tin, metal, and inorganic compounds:** Dusts irritating to the eyes, nose, throat, and skin. Prolonged inhalation may cause chest x-ray abnormalities. Some compounds react with water to form acids (tin tetrachloride, stannous chloride, and stannous sulfate) or bases (sodium and potassium stannate). | 2 mg/m$^3$ (as Sn) | 100 mg/m$^3$ (as Sn) | | Metallic tin is odorless with a dull, silvery color. |
| **Tin, organic compounds:** Highly irritating upon direct contact; burns may result. Dusts, fumes, or vapors highly irritating to the eyes and respiratory tract. Triethyltin is a potent neurotoxin; triphenyltin acetate is highly hepatotoxic. Trialkyltins are the most toxic, followed in order by the dialkyltins and monoalkyltins. Within each of these classes, the ethyltin compounds are the most toxic. All are well absorbed dermally. | 0.1 mg/m$^3$, S (as Sn) | 25 mg/m$^3$ (as Sn) | | There are many kinds of organotin compounds: mono-, di-, tri-, and tetra-alkyltin and -aryltin compounds exist. Combustible. Organic tin compounds are used in some polymers and paints. |
| **Titanium dioxide (CAS: 13463-67-7):** A mild pulmonary irritant. IARC 3. | 10 mg/m$^3$ NIOSH CA | 5000 mg/m$^3$ | | White odorless powder. Rutile is a common crystalline form. Vapor pressure is negligible. |
| **Tolidine (o-tolidine, 3,3'-dimethylbenzidine [CAS: 119-93-7]):** A carcinogen in test animals (IARC 2B). | S, A3 NIOSH CA | | | White to reddish solid. Oxides of nitrogen are among thermal breakdown products. |
| **Toluene (toluol, methylbenzene [CAS: 108-88-3]):** Vapors mildly irritating to eyes and respiratory tract. A CNS depressant; may cause brain, kidney and muscle damage with frequent intentional abuse. May cause cardiac arrhythmias. Liver and kidney injury with heavy exposures. Abusive sniffing during pregnancy associated with birth defects. See also p 358. (IARC 3). | 50 ppm, S | 500 ppm ERPG-1: 50 ppm ERPG-2: 300 ppm ERPG-3: 1000 ppm | 2 3 0 | Colorless liquid. Aromatic, benzene-like odor detectable at very low levels. Irritation serves as a good warning property. Vapor pressure is 22 mm Hg at 20°C (68°F). Flammable. |

| | | | | |
|---|---|---|---|---|
| **Toluene 2,4-diisocyanate (CAS: 584-84-9):** A potent respiratory tract sensitizer (asthma) and potent irritant of the eyes, skin, and respiratory tract. Pulmonary edema has resulted with higher exposures. A carcinogen in test animals (IARC 2B). See also p 358. | 0.005 ppm, SEN<br>NIOSH CA | 2.5 ppm<br>ERPG-1: 0.01 ppm<br>ERPG-2: 0.15 ppm<br>ERPG-3: 0.6 ppm | 3 1 3<br>W | Colorless needles or a liquid with a sharp, pungent odor. Vapor pressure is approximately 0.04 mm Hg at 20°C (68°F). Combustible. |
| ***o*-Toluidine (2-methylaniline [CAS: 95-53-4]):** A corrosive alkali; can cause severe burns. May cause methemoglobinemia (see p 262). Dermal absorption occurs. A carcinogen in test animals. (IARC 2A). | 2 ppm, S, A3<br>NIOSH CA | 50 ppm | 3 2 0 | Colorless to pale yellow liquid. The weak aromatic odor is thought to be a good warning property. Vapor pressure is less than 1 mm Hg at 20°C (68°F). |
| ***m*-Toluidine (3-methylaniline [CAS: 108-44-1]):** A corrosive alkali; can cause severe burns. May cause methemoglobinemia (see p 262). Dermal absorption occurs. | 2 ppm, S | | | Pale yellow liquid. Vapor pressure is less than 1 mm Hg at 20°C (68°F). |
| ***p*-Toluidine (4-methylaniline [CAS: 106-49-0]):** A corrosive alkali; can cause severe burns. May cause methemoglobinemia (see p 262). Dermal absorption occurs. A carcinogen in test animals. | 2 ppm, S, A3<br>NIOSH CA | | 3 2 0 | White solid. Vapor pressure is 1 mm Hg at 20°C (68°F). |
| **Tributyl phosphate (CAS: 126-73-8):** Highly irritating upon direct contact; causes severe eye injury and skin irritation. Vapors or mists irritating to the eyes and respiratory tract; high exposure in test animals caused pulmonary edema. Weak anticholinesterase activity. Headache and nausea are reported. | 0.2 ppm | 30 ppm | 2 1 0 | Colorless to pale yellow liquid. Odorless. Vapor pressure is very low at 20°C (68°F). Combustible. Thermal breakdown products include phosphoric acid fume. |
| **Trichloroacetic acid (CAS: 76-03-9):** A strong acid. A protein denaturant. Corrosive to eyes and skin upon direct contact. IARC 3. | 1 ppm, A3 | | | Deliquescent crystalline solid. Vapor pressure is 1 mm Hg at 51°C (128.3°F). Thermal breakdown products include hydrochloric acid and phosgene. |
| **1,2,4-Trichlorobenzene (CAS: 120-82-1):** Prolonged or repeated contact can cause skin and eye irritation. Vapors irritating to the eyes, skin, and respiratory tract. High-dose animal exposures injure the liver, kidneys, lungs, and CNS. Does not cause chloracne. | 5 ppm (C) | | 2 1 0 | A colorless liquid with an unpleasant, mothball-like odor. Vapor pressure is 1 mm Hg at 38.4°C (101.1°F). Combustible. Thermal breakdown products include hydrogen chloride and phosgene. |

(C) = ceiling air concentration (TLV-C); S = skin absorption can be significant; SEN = potential sensitizer; A1 = ACGIH-confirmed human carcinogen; A2 = ACGIH-suspected human carcinogen; NFPA Hazard Codes: H = health, F = fire, R = reactivity, Ox = oxidizer, W = water-reactive, 0 (none) <—> 4 (severe). ERPG = Emergency Response Planning Guideline. See p 539 for an explanation of definitions.

(*continued*)

TABLE IV–4. HEALTH HAZARD SUMMARIES FOR INDUSTRIAL AND OCCUPATIONAL CHEMICALS (CONTINUED)

| Health Hazard Summaries | ACGIH TLV | IDLH | NFPA Codes H F R | Comments |
|---|---|---|---|---|
| **1,1,1-Trichloroethane (methyl chloroform, TCA [CAS: 71-55-6]):** Vapors mildly irritating to eyes and respiratory tract. A CNS depressant. May cause cardiac arrhythmias. Some dermal absorption occurs. Liver and kidney injury may occur. See also p 360. IARC 3. | 350 ppm | 700 ppm<br>ERPG-1: 350 ppm<br>ERPG-2: 700 ppm<br>ERPG-3: 3500 ppm | 2 1 0 | Colorless liquid. Vapor pressure is 100 mm Hg at 20°C (68°F). Not combustible. Thermal breakdown products include hydrogen chloride and phosgene. Widely used chlorinated solvent. |
| **1,1,2-Trichloroethane (CAS: 79-00-5):** Dermal absorption may occur. Vapors mildly irritating to eyes and respiratory tract. A CNS depressant. May cause cardiac arrhythmias. Causes liver and kidney injury in test animals. Limited evidence for carcinogenicity in test animals (IARC 3). See also p 360. | 10 ppm, S<br>NIOSH CA | 100 ppm | 2 1 0 | Colorless liquid. Sweet, chloroform-like odor is of unknown value as a warning property. Vapor pressure is 19 mm Hg at 20°C (68°F). Not combustible. Thermal breakdown products include phosgene and hydrochloric acid. |
| **Trichloroethylene (trichloroethene, TCE [CAS: 79-01-6]):** Dermal absorption may occur. Vapors mildly irritating to eyes and respiratory tract. A CNS depressant. May cause cardiac arrhythmias. May cause cranial and peripheral neuropathies and liver damage. Has a disulfiram-like effect, "degreasers' flush" (see p 184). Reported to cause liver and lung cancers in mice (IARC 2A). See also p 360. | 50 ppm<br>NIOSH CA | 1000 ppm<br>ERPG-1: 100 ppm<br>ERPG-2: 500 ppm<br>ERPG-3: 5000 ppm | 2 1 0 | Colorless liquid. Sweet chloroform-like odor. Vapor pressure is 58 mm Hg at 20°C (68°F). Not combustible at room temperature. Decomposition products include hydrogen chloride and phosgene. |
| **Trichlorofluoromethane (Freon 11 [CAS: 75-69-4]):** Vapors mildly irritating to eyes and respiratory tract. A CNS depressant. May cause cardiac arrhythmias. See also p 208. | 1000 ppm (C) | 2000 ppm | | Colorless liquid or gas at room temperature. Vapor pressure is 690 mm Hg at 20°C (68°F). Not combustible. Thermal breakdown products include hydrogen chloride and hydrogen fluoride. |
| **Trichloronaphthalene (Halowax [CAS: 1321-65-9]):** Causes chloracne. A hepatotoxin at low doses, causing jaundice. Stored in body fat. Systemic toxicity may occur after dermal exposure. For chloracne see also dioxins, p 183. | 5 mg/m$^3$, S | 20 mg/m$^3$<br>(effective IDLH) | | Colorless to pale yellow solid with an aromatic odor of uncertain value as a warning property. Vapor pressure is less than 1 mm Hg at 20°C (68°F). Flammable. Decomposition products include phosgene and hydrogen chloride. |

| | | | | |
|---|---|---|---|---|
| **2,4,5-Trichlorophenoxyacetic acid (2,4,5-T [CAS: 93-76-5]):** Moderately irritating to eyes, skin, and respiratory tract. Ingestion can cause gastroenteritis and injury to the CNS, muscle, kidney, and liver. A weak uncoupler of oxidative phosphorylation. Polychlorinated dibenzodioxin compounds are contaminants (see p 163). There are reports of sarcomas occurring in applicators. Adverse effects on fetal development in test animals. | 10 mg/m$^3$ | 250 mg/m$^3$ | | Colorless to tan solid. Appearance and some hazardous properties vary with the formulation. Odorless. Vapor pressure is negligible at 20°C (68°F). Not combustible. Thermal breakdown products include hydrogen chloride and dioxins. A herbicide once widely used as a defoliant and in Vietnam, "Agent Orange." |
| **1,1,2-Trichloro-1,2,2-trifluoroethane (Freon 113 [CAS: 76-13-1]):** Vapors mildly irritating to eyes and mucous membranes. Very high air levels cause CNS depression and may injure the liver. May cause cardiac arrhythmias at air concentrations as low as 2000 ppm in test animals. See also p 208. | 1000 ppm | 2000 ppm | | Colorless liquid. Sweetish, chloroform-like odor occurs only at very high concentrations and is a poor warning property. Vapor pressure is 284 mm Hg at 20°C (68°F). Not combustible. Thermal breakdown products include hydrogen chloride, hydrogen fluoride, and phosgene. |
| **Triethylamine (CAS: 121-44-8):** An alkaline corrosive; highly irritating to eyes and skin; severe burns may occur. Vapors very irritating to eyes and respiratory tract; pulmonary edema may occur. High doses in animals cause heart, liver, and kidney injury. CNS stimulation possibly resulting from inhibition of monoamine oxidase. | 1 ppm, S | 200 ppm | 3 3 0 | Colorless liquid with a fishy, ammonia-like odor of unknown value as a warning property. Vapor pressure is 54 mm Hg at 20°C (68°F). Flammable. |
| **Trifluorobromomethane (Halon 1301; Freon 13B1 [CAS: 75-63-8]):** Extremely high air levels (150,000–200,000 ppm) can cause CNS depression and cardiac arrhythmias. See also p 208. | 1000 ppm | 40,000 ppm | | Colorless gas with a weak ether-like odor at high levels and poor warning properties. Not combustible. |
| **Trifluoromethane (Freon 23 [CAS: 75-46-7]):** Vapors mildly irritating to the eyes and mucous membranes. Very high air levels cause CNS depression and cardiac arrhythmias. See also p 208. | | | | Not combustible. |
| **Trimellitic anhydride (TMAN [CAS: 552-30-7]):** Dusts and vapors extremely irritating to eyes, nose, throat, skin, and respiratory tract. Potent respiratory sensitizer (asthma). Can also cause diffuse lung hemorrhage (pulmonary hemosiderosis). | 0.04 mg/m$^3$ (C) | | | Colorless solid. Hydrolyzes to trimellitic acid in aqueous solutions. Vapor pressure is 0.000004 mm Hg at 25°C (77°F). TMAN is an important component of certain epoxy coatings. |

(C) = ceiling air concentration (TLV-C); S = skin absorption can be significant; SEN = potential sensitizer; A1 = ACGIH-confirmed human carcinogen; A2 = ACGIH-suspected human carcinogen; NFPA Hazard Codes: H = health, F = fire, R = reactivity, Ox = oxidizer, W = water-reactive, 0 (none) <—> 4 (severe). ERPG = Emergency Response Planning Guideline. See p 539 for an explanation of definitions.

(*continued*)

TABLE IV–4. HEALTH HAZARD SUMMARIES FOR INDUSTRIAL AND OCCUPATIONAL CHEMICALS (CONTINUED)

| Health Hazard Summaries | ACGIH TLV | IDLH | NFPA Codes H F R | Comments |
|---|---|---|---|---|
| **Trimethylamine (CAS: 75-50-3):** An alkaline corrosive; highly irritating upon direct contact; severe burns may occur. Vapors very irritating to respiratory tract. | 5 ppm | ERPG-1: 0.1 ppm<br>ERPG-2: 100 ppm<br>ERPG-3: 500 ppm | 3 4 0 | Highly flammable gas with a pungent, fishy, ammonia-like odor. May be used as a warning agent in natural gas. |
| **Trimethyl phosphite (phosphorous acid trimethylester [CAS: 121-45-9]):** Very irritating upon direct contact; severe burns may result. Vapors highly irritating to respiratory tract. Cataracts have developed in test animals exposed to high air levels. Evidence for adverse effects on fetal development in test animals. | 2 ppm | | 0 2 0 | Colorless liquid with a characteristic, strong, fishy, or ammonia-like odor. Hydrolyzed in water. Vapor pressure is 24 mm Hg at 25°C (77°F). Combustible. |
| **Trinitrotoluene (2,4,6-trinitrotoluene, TNT [CAS: 118-96-7]):** Irritating upon direct contact. Stains tissues yellow. Causes sensitization dermatitis. Vapors irritating to respiratory tract. May cause liver injury, methemoglobinemia (see p 262). Occupational overexposure associated with cataracts. Causes vasodilation, including coronary arteries. Headache and drop in blood pressure are common. Well absorbed by all routes. Tolerance to vasodilation can occur; cessation of exposure may precipitate angina pectoris in pharmacologically dependent workers. See also nitrates, p 279. IARC 3. | 0.1 mg/$m^3$, S | 500 mg/$m^3$ | | White to light yellow crystalline solid. Odorless. Vapor pressure is 0.05 mm Hg at 85°C (185°F). Explosive upon heating or shock. |
| **Triorthocresyl phosphate (TOCP [CAS: 78-30-8]):** Inhibits acetylcholinesterase (see p 292). Potent neurotoxin causing delayed, partially reversible peripheral neuropathy by all routes. | 0.1 mg/$m^3$, S | 40 mg/$m^3$ | | Colorless viscous liquid. Odorless. Not combustible. Although an anticholinesterase inhibitor, it is widely used as a chemical additive and in chemical synthesis. |
| **Triphenyl phosphate (CAS: 115-86-6):** Weak anticholinesterase activity in humans (see p 292). Delayed neuropathy reported in test animals. | 3 mg/$m^3$ | 1000 mg/$m^3$ | 2 1 0 | Colorless solid. Faint phenolic odor. Not combustible. Thermal breakdown products include phosphoric acid fumes. |

| | | | | |
|---|---|---|---|---|
| **Tungsten and compounds:** Few reports of human toxicity. Some salts may release acid upon contact with moisture. Chronic exposure to tungsten carbide–cobalt amalgams in the hard-metals industry may be associated with fibrotic lung disease. | 5 $mg/m^3$ (insoluble compounds)<br>1 $mg/m^3$ (soluble compounds) | | | Elemental tungsten is a gray, hard, brittle metal. Finely divided powders are flammable. |
| **Turpentine (CAS: 8006-64-2):** Irritating to eyes upon direct contact. Dermal sensitizer. Dermal absorption occurs. Vapors irritating to respiratory tract. A CNS depressant at high air levels. See also hydrocarbons, p 219. | 20 ppm, SEN | 800 ppm | 1 3 0 | Colorless to pale yellow liquid with a characteristic paint-like odor that serves as a good warning property. Vapor pressure is 5 mm Hg at 20°C (68°F). Flammable. |
| **Uranium compounds:** Many salts are irritating to the respiratory tract; soluble salts are potent kidney toxins. Uranium is a weakly radioactive element (alpha emitter); decays to the radionuclide thorium 230. Uranium has the potential to cause radiation injury to the lungs, tracheobronchial lymph nodes, bone marrow, and skin. | 0.2 $mg/m^3$ (soluble and insoluble compounds, as U), A1<br>NIOSH CA | 10 $mg/m^3$ | | Dense, silvery-white, lustrous metal. Finely divided powders are pyrophoric. Radioactive. |
| **Valeraldehyde (pentanal [CAS: 110-62-3]):** Very irritating to eyes and skin; severe burns may result. Vapors highly irritating to the eyes and respiratory tract. | 50 ppm | | 1 3 0 | Colorless liquid with a fruity odor. Flammable. |
| **Vanadium pentoxide (CAS: 1314-62-1):** Dusts or fumes highly irritating to eyes, skin, and respiratory tract. Acute overexposures have been associated with a persistent bronchitis and asthma-like responses, "boilermakers' asthma." Sensitization dermatitis reported. Low-level exposure may cause a greenish discoloration of the tongue, metallic taste, and cough. IARC 2B. | [proposed: 0.01 $mg/m^3$ (inhalable fraction), A3] | 35 $mg/m^3$ (as V) | | Yellow-orange to rust-brown crystalline powder or dark gray flakes. Odorless. Not combustible. |
| **Vinyl acetate (CAS: 108-05-4):** Highly irritating upon direct contact; severe skin and eye burns may result. Vapors irritating to the eyes and respiratory tract. Mild CNS depressant at high levels. Limited evidence for adverse effects on male reproduction in test animals at high doses. IARC 2B. | 10 ppm, A3 | ERPG-1: 5 ppm<br>ERPG-2: 75 ppm<br>ERPG-3: 500 ppm | 2 3 2 | Volatile liquid with a pleasant fruity odor at low levels. Vapor pressure is 115 mm Hg at 25°C (77°F). Flammable. Polymerizes readily. Must contain inhibitor to prevent polymerization. |

(C) = ceiling air concentration (TLV-C); S = skin absorption can be significant; SEN = potential sensitizer; A1 = ACGIH-confirmed human carcinogen; A2 = ACGIH-suspected human carcinogen; NFPA Hazard Codes: H = health, F = fire, R = reactivity, Ox = oxidizer, W = water-reactive, 0 (none) <—> 4 (severe). ERPG = Emergency Response Planning Guideline. See p 539 for an explanation of definitions.

(*continued*)

TABLE IV–4. HEALTH HAZARD SUMMARIES FOR INDUSTRIAL AND OCCUPATIONAL CHEMICALS (CONTINUED)

| Health Hazard Summaries | ACGIH TLV | IDLH | NFPA Codes H F R | Comments |
|---|---|---|---|---|
| **Vinyl bromide (CAS: 593-60-2):** At high air levels, an eye and respiratory tract irritant and CNS depressant; a kidney and liver toxin. Animal carcinogen (IARC 2A). | 0.5 ppm, A2<br>NIOSH CA | | 2 0 1 | Colorless, highly flammable gas with a distinctive odor. |
| **Vinyl chloride (CAS: 75-01-4):** An eye and respiratory tract irritant at high air levels. Degeneration of distal phalanges with "acroosteolysis," Raynaud's disease, and scleroderma have been associated with heavy workplace overexposures. A CNS depressant at high levels, formerly used as an anesthetic. May cause cardiac arrhythmias. Causes angiosarcoma of the liver in humans (IARC 1). | 1 ppm, A1<br>NIOSH CA | ERPG-1: 500 ppm<br>ERPG-2: 5000 ppm<br>ERPG-3: 20000 ppm | 2 4 2 | Colorless, highly flammable gas with a sweet ether-like odor. Polymerizes readily. Current potential exposure is limited to vinyl chloride synthesis and polymerization to PVC. |
| **Vinyl cyclohexene dioxide (vinylhexane dioxide [CAS: 106-87-6]):** Moderately irritating upon direct contact; severe burns may result. Vapors highly irritating to eyes and respiratory tract. Testicular atrophy, leukemia, and necrosis of the thymus in test animals. Topical application causes skin cancer in animal studies. IARC 2B. | 0.1 ppm, S, A3<br>NIOSH CA | | | Colorless liquid. Vapor pressure is 0.1 mm Hg at 20°C (68°F). |
| **Vinyl toluene (methylstyrene [CAS: 25013-15-4]):** Vapors irritating to eyes and respiratory tract. A CNS depressant at high levels. Hepatic, renal, and hematologic toxicities observed at high doses in test animals. Limited evidence for adverse effects on the developing fetus at high doses. IARC 3. | 50 ppm | 400 ppm | 2 2 2 | Colorless liquid. Strong, unpleasant odor is considered to be an adequate warning property. Vapor pressure is 1.1 mm Hg at 20°C (68°F). Flammable. Inhibitor added to prevent explosive polymerization. |
| **VM&P naphtha (varnish makers' and printers' naphtha; ligroin [CAS: 8032-32-4]):** Vapors irritating to eyes and respiratory tract. A CNS depressant at high levels. May contain a small amount of benzene. See also hydrocarbons, p 219. | 300 ppm,<br>A3 | | | Colorless volatile liquid. |
| **VX (CAS 50782-69-9):** Extremely toxic chemical warfare nerve agent (see p 373) by all routes of contact. Readily absorbed via respiratory tract and skin and eyes. A potent cholinesterase inhibitor with rapid onset of symptoms. Vapors highly irritating. | | | 4 1 1 | Colorless or amber liquid. Least volatile of the chemical nerve agents: vapor pressure is 0.007 mm Hg at 25°C (77°F). Odor is not an adequate warning of exposure. Flammability unknown. |

| | | | | | | |
|---|---|---|---|---|---|---|
| **Warfarin (CAS: 81-81-2):** An anticoagulant by ingestion. Medicinal dosages associated with adverse effects on fetal development in test animals and humans. See also p 379. | 0.1 mg/$m^3$ | 100 mg/$m^3$ | | | | Colorless crystalline substance. Odorless. Used as a rodenticide. Exposure is typically from inadvertent or deliberate ingestion rather than through workplace contamination. |
| **Xylene (mixture of *o*-, *m*-, *p*-dimethylbenzenes [CAS: 1330-20-7]):** Vapors irritating to eyes and respiratory tract. A CNS depressant. By analogy to toluene and benzene, may cause cardiac arrhythmias. May injure kidneys. Limited evidence for adverse effects on fetal development in test animals at very high doses. See also p 358. IARC 3. | 100 ppm | 900 ppm | 2 | 3 | 0 | Colorless liquid or solid. Weak, somewhat sweet aromatic odor. Irritant effects are adequate warning properties. Vapor pressure is approximately 8 mm Hg at 20°C (68°F). Flammable. |
| **Xylidine (dimethylaniline [CAS: 1300-73-8]):** May cause methemoglobinemia (see p 262). Dermal absorption may occur. Liver and kidney damage seen in test animals. | 0.5 ppm (inhalable fraction and vapor), S, A3 | 50 ppm | 3 | 1 | 0 | Pale yellow to brown liquid. Weak, aromatic amine odor is an adequate warning property. Vapor pressure is less than 1 mm Hg at 20°C (68°F). Combustible. Thermal breakdown products include oxides of nitrogen. |
| **Yttrium and compounds (yttrium metal; yttrium nitrate hexahydrate; yttrium chloride; yttrium oxide):** Dusts may be irritating to the eyes and respiratory tract. | 1 mg/$m^3$ (as Y) | 500 mg/$m^3$ (as Y) | | | | Appearance varies with compound. |
| **Zinc chloride (CAS: 7646-85-7):** Caustic and highly irritating upon direct contact; severe burns may result. Ulceration of exposed skin from exposure to fumes has been reported. Fumes extremely irritating to respiratory tract; pulmonary edema has resulted. | 1 mg/$m^3$ (fume) | 50 mg/$m^3$ | | | | White powder or colorless crystals that absorb moisture. The fume is white and has an acrid odor. Exposure is principally through smoke bombs. |
| **Zinc chromates (basic zinc chromate, $ZnCrO_4$; zinc potassium chromate, $KZn_2(CrO_4)2(OH)$; zinc yellow):** Contains hexavalent chromium, which is associated with lung cancer in workers. See also p 166. | 0.01 mg/$m^3$ (as Cr), A1 | | | | | Basic zinc chromate is a yellow pigment; dichromates are orange. |

(C) = ceiling air concentration (TLV-C); S = skin absorption can be significant; SEN = potential sensitizer; A1 = ACGIH-confirmed human carcinogen; A2 = ACGIH-suspected human carcinogen; NFPA Hazard Codes: H = health, F = fire, R = reactivity, Ox = oxidizer, W = water-reactive, 0 (none) <—> 4 (severe). ERPG = Emergency Response Planning Guideline. See p 539 for an explanation of definitions.

(*continued*)

TABLE IV–4. HEALTH HAZARD SUMMARIES FOR INDUSTRIAL AND OCCUPATIONAL CHEMICALS (CONTINUED)

| Health Hazard Summaries | ACGIH TLV | IDLH | NFPA Codes H F R | Comments |
|---|---|---|---|---|
| **Zinc oxide (CAS: 1314-13-2):** Fumes irritating to the respiratory tract. Causes metal fume fever (see p 259). Symptoms include headache, fever, chills, and muscle aches. | 2 mg/m$^3$ (respirable fraction) | 500 mg/m$^3$ | | A white or yellowish-white powder. Fumes of zinc oxide are formed when elemental zinc is heated. Principal exposure is through brass foundries or welding on galvanized steel. |
| **Zirconium compounds (zirconium oxide, $ZrO_2$; zirconium oxychloride, ZrOCl; zirconium tetrachloride, $ZrCl_4$):** Zirconium compounds are generally of low toxicity. Some compounds are irritating; zirconium tetrachloride releases HCl upon contact with moisture. Granulomata caused by the use of deodorants containing zirconium have been observed. Dermal sensitization has not been reported. | 5 mg/m$^3$ (as Zr) | 50 mg/m$^3$ (as Zr) | | The elemental form is a bluish-black powder or a grayish-white, lustrous metal. The finely divided powder can be flammable. |

(C) = ceiling air concentration (TLV-C); S = skin absorption can be significant; SEN = potential sensitizer; A1 = ACGIH-confirmed human carcinogen; A2 = ACGIH-suspected human carcinogen; NFPA Hazard Codes: H = health, F = fire, R = reactivity, Ox = oxidizer, W = water-reactive, 0 (none) <—> 4 (severe). ERPG = Emergency Response Planning Guideline. See p 539 for an explanation of definitions.

## REFERENCES

American Conference of Governmental Industrial Hygienists (ACGIH): *Guide to Occupational Exposure Values 2002*. Cincinnati, OH: ACGIH, 2002. Available for purchase at http://www.acgih.org/store/.

Emergency Response Planning Committee: *Emergency Response Planning Guidelines*. American Industrial Hygiene Association, 2002. Cincinnati, OH: ACGIH, 2002.

*Fire Protection Guide on Hazardous Materials*, 11th ed. National Fire Protection Association, 2001. Batterymarch Park, MA, 2001.

Hathaway G et al: *Proctor and Hughes' Chemical Hazards of the Workplace*, 4th ed. New York: Wiley, 1996.

Hayes WJ Jr: *Pesticides Studied in Man*. Baltimore: Williams & Wilkins, 1982.

*IARC Monographs on the Evaluation of the Carcinogenic Risk of Chemicals to Humans*. International Agency for Research on Cancer, 1987–2001. Available online at http://193.51.164.11/monoeval/grlist.html.

National Technical Information Service: Documentation for Immediately Dangerous to Life or Health Concentrations (IDLH). NTIS Pub. No. PB-94-95-195-047. Available online at http://www.cdc.gov/niosh/idlh/idlh-1.html.

National Toxicology Program: *Sixth Annual Report on Carcinogens*. Bethesda, MD: US Department of Health and Human Services, 1991. Also available online at: http://ntp-server.niehs.nih.gov/NewHomeRoc/AboutRoC.html.

*NIOSH Pocket Guide to Chemical Hazards*. DHHS Pub. No. 97-140. Available online at http://www.cdc.gov/niosh/npg/npgd0000.html.

Schardein JL: *Chemically Induced Birth Defects*. New York: Marcel Dekker, 1985.

US Department of Labor, OSHA, Title 29, Code of Federal Regulations, Part 1910.1000-1910.1200. Table Z-1: Limits for Air Contaminants. Available online at http://www.osha-slc.gov.

# Subject Index



NOTE: A *t* following a page number indicates tabular material and an *f* following a page number indicates an illustration. Both proprietary and generic product names are listed in the index. When a proprietary name is used, the reader is encouraged to review the full reference under the generic name for complete information on the product.